GOLDEN'S DIAGNOSTIC RADIOLOGY

Section 3:
RADIOLOGY OF THE CHEST

SECOND EDITION

VOLUMES OF
GOLDEN'S DIAGNOSTIC RADIOLOGY SERIES

RADIOLOGY OF THE CHEST

SECOND EDITION

COLEMAN B. RABIN, M.D.

Emeritus Clinical Professor of Medicine and Lecturer in Radiology,
Mount Sinai School of Medicine of the City University of New York.
Consulting Physician for Chest Diseases and Consulting Radiologist,
The Mount Sinai Hospital, New York, New York

MURRAY G. BARON, M.D.

Chairman, Department of Radiology,
The Long Island Jewish-Hillside Medical Center,
New Hyde Park, New York
Professor of Radiology,
School of Medicine, Health Sciences Center,
State University of New York at Stony Brook, New York

WILLIAMS & WILKINS
Baltimore/London

SECTION 3

GOLDEN'S DIAGNOSTIC RADIOLOGY
Laurence L. Robbins, M.D., Series Editor

Copyright ©, 1980
The Williams & Wilkins Company
428 E. Preston Street
Baltimore, Md. 21202, U.S.A.

Made in the United States of America

Library of Congress Cataloging in Publication Data

Rabin, Coleman Berley, 1900-
   Radiology of the chest.

   (Golden's diagnostic radiology; section 3)
   Includes index.
    1. Chest—Radiography.   I. Baron, Murray G., joint author.   II. Title.   III. Series.
RC78.G6 sect. 3 [RC941] 616.07'572'08s   79-25778
ISBN 0-683-07103-3   [617'.54'07572]

Composed and printed at the
Waverly Press, Inc.
Mt. Royal and Guilford Aves.
Baltimore, Md. 21202, U.S.A.

DEDICATION

To Janice Rabin and Eva Chajmovitz Baron, whose encouragement and patient forbearance contributed so much to this work.

Preface

The x-ray examination is the single most important technique for the diagnosis and evaluation of diseases of the chest. Often, it is the only means by which silent lesions of the lungs can be detected. Even with diseases that are clinically evident, the roentgen examination is essential for localization of lesions and determination of their extent and, at times, for identification of the underlying cause. In many instances the chest radiograph serves as a guide to treatment and provides a means of monitoring its success or failure.

To those whose special interest has been the pathogenesis and epidemiology of lung diseases, the roentgen examination has provided information that cannot be gotten by any other means. The pathologist usually sees only the end stage of a disease and must deduce the manner in which the disease developed from these terminal findings. Only occasionally does he discover, as an incidental finding, an example of an early or intermediate stage. He never has the opportunity to observe a disease as a continuum but must integrate the whole from multiple specific bits of information, each derived from a different patient.

The roentgenologist is not limited in this way. He can follow the changes that occur at every stage of the pathologic process. Equipped with a knowledge of the pathologic significance of the different roentgen shadows and certain clinical data, he is able to unravel the pathogenesis of many diseases. The natural histories of pulmonary tuberculosis, putrid lung abscess and bronchiectasis, to name but a few, have been uncovered in this manner.

Although the roentgen manifestations are constantly changing during the course of a disease, the appearance on any one examination is static and corresponds to the gross pathologic picture at that specific time. By closely correlating the roentgen appearances with the anatomic findings, the significance of the shadows on the film can often be appreciated in terms of underlying pathologic processes. From the virtually unlimited number of roentgen observations that are available it is possible to recognize the progression of the gross anatomic changes throughout the disease. This anatomic approach to the study of roentgen films is a most fruitful method for the diagnosis and understanding of thoracic diseases.

Before attempting to interpret films of the chest, it is essential to have a thorough knowledge of the anatomy of the thorax from a radiologic standpoint and an understanding of the principles underlying the various techniques employed in the roentgen examination. An appreciation of the uses of these "tools of the trade" and their limitations is vital because the process of arriving at a correct diagnosis often depends as much on the design of the x-ray study as on the skill and acuity of the interpreter. These subjects are considered in Part I, *General Considerations*. Fluoroscopy is discussed at some length even though there is a tendency to utilize it infrequently in the examination of the chest. However, fluoroscopy has considerable diagnostic value because it discloses the motion of the different thoracic structures as well as allowing them to be viewed in an almost infinite number of projections. When necessary, fluoroscopy can be used to determine the optimal positions of the patient and the x-ray tube for making the radiographs.

The correlation between the appearance of the roentgen shadows and the individual pathologic processes that they represent is discussed in Part II, *General Roentgen Pathology*. These form the basis for a logical approach to roentgen interpretation instead of relying only on memorization and pattern recognition.

Part III, *Regional Roentgen Pathology*, consists of a description of the changes in the thoracic organs during the course of specific diseases, changes that are determined by the combination and distribution of the multiple pathologic processes that are present at any given stage. Although the basic concepts of pathology can be applied in the elucidation of the x-ray appearances of chest diseases, roentgen interpretation often cannot be divorced from clinical findings. In some cases this information is provided by the patient or the referring physician but in other instances the relevant data are not volunteered. However, the correct path of questioning and study can be developed from the differential diagnostic considerations derived from the roentgen shadows. No attempt has been made to detail the purely clinical aspects of chest diseases because this would have meant curtailment of the discussion of the roentgenological material and would provide an incomplete and misleading picture of the disease. But, these aspects have been stressed wherever they assist in interpreting the films or when the roentgen findings serve to explain the clinical features of a disease.

The discussion of abnormalities of the great vessels has been limited to those that can simulate disease of the mediastinum or lungs. Similarly, consideration has been given to only those cardiac conditions which cause changes in the lungs or which are the result of pulmonary disease.

Numbered references and footnotes have been omitted from the text because it was felt that they would interfere with the primary purpose of the book—to provide a lucid and readable exposition of the roentgen manifestations of chest diseases. The references that are appended are meant to provide sources of additional detail when desired. The bibliography is not comprehensive. The articles were chosen either because of their contribution to an appreciation and understanding of the subject material or because of the completeness of their bibliography.

The preparation of this work has required the help of many associates to whom we are indebted. We wish to thank particularly Dr. Oscar H. Friedman who spent many hours selecting and cataloging the material for the illustrations, Miss Nette Rabin who made most of the diagrams and Miss Deborah Taylor who did the drawings of the bronchi and the bronchopulmonary segments. We also wish to thank Mr. Michael Carlin, and Mr. Fred Liebman and the Audiovisual Resources Department of the Long Island Jewish Hillside Medical Center for the photography and Miss Linda Dubester and Mrs. Ann Duncan for typing the manuscript.

We are greatly indebted to Dr. Laurence L. Robbins for his many suggestions and critique of the manuscript and to Mrs. Ruby Richardson for her painstaking efforts in the production of this volume.

Contents

Part I

General Considerations

Uses of Roentgen Examination of the Chest

The importance of the roentgen-ray examination of the chest as part of a general diagnostic investigation is now generally appreciated. It is well known that this examination will disclose lesions in the lungs which can be found in no other way, and that it will often disclose evidence of disease in patients who have no pulmonary symptoms. The roentgen findings aid not only by confirming the clinical diagnosis of pulmonary disease but also, in many cases, by firmly establishing a diagnosis which can only be suspected from the clinical examination (Fig. 1). In many instances, the results of the roentgen examination determine the diagnosis with as much finality as any laboratory procedure; in fact, the roentgen examination may reach this objective when there is no other laboratory procedure which can do so. In addition, the physician is enabled by the roentgenographic examination to follow and to record permanently the course of a pulmonary disease from the beginning to the end.

The findings on the films, if properly interpreted, disclose the pathology of the disease in all of its stages. In previous years our knowledge concerning the pathogenesis of pulmonary disease depended largely on an interpretation gained from the appearance of the organs at the end stage as seen by the pathologist at postmortem examination. The pathologist was indeed fortunate who had the opportunity of observing the early or intervening stages when the patient died of some other condition. The formulation of concepts concerning the pathogenesis and course of pulmonary disease was slow, painstaking and fraught with error before the interpretation of roentgen films of the chest became accurate. Eventually the clinician with the help of the radiologist was able to supply to the pathologist the missing links which enabled him to understand the evolution of the final picture as he saw it.

Roentgen techniques have made it possible to recognize diseases in the early stages and thus have made them more amenable to cure. Proper medical treatment can now be instituted promptly whereas previously it was often withheld because of inability to ascertain the nature of the disease. The roentgen examination has also made possible the accurate localization of diseases, permitting a definitive surgical approach.

The need for roentgen examination is obvious in patients who have symptoms referable to the lungs. However, the indications for the study of the chest have a much wider range. X-ray examination of the chest is an indispensable part of the physical examination which precedes any operation. It is the only method by which one can exclude the presence of pulmonary tuberculosis (Fig. 2). In the patient with a brain tumor, it may be the only way to determine that the tumor is secondary to a carcinoma arising in a bronchus. In the patient who is to be operated on for a malignant neoplasm anywhere in the body, the chest film is the only reliable means by

1

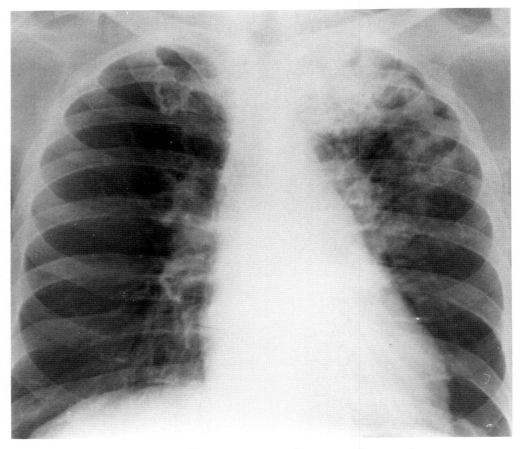

FIG. 1. PULMONARY TUBERCULOSIS WITH MISLEADING PHYSICAL SIGNS

The exudative tuberculous lesion in the left upper lobe is extensive and contains a number of small cavities. Nevertheless, no abnormal physical signs could be detected over the diseased lobe despite repeated examinations. On the other hand, subcrepitant rales, seemingly characteristic of tuberculosis, were found at the right apex. This area is perfectly clear on the roentgenogram. The shadow over the mesial portion of the right first rib is due to calcification of the first costal cartilage.

which one can exclude even extensive, large metastases in the lungs (Fig. 3). The roentgen examination of the chest is so important a part of the preoperative study that it should never be omitted before any major surgical procedure, or a minor one under general anesthesia. X-ray examination of the chest can also be of critical importance in the postoperative period. In a patient who has fever after an operation, films are useful even when they prove to be negative, for this excludes a postoperative pneumonia and directs the attention elsewhere.

Because tuberculosis and neoplasm occur so often without any pulmonary symptoms, a roentgenogram of the chest should be part of the routine physical examination. This has been recognized by the many agencies which require a roentgen examination of the chest before employment. In occupations in which there is exposure to dust or chemicals which may possibly produce pulmonary disease, chest films should be made periodically so that the patient as well as his employer may be informed concerning the inception of an industrial disease. Study of roentgen surveys in occupations involving exposure to dust or other irritants provides a truer picture of the hazards involved and serves as a guide to the efficacy of measures taken to prevent industrial disease.

Public health agencies have discovered the value of x-raying all contacts of patients with open pulmonary tuberculosis. In this way, many cases of early tuberculosis are found in a stage where treatment offers the best chance of cure. The routine examination of tuberculous contacts has not only yielded information concerning individual persons who have been exposed but also has immeasurably increased our knowledge of the epidemiology of this disease.

Perhaps not so fruitful as the examination of

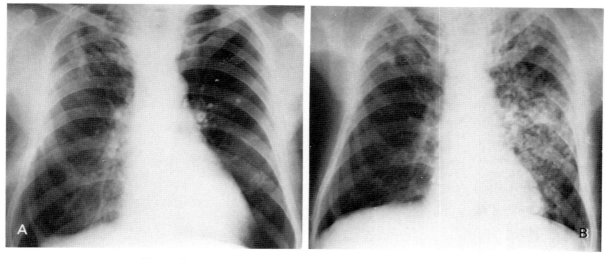

FIG. 2. POSTOPERATIVE SPREAD OF UNSUSPECTED TUBERCULOSIS

A: Preoperative film. The patient had no pulmonary symptoms and examination failed to disclose any abnormal physical signs in the chest. The routine film was overlooked before a cholecystectomy was performed under general anesthesia. Interstitial infiltrations are present in the outer portion of the right upper lobe together with streak-like shadows indicating focal areas of atelectasis. This combination of shadows beneath the outer portion of the clavicle is highly suggestive of exudative tuberculosis. The linear shadow above the right costophrenic sinus represents an area of discoid atelectasis and fibrosis. The entire right pulmonary field is grayer than the left because of diffuse pleural thickening. The calcific deposit in the left upper lobe, together with the one at the left root, represents a healed tuberculous primary complex. *B*: Film, 15 days postoperative. The patient had persistent fever without localizing signs after the operation. There are small, irregular nodular shadows, typical of acinar-nodose tuberculosis throughout most of the left lung. These are the result of bronchial spread of the disease. Changes have also occurred in the lesion in the right upper lobe, indicating activity of the disease.

contacts but nevertheless important, have been the results of survey examinations of the chest of large segments of the population. These have disclosed the presence of some form of pulmonary disease in as many as 10% of certain groups of people. Whereas in many of these cases, the abnormal findings are not of any great clinical importance, the number of cases with important and remediable pulmonary lesions is an impressive one. The practical importance of the findings in these surveys has led not only public agencies but also many business organizations and labor unions to employ them.

Among hospital employees, who are often unknowingly exposed to tuberculosis, routine roentgen examinations of the chest aid in the early discovery of the disease. Moreover, examinations at frequent intervals may determine the time at which the disease was contracted and thus settle legal responsibility which otherwise might not be clear.

Limitations of Roentgen Examination of the Chest

In interpreting roentgen films of the chest, the limitations of the procedure should be borne in mind. Inflammatory diseases of the bronchi are not visible on the film unless they produce a

secondary change in the lungs. Bronchial ulcerations and narrowing of the bronchi short of obstruction are usually not visible without special techniques. Small foci of the first infection type of tuberculosis may not be seen. The change from a negative to a positive tuberculin test is more reliable than the roentgen film for the detection of a primary tuberculous infection. Fortunately, such tuberculous foci are relatively unimportant and rarely give rise to clinical tuberculosis. On the other hand, as important and extensive a disease as miliary tuberculosis of the lungs, because of the small size of the lesions, shows no change in the film until as late as $2^{1}/_{2}$ weeks after its onset.

Dry pleurisy may not be recognizable roentgenologically, and small effusions are not always visible. Even larger effusions which are sometimes detected on physical examination may cast no visible shadow on the frontal projection. However, they may be seen on oblique or lateral views. The same holds true for lesions in that large portion of the lung which is hidden by the domes of the diaphragm or by the heart.

Early metastases from malignant tumors are often so minute that they can be seen only microscopically, and they may remain this small for many years before they begin to grow to macro-

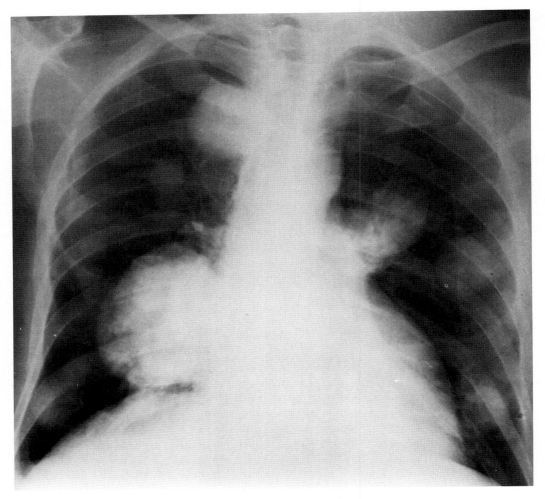

FIG. 3. LATENT METASTASES FROM SEMINOMA

The pulmonary metastases were discovered on the preoperative chest film prior to resection of a seminoma of the testicle. The large, round, sharply demarcated densities are often described as "cannon ball" shadows. Despite the large size of some of the masses, there were no abnormal physical signs.

scopic proportions. It is sometimes embarrassing for a surgeon to remove a malignant neoplasm after having been assured that the roentgenogram of the chest is negative, only to find the lungs studded with metastatic tumors a few months later. However, this limitation of the examination must be accepted.

In certain cases of bronchopneumonia in which the lesions are of the interstitial type, the infiltration about the bronchi and the interlobular septa cannot be detected on the roentgen film. This is also true in lymphangitic carcinosis when the infiltrations are very fine. Even fairly extensive carcinomas of the large bronchi may not be visible if they do not cause bronchial obstruction.

In dry bronchiectasis where there is little active inflammation, the roentgen films may be negative. However, even in the absence of any visible infiltration, there is usually a recognizable distortion of the bronchi and blood vessels. Pulmonary emboli which do not cause infarction may also cause no roentgenographic changes. Emphysema of considerable degree, even though perfectly obvious on physical examination, may be undetectable on the roentgen film, particularly in sthenic or obese persons.

Moderate enlargement of the mediastinal lymph nodes cannot be detected on roentgen examination. In many cases of pneumonia, particularly of the suppurative variety, the lymph nodes are considerably enlarged but they rarely can be seen on the films. Because of the difficulty in disclosing enlargement of these nodes, it is impossible to exclude the presence of mediastinal lymph node metastases by roentgen examination. Small anterior mediastinal tumors may also be hidden completely by other mediastinal structures on the frontal view. However, they may be disclosed on the lateral projection or by tomography.

As in the case of bones elsewhere in the body, metastatic tumors of the ribs or shoulder girdle are usually not visible roentgenologically in the early stages, before the cortex is involved, even though the lesions are widespread. In the ribs, there may be no indication of the metastatic neoplasm until it causes a pathologic fracture. Osteochondritis of the ribs, a common cause of chest pain, rarely produces visible changes at the costochondral junction. Even tuberculous osteochondritis involving many of these junctions, and complicated by cold abscesses in the adjacent chest wall, may not cause any alteration on the roentgen film.

The possibility that all of these pathologic conditions may be present without any roentgenologic evidence must be recognized. In certain cases the negative roentgen film should be disregarded and the diagnosis made by the clinician from the history and the findings on physical examination. Fortunately, in many of these diseases, the clinical findings are perfectly adequate for the diagnosis. In others, there is sufficient clinical evidence to warrant reexamination with films made in special positions and by special technics which may disclose the disease.

It should always be remembered that the roentgen films depict only the *shadows* of the pathologic process in the chest, and that the nature of the disease is only *inferred* in each individual case from the density, conformation, delineation, position, extent, and distribution of the shadows that it causes. Thus, it is usually impossible to differentiate between pneumonia and infarction and it may be difficult to differentiate between consolidation and an effusion. Solitary nodular shadows in the lungs can be caused by a variety of conditions which are indistinguishable from each other from a consideration of the roentgen shadows alone.

Although, in a great many cases, the roentgen characteristics permit the diagnosis of a specific disease without fear of error, there are many instances in which this cannot be done. However, narrowing down the possibilities to a few diseases is still of considerable assistance to the clinician, who may then be in a position to differentiate them easily by other means.

Technique

It is, of course, necessary to have films which are made properly if maximum information is to be obtained from them. Good films show clear definition of the shadows of the structures in the chest, even of the small blood vessels. Visualization of these structures depends upon differences in the density of their shadows (contrast). Where there is insufficient contrast, the films have an overall grayness so that the shadows of the smaller structures do not stand out clearly. With too high a degree of contrast, black and white are accentuated with a loss of the gray tones between them. Such films fail to show variations in shades produced by structures or lesions which do not differ widely in density. They also tend to obscure details within the shadow of the lesion—details required for proper interpretation. The good film, therefore, shows the shadows with sufficient contrast to enable them to be seen clearly, but at the same time exhibits a wide range of shades corresponding to the densities of the structures traversed by the rays.

The factors involved in the production of a film are the position of the patient, the voltage, the amperage, the exposure, time, and the phase of respiration. These, together with the speed of the film and intensifying screen and the process used in developing, will determine the appearance of the films. It is difficult to make a comparison of films, so often necessary in observing the course of a disease, unless the same technique is used at the various examinations. Films are made in full inspiration unless otherwise indicated. A standard scale of exposure should be adopted for individuals of different sizes and muscular development. If for some reason there is deviation from these standards, a record should be kept of it, so that a subsequent examination can be made in exactly the same manner. It is only in this way that one film in the series can be reliably compared with another for evaluating spread or regression of the disease. Such comparisons are often of utmost importance from the standpoint of diagnosis or treatment.

Position of the Patient and Tube. The alignment of the tube with the patient determines the relative position of the shadows of the structures of the chest on the roentgen film. It also influences the sharpness with which the shadows are depicted.

POSITION OF PATIENT. *Posteroanterior View.* For ordinary routine examinations the patient is placed in the erect position with the anterior portion of the chest in contact with the cassette. Because the rays travel through the patient from behind forward, this is called the posteroanterior or dorsoventral view. The arms should be placed in such a position that the scapulae are drawn forward and outward, so that they are removed from the pulmonary field. This is best accomplished by rotating the arms inward as far as possible and pointing the elbows forward as far as they will go.

It is important, particularly in the case of females, for the patient to exert firm pressure against the cassette. Otherwise, the breasts are not flattened, and may produce shadows suggesting disease in the underlying lung (Fig. 4).

Anteroposterior View. The anteroposterior view may be used where it is desired to outline more clearly the structures in the posterior part of the chest. It is used particularly in conjunction with the lordotic position for the demonstration of tuberculous cavities which are situated posteriorly, and which are often hidden by the clavicle and the first rib in the ordinary posteroanterior projection. In this position only the upper posterior part of the chest and the shoulders are in contact with the cassette, while the lower part of the chest is separated from it by a considerable distance.

Lateral View. In placing the patient for examination in the lateral view, it is essential that the shoulders and hips lie in a plane which is absolutely perpendicular to the film and parallel to the rays. Ordinarily, the position is checked by observing the patient from a vantage point behind the tube. However, time may be saved and the position of the patient in relation to the cassette may be made more perfect by aligning the patient with the aid of a right-angled instrument. There is a tendency for the arms and

shoulders to obscure a portion of the chest on the lateral view if care is not taken to remove them from the path of the rays. One way to accomplish this is to place the patient's hands on his head. Still, the arms may remain in the way if the elbows are not sufficiently elevated. A good plan is to cross the forearms of the patient over the head so that the arms lie alongside the face in a vertical direction. The chin should then be elevated. This will ensure raising of the shoulders and removal of the arms from the pulmonary field and upper anterior mediastinum.

If the patient cannot raise his arms to the desired degree, a satisfactory view of the anterior mediastinum can be obtained by placing his arms behind him and asking him to throw his shoulders back. An unobstructed view of the posterior mediastinum may be obtained by having the patient cross his arms in front of him (Fig. 448).

In placing the patient in position for the lateral view, it is important to have the side involved by the lesion as close to the cassette as possible. This produces clearer definition of the shadows on the affected side. In addition, it exposes the lung on that side completely. The lower part of the opposite lung is hidden by the abdominal structures because it is projected below the diaphragmatic leaf on the side adjacent to the film (Fig. 5).

Inclined Lateral View. When a lateral view of structures high in the superior mediastinum is required, the conventional lateral view is gener-

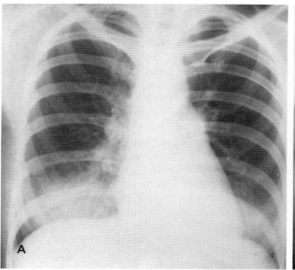 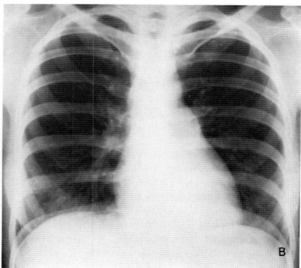

FIG. 4. BREAST SHADOWS SIMULATING PNEUMONIA

A: The homogeneous shadow at each base suggests lobar pneumonia. However, the patient, who had leukemia, was not acutely ill and had no respiratory symptoms. *B:* When the examination was repeated with the patient pressed firmly against the cassette, the lungs appeared clear. The shadows were caused by the breasts which are now flattened and displaced laterally.

ally unsatisfactory, since this region is hidden by the shoulders. In this case, the inclined lateral view is helpful (Fig. 6). The superior mediastinum may be projected through the supraclavicular fossa by inclining the patient toward the

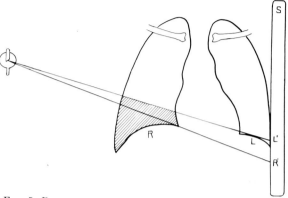

FIG. 5. PROJECTION OF DIAPHRAGM ON LEFT LATERAL VIEW

With the left side of the chest against the screen (S), the left leaf (L) of the diaphragm is projected above the right. The entire left lung is viewed on the film, clouded only by the shadows of the heart and the chest wall. All of the shaded area at the base of the right lung is projected below the left leaf of the diaphragm and is, therefore, obscured by the abdominal contents.

cassette while he maintains a lateral position. The side of the head and the shoulder, which is depressed as much as possible, are then in contact with the cassette, while the lower part of the chest is at a distance from it. The rays are directed from below upward, from the lower axilla on the side away from the film in the direction of the supraclavicular fossa on the opposite side. The shadow of the superior mediastinal lesion will then be projected by rays which pass successively under one shoulder, through the mediastinum, and out through the opposite superior clavicular fossa. The position of structures high in the mediastinum may also be disclosed by transverse laminagraphy.

Oblique Views. The oblique views, conventionally, are obtained with the patient's body at an angle of 45 degrees to the film. They may be made either in the posteroanterior or the anteroposterior positions, and with either the right or the left shoulder to the film. Usually, the posteroanterior position is used, and the films are said to be made in the anterior oblique position. If the anteroposterior position is used, i.e., with the back of one shoulder against the film, the position is called the posterior oblique. Regardless of whether the film is made in the anterior or the posterior oblique position, it is designated

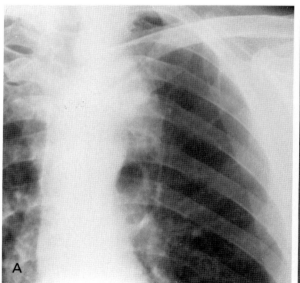
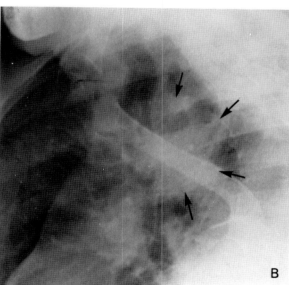

FIG. 6. INCLINED LATERAL VIEW OF POSTERIOR MEDIASTINAL TUMOR

A: The mass on the left side of the mediastinum obliterates the upper border of the aortic knob and is therefore situated posteriorly. The trachea is displaced slightly to the right, indicating that the mass extends to the middle mediastinum. On the lateral view the mass was hidden by the shoulders and it could not be localized on the ordinary oblique projections. *B:* The inclined left lateral view discloses the mass (arrows) in the posterior mediastinum, pushing the trachea forward. This view is made by depressing the left shoulder, raising the right shoulder, and tilting the tube upward. The tumor proved to be a lymphosarcoma.

in accordance with the shoulder that is in contact with the cassette. Thus, if the right shoulder is in contact with the film, the term right oblique is used, and if the left shoulder is in contact, the position is called the left oblique. There are, therefore, four positions which are possible with the patient at a 45 degree angle: the right and left anterior obliques and the right and left posterior obliques. The posterior oblique view is sometimes used when it is desired to show lesions in the posterior part of the chest with the better definition which is obtained when the pulmonary lesion is closer to the film.

Oblique views are made at angles other than 45 degrees when they are especially indicated. Only a 10 or a 20 degree angle of inclination of the patient on the film is required to expose the left lower lobe from behind the heart. The lesser angle is advisable because it exposes this region without superimposing the shadows of the spine and mediastinal structures. Various angles of obliquity are used in localization or in separating superimposed shadows for detailed study. The proper angle for the exposure in each case is best determined from a preliminary fluoroscopic examination.

As in the lateral view, care must be taken to prevent the arms from obscuring the chest on the film. Again, this is done best by placing the arms over the head. Some technicians prefer to displace backward the arm that is closer to the film. Usually, the arm clears the chest even though it is not elevated, but frequently its shadow will overlap the lung on that side if care is not taken to see that there is a clear space between the arm and the chest wall. This position is necessary if there is difficulty in raising the arm.

In the case of females, the shadow of the breast may obscure an important portion of the lung in the oblique projection. This occurs particularly when the breasts are heavy and when the breast which touches the film is displaced towards the midline while positioning the patient. The mediastinum and the adjacent portion of the opposite lung can then be obscured. This is obviated by displacing the breast in contact with the film, laterally rather than medially. It is kept in this position by the pressure of the patient against the cassette (Fig. 7).

Horizontal Positions. All exposures should be made with the patient erect unless there is a special reason for using the recumbent position. Two disadvantages of the recumbent position are the limitation of inspiration and the increase in distortion which results from the diminished tube distance that is usually employed. The recumbent positions are necessary when the patient cannot remain upright and when it is desirable to demonstrate the shift of a collection of

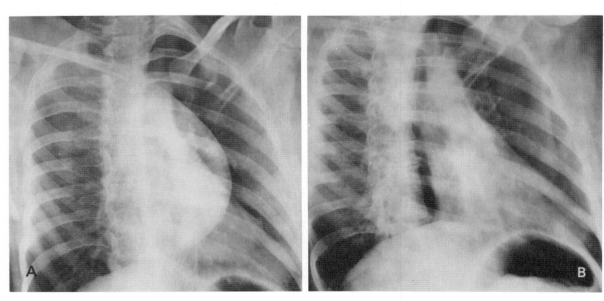

FIG. 7. SHADOW OF PENDULOUS BREAST

A: The shadow of a pendulous breast can obscure the mediastinum in the oblique view when the breast is trapped between the patient and the cassette. The large sharply demarcated density in this right oblique view represents the right breast. *B*: When the breast is displaced laterally before the patient leans against the cassette, its shadow is thrown off the pulmonary field and no longer creates any problem.

fluid in the lung, pleura, or subphrenic region. The position most commonly used for the latter purpose is the lateral decubitus, either right or left depending on which side the patient lies, using horizontal rays.

When placing the cassette in relation to the patient who is in the lateral decubitus position, care should be taken that the entire chest is projected on the film. The patient should be placed on a light pillow on the very edge of the table so that the film extends beyond the silhouette of the chest, or the shoulder and hip should be elevated on firm pillows or sandbags so that the chest hangs free above the table.

Patient-Film Distance. It has been mentioned that sharper roentgen images are produced when the lesion is situated closer to the film. This is true particularly if the tube is less than 6 feet from the film. The size of the image also depends on the distance between the lesion and the film if the tube film distance is short. The closer the lesion lies to the film, the smaller its shadow, but this can never be smaller than the actual size of the lesion (Fig. 8). On the other hand, magnification of the image is produced as the distance between the lesion and the film increases. Thus the image can be magnified at will by placing the patient at a distance from the film. However, with the x-ray tubes generally used in chest radiography, this is not desirable because the resulting degradation of the image nullifies the advantage of its enlargement.

There is an additional factor which determines the definition of lesions. This is the size of the focal spot of the x-ray tube. The smaller the focal

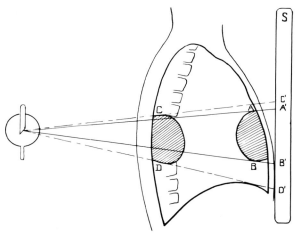

FIG. 8. MAGNIFICATION OF IMAGE AT A DISTANCE FROM THE SCREEN

In the posteroanterior projection the mass (AB) in the anterior part of the chest, nearer the screen, is projected as a smaller shadow than the mass of similar size (CD) in the posterior part, at a distance from the screen.

spot, the sharper the definition of the shadows. With currently available tubes, it is possible to picture lesions in the chest as well-defined shadows with two- or threefold magnification, by placing the patient at a distance from the film.

POSITION OF THE TUBE. Different effects may be produced by varying the position of the roentgen tube. The factors that can be changed are the distance of the tube from the film, its height and its inclination.

Tube-Patient Distance. Because lesions in the lung are necessarily separated by some distance from the roentgen film and because the image is produced by rays which diverge from the tube, there is always some magnification and loss of definition in their images. The more distant the tube is from the film, the less the rays diverge, and consequently, the image will be more sharply defined. At a distance of 8 feet, the rays are practically parallel and little further definition is produced by increasing the distance beyond this. For ordinary purposes, a distance of 6 feet between the tube and the film is sufficient for clarity of the image and this is the distance adopted for routine chest radiography. When an extremely short exposure is necessary, particularly in the examination of patients who have difficulty in holding their breath, or if the output of the x-ray equipment is insufficient, shorter distances may be used. In general, the resolution of films made at a distance of less than 3 feet is unsatisfactory.

Height of the Tube. Position of shadows in the lung relative to the clavicle, the anterior and posterior portions of the ribs and the dome of the diaphragm is affected by the height of the x-ray tube. For routine purposes, satisfactory views are obtained if the central ray is at the level of the spine of the scapula. It is advisable to set the tube at the same height at successive examinations of the same patient in order to facilitate comparison of the films. With older equipment, without a light collimator, visual estimation of the tube height is not sufficiently accurate to produce comparable results consistently. This can be accomplished if the distance from the spine of the scapula to the floor is measured and the tube height adjusted accordingly. A record is kept of this measurement so that the tube position can be duplicated whenever the patient is re-examined. This is unnecessary if the x-ray unit is equipped with a light collimator that indicates the center of the beam.

In some cases it is desirable to vary the height of the tube from the adopted standard. Thus, if it is wished to expose the anterior costophrenic sinus completely in the posteroanterior view, the tube should be elevated. Elevation of the tube in this view will also bring shadows in the posterior portion of the upper part of the lung, which are partially obscured by the clavicle, into view below this bone (Fig. 9A). Similarly, elevation of the tube in the anteroposterior projection will disclose that large portion of the lung which is hidden by the posterior costophrenic sinus (Fig. 9B). Depression of the tube in this view displaces the shadow of the clavicle upward above lesions in the upper posterior chest and produces a film similar to one made with the patient in the lordotic position.

The same effect that is produced by lowering or elevating the tube can be obtained by having the patient bend forward (kyphotic position), or slightly backward (hypererect position). In the posteroanterior view, with the patient kyphotic, the lung in the posterior costophrenic sinus is projected above the dome of the diaphragm and the posterior part of the upper lobe, ordinarily hidden by the clavicle, is projected above this bone. Conversely, in the hypererect position, lesions behind the clavicle are projected below it and the lung in the anterior costophrenic sinus is more completely exposed.

Angulation of the Tube. When the tube is placed either high or low, it should be angulated so that the central beam passes approximately through the center of the chest. This not only

produces clearer films, but also prevents cutting off a portion of the chest.

The tube may be angulated from side to side, as well as in a vertical direction. If the tube is displaced to one side, the rays pass obliquely through the chest in a horizontal direction and produce an effect similar to that of a partial oblique view. This is sometimes called the lateral eccentric projection. It is useful particularly in exposing the left lower lobe behind the heart (Fig. 10). Two views made by shifting the tube first to one side and then to the other, with a corresponding tilt in the tube to bring the central ray over the center of the chest are also useful in producing parallax which aids localization of lesions in the chest. If the shift of the tube, either horizontally or vertically, is about one-tenth of the tube-film distance, the films are suitable for stereoscopy.

A lateral eccentric position of the tube without angulation is sometimes useful in making films in the lateral projection, particularly if it is necessary to place the tube at a comparatively short distance from the film. The tube may be shifted toward the anterior part of the chest if a lateral view of the sternum or anterior mediastinum is required.

Roentgen Exposure. The amount of exposure a film receives in a given patient using a

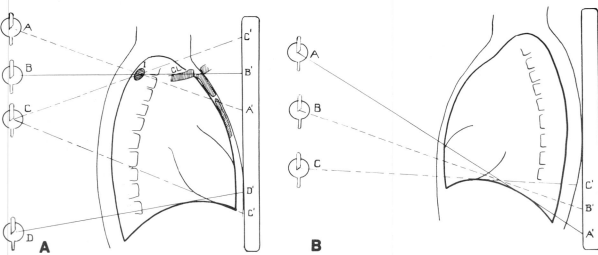

FIG. 9. EFFECT OF VARYING HEIGHT OF TUBE

A: Posteroanterior projection. The image of the lesion (I) in the posterior part of the right upper lobe is obscured by the clavicle (CL) when a horizontal ray (B) is used. If the tube is elevated (A), the image is projected below the clavicle. If the tube is depressed (C), it is projected above the clavicle. With the tube in any of these positions the anterior costophrenic sinus is completely exposed but a considerable portion of the lower posterior part of the lung is projected below the diaphragm and is obscured by the abdominal contents. When the tube is lowered further (D) most of the lower part of the lung in the posterior costophrenic sinus is projected above the diaphragm and is clearly visualized. Only the small portion of lung in the anterior costophrenic sinus is hidden. *B*: Anteroposterior projection. With the tube high (A), a portion of the lower anterior part of the lung is projected below the diaphragm, but practically all of the posterior portion is clearly exposed. As the tube is lowered (B and C), more of the lower anterior part of the lung is projected above the diaphragm, but an increasing portion of the posterior part becomes hidden by the abdominal organs.

standard focal spot, is a product of three factors: the voltage, milliamperage, and length of exposure. A properly exposed frontal film should permit faint visualization of the structures of the

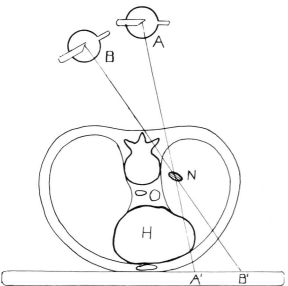

FIG. 10. LATERAL ECCENTRIC PROJECTION

Cross section of patient in the posteroanterior position, viewed from above. With the tube in the usual position at A, the image of the nodule (N) is obscured by the heart (H). However, if the tube is shifted laterally to position B, the image of the nodule is projected lateral to the heart and is therefore brought clearly to view.

chest through the heart (Fig. 11).

VOLTAGE. Variation in the voltage changes the penetrating quality of the rays. In general, the higher the voltage, the greater the penetration; and the greater the anteroposterior diameter of the chest, the higher the voltage that is required. The thickness of the chest is usually measured with calipers as a guide to the proper voltage.

The voltage should be sufficient to cause enough penetration of the heart to permit faint visualization of the spine and recognition of the vascular pattern through the cardiac shadow. The shadows of the breasts then, as a rule, will not obscure the lower pulmonary fields. On the other hand, the voltage should not be so great as to overexpose the outer portions of the lungs and obscure the small blood vessels in the periphery.

The voltage required is also modified by factors other than the depth of the chest. The density of the tissues of the chest wall must be taken into account. Thus, in muscular people, the voltage must be raised. Less allowance is made in the case of obesity since adipose tissue is easily penetrated by the rays.

Conditions inside the chest should be taken into account in estimating the voltage. Fluid or dense exudate in the pleura must be penetrated sufficiently to disclose abnormalities in the underlying lung. Similarly, in the case of dense lesions within the lungs, higher voltage is required to penetrate through the lesions to dis-

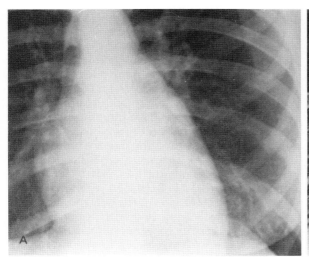
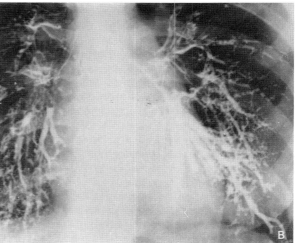

FIG. 11. RETROCARDIAC SHADOW IN BRONCHIECTASIS

A: The film, which was made with sufficient exposure to disclose the ribs and the spine behind the cardiac shadow, should show the vessels in the left lower lobe through the heart. Although the characteristic branching shadows of the vessels are visible within the cardiac shadow on the right side, they are not delineated on the left. This indicates the presence of disease in the left lower lobe. *B*: The bronchogram shows cylindric dilatation of the basal bronchi of the left lower lobe. These are drawn together behind the heart, indicating shrinkage of the basal segments. The incomplete filling of the distal portion of the dilated bronchi is due to retained secretion. A more complete bronchogram could have been obtained if postural drainage had been performed before bronchography.

close details within them. On the other hand, the emphysematous lung is easily penetrated by the rays. The marked increase in the anteroposterior diameter of the chest in patients with severe emphysema is no index as to the voltage that is required. The musculature of the chest wall in these patients is usually poorly developed. Because of this and the increased radiability of the lungs, a comparatively low voltage usually proves more suitable.

The use of low voltage produces films of greater contrast. Whereas contrast is desirable, it diminishes the range of shades from black to white which help in the interpretation of the roentgen film. The use of excessively low voltage, therefore, is not advisable. While films made with higher voltage appear generally more gray and less striking, the shadows of the structures in the chest are usually more sharply defined even though they may not be so obvious.

TIME AND MILLIAMPERAGE. Because there is always some movement of the structures in the chest, the clearest definition is obtained on films made with short exposures. Adequate films can be obtained with exposures as long as $1/5$ second if the patient can cooperate. However, shorter exposures are required in young children and in patients who have difficulty in holding their breath.

The length of exposure also depends upon the voltage and milliamperage; the higher these factors, the shorter the exposure. The intensity of radiation varies inversely as the square of the distance from its source. The time required for the exposure, therefore, varies as the square of the distance between the tube and the film. If the voltage is raised, either the exposure time or the milliamperage must be lowered.

Because of the diminution in contrast when high voltage is used, there is more leeway in the time-milliamperage factor. Errors as high as 50% in estimating the latter may not interfere with the interpretation of the film. However, when low amperage is used, this degree of error produces a film that is unsatisfactory from a diagnostic standpoint.

Automatic Exposure. The exposure time may be regulated automatically by means of a phototimer. This will terminate the exposure once sufficient x-rays have passed through the patient to produce a proper image on the film. When a standard exposure is not desired, the phototimer can be defeated and the technique determined by measuring the patient and observing his muscular development. In the great majority of cases, a well-calibrated phototimer ensures perfectly adequate films and, in addition, shortens the time required for the examination.

Portable Films. Films made with a portable x-ray machine are often not entirely satisfactory because the available milliamperage is lower than with most stationary machines and, therefore, requires longer exposure times. The exposure can be shortened by moving the tube closer to the patient but this increases distortion and lowers the quality of the picture.

The restriction in milliamperage is only partly due to the x-ray equipment itself. Most often the current must be kept at a low level because of the limitation imposed by the type of wiring where the examination is performed. Hospitals should be equipped with readily available outlets leading to heavy wiring and fuses to permit delivery of 220 volts so that sufficient amperage and voltage can be used. The difficulty in obtaining good films, however, is further accentuated by the fact that the patients are so ill that it is difficult for them to maintain the upright position or to hold their breath even for a comparatively short exposure. For these reasons, it is best, whenever possible, to transport the patient to the x-ray department for the examination.

Value of Special Examinations

Fluoroscopy. Fluoroscopy is helpful in the radiologic examination of the chest because of the dynamic factor that it affords. By means of fluoroscopy one is able to study the motion of the diaphragm and rib cage during respiration and to recognize pendular movement of the mediastinum, an important sign of bronchial obstruction. The vascular nature of certain shadows may be disclosed by observing their pulsations and the effect of the Valsalva and Mueller maneuvers. Ventilatory function of the lung may be studied by observing its clouding during expiration and its illumination during inspiration. By rotating the patient and moving the tube during fluoroscopic observation it is possible to accurately localize lesions in the thorax, either preoperatively or as a guide to needle biopsy. Shadows cast by lesions in the soft tissues of the chest wall, easily confused with lesions within the chest, are readily recognized by manipulating the soft tissues in the region of the shadow during fluoroscopy. Finally, fluoroscopy will often disclose the need for special positions in which additional films should be made.

Special Positions. LATERAL VIEW. The lateral view is used for several reasons. This view will determine whether a lesion is situated in front or in back and whether it is in approximation with the anterior or posterior chest wall. It may be the only view in which a small tumor of the anterior mediastinum is visible, and it is the only film on which one can accurately judge anterior or posterior displacement of the trachea or esophagus (see Fig. 457). Both the long and short fissures lie in planes which are parallel to the rays in this view and they are clearly outlined when they are the site of adhesions. The presence of an effusion in the long fissure can be determined with certainty only on the lateral projection (see Fig. 529). This view is also best for delineation of the middle lobe (Fig. 12).

The lateral projection reveals the lobar distribution of disease and the relation of lesions to the interlobar fissures. Certain segments of the lungs, notably the posterior and anterior segments of the upper lobes and the anterior and lateral basal segments of the lower lobes, are best outlined in this projection because their borders lie parallel to the x-ray beam. The exact relationship of lesions in the mid and posterior axillary regions to the ribs can be determined only on the lateral view.

The lateral view has the following limitations:

the lungs are projected over each other so that it is difficult, and sometimes impossible, to differentiate lesions in one lung from those in the other. Even when the disease is confined to one side of the chest, the lateral view may be entirely uninformative because the lucency of the opposite lung can eradicate the shadow of the lesion. This occurs in some cases of atelectasis and in some pleural effusions, particularly those situated in the axillary portion of the chest. In the latter, the aeration of the lung mesial to the effusion on the same side, as well as the aeration of the opposite lung, serves to obliterate the shadow of the fluid.

OBLIQUE VIEWS. The oblique views are particularly valuable in disclosing the position of those lesions which cannot be seen well on the lateral view. In the right anterior oblique position (right shoulder to the film), the posterior portion of the right chest and the anterior portion of the left chest are disclosed clearly because they are not overlapped by the opposite aerated lung or by the dense mediastinal structures. Similarly, in the left anterior oblique view (left shoulder to the film), lesions in the posterior part of the left lung and the anterior part of the right lung are

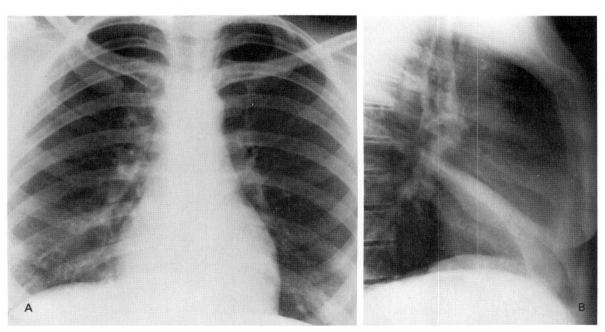

FIG. 12. ATELECTASIS OF MIDDLE LOBE

A: The patient had cough and fever and expectorated tenacious, nummular sputum. There is a nondescript shadow in the right paracardiac region. This obscures a portion of the right border of the heart, indicating that the disease involves the middle lobe. The appearance is most suggestive of a pneumonia. *B*: The lateral view shows a thin, triangular shadow running downward and forward from the lower portion of the root of the lung to the anterior costophrenic sinus. This is characteristic of atelectasis of the middle lobe. Bronchoscopy disclosed a purulent bronchitis with obstruction of the orifice of the middle lobe bronchus by thick secretion. The lobe reexpanded and appeared normal after the secretion was removed.

clearly delineated. Only rarely are the posterior oblique views preferable to the anterior obliques.

The oblique views are particularly valuable in disclosing the retrocardiac region (Fig. 13). They also bring into view the posterior costophrenic sinuses which contain a considerable portion of the lung hidden by the dome of the diaphragm in the ordinary posteroanterior projection. Small

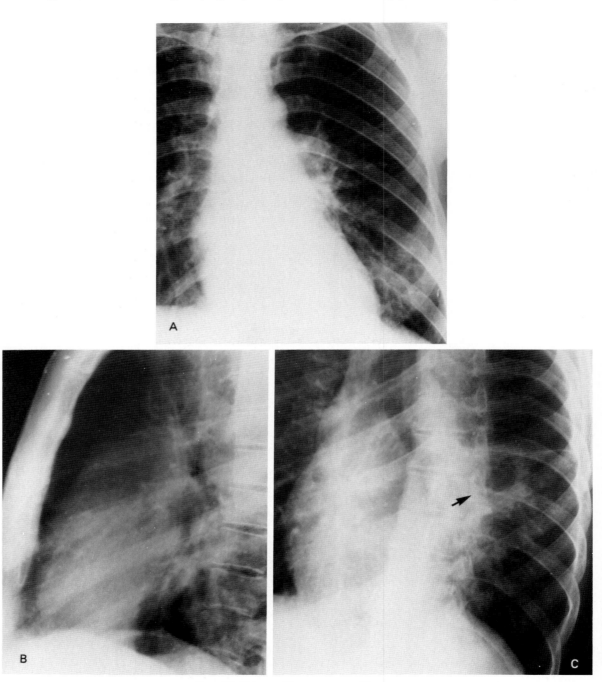

FIG. 13. HIDDEN TUBERCULOUS CAVITY

A: Frontal view. The only abnormality noted is an increase in the density of the root of the left lung. *B*: Lateral view. Except for questionable clouding over the posterior mediastinum, the film appears normal. Additional films were obtained because the patient had a persistent cough and the sputum contained tubercle bacilli. *C*: Left anterior oblique view. A well-defined empty cavity (arrow) is visualized in the superior segment of the left lower lobe. There are several faint, satellite nodules, peripheral to the cavity, suggesting that it is tuberculous.

effusions usually are better delineated on the oblique than on the frontal view, because it provides an unobstructed view of the deep posterior costophrenic sinus.

Slight oblique projections, from 5 to 10 degrees, may prove most useful in differentiating the vascular shadows at the lung roots from a density caused by a lesion in the lung or mediastinum (see Fig. 33). A lesion in the lung situated anterior or posterior to the lung root is separated from the hilar vessels in this projection. A rather prominent blood vessel, which appears as a round shadow in the frontal view suggesting a neoplasm or large lymph node at the hilum, may appear entirely different in the slight oblique projection. This view may disclose its true linear shape and its branching, leaving no doubt as to the vascular nature of the shadow.

A slightly more pronounced oblique projection, perhaps 15 or 20 degrees, is frequently useful in disclosing the details of a small lesion partly obscured by the lateral portion of the clavicle and the ribs in the upper, outer part of the chest. Since the early lesion of reinfection tuberculosis is located posteriorly in this region in most instances, the left oblique projection displaces the focus in the right upper lobe mesially to the anterior portion of the first rib, where it is seen more clearly. A slight right oblique projection is used to reveal the details of small tuberculous lesions in the left upper lobe. Bending the patient somewhat forward and lowering the roentgen tube in conjunction with the oblique projection, will also aid in bringing the lesion to view above the clavicle.

A left anterior oblique projection of about 25 degrees is often useful in disclosing the trachea and main bronchi. The manubrium and body of the sternum are projected away from the mediastinum in this projection.

The oblique views are also useful in the localization of lesions situated in the outer third of the chest (Fig. 14). One of the oblique projections may show an approximation of the lesion to the chest wall. It is the opposite oblique which shows the overlying ribs in their true length and without distortion of their relationship to the underlying lesion. It is in this view that the ribs are counted to determine the vertical level of a peripheral pulmonary lesion in relation to the thoracic cage. This is also the projection in which points of reference on the chest wall are studied for localization of the focus.

LORDOTIC VIEW. This view is valuable in revealing the apical regions and in delineating a diseased or collapsed middle lobe. The apex of the lung is partly hidden by the clavicle and the posterior portions of the first three ribs on the frontal projection. Because of the forward curve of the spine, the upper rib spaces are foreshortened and narrowed in this view. This is more marked in older people who have a tendency to a dorsal kyphosis. The lordotic view brings the upper posterior chest wall to a position parallel to the film and thus shows the intercostal spaces in their full width, making for a clearer view of the pulmonary apices.

The lordotic view is generally made in the anteroposterior projection. The patient stands at a distance from the film and leans backward until his shoulders are against the cassette. The roentgen tube is positioned low and tilted upward. The shadow of the clavicle is projected upward in relation to the posterior ribs. In the extreme lordotic position, the shadow of the clavicle is displaced above the posterior part of the first rib. However, this is usually not necessary because in most cases the lordotic view is used to uncover lesions behind the clavicle at the level of the second, third or fourth posterior intercostal spaces. The lordotic projection is especially useful in demonstrating the details of tuberculous lesions (Fig. 15), and in differentiating a carcinoma at the apex of the lung from inflammatory thickening of the pleura (see Fig. 407).

When the middle lobe is contracted, the anterior portion of the short fissure is usually displaced downward. The fissure then extends downward and forward instead of in a horizontal direction and is no longer parallel to the x-ray beam in the frontal projection. The upper border of the collapsed middle lobe, therefore, is not well delineated in this view. Since the long fissure also lies in an oblique plane, the shadow of a collapsed middle lobe is poorly demarcated on the ordinary frontal view.

The lordotic position brings both fissures that bound the middle lobe more parallel to the path of the rays. The collapsed middle lobe then casts a characteristic, sharply marginated, triangular shadow (Fig. 16). Since the middle lobe is situated anteriorly, it is somewhat better outlined if the lordotic view is made in the posteroanterior projection with the lower part of the chest close to the cassette and the upper part of the chest bent backward. The tube should be elevated and tilted downward so that the rays are more or less parallel to the fissures that bound the collapsed middle lobe.

The posteroanterior lordotic view is also useful in delineating the characteristic shadow of a hyperplastic thymus gland. The lower border of the hyperplastic thymus sometimes projects outward from the mediastinum in an angular manner, like a sail, producing a notch between it and the cardiac border below it (thymic notch). The

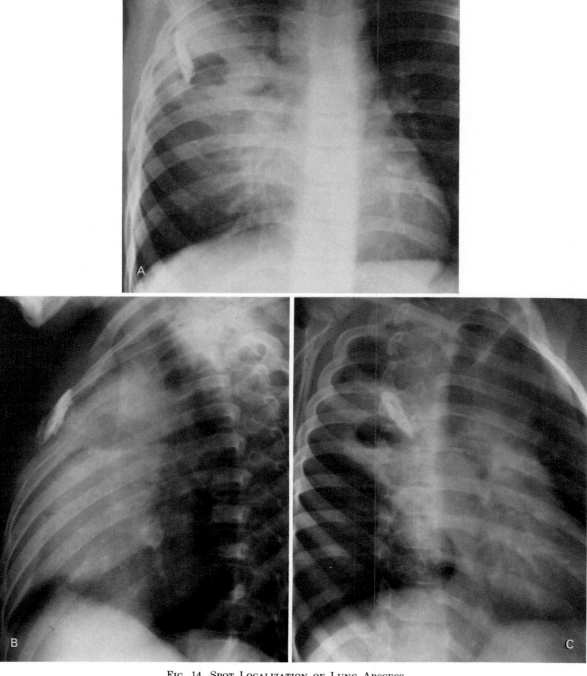

FIG. 14. SPOT LOCALIZATION OF LUNG ABSCESS

A: Frontal projection. Subacute putrid lung abscess in the outer part of the right upper lobe with extension of infection into the middle lobe. The elongated density lateral to the upper part of the cavity represents a mixture of Lipiodol and methylene blue, injected into the intercostal muscle for purposes of localization preliminary to operation. *B*: Touching oblique. The lesion is seen to approximate the chest wall in the left oblique view, indicating that it is situated beneath the anterior bend of the ribs. *C*: Counting oblique. The right oblique view is the projection in which there is the least distortion of the anterior bend of the ribs on the right side and is the position in which the true relationship of the lung, the overlying ribs and the material injected into the intercostal muscle is seen. In this projection the injected material is seen to be in the second intercostal space above and slightly anterior to the center of the abscess.

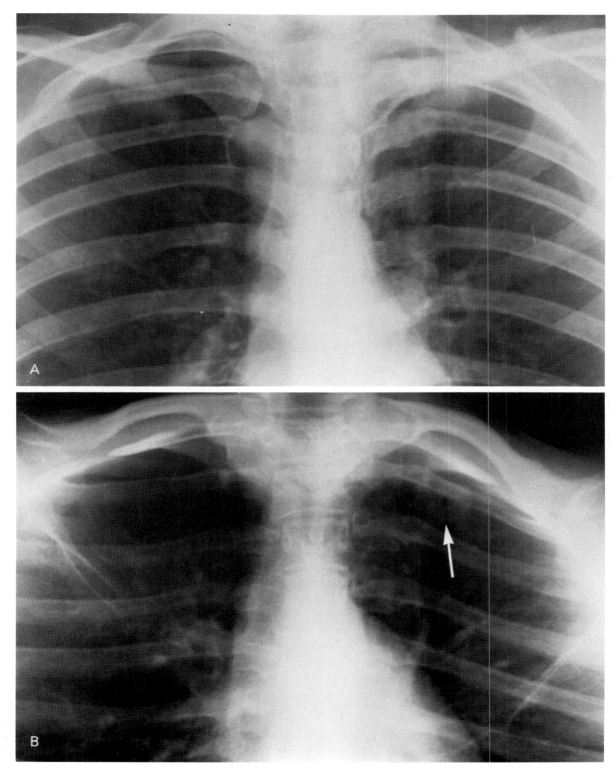

FIG. 15. USE OF LORDOTIC VIEW

A: On the frontal projection, there is an indistinct shadow at the left apex, mostly hidden by the first rib and the clavicle. *B*: Because the sputum was positive for tubercle bacilli, a lordotic view was obtained. The shadows of the clavicle and first rib are displaced upward, exposing the lesion in the posterior portion of the upper lobe. This contains a thick-walled cavity (arrow), representing an active tuberculous lesion.

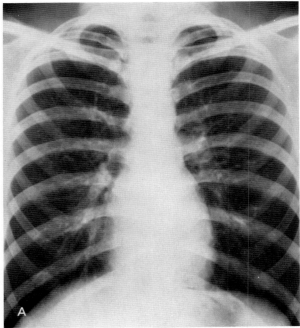

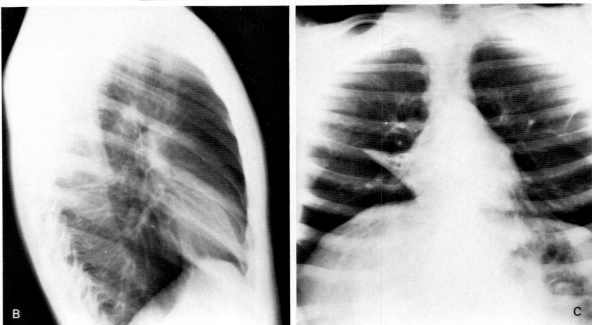

FIG. 16. MIDDLE LOBE ATELECTASIS: USE OF LORDOTIC VIEW

A: Frontal view. The only visible abnormality is an indistinctness of the right cardiac border suggesting disease of the middle lobe. *B*: Lateral view. There is a faint density within the cardiac shadow in the general region of the middle lobe. *C*: Lordotic view. The sharply demarcated triangular shadow adjacent to the heart represents the completely atelectatic middle lobe. The lucencies within the lobe are due to bronchiectases.

thymic notch and the sail sign are almost always more evident on the lordotic view (see Fig. 474). Not infrequently, the notch is visible on this view when only a diffuse, nondescript widening of the mediastinal shadow can be observed on the ordinary film.

In some instances, the thymic notch is more clearly demonstrated in the oblique projection (see Fig. 45). However, there are cases in which the only way to demonstrate the characteristic shadow of the hyperplastic thymus is by making the oblique projection while the patient maintains a lordotic position.

HYPERERECT POSITION. An effect somewhat similar to that obtained from the lordotic position can be obtained on the ordinary posteroanterior view if the patient stands erect and the tube is elevated. Ordinarily, in exposing a film in this projection, the patient's chin is placed over the cassette and he is bent forward in order to maintain close contact between the upper part of the chest and the cassette. When using the hypererect position, it is best to elevate the cassette so that the chin touches the face of the cassette, to ensure a vertical position of the body. The patient may even be instructed to bend slightly backward. This raises the clavicle and permits the rays to cast the shadow of the posterior part of the third rib beneath it. This position combines the advantages of the lordotic view and the posteroanterior projection of the chest. It is valuable when a smaller degree of angulation than that provided by the lordotic view is required.

APICAL VIEWS. The apices may be disclosed more completely by projecting the clavicle downward rather than upward as is done in the lordotic view. This is accomplished by making a posteroanterior projection with the patient bent forward. In essence, this is a *kyphotic* rather than a lordotic position.

Superior mediastinal masses which cannot be well delineated on the ordinary lateral view because of the intervention of the shoulders, may be more clearly disclosed by utilizing the inclined lateral position (see p. 6). In this view the shoulder, rather than the clavicle, is depressed and the mediastinal mass is projected through the apex of the lung.

KYPHOTIC VIEW. Not only is the kyphotic position useful in disclosing lesions at the pulmonary apices, but it is also helpful in bringing into view lesions of the posterior costophrenic sinus which are hidden by the subphrenic structures in the standard projections. The films are best made with the patient's back against the cassette. He is bent either directly or obliquely forward and the tube elevated and angled downward.

LATERAL DECUBITUS. The lateral recumbent position, using horizontal rays, is sometimes required to detect a pleural effusion (see Fig. 521) or to confirm the presence of a fluid level in the lung, pleural cavity, or subphrenic region (see Fig. 566). Similar information may be obtained by simply tilting the patient to one side, but the demonstration of fluid by this means is not so striking. The lateral decubitus position is helpful in demonstrating fluid or air in a cavity when there is very little air or when the fluid content is extremely small. The lateral decubitus position may be the only one in which an extremely small pleural effusion can be demonstrated. In some cases, it is impossible, from the ordinary roentgen examination, to differentiate between consolidation at the base of the lung and a collection of fluid in the lower part of the pleural cavity. In such instances, the lateral decubitus position will cause the fluid to gravitate from its original location if it is not completely loculated by adhesions. In addition, displacing the fluid will expose the diaphragm so that its position can be determined.

TRENDELENBURG POSITION. This position is particularly useful in bronchography when it is necessary to obtain complete filling of the upper branches of the upper lobes, or when an attempt is made to fill cavities at the apex and the bronchi in this region cannot be outlined well in the ordinary recumbent position. Obstruction of the apical or posterior branches, inferred from lack of filling on films made in the flat position, often requires confirmation by reexamination with the upper part of the body tilted downward in the Trendelenburg position. If the passage of oil into the upper bronchial branches is blocked with the patient in this position, the presence of an obstruction is substantiated.

Examination in the Trendelenburg position may aid in the diagnosis of a parapericardial cyst. A large parapericardial cyst tends to change its shape when the patient is shifted from the erect to the Trendelenburg position, while a properitoneal fat herniation through the foramen of Morgagni maintains its original shape. A small parapericardial cyst remains round no matter what position is used. However, if it is pedunculated, it will change its position on shifting the patient.

Stereoscopy. There is considerable disagreement among radiologists concerning the value of stereoscopic examination of the chest. This method is favored by those who are accustomed to using it frequently and who find no difficulty in obtaining a stereoscopic image.

Stereoscopy can be useful in several ways. An important point in its favor is that it supplies two roentgen films of the chest. Artifacts are easily recognized because they are evident on only one of the films. Furthermore, since these films represent projections from two different points, they show the effects of parallax. Careful study of the difference in relationship of the lesion to anatomic landmarks on the two films aids in localization even without the use of stereoscopic viewing apparatus. However, the use of this apparatus often discloses the location of the disease more accurately.

Aside from its value in localization, the view in depth afforded by stereoscopy, aids in the interpretation of the shadow by demonstrating its topography more clearly than a single film. Overlapping shadows can be separated to disclose the shape, extent, and variations in density of each of the shadows.

Stereoscopic examination is useful particularly in the localization of lesions in the lung or bronchi where a contrast medium is used as a point of reference. This applies particularly in bronchography, where the three-dimensional view serves to separate overlapping bronchi from each other, simplifying their identification.

Examination after Sedation. Abolition of the cough reflex for a time previous to the examination is sometimes useful in demonstrating pulmonary cavities. Most tuberculous cavities are supplied by a wide open bronchus which drains the cavity so well that no fluid level is seen, and in the absence of a fluid level it is often difficult to demonstrate the cavity on the ordinary film. If the secretions are permitted to accumulate by abolishing the cough reflex for a period of time, they may produce a visible fluid level which proves the presence of a cavity.

Postural Drainage. In some cases of lung abscess and, more rarely, in bronchiectasis, the cavities are filled with fluid exudate and secretions, and are represented by solid shadows on the film.

A filled lung abscess may simulate a neoplasm or pneumonia. Filled, widened bronchi in bronchiectasis may appear as finger-like projections, spreading out from the root of the affected lobe, producing a bizarre, although characteristic, picture. Proof that these shadows are due to retained secretion is afforded by reexamination after postural drainage, which causes the disturbing shadows to disappear. In the case of a filled lung abscess, evidence of cavitation can be obtained after postural drainage when some or all of the contents of the abscess are evacuated and replaced by air.

Where postural drainage fails to drain the cavity and permit the ingress of air to disclose a fluid level, bronchoscopy may accomplish this change. It is, therefore, advisable in cases of a solid shadow which may be due to an abscess of the lung, to repeat the roentgen examination after bronchoscopy in an attempt to demonstrate a fluid level that would establish the diagnosis.

Inspiration and Expiration. Films made in full inspiration and full expiration provide information regarding aeration of the lungs and motion of the diaphragm, the mediastinum and chest wall. This knowledge is important in evaluating the function of each lung preliminary to resective surgery.

The presence of obstruction of one of the larger bronchi can be demonstrated even in the absence of atelectasis. The inability of one lung, or of a single lobe to empty itself of air can be determined by the absence of clouding of that portion on expiration and displacement of the mediastinum to the opposite side (see Figs. 17 and 43). In obstructive emphysema, the blood vessels remain separated during expiration and the mediastinal structures are displaced toward the opposite side. Diminished excursion of the chest wall and diaphragm during respiration are depicted on the films for permanent record.

Films made in both inspiration and expiration are particularly helpful in the detection of obstruction of the smaller bronchi supplying a portion of a lobe. The normal fanning out of the blood vessels in the obstructed segment does not occur during inspiration, and the obstructed portion does not change its degree of aeration.

Relative motion is visible between a lesion in the lung and the overlying ribs during respiration if there are no adhesions over the diseased area. If the shadow of the lesion does not move independently of the ribs, it may be assumed that the pleura is adherent over it. However, to be certain of the presence of adhesions, the examination should be made in the recumbent as well as in the erect position. We have observed a case of subpleural fibroma that simulated an adherent peripheral carcinoma of the lung or a tumor of the parietal pleura. No motion could be detected between the lesion and the overlying ribs even during forced respiration when the patient was fluoroscoped in the erect position. However, there was a considerable excursion of the shadow during respiration when the patient was recumbent.

The expiratory film is superior to the film made in inspiration for the detection of a small pneumothorax. It is important to bear in mind that a small pneumothorax may easily be overlooked in films made only in inspiration (see Fig. 32). The expiratory film may also be useful in disclosing the shadows of interstitial infiltrations which cannot be recognized on the ordinary inspiratory film, or to accentuate the shadows of these lesions in questionable cases. The expiratory film will frequently show a dense clouding

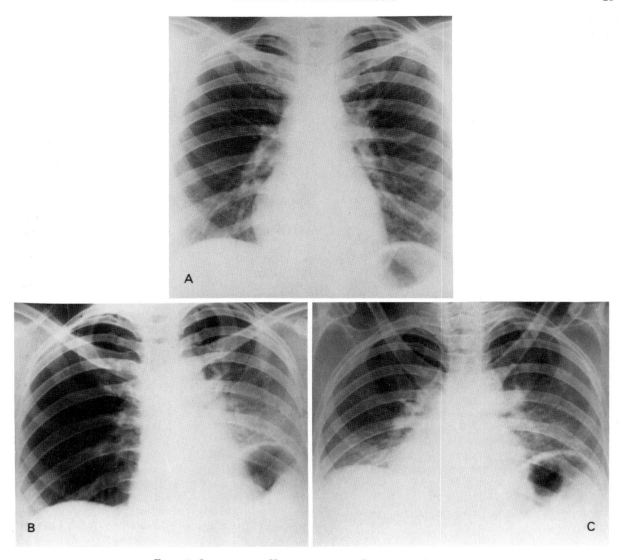

FIG. 17. OBSTRUCTIVE HYPERINFLATION: BRONCHIAL ADENOMA

A: The film made in inspiration shows the pulmonary field on the right side to be somewhat darker and the vascular shadows less prominent than on the left. The heart and mediastinum are in their normal positions. The same changes were noted on previous films, all of which had been made in inspiration. The cause for the difference in the appearance of the two lungs is not apparent. *B*: Because of a persistent wheeze, a film was made in expiration. The right lung remains aerated. The left lung, which was able to expel its air, is now clouded. The left leaf of the diaphragm is at a much higher level and the heart has shifted toward the left side. These changes are diagnostic of obstructive hyperinflation of the right lung which, in this case, was due to an adenoma in the right main bronchus. *C*: The film made in expiration after bronchoscopic removal of the adenoma shows both lungs to be equally deflated. There is no longer a shift of the mediastinum. The left lung is less clouded than on the previous film because it is not compressed by the heart.

of the lower third of the pulmonary field in such instances. The increased clouding during expiration, however, does not occur when the infiltrative disease is complicated by emphysema.

Valsalva Maneuver. Valuable information may be obtained by comparing a film made in the ordinary way with one made while the patient is straining (Valsalva maneuver). During constant straining against the closed glottis, diminished blood flow through the heart results in a narrowing of the pulmonary blood vessels which can be demonstrated on film. This aids in differentiating between the shadows of distended pulmonary arteries and veins at the lung roots and large lymph nodes or neoplastic infiltrations in that region. A diminution in the size of the shadow indicates that it is produced by blood vessels rather than by enlarged lymph nodes or infiltrations. The manuever is also helpful when there is difficulty in differentiating between distended peripheral vessels and interstitial infiltrations of the lung. Diminution in the width of the shadows on straining leads to the conclusion that the prominent pulmonary markings are due to widening of the blood vessels rather than to infiltrations of the interlobular septa or perivascular and peribronchial connective tissue.

Special Techniques

A large variety of roentgen methods has been developed involving the use of special apparatus.

This has resulted in increasing the rate at which films can be made, improvement in the delineation of pathologic processes in the lungs, more precise localization of these lesions, better demonstration of the respiratory movements and pulsations of structures within the chest, correlation of these movements with pulsations elsewhere in the cardiovascular system, and the differentiation of mediastinal and pulmonary lesions from diseases of the vascular system.

Examination of Young Children and Very Sick Adults. The use of high milliamperage equipment has made it possible to obtain clear films in children and patients who are too ill to hold their breath for the time involved in ordinary exposures. The rapid exposures afforded by

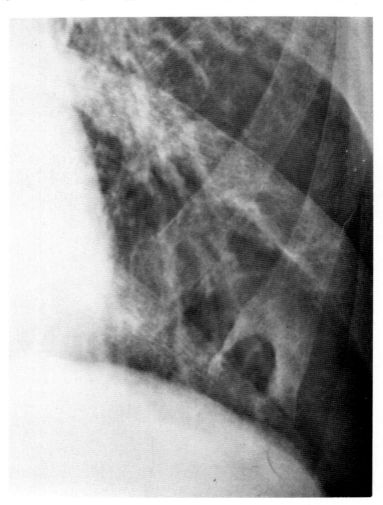

FIG. 18. TUBERCULOUS OSTEOCHONDRITIS OF THE RIB

There is a semicircular defect with a sclerotic margin in the anterior portion of the sixth rib adjacent to the costochondral junction. The rib is widened in this region. The lesion was associated with a cold abscess in the overlying chest wall. The patient had active pulmonary tuberculosis at this time.

modern x-ray apparatus result in sharply defined shadows even though the patient breathes during the examination. Children and sick adults are helped to maintain the upright position during filming by special supports, so that the undesirable recumbent position is rarely necessary. Patients too ill to be transported to the x-ray department can be examined in bed with portable x-ray apparatus.

Film Changers. Rapid sequential films are essential for angiocardiography. This is accomplished through the use of automatic film changers which are designed so that exposures can be made at stated time intervals or in relation to selected phases of the cardiac cycle. Ciné equipment can provide 60 or more films per second, but the delineation of the structures is not so sharply defined as in the larger standard films. Better definition can be obtained by recording the output from the image intensifier tube on serial 105 mm films.

Grids. The grid consists of a series of alternating strips of lead and radiolucent material arranged on end and placed between the patient and the film. The lead strips are relatively deep and the spaces between them are narrow. Therefore, rays which are deflected in passing through the patient strike the sides of the lead strips and are absorbed so that only parallel rays pass through the grid to the film. Contrast is therefore increased with a minimum loss of definition of the shadows.

A grid is useful where increased penetration is required as in the examination of heavy patients, especially in the lateral and oblique views. It is particularly useful in disclosing cavities in fibrotic or densely infiltrated lungs, and in showing the condition of the lung which is masked by an effusion. It is helpful in disclosing the architecture of the bones of the thoracic cage (Fig. 18), and lesions behind the heart. Radiopaque foreign bodies, areas of calcification and injected contrast material are more sharply delineated (Figs. 19, 140, and 160), as is the lucent air column in the trachea and bronchi.

The stationary grid has the disadvantage of showing striped shadows on the film, but the grids are so fine that the lines are not disturbing.

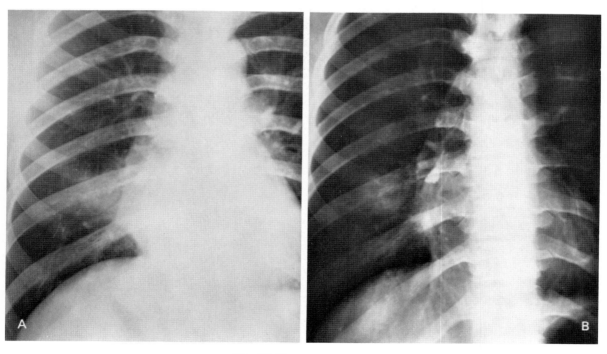

FIG. 19. BRONCHOLITHIASIS

A: There is an area of consolidation adjacent to the heart. The right cardiac border is obliterated, indicating that the lesion is situated in the middle lobe. The picture is that of a nonspecific pneumonia. However, because of a faint shadow at the hilum, the possibility of underlying broncholithiasis was considered. *B:* The film made with a Bucky grid shows the hilar shadow to represent a calcified lymph node. This is situated adjacent to the intermediate bronchus at the origin of the bronchus to the middle lobe. The stone was removed through the bronchoscope.

The movable grid or Potter-Bucky diaphragm does away with the stripes, but it requires a greater exposure.

Kymography. Roentgen kymography is a method which depicts the movements of structures on a single film. A lead screen with fine parallel slits, 12 to 18 mm apart, is placed between the patient and the film. An exposure is made while the film moves for a distance corresponding to that between the slits, in a direction perpendicular to them. In this way the pulsation, or movement, of structures seen through the slits is demonstrated. The amplitude, speed, and character of their motion can be determined from the curves on the film. Although these move-ments can be seen by fluoroscopy, the kymogram is useful for the analysis of the movement as well as for future record. Movements of the chest wall, the diaphragm, and the mediastinum can be recorded. In addition, the pulsation of the pulmonary arteries and of pulsatile masses in the lungs or mediastinum can be analyzed. The difference between *expansile* pulsation indicating a vascular mass and pulsation *transmitted* to a solid mass from the heart or great vessels can be determined in some cases, if the kymogram is made in the transverse, as well as in the vertical direction.

A clearer delineation of the curve of pulsation may be obtained by *electrokymography*. Instead

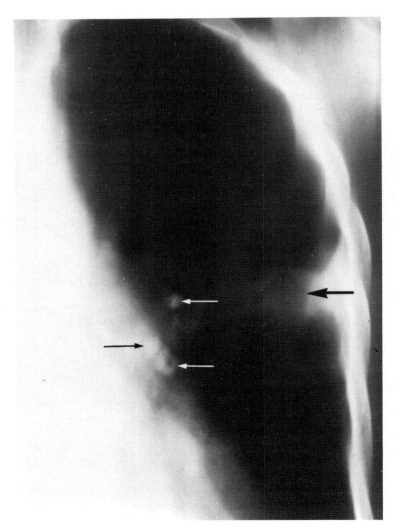

Fig. 20. Broncholithiasis: Tomography

Three calcific deposits (arrows) are visualized at the left hilum. The uppermost one lies in the same plane as the root of the collapsed anterior segment of the upper lobe. There are at least two cavities within this segment, one of which is visible (lateral arrow) in this plane.

of recording the movement of the borders of the structures on an x-ray film, a photomultiplier tube scans the fluoroscopic image of the moving borders and records the characteristics of their motions as a linear curve. The curve of the pulsation of a structure in the chest may be correlated with the pulsations of the heart, arteries, and veins outside the chest, and with the movements of respiration, by apparatus which makes simultaneous recordings of all of them. Thus, the pulsation of structures in the lungs or mediastinum may be related to the cardiovascular cycle, and the effects of respiration on cardiovascular dynamics may also be studied.

Biplane Examinations. Equipment is available for fluoroscoping simultaneously in two planes at right angles to each other. Biplane serial or ciné films can also be obtained. This method is particularly useful for angiocardiography. Biplane fluoroscopy is useful for the localization of foreign bodies and obtaining biopsies through the flexible bronchoscope or percutaneously through the chest wall.

Body Section Radiography. Body section radiography, which includes the terms planigraphy, stratigraphy, laminagraphy and tomography, is a method by which the structures lying in a single plane of the chest are sharply delineated, while structures in other planes are blurred. The roentgen tube and the film holder are connected so that they can be moved in opposite directions during the exposure. In essence, this creates a lever with the film at one end and the tube at the other. When this lever is moved during the exposure, objects in a plane corresponding to the level of the fulcrum are constantly projected on the same point on the roentgen film. These, therfore, remain sharply outlined. The shadows of objects outside the plane move in relation to the film and are blurred so that their outlines are indiscernible. In this way an image is produced in which only the structures in one plane are clearly demonstrated (Fig. 20). By changing the height of the tube-film complex, thus altering the relationship of the fulcrum to the patient, sections at different levels are obtained. Tomograms are most commonly made in the frontal, lateral and oblique planes. They can also be made in the horizontal, or cross-sectional plane (transverse laminagraphy), by the use of special equipment.

Lesions in the chest are often obscured by the shadows of overlying structures so that tomography is frequently essential for diagnosis and treatment. It is often required for the demonstration of cavities (Fig. 21) or calcific deposits (see Fig. 137) and the visualization of lesions in the lung hidden by diseased pleura. Tomograms can

demonstrate pulmonary metastases so small that they cannot be visualized on conventional films. Therefore, tomography of the lungs should be performed before operation for a metastatic tumor that is presumed to be single.

The air column in the bronchi and trachea can be sharply defined by tomography, permitting the demonstration of lesions encroaching on the lumen (Fig. 22). This method can also disclose sacculated and cylindrical bronchiectases.

The size, shape and position of the blood vessels are more clearly shown on tomograms than on conventional films. Observation of the distribution of the blood vessels on the lateral as well as on the frontal projections aids in determining the size and position of the lobes when the pleural fissures cannot be visualized. This is useful not only in determining the presence of partial atelectasis or of obstructive emphysema, but also in determining the segment in which a pulmonary lesion lies.

Tomograms are commonly made in the frontal and lateral projections. These provide the necessary detail of most lesions and have the advantage of being easily reproducible. This is important when serial studies are needed as the patient can be placed in the same position time after time allowing a valid comparison between films from different examinations. However, in some cases, a lesion is best demonstrated on tomograms made in an oblique projection. The optimal degree of obliquity can be determined from routine films or by preliminary fluoroscopic examination.

With the patient in a 55-degree posterior oblique position, a standard tomographic projection is obtained that is extremely useful for evaluation of the major bronchi, the pulmonary hila and the posterior segments of the upper and lower lobes. In this view, the main bronchus on the side closest to the film lies in a plane that is essentially parallel to that of the tomogram. The bronchus therefore is seen in its entire length and endobronchial lesions are easily identified. In addition, these oblique sections are of extreme value in the identification of enlarged hilar nodes and in differentiating prominent hilar vessels from such nodes. The main pulmonary artery is viewed in cross section and appears as a circular density within the area circumscribed by the trachea mesially, the main bronchus below and the upper lobe bronchus on the lateral side. Densities outside of these structures almost always represent enlarged hilar nodes (Fig. 23).

CALCIFIC DEPOSITS. Tomography is the best available method for determining the presence of calcific deposits within nodular shadows in the

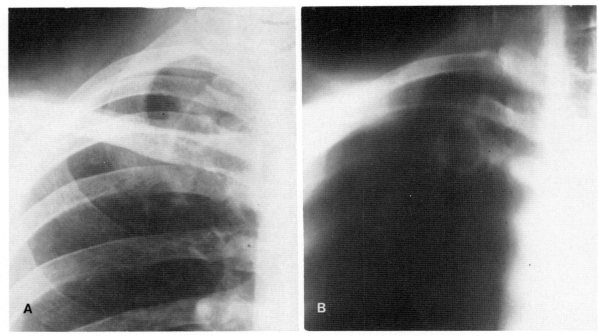

FIG. 21. TUBERCULOSIS WITH CAVITATION

A: Conventional film. A cavity on the left side had been obliterated by pneumothorax therapy but the sputum remained positive for tubercle bacilli. There is an irregular density with nodular infiltration in the upper part of the right upper lobe. *B*: Tomography. The disturbing shadows of the clavicle and the fourth rib have been blurred out, exposing a sharply circumscribed, round cavity. The posterior portions of the second and third ribs are clearly outlined in the same section, indicating that the cavity is situated posteriorly.

lung. These may not be recognizable on Bucky films although they are clearly outlined on to-mograms. This is of the utmost value in differential diagnosis because the presence of calcification within a nodule, in a definite pattern, indicates that it does not represent a malignant neoplasm (see Fig. 410). The relationship of calcified lymph nodes to adjacent bronchi may be difficult to determine with acceptable accuracy by any means other than tomography. Moreover, calcifications can be differentiated from the shadows of blood vessels viewed on end. The diagnosis of broncholithiasis can be established by tomography if the stones are demonstrated to lie within the bronchi or in relation to an atelectatic or infected area (Fig. 20).

CAVITIES. The demonstration of a cavity within a lesion of the lung may be crucial in the diagnosis of pulmonary tuberculosis or lung abscess. In tuberculosis, the cavities usually do not have a fluid level to indicate their presence and the cavity wall itself is frequently hidden by the overlying densely infiltrated pulmonary tissue. While films made with increased exposure, as well as those made in the slight oblique projection or in the lordotic position may disclose some of the cavities, many cavities are detectable only by tomography (Fig. 21). This method of exami-

nation is therefore indispensable whenever a tuberculous lesion is suspected.

Tomography is essential in following the course of a tuberculous infection and in determining the effectiveness of treatment. This is especially true in evaluating closure of a tuberculous cavity since persistence of the cavity may signify the need for resective surgery. It is common to have all evidence of cavitation disappear on ordinary films, only to have the cavity demonstrated by tomography.

A lung abscess almost completely filled with exudate usually fails to show a fluid level on conventional radiography. The shadow may have the appearance of a round tumor. Tomography can disclose small amounts of air within the lesion, not demonstrable in any other way.

LOCALIZATION. Sectional radiography is also valuable in localization of lesions in the chest. Occasionally one is seen on the frontal view but is not visualized clearly enough on the lateral or oblique views or on fluoroscopy, to determine its location. In such cases, sections at different levels will disclose the lesion in a plane whose location is known. Lateral sections are also helpful for this purpose. These also serve to demonstrate the relation of the disease to the lobes and fissures and are therefore important as a prelimi-

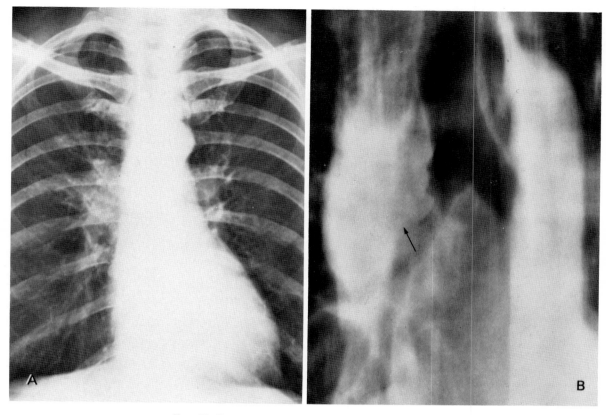

FIG. 22. BRONCHOGENIC CARCINOMA: TOMOGRAPHY

A: The conventional film of a 51 year old female who was coughing bloody sputum, shows an indistinct density at the right hilum. A lesion could be seen in the right main bronchus on a film made in the left anterior oblique projection. *B*: The tomogram in the right posterior oblique position reveals a sharply demarcated, lobulated mass intruding into the lumen of the right main bronchus. Its upper limit is slightly below the tracheobronchial angle and its lower border (arrow) reaches the beginning of the intermediate bronchus. Because of the circumscription of the tumor as determined from the tomograms, it was possible to avoid pneumonectomy by resecting the right main bronchus together with the right upper lobe and anastomosing the intermediate bronchus to the trachea.

nary to resective surgery for tuberculosis. Transverse, or horizontal sections of the chest may be definitive in localization where the usual measures are inconclusive.

The Use of Contrast Media

The roentgen visualization of the structures of the chest in health and disease depends, in the main, on the contrast between the soft tissues and the radiolucent air in the lungs, trachea and bronchi. Further contrast may be produced by introducing materials to alter the density of structures whose outlines are otherwise not well visualized.

Air as a Contrast Medium

Where solid shadows of adjacent structures merge, there is no natural demarcation by which their boundaries can be determined on the roentgen film. Introduction of air between these structures separates them and allows their outlines to be sharply defined against the intervening radiolucent gas. The air may be injected into the pleural cavity to separate dense shadows of the lung from the chest wall, and into the peritoneal cavity to bring the undersurface of the diaphragm into view by separating it from radiopaque structures in the abdomen. The mediastinal organs may be separated from each other by pneumomediastinography.

Preexisting Air. BRONCHI. Ordinarily only the largest bronchi can be visualized on the roentgen film. However, if there is solidification of the surrounding lung, the smaller bronchi may be seen, outlined by the air within them.

In bronchiectasis, the widened, air-filled bronchi are often visible on ordinary films for the same reason. The dilated bronchi are shown

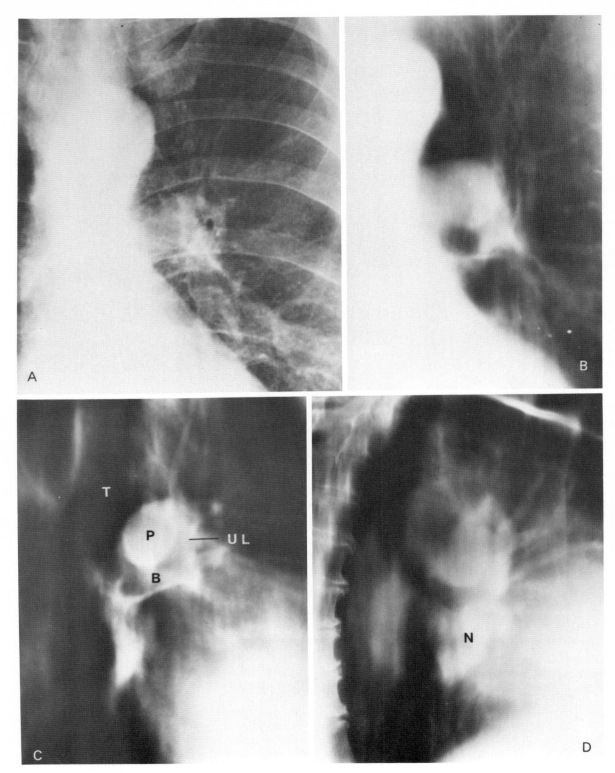

FIG. 23. POSTERIOR OBLIQUE TOMOGRAPHY

A: On the frontal film, the left hilar shadow appears abnormally prominent and dense. It was thought to be caused by a bronchogenic carcinoma or an enlarged hilar node. However, the possibility that the shadow was due only to the left main pulmonary artery could not be excluded. *B*: A frontal tomogram shows a shadow at the hilus curving downward and appearing to branch. This suggests that it represents only a prominent main pulmonary artery. However, it was felt that this could not be stated with certainty. *C*: A tomogram in the left posterior oblique reveals the smooth shadow of the left main pulmonary artery (P) seen in cross section, between the trachea (T), the left main bronchus (B) and the bronchus to the upper lobe (UL). There are no densities beneath the main bronchus, indicating that the hilar shadow was due solely to the pulmonary artery. *D*: Posterior oblique tomogram in a patient with sarcoidosis. The lobulated mass (N) beneath the left main bronchus represents enlarged hilar lymph nodes.

more clearly on overpenetrated or Bucky films or by tomography.

When dilated bronchi are filled with secretion, they appear as finger-like shadows radiating from the root of the lung (see Fig. 202). Disappearance of the shadows after postural drainage confirms the diagnosis of bronchiectasis. When the secretions are only partly eliminated, fluid levels may be demonstrated in dilated bronchi.

ABSCESS CAVITIES. Difficulty is encountered in the diagnosis of a lung abscess when it is filled with exudate. It may be impossible, even with the aid of clinical information, to differentiate between a lung abscess, a tumor of the lung, pneumonia, and an infarct. If some of the pus from the abscess can be eliminated through the bronchi and air is permitted to enter the cavity, a fluid level appears. This proves that the dense shadow was not cast by solid lung or a tumor.

If one waits long enough and repeats the roentgenographic examination periodically, a fluid level may eventually become demonstrable spontaneously. However, the same end may be accomplished more quickly by simple postural drainage or bronchoscopic aspiration. Here again, examination with increased penetration, Bucky films or sectional radiography may be necessary to disclose the air by which the abscess is recognized.

MEDIASTINAL EMPHYSEMA. Pneumomediastinum occurs secondarily as a result of dissection of air into the mediastinum from interstitial emphysema of the lung. Air can also enter the mediastinum directly during tracheotomy or during operations in which the mediastinum is opened. In any case, the air serves to outline the mediastinal structures (Fig. 24) and may displace the thymus gland. The changes on the roentgen film are the same as those produced by the deliberate injection of air into the mediastinum (p. 30).

Injected Air. INDUCED PNEUMOTHORAX. Air injected after withdrawal of fluid from the pleural cavity will outline more accurately the extent of the effusion. In encapsulated effusions particularly if films are made in the lateral recumbent, as well as the upright position, the borders of the loculation are clearly outlined.

The separation of the lung from the parietal pleura by an induced pneumothorax after removal of the pleural effusion may disclose nodules projecting from either the parietal or the visceral pleura into the air-filled pleural space (Figs. 25 and 562). It may be necessary to make oblique as well as frontal views to demonstrate the nodules on the pleura clearly. The position required depends on the location of the nodules.

A circumscribed neoplasm of the lung may grow through the pleura to involve the chest wall. The only radiologic method by which such a primary neoplasm can be differentiated with certainty from a tumor originating in the chest wall itself is by examination after induction of a pneumothorax. Complete separation of the lung from the tumor indicates that the neoplasm originates in the chest wall. Lack of separation of the pleura in the region of the shadow does not prove conclusively that the tumor is primary in the lung because it is possible that the lung may be bound to the chest wall simply by inflammatory adhesions.

Separation of the mesial surface of the lung from the mediastinum by a pneumothorax is unusual even in the absence of adhesions. Moreover, mediastinal neoplasms often become adherent to the mesial surface of the lung and, in fact, actually infiltrate the lung. Therefore, a pneumothorax is generally of little use in determining the origin of a growth in this region. However, if the mesial surface of the lung can be separated from the mediastinum by the pneumothorax, the position of the tumor, whether in the lung or in the mediastinum, becomes evident.

An induced pneumothorax may be helpful in the diagnosis of lesions in relation to the diaphragm. It is useful in the differentiation between an infrapulmonary empyema and a subphrenic abscess, both of which may cause identical shadows. If air can be demonstrated between the lower surface of the lung and the diaphragm, the possibility of an infrapulmonary empyema is excluded. The diaphragm can be separated from the lung only by the induction of a fairly large pneumothorax, and even then examination in the lateral recumbent position, using horizontal rays, may be required. The inability to separate the lung from the diaphragm does not exclude a subphrenic abscess from consideration. Adhesions of the lung to the diaphragm are often present in association with a subphrenic abscess and prevent the air from entering the infrapulmonary space.

The differentiation between a tumor of the lung and a bulge of the diaphragm may be made after the induction of a pneumothorax. If the lesion can be separated from the diaphragm by the air, it must be situated in either the lung or the visceral pleura. However, as in the case of the mediastinal surface of the lung, the base may not separate from the diaphragm even in the absence of adhesions. This occurs particularly in its mesial portion. Oblique, lateral, and lateral decubitus views are often required to disclose separation of these structures. In one of our cases

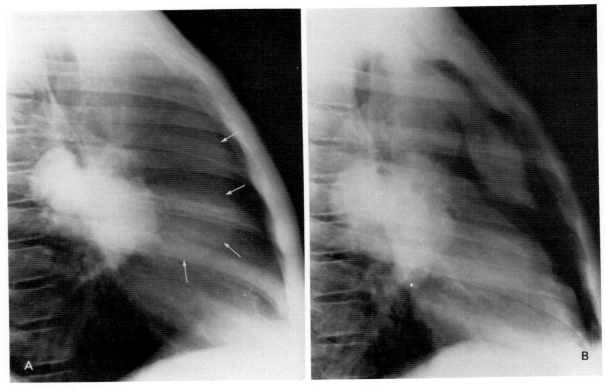

FIG. 24. DEMONSTRATION OF THYMUS GLAND BY PNEUMOMEDIASTINUM

A: Lateral view of a patient with Hodgkin's disease shows a mass of large nodes at the hilum. There is a faint shadow over the anterior mediastinum whose anterior border is marginated (arrows). Infiltration of the anterior mediastinum by Hodgkin's disease usually causes a more diffuse shadow. *B*: Injection of air into the mediastinum shows a large thymus gland to be the cause of the anterior mediastinal shadow. This represents a hyperplastic thymus. There is no evidence of invasion of the anterior mediastinum by the Hodgkin's disease, as evidenced by the free dissection of the air about the thymus.

this was accomplished only by the use of the Trendelenburg position.

PNEUMOPERITONEUM. Examination after the injection of air into the peritoneal cavity is generally more useful than an induced pneumothorax in delineating the diaphragm.

Localized Diaphragmatic Elevations. A localized eventration of the diaphragm or a diaphragmatic hernia can cause a solid shadow at the base of the lung which can be confused with an intrathoracic neoplasm. Air injected into the peritoneum will outline the undersurface of the elevated portion of the diaphragm or the hernial sac. In mammilation of the diaphragm the air enters small pockets on its undersurface where the musculature is not well developed and outlines the corresponding protuberances and depressions in the upper surface of the liver.

Diaphragmatic Tumors. It is impossible to make an accurate diagnosis of a diaphragmatic tumor by ordinary methods. To do this, it is necessary to induce both a pneumothorax and a pneumoperitoneum. These will separate the dia-

phragmatic tumor from the lung above and the abdominal viscera below. A neoplasm of the liver causing a bulge in the diaphragm can be separated from the lung by a pneumothorax. It is usually fixed to the diaphragm by adhesions or direct invasion of the tumor.

Subphrenic Abscess. A subphrenic abscess is always shut off from the free peritoneal cavity. Therefore, air injected into the peritoneal cavity will not enter the region of the abscess. If the air outlines the entire subphrenic space, as determined in both frontal and lateral projections, the possibility of subphrenic abscess can be excluded. On the other hand, the failure to demonstrate a completely free subphrenic space does not prove the presence of an abscess because the spread of the air may be limited by preexisting adhesions.

PNEUMOMEDIASTINOGRAPHY. A pneumomediastinum is produced by injecting air through a needle inserted behind the sternum in the jugular notch. A curved needle is used and advanced into the mediastinum along the posterior surface of the sternum, keeping as close to the bone as possible. The procedure is not without danger and therefore its indiscriminate use is not to be recommended. A pneumothorax can result from perforation of the pleura by injection of the air into the mediastinum under too great a pressure. Another danger is perforation of an aortic aneurysm, mistaken for a tumor.

In some cases pneumomediastinography is helpful in differentiating between benign and malignant neoplasms of the thymus. Malignant tumors are usually adherent to the parietal pleura, preventing the air from dissecting this layer from the growth. On the other hand, the injected air can usually separate a benign tumor completely from the overlying pleura.

The thymus gland is especially well demonstrated by mediastinography. Beautiful demonstrations of the gland are obtained in the lateral view (Fig. 24). However, care must be taken to differentiate the thymus from ordinary fat in the mediastinum. In the frontal projection, the lobes of the thymus tend to become separated from the remainder of the mediastinum and their appearance has been likened to that of a spinnaker sail. This is seen especially in children, or in adults when the thymus gland is enlarged.

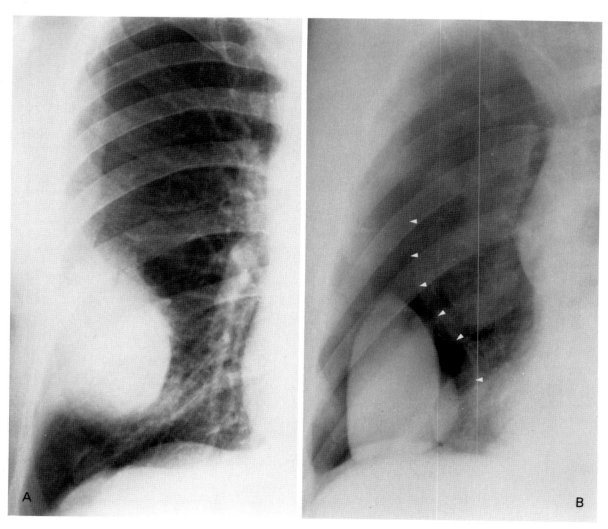

FIG. 25. DIAGNOSTIC PNEUMOTHORAX

A: The mass in the lower part of the right hemithorax abuts on the chest wall. It is impossible from this film to differentiate between a neoplasm of the lung, the pleura, or extrapleural tissues. *B:* Left anterior oblique view after induction of pneumothorax. The lung is partially collapsed (arrows) and is separated from the tumor. Because the tumor was surrounded by air on this, as well as on other views, a lesion of the parietal pleura or chest wall could be excluded. At operation the neoplasm proved to be a fibroma of the visceral pleura attached to the upper lobe by an elongated pedicle.

We once inadvertently entered a mediastinal cyst when inserting the needle for the introduction of air into the mediastinum. After the withdrawal of clear fluid, air was injected. The films made after this procedure gave a remarkable demonstration of the interior of the cyst. The films were relatively unimportant once the presence of clear fluid had been demonstrated. However, the procedure may demonstrate whether the cyst is a simple, thin-walled one or whether its walls are thick and irregular, as in the case of a dermoid.

The lower limit of a substernal thyroid is difficult to determine on ordinary roentgen films, but it can be demonstrated clearly by pneumomediastinum.

The roentgen examination after the injection of air often discloses the aorta and its larger branches clearly. It may serve for the recognition of a dilated tortuous innominate artery whose shadow might otherwise be confused with a mediastinal or a pulmonary tumor.

A more detailed picture of the mediastinal structures may be obtained by tomography after the air has been injected. This can disclose a coarctation of the aorta or even patent ductus arteriosus.

Radiopaque Materials

As in other parts of the body, the hollow organs, sinuses, fistulas, and drained foci in the chest may be outlined by opaque material. The esophagus, bronchi, and blood vessels, as well as sinuses in the chest wall, empyema cavities, and bronchopleural fistulas, are demonstrable by this means. The extent of drained cavities can be determined, and the relationship of these cavities to the disease in the surrounding lung demonstrated. Long and tortuous sinus tracts leading to the mediastinum can also be delineated. In addition, a mixture of radiopaque material and methylene blue can be injected into an intercostal muscle to serve as a landmark for the surgeon in approaching a lesion.

Ingestion of Barium. The dilated esophagus in cardiospasm often simulates a mediastinal tumor or an aneurysm (see Fig. 497). A similar shadow can be produced by the stomach or colon which has been brought up into the chest following resection of the esophagus. Examination following the ingestion of barium readily discloses the cause of the shadow. Occassionally a hiatus hernia or a large epiphrenic diverticulum can create the appearance of a mediastinal mass (Fig. 26). These are clearly demonstrated on barium studies.

Displacement of the esophagus by a mediastinal mass indicates that it is situated in the posterior mediastinum or, at least, extends into this region. Displacement, distortion, or obstruction of the esophagus in a patient with a tumor of the lung indicates that the mediastinum has been secondarily involved.

Acquired bronchoesophageal fistulas can be easily demonstrated by ingestion of opaque material. Most commonly, these result from perforation of an esophageal neoplasm into a bronchus, although the reverse may be the case. When such a fistula is suspected it is preferable to use iodized oil or a water-soluble contrast medium instead of barium.

The aspiration of ingested barium into the trachea and bronchial tree, or its retention in the pyriform fossae, may serve as an indication of the cause of a cough of obscure origin. The cough which occurs after swallowing may be due to anesthesia of the hypopharynx or to poor muscular control of the pharyngeal muscles. This occurs in neurologic disturbances associated with incoordination of the swallowing mechanism and in myasthenia gravis. Retention of the barium in one pyriform fossa is often due to paralysis of the recurrent nerve which can be caused by a neoplasm in the mediastinum, not visible on the films.

Congenital tracheo- or bronchoesophageal fistulas can sometimes be demonstrated by the ingestion of radiopaque material. However, in the majority of cases, there is atresia of the esophagus above the level of the fistula. The bronchus then communicates with the distal portion of the esophagus, and the fistula can be demonstrated only by injecting the contrast agent into the lower esophagus by means of a tube inserted through a gastrostomy.

Not infrequently a shadow in the lower mesial portion of the chest is caused by a diaphragmatic hernia. Most often this contains stomach and is made evident by a barium meal. If the stomach is demonstrated in its normal position, late films must be obtained to exclude the possibility of the hernia containing intestine. Since the hernia may reduce itself when the patient is erect, it is necessary to perform the examination while he is recumbent. Failure to disclose a portion of the gastrointestinal tract within the lesion does not exclude the possibility of a diaphragmatic hernia since the latter may contain omentum, spleen, kidney, or properitoneal or retroperitoneal fat.

Injection of Sinuses and Fistulas. The course of sinus tracts whose origin and extent are unknown should be studied radiologically after

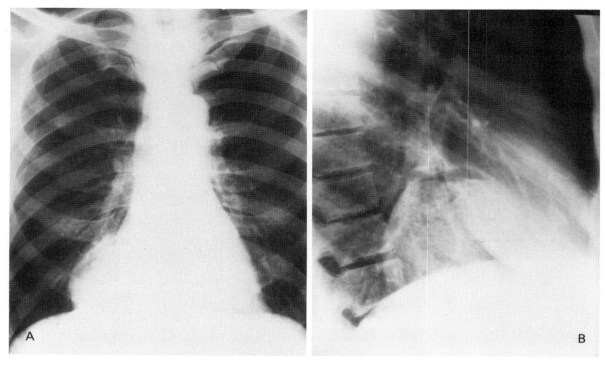

FIG. 26. EPIPHRENIC DIVERTICULUM OF THE ESOPHAGUS

A: The frontal projection shows a sharply demarcated density with a curved border in the region of the right cardiophrenic angle. There is a suggestion of irregular lucency in its upper portion, possibly due to air within it. Although the lateral film showed the lesion to be situated posteriorly, the right border of the heart is obscured. This is due to the high contrast of the film and inadequate penetration of the heart. *B*: The lateral view demonstrates an air-fluid level within the lesion. The irregular mottling of the shadow beneath the fluid level is due to admixture of air with liquid and food. The posterior location of the shadow excludes a hernia through the foramen of Morgagni. The two possibilities to be considered are a hiatus hernia and an esophageal diverticulum. Hiatus hernias rarely project only on the right side of the mediastinum. The barium swallow showed a diverticulum at the lower end of the esophagus.

their injection with contrast material (see Fig. 567).

The type of sinus or its origin usually cannot be determined by external examination nor by probing with an instrument. After injection of radiopaque material, the sinus tract can be traced to its origin. Termination in the region of the costochondral junctions indicates that the source is an osteochondritis of the ribs. It may lead to the bony part of the ribs or to the sternum, to indicate osteomyelitis of these bones.

In other instances the sinus tract originates from a large empyema cavity that has not been completely drained. A water-soluble contrast agent usually will outline the residual cavity but the shadow may be faint because it is diluted by the exudate within it. Not infrequently an oily substance will not outline the cavity. However, division of the oil into small globules denotes that it is lying within liquid exudate and therefore indicates the presence of a cavity. A persist-

ent tract following drainage of an empyema may communicate with a bronchus even though there is no other sign of bronchopleural fistula.

The tract may extend from the pleura to the mediastinum (Fig. 27). This indicates that the empyema was secondary to the mediastinal abscess. We have seen two cases in which a persistent sinus, associated with an empyema, not only entered the mediastinum but extended in the posterior mediastinal space upward to the base of the skull and downward to the diaphragm. In another case, the fistulous tract could be traced to an old perforation of the esophagus which had been entirely unsuspected.

Following drainage of a mediastinal abscess through a cervical incision, the extent of the lesion should be determined by injection of a contrast substance. In almost all cases the abscess will not reach beyond the tracheal bifurcation. If it does extend below this point, simple cervical drainage is usually not adequate. If a

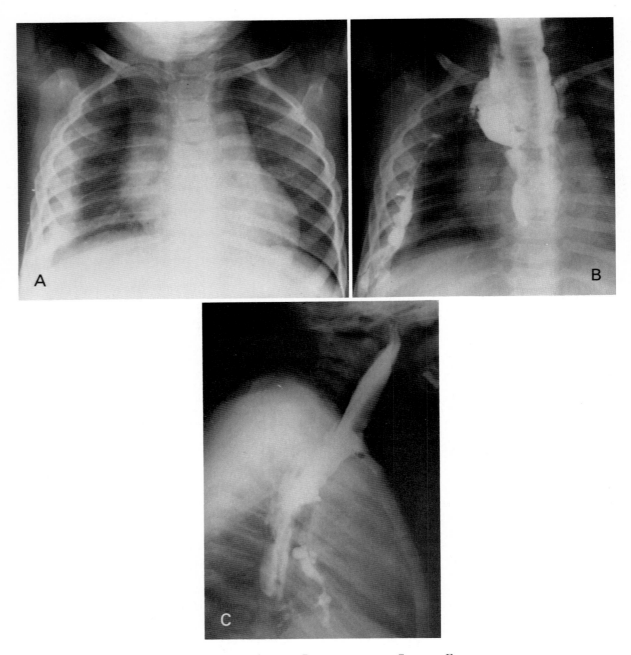

FIG. 27. MEDIASTINAL ABSCESS PRESENTING AS A CHRONIC EMPYEMA

A: An empyema had been drained 2 years previously, but a recurrently draining sinus remained. A band of density with a poorly demarcated mesial border is seen along the outer part of the right chest. The mediastinal shadow is widened. *B*: Lipiodol injected into the sinus in the lower right chest discloses a tract ascending upward and inward in the right pleural space, communicating with a large cavity in the superior mediastinum. This represents an unsuspected mediastinal abscess which was the cause of the empyema. *C*: The lateral view shows the abscess to be localized to the posterior mediastinum, extending from the base of the skull almost to the diaphragm. The infection originated in the adenoid tissue of the nasopharynx.

fistula persists after drainage of a lung abscess or an empyema, it should be opacified to determine the condition of the underlying lung. Even though a pulmonary abscess was not demonstrated at the time of drainage, it may be disclosed by the injected radiopaque material. Where an abscess has already been drained fistulography may demonstrate a neighboring abscess which requires drainage, or surrounding bronchiectasis for which resective surgery may be required.

Delineation of Empyemas. After drainage of an empyema, it is good practice to demonstrate the extent of the drained area by the introduction of radiopaque material. When the wound is large, this may be done by filling the cavity with radiopaque gauze. Iodoform gauze casts a satisfactory shadow for this purpose. Films are then made in various positions to make certain that no shadow remains outside the drained area. An additional shadow may be caused by a loculation of pus in the pleura, not found during the course of the operation. This occurs more frequently with recurrent than with acute empyemas.

The empyema may have ramifications that cannot be packed completely. Under such circumstances, liquid contrast material may be instilled into the region that cannot be packed, in order to determine their extent and position. The contrast material may pass through a narrow channel to enter a distant part of the pleural cavity, almost completely separated from the drained area by intervening lung. Counterdrainage is indicated if subsequent examinations do not show clearing of this portion of the empyema.

Packing of Drained Pulmonary Cavity. One of the difficulties encountered with the drainage operation for lung abscess, particularly after the acute stage has passed, is the presence of one or more residual undrained foci adjacent to the drained abscess. On postoperative films, the region is largely obscured partly by the packing within the wound and partly by thickening of the pleura. If a persistent shadow is seen in the region of the drained cavity, it must not be assumed that this is simply due to a persistent inflammatory reaction about the cavity and that it will eventually resolve. Such residual shadows usually connote an additional undrained focus (see Fig. 273).

The relationship of the undrained area to the original abscess may be determined by reexamination in various positions after insertion of radiopaque packing into the drained cavity. Iodoform gauze or gauze soaked in iodized oil is placed in the cavity of the lung, but not in the wound since this interferes with interpretation. It may be held in place by plain gauze, which will not cast a disturbing roentgen shadow, packed into the wound. Once the relationship of the residual shadow to the drained area is known, the lesion may be found either by careful inspection or by aspiration in the place indicated by the films.

Angiography. The blood vessels within the mediastinum are not well visualized on ordinary films because their shadows are of the same density as those of the other mediastinal structures, and merge with them. However, the vessels can be clearly delineated if the radiodensity of the blood within them is increased by rapid injection of contrast material into the blood stream. The injected material forms a radiopaque bolus which courses in the direction of the blood flow, sequentially opacifying the vessels and the cardiac chambers.

Almost every vessel in the chest can be well visualized by one or another technique of angiography. Good visualization of the systemic veins, the right side of the heart and the main pulmonary arteries is obtained by injecting the contrast material rapidly through a large bore cannula into a peripheral vein or through a catheter into the superior or inferior vena cava. If the circulation time is not too prolonged, the pulmonary veins, the left heart and the aorta are opacified on later films.

Because the contrast material is diluted by the blood in the heart, the systemic arteries are not well delineated by a venous injection. Selective arteriography provides the best visualization of the arteries and their branches. A catheter is inserted percutaneously into a peripheral artery and guided through the aorta into the branch to be investigated. In experienced hands, the risk of this procedure is minimal even when there is extensive disease of the aorta. Any of the arteries arising from the aorta or from its major branches can be opacified in this way with little difficulty.

The azygos venous system is opacified by injecting the contrast material directly into the marrow of a rib or the spinous process of one of the vertebrae. The material flows rapidly from the point of injection into the intercostal veins or the paravertebral and ascending lumbar veins, and from these, into the azygos system.

A rapid serial film changer is indispensable for all forms of angiography. If the procedure is carried out by direct injection into a peripheral vein, little additional specialized equipment is required. However, catheterization requires fluoroscopy for monitoring the position of the catheter. Image intensification, television monitoring and ciné recording are useful adjuncts. In most instances a pressure injector is required to ensure rapid introduction of the contrast material.

All of the contrast materials in current use are water-soluble solutions of an organic iodine compound. Sensitivity to the iodine occasionally results in mild urticaria. Serious reactions are rare. Side effects, such as a sensation of heat or nausea may occur, but are usually short-lived and not troublesome. Bleeding or occlusion of the artery at the puncture site occurs in somewhat less than 1% of the cases but responds well to prompt local surgical intervention.

ANEURYSMS. It would appear to be a simple matter to differentiate between an aneurysm and other mediastinal masses by the presence or absence of expansile pulsations. Unfortunately, this is often not the case. If the wall of an aneurysm is lined by a thick layer of thrombus, the aneurysm will not pulsate. Conversely, me-

diastinal tumors that are closely related to the aorta transmit the pulsations of this vessel, and it is frequently impossible to distinguish between transmitted and expansile pulsations. It is a safe rule that angiography should be performed whenever a sharply outlined mass with a convex outer margin is found in relation to the course of the aorta or innominate artery before an aneurysm is exluded (Fig. 28). Certainly, every patient with evidence of syphilis, who has a mediastinal tumor the nature of which is unknown, should be investigated in this way. The same is true whenever the ascending aorta is abnormally prominent or shows evidence of calcification in a patient with such a mediastinal mass.

Venous angiocardiography, properly performed, will produce some opacification of practically every aneurysm, even though it is almost completely filled with blood clot. Even in luetic

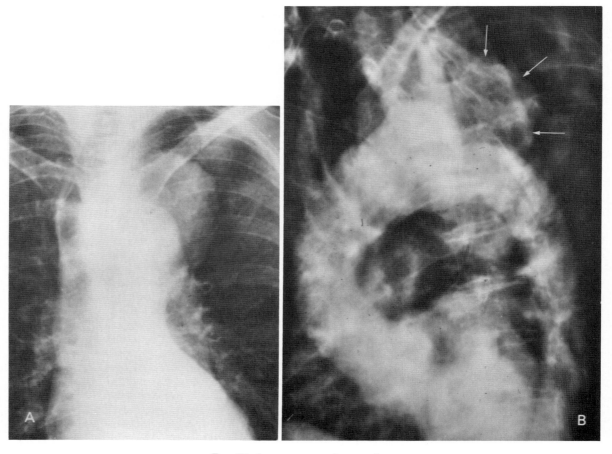

FIG. 28. ANEURYSM OF AORTIC ARCH

A: The large mass which projects from the left side of the mediastinum does not obliterate the silhouette of the aortic knob. The trachea is displaced to the right. The film made 2 years previously was negative and therefore a presumptive diagnosis of bronchogenic carcinoma was made. *B*: Because the mass could not be separated from the aorta on any projection, angiography was performed. A late film of a venous angiogram in the right posterior oblique view shows an outpouching of the lumen of the midportion of the aortic arch. The shadow around it (arrows), represents thrombus within the aneurysm.

aneurysms of the innominate artery completely filled with clot, the irregularity of the aortic lumen resulting from the accompanying syphilitic aortitis, will suggest the presence of an aneurysm. However, aortography is often required for a definitive diagnosis.

In the absence of associated aortic insufficiency, venous angiography may provide adequate opacification of the aorta. However, aortography is the method of choice for the diagnosis and determination of the extent of a dissecting aneurysm. The lumen of the aorta is usually compressed by the blood within the aortic wall. Frequently, both the true and false channels are opacified when contrast material is injected into the ascending aorta. The two channels are separated by a radiolucent line which represents the inner portion of the dissected aortic wall. This appearance is pathognomonic of dissecting aneurysm. If the false channel is not opacified, it may be difficult to differentiate between a dissection and a fusiform aneurysm lined by thrombus.

PULMONARY NEOPLASMS. The blood supply of pulmonary neoplasms can often be outlined by selective bronchial arteriography. However, the similarity between the vascular pattern of neoplasms and that of inflammatory lesions greatly limits the diagnostic value of this procedure.

Pulmonary angiography has a place in determining that a carcinoma of the lung is not resectable (see Fig. 415). Invasion of the main pulmonary artery, evidenced by narrowing of the vessel or irregularity of its wall indicates that the tumor cannot be completely removed. However, care must be taken in the interpretation of a venous angiogram because poor filling of the pulmonary artery on the side of the lesion does not necessarily indicate that it is obstructed. Lack of opacification of the vessel may be due simply to poor flow of blood through the lung from interference with the mechanics of breathing, rather than to organic obstruction of the vessel (see Fig. 313). The caliber of the vessel can be demonstrated by selective pulmonary arteriography.

Occlusion of the azygos vein or its major tributaries in a case of bronchogenic carcinoma signifies involvement of the posterior mediastinum by the tumor (Fig. 29). Occlusion or marked narrowing of the superior vena cava indicates involvement of the mediastinal lymph nodes. In either instance, it may be concluded that the tumor cannot be resected in its entirety.

PULMONARY EMBOLISM. Emboli or thrombi within the main pulmonary artery or its branches are easily visualized as relatively lucent filling defects when these vessels are opacified. While the pulmonary arteries can be demonstrated by venous angiography, not uncommonly the opaque material becomes too dilute to provide optimal visualization. This is especially true in the presence of heart failure. In addition, opacification of the right atrium and superior vena cava may obscure a portion of the right pulmonary artery. For these lesions, selective pulmonary arteriography is preferred.

By advancing the catheter into a lobar artery or into one of its divisions, emboli in relatively small arteries can be recognized. However, peripheral emboli are difficult to demonstrate because the individual vessels in this portion of the lung are partly obscured by overlapping shadows of other branches.

ARTERIOVENOUS FISTULAS. Arteriovenous aneurysms produce nonspecific shadows which are easily confused with neoplasms. Frequently, dilated arteries and veins are seen extending from the lesion in the direction of the hilum. These indicate the presence of an arteriovenous communication, but they cannot always be visualized even with the aid of tomography. In some cases, fluoroscopy reveals pulsations of the lesion, and the Valsalva maneuver may cause diminution in its size, excluding the possibility of neoplasm. An unequivocal diagnosis can be made by angiography (Fig. 30). It is especially important to study the pulmonary vasculature by this method if surgical excision is contemplated because the aneurysms are frequently multiple and smaller lesions can otherwise escape detection.

Bronchography. The bronchi are poorly visualized on standard roentgen films, and only the larger branches can be satisfactorily studied by tomography. Radiopaque material instilled into the tracheobronchial tree coats the mucosa and affords clear visualization of even the small peripheral bronchial branches. Bronchopulmonary malformations, and widening, stenosis and irregularities of the bronchial lumen become evident. Bronchography is indispensable in the evaluation of bronchiectasis, not only to establish the diagnosis, but to map out the distribution of the diseased bronchi prior to surgical resection. Moreover, it is of use in demonstrating bronchial communications with cavities, communications between cavities in the lung, and in localizing fistulous tracts arising from the bronchi. Ciné bronchography is an invaluable tool for the study of bronchial physiology in normal and diseased states.

The instillation of any foreign material into the bronchi excites a strong cough reflex. It is necessary, therefore, to obtain satisfactory local anesthesia of the tracheobronchial tree before the contrast material is introduced. Except in

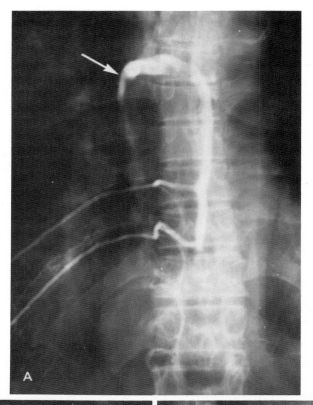

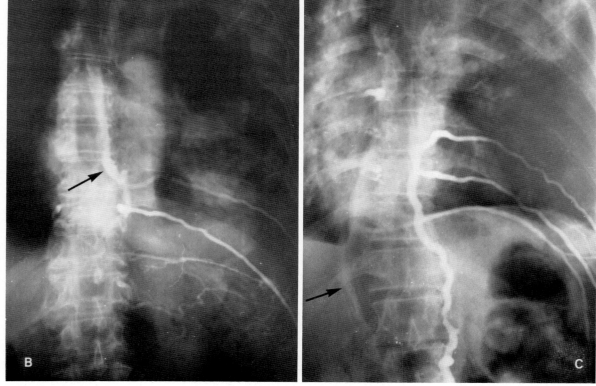

infants and young children, in whom a general anesthetic is required, topical anesthesia is sufficient for this purpose. Cocaine and Pontocaine have been the anesthetic agents of choice for many years but are gradually being supplanted by newer compounds, such as Xylocaine, which produce less frequent and less severe side reactions.

Many contrast materials are available for bronchography, all of them with certain advantages and disadvantages. With the exception of barium sulfate suspension and tantalum powder, the contrast agents in use today are radiopaque because of their iodine content. The iodine is organically bound and allergic reactions are rare. Most are used in oily suspensions which are relatively nonirritating to the bronchial mucosa. Following bronchography, the iodine usually disappears from the lungs within a few days, although the oily vehicle remains for a longer period of time and, in rare instances, leads to granuloma formation or lipid pneumonia. Aqueous suspensions are more rapidly excreted and absorbed but are more irritating to the bronchi than the oily contrast media and often necessitate the use of excessive amounts of local anesthetic.

Bronchography can be performed by several routes: the contrast material may be injected directly through a needle into the trachea or inserted into the bronchi through a bronchoscope; it can be inhaled from the nasopharynx or injected through a catheter into the trachea, or directly into one of the bronchi. Regardless of the route chosen, the bronchographic examination should be preceded by postural drainage to clear the bronchi of as much mucus and exudate as possible.

TRANSGLOTTIC ROUTE. This is the most commonly used method and the one to be preferred, especially in cooperative patients. Anesthesia of the nasopharynx, palate and hypopharynx is obtained by spraying these regions with a local anesthetic. Using a curved cannula, the anesthetic agent is then dripped over the back of the tongue to the epiglottis and valleculae and directly into the larynx. Satisfactory anesthesia can also be obtained by inhalation of an aerosol. Once the upper airway is anesthetized, it is relatively simple to pass a catheter, inserted through a nostril or the mouth, between the vocal cords into the trachea. This can be done blindly with the patient's head extended, under visualization with a laryngeal mirror, or under fluoroscopic control. Specially curved catheters or guide systems can be used to enter any of the major bronchial branches in order to obtain selective bronchograms.

The order in which the bronchi are filled and the positioning of the patient to accomplish this varies with the individual examiner. When the contrast material is injected, the patient should be positioned so that the portion of the lung to be opacified is dependent. The bronchi of either upper lobe are filled with the patient lying on the corresponding side. Rotating the patient into the prone and then to the supine position will help assure good distribution throughout the upper lobe. It may be necessary to place him into the Trendelenburg position to delineate the bronchi in the apical regions. About 5 cc of contrast material are sufficient for an upper lobe.

To visualize the lower lobe bronchi, the patient is brought to the upright position and 5 to 10 cc of contrast material are injected. The patient is then placed on his back to fill the superior segment. The middle lobe is filled by turning the patient on his abdomen. Often no more oil is required, but an additional 2 or 3 cc may be needed. Usually 15 to 20 cc are adequate to completely outline the bronchial tree of one lung.

It is best to inject the contrast material under fluoroscopic control. Spot or ciné films are made in the frontal, lateral and oblique projections while the bronchi are being filled, before they are obscured by superimposition of other bronchi or by contrast material in the alveoli. At the end of the injection, standard films are made, first in the recumbent and then in the erect positions. The opposite lung may be injected at the same

FIG. 29. AZYGOS VENOGRAPHY

Injection of contrast material into the marrow space of a rib results in opacification of the draining intercostal vein and the veins at adjacent levels. The contrast material flows into the azygos vein or the hemiazygos depending on which side is injected. It then flows cephalad into the azygos vein which empties into the superior vena cava. A: Normal azygos venogram. The contrast material has been injected into the ninth rib on the right side. The arrow indicates the point of entry of the azygos vein into the superior vena cava. B: Normal azygos venogram. Contrast material has been injected into the left ninth rib and fills a short segment of the hemiazygos vein before it crosses over (arrow) to join the azygos. C: Obstruction of the azygos vein. The patient had a carcinoma in the left upper lobe. Contrast material injected into the left ninth rib courses retrograde in the hemiazygos vein which is continuous with the left ascending lumbar vein in the abdomen. The lumbar vein communicates with the common iliac vein so that the contrast material enters the inferior vena cava (arrow).

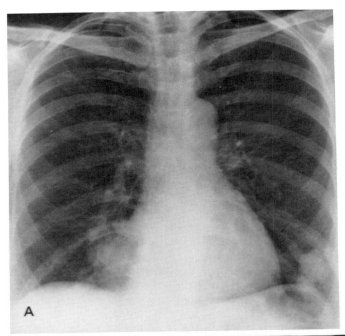

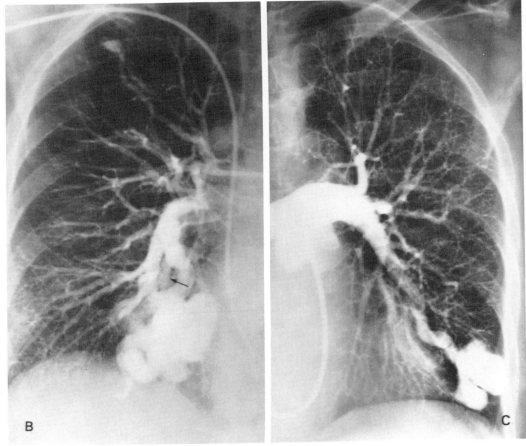

sitting, if desired. If both lungs are injected, it is essential to obtain both oblique views if errors in identification of the bronchi are to be avoided. Stereoscopic films are helpful.

Immediately after the procedure, postural drainage should be performed in conjunction with forcible coughing to get rid of as much of the contrast material as possible. It is advisable to obtain additional films after coughing, as bronchi not previously visualized may then be filled.

NASOPHARYNGEAL ROUTE. In young children, the necessity for a general anesthetic may be avoided by injecting the oil through a catheter passed through the nose into the nasopharynx. A local anesthetic is dripped into the nasopharynx, followed by the injection of contrast material. If it is instilled intermittently during inspiration, enough of the contrast material will be aspirated for good visualization of the bronchial tree, even though some of it is swallowed.

TRANSTRACHEAL INJECTION. Injection of the contrast material directly into the trachea through a needle is a common practice in some clinics. This method is particularly useful in patients in whom it is not possible to pass a catheter through the larynx. In general, it is more rapid than the transglottic method since the pharynx and larynx need not be anesthetized.

The patient's head is hyperextended and, after the skin has been anesthetized, a needle is inserted in the midline through the cricothyroid membrane. A local anesthetic is injected to inhibit the cough reflex of the bronchi. The contrast material is then instilled and the patient positioned so as to fill the bronchi in the order desired. The Trendelenburg position cannot be used because severe coughing occurs when the contrast material runs up to the unanesthetized larynx.

Selective bronchograms can be obtained if a catheter is introduced into the tranchea and bronchi by means of the Seldinger technique. A guide wire is passed through the needle which has been inserted into the trachea, removing the needle while the guide wire remains in place and advancing a catheter over the wire.

Ciné studies can be performed with any of these methods, filming the image from the intensifier during fluoroscopy. These can be used in place of spot films. The motion of the bronchi can then be studied during respiration and coughing, and the effects of various drugs upon the bronchi can be evaluated.

Fluoroscopy

In general, the information afforded by a general fluoroscopic survey of the chest is available in more accurate and permanent form on standard roentgen films. However, in specific instances, fluoroscopy can yield important information that is difficult to obtain from the films. This applies to regions that are not clearly visualized on ordinary films, to the study of movements of the structures in the chest, and for observation of ventilation of the lungs, the lobes and their segments during respiration. In addition, fluoroscopy is useful for the selection of the optimal position in which films should be made in special cases.

Limitations of Fluoroscopy. Fluoroscopy has its limitations, and they must always be kept in mind if serious errors are to be avoided. These may have such serious implications that a knowledge of the limitations of fluoroscopy should be a prerequisite to the use of the instrument.

Single or discrete infiltrations measuring less than 1 cm in diameter are easily overlooked at routine fluoroscopy and they may be invisible even if they are searched for carefully by closing down the diaphragm and concentrating on each portion of the pulmonary field. Fine infiltrations or nodules may be visible if they are close to each other, but, generally, they are not discernible if they are more widely separated, even though they cover a large area of the lung. Therefore, one can place no reliance on fluoroscopy in excluding small tuberculous lesions, small metastases, and the fine infiltrations of certain types of bronchopneumonia.

Accommodation. If an image intensifier is not used, the eyes must be accommodated properly. The time required for this varies with the individual, the intensity of light to which he has been exposed prior to the examination, and the type of fluoroscopic screen, as well as the milliamperage that is used.

FIG. 30. PULMONARY ARTERIOVENOUS FISTULA

A: The conventional film shows a lobulated density in the lower part of each lung. A large blood vessel extends from the mass on the left side toward the hilum. This appearance is characteristic of an arteriovenous fistula. *B:* Right pulmonary arteriogram. An early film shows the mass in the lower lobe to be composed of dilated, tortuous vessels. Even though the contrast material has not yet reached the arteriolar branches in the remainder of the lung, the vein (arrow) draining the lesion is opacified. This indicates the presence of an arteriovenous shunt. A small fistula is seen in the upper lobe. This is barely visible on the conventional film even in retrospect. *C:* Left pulmonary arteriogram. (Courtesy of E. E. Rockey, New York City.)

Protection of the Patient. Protection of the patient against unnecessary exposure should be constantly kept in mind. A major factor in determining exposure is the duration of the fluoroscopic examination. This will be kept to a minimum if the examiner has a clear idea of exactly what he is looking for prior to the fluoroscopy. For this reason, standard films should be reviewed first. A competent fluoroscopic examination is usually of such short duration that the patient suffers little exposure to the roentgen rays. However, in cases involving localization of lesions and during the performance of special procedures, the patient exposure may be considerable even with image intensification. It is important in these cases to keep a record of the length of the fluoroscopy. In patients who are examined repeatedly, particularly those who have received radiotherapy, the exposure should be sharply limited. In the latter it is usually best to avoid fluoroscopy altogether.

To avoid unnecessary exposure, the fluoroscope should be calibrated periodically and the collimation checked to ensure that, whenever possible, the maximum opening does not allow the beam to reach the edges of the fluoroscopic screen. During the procedure, the shutters should be closed down to the field of interest. The lowest milliamperage, consistent with the production of an adequate image, should be employed. It should be borne in mind that intensifying screens deteriorate with time. They should be checked periodically.

Protection of the Observer. Because the exposure in fluoroscopy of the chest is usually not great, the fluoroscopist may have a tendency to be careless concerning his personal exposure to the rays. The danger of cumulative exposure over a period of many years should be constantly kept in mind. A lead-backed chair, a leaded screen, or a leaded apron should always be used during the performance of fluoroscopy. In addition, protective gloves should be worn routinely, because the temptation to put the hands in the path of the rays is too great for most of us to avoid consistently.

Detailed Fluoroscopic Examination

Lungs. APICES. If the apices are not clearly visualized, a comparison of their illumination on inspiration and expiration should be made. This is done after narrowing the shutters from above downward so that only the apices are in view. If they both illuminate well on inspiration, the possibility of a lesion in this region is unlikely. Increased aeration of the apices may be produced by coughing.

The portion of the lung visible above the clavicle may be increased by having the patient bend forward. Displacing the clavicle downward by this maneuver brings the posterior part of the apex into view down to the level of the posterior portion of the fifth rib. In this way, small lesions hidden by the first rib or the clavicle can be exposed. Bending the patient backward elevates the clavicle, uncovering a lesion that is hidden by this bone in the ordinary frontal view.

SMALL NODULES AND INFILTRATIONS. If, in the routine survey, there is suspicion of one or more nodules or infiltrations in the lung, they can be visualized more clearly by closing the diaphragm to a space not much larger than the suspected lesion. It is remarkable how much better the lesions can be seen when light from the neighboring pulmonary field is excluded. Small foci may be obscured by the ribs on ordinary inspection, but their shadows can be separated from these bones by moving the tube upward or downward or bending the patient backward or forward. Lesions may thus be projected into the intercostal spaces where they can be seen more clearly.

Often the abnormality may be made to stand out more clearly by either raising or lowering the voltage. It should be borne in mind, however, that excessive illumination tends to eliminate the shadow of a small lesion.

If the nodules or infiltrations are situated posteriorly, they are usually more clearly visualized by turning the patient around so that his back is nearer the screen. Nodules in the posterior portion of the chest may appear somewhat smaller but they are much more sharply defined.

HIDDEN AREAS. Most of the posterior costophrenic sinus and the region behind the heart are largely hidden unless the oblique position is used. The area behind the heart is best studied by rotating the patient from 10 to 20 degrees toward the left anterior oblique position. The exact angle to which the patient is turned is that which is just sufficient to displace the left border of the heart to the spine (Fig. 13). More rotation brings a considerable portion of the anterior part of the lower lobe over the spine and obscures the lesions in this part of the lung.

Turning the patient to the full left oblique postion will disclose the entire left posterior costophrenic sinus and the lowermost portion of the left lower lobe ordinarily hidden by the dome of the diaphragm. Small effusions, which are not well visualized either fluoroscopically or on the roentgen films in the frontal projection, can be clearly outlined in the full oblique view. Such effusions are better demonstrated during expiration because the fluid is forced up higher in the pulmonary field. Tilting the patient toward the side of the effusion causes the fluid to rise still higher and results in a more striking demonstration of the effusion.

The right anterior oblique position is used to study the lowermost portion of the right lower lobe and the posterior costophrenic sinus on this side.

RADIOLUCENCY OF THE LUNG. Any marked change in the lucency of the lung is evident at the preliminary survey. A slight degree of lessened illumination of both lungs occurs in pulmonary congestion and in the case of fine infiltrations distributed diffusely throughout the lungs as in pneumoconiosis, sarcoidosis and lymphangitic carcinosis. By closing down the shutters it may be possible to see the individual infiltrations which cause the generalized clouding, but in many cases the lesions are so fine that they cannot be delineated. In these conditions the lessened illumination involves both lungs, and it may be ascribed erroneously to the thickness of the patient. Thus, these diseases may be overlooked on fluoroscopy.

Diminished Lucency. Decreased lucency of one of the lungs or part of a lung is judged by comparing it with the well-illuminated normal lung. Diminished lucency is often due to a decrease in ventilation of the alveoli. This may be caused by obstruction of the bronchus leading to that region, or to inability of the lung to expand even though its airway is open. In the latter instance, the interference with expansion may be due to infiltration or fibrosis of the affected portion of the lung or to its encasement by a thick, inexpansile pleura.

One of the causes for imprisonment of the lung is the thickening of the pleura that occurs in prolonged artificial pneumothorax. The pleura need not be much thickened to prevent complete pulmonary expansion, particularly if it had been the seat of a mild pleuritis while the lung was contracted by the pneumothorax. Because of the inability of the lung to expand, the mediastinum is drawn to the affected side, the diaphragm is elevated, and the chest wall is flattened by an increased obliquity of the ribs.

Another cause for imprisonment of the lung in a partially contracted state, preventing increased illumination on inspiration, is an old hemothorax, either traumatic, spontaneous, or the result of previous pulmonary infarction (Fig. 31). An old empyema or a chronic tuberculous pleuritis may have a similar effect on the pleura. In this connection it should be emphasized that the filmy adhesions which are present after complete resolution of a pleuritis do not interfere with proper aeration and illumination. This is the case after

proper drainage and cure of even old, thick-walled empyemas (see Fig. 540).

Increased Illumination. The lungs may appear to be abnormally lucent in thin people, but their illumination changes during inspiration and expiration. On the other hand, there is little change with the phase of respiration of the hyperlucent lungs in emphysema. The emphysema may be either diffuse or local, it may involve only one lung or part of a lung. Local emphysema that does not change with respiration, is of the obstructive type. The obstruction may involve the main bronchus to the lung, one of the lobar bronchi, or only the smallest bronchi. In the last instance, the emphysema is often of the bullous variety.

Difficulty may be experienced in differentiating between emphysema of one lung and a pneumothorax because both conditions are characterized by increased lucency, and because the border of the lung adjacent to the pneumothorax often is not easily visualized. Contrast between the lung and the pneumothorax may be increased by examining the patient during expiration (Fig. 32). The area of pneumothorax retains its lucency while the lung becomes somewhat clouded. The separation of the visceral pleura from the chest wall, which indicates the presence of a pneumothorax, is best demonstrated by closing down the shutters and observing the area during complete expiration.

In the acute emphysema which occurs during an attack of asthma, in acute tracheobronchitis, or in ball-valve obstruction of the trachea or glottis, both lungs are abnormally lucent. Both leaves of the diaphragm are depressed and are relatively immobile. Little clouding occurs during expiration. Because of the bronchial obstruction, an attempt at complete expiration raises the intrathoracic pressure considerably. This interferes with the passage of blood from the vena cavae into the heart. The cardiac silhouette therefore becomes smaller as in the Valsalva maneuver.

LUNG ROOTS. *Blood Vessels and Lymph Nodes.* The region of the lung roots requires special attention when the hilar shadows appear abnormally prominent. The shadows of dilated vessels may be differentiated from those of enlarged lymph nodes by noting their pulsations. The pulsation of the vessels is especially marked in patients who have an atrial septal defect or an arteriovenous fistula in the general circulation. Even in the absence of these conditions, careful observation, after closing down the diaphragm often will disclose pulsation of the vessels. In the absence of visible pulsations, it is necessary to examine the patient in the oblique projection.

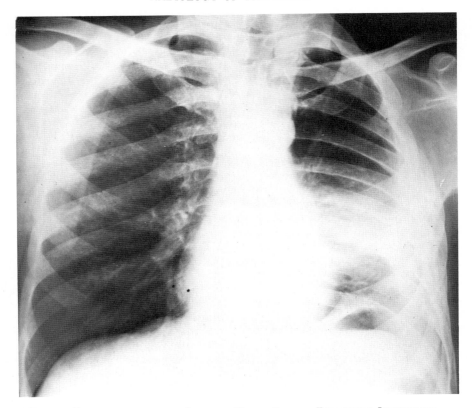

FIG. 31. ENCASEMENT OF THE LUNG BY THICK PLEURA FOLLOWING INFARCTION

The left chest is smaller than the right, the diaphragm is elevated, and the ribs are drawn together. The density over the lower part of the left lung is largely due to carnification of the pleura. This followed extensive pulmonary infarction complicated by a clotted hemothorax. The dense fibrosis of the pleura that resulted from organization of the hemothorax prevented complete reexpansion of the lung.

The right anterior oblique is used for observation of the right lung and the left anterior oblique for the left root. The shadows of the vessels, which often appear oval in shape and simulate large lymph nodes on the frontal projection, become elongated in the oblique view and often show characteristic branching which proves their vascular origin.

Calcified Nodes. In certain cases it is necessary to differentiate between calcified lymph nodes and blood vessels that are viewed on end. This is especially important when broncholithiasis is suspected or when it is necessary to know if the patient has an old healed primary tuberculous infection. It may be difficult to make this differentiation by examination of the roentgen film alone. If the shadows are caused by blood vessels viewed head-on, their shape may change when the patient is rotated slowly for a few degrees (Fig. 33). The round shadows become elongated, and often, branching of the shadows can be observed, indicating that they represent blood vessels rather than calcific deposits.

Pseudocavity. The differentiation between a true cavity and an annular shadow caused by crossing blood vessels may also be made by fluoroscopy. Here again, turning the patient a few degrees will separate the blood vessels from each other, causing the annular shadow to disintegrate.

Calcified Pleura. The shadow caused by calcification of the pleura may be recognized fluoroscopically by turning the patient into the oblique position. When seen *en face,* calcified pleura may present a rather faint shadow. However, in the oblique view, this is transformed into a thin, dense line, adjacent and parallel to the rib cage.

LUNG BASES. Fluoroscopically, one can often differentiate between obliteration of a costophrenic sinus by adhesions and blunting by a small collection of fluid. This differentiation may be impossible from the ordinary frontal film. If examination in the oblique view in full expiration, or while the chest is tilted shows a change in the configuration of the costophrenic sinus, it indicates that the blunting is due to fluid. In other cases, fixation of the outer part of the diaphragm can be recognized during respiration, signifying the presence of adhesions. Infiltrations or nodules at the extreme base of the lung, in the posterior costophrenic sinus, a region hidden by the diaphragm on the frontal film, are disclosed by turning the patient to the proper oblique position during fluoroscopy.

Diaphragm. Fluoroscopy is the best method for examination of the diaphragm, especially because it permits observation of its movement. The motion of the diaphragm may also be studied on films made in expiration as well as inspiration. Both of these exposures may be made on the same film. However, fluoroscopy has the advantage of disclosing the motion of the diaphragm throughout the entire course of respiration and during forceful as well as quiet breathing.

In studying the diaphragm, its position is first noted. It is then examined for irregularities in contour. The motion of the diaphragm is then studied and finally the subphrenic regions are observed.

The height of the diaphragm varies in normal individuals in accordance with the contour of the chest. In the long, narrow person, the diaphragm is lower than in the one who is squat and heavyset. In the former, on inspiration, it reaches the level of the sixth costal cartilage in front and the tenth rib behind, while in the latter, it is usually situated at about the height of the fifth rib or fifth intercostal space anteriorly and the ninth rib or ninth space posteriorly. When the rays pass from back to front, the dome of the diaphragm appears higher in relation to the anterior ribs if the tube is low. It appears lower in relation to the posterior ribs when the tube is in this position so that a larger part of the posterior

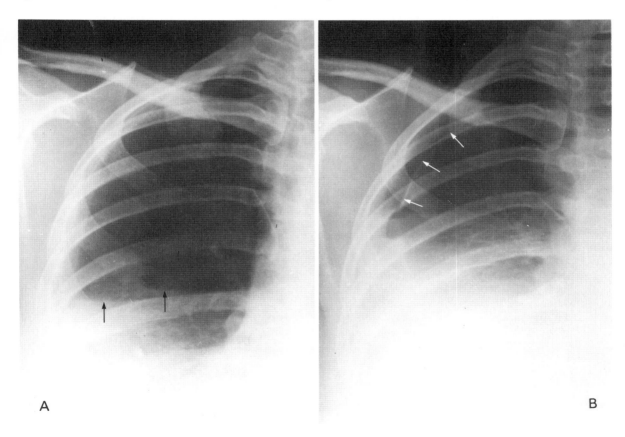

A   B

FIG. 32. HYDROPNEUMOTHORAX

A: Film made in inspiration. Air-fluid levels (arrows) are seen at the upper border of the effusion. There is no other indication of pneumothorax because the lung appears to touch the lateral chest wall. *B*: Film made in expiration. With the rise of the diaphragm, the fluid is displaced upward. Since there is no change in the volume of the collection of air in the pleura, as its height decreases its width must increase. The separation of the lung (arrows) from the chest wall, therefore, becomes more marked.

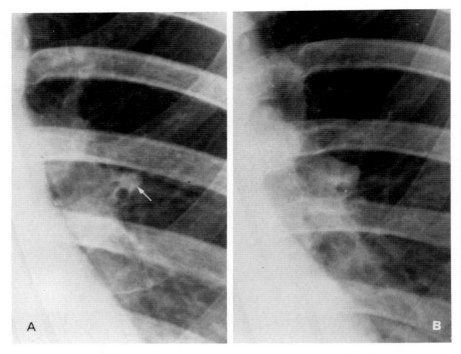

FIG. 33. PULMONARY BLOOD VESSEL SIMULATING CALCIFICATION

A: Frontal Projection. The small, round, dense shadow (arrow) at the root of the left upper lobe represents the artery supplying the anterior segment. Immediately beneath it is the accompanying bronchus seen in cross section. The shadow of a blood vessel projected on end is often dense enough to simulate calcification. *B*: Partial right oblique view. The patient was rotated a few degrees to the right oblique position. The vessel, which is no longer seen in cross section, appears less dense and is not sharply delineated. The shadow of the bronchus is not circular because it is viewed obliquely.

chest is seen. Conversely, if the tube is elevated, more of the anterior chest can be visualized. The opposite is true if the rays pass from front to back (Fig. 9). The right leaf of the diaphragm is generally 1 to 2 cm higher than the left.

ELEVATION. Both leaves of the diaphragm are often higher than the average in obese persons, in pregnancy, and in association with ascites or generalized intestinal distension. Judgment as to whether the position of the diaphragm is clinically important must be made with due consideration to the habitus of the patient and his manner of breathing. The diaphragm may appear to be high if the breathing is mainly costal in character. The association of elevation of both leaves of the diaphragm with a crescentic shadow between the stomach bubble or colon and the left leaf of the diaphragm suggests the presence of ascites. However, bilateral infrapulmonary effusions or a bilateral subphrenic abscess may produce the same roentgen appearance.

Elevation of one leaf of the diaphragm may be due to weakness or paralysis of this organ (Figs. 34 and 442), or to an abnormality above or below it (see Figs. 102 and 565). Contraction of the lung, either as a result of bronchial obstruction and

atelectasis, or imprisonment of the lung by dense pleura can elevate the diaphragm to a considerable degree. The diaphragm can also be elevated in pleuritis because of reflex limitation of its downward motion, or because of adhesions which bind its outer part to the chest wall.

Abdominal conditions that cause elevation of the diaphragm are subphrenic abscess, enlargement of the liver or spleen, a large abdominal neoplasm, or distention of the colon or stomach (Fig. 35).

DEPRESSION. Depression of both leaves of the diaphragm beyond that which would be expected from the habitus of the patient is usually due to diffuse obstructive emphysema. It also occurs in the more acute, evanescent hyperinflation of the lungs caused by incomplete obstruction of the trachea, attacks of bronchial asthma and acute diffuse tracheobronchitis (see Fig. 192), and is present in the rare case of bilateral diaphragmatic spasm.

Depression of one leaf of the diaphragm is the result of more local disease. The most common cause is a large pleural effusion, although a smaller collection of fluid may depress the diaphragm if it is loculated between this organ and

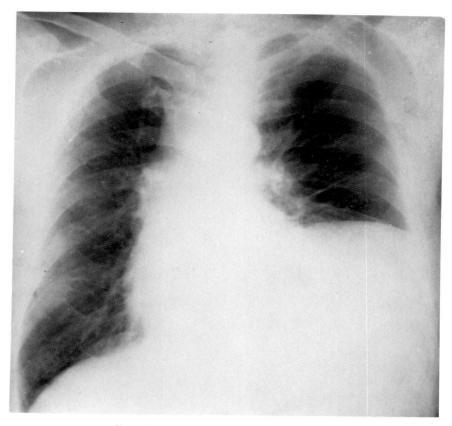

FIG. 34. EVENTRATION OF THE DIAPHRAGM

The left leaf of the diaphragm is markedly elevated. The fact that the entire leaf is affected was confirmed on the lateral view. The heart and mediastinal structures are displaced to the right. The involved diaphragm moved paradoxically during sniffing. Similar findings occur in diaphragmatic paralysis, but the degree of elevation is not so great until atrophy of the muscle has taken place.

the lower surface of the lung (see Fig. 539). It may be impossible to differentiate the latter from elevation of the diaphragm by a subphrenic abscess. A large tumor at the base of the lung or hyperinflation of the lung caused by partial bronchial obstruction can also depress the diaphragm. A low position of one leaf of the diaphragm may be caused by large bullae at the base of the lung or by a tense pneumothorax. These two conditions can be differentiated if the outline of the lung, collapsed by the pneumothorax, can be clearly visualized. However, it is often impossible to recognize the border of the lung on fluoroscopic examination.

IRREGULARITIES. Small, tent-like elevations of a portion of the diaphragm are generally of little significance (see Figs. 160 and 322). It has been assumed that they are due to pleural adhesions which draw up a small segment of the diaphragm. However, our observations indicate that this is probably not the correct explanation. We have

seen these small triangular shadows disappear after the occurrence of a pneumothorax and reappear promptly when the pneumothorax was absorbed. Most likely they represent a portion of the diaphragm or diaphragmatic pleura that has invaginated to fill a cleft in the undersurface of the lung caused by a focal area of atelectasis (see Figs. 307 and 516). The pulmonary lesion may or may not be associated with an overlying adhesive pleuritis.

Local elevation of the outer portion of the diaphragm with obliteration of the costophrenic sinus is due to dense adhesions between the diaphragm and the lateral chest wall. It is sometimes difficult to distinguish this from a small pleural effusion (see Fig. 75). The differentiation can often be made by examining the patient in the oblique position, particularly during expiration. The typical shadow of an effusion usually becomes evident. Occasionally, tilting the patient toward one side produces a shift of an effusion

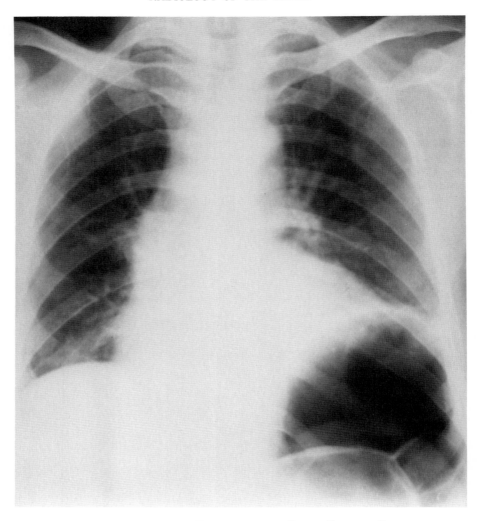

FIG. 35. ELEVATION OF THE DIAPHRAGM BY A LARGE STOMACH BUBBLE
The stomach is markedly distended with air and has displaced the left diaphragm upward. Motion of the left leaf of the diaphragm was somewhat restricted but it moved in a normal direction on sniffing as well as during quiet respiration. The splenic flexure, which is recognizable because of its haustrations, lies beneath the fundus of the stomach.

while there is no change when the shadow is due to adhesions of the diaphragm to the lateral chest wall.

An adhesion of the diaphragm localized to one point on the undersurface of the lung can produce a localized straightening of the diaphragm which simulates an air-fluid level in a pulmonary cavity or a pneumothorax (see Fig. 111). An extensive adhesion between the diaphragm and the lateral chest wall can cause a straightening of the entire leaf of the diaphragm to create an appearance that may be indistinguishable from a collection of fluid and air in the pleura on the frontal projection. This poses a problem particularly after resective surgery.

The most common type of irregularity of the diaphragm is that which is characterized by the presence of one or more scalloped elevations. When these occur on the left side, their undersurface is outlined by gas in the colon or stomach so that the cause of the shadow is evident. However, on the right side the appearance is that of a solid projection into the chest because the space beneath the diaphragmatic protuberance is occupied by a portion of the liver. The shadow may be confused with a tumor of the diaphragm, lung or liver.

This abnormality is caused by incomplete development of a localized portion of the diaphragmatic musculature. The weakened part of the diaphragm becomes elevated because the intraabdominal pressure is greater than that in the pleura. It is best visualized during inspiration when the diaphragmatic muscles contract and cause the diaphragm to descend. The weak portion remains elevated and forms a localized protrusion from the diaphragmatic contour (Fig. 36). The developmental defect in the diaphragm is practically always situated anteriorly. It can be differentiated from a tumor when the elevations are multiple and give the appearance of interlacing scallops or when it does not descend with the rest of the diaphragm on respiration. A diaphragmatic tumor will move together with the remainder of the organ.

MOVEMENTS. The motion of the diaphragm is best studied by fluoroscopy. It should be observed in quiet and in deep respiration and, in special cases, during sudden forced inspiration as when the patient sniffs.

When the patient's breathing is predominantly costal in type it is best for routine purposes to confine the examination to ordinary quiet respiration in which there is more tendency to use the diaphragm. When instructed to breathe deeply or forcibly, the patient often employs only costal respiration and does not move the diaphragm at all. If it is essential to study the movement of the diaphragm in deep respiration, two methods may be employed to teach the patient to breathe with his diaphragm. First, with the room lights on, the examiner's hand is placed about 1 cm from the abdominal wall and the patient is asked to get his abdomen to touch the examiner's finger while making a deep inspiration. Usually this is easily learned. The maneuver is accomplished by pulling down the diaphragm. After the room is darkened, the patient may revert to costal respiration when asked to breathe deeply and it may be necessary to repeat the procedure several times. If the patient cannot learn to do this, it is best to have him make a forced expiration by humming as long as he can without interruption. The diaphragm will ascend markedly and at the next inspiration a sharp descent will occur automatically. Another method that we have found useful in teaching patients to use the diaphragm during respiration is to press the hand against the abdomen and ask the patient to push the hand away as he breathes in. This is done best if he is told to suck in air through his teeth while making the forced inspiration.

Downward motion of the diaphragm of 1 cm or more is satisfactory. Increased motion is of no clinical significance. It is produced largely by increased elevation of the diaphragm during expiration and is usually due to a voluntary large exhalation. An increase in the mobility of the diaphragm may be produced by placing the patient in the supine or prone position. When

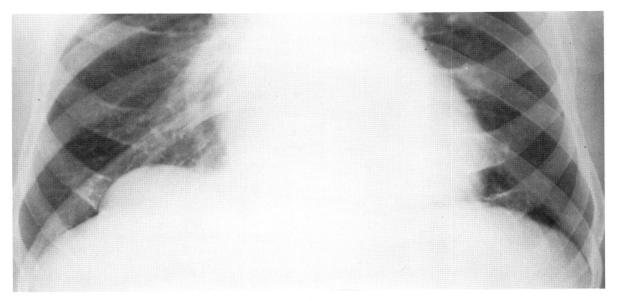

FIG. 36. LOCAL EVENTRATION OF THE DIAPHRAGM

There is a protuberance of the mesial portion of the right leaf of the diaphragm. The entire diaphragm descended during slow inspiration. However, on sniffing, the bulging portion moved paradoxically upward while the remainder of the diaphragm moved in the normal downward direction. This indicates a weak area in the diaphragm rather than a tumor in the lung or pleura. As is usual, the eventration was situated anteriorly.

viewed with vertical rays, both leaves of the diaphragm are seen to ascend to a greater degree because of the pressure of the viscera on the relaxed organ during expiration. If the patient is fluoroscoped in the lateral recumbent position, using horizontal rays, the increased elevation during expiration occurs on the side on which he is lying. This is due to transmission of the abdominal pressure to this side by gravity. The descent during inspiration is not impeded. There is, therefore, an increased excursion of the diaphragm on the side on which the patient lies. This explains the increase in pain on respiration in some cases of diaphragmatic pleurisy when the patient lies on the affected side (Fig. 37).

Diminished Mobility. One must differentiate between diminished mobility of the diaphragm in a normal direction and absent or paradoxical movement of this organ. Partial limitation in the movement of one of the leaves of the diaphragm is not rare in normal persons and occurs more frequently on the right side. Since a forced inspiration can be almost entirely costal on this side, this leaf of the diaphragm may seem to be

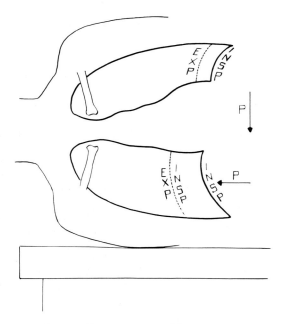

FIG. 37. DIAPHRAGMATIC MOVEMENT IN
THE LATERAL DECUBITUS POSITION

The patient is shown lying on his right side. On inspiration (INSP), the right leaf of the diaphragm descends to its normal level because the force of the diaphragmatic contraction is sufficient to overcome the pressure (P) of the abdominal viscera. However, when the diaphragm is relaxed during expiration (EXP), the weight of the abdominal organs, which is greater on the dependent side, forces the right leaf to a higher level than the left.

immobile. However, a good downward movement may be observed on ordinary inspiration. Quiet breathing, therefore, brings out the normal motion and is useful for proving that the diaphragm is not completely paralyzed.

Sometimes diminished movement is localized to the anterior portion of the diaphragm. This is obvious in the oblique view which exposes the posterior, as well as the anterior portion of the diaphragm. Perfect movement of the posterior portion may then be seen although the entire diaphragm appears paralyzed in the frontal view.

As a rule, diminished motion of both leaves of the diaphragm occurs in most conditions in which the diaphragm is abnormally elevated or depressed. Restriction in the movement of the diaphragm is common in association with chronic bronchitis and emphysema (diffuse obstructive emphysema). This is characterized by interference with expiration, causing a considerable amount of air to be trapped in the lung, increasing its volume and depressing the diaphragm. The diminution in diaphragmatic movement usually parallels the degree of functional impairment of the lungs. Films made during inspiration and expiration are useful as a permanent record of the degree of functional impairment.

Motion of both leaves of the diaphragm is also limited when they are elevated as the result of diffuse fibrotic pulmonary disease. Elevation of both leaves may also be due to distention of the abdomen from various causes. In peritonitis, diaphragmatic motion may be absent.

Absent Movement. It is rather difficult to determine if the diaphragm is immobile from casual inspection. The elevation of the ribs during inspiration may suggest that the diaphragm has descended, even though it remains stationary. Placing the finger on the fluoroscopic screen or television screen at the level of the dome of the diaphragm is helpful as a marker in determining its mobility. Complete absence of diaphragmatic movement during ordinary respiration occurs particularly in diaphragmatic paralysis and in subphrenic abscess. In the latter, this sign is essential for the diagnosis. It is so rare for there to be any movement of the diaphragm in the presence of a subphrenic abscess that even slight motion usually suffices to exclude the diagnosis. Frequently the diaphragm also remains immobile in pleurisy and particularly with a chronic empyema.

Paradoxical Movement. Paradoxical movement of an entire leaf of the diaphragm is characteristic of phrenic paralysis. The completely relaxed leaf of the diaphragm moves upward instead of downward during inspiration. When both leaves of the diaphragm are observed, they exhibit a see-saw motion. The upward movement of the paralyzed diaphragm during inspiration is caused by the pressure of the abdominal viscera. The downward motion of the normal diaphragm increases the intraabdominal pressure which is transmitted to the paralyzed side. The paralyzed diaphragm moves paradoxically downward during expiration because of the release of this pressure (Fig. 38).

Paradoxical movement may not occur in quiet respiration because the abdominal pressure is not raised sufficiently by the slow downward movement of the opposite leaf of the diaphragm. However, the paradoxical movement becomes evident when the patient makes a sudden forced inspiration. This is best accomplished by sniffing. The sudden forceful downward movement of the healthy diaphragm causes sufficient pressure on the abdominal viscera to force the paralyzed leaf upward. Here again, there may be some doubt as to the movement of the affected leaf of the diaphragm from casual inspection. It is wise, therefore, to place a finger on the screen as a marker over the shadow of the diaphragm to define its movement.

The paradoxical movement may be confined to only that portion of the diaphragm where its muscle is undeveloped and weak. The movement is accentuated by sniffing (Fig. 39). This maneu-

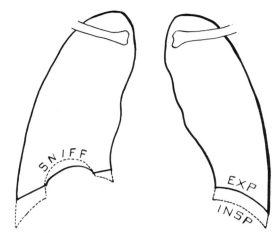

FIG. 39. PARADOXICAL MOTION OF A
PORTION OF THE DIAPHRAGM

The effect of a sudden forced inspiration on a weak portion of the right diaphragm is depicted by the broken line. The bulge is due to a local deficiency of the musculature of the diaphragm, and its characteristic elevation during sniffing is brought about in the same way as the paradoxical motion in diaphragmatic paralysis.

ver is particularly useful in differentiating the rounded protuberance produced by weak portions of the diaphragm from tumors in the adjacent lung. The latter descend with the diaphragm if they are not adherent to the chest wall. If they are fixed, they fail to exhibit any movement on sniffing.

There is a possibility of error in concluding that a patient has paralysis of the diaphragm because of the occurrence of paradoxical motion on sniffing. A diaphragm whose downward movement on inspiration is limited because of weakness of the organ, as a result of pleuritis, or by increased negative pressure in the pleural cavity resulting from atelectasis of the lung, may also show paradoxical movement when the abdominal pressure is suddenly increased. In such cases some movement of the diaphragm in the normal direction is usually demonstrable by less forceful inspiration and this excludes the possibility of complete paralysis.

Paradoxical movement of the diaphragm can also occur when the diaphragm is inverted by the weight of a large pleural effusion. An infrapulmonary effusion of only moderate size can produce the same effect. If the diaphragm is inverted, its contour is concave with the curve directed downward. As the diaphragm contracts during inspiration, it tends to straighten out and its dome therefore moves upward.

Diaphragmatic Tic, Spasm and Flutter. These abnormalities of the diaphragm are ade-

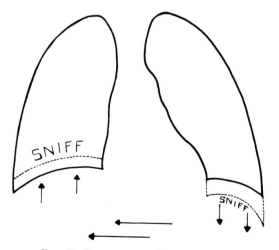

FIG. 38. PARADOXICAL MOTION OF THE
DIAPHRAGM

The solid line indicates the position of the diaphragm during expiration. The dotted line shows the position of the diaphragm on forced inspiration as in sniffing. The left leaf, which is normal, moves downward during inspiration. The right leaf of the diaphragm, which is paralyzed, moves suddenly upward. This is due to transmission of the abdominal pressure caused by the downward thrust of the left leaf of the diaphragm.

quately described by the names applied to them. They are the result of either a local reflex or abnormal impulses descending from the brain. Diaphragmatic tics may be caused by acute distention of the stomach as well as cerebral disturbances. They produce the characteristic hiccough. Diaphragmatic flutter is extremely rare. It is bilateral and causes marked dyspnea. It may be psychogenic or result from an intracranial lesion. Unilateral spasm of the diaphragm results from irritation of the pleura above the organ or irritation of the peritoneum beneath it. Bilateral spasm is rare. The diaphragm is fixed in the inspiratory position and respiration is entirely costal in type. It is sometimes associated with asthma.

SUBDIAPHRAGMATIC SHADOWS. Special attention should be paid to the subphrenic region when fluoroscoping the diaphragm. The presence of free air in the peritoneal cavity is evidenced by a crescentic area of radiolucency immediately beneath the diaphragm (Fig. 40). There is usually no difficulty in differentiating this from air in the colon or the stomach. Gas confined to the colon usually does not extend the entire width of the diaphragm and, when it does, the haustral stria-

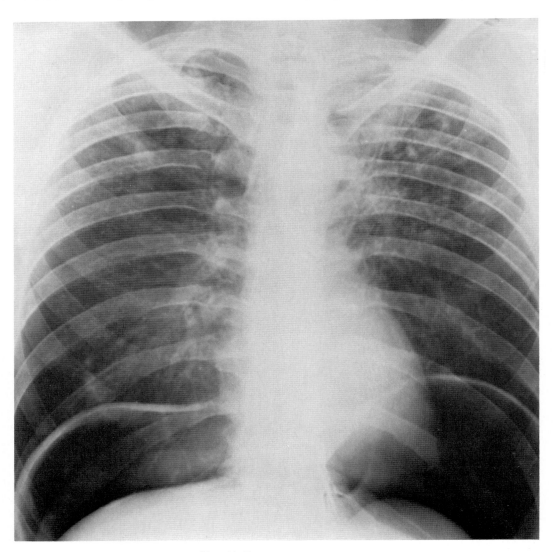

FIG. 40. PNEUMOPERITONEUM

A pneumoperitoneum had been induced for the treatment of bilateral hematogenous tuberculosis. The upper surface of the diaphragm is delineated by the contrasting air in the lungs. Its lower border, which is usually hidden by the shadows of the abdominal viscera, is now outlined by the air in the peritoneal cavity. The tuberculous lesions are represented by numerous indistinct small nodules, predominantly in the upper half of each lung.

tions in the colon are clear. A large stomach bubble is recognized by the fluid level in the stomach beneath it. That the air is really in the stomach and not in the peritoneal cavity can be determined in several ways (see p. 705).

On the right side, it is possible to confuse air in a distended colon interposed between the liver and diaphragm with air in the peritoneal cavity (Fig. 41). If any air is seen immediately beneath the right diaphragm it is advisable to close down the shutters and observe that region carefully for colonic haustrations.

Air is present directly beneath the diaphragm for a number of days following an abdominal operation and after the introduction of air into the peritoneum in the course of tubal insufflation. After perforation of a hollow viscus, the subphrenic air usually can be seen for a longer period. A marked elevation of the left leaf of the diaphragm is commonly associated with a large stomach bubble that results from aerophagia or the marked gaseous distention of the splenic flexure that appears to be constantly present in certain patients. It is usually impossible to dif-

ferentiate between elevation of the diaphragm by the pressure of these air-distended structures and paralysis of the diaphragm, from study of roentgen films alone. However the differentiation is simple on fluoroscopy. Even marked elevation of the diaphragm does not interfere greatly with its mobility.

Elevation of the left leaf of the diaphragm with a solid shadow beneath it suggests a more important abnormality. This may be due to subphrenic abscess or a large mass in the left upper abdomen. The latter can be a large spleen or kidney, a pancreatic cyst or a retroperitoneal neoplasm. Elevation of the right leaf of the diaphragm is somewhat different because the liver lies immediately beneath it. If this part of the diaphragm is elevated and the lower border of the liver depressed, the disease process lies in the subdiaphragmatic region or within the liver. If, on the other hand, the lower border of liver is elevated as well as the diaphragm, the most likely diagnosis is diaphragmatic paralysis or eventration.

At the time of fluoroscopy, the appearance of

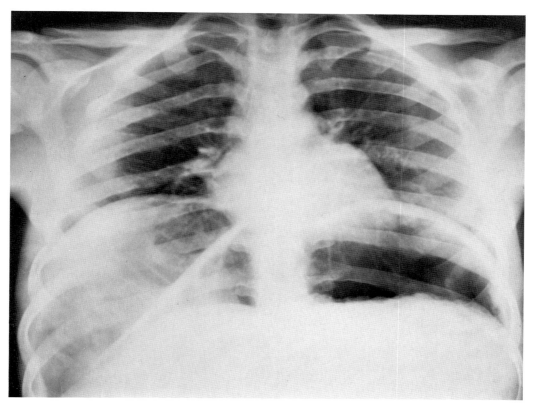

FIG. 41. INTERPOSITION OF THE COLON

Both leaves of the diaphragm are elevated by the markedly distended colon in a case of Hirschsprung's disease. The liver is depressed by the colon which is interposed between it and the diaphragm. The picture of the distended colon is differentiated from that of a pneumoperitoneum because of the haustral markings crossing the air shadow.

the stomach bubble should be noted. A shadow in its medial portion may represent a carcinoma of the cardia (Fig. 42), although it can also be caused by a large left lobe of the liver, a hiatus hernia or a retroperitoneal neoplasm. The shadow cast by the left lobe of the liver is characteristically oblique and has a sharply defined lower border. A fluid level immediately beneath the right leaf of the diaphragm is almost always due to a subphrenic abscess. It can also be caused by a large liver abscess or an echinococcus cyst which has perforated into one of the bile ducts.

Mediastinum. Fluoroscopy often supplies information regarding abnormalities of the mediastinum that is difficult or impossible to obtain from films alone. Not only can mediastinal movement be best evaluated by this means but pulsation of masses and the effects of changes in the intrathoracic pressure during respiration or the Valsalva maneuver can be studied.

MOVEMENT OF THE MEDIASTINUM. Under normal circumstances no movement of the mediastinum to either side can be detected except for the beating of the heart and the associated pulsation of the aorta and pulmonary arteries. No lateral movement of the mediastinal structures is visible even with deep and forced respirations. The only change that occurs is a narrowing of the mediastinal shadow on inspiration and a widening on expiration. Movement of the mediastinum from side to side with breathing indicates unequal expansion of the lungs during inspiration or unequal contraction during expiration. The latter may be due to a valve-like obstruction of a large bronchus which permits air to enter the lung but interferes with its expulsion. The ordinary roentgen film of the chest, which is made in complete inspiration, may appear entirely normal even though there is partial obstruction of a main bronchus by a tumor or

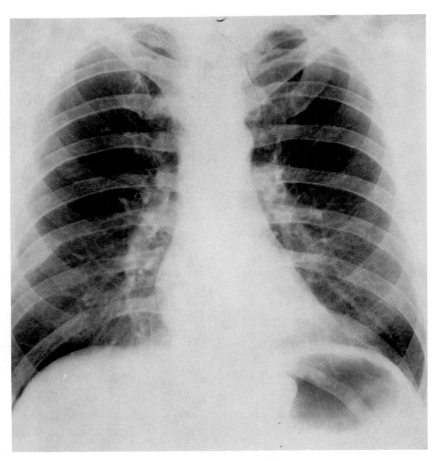

FIG. 42. CARCINOMA OF THE STOMACH

Except for emphysema involving the upper part of each lung the chest appears normal. However, a mass is seen encroaching on the mesial border of the stomach bubble. Barium study showed this to be a carcinoma of the cardia. The apex of the heart is obscured by an epicardial fat pad.

foreign body. For the roentgen demonstration of such an obstruction it is necessary to examine the patient in expiration as well as in inspiration. This is most easily done by fluoroscopy (Fig. 43).

Both lungs are equally inflated during inspiration and the mediastinum remains in its normal position during this phase. Failure of the obstructed lung to empty itself during expiration results in a positive pleural pressure on that side and displaces the mediastinum in the opposite direction. The to-and-fro movement of the mediastinum, with return toward the midline in inspiration, is characteristic of obstructive emphysema (Fig. 44A). The obstructed side is indicated by the direction of movement of the mediastinum during inspiration. It is not necessary for the obstruction to be in the main bronchus or one of the larger bronchi to produce this phenomenon. It can also be seen when many of the smaller bronchi are partially obstructed and prevent egress of air from one lung. This occurs particularly in the unilateral emphysema associated with an atrophic, bullous lung (so-called

vanishing lung). A similar pendular movement of the mediastinum occurs in association with a pneumothorax, particularly when large.

Pendular movement of the mediastinum also occurs when the expansibility of one lung is limited. Although the mediastinum tends to remain on the incompletely expanded side during both phases of respiration, it swings toward the affected lung during inspiration.

Limitation of expansion of the lung may be due to pulmonary fibrosis, but is more commonly due to bronchial obstruction (Fig. 44B). In both instances, the mediastinum shifts toward the diseased side during inspiration. On the other hand, when the limitation is caused by marked thickening of the pleura, the mediastinum usually does not move with respiration. This is due partly to fixation of the mediastinum by the inflammatory process and partly to restriction of the movement of the chest wall and diaphragm.

Minor lateral movements of the mediastinum are extremely significant in the diagnosis of bronchial obstruction, particularly in the absence of

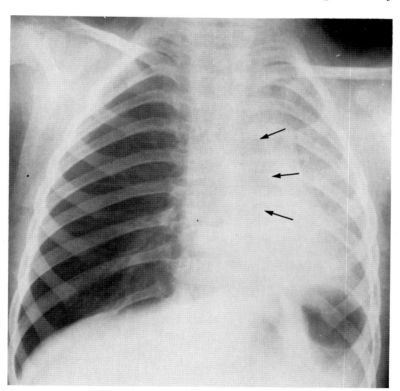

FIG. 43. OBSTRUCTIVE EMPHYSEMA WITH MEDIASTINAL HERNIATION

A three year old child aspirated a pumpkin seed. The film made in expiration shows exaggerated clouding of the left lung. The right lung remains fully aerated because of a valve-like obstruction of the right main bronchus. The heart is displaced to the left and the right lung has herniated (arrows) across the mediastinum. The picture is identical to that of atelectasis of the left lung on films made during inspiration. However, here, the left lung became fully aerated during inspiration and the heart and mediastinum returned to their normal position.

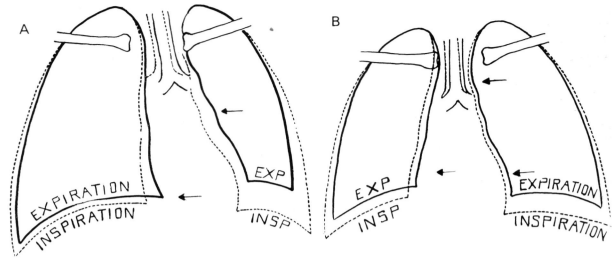

FIG. 44. PENDULAR MOVEMENT OF THE MEDIASTINUM

A: Obstructive emphysema of right lung. On inspiration (broken line), the chest appears approximately normal. On expiration (solid line), the right leaf of the diaphragm ascends only slightly in comparison with the marked upward excursion of the left side. The abdominal pressure together with the inward motion of the chest wall during expiration causes an increase in the pressure on the right lung because its bronchus is obstructed. This displaces the heart and trachea to the left. On inspiration, the mediastinal structures return to their former position. The direction of mediastinal shift during inspiration is toward the side of the obstruction. *B*: Atelectasis of right lung. The heart and mediastinal structures are approximately in their normal position at the end of expiration (solid line). During inspiration (dotted line), the chest wall moves outward and both leaves of the diaphragm descend. The resulting negative intrathoracic pressure is largely neutralized on the left side because of the influx of air into the lung. Because its bronchus is obstructed, air cannot enter the right lung so that the intrathoracic pressure on that side remains highly negative. This causes the heart and mediastinal structures to shift to the right. As the chest wall falls inward and the diaphragm rises during expiration, the negative pressure on the right side diminishes and the mediastinum moves back to its former position. As in obstructive emphysema, the mediastinal shift during inspiration is toward the abnormal side. However, in atelectasis the mediastinum is not displaced past the midline during expiration.

extensive fibrosis or infiltration of the lung. The small excursion of the mediastinum may not be noted on casual examination. A deep, quick inspiration is often necessary to produce sufficient differential between the pressures on the two sides to cause an appreciable mediastinal shift. It is therefore a good plan to have the patient breathe out completely in order to ensure a deep sudden inspiration. If he seems unable to do this consciously, the same effect may be obtained by having him make a humming sound and maintain it as long as he can and then take a deep breath. An additional effort may also be required to demonstrate the shift of the mediastinum in unilateral obstructive emphysema. In this case it is easier to recognize the shift of the mediastinum toward the *opposite* side on *expiration*. The patient should be instructed to take in a deep breath and breathe out suddenly and forcibly. This will accentuate any tendency of the mediastinum to shift to the opposite side.

The upward movement of the diaphragm during expiration causes an increase in the width of the cardiac and mediastinal shadows. This may make it difficult to detect lateral movement of the mediastinum. The difficulty can be obviated by placing a finger alongside each cardiac border at the end of expiration, and noting displacement of the heart in relation to the fingers during inspiration. In some cases, the mediastinal movement is detected more easily by using the position of the trachea as a guide. The trachea is seen quite clearly under the fluoroscope, particularly if the voltage is raised. In fact, it is usually seen more clearly than on ordinary roentgen films, and even slight movements of the trachea can be detected by placing the finger on the screen over the lateral border of its shadow. A shift of the trachea from side to side during respiration is most noticeable in obstruction of the upper lobe or main bronchi and may not be evident when there is obstruction only of the lower lobe bronchus.

Vertical Movement: (Swallowing Sign). Little vertical movement of the mediastinal structures is noted on ordinary respiration. However, on deep inspiration the heart may be pulled downward and its transverse diameter narrowed as the diaphragm descends. A similar downward movement may be noted in the ascending aorta, and occasionally at the lung roots, but there is no apparent clinical application to the study of the vertical movement of the mediastinum during respiration. There is, however, clinical significance to the movement of the mediastinal structures during the act of swallowing.

During swallowing the larynx is always raised upward by the contraction of the constrictor muscles of the pharynx. The upward motion is transmitted from the larynx to the trachea. Large paratracheal lymph nodes and the thyroid gland, both in the neck and in the substernal region, are attached to the trachea and therefore rise on swallowing.

The tracheal bifurcation and the left main bronchus are attached to the arch of the aorta by loose areolar tissue. This is sufficiently elastic to prevent transmission of the upward movement on swallowing from the trachea to the aorta, provided that the head is held erect or bent forward. If the head is bent backward, however, the larynx and, consequently, the trachea are elevated, so that the areolar tissue between the trachea and the aorta is stretched to its full extent. Under these circumstances, therefore, swallowing often causes elevation of the aortic arch. Upward motion of the arch of the aorta on swallowing while the head is extended is, therefore, a normal fluoroscopic finding.

On the other hand, upward motion of the aortic arch on swallowing while the head is in the natural position, is abnormal and indicates a pathologic relationship between the aortic arch and the trachea at the origin of the left main bronchus. This may occur under several circumstances. In emphysematous patients with marked depression of the diaphragm, the heart and the aorta are pulled downward. The loose areolar tissue connecting the aorta and the trachea is then under tension, producing a rigid connection between these structures. The rise of the trachea on swallowing, therefore, causes a simultaneous rise of the aortic arch. Similarly, a greatly widened aortic arch in arteriosclerosis may also produce a positive swallowing sign.

When the loose areolar tissue is transformed into firm fibrous tissue as a result of an inflammatory process in the mediastinum, a distinct rise of the arch of the aorta is usually noted during the act of swallowing. This may occur in aneurysms or luetic aortitis, which result in adhesion of the aorta to the trachea and left main bronchus from periaortic inflammation. In the absence of these diseases of the aorta and of emphysema, a rise of the aortic arch on swallowing, while the head is in the natural position, is indicative of an adhesive process in the medias-

tinum. In some cases the adhesion is caused by an invading neoplasm. In the absence of this, one must consider the possibility of adhesive mediastinitis. The sign is of particular value in the differential diagnosis of constrictive pericarditis. In this disease there is invariably an adhesive mediastinitis and in practically all of the cases that we have observed, this sign was present.

Fluttering Movement. A fluttering movement of the heart, notably of the atrium is often visible in pneumothorax. This is an important fluoroscopic sign because it calls attention to the possibility of a pneumothorax which otherwise might be overlooked. Whenever this unusual movement is noted, a careful inspection should be made of the pulmonary field in a search for a small pneumothorax. This should be done particularly during expiration, in which phase the pneumothorax is recognized more easily. Especially pronounced fluttering movement of the heart occurs in congenital absence of the pericardium.

GENERALIZED WIDENING. A generalized widening of the mediastinal shadow is seen in many abnormal conditions. However, because a widened mediastinum can be normal in short, heavy-set persons, allowance must be made for the habitus of the patient in evaluating whether or not the mediastinum is abnormal. The mediastinal shadow also becomes broader when the diaphragm is elevated. This occurs normally when the patient is recumbent and during expiration even in the erect position.

Simple hyperplasia of the thymus gland produces diffuse widening of the mediastinal shadow in the frontal projection. On the oblique and lateral views, however, it may be observed that the widening is confined to the anterior mediastinum. In addition, examination in the oblique or lordotic position, particularly in deep inspiration, may disclose the presence of an abrupt cessation of the shadow just before it comes in contact with the cardiac silhouette. Here the lower border of the mediastinal shadow often has an angular shape and makes a notch with the cardiac border, the appearance being not unlike the shape of a sail. This "sail sign" is rather characteristic of a hyperplastic thymus gland (Fig. 45).

Of the neoplastic diseases, the one which most frequently produces a generalized widening of the mediastinal shadow is Hodgkin's disease. Occasionally a similar widening of the mediastinum occurs in lymphosarcoma, in metastasis to the mediastinal lymph nodes, or invasion of the mediastinum by a carcinoma of the lung even when the primary tumor is not visible. However, in these cases, the neoplastic nature of the disease

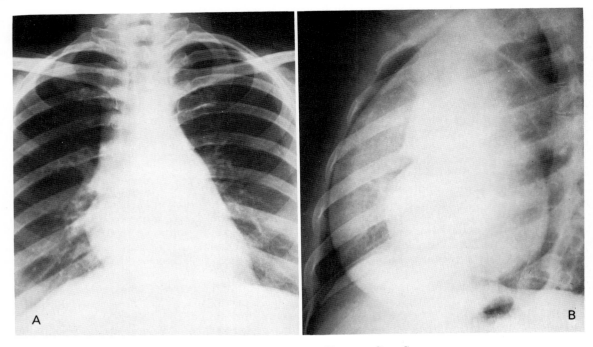

FIG. 45. HYPERPLASIA OF THE THYMUS: SAIL SIGN

A: The frontal view shows a fullness of the superior mediastinum. Although a definitive diagnosis is not warranted, the sharp indentation between the right border of the mass and the cardiac contour suggests an enlarged thymus. *B*: Left oblique view. The sharp incisura in the right border of the mediastinum delimits the anterior mediastinal mass from the heart. The conformation of the mass resembles a sail, an appearance characteristic of an enlarged thymus gland.

may be inferred from an irregularity of the borders of the mediastinum, best appreciated in the oblique position.

Widening of the superior mediastinal shadow to the right may be due to distention of the superior vena cava. This generally occurs in cardiac failure. The associated enlargement of the heart and distention of the pulmonary vessels indicate that the superior vena cava is the cause for the abnormal mediastinal shadow. The superior vena cava is also widened in association with various congenital lesions, such as anomalous drainage of the pulmonary veins into the vena cava (see Fig. 219) and cardiac anomalies associated with elevation of the pressure in the right atrium. Thrombosis of the superior vena cava may also be manifested by widening of the superior mediastinal shadow. In rare instances, the widening of the superior mediastinum develops gradually following the thrombosis. This results from the development of cavernous transformation of the vein similar to that which occurs in thrombosis of the portal vein. The obliterated vena cava is replaced by a spongy, vascular network formed by collateral circulation about and within the wall of the vein together with the recanalized thrombus.

A right aortic arch may also produce widening of the right side of the mediastinum. It is recognized by observing the course of the aorta and its indentation on the esophagus (see Fig. 502). In most cases, the shadow of the descending aorta is seen to be situated alongside the right of the spine, although in some it descends on the left side. In either instance, the aortic arch indents the right posterior border of the esophagus rather than the left anterior border as it does when the aorta develops normally.

Diffuse widening of the mediastinum occurs in acute mediastinitis. In this disease, the clinical condition of the patient in conjunction with the widened mediastinum usually makes the diagnosis perfectly clear. In doubtful cases, observation of the neck in the lateral view is helpful. A concomitant widening of the retrotracheal space is indicative of mediastinitis (Fig. 46).

The shadow of the dilated esophagus in cardiospasm can cause a puzzling appearance on fluoroscopy. The esophagus projects to the right and widens the mediastinal shadow from the clavicle to the diaphragm (see Fig. 497). However, when the shutters are closed down so that details are seen more clearly, mottling of the shadow may become evident. This is character-

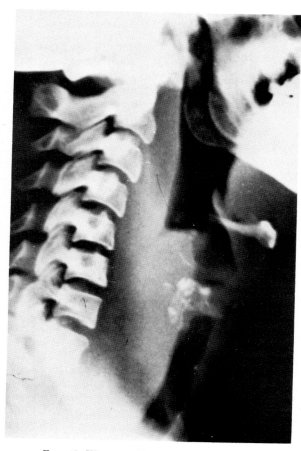

FIG. 46. WIDENED RETROTRACHEAL SPACE
IN MEDIASTINITIS

The anterior displacement of the trachea and the wide space between the trachea and the spine are due to suppuration in the prevertebral space. The trachea is displaced forward as far down as the jugular notch by the suppurative process which extends into the posterior mediastinum. Widening of the retrotracheal space is one of the most important roentgen signs of mediastinitis.

istic of cardiospasm and is caused by frothy fluid and food within the dilated esophagus. Sometimes a fluid level is present. If there is any possibility that the shadow is due to cardiospasm, the esophagus should be outlined with barium.

MEDIASTINAL MASSES. Localized bulges of the mediastinum, or irregular widening of the mediastinum indicating the presence of mediastinal masses are generally quite evident at fluoroscopic examination. However, they may be obscured by the normal mediastinal structures in the frontal view and found only on the oblique projections. In general, a mediastinal mass is seen with considerably more detail on films and therefore the differential diagnosis is best made from radiographic rather than fluoroscopic examination. However, fluoroscopy can be helpful in determining the positions in which films should be made and by disclosing evidence pointing to a vascular origin of the mass in some instances.

Hidden Masses. The chest should always be examined in the oblique view at fluoroscopy, not only to uncover unseen shadows in the posterior costophrenic sinuses and the region behind the heart, but also because the oblique view may disclose a mass in the mediastinum which otherwise would be missed. A small, hidden dermoid or thymus tumor in the anterior mediastinum may be brought into view by simply rotating the patient a few degrees to either side. Examination in the full oblique position may disclose a large mass of lymph nodes at the tracheal bifurcation which cannot be visualized in the frontal view, even on films. The lateral view is also useful for disclosing abnormalities in the mediastinum, but visualization is not always satisfactory in heavy persons.

Substernal Thyroid. Mediastinal masses in the region of the superior thoracic aperture should always be observed during the act of swallowing. A sharply demarcated tumor in this location which rises on swallowing usually proves to be a tumor of the thyroid gland. If the mass fails to rise on swallowing, a substernal thyroid may be excluded from consideration.

By increasing the voltage, one can often determine the effect of a thyroid mass on the trachea more clearly by fluoroscopy than on ordinary roentgen films. Sometimes the superior mediastinal shadow of a substernal thyroid is not noted on casual examination, but the associated displacement of the trachea should not be overlooked, for no fluoroscopic examination of the chest is complete without examining this organ. It may be necessary to close down the vertical shutters and to increase the voltage, to get a good view of the trachea. If there is no evidence of disease in the upper lobe to account for the tracheal displacement, an enlarged thyroid gland should be searched for by "diaphragming" down. Almost invariably this will be found to be present when the trachea is displaced without apparent cause.

Pulsatile Masses. Every mediastinal mass should be observed for pulsations. This is done by closing down the diaphragmatic shutters to the edge of the mass to outline it sharply and to provide a straight contrasting frame in relation to which the pulsations can be seen clearly. Pulsations in a lateral direction only may be due simply to transmission of the movements of the heart or aorta (transmitted pulsation). But if the pulsation is seen in other directions as well (expansile pulsation), it may be assumed that the pulsation is intrinsic and that the shadow is vascular in origin. A pulsating mass on the right side of the superior aperture of the chest, simulating a substernal thyroid, usually represents a tortuous, dilated or aneurysmal innominate artery. It should be borne in mind that absence of pulsation does not exclude an aneurysm, since the walls of an aneurysm are often lined by a thick, lamellated clot which effectively prevents pulsatile movement.

One can usually determine by fluoroscopy whether large shadows at the root of the lung are due to large lymph nodes or wide pulmonary arteries. The presence of expansile pulsation indicates that the shadows are vascular in origin.

Where there is doubt concerning the differentiation between vascular and lymph node shadows, the question may often be resolved by resorting to the Valsalva maneuver. If the shadows become smaller after the patient strains for a few seconds, it is safe to conclude that they are vascular in origin. The vascular origin of the shadow may also be determined by examination in the oblique view. What appears as a round mass near the root of the lung in the posteroanterior view may then be demonstrated clearly to be a branching pulsating blood vessel.

Cardiophrenic Angle Shadows. A sharply demarcated mass in the right cardiophrenic angle in the shape of a quarter circle usually represents properitoneal fat that has herniated through the foramen of Morgagni into the mediastinum anterior to the heart. Occasionally the hernia contains omentum.

Other abnormalities which produce shadows in the anterior cardiophrenic angle are large epicardial fat pads, pericardial cysts, and low lying thymic tumors. The epicardial fat pad is usually seen in the angle between the apex of the heart and the diaphragm. Here it produces a hazy density which obliterates the border of the cardiac apex and fades off gradually into the pulmonary field, although it occasionally is well demarcated. The fat pad tends to be triangular in shape. An epicardial fat pad is occasionally visible on the right side, but rarely without a similar one on the left.

A parapericardial cyst may occupy either cardiophrenic angle. Its outer border is curved and extremely well demarcated on the frontal projection but is usually lost within the cardiac shadow on the lateral view. The cyst has a tendency to change its shape somewhat during respiration and it may be observed to alter its position as

well as its shape when the patient assumes the recumbent or Trendelenburg position.

Occasionally a thymoma originating from the lower part of the thymus or one extending downward from the thymus by a long stalk, is situated immediately above the diaphragm, and appears as a cardiophrenic angle shadow. The ones that we have seen have all been on the right side. It is usually impossible, from the fluoroscopic examination, to differentiate between such a thymus tumor, properitoneal fat herniation, and a parapericardial cyst.

The shadow of a hiatus hernia or an esophageal diverticulum may appear to be situated in the cardiophrenic angle on the frontal projection. However, the abnormal density is demonstrated to be situated behind the heart by turning the patient to the oblique position. Its nature is easily determined by fluoroscopy after the administration of barium.

Spine. It is evident that fluoroscopy is not especially useful in examination of the spine. Scoliosis and extensive bridging of the vertebrae occasionally cause confusing shadows in the mediastinal region, but are easily recognizable on properly exposed films. In scoliosis of the dorsal spine, the convexity is usually directed to the right. At the preliminary survey of the chest the shadow of the curved spine often suggests enlargement of the right side of the heart. That the convex shadow in this region is not related to the heart is quickly determined by turning the patient to the right oblique view. The spine then projects further to the right and the right cardiac border is displaced to the left, thus separating the two structures. Furthermore, by closing down the diaphragm, one can outline the individual vertebrae and identify the cause of the unusual shadow.

Prominent bony projections bridging the bodies of the vertebrae in hypertrophic spondylitis may simulate a mediastinal tumor at first glance. Here again, the cause of the shadow can be determined by careful inspection after cutting down the field. Turning the patient slightly to either oblique position is also helpful.

The shadow of a Pott's abscess may simulate either an aortic aneurysm or a mediastinal tumor. Here also, cutting down the shutters will usually define the shadow sufficiently to enable recognition of its source. Most often the shadow will be seen to be fusiform in shape, gradually flattening out along the spine on each side. This appearance is characteristic of an abscess originating in the spine. Examination in the oblique position may also disclose collapsed vertebrae and absence of the intervertebral spaces.

Ribs. The observer should not be confused by

calcification of the costal cartilages. This occurs particularly in the cartilage of the first rib and, at first glance, the shadow suggests an infiltration or a nodule within the lung. By moving the screen, and consequently the tube, up and down and by turning the patient slightly from side to side the continuity of the shadow with that of the first rib is demonstrated. The character of the shadow then becomes clear. In some cases it may be necessary to close down on the first rib to clarify the picture.

Calcification of the lower costal cartilages may be confused with infiltrations of the lung, but careful observation of the course of the shadows will show that these, which are also situated anteriorly, are connected with the ribs.

Well-developed cervical ribs are seen quite clearly if the diaphragmatic shutters are closed down. If they are small, considerable experience may be required to recognize them. However, the shape of small cervical ribs is so characteristic that their recognition is not difficult. They present as sharply defined, acute triangles with the base at the transverse process of the lowermost cervical vertebra and the apex directed over the shadow of the paravertebral part of the first and second ribs.

Synchondroses of the ribs and bifid ribs may also cause confusing shadows. Here also the nature of the shadows can be determined by diaphragming down over the shadows (Fig. 47).

Special Uses of Fluoroscopy

In addition to serving as a preliminary procedure in the roentgen examination of the chest, fluoroscopic examination may yield information not provided by the roentgen films. Fluoroscopy serves as a guide in the performance of certain procedures such as pneumothorax therapy, bronchography and percutaneous or transbronchial lung biopsy. It is extremely useful in localizing lesions within the chest and is required for the proper placement of the catheter for aspiration of a lung abscess and the injection of antibiotics directly into the lesion.

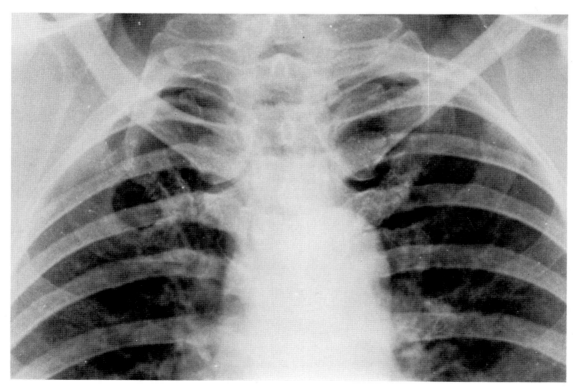

FIG. 47. PSEUDOCAVITY: RIB ANOMALY

A sharply defined, round area of lucency in the upper part of the right chest was wrongly interpreted as a pulmonary cavity on a film made with less exposure. On this film the cause of the lucency is seen to be a synchrondrosis of the anterolateral portions of the first and second ribs and a synostosis of the anterior extremities of these ribs. On fluoroscopic examination, the outlines of the ribs were not so clearly visualized. However as the patient was turned from the frontal to the left oblique position, the area of lucency was found to be situated anteriorly and became progressively narrower until eventually, on rotating the patient further, the lucency disappeared entirely. These findings indicated that its origin was outside the lung.

Interpretation of Obscure Shadows. It is often difficult to determine from the roentgen film whether a small nodule in the lower part of the chest is situated in the lung, or whether it represents the shadow of a nipple. Even the male nipple may cast a shadow simulating a metastatic tumor. The nipple may be visible on only one side of the chest. It is a simple matter to locate the shadow under the fluoroscope and determine whether it really represents a nipple by moving the breast and noting whether the shadow moves. The shadow of a nevus or of a pedunculated tumor of the skin can be displaced and identified in the same manner.

In similar fashion, fluoroscopy permits the differentiation between a calcified lymph node in the lower part of the mesial portion of the neck and a calcific focus in the apex of the lung. An attempt is made to move the calcified area with the examining finger while the patient is behind the fluoroscopic screen. If the nodule can be moved, it may be concluded that it represents a calcified lymph node.

Sometimes it is difficult, from the roentgenographic examination alone, to differentiate the shadow cast by heavy pectoral muscles or breasts from consolidation in the lung. Movement of these superficial structures during fluoroscopic observation will usually make the differentiation clear. If there remains any doubt after fluoroscopy, the roentgenographic examination may be repeated using higher voltage which tends to eliminate the shadows of the structures on the chest wall (Fig. 4).

Fluoroscopy is a rapid method for confirming or negating the possibility of an artifact which simulates a lesion in the chest on the roentgen film. If there is a well-demarcated shadow, measuring more than 1 cm in diameter on the film, which cannot be seen fluoroscopically, it is safe to conclude that it represents an artifact.

Bronchoesophageal Fistula. Cough on the ingestion of fluids may be due to a bronchoesophageal fistula, and this may be demonstrated by roentgen examination after the ingestion of iodized oil or a thin mixture of barium. However, the diagnosis of a bronchoesophageal fistula is not justified simply because the bronchi are outlined on films following the ingestion of radiopaque material, as it is possible for the barium to be aspirated into the bronchial tree from the pharynx. Therefore, it is necessary to demonstrate the passage of the barium directly from the esophagus into the bronchi. This is best done by fluoroscopic observation with spot filming or ciné recording.

Aspiration of barium through the glottis occurs when there is anesthesia of the pharynx and larynx in association with a lesion near the base of the brain, or when there is poor coordination of the swallowing mechanism from other causes. It is surprising how little cough may be occasioned by the passage of barium into the bronchial tree in such cases. It is also remarkable that patients with this condition so often avoid aspiration pneumonia.

Retention of Barium in Pyriform Fossae. In some cases no barium enters the bronchi even though the patient complains of severe cough after the ingestion of fluids. This is usually due to improper functioning of the muscles of the hypopharynx. Ingested fluid fills the pyriform fossae and eventually overflows into the larynx, initiating a spell of coughing. Depending upon the amount of barium that is given, retention in the pyriform fossae may be the only abnormal sign. Dyskinesia of the pharyngeal muscles may be due to a lesion in the central nervous system. Unilateral retention of barium in a pyriform fossa can occur in paralysis of a recurrent laryngeal nerve. The absence of movement of the vocal cords and the arytenoid cartilage on that side may be observed by diaphragming down on the larynx and having the patient phonate.

Retention of barium in the pyriform fossae and in the vallecular spaces also occurs in some cases of myasthenia gravis. Here it is due to weakness of the muscles of deglutition. A diagnosis of myasthenia gravis can be made in such cases if swallowing is completed without retention of the barium after injection of Tensilon.

Control of Pneumothorax Treatment. Fluoroscopy was generally used for the control of pneumothorax treatment for tuberculosis. Patients were routinely fluoroscoped before and after each injection of air. This form of therapy has been almost completely abandoned. Even in the rare instances when it is employed, it is preferable to monitor the procedure with films rather than fluoroscopy, avoiding unnecessary irradiation. Occasionally fluoroscopy is required for the discovery and localization of pleural adhesions which require lysis.

In a patient who has developed thickening of the pleura during the course of pneumothorax treatment, limitation of pulmonary expansion is easily recognizable by fluoroscopy. If the mediastinum shifts into the side of the pneumothorax during inspiration, it is justifiable to conclude that the lung is unable to expand properly. While this may be due to pulmonary fibrosis or bronchial obstruction, the most common cause in patients with prolonged pneumothorax treatment, or in those who have developed a small pleural effusion, is encasement of the lung by thickened pleura. The fluoroscopic findings may be the determining factor in deciding the need for decortication. Shift of the mediastinum during respiration indicates that this region is not involved by the inflammatory process.

Aspiration under Fluoroscopic Control. Needling of the chest is not without its dangers. These consist essentially of the production of a pneumothorax as a result of a tear in the pleura and the much more important complication of air embolism to the brain or to a coronary artery. Both of these complications can arise from puncture of the lung. Only rarely is the technique so faulty that air is permitted to enter the pleura through the aspirating needle and the sudden deaths which occur after aspiration of the chest can no longer be attributed to so-called pleural shock.

In the aspiration of pleural effusions both of these dangers may be avoided if the needle is inserted into the effusion without transversing lung tissue. The generalization that it is the dry tap which results in complications usually holds. It is, therefore, necessary to precede the aspiration by careful roentgen examination, particularly with respect to the localization of the suspected effusion. At this time it is also noted whether there is a fluid level which would indicate the presence of air as well as fluid in the chest. This will be decisive in determining whether air found in the chest after aspiration was due to the aspiration or whether it had been there previously, a question which is most important not only from a diagnostic, but also from a therapeutic standpoint.

As a rule, the preliminary roentgen findings suffice for adequately accurate localization of the effusion for aspiration. However, when the collection of fluid is small, particularly when it is mainly within an interlobar fissure, the aspiration had best be done under direct fluoroscopic control.

Since there is always the danger of penetrating the lung with a needle in the search for a small collection of fluid, precautions should be taken to prevent air embolization to the brain during the procedure. When the lung is punctured bubbles of air may enter a branch of the pulmonary vein and travel through the left side of the heart to the aorta. The carotid arteries arise and ascend vertically from the summit of the aortic arch. Therefore, the air bubbles have a tendency to rise within them and enter the brain if the patient is in the erect position. If the patient is lying down, these bubbles are more apt to follow the course of the blood stream to the lower branches of the aorta where they are relatively harmless. It is wise, therefore, never to aspirate the chest with the patient upright when there is any question concerning the entry of the needle into the lung. The horizontal fluoroscope is, therefore, used during chest aspirations done under fluoroscopic control.

Fluoroscopic control is required particularly during aspiration biopsy of the lung, even if the nodule is fairly large. Only its midportion may be in contact with the chest wall and there may be a considerable amount of pulmonary tissue between the other parts of the periphery of the tumor and the pleura. The aspiration should be carried out at a point as near as possible to the center of the shadow of the tumor with the fluoroscopic screen tangential to the point where the lesion is most superficial.

It is only rarely that one would attempt aspiration of a cavity in the lung. In the case of a pulmonary abscess the dangers of infection of the pleura are so great and the gain from aspiration so little, that this procedure is contraindicated. However, it may be desirable to insert a needle into an air cyst of the lung, possibly for the injection of sclerosing solutions in an attempt to obliterate the bronchial opening into the cyst. In such cases, it is essential that the irritating substance be introduced into the cavity and not into the adjacent lung. The safest way to perform this is under the fluoroscope and here again, the maneuver should be carried out with the patient in the horizontal position. The same precaution should be taken in the needling of tense cavities in the Monaldi procedure.

Localization with the Fluoroscope. Fluoroscopy is the most rapid method by which accurate localization of lesions within the chest can be carried out and, in some cases, it is an indispensable procedure for the determination of the exact position of the lesion. Films are required for localization when the shadow of the lesion is very faint, or when it is partly obscured by other shadows. In occasional cases, the lesion is not clearly seen on the oblique or the lateral views even on the roentgen films, and in such cases sectional radiography is required for localization.

Localization of the lesion is important both for diagnostic and therapeutic purposes. The reinfection type of tuberculosis almost always occurs in the posterior part of the upper lobe. A shadow in the anterior part of this lobe, even though it simulates tuberculosis in all other respects, is more apt to represent a neoplasm or a nonspecific inflammatory mass. A bizarre shadow in the pulmonary field may be extremely difficult to interpret until fluoroscopy in the proper view shows it to be thin and shell-like, characteristic of pleural calcification.

Lesions requiring diagnostic aspiration or biopsy such as small loculated collections of fluid, peripheral pulmonary masses, cysts in the lung or mediastinum and, occasionally, mediastinal tumors, must be localized accurately before the needle is inserted. Precise localization is also necessary before drainage of a lung abscess. Exact localization of tumors of the lung or ribs is required preliminary to radiotherapy in order to keep the field of radiation as small as possible and to administer maximum dosage with a minimum of secondary effects.

Several types of procedures are used in localization and these involve different principles. The location of the lesion must be related to one or more points on the chest wall. Briefly, localization is achieved by using the central ray to determine the height of the lesion and by using the phenomenon of parallax or two or more views to determine its depth and its relationship to the chest wall. The points of reference are the anterior and posterior ribs, the costochondral junctions, the sternum, the spine and transverse processes, radiopaque markers on the chest wall or in an intercostal muscle and radiopaque materials inserted either in the bronchi, the pleural cavity or a drained focus in the lung. An additional lesion in the lung may also serve as a point of reference.

It is important, at the outset, to decide whether or not the lesion is adherent to the chest wall. This can be determined by noting whether there is a change in the relationship of the shadow to the adjacent ribs when the patient breathes or when he lies down. If the pleura is not adherent, the lesion will be displaced downward with inspiration and upward when the patient is placed in the recumbent position. The anterior portions of the ribs are usually raised during inspiration. If the lesion is situated posteriorly, it will move in relation to the anterior ribs even if it is adherent to the posterior chest wall. It is necessary, therefore, to determine which portion of the ribs is adjacent to the lesion before deciding whether or not there are pleural adhesions over the diseased area.

CENTRAL RAY. In order to determine the height of the lesion in the chest it is necessary that the lesion be projected on the screen by rays that are truly horizontal. If the tube is situated above a lesion in the posterior part of the chest and if the patient is examined in the ordinary posteroanterior position, the shadow of the lesion will be projected too low, while if the tube is situated below the lesion, it will be projected too high (Fig. 9).

The error in determining the level of the lesion can be minimized by positioning the patient so that the lesion is closest to the screen. The greater the distance between the x-ray tube and the screen, the less the distortion. In radiography, the 6-foot distance between the tube and the film brings all the rays nearer to the horizontal. Even here, however, the error in determining the height of a lesion is considerable if the tube is not positioned properly or if the lesion is at a distance from the film. The distance between the tube and the screen is so short in fluoroscopy that any deviation in the height of the tube may displace the shadow upward or downward for a distance of as much as 2 inches.

In order to determine the correct height of the lesion, the central ray, which is horizontal, is used. This is done by closing down the shutters to a square of about 1 cm in width and centering this over the midpoint of the lesion. A radiopaque pointer is then placed on the side of the chest nearest the screen within the center of this square and held tightly against the patient's skin. This point is then marked either with ink or a wax pencil. A line drawn horizontally across the chest at this level indicates the height of the lesion. Since the skin which bears the mark often shifts in relation to underlying structures as the position of the patient's arm is changed or when he lies down, it is necessary that the same position be maintained during the remainder of the examination. Various factors are to be considered in localizing the exact position of the lesion within the horizontal plane which has been marked out on the patient's chest.

MAGNIFICATION AND DEMARCATION OF SHADOW. As in the case of shadows produced by any small light source, the size of the image on the fluoroscopic screen and its demarcation depend on the distance between the lesion and the screen (Fig. 8). If the lesion were touching the screen, the size of its image would be identical to that of the lesion and it would appear sharply demarcated. As the distance between the lesion and the screen increases, its shadow becomes larger and its border less distinct.

These characteristics of the shadow serve as a rough but useful method of localization. The size and demarcation of the lesion are noted in both the posteroanterior and the anteroposterior positions. The lesion is considered to be more anterior when it appears smaller and more sharply demarcated in the posteroanterior view and vice versa.

PARALLAX. *Rotation of Patient.* The phenomenon of parallax as applied to localization of lesions in the chest may be demonstrated by simply turning the patient slightly toward the right oblique position while he is behind the fluoroscopic screen facing the observer. The heart, which is situated nearer the screen, is seen to be displaced to the patient's left, and the spine, which is situated posteriorly, is displaced to his right (Fig. 48). The shadow of a lesion in the chest moves accordingly. Thus, the shadow of an anterior lesion moves with the heart, and one that is situated posteriorly moves with the spine.

So much for the direction of the movement of shadows on the fluoroscopic screen while the patient is being rotated. The speed of the movement of shadows is also important in localization. The closer the lesion is to the surface of the chest, the more rapid the motion of its shadow. Thus, if one should place a metal marker over the costochondral junction of an obese patient and then rotate him, both the marker on the skin and the edge of the bony part of the rib will be seen to move in the same direction. However, the motion of the marker, which is closer to the screen, is more rapid than that of the costochondral junction, so that the two points, which at first were superimposed on each other, gradually become separated. The separation reaches its maximum when the patient is in the lateral position. If the marker on the skin were placed over

a lesion more deeply situated, the rate of separation would be greater. Therefore, if a radiopaque pointer placed over a lesion becomes separated only slightly from the shadow of the lesion as the patient is being rotated, it may be concluded that the lesion is situated close to the surface.

The lesions which most frequently require localization—small collections of fluid in the pleura, peripheral neoplasms and lung abscesses—lend themselves to this method of localization. The metal pointer is placed directly over the lesion with the patient in the postero-anterior position and he is then rotated. The degree of relative movement is observed. He is then placed in the anteroposterior position and the process is repeated, noting in which position there is less relative movement between the pointer and the shadow of the lesion.

The problem is to find the position in which there is the least parallax. When the lesion is in the mesial portion of the chest this is a relatively simple matter, provided that it is located superficially, as are almost all of the lesions requiring accurate localization. Both the anterior and posterior surfaces of the mesial portion of the chest

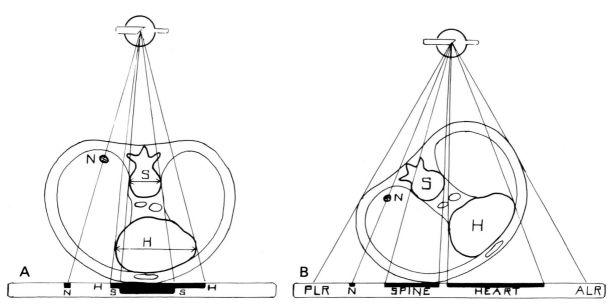

FIG. 48. FLUOROSCOPIC LOCALIZATION: EFFECT OF TURNING PATIENT

A: Posterior view with tube centered: cross section of patient viewed from above. The shadow of the spine (S) is superimposed upon the shadow of the heart (H), and the shadow of the nodule (N) is projected to its right. *B*: The patient is turned to the right oblique position. The shadow of the heart is projected into the left chest while the projection of the spine is on the right. The shadow of the nodule in the posterior part of the right lung maintains its relationship to the shadow of the spine which becomes increasingly separated from the cardiac shadow as the patient continues to be turned toward the right lateral position. The shadow of a lesion in the posterior part of the chest moves with the shadow of the spine on rotating the patient while lesions in the anterior part of the chest appear to move together with the heart. In the right oblique view, which is depicted, the silhouette of the right side of the thorax corresponds to the posterolateral region while the silhouette of the left side of the chest corresponds to the anterolateral region.

are roughly parallel to the screen, and hence there remains only the necessity of determining whether the lesion is situated anteriorly or posteriorly. In one of these two positions there will be practically no parallax. It is in this position that the pointer lies in direct approximation to the underlying lesion.

Lesions situated in the lateral third of the chest are more difficult to localize. Because of the curve of the ribs in the outer part of the thorax, these lesions, even though superficial, are separated from the screen in both frontal projections. Parallax is therefore present between the shadow of the pointer and that of the lesion whether the examination is made in the postero-anterior or the anteroposterior position.

The position in which least parallax occurs will be the lateral or either oblique, depending upon the location of the lesion in relation to the chest wall. The patient is therefore fluoroscoped in all three positions, and the degree of parallax is noted in each one by placing the pointer over the center of the shadow and rotating the patient to and fro. When the position causing the least parallax is found, the shutters are narrowed down over the lesion in order to utilize the central ray. The point of localization is then marked on the skin. It is essential when marking the position of the lesion that the patient's arm be in the same position in which any anticipated aspiration or operation is to be performed. If the position of the arm is changed, there may be a considerable shift between the mark on the skin and the underlying lesion.

Movement of Tube. Localization is best carried out with the patient in the upright position because the shadows in the lungs are seen more clearly when the subject is erect. If the patient is too sick to stand, a high swivel stool is usually helpful. In patients who cannot cooperate, the phenomenon of parallax may be utilized by moving the tube instead of rotating the patient.

It will be found that shadows of objects in the same plane parallel to the screen, move together as the tube moves. The shadows of objects closest to the screen seem to move with it, whereas those situated farther away seem to move in the opposite direction. Thus, on moving the tube from the midline to either side, the heart and spine become separated from each other (Fig. 49). The costochondral junctions appear to move together with the heart while a radiopaque object placed on the posterior part of the chest moves with the spine. If the tube is moved upward with the patient in the posteroanterior position, the anterior ribs appear to rise and the posterior ribs appear to move downward across them.

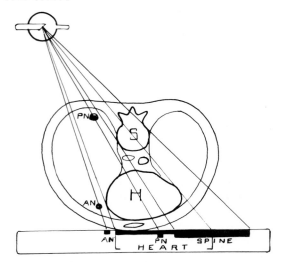

FIG. 49. FLUOROSCOPIC LOCALIZATION: LATERAL SHIFT OF TUBE

The tube, which was centered in Fig. 48A, has now been shifted to the patient's right. Although the shadow of the heart has moved somewhat toward the right of the screen, the shadow of the spine has moved farther to that side. The cardiac shadow moves slowly during the shifting of the tube, while the movement of the shadow of the spine is rapid. The shadows, therefore, appear to move in opposite directions, the heart with the tube, and the spine, against it. The shadow of the nodule in the posterior part of the chest (PN) maintains its relationship to the spine, while the image of the nodule in the anterior part of the chest (AN) appears to move with the heart.

As in determining parallax by rotation, the patient is viewed in several different degrees of obliquity. In each position, a radiopaque marker is placed over the shadow of the lesion and the relative motion between the lesion and the marker is noted as the screen is moved. When there is no apparent movement between the two as the tube is shifted, it can be concluded that the pointer is situated immediately over the lesion where it is closest to the chest wall. This point is then marked on the skin for future reference.

POINTS OF REFERENCE. Mention has been made of the use of a radiopaque pointer over the skin and the marking of the skin as a point of reference to the lesion. Other points of reference are also used, namely, the spine, the ribs, radiopaque materials placed into a cavity in the lung or pleura, and radiopaque materials which are injected into an intercostal muscle. In addition, the spatial relationship of a lesion in the chest may be determined in relation to another lesion within the lung, in relation to the bronchi which have been filled with iodized oil or to a bronchoscope within one of the bronchi.

Bony Landmarks. The costochondral junctions and the transverse processes of the spine are useful as points of reference to determine the lateral relationship of shadows which lie in the same coronal plane. These landmarks are particularly useful because, unlike skin markers, they remain fixed and are visible to the surgeon throughout the operation. The ribs may be used as reference points to determine the vertical relationship of an intrathoracic lesion. However, their practical use in this regard is limited by the ability of the surgeon to identify them at operation.

The surgeon often uses the angle of Louis, i.e., the prominence of the second chondrosternal junction, as a starting point for identifying the ribs. However, not infrequently, this prominence is lacking and sometimes the prominence represents the junction of the third rib cartilage with the sternum. Thus an error may be made in identifying the ribs used as points of reference. By fluoroscopy, the roentgenologist can identify the rib causing the prominence at the angle of Louis and thus provide a precise landmark for the surgeon. It is often difficult for the surgeon to recognize the twelfth rib and to count the ribs in the interscapular area so that the ribs in these regions are not helpful to him as points of reference at operation. There is no exact landmark which can be used for this purpose in the outer part of the chest.

Intercostal Spot. To supply an immovable reference point visible to both the roentgenologist and the surgeon, the *spot method* has been devised: 0.5 cc of a mixture of methylene blue and Lipiodol is injected into the intercostal muscle over the general region of the lesion (see Figs. 14 and 567). The relationship of the underlying lesion to this point of reference is then determined on films made with a cassette tangential to the point of injection. The stained area in the intercostal muscle is visible to the surgeon who uses this spot as a guide to the lesion in the underlying lung. The details of this procedure are discussed more fully in the section on lung abscess.

Neighboring Lesions. It is sometimes necessary to localize a pulmonary lesion in relation to another one whose position is known. This may be required in multiloculated abscesses which have not been completely drained or in inflammatory lesions associated with calcific foci in which the diagnosis of broncholithiasis is suspected. By rotating the patient to the right and to the left, and by shifting the fluoroscopic screen either from side to side or in a vertical direction their relative positions can be determined.

If, after drainage of an empyema or a lung abscess, a residual focus remains, radiopaque packing placed in the drained area can be used as the reference. The packing, usually iodoform gauze, or gauze soaked in Lipiodol, is held in place by plain packing.

Bronchi. The relationship of pulmonary lesions to the bronchi can be determined by bronchography. The fluoroscopic examination will indicate the best position in which films should be made to determine the relative position of the bronchial branches to the pulmonary lesion. In this way, the exact segment of lung which is involved by the disease may be determined despite distortion and displacement caused by fibrosis, atelectasis, a pneumothorax, pleural effusion or the pressure of neighboring masses.

The Bronchoscope. The relationship of a radiopaque foreign body or a mass in the lung to the bronchoscope can be determined by noting the parallax produced when the tube is shifted up and down and from side to side, or when the patient is rotated. Biplane fluoroscopy eliminates the necessity for relying on parallax. It is performed by means of two image intensifiers aligned at right angles to each other.

Injection of Sinuses. In persistently draining sinuses of the chest wall, it is advisable to outline the tract with radiopaque contrast material to determine its extent and direction, to discover communications with poorly draining foci in the lung or pleura, and to demonstrate the presence of a bronchial fistula. A catheter is inserted into the sinus tract and wedged in tightly by packings so that there is no leakage of the contrast material. The procedure is best performed under fluoroscopic vision. After complete filling of the tract, the patient is examined in various positions so that films can be made in those projections which best demonstrate the tract.

Study of Hiccough and Diaphragmatic Spasm. Usually hiccough and other diaphragmatic spasms are associated with an abnormal movement of both leaves of the diaphragm. However, at times, only one leaf of the diaphragm is involved and, in such cases it may be desirable to anesthetize the phrenic nerve to determine whether this allays the spasm. Fluoroscopy is the method by which one can determine the rare instance in which the condition is unilateral and, therefore, amenable to this type of treatment.

Anatomy of the Lungs

The boundaries of the lobes of the lungs and the borders of the bronchopulmonary segments which comprise these lobes, as well as the bronchi that supply them, usually cannot be identified on the ordinary chest film. However, proper interpretation of the shadows caused by pulmonary disease requires a detailed knowledge of the anatomic relationships of these structures to the roentgen image.

Since the original description and naming of the bronchopulmonary segments by Glass, two systems of nomenclature have been adopted by important organizations and are in general use. These are closely enough related so that both may be followed if one of them is known. The first is the one proposed by Jackson and Huber and accepted by the American Association for Thoracic Surgeons. The second is a modification of this nomenclature which was adopted at the International Congress of Otolaryngologists in London in July, 1949. Both systems of nomenclature will be outlined and alternate names in more or less common use will be mentioned in conjunction with them so that the reader can follow the literature.

Various numbered designations of the bronchial branches are used for labeling films and diagrams. Our illustrations are numbered according to the pattern set by Huizinga and Smelt. In some instances letters have been appended to designate important parts of segments.

The Interlobar Fissures. Each lung is divided into an anterior superior and a posterior inferior portion by a *long fissure.* The fissure lies in an oblique plane, perpendicular to the lateral chest wall and the lateral surface of the spine and mediastinum. The plane runs downward and forward, cutting through the posterior surface of the lung at a level varying from the posterior portion of the fourth to the sixth rib. As a rule the upper border of the fissure is higher on the left side than on the right. The lower border extends to the junction of the diaphragm and the anterior chest wall on the right side. On the left, it reaches the diaphragm 2 to 4 cm behind the anterior costophrenic sulcus (Fig. 50). The long fissure is therefore more steeply inclined on the left side.

Because of the obliquity of the fissure, a lesion in the posterior portion of the upper lobe may have only its uppermost portion in contact with the chest wall. Its lower portion, which extends downward and forward, is in contact with the long fissure and is separated from the chest wall by the intervening superior segment of the lower lobe. Obviously, it is necessary to drain an abscess in the posterior segment of the upper lobe through its upper portion where it is in contact

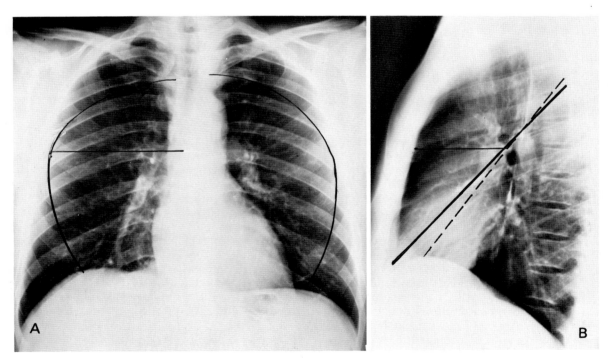

FIG. 50. INTERLOBAR FISSURES

A: Frontal view. The long fissure lies in an oblique plane, coursing downward and forward. The curved lines indicate the outer margin of the long fissures, the horizontal line represents the short fissure. *B*: Lateral view. The solid lines indicate the long and short fissures of the right lung. The long fissure on the left side is represented by the dotted line.

with the chest wall and where adhesions are present (see Fig. 276).

The long fissure is displaced backward when the lower lobe is atelectatic, and it is displaced forward when the upper or middle lobe is shrunken. There is some variation in the position of the normal long fissure so that it may be difficult to determine whether or not it is displaced. If there is any question, an abnormality of the adjoining lobes should be looked for.

The position of the *short fissure* is less variable. It is generally described as lying in a horizontal plane at the level of the anterior portion of the fourth rib. However, more often than not, its plane is not horizontal but slopes downward as it proceeds forward from the root of the lung. The short fissure meets the long fissure in the axilla. The triangular portion of lung delimited by the short fissure above and the long fissure below represents the middle lobe (Figs. 51 and 534).

It is useful to recognize landmarks in the chest wall which are crossed by the fissures so that the

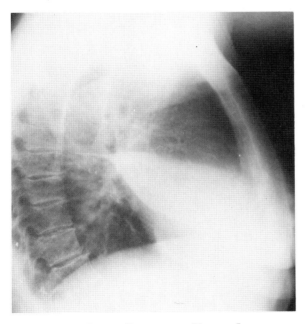

FIG. 51. LOBAR PNEUMONIA, MIDDLE LOBE

In the lateral view, the consolidated middle lobe appears as a triangular shadow with its apex at the root of the lung. The lower border is formed by the lower half of the long fissure while the upper border corresponds to the short fissure. The latter slants slightly downward because of partial atelectasis due to plugging of peripheral bronchi by fibrinous exudate. The streak-like shadow behind the junction of the two fissures represents an anomalous fissure between the superior segment and the rest of the lower lobe. It is thickened by fibrinous exudate.

lobes may be delineated in relation to the surface anatomy and to the anatomy of the chest when the ribs are exposed by the surgeon. In our experience the upper or paravertebral portion of the long fissure has generally been situated at the height of the fourth intercostal space. The outer border of the fissure then proceeds downward and outward across the fifth rib to reach the fifth intercostal space in front of the scapula. In the axillary region, the long fissure crosses the sixth rib at a shallow angle and runs anteriorly almost parallel to this rib to reach the diaphragm just mesial to the sixth costochondral junction.

The short fissure joins the long fissure in the axillary region at about the level of the fifth space or sixth rib on the frontal projection. As the outer border of the short fissure extends mesially, it crosses the fifth rib, the fourth intercostal space and the fourth rib, reaching the mediastinum at the level of the lower border of the anterior portion of the third rib.

Most often the long fissure lies in a flat plane and is projected on the lateral view as a straight line. Occasionally the plane of the fissure is somewhat curved. It then presents as a linear shadow with a slight S-shaped conformation on the left side, and a reverse S shape on the right.

The Bronchial Tree. Although there is agreement as to the anatomy of the bronchi, there is some difference in the terminology applied to the various branches. The nomenclature used here will be that adopted by the International Congress of Otorhinolaryngology (Fig. 52).

TRACHEA AND MAIN BRONCHI. The trachea divides into two major bronchi at about the level of the body of the sixth dorsal vertebra. The tracheal bifurcation is called the carina. From this point the main bronchi course downward and outward. The main bronchus is considered to end at the spur formed by the lower lip of the upper lobe bronchus. The right main bronchus descends at a more vertical angle than the left and is shorter, measuring only about 2.5 cm in length.

RIGHT UPPER LOBE. From its origin, the right upper lobe bronchus runs forward and outward for a distance of about 1 cm. It then trifurcates, one branch going upward, one backward and upward, and a third running in an anterior and slightly downward direction.

The uppermost branch is called the *apical* and pursues a course in the general direction of the apex of the lung which it supplies by several branches.

The second, or *posterior* division, courses behind and somewhat lateral to the apical division. It supplies the posterior part of the upper lobe

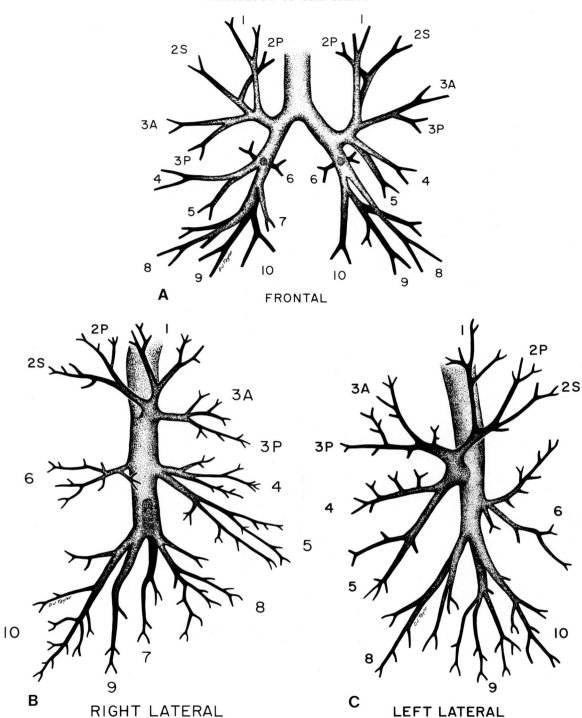

FIG. 52. THE BRONCHI

The bronchial pattern in the two lungs is essentially the same except for three major differences. In the left upper lobe, the apical and posterior divisions arise as a common trunk; the lingular bronchus, which corresponds to the middle lobe bronchus on the right side, arises from the left upper lobe bronchus and there is no medial basal division of the left lower lobe bronchus. Upper lobe: (1) apical division; (2) posterior division, (P) paravertebral branch, (S) subscapular branch; (3) anterior division, (A) axillary branch, (P) pectoral branch. Right middle lobe: (4) lateral division; (5) mesial division. Lingula: (4) superior division; (5) inferior division. Lower lobe: (6) superior division; (7) medial basal division; (8) anterior basal division; (9) lateral basal division; (10) posterior basal division.

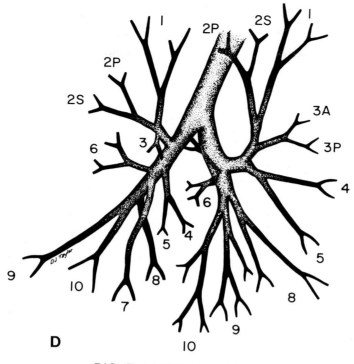

D

RIGHT ANTERIOR OBLIQUE

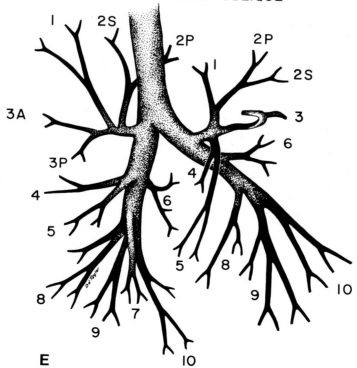

E

LEFT ANTERIOR OBLIQUE

Fig. 52 (*cont.*)

together with most of the mesial surface of this lobe below the apex, and the posterolateral part of the lobe lateral to the vertebral border of the scapula. It also supplies the posterior portion of the lobe abutting on the long fissure. This bronchial division is called the *subapical* by Brock. It divides into two important branches: one which runs medially and backward to supply the paravertebral portion of the right upper lobe, and one which pursues a lateral direction to supply the scapular portion of this lobe. The former branch can best be termed the *paravertebral* branch. The latter, which is spoken of as the *axillary* branch by the British, is better called the *subscapular* because its main distribution is to the region hidden by the scapula and it reaches only a small portion of the posterior axillary region.

The third and final division of the right upper lobe bronchus is the *anterior*. This supplies the entire anterior portion of the right upper lobe from the region beneath the clavicle to the short fissure and also the outer portion of the lobe which is covered by the axilla. The British call the entire anterior division the pectoral, but it appears more reasonable to use the term *pectoral* to designate only the anterior branch of this bronchus which supplies that portion of the lobe covered by the pectoral muscle. The outer branch of the anterior division is directed toward the axilla, and is best termed the *axillary* branch.

The right upper lobe, then, has three main divisions, the apical, the posterior, and the anterior. The posterior divides into the paravertebral and the subscapular branches, and the anterior divides into the pectoral and axillary branches.

LEFT UPPER LOBE. The left main bronchus is longer than the right main bronchus and pursues a more horizontal course. Its total length, from the carina to the lower margin of the left upper lobe orifice, is about 5 cm.

Within 1 cm of its origin, the left upper lobe bronchus gives off a large division from its inferior anterior wall. This supplies the lingular portion of the lobe which lies between the left cardiac border and the lower part of the long fissure. This anterior descending or *lingular* division then divides into two branches, a superior and an inferior. The inferior branch is distributed to the lower, tongue-like portion of the lobe adjacent to the heart, while the superior supplies the upper portion of the lingula.

Beyond the origin of the lingular division, the left upper lobe bronchus divides into an upper and a lower branch. The lower one proceeds anteriorly and is the counterpart of the *anterior division* of the right upper lobe. Like the anterior division of the right upper lobe bronchus, the left anterior segmental bronchus is projected on end, and often appears on the frontal film as a small annular shadow adjacent to a round opacity which represents the corresponding blood vessel (Fig. 33). It also divides into an axillary and a pectoral branch. The upper division supplies the remainder of the left upper lobe. It corresponds to both the apical and posterior branches on the right side and is called the *apical posterior* division. It measures about 1 to 2 cm in length, runs in an upward direction and divides into an ascending, *apical* branch and a *posterior* branch. The posterior divides, as on the right side, into a paravertebral and a subscapular branch. The latter is called the posteroaxillary by the British.

INTERMEDIATE BRONCHUS. Beyond the spur which represents the lower lip of the right upper lobe bronchus is the *intermediate* bronchus, previously known as the stem bronchus. This represents the downward extension of the main bronchus.

MIDDLE LOBE. The intermediate bronchus terminates by dividing into the middle lobe bronchus and the bronchus to the right lower lobe. The middle lobe bronchus runs anteriorly downward and laterally. About 1 cm from its origin it divides into a *lateral* and a *mesial* division. The lateral division supplies the outer and superior portions of the lobe, while the mesial division proceeds downward and forward to supply the mesial, anterior and lower portions of the middle lobe adjacent to the heart.

RIGHT LOWER LOBE. The right lower lobe bronchus, which begins at the lower lip of the middle lobe orifice, proceeds downward and very slightly outward. Immediately at its origin, directly opposite or slightly below the middle lobe orifice, it gives off from its posterior wall a *superior,* or *apical* division which soon divides into several branches. One pursues an upward course to supply the apical portion of the lobe, and the lower branch proceeds downward and posteriorly to supply that portion of the lung below the apex of the lobe. The British refer to the latter as the *subapical* branch. Not infrequently this arises as a separate branch from the posterior surface of the lower lobe bronchus about 1 cm below the origin of the apical branch. A third branch of the superior division courses laterally and posteriorly to supply the outer portion of the superior segment.

Within a centimeter below the origin of the superior division, a branch arises from the mesial wall of the lower lobe bronchus and proceeds downward toward the mesial portion of the diaphragm, giving off branches to supply the mesial surface of the lobe. This has been called the *cardiac* division. However, the term *medial basal* is preferable because the portion of lung that it supplies is not entirely adjacent to the heart.

About 1.5 cm below the origin of the medial division the right lower lobe bronchus divides into three branches which supply the lower or *basal* part of the lobe. These are the anterior basal, the lateral basal and posterior basal divisions. The *anterior basal* bronchus proceeds downward, outward and forward to supply the anterior surface of the lower lobe immediately behind the middle lobe, the lateral surface of the lower lobe and the anterolateral portion of its diaphragmatic surface. The *lateral basal* bronchus proceeds in a more posterior direction. It supplies the posterolateral portion of the lobe and the corresponding portion of the base. The *posterior basal* division, sometimes called the paravertebral division of the lower lobe, runs directly downward and backward. It supplies the lower part of the lobe adjacent to the spine and the mesial portion of its posterior surface, together with the corresponding portion of the basal surface of the lung.

LEFT LOWER LOBE. The left lower lobe bronchi are similar to those of the right lower lobe except that there is usually no separate medial basal division. According to Boyden, the left lower lobe bronchus ends in a bifurcation. This occurs about 2 cm below the origin of the superior segmental division. One of the two radicles divides into an anterior basal division and a medial basal division as on the right side. This radicle has been termed the *anterior medial basal* by Jackson and Huber (American Association of Thoracic Surgeons). The other radicle divides into the *lateral* and *posterior basal* divisions.

TERMINOLOGY OF BROCK. For the convenience of those who wish to refer to the classical exposition of Brock on the anatomy of the bronchial tree, the following comparison of nomenclature will prove useful. In the right upper lobe, the posterior division is termed the *subapical* and the anterior division is called the *pectoral*. The branches on the left side have the same terminology as on the right. The apical and the subapical divisions are considered to arise from a common stem and the pectoral and lingular divisions by separate stems. The middle lobe bronchus divides into the lateral and medial divisions as mentioned above. The only difference in the terminology in the left lower lobe is the appellation of *middle basal* for the lateral basal division. Brock divides the apical division into three con-

stant branches, a *superior* which runs upward, a *paravertebral* which runs downward and slightly medially, and an *axillary* branch which runs downward and laterally. The terminology of the right lower lobe is the same, but the medial branch is called the *cardiac* bronchus.

NUMERICAL SYSTEMS. For labeling diagrams, photographs and films, numerical designations have been applied to the segmental bronchi. While there has been no uniform adoption of these numbers, those used in our illustrations are the ones most frequently applied. The numbers run from 1 to 10, and correspond to the main divisions on each side, proceeding from above downward. The apical, posterior and anterior branches of both upper lobes are labeled 1, 2 and 3 respectively, and the lateral and mesial divisions of the right middle lobe bronchus are labeled 4 and 5, as are the superior and inferior branches to the lingular segment of the left upper lobe. The superior, medial, anterobasal, laterobasal and posterobasal divisions of the lower lobes are labeled 6, 7, 8, 9 and 10, in that order. In addition to these numbers we have appended letters to denote certain important subsegmental branches. The subdivisions of the posterior branch of the right upper lobe have been labeled 2S and 2P to denote the subscapular and the paravertebral branches. The axillary and pectoral branches of the anterior segmental division of each upper lobe have been labeled 3A and 3P. The branches of the superior segment of each lower lobe are designated as 6A, 6P and 6L to denote the branches which supply the apical, paravertebral and lateral portions of this segment. These subdivisions are made because of the importance of the subsegments in cases of abscess of the lung. Where there is a subapical division it is called 6S.

Bronchopulmonary Segments. The concept of the bronchopulmonary segment, originated by Glass, together with the development of a terminology for these segments, has proved most useful to the clinician, thoracic surgeon, and endoscopist, as well as to the radiologist. It is necessary for the radiologist to be thoroughly acquainted with the bronchopulmonary segments so that he can designate them by name in referring to the distribution of lesions seen on the roentgen films.

The bronchopulmonary segment is that portion of the lobe of a lung which is supplied by a major branch of one of the lobar bronchi. This bronchial division is accompanied by a corresponding branch of the pulmonary artery and pulmonary vein. Thus, each of the segments has its own blood and air supply, independent of the adjacent segments. The individual segment therefore, constitutes a functional as well as an anatomic unit.

The boundaries of the segments are not traversed by bronchi or blood vessels of any consequential size. The shape of the bronchopulmonary segment is either conical or pyramidal with the apex toward the root of the lobe where its bronchus originates. From this point the bronchial branches spread out to the base of the segment which is situated in the periphery of the lobe.

The bronchopulmonary segments are named in accordance with the bronchi that supply them. The latter have been described and their nomenclature has been discussed. However, it is well to consider the segments themselves with reference to their topographic relationships, particularly from the viewpoint of their position on the roentgen film in the various projections (Fig. 53).

RIGHT UPPER LOBE. The right upper lobe is made up of three segments, the apical, the posterior, and the anterior.

The *apical* segment extends from the extreme apex to the level of the first intercostal space anteriorly. Its posterior surface extends from the apex to about the level of the third dorsal vertebra.

The *posterior* segment occupies the posterior half of the upper lobe immediately below the apical segment. Mesially it is bounded by the spine, and laterally it extends along the posterior outer surface of the upper lobe, to about the midlateral line. Its upper posterior surface is in

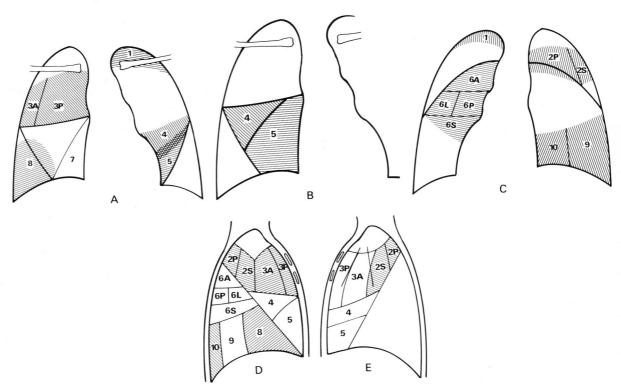

FIG. 53. BRONCHOPULMONARY SEGMENTS

Numerical terminology. *Upper lobe*: apical segment (1); posterior segment, paravertebral subsegment (2P), scapular subsegment (2S); anterior segment, pectoral subsegment (3P), axillary subsegment (3A); lingula of left upper lobe, superior lingular segment (4), inferior lingular segment (5). *Middle lobe*: lateral segment (4), mesial segment (5). *Lower lobe*: superior segment, apical subsegment (6A), paravertebral subsegment (6P), lateral subsegment (6L), subapical subsegment (6S); mesial segment of right lower lobe (7); anterior basal segment (8); lateral basal segment (9); posterior basal segment (10). *A*: segments with anterior representation. The mesial segment of the right lower lobe (7) is in the middle of the chest. It does not reach the anterior or posterior surface of the lung. The upper part of the anterior basal segment (8) extends behind the middle lobe. The segments of the lingula overlap each other in the frontal view. The middle lobe segments are omitted for clarity. *B*: Segments of the middle lobe. *C*: Segments having a posterior representation. *D*: Lateral view of segments of the right lung. The medial segment of the lower lobe is not indicated. Its position is shown on Fig. 54*B*. *E*: Lateral view of segments of left lung. The two oblique lines over the upper lobe indicate the projection of the anterior and posterior borders of the axilla with the patient's arms extended over the head.

contact with the chest wall, high in the interscapular region. The parietal representation here is quite small. Below this, it faces on the upper part of the long fissure. As the fissure slopes downward and forward, this part of the posterior segment is separated from the chest wall by the intervening apex of the lower lobe (see Figs. 276 and 282).

More laterally, the posterior surface of the posterior segment abuts on the chest wall as far forward as the middle of the lateral surface of the lobe (posterior axillary line). It is covered by the scapula and the latissimus dorsi muscle. This portion of the posterior segment is usually referred to as the axillary subsegment. Since the axilla lies almost entirely anterior to the outer border of the posterior segment (Fig. 53E), this is not an accurate term. It is better, therefore, to call the outer part of the posterior segment the *scapular* or *subscapular* portion. The mesial portion of the posterior segment may well be termed the *paravertebral* portion, since it lies adjacent to the bodies of the vertebrae as well as the chest wall.

In the frontal view, the posterior segment of the right upper lobe extends from the spine to the lateral border of the chest. Its upper margin is situated below the clavicle. The segment is bounded below by a curved line, sloping downward and outward from the level of the fourth space or fifth rib near the spine to about the level of the anterior part of the third rib in the outer part of the chest. On the lateral view, the posterior border extends upward from the long fissure for a distance of 2 to 4 cm to reach the posterior portion of the lower border of the apical segment. The lower border extends anteriorly along the long fissure and the short fissure to the midlateral line of the chest which is situated near the posterior border of the axilla. The anterior border extends upward from this point to the lower limit of the apical segment. On the right anterior oblique view the subscapular part of the posterior segment is in approximation with the chest wall over a distance of 5 to 6 cm.

The anterior segment makes up the rest of the upper lobe. It is bounded below by the short fissure at the level of the fourth rib on the frontal view, and above by the first intercostal space (see Figs. 226 and 239). It extends from the sternum to the lateral border of the chest. On the lateral view it is roughly quadrilateral in shape, being bounded anteriorly by the sternum, posteriorly by the posterior segment which meets it in the midlateral line, below by the short fissure, and above by the lower border of the apical segment. On the left anterior oblique view the

axillary portion of the anterior segment is in approximation to the chest wall.

MIDDLE LOBE. The middle lobe is bounded above by the short fissure at the height of the fourth rib anteriorly. The lower border is oblique and corresponds to the lower part of the long fissure. It extends upward and outward from the level of the sixth costochondral junction at the dome of the diaphragm to about the level of the fourth space or fifth rib in the axillary portion of the chest. The mesial border of the middle lobe corresponds to the right border of the heart from the level of the third space or fourth rib to the diaphragm (Fig. 50).

The lateral and upper portions of the lobe are made up of the *lateral* segment, and its lower mesial portion comprises the *medial* segment. On the lateral view, the lateral or axillary segment of the middle lobe is triangular in shape and is situated in the angle of the confluence of the long and short fissures, with a longer representation on the short, than on the long fissure. The medial segment is projected in triangular contour on the lateral view, occupying the area anterior to and below the lateral segment.

RIGHT LOWER LOBE. This lobe is divided into an upper portion comprising the superior segment, and a lower portion made up by the basal segments (see Fig. 237). The superior segment of the lower lobe is represented on both the frontal and lateral views as a triangular area enclosed in the angle made by the long fissure and the spine in the interscapular region (see Fig. 134). When there is a *subapical* segment, it occupies the area immediately beneath this, adjacent to the spine, extending down to the ninth rib or ninth intercostal space posteriorly (see Fig. 284).

The *anterior basal* segment consists of a triangular portion of lung, well outlined on the lateral view immediately behind the lower part of the long fissure. Its anterior surface faces the middle lobe and its lower surface is in contact with the diaphragm. On the frontal view, it extends below and lateral to the lower border of the middle lobe to the base of the costophrenic sinus.

The *lateral basal* segment is situated directly behind the anterior basal segment in the outer portion of the lower lobe, above the diaphragm. On the frontal view, its outer margin does not quite reach the lateral border of the chest. However, on the right anterior oblique projection it does abut on the chest wall. Its posterior border touches the posterior chest wall on the lateral view.

The *posterior basal* segment occupies the inferior posterior part of the lower lobe, mesial to the lateral basal segment. It extends from this segment to the spine and is largely overlapped by the lateral basal segment on the lateral view.

The *medial basal* or *cardiac* segment is situated adjacent to the posterior mediastinum and is conical in shape. On the lateral view it is projected as a triangle with its apex at the root of the lower lobe and its base at the diaphragm. Its posterior border extends downward and backward from the lung root just in front of the anterior border of the bodies of the vertebrae, and its anterior border is situated a short distance in front of the posterior margin of the heart. On the frontal view it is projected as a right angle triangle. The vertical part of the triangle is situated along the border of the spine and the horizontal portion over the mesial part of the diaphragm. Its lateral border, which is the hypotenuse of the triangle, runs downward and outward from the root of the lower lobe to a point about one-third the distance from the right cardiac border to the lateral chest wall. The base of the segment, adjacent to the diaphragm, is semicircular in shape with the flat border against the mediastinum (Fig. 54). The outer surface is at a distance from the chest wall, separated from it by the other basal segments.

LEFT UPPER LOBE. Because the apical and posterior segments of this lobe are supplied by a common bronchial stem, they are considered as a single unit, the *apicoposterior* segment. Its projection on the film is roughly the same as that of the two corresponding segments on the right side. The *anterior* segment of the left upper lobe is similar in distribution to that of the right upper lobe (Fig. 20).

The location and shape of the *lingular* division of the left upper lobe is similar to the middle lobe of the right lung (Fig. 53A) except that its mesial portion is abbreviated because of the space occupied by the heart. The lingular division is quite large and is divided into *superior* and *inferior* segments. The superior lingular segment is the larger of the two and is bounded above by the anterior segment of the upper lobe and below by the inferior lingular segment. The latter extends downward and makes contact with the diaphragm. In the lateral view, the lower border of the lingula is continuous with the anteriormost 2 to 3 cm of the diaphragm. Behind and laterally, the lingula is bounded by the long fissure.

LEFT LOWER LOBE. The distribution and position of the segments of the left lower lobe are similar to that of the right (Figs. 13, 69, 229 and 270). Commonly, the mesial basal segment is missing on the left side. Most of the lung normally comprising this segment is usually incorporated into the anterior basal segment. Sometimes, however, it is represented by an anterior extension of the posterior basal segment and a mesial extension of the lateral basal segment.

IMPORTANCE OF THE SEGMENTS. Because the bronchopulmonary segments and subsegments represent anatomic and physiologic units of the

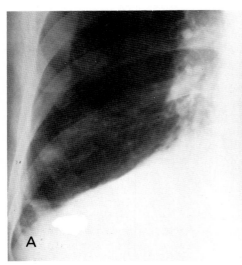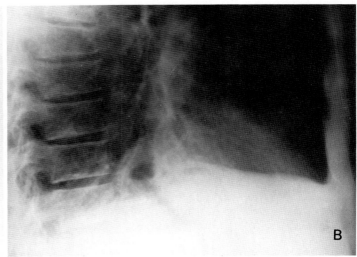

FIG. 54. LUNG ABSCESS, MESIAL BASAL SEGMENT RIGHT LOWER LOBE

A: Frontal projection. The cardiophrenic angle is obliterated by a dense shadow in the mesial segment of the right lower lobe. There is a faint infiltration in the lung just above it. Horizontal streaks in the costophrenic sulcus represent atelectatic foci. *B*: Lateral projection. In this view, the density in the mesial basal segment is seen to be caused by an abscess containing air and fluid. The abscess lies immediately above the diaphragm and is projected over the posterior mediastinum and the posterior border of the heart. The air-fluid level was completely obscured on the frontal film by the shadow of the infiltrated lung anterior to the abscess.

lobe, they are not only of academic interest but are extremely important from the clinical standpoint. The pathogenesis of many pulmonary diseases is intimately related with involvement of the segmental bronchi. In these conditions, such as suppurative bronchopneumonia, bronchiectasis, lung abscess, foreign bodies, and bronchial strictures and neoplasms, the lesions are of segmental distribution.

Obviously, the surgeon must have a comprehensive understanding of the segmental anatomy because his operations are often localized to one of them. The bronchoscopist must be able to correlate the pulmonary segments with their corresponding bronchi in order to perform an adequate and accurate examination. The same applies to the pathologist if he is to demonstrate the bronchial disease underlying pulmonary lesions. To the clinician who has the responsibility for the final diagnosis and the choice of treatment, a thorough knowledge of the pulmonary segments and their bronchi is essential for understanding the disease and for discussion with other specialists concerned with the case.

Among all of these, the radiologist occupies a key position because he can provide this information concerning the lungs and bronchi that is required by the other specialists. In many instances, this knowledge is of considerable help in determining the correct diagnosis because certain diseases have a marked predilection for specific segments. In addition, it is necessary for him to transmit his judgment as to the anatomic distribution of the disease in a precise manner to the endoscopist, surgeon, pathologist and clinician. This is best done in terms of the bronchopulmonary segments whose exact location and terminology should be known by all concerned.

General Roentgen Pathology: The Roentgenologic Manifestations of Single Pathologic Processes

Diseases consist of a combination of pathologic changes involving one or more organs and practically always affecting more than one tissue. Knowledge of a disease from a clinical and diagnostic standpoint presupposes an understanding of the component pathologic changes in the tissues and organs and the sequence in which these changes occur. This knowledge is also basic for the roentgenologic recognition of diseases of the chest, as well as for the discovery of their complications. The pathologic processes are reflected roentgenologically by abnormal shadows or altered function. The shadows vary in size, shape, density, demarcation, distribution, and homogeneity or lack of homogeneity, according to the nature of the pathologic process. Disturbances of the mechanics of respiration and circulation cause alterations in the movement of the thoracic structures of the chest wall, diaphragm, the mediastinum, the bronchi and blood vessels.

Before embarking on a description of the roentgenologic changes which characterize the specific diseases, it is necessary to have a thorough understanding of the roentgenologic changes produced by each of the individual pathologic processes whose combination forms the disease in question. For example, in the case of a bronchial neoplasm, the chest films may show the shadow of the neoplasm itself, the infiltration of the lung by the spreading growth, enlarged lymph nodes involved by metastases, a pleural effusion, or the shadows of changes secondary to the tumor, such as atelectasis, emphysema, infection, and cavitation. All the shadows related to these individual pathologic changes should be evaluated in arriving at a diagnosis.

This section will consist of a description of the manifestations of each pathologic change that can be recognized on the roentgen film. The various combinations of shadows and abnormalities due to individual diseases will be discussed in the section on Regional Roentgen Pathology (Part III), where the diseases are considered as whole entities.

It should be stated at the outset that different individual pathologic changes can produce similar shadows so that it may not be possible to establish a specific diagnosis from the appearance of a single lesion. However, in some instances, when all of the pathologic changes are considered in relation to each other, an accurate roentgen diagnosis can be made. In other cases, the evolution of changes in the shadows over a period of time or the occurrence of new shadows or the disappearance of old ones may yield information which will indicate a definitive diagnosis.

THE NORMAL CHEST

Films of the chest vary as much as the individuals whose chests are represented. Before one can begin to interpret pathologic conditions from chest films, it is essential to have a thorough appreciation of the limits of the normal roentgen image. Even then, the possible variations in the appearance of the thoracic structures in normal subjects is so great that drawing the line between the normal and abnormal will often tax the most experienced radiologist.

Certain minor pathologic changes are considered within the range of normal. Few of us go through life without showing the marks of wear and tear that take place through the years. Moreover, all of us are exposed to pathogenic influences which leave their traces, even though they do not produce serious disease. These are the changes which must be considered normal if we are to be practical in our interpretation of disease from the roentgen film.

Method of Examination of the Film. It is advisable for the beginner to train himself to examine the chest film in a systematic fashion. First, it is necessary to evaluate the quality of the film so that allowances can be made for variations in technique. It is then best to focus attention on the heart and mediastinum because abnormalities in these structures will influence the interpretation of the shadows within the lungs. The size, shape and position of the heart and aorta are observed. The course of the trachea is noted and the borders of the mediastinum are then scanned, carefully differentiating them from the overlying bony structures. Next, the lungs are inspected, first above and then below the clavicles, noting the general tone of the pulmonary field, the variations in tone within each lung, and comparing the overall density of one side with the other. The size, shape, and position of the lung roots are carefully observed, as well as the pulmonary markings which fan out from the roots and represent chiefly the blood vessels and their branches within the lung. Distortions of the vascular shadows are searched for, as well as abnormal densities between and overlying them.

In this manner, each lung is thoroughly inspected from apex to base, taking care not to omit those areas covered by the ribs or scapulae. The region of the left lower lobe, which can be seen through the shadow of the heart on a properly exposed frontal film, must not be neglected. The curve of the diaphragm on each side is followed from the region of the costophrenic sinus to the spine. Its height is noted in relation to the anterior and posterior portion of the ribs. At this time, it is well to note the subdiaphragmatic region, looking for air or calcifications on the right side in the position normally occupied by the liver, and observing the left side for overdistention of the stomach or colon by gas, irregularities of the stomach bubble and enlargement of the spleen.

Finally, the structures of the chest wall are examined. The clavicles are scanned from one end to the other. The relation of the mesial margins of the clavicles to the midline is used to evaluate whether the film represents a true frontal projection or if the patient was rotated, however slightly. A vertical line drawn through the shadows of the vertebral spines is considered to represent the midline, assuming there is no scoliosis. If the spine is curved, the trachea is used to determine the midline. The general course of the ribs is noted, paying particular attention to the inclination of the anterior and posterior portions of the ribs, and whether or not the two sides of the chest are symmetrical. The widths of corresponding intercostal spaces on the two sides are compared and then each rib is examined from the spine to the costochondral junction. Each scapula and the head of each humerus is inspected and as much of the cervical and thoracic spine as can be seen. Lastly, the soft tissues of the neck and chest are examined.

If a systematic approach such as this is used time after time, the allowable normal variation in the appearance of the different structures will become evident with increasing experience. At the same time, few changes of importance will be overlooked. Eventually, such familiarity with the normal structures is acquired that a glance at a film suffices to detect an abnormality as readily as one notes a change in a familiar room. Those who intend to make a practice of interpreting chest films are advised, after a while, to train themselves to view the film as a whole rather than one part at a time. Abnormalities eventually obtrude themselves on the observer so that, strange to say, one may detect with one glance at the entire film what may be missed by a minute inspection of its parts. It must be realized that this can be accomplished only after long practice and should not be attempted by the beginner.

It is necessary to have a thorough knowledge of the appearance of the normal chest in the lateral and oblique views as well as the frontal, if one is to have a proper basis for detecting the presence of disease and to determine its location.

Frontal View. The film made in the postero-anterior direction represents a silhouette of the maximal breadth of the chest, containing within it a summation of the shadows of all of the structures of the chest in the coronal planes (Fig. 55). In the midportion is the shadow of the mediastinal structures separating the lungs. The latter are bounded laterally and above by the ribs, and below by each leaf of the diaphragm. Outside the ribs are the shoulder girdles and the

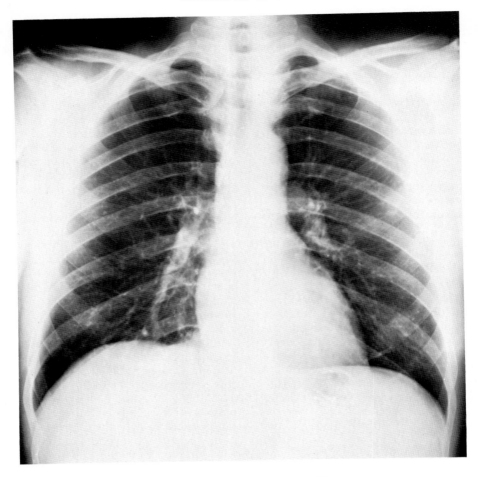

FIG. 55. NORMAL CHEST: FRONTAL VIEW

soft tissues of the chest wall. Variations in the thickness of the anterior and posterior chest wall modify the appearance of the intrathoracic structures in this view.

MEDIASTINUM. The mediastinum is of variable width. Generally speaking, its borders are limited by definitely recognizable structures. On the right these are the superior vena cava, the ascending aorta and the right border of the heart; on the left, the aortic knob, the root of the pulmonary artery and the left side of the heart. The shadow of the sternum overlies the structures above the aortic knob. Projecting from the middle of each lateral border of the mediastinum are the shadows of the pulmonary vessels, the bronchi and the hilar lymph nodes.

The borders of the mediastinum correspond to the mediastinal pleura. When the latter is thickened, it obliterates the angles between the structures that form the boundary of the mediastinum. Such ironing out of the contours is abnor-

mal (see Fig. 75). The angles between the heart and the diaphragm should be sharp.

Within the mediastinum the trachea is usually visible as a longitudinal lucent strip bounded on each side by a fine linear stripe formed by the tracheal wall. The tracheal air column should be straight and practically in the midline, although moderate deviation to the right in older persons may be normal. The tracheal bifurcation is situated at approximately the level of the sixth dorsal vertebra. The two main bronchi form an angle of about 75 degrees. The right bronchus extends more directly downward than the left. The course of each of the bronchi should be relatively straight and uniform. Distortions of the main bronchi indicate pathologic processes which may be of great clinical significance.

LUNGS. On either side of the mediastinum are the darker areas occupied by the lungs. These are partly obscured by the shadows of the overlying ribs. However, on films made with proper exposure, the lungs can be seen through the ribs in sufficient detail for the detection of pulmonary abnormalities.

The hilum of each lung is represented by the shadows of the main pulmonary blood vessels, the arteries and the veins, together with the much more delicate shadows of the bronchi, the lymph nodes and connective tissue in this region. In the main, root shadows are due to blood vessels. The branches of the main pulmonary vessels radiate outward from the hilum and continue to spread, as they divide in their course, to the periphery of the lung.

It is most difficult to differentiate between the pulmonary arteries and veins on conventional films except in the case of the vessels supplying the basal segments of the lower lobes. The course of the veins of these segments is directed toward the left atrium, below the position of the pulmonary arteries at the root of the lung. In general, the veins in the upper lobes are situated lateral to their accompanying arteries, and may sometimes be recognized as structures which lie parallel to the pulmonary artery branches. These relationships are more clearly visualized on tomograms. The pattern of the blood vessels is well delineated on sections made in the lateral view. Study of the blood vessels in these sections may be helpful in determining the boundaries of the lobes when the fissures are not visible.

Where the shadows of the blood vessels are projected perpendicular to the film (parallel to the rays), the vessels appear as circular, homogeneous shadows. They are largest at the root of the lung and are of lesser size in the periphery where the branches are smaller. The shadows may be quite dense and are often confused with calcified lymph nodes or calcific deposits within the lungs (Fig. 33). However, calcified lymph nodes are practically always irregular in outline and of uneven density because of the irregular deposition of calcium within them. The shadows of the blood vessels are cast not only by the vessel walls but also by the blood within them. The shadow of the cylindrical column of blood coursing perpendicular to the film is round, sharply outlined and homogeneous.

Near the root of the upper lobe a small, sharply outlined, perfectly round, annular shadow is often seen adjacent to a smaller circular but solid shadow of a branch of the pulmonary artery. The hollow circle represents the anterior segmental bronchus of the upper lobe, seen on end (Fig. 33).

Normally, the shadows of the blood vessels and bronchi are most dense and close together at the hilum, and in the mesial third of the lungs where they extend almost to the apex and to the

base. They are usually not prominent in the lateral third of the chest.

The curved branches of the vessels are sometimes projected so that their shadows cross each other in such a manner as to simulate a ring-like cavity. Before deciding that an annular shadow represents a cavity, it is wise to examine its borders carefully to determine whether they form a continuous margin, and whether the annular shadow can possibly represent the outlines of overlapping blood vessels. If there is any doubt, films should be made in a partial oblique position. Overlapping blood vessels will now be separated, while a cavity will still cast a complete annular shadow.

Films made with proper exposure disclose the branching pulmonary vessels through the shadow of the heart. These pursue a regular downward and outward course, spreading apart gradually as they extend to the diaphragm. An irregularity in the density of the cardiac shadow, obscuration of the vessels, or alteration in their course, indicates an abnormality in the left lower lobe (see Fig. 69).

The position of the lung roots varies somewhat in different individuals. Generally, the right root is situated at about the level of the upper border of the anterior portion of the third rib and the seventh posterior intercostal space. The left is somewhat higher. Any displacement of the lung root should be noted carefully as it may be extremely significant (see Fig. 80).

DIAPHRAGM. The leaves of the diaphragm are depicted as curved structures. They extend outward from the base of the cardiac shadow and, after a short horizontal course, curve downward over the liver on the right side and the stomach and spleen on the left. Here they form the costophrenic sinuses as their shadows join those of the lower outer boundaries of the chest wall at an acute angle. The diaphragmatic shadow makes an acute angle with that of the heart during expiration.

The height of the diaphragm varies in accordance with the general contour of the chest. In the broad, sthenic individual and in obese persons it is situated higher than in the patient with a long narrow chest. The diaphragm is 0.5 to 1.5 cm higher on the right side than on the left. The mesial border of the right leaf of the diaphragm usually joins the cardiac shadow at the level of the fifth intercostal space and on the left side at the level of the sixth costal cartilage. The dome of the diaphragm on the right side usually corresponds to the tenth intercostal space near the spine and the lower border of the tenth rib more laterally. On the left side the outer portion of the diaphragm is usually situated at the height of the tenth intercostal space and its mesial portion crosses the eleventh rib near the spine.

SOFT TISSUES. The soft tissues cast a homogeneous shadow outside of the rib cage. The intensity of the shadow depends on the factors used in making the roentgen exposure.

In the female, the rounded outline of the outer border of the breast is usually seen lateral to the ribs. The breast casts a rather faint shadow over the lower outer portion of the lung, most dense in the periphery, gradually fading out mesially. A round, homogeneous density, about 1 cm in diameter, representing the nipple, is occasionally seen within the breast shadow (see Fig. 525). When the breast is small and its lower border poorly demarcated, the shadow of the nipple can be easily mistaken for an intrapulmonary lesion.

In the young female, whose breast is not completely developed, the organ casts an indistinct shadow. This does not extend beyond the chest wall. On films made with low voltage or with insufficient exposure, the density may be mistaken for a lesion in the lung (Fig. 4). However, the presence of a similar shadow on the other side should suggest that it represents the breast. This may be proved by manipulating the breast during fluoroscopy.

More difficulty is encountered when the shadow is seen only on one side. This occurs occasionally in males who are obese or whose breasts are overdeveloped. If the patient presses one side of the chest more forcefully against the cassette, the flattening of the breast tends to eliminate the shadow on that side, and the faint shadow of the breast on the opposite side then simulates a lesion in the lung. The effect of pressure against the screen can be strikingly demonstrated during fluoroscopy. Applying pressure against even a rather large breast will tend to eliminate its shadow.

The male nipple can cast a shadow several millimeters is diameter, so sharply demarcated that it mimics a nodule in the lung. The nipple is seen on the film only when it is of the protuberant type. Here again, pressure against the screen on one side may flatten out one nipple so that a small, well-demarcated, round density is seen on only one side. The possibility of a nipple shadow should be considered whenever a small round density is seen at the level of the fourth or fifth space near the outer part of the chest. If a similar density is seen in exactly the same position on the opposite side, one may be quite certain that this is the case. If a nodule is seen on only one side, it is necessary to fluoroscope the patient or repeat the x-ray examination with

a metallic marker about the nipple to determine whether or not this structure is responsible for the shadow (see Fig. 148).

The anterior axillary fold often casts a curvilinear shadow running obliquely downward and inward over the outer part of the pulmonary field. This is continuous with the shadow of the arm (see Fig. 144). Within it there may be a faint, homogeneous density cast by the pectoral muscle.

The shadow of the sternomastoid muscle can often be seen at the root of the neck (see Fig. 172). Its lower portion overlies and may partially obscure the apex of the lung. It can be recognized by its straight, vertical borders. The skin over the clavicle often produces a faint shadow which has a straight, sharply outlined, horizontal border, a few millimeters above the bone. Usually, a triangular area of lucency is seen above the calvicle, demarcated by the muscles in the supraclavicular region. The areas on the two sides are more or less symmetrical. If either is absent or appears irregular in comparison with the opposite one, the presence of a mass in the supraclavicular region should be suspected (see Fig. 407).

Lateral View. The lateral view of the chest shows a summation of the shadows of both lungs (Fig. 56). If the patient is properly positioned, an exact profile of the sternum is obtained and the synchondrosis between the manubrium and the body of the sternum is clearly visualized.

The cardiac shadow and the shadow of the ascending aorta are continuous with each other. The long axes of their shadows are directed obliquely downward and forward and they extend from the middle of the upper chest to the anterior portion of the diaphragm. Between the heart and the underside of the aortic arch is a dense area which often appears rounded, and from which blood vessels appear to radiate in all directions. This shadow represents the lung root and is made up largely by the pulmonary artery above and the pulmonary veins below.

Anterior to the shadows of the heart and the ascending aorta, and behind the sternum, is a radiolucent area, the *retrosternal space*. This includes the anterior mediastinum and the anterior portions of the upper lobes and middle lobe. A strip of radiolucency ascending vertically in the middle mediastinum from above the lung root to the neck represents the air-filled trachea. The left upper lobe bronchus is often viewed on end and casts a round, lucent shadow within the lower end of the tracheal air column near the lung root.

The *retrocardiac space* lies behind the heart and below the lung root, extending backward to

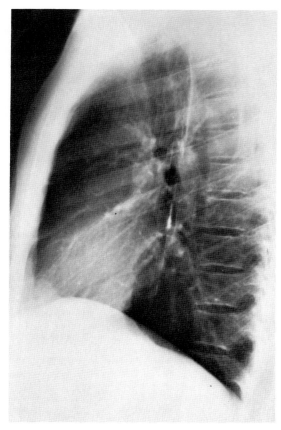

FIG. 56. NORMAL CHEST: LEFT LATERAL VIEW

the anterior borders of the vertebrae. This is usually quite lucent, although the descending aorta may cast a broad, vertical strip of faint density in front of the vertebral column. The pulmonary veins, as they enter the left atrium, cause a bulge on the posterior border of the cardiac shadow extending into the retrocardiac space. Behind and below this bulge a faint density with poorly outlined, irregular borders may be seen. This is caused by a summation of the shadows of the aorta and the arteries and veins near the roots of the lower lobes. The resulting shadow may be fairly dense and is easily mistaken for a pathologic process.

Behind the retrocardiac space, the vertebrae are seen in profile. The density of their shadows varies with the type of exposure and the thickness of the patient, and is modified by the air in the lungs which extends into the thoracic gutters on either side of the spine. The vertebrae appear more dense in the upper portion of the chest down to the angles of the scapulae because of the shadows of these bones and the heavy musculature in this region. Below this level, the bodies of the vertebrae appear less dense down to the diaphragm.

An increase in the density of one or more of the vertebral bodies may be caused by any lesion projected over the spine on the lateral view of the chest as well as by disease of the spine itself. A significant difference in the density of adjacent vertebral bodies requires careful investigation if an important lesion is not to be overlooked (see Fig. 91).

Behind the borders of the vertebrae are the pedicles which are continuous with the posterior parts of the ribs. The posterior border of the chest is outlined by these portions of the ribs, which extend for a variable distance behind the posterior borders of the vertebral bodies. The entire pulmonary field is crossed by the ribs of both sides of the chest. These extend downward and forward and cause oblique, sharply margin-ated, strip-like densities. The ribs that are in contact with the film appear denser and narrower and with more sharply outlined borders than do the ribs on the side facing the roentgen tube.

The posterior border of the lungs is bounded by the posterior part of the rib cage. Since the side of the chest that is farthest from the film is enlarged because of the divergence of the rays, the lung on that side extends beyond the posterior ribs on the side which is in contact with the film (Fig. 57).

The diaphragm arches slightly upward from the anterior costophrenic sinus to the high point of its dome at the posterior border of the heart. It then slopes sharply downward and backward to make an acute angle with the posterior ribs at the base of the chest, thus forming a deep posterior costophrenic sinus which is situated at a lower level than the anterior one.

The normal interlobar fissures are occasionally represented by thin, fine lines which are produced by the subpleural connective tissue. These lines are accentuated if there are pleural adhesions within the fissures, if the subpleural connective tissues are thickened, or if the fissures contain a small amount of fluid.

The long fissure extends from the upper posterior chest at about the level of the fifth dorsal vertebra, downward and forward to the general region of the anterior costophrenic sinus. The short fissure extends forward to the sternum from a point on the long fissure where the latter crosses the lung root. The short fissure usually slopes slightly downward and forward from this point (Fig. 50B).

Because the lateral film is made with the x-ray tube higher than the diaphragm, the leaf of this organ closest to the film is projected above the one on the opposite side (Fig. 58). If the film is

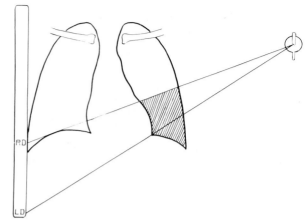

Fig. 58. Projection of the Heart over the Liver in
Right Lateral View

In the right lateral view the right leaf of the diaphragm is
projected higher than the left. Practically the entire right
lung is clearly exposed while the lower part of the left lung
and heart are projected beneath the right diaphragm. The
crossing of the shadow of the liver and the heart produces an
area of greater density which is delineated posteriorly by the
posterior border of the heart and anteriorly by the diaphragm, and may simulate an interlobar effusion (see Fig.
59). This shadow is more prominent when the tube is high.

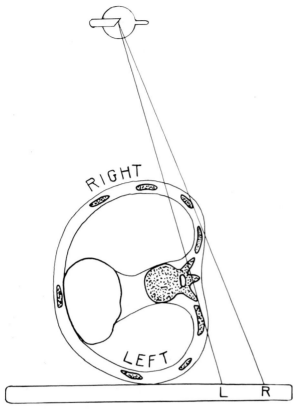

Fig. 57. Projection of Posterior Ribs on the Lateral
View.

The patient is depicted in cross section, viewed from
above, with the left side of the chest against the film (left
lateral view), and the tube centered. The right posterior ribs,
which are at a distance from the screen, are projected lateral
to those on the left, which are closer to the screen. The
posterior boundary of the thorax on the lateral view, corresponds to the side away from the film.

made with the *right* side of the body against the
cassette, the right diaphragm is at a higher level
and the region beneath it, occupied by the liver,
appears homogeneously dense. The superimposition of this subdiaphragmatic shadow on the
cardiac silhouette often produces a dense, fusiform shadow. The long axis of this shadow is
oriented in line with the long fissure. Its supe-
roanterior border is formed by the sharp, curved
margin of the diaphragm and its posterior border
corresponds to the lower posterior contour of the
heart. The shadow is sometimes confusing because its shape and position suggest an interlobar
effusion (Fig. 59). It is seen only on the right
lateral projection.

In the *left* lateral view, which is made with the
left side of the chest against the film, the left leaf
of the diaphragm is situated at a higher level

then the right. Beneath it there may be radiolucent areas caused by gas in the stomach and/or
splenic flexure. The leaf of the diaphragm is then
seen as a sharp, curvilinear density outlined by
the bowel gas below and the air in the lung
above.

Oblique Views. These views are most useful
for the localization of lesions and for the disclosure of shadows hidden by the domes of the
diaphragm and the heart in the frontal and lateral projections. They have an advantage over
the lateral view because there is less superimposition of the two lungs. The oblique projections
are made with the patient at an angle to the film,
either facing the cassette or with his back to it.
The former are the anterior oblique projections
and the latter the posterior obliques. The anterior oblique projections are the most commonly
used and, unless otherwise stated, it is to be
assumed that all references to oblique views signify the anterior obliques. Our own preference in
viewing the film is to place it so that the image
appears the same as on the fluoroscopic screen,
i.e., with the patient facing the observer.

Right Oblique. This view is made with the
patient's right shoulder to the film or fluoroscopic screen. In this projection, the left border
of the chest corresponds to the anterior axillary
line and the border of the right side of the chest
corresponds to the posterior axillary line (Figs.

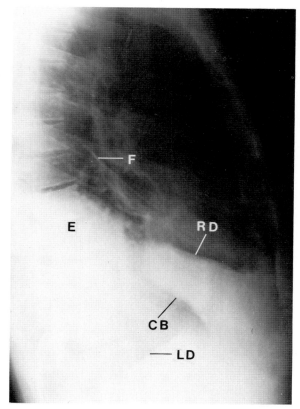

FIG. 59. SUPERIMPOSITION OF SHADOWS OF LIVER AND HEART SIMULATING INTERLOBAR EFFUSION

The right lateral view shows an encapsulated effusion (E) in the lower posterior part of the right pleural cavity. The triangular shadow extending downward and forward from this suggests an effusion in the long fissure. However, the fissure (F) can be identified at a distance above the shadow. The triangular shadow is formed by the superimposition of the shadows of the liver and the heart. The upper border (RD) corresponds to the right leaf of the diaphragm and the lower border (CB) represents the lower posterior margin of the heart. The posterior portion of the right leaf of the diaphragm is obscured by the effusion immediately above it. The left leaf of the diaphragm (LD), as is to be expected in the right lateral view, is projected below. At operation, only a basal empyema was found. There was no fluid in the long fissure.

48 and 60). The spine runs vertically in a curved fashion with the convexity more or less parallel to the border of the right chest. The axillary and posterior portions of the right lung lie between the margin of the spine and the right border of the chest. The right posterolateral costophrenic sinus is best seen in this view.

Between the heart and the left border of the spine is a radiolucent space. Within it is the faint, broad, elongated shadow of the descending aorta

which, in its upper portion, forms the aortic arch. The lower border of the retrocardiac space in this view is defined by the anterior part of the right leaf of the diaphragm.

The sternum is projected over the shadow of the heart. The space between the sternum and the spine is occupied by the anterior part of the right lung and the posterior part of the left lung. The clear space beyond the left border of the sternum is occupied by the anterior and axillary portions of the left lung, bounded laterally by the left anterior axillary line. The anterior portion of the left leaf of the diaphragm is visualized in this view. The posterior part of the left diaphragm is situated mesially at a somewhat lower level than the right and is partially obscured by the liver.

The trachea is well outlined, running downward in front of the spine. Soon after it crosses the arch of the aorta the trachea bifurcates. The proximal portion of the main bronchi can be visualized in this view.

LEFT OBLIQUE. The appearance of the lungs is similar to that in the right oblique. The two projections can be distinguished by the difference in the appearance of the cardiac contour. In the left oblique, the bulge of the left ventricle extends more sharply backward and almost obliterates the lower part of the retrocardiac space.

In this view, the right border of the chest is bounded by the anterior axillary line and a clear view of the anterior and axillary portions of the right lung is obtained to the right of the shadows of the heart and ascending aorta. The left border of the chest is outlined by the chest wall in the posterior axillary line (Figs. 61 and 62). The posterior portion of the left lung is visualized between it and the spine. The convexity of the spine is now to the left. The space between the spine and the sternum, which is projected over the ascending aorta, contains portions of both lungs. Here the anterior portion of the left lung and the posterior portion of the right are superimposed.

The lower border of the right chest is bounded by the anterior part of the right diaphragm beneath which is the dense shadow of the liver. The lower border of the left chest is bounded by the posterior part of the left diaphragm and, directly beneath this, radiolucent gas in the stomach or splenic flexure. The shadows of the posterior part of the right diaphragm and the anterior part of the left diaphragm cross each other. The trachea runs downward and somewhat backward behind the sternum and its bifurcation as well as both main bronchi are usually clearly depicted.

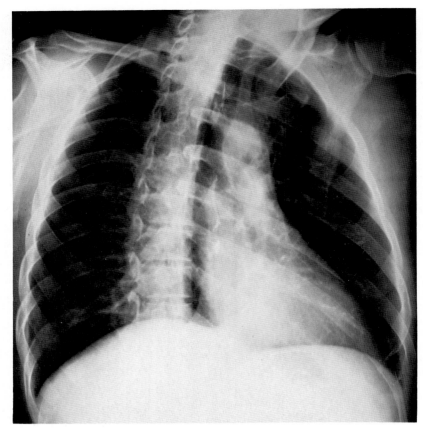

FIG. 60. NORMAL CHEST: RIGHT OBLIQUE VIEW

Conditions Bordering on the Normal

With advancing years, changes take place in the organs as a result of influences to which the body is more or less constantly exposed. Some of these may be termed physiologic since they occur when the body is functioning under relatively normal conditions. Arteriosclerosis in older people is an example. Other influences, external in origin, often cause changes in structure which are insufficient to result in any significant disturbance in function. This is true of the lungs as well as of other organs. Some of these minor changes represent the residua of disease important during its active stage, but not at the time of the examination. These changes, although departures from the normal, may usually be disregarded in the interpretation of the films.

Lymph Nodes. The mediastinal and bronchopulmonary lymph nodes are continually exposed to many irritating substances breathed into the lungs. Infections of the lungs and bronchi, whether of major or minor importance, may also leave a trace of their existence in these nodes. It is natural, then, that they should vary in their appearance on roentgen films. The nodes may be somewhat, though not notably, enlarged in nonspecific respiratory infections or when they are involved by anthracosis. Childhood tuberculosis, almost always of no importance in later life, leaves its mark in the form of areas of calcification within the lymph nodes.

Pleura. Pleural adhesions resulting from old infections may practically always be disregarded from the standpoint of interpretation of symptoms (see Fig. 537). Retraction or thickening of the pleura at the apex of the lung may be due to a small, healed tuberculous lesion. In previous years undue importance was attached to this finding but today we know that this pathologic change may be disregarded as far as clinical tuberculosis is concerned. Thickening of the apical pleura due to tuberculosis is almost always bilateral (see Fig. 495).

Lung Roots. The hilar shadows are composed of the overlapping shadows of the large bronchi, pulmonary blood vessels, lymph nodes and the pleural reflections over the roots of the lungs.

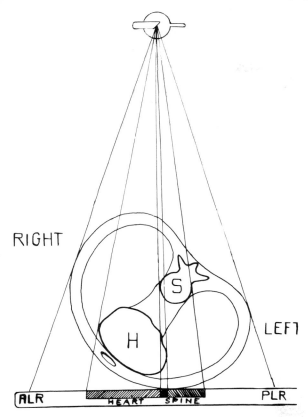

RIGHT

LEFT

<table>
<tr><td>ALR</td><td>HEART   SPINE</td><td>PLR</td></tr>
</table>

FIG. 61. THE LEFT ANTERIOR OBLIQUE PROJECTION

The patient is seen in cross section, viewed from above, with the left shoulder to the film. The thoracic silhouette on the right side corresponds to the anterolateral region (ALR), and the left border corresponds to the posterolateral region (PLR). The spine is projected into the left pulmonary field while the shadow of the heart is on the right. There may be slight overlapping of the apex of the heart over the spine, depending on the thickness of the chest and the degree of rotation.

Their size and conformation vary not only because of the pathologic changes in these structures but also because of normal variations in the width of the pulmonary vessels and the density of the bronchial walls and interstitial connective tissues. There is, then, a considerable range to the appearance of the normal lung roots.

Differences in the density of the root shadow can also be due to pathologic conditions of minor importance which may be disregarded. Old pulmonary or bronchial infections, anthracosis and pleural adhesions will thicken the structures at the roots of the lungs and intensify their shadows. Occasionally, these changes reflect important pathologic conditions but then they are usually associated with additional changes in the lungs or mediastinum.

Calcific Deposits and Fibrous Strands. Small areas of calcification in the lungs are usually due to the tuberculosis of childhood and are found at necropsy in a large percentage of the urban population. In the Mississippi Valley they are often the result of healed histoplasmosis (see Fig. 143). Since they occur so frequently without giving rise to secondary lesions, they may be considered of no clinical significance. Similarly, the presence of a few localized, sharply defined, streak-like shadows may be disregarded. In the upper lobes these shadows usually represent completely healed tuberculous lesions which do not tend to reactivate. In the lower lobes they most frequently represent the residua of nonspecific inflammatory disease which has undergone organization.

Epicardial Fat Pads. Large epicardial fat pads occur particularly in obese people and those who were formerly obese. The fat pad is represented by a triangular shadow at the cardiophrenic angle and is seen more commonly on the left side than on the right. The fat pad on the left tends to obscure the silhouette of the apex of the heart. However, on careful inspection of properly exposed films, the curve of the cardiac apex can usually be recognized because the fat is less dense than the heart.

Because of its triangular shape, a large epicardial fat pad on the left side may suggest the possibility of atelectasis of the left lower lobe. However, the latter is situated posteriorly and is recognizable on lateral or oblique films. In addition, it does not interfere with the silhouette of the apex of the heart on the frontal projection. Epicardial fat pads are less frequently seen on the right side. Here, they may be confused with a parapericardial cyst or properitoneal fat herniation. Their straight, oblique border helps to differentiate them from parapericardial cysts, while the absence of a well-defined quadrantic border on the lateral view serves to distinguish them from properitoneal fat herniations. Furthermore, it is uncommon for an epicardial fat pad to be visible on the right side without a concomitant one on the left. The presence of such triangular shadows on both sides is indicative of epicardial fat pads (Fig. 63).

Actually, the term epicardial fat pad is a misnomer. The epicardial fat lies deep to the visceral layer of pericardium, between it and the myocardium. The collections of fat that are seen in the cardiophrenic angles have nothing to do with the epicardium but are located in the mediastinum outside of the parietal pericardium and beneath the mediastinal pleura. This becomes obvious when air is injected into the pericardial space.

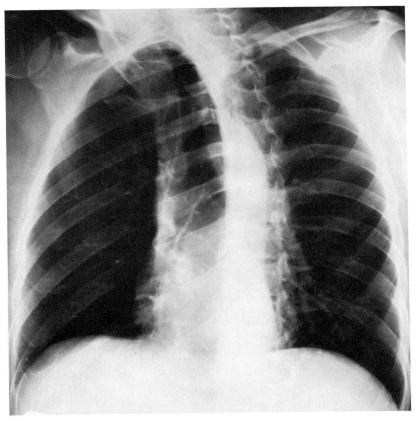

FIG. 62. NORMAL CHEST: LEFT OBLIQUE VIEW

Roentgen Artifacts

On occasion, extraneous shadows appear on the chest film superimposed on the thoracic structures. In some cases the artifact has a characteristic appearance and is easily recognized but, not uncommonly, it cannot be distinguished on a single film from the shadow of a pathologic process. In these instances failure to consider an artifact in the differential diagnosis can lead to serious errors in interpretation. Artifacts can be divided into three groups: shadows cast by objects interposed between the x-ray tube and the film, defects related to the film, the intensifying screen or the cassette and, lastly, aberrations resulting from misalignment of the x-ray tube.

Articles of clothing, especially when the material contains lead salts, can cast bizarre shadows. The only certain way to avoid this problem is to bare the chest completely when making the exposure. If it is preferred that the patient wear a gown or drape, care should be taken to see that the garment is not folded or crumpled between the patient and the cassette.

Ornaments about the neck are usually not difficult to recognize but create problems because they can obscure an important area of the lung. Hair drooping down over the lower part of the neck, particularly if braided, can give rise to shadows that are almost indistinguishable from the early infiltrate of tuberculosis (Fig. 64). It is essential that hair long enough to reach the field of exposure be pinned up before the examination. Simple dressings usually do not cast disturbing shadows, but the sharp edge of adhesive tape is often visible and may simulate an air-fluid level. Some dressings, especially those that contain iodine, e.g. iodoform gauze, can create a shadow on the film that resembles fluid or consolidation. This is especially true when the film is underexposed.

The skin of infants and emaciated patients is very lax. When the patient is in the recumbent position, it is possible for the skin to be thrown into folds. The double layer of skin and subcutaneous tissue casts a faint shadow which often has a sharply defined outer border and can simulate a pneumothorax (Fig. 65). If this is kept in mind, the possibility of a skin fold is easily con-

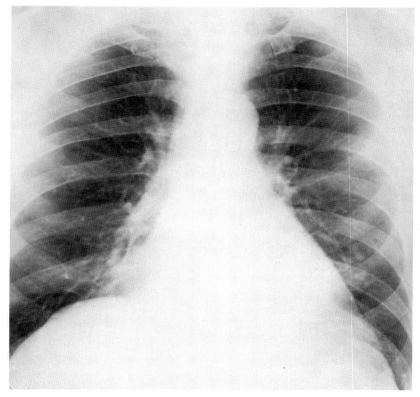

FIG. 63. EPICARDIAL FAT PADS

Each cardiophrenic angle is filled in by a triangular shadow which is less dense than that of the heart. Because of this, the cardiac borders, although faint, can be recognized. These shadows are characteristic of extrapleural fat adjacent to the heart.

firmed by repeating the examination in the erect position or with the patient turned slightly toward the opposite side.

When a patient is positioned for a posteroanterior film of the chest, the wrists should be flexed and the dorsum of the hands placed against the waist. If the patient is allowed to grab his waist, the fingers may be projected over the pulmonary field. We have observed three cases in which the shadow of a thumb was misdiagnosed as a tumor of the lung (Fig. 66). One of the patients was already scheduled for thoracotomy before the true nature of the shadow was appreciated.

In most of these cases, the extraneous nature of the shadow can be readily recognized because it extends beyond the boundary of the thorax (see Fig. 373). This may be difficult to detect when the artifact is caused by hair. Hair is not particularly radiopaque and, especially if the film is overexposed, its shadow outside of the chest may be burned out. Streaky densities that are most dense at the lateral border of the chest and rapidly fade an inch or two inside the pulmonary field, can be caused by scatter of the x-rays from lead markers used to identify the film. These shadows will be continuous with those of the marker.

Incomplete development or fixing of portions of a film can cause disturbing shadows. This was quite common with hand development when two films touched each other in the developer or the hypo tanks. Naturally, the adjacent film will show a similar artifact. Although this type of artifact has almost disappeared with the advent of automatic processers, it still does occur sporadically. The shadow of such a "kissing artifact" is usually faint but at times is quite dense (see Fig. 202). When the shadow extends beyond the lung, its recognition is simple. When it is entirely confined to the pulmonary field, it may be erroneously interpreted as representing an area of consolidation or a neoplasm (Fig. 67). The real nature of the shadow can usually be recognized because it is characteristically homogeneous, it fades uniformly in all parts of the periphery, and the undisturbed pulmonary vascular pattern may be seen through it.

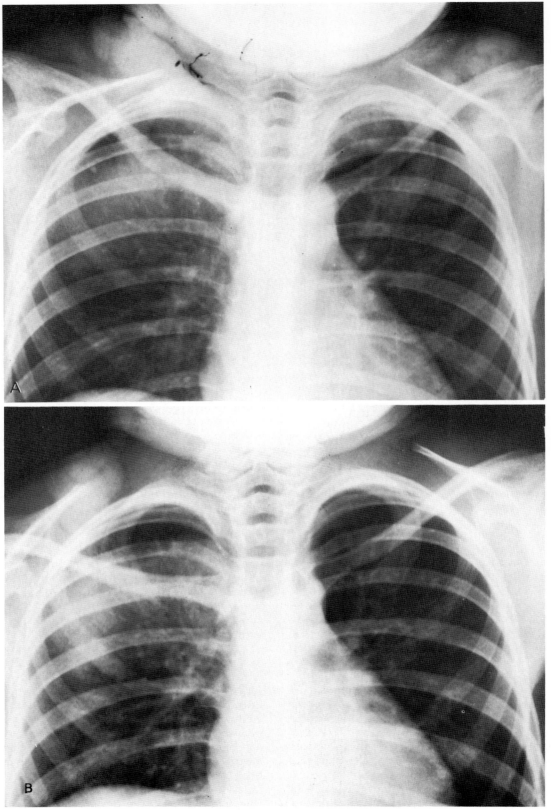

Fig. 64. Artifact Due to Hair

A: The frontal film of a young girl with symptoms of pneumonia shows an area of consolidation in the right upper lobe and a shadow at the apex of the left lung. The latter suggests the possibility of a tuberculous lesion. However, convoluted shadows caused by braids are seen above both shoulders. On the left side there is a possibility that the shadow in the lung is due to the braid and not to pulmonary disease. *B:* The left braid was pinned up and the left apex and supraclavicular regions are now clear. The braid on the right side has fallen down and is now projected over the outer part of the right lung.

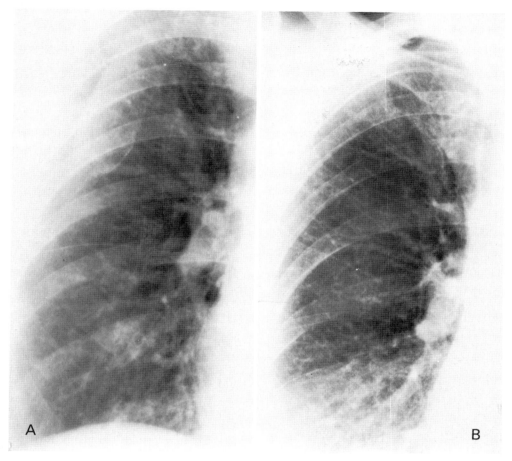

FIG. 65. SKIN FOLD

A: A portable film shows a faint density in the outer part of the right chest with a sharp lateral margin, simulating a pneumothorax. The patient was emaciated and the film was made in the supine position. *B*: A film repeated on the same day, but in the erect position, no longer shows the shadow.

Black zig-zag, forked or stellate streaks which obviously represent artifacts are caused by static electricity that is generated when one undeveloped film rubs against another. These artifacts are most common during the winter months when the humidity is low. Irregular, nondescript shadows may be due to defects in the film emulsion. A fault in this layer can usually be identified by sighting along the surface of the film away from the view box and looking for irregularities in the pattern of reflected light.

Bending of an undeveloped film can cause a short, black, crescent-shaped shadow, often called a "pinch mark" (see Fig. 521). The shadow is frequently surrounded by an ill-defined white halo. Poor contact between the film and the intensifying screens in the cassette can result in areas of unsharpness or a faint, indistinct area of increased density. When such a shadow is situated over the upper portion of the lung, it may be confused with a tuberculous lesion.

Errors in tube alignment result in misdirection of the central ray of the x-ray beam. When this is pointed to one side of the patient, that portion of the chest will be slightly darker than normal, while the opposite side will be underexposed. This may suggest pleural thickening on one side or hyperaeration of the lung on the other. The absence of other evidences of pleural disease on the light side or of overexpansion of the lung on the dark side should make one suspicious of an artifact. This is confirmed if the ribs on the lighter side appear less dense than those on the overexposed side.

ATELECTASIS

The word atelectasis simply means incomplete expansion of the lung or of a portion of the lung. It is a precise word whose meaning follows directly from its derivation and its connotation does not extend any further than the above definition. The term atelectasis is applied to the incomplete distention of the alveoli that occurs as a result of compression of the lung as well as from bronchial obstruction. The term should not be confused with apneumatosis which signifies only the absence of air in the alveoli. Apneumatosis may be present even when the alveoli are widely distended or overdistended if they are filled with exudate or other substances to the exclusion of air. Apneumatosis may also refer to complete atelectasis.

Atelectasis is complete when the alveolar walls are apposed to each other and no air, exudate, or edema fluid separates them. It is incomplete when the alveoli are partly distended. The partially atelectatic alveoli may contain air or they may contain exudate, but in any case their volume is diminished. If one adheres to this definition of atelectasis, all cases are included in which the volume of the lung or a portion of the lung is diminished either because of bronchial obstruction, external pressure, or any disease which prevents the affected portion from expanding to its full volume in inspiration. The term applies whether or not air, exudate, edema fluid, or other substances are present in the alveoli.

The word collapse is often used to denote complete atelectasis, and massive collapse denotes complete atelectasis of a large portion of a lung, either of a lobe or of the entire lung. The term should not be used if the atelectasis is incomplete, even though the entire lung is involved. The term massive collapse of the lung as used clinically is a poor one. It refers to a clinical picture with a dramatic onset, secondary to more or less sudden bronchial obstruction. In the earliest, or acute, phase, the roentgen film is likely to show emphysema rather than atelectasis. Because of this, the term is confusing and had better be replaced by the designation acute bronchial obstruction. Since the word represents a clinical picture which has no precise roentgenologic counterpart, it is best omitted from roentgenologic terminology. It is preferable in describing and interpreting roentgen films in this clinical state, to indicate the extent and degree of atelectasis, the evidences of bronchial obstruction and the presence or absence of infection in the involved lung.

General Roentgen Changes. The roentgen film may disclose only the evidences of atelectasis or it may show in addition, the shadows of other changes in the lung. These may represent the cause of the atelectasis or they may depict complications. Thus, one may observe on the film the shadow of an intrabronchial foreign body or a bronchial neoplasm that has extended through the wall into the surrounding pulmonary tissue, infiltrating the atelectatic lung. Furthermore, the atelectatic area may also be involved by an inflammatory process resulting from infection distal to the obstruction. These additional changes serve to complicate the roentgen picture.

Since the purpose of this chapter is to consider one specific pathologic change at a time, the associated abnormalities will be disregarded. Only a description of the various types of atelectasis as they are manifested at the roentgen examination will be considered.

Because the atelectatic lung contains less air than the normal, it is less radiolucent and there-

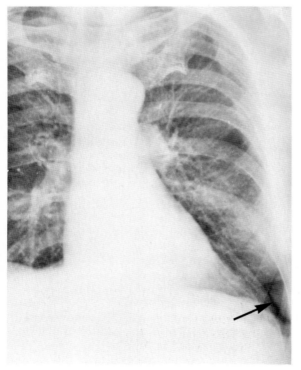

Fig. 66. Artifact

The shadow above the left costophrenic sinus (arrow) was considered to represent a mass involving the pleura. However, the shape of the shadow suggested the possibility that it might represent the patient's thumb. The examination was repeated with the patient's hand lower down and the shadow disappeared.

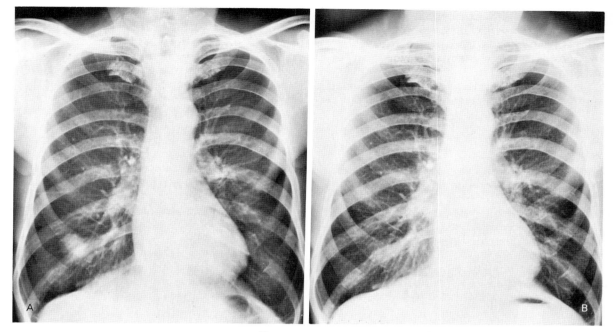

FIG. 67. ARTIFACT

A: The shadow over the lower part of the right lung was found on a routine examination. Because of its nodular character and indistinct margin it was thought to represent either a malignant neoplasm or a chronic inflammatory process. *B*: The examination was repeated 2 days later to exclude the possibility of an artifact. The lung now appears normal.

fore appears lighter on the film than the well aerated lung. This, in itself, is a nonspecific change, for diminished radiolucency of the lung occurs in a great variety of pathologic processes.

Specific Roentgen Changes. More specific changes from which the diagnosis of atelectasis can be made are dependent on the effect of the shrinkage of the involved lung tissue on the blood vessels within it and on the surrounding structures. The pleural fissures, adjacent lung, heart, mediastinum, chest wall and diaphragm may change their positions to conform to the space relinquished by the shrunken lung. In addition, abnormalities in the movement of the chest wall, mediastinum, blood vessels and diaphragm may be noted.

The lateral view often provides the most important information regarding atelectasis since it is in this projection that the position of the fissures is best determined. Fluoroscopy or films made in inspiration and expiration are required for the detection of the abnormal mediastinal movement caused by the inexpansile lung.

BLOOD VESSELS. In lobar atelectasis, the lung roots, which contain the main pulmonary blood vessels, are elevated or depressed depending upon the lobe that is involved. The smaller blood vessels within the atelectatic lung may not be visualized if the atelectasis is complete because

the density of the collapsed lung is the same as that of the blood vessels and their shadows merge imperceptibly.

The same principle can be used when examining the frontal projection to provide a clue as to the part of the lung involved. In general, the shadow of a lesion in the anterior portion of the chest merges with the shadow of the anterior mediastinum, so that the boundary between the two is not seen. Thus, the shadow of a collapsed middle lobe tends to obliterate that portion of the right heart border that lies adjacent to it. Similarly, in atelectasis of the lingula, the corresponding portion of the left border of the heart loses its delineation. In atelectasis of the anterior segment of the upper lobe there is a tendency to obliteration of the border of the ascending aorta on the right side (see Fig. 94), and of the pulmonary artery segment on the left. Conversely, in atelectasis of the lower lobes, the cardiac borders remain sharply outlined. In these cases, however, the silhouette of the diaphragm is usually lost.

If the atelectasis is incomplete, the vessels may be discerned within the clouded lung which covers them with a diffuse, veil-like shadow. However, the vessels appear closer together than normal. This approximation or condensation of the vascular shadows is characteristic of atelectasis (Fig. 68). On fluoroscopy, these vessels are seen to maintain their relative position during respiration and do not show the normal fanning out on inspiration and approximation during expiration.

FISSURES. The position and course of the short fissure on the frontal view and both the short and long fissures on the lateral view, are most helpful in determining the presence of atelectasis (see Figs. 96 and 226). When the fissures are visible, the presence of atelectasis of a lobe or even of a segment abutting on a fissure is quite clear. If the fissure is not visible, the recognition of atelectasis may be more difficult. However, the density of the affected lobe or segment may be sufficiently increased so that its boundary is well delineated, making the displacement of the fissure obvious (Fig. 69).

ADJACENT LUNG. The lung next to an atelectatic area tends to become overexpanded and to take up the space relinquished by the collapsed portion of the lung (Fig. 70). The development of this *compensatory hyperinflation* is a passive process and results from an increase in the negative pressure in the pleura due to shrinkage of the involved portion of the lung. The emphysema is manifested by an increased radiolucency caused by the hyperexpanded alveoli. The emphysematous lung, therefore, appears darker than the rest of the pulmonary field. Its blood vessels may be spread apart and straightened.

MEDIASTINUM. *Displacement.* In the case of atelectasis of a large portion of a lung, the mediastinum is displaced toward the side of the lesion (Figs. 71 and 175). This displacement is caused by the diminution in pressure on the affected side which results from incomplete expansion of the lung. The extent of the mediastinal displacement depends on the mobility of the mediastinum and the presence or absence of pleural adhesions, as well as on the degree of atelectasis. During inspiration there is a greater

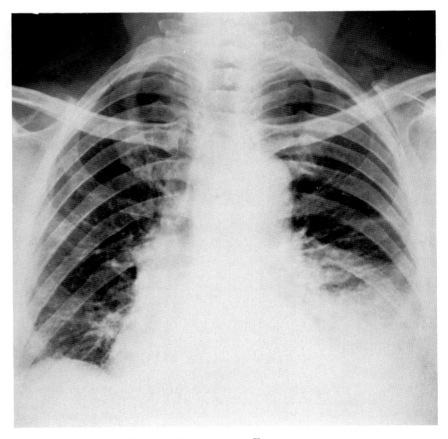

FIG. 68. ATELECTASIS IN EMBOLIZATION
There is an effusion at the left base as the result of pulmonary infarction. The left lung root is depressed and the vessels immediately above the fluid are drawn together and directed horizontally. Approximation of blood vessels is an important sign of atelectasis. The diaphragm is elevated because chest pain prevented the patient from taking a deep breath.

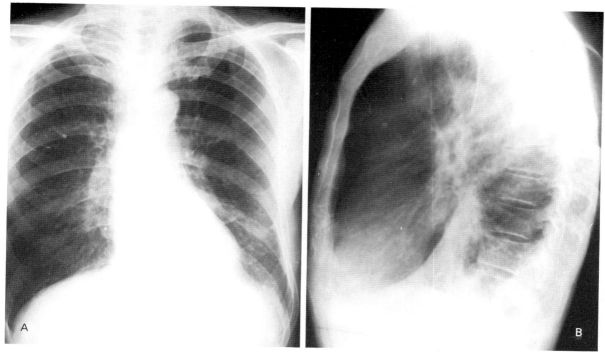

FIG. 69. SEGMENTAL ATELECTASIS IN BRONCHIAL CARCINOMA

A: The frontal film, made after a few months of low grade fever, shows no apparent abnormality. However, the heart is not adequately penetrated so that the left lower lobe cannot be evaluated. The presence of disease in this region was detected on a film of the abdomen. *B*: The lateral view shows a triangular density behind the long fissure which is bowed backward. This is due to atelectasis and infiltration of the anterior and lateral basal segments of the left lower lobe. These segments were retracted mesially as well as posteriorly so that they were hidden by the heart on the frontal film.

increase in the negative pressure on the affected side than on the healthy side. This is due to the limited ability of the lung to expand in response to the downward motion of the diaphragm and the outward motion of the chest wall. The increased size of the thoracic cavity that results from these movements is taken up partly by the shift of the mediastinal structures to that side.

The change in the position of the mediastinum during respiration is easily noted on fluoroscopy, although it can also be observed on films made in inspiration and expiration. The mediastinum may be situated in its normal position during expiration but on inspiration it will usually move toward the abnormal side. At the beginning of expiration the direction of the shift is reversed as the mediastinum moves towards its normal position. This has been described as *pendular movement* of the mediastinum. It may not be apparent on quiet respiration but becomes quite clear when the subject makes a sudden, strong, short inspiration as in the act of sniffing. The movement of the mediastinum toward the side of the obstruction is especially well seen in children during the sudden, sharp inspiration follow-

ing the prolonged expiration that occurs during a spell of crying.

Pendular movement of the mediastinum is not pathognomonic of atelectasis. It also occurs in obstructive emphysema and is not uncommon in pneumothorax. In atelectasis, however, the mediastinum is never displaced into the opposite pulmonary field during expiration (Fig. 44*B*). There is little or no lateral movement of the mediastinum in the normal chest. In older persons, however, slight movement of the aortic arch to the right may occur during inspiration.

Herniation. When the shrinkage of the lung produces a very marked negative pressure in the pleura, not neutralized by a shift of the entire mediastinum, herniation of a portion of the mediastinum may occur. The lucent contralateral lung then extends across the midline to the diseased side. This takes place where the mediastinum is narrow, particularly in patients in whom the pleural layers on each side of the mediastinum are separated only by a thin layer of connective tissue (see Fig. 83). It may also occur when one portion of the mediastinum is free while the remainder is fixed. The most common

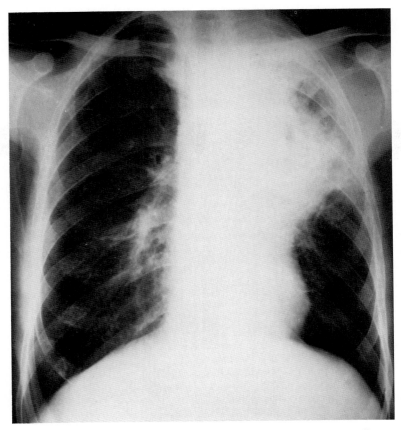

FIG. 70. ATELECTASIS AND INFECTION OF LEFT UPPER LOBE: BRONCHOGENIC CARCINOMA

There is opacification of the left upper lobe with lucencies in the lateral portion, indicating inflammation with cavitation. The flattening of the left hemithorax and compensatory hyperinflation of the left lower lobe signify that the upper lobe is atelectatic as well as inflamed. The paradoxical displacement of the trachea to the right side was due to the presence of mediastinal metastases from the carcinoma which obstructed the left upper lobe bronchus.

site for the herniation is in the upper anterior mediastinum. Less commonly, it occurs in the posterior mediastinum in the lower part of the chest, behind the heart (Fig. 71).

It is customary to observe mediastinal herniation in patients receiving pneumothorax treatment for tuberculosis. The herniation in these cases is practically always to the side opposite the pneumothorax. However, particularly when the pneumothorax is being discontinued and some of the air has been absorbed from the pleural cavity, a hernia may develop *toward* the side of the pneumothorax. This occurs because of the high degree of negative pressure that develops in the involved pleural space as the pneumothorax absorbs. However, absorption of the air alone cannot explain the excessive negative pressure. This can be accounted for only by the inability of the diseased lung to expand in response to the negative pressure, either because of the presence of inelastic fibrous tissue within

the lung, imprisonment of the lung by a thickened visceral pleura or the presence of a complicating bronchial stricture. Persistence of atelectasis of the diseased lung while the air in the pleura is being absorbed, is the reason for the paradox of mediastinal displacement or herniation toward the side of a pneumothorax (Fig. 72).

CHEST WALL. In atelectasis of a single lobe or a portion of a lobe, there is usually no flattening or restriction of the movement of the chest wall unless there are complicating factors. The shift of the mediastinum and overexpansion of the remaining lobe of the lung is usually sufficient to fill the additional space in the thorax created by the outward and upward movement of the chest wall during inspiration. However, if these structures are fixed because of fibrous tissue deposition, atelectasis of even a moderate portion of the lung is sufficient to restrict the movement of the chest wall.

In most patients with a considerable degree of

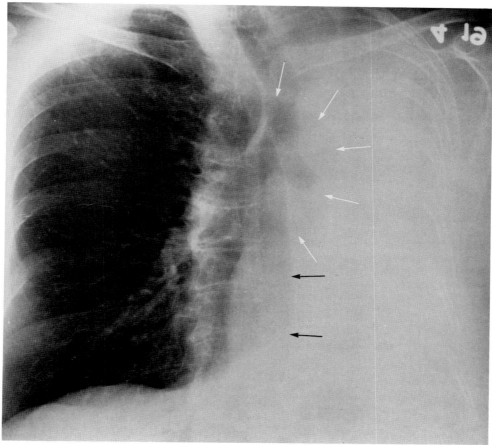

FIG. 71. ATELECTASIS OF LEFT LUNG

The left lung is completely opacified so that its blood vessels and the left cardiac border cannot be visualized. All the mediastinal structures are shifted markedly to the left. The right lung is hyperinflated and the lower lobe extends across the midline behind the heart (black arrows). The anterior lappet of the upper lobe (white arrows) has herniated through the anterior part of the superior mediastinum. The left main bronchus is sharply cut off by a mass in its lumen representing the carcinoma responsible for the atelectasis.

atelectasis of an entire lung, there is well-marked diminution in the movement of the ribs on the affected side. This restriction can be noted on fluoroscopy and on films made on inspiration and expiration. The effect on the chest wall is studied by comparing the two sides of the thorax. The width of the diseased side can usually be found to be diminished by actual measurement of the distance from the lateral chest wall to the spinous processes of the vertebrae. In the upper part of the chest, the effect of atelectasis on the chest wall is often manifested by a flattening of the curve over the outer part of the dome of the thorax (see Fig. 78).

When the volume of thoracic cavity is diminished, the course of the ribs changes. Normally the ribs are elevated during inspiration. This elevation is most pronounced in the anterior portion of the ribs and diminishes progressively toward the posterior portion where the ribs are pivoted at their costovertebral articulations. If the motion of the chest is restricted because the lung is unable to expand properly, the anterior portions of the ribs are depressed to a considerable degree. Therefore, they slant downward more than normally, particularly during inspiration. The difference in the movement of the anterior portions of the ribs on the two sides in some patients with atelectasis is quite striking during fluoroscopy.

Narrowing of the intercostal spaces, a common finding in atelectasis, is best observed in the outer portion of the chest. Here, the spaces may become so narrow, that the ribs seem to overlie each other in the manner of shingles (Fig. 31). In the absence of scoliosis or chronic peripleuritis, which also causes this change, shingling of the ribs indicates atelectasis of long duration.

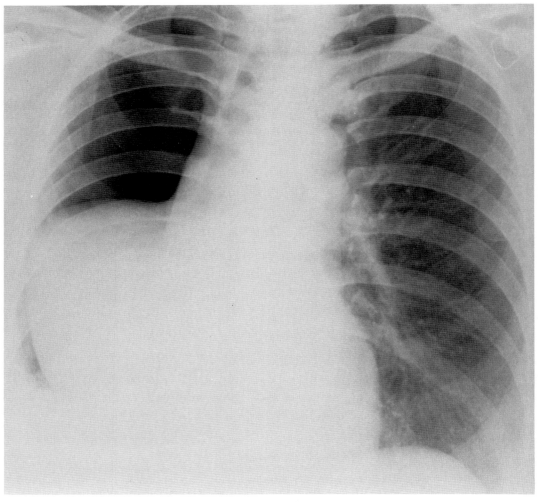

FIG. 72. OBSTRUCTIVE ATELECTASIS WITH PNEUMOTHORAX

The patient, who was receiving pneumothorax treatment, suddenly became dyspneic. The right lung, which previously had been fairly well aerated, became completely collapsed and the heart and mediastinum were displaced to the right despite the pneumothorax. The picture of a "white lung" with displacement of the mediastinum to the side of the pneumothorax is indicative of bronchial obstruction. The lung reexpanded and the mediastinum returned to its normal position following bronchoscopic aspiration of mucoid secretion from the right bronchus.

DIAPHRAGM. The diaphragm is often elevated when there is considerable shrinkage of the lung. The elevation of this organ in atelectasis is largely due to a diminution in its downward movement during inspiration. This is clearly observed on fluoroscopy. The failure of the diaphragm to contract in the face of the increased negative pressure in the pleura is most evident during sudden inspiration, for this causes a marked increase in the negative pleural pressure. The diaphragm is rarely immobilized completely as the result of atelectasis alone. In ordinary respiration and during a slow, deep inspiration, the diaphragm descends in the normal direction although its excursion may be limited. However, if the patient makes a sudden, forced inspiration, as in sniffing, a quick upward or paradoxical movement of the diaphragm may occur. This movement is the same as that which occurs in diaphragmatic paralysis.

Differentiation between the paradoxical movement of paralysis of the diaphragm and that which occurs in atelectasis can be made by observing the diaphragm as the patient takes a slow, deep breath. In the case of atelectasis the negative pressure is partly neutralized by expansion of adjacent portions of the lung and by movement of the mediastinum toward the affected side, enabling the diaphragm to move in a normal, downward direction. In paralysis of the diaphragm little downward motion is visible.

The differentiation can also be made by fluoroscopy in the lateral decubitus position by observing the diaphragmatic motion with the patient lying on the side of the lesion. The high negative pleural pressure in the case of atelectasis is neutralized by the weight of the mediastinum and limitation of outward movement of the chest wall. The diaphragm is then enabled to move downward during inspiration for a considerable distance. Of course, if the diaphragm is paralyzed, little or no downward movement will occur.

The movement of the diaphragm in atelectasis does not differ from the movement of a weakened or paretic diaphragm, i.e., one which is not completely paralyzed. The impairment of diaphragmatic motion due to atelectasis must be differentiated from that caused by paralysis of the diaphragm. This is particularly important in patients with an obstructing bronchial neoplasm because diaphragmatic paralysis indicates invasion of the phrenic nerve and suggests that the neoplasm is not resectable. It is apparent that a grave error may be made if one should wrongly infer that the diaphragm is paralyzed in such a case, when in fact, the paradoxical movement produced by sniffing is due solely to the atelectasis caused by the obstructing growth.

EFFECT OF PLEURAL ADHESION AND MEDIASTINAL FIXATION. When there are no pleural adhesions, the healthy portion of lung shifts to take up the space relinquished by a collapsed lobe. There is then little increase in the negative pressure in the pleura, and the trachea and the mediastinal structures may remain in the midline (see Fig. 186). Considerable displacement of the pulmonary fissure bordering the atelectatic lobe is usually demonstrable (Fig. 73). If, on the other hand, there are adhesions which fix the parietal border of the fissure, this shift cannot take place. The fissure then only bulges in the direction of the atelectatic area (Fig. 73B). Since the increased negative pressure is not completely neutralized by the limited expansion of the neighboring portion of the lung, the mediastinum shifts toward that side. In addition, the increased negative pressure in the pleural cavity may cause flattening of the overlying chest wall.

If the mediastinum is fixed by inflammatory or neoplastic disease so that it cannot shift freely to the affected side, the flattening of the chest wall is more pronounced and the diaphragm is often elevated. This is most marked in atelectasis of

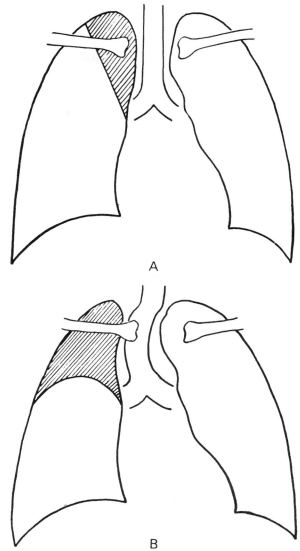

A

B

FIG. 73. UPPER LOBE ATELECTASIS: EFFECT OF PLEURAL ADHESIONS

A: In the absence of adhesions the short fissure is able to shift toward a vertical position. The middle and lower lobes are able to take up the space relinquished by the collapsed upper lobe so that there is little or no shift of the mediastinum. *B*: When the circumference of the fissure is fixed by adhesions the upward retraction of the collapsed lobe is limited so that only the central portion of the short fissure is elevated. The space relinquished by the collapsed upper lobe is largely occupied by the mediastinum which has shifted toward the involved side. This is easily recognized by bowing of the trachea.

the entire lung (see Fig. 423) but it can occur with atelectasis of a single lobe.

Types of Atelectasis. It is useful to classify atelectasis of the lung according to its cause. Not only does this type of classification aid in understanding the pathogenesis of atelectasis but it also aids in the roentgen interpretation. There are four etiologic types of pulmonary atelectasis.

First, there is the atelectasis due to failure of the extrapulmonary respiratory system. In this, there is absence of movement of the chest wall and diaphragm so that little or no negative pressure is established in the lung. In the absence of an expansive force, the lung is atelectatic. This may be classified as *adynamic* atelectasis.

The second type is due to *external pressure* which interferes with expansion of the lung. Pressure atelectasis is most commonly caused by a pleural effusion or pneumothorax, but it may also be caused by large neoplasms and by elevation of the diaphragm resulting from increased intraabdominal pressure.

The third type of atelectasis is that which is due to the presence of a thick, inelastic pleura over the lung or of fibrous tissue within the lung, preventing its expansion, even though the bronchi are free. This type of atelectasis may best be called *restrictive atelectasis*.

The fourth type of atelectasis, and the most common, is that due to *bronchial obstruction*.

ADYNAMIC ATELECTASIS. The classic example of adynamic atelectasis is atelectasis of the stillborn. The lungs are practically airless and appear as solid structures which have the same density as the other soft tissues of the body. They are uniformly opaque and their shadows merge imperceptibly with those of the diaphragm and the heart.

The chest wall has a characteristic bell shape. The dome of the chest retains its natural curve because it is supported by the arch of the upper ribs while the lowermost ribs flare out because of the pressure of the abdominal contents. A sinking in of the intermediate portion of the lateral wall of the chest completes the bell-like contour.

Partial atelectasis due to paralysis of the musculature of the chest wall and of the diaphragm occurs particularly in poliomyelitis. The diaphragm is elevated and the pulmonary fields have a grayish tone because of diminished aeration of the lung. If the diaphragm alone is paralyzed, there may be only a slight loss of illumination of the lower lobe. In some cases, the upper lobe also is slightly clouded since normally the downward movement of the diaphragm during inspiration tends to affect the expansion of the upper as well as the lower lobes. Clouding of the upper lobes occurs particularly when the diaphragm is markedly elevated.

ATELECTASIS FROM EXTERNAL PRESSURE. The effect of the pressure of large collections of fluid and of large masses in the chest on the aeration of the lung is usually not notable on the roentgen films because it is overshadowed by the effusion or the tumor. However, there may be noted, particularly in the larger circumscribed tumors of the lung, a condensation of the shadows of the adjacent pulmonary vessels which are displaced by the neoplasm. In this region there may also be noted some haziness of the pulmonary field as a result of diminished aeration of the compressed portion of the lung. Compression of the lung is particularly well illustrated when there is marked bullous emphysema of a neighboring lobe.

Increased abdominal pressure, as a result of gaseous distention, ascites, or a subphrenic abscess, interferes with the aeration of the lung, particularly of the lower lobe. Here, there is often a diffuse graying of the pulmonary field as a result of partial atelectasis. The clouding of the lung and the approximation of the vessels that occur in atelectasis are well depicted in the lung on the side of a pneumothorax. One portion of the lung may be collapsed to a greater degree than the rest of the lung (*selective collapse*). This is often due to bronchial obstruction (Fig. 74).

RESTRICTIVE ATELECTASIS. Partial atelectasis due to restriction of pulmonary expansion without bronchial obstruction occurs when there is marked thickening of the pleura, fixation of the chest wall, or fixation of the tissues within the lung.

Fixation of the chest wall occurs particularly after thoracoplasty, but the diminished radiolucency of the pulmonary field in these cases is largely due to the underlying lesion and the close approximation of the ribs and their bony bridges. Less interference with visualization of the lungs is produced when the chest wall has been collapsed by multiple fractures. After the disappearance of a complicating effusion which may have been present soon after the injury, only a moderate graying of the pulmonary field remains as an expression of the diminished aeration of the lung.

If a pleuritis occurs during the course of pneumothorax treatment and the lung is not reexpanded promptly, it may become enveloped in a thick fibrous membrane while it is still collapsed by the pneumothorax. This used to occur frequently when the pneumothorax was complicated by a large effusion which was treated by aspiration of the fluid and replacement by air.

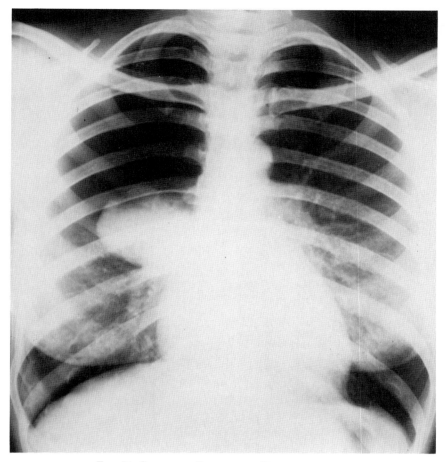

FIG. 74. SELECTIVE COLLAPSE IN PNEUMOTHORAX

The patient, who had diffuse bronchitis, developed a spontaneous pneumothorax. The shadow at the right root represents a completely collapsed upper lobe while the middle and lower lobes remain expanded. The pneumothorax was limited to the upper part of the chest, occupying the space relinquished by the collapsed lobe. The selective collapse of the upper lobe was due to obstruction of its bronchus by secretions. The lobe reexpanded promptly after the mucus was expectorated.

After the lung was maintained in the collapsed state for a considerable length of time in this way, it could no longer reexpand after the pneumothorax was discontinued. In such cases, the pulmonary field often remains somewhat gray because of the partial atelectasis and the thickening of the pleura. The chest wall usually is flattened, the diaphragm elevated, and the mediastinum displaced somewhat to the involved side (Fig. 75). This uniform contraction of the lung in association with other evidences of thickening of the pleura is so characteristic of imprisonment of the lung in the postpneumothorax state, that the diagnosis can usually be made simply from inspection of the film. The constriction of the lung that results from organization of an old hemothorax or from carnification of the pleura in an old tuberculous pleuritis, is usually localized to the lower portion of the chest. Here, the poor aeration of the lung is overshadowed by the extensively thickened pleura. In some cases of tuberculous pleurisy, the thickening of the pleura is more extensive and causes extreme restriction of the lung. The pleura may be calcified (see Fig. 133). A similar imprisonment of the lung from pleural thickening can follow a hemothorax which may be due to infarction or trauma (Fig. 31).

Restrictive atelectasis occurs quite regularly as the result of deposition of fibrous tissue in the lung while it is in a contracted state. In various inflammatory diseases there is atelectasis in the involved portion of the lung because of obstruction of larger or smaller bronchi while the lung is acutely inflamed. If the disease is accompanied by destruction of pulmonary tissue, fibrosis takes

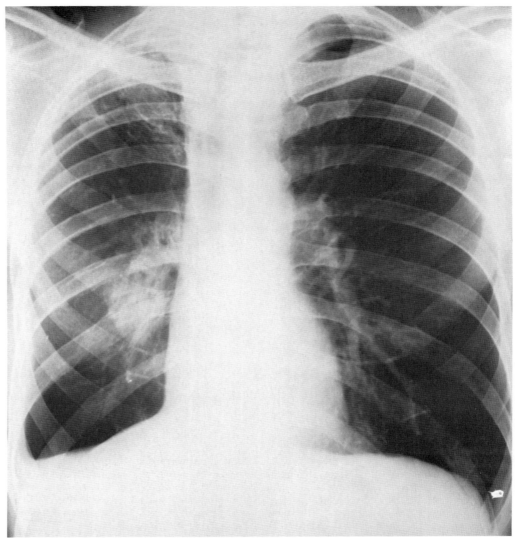

FIG. 75. RESTRICTIVE ATELECTASIS: POSTPNEUMOTHORAX LUNG

There is marked diminution in the volume of the right lung. The right chest is flattened, the intercostal spaces are narrowed, and the heart and trachea are displaced to the right side. The right costophrenic sinus is obliterated and there is blunting of the cardiophrenic angle and retraction of the apex. The changes are due mainly to imprisonment of the lung by pleura which became thickened while the lung was collapsed during pneumothorax therapy for tuberculosis. The remains of the tuberculous process are seen in the form of fibrous strands at the right apex and the dense shadow near the root of the right lower lobe. Despite the considerable thickening of the pleura and diminution in the size of the right lung, the right pulmonary field is only slightly grayer than the left.

place. This usually occurs rather early, when the involved lung is more or less atelectatic. Once the inflammation resolves, the fibrous tissue prevents the lung from reexpanding completely and it remains permanently collapsed. The marked elevation of the lung roots that occurs so frequently in tuberculosis, even when there is little fibrous tissue to be seen, is largely due to this cause.

The atelectasis that occurs in some cases of bronchiectasis is usually due to a combination of factors (see Figs. 90 and 201). It results, in part, from destruction and stricture of the smaller bronchial branches which prevents aeration of the diseased lung, as well as from the deposition of fibrous tissue during the phase of suppurative bronchopneumonia which precedes the bronchiectasis. At the time of the pneumonia the lung is collapsed because the bronchi are obstructed by exudate and swelling of the mucous membrane.

Although many of the bronchi become strictured in the process of healing, a considerable number of them regain their patency. However, the lung tissue they supply cannot expand because of restriction by scar tissue (see Fig. 241). This is the cause of continued atelectasis in old inflammatory diseases in which there is no bronchial obstruction at the time of examination.

The explanation often given for the atelectasis associated with fibrosis is that the scar tissue, once it is formed, contracts and draws the lung together. While it is true that scar tissue does contract during its development, this does not appear to be an adequate explanation. In patients who are carefully studied from the onset of their disease, it is observed that the atelectasis occurs rapidly during the acute stage of bronchopulmonary inflammation when the bronchi are obstructed, before the deposition of fibrous tissue. It is logical, therefore, to conclude that the fibrous tissue simply keeps the affected lung in the contracted state by restricting its expansion rather than by actively constricting the lung.

The conformation of the atelectatic area, the approximation of the blood vessels within it, and the effect of the atelectasis on the pulmonary fissures, the neighboring lung and the mediastinum are similar to the changes that occur in atelectasis from bronchial obstruction. This is not surprising since the atelectasis was originally due to this cause.

In restrictive atelectasis associated with fibrosis of the lung, whether it be due to tuberculosis, bronchiectasis or some other disease, the density and extent of the shadow of the abnormal lung is caused mainly by the inflammatory process. When there is little inflammation, the change in tone of the affected pulmonary field may be quite small. For example, in neoplastic lymphangitis, the lung between the strands of neoplastic tissue shows only a faint, diffuse graying (see Fig. 390). This is due to the poor aeration of the lung rather than to the tumor tissue. The latter is in the form of rigid cords situated in and about lymphatic channels. These prevent complete expansion of the lung because they act as guy ropes which hold it in a partially collapsed state (see Fig. 411).

OBSTRUCTIVE ATELECTASIS. The most important form of atelectasis, from the clinical standpoint, is the one due to bronchial obstruction. This is usually associated with a characteristic

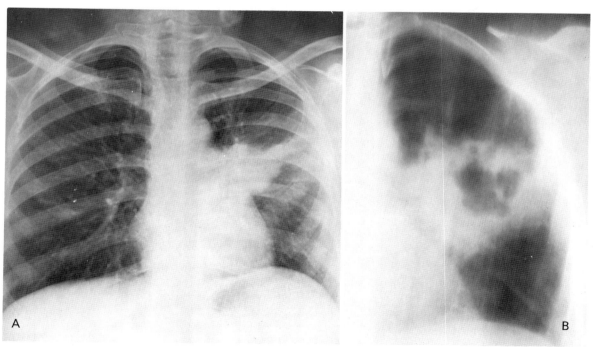

FIG. 76. HODGKIN'S DISEASE OF THE LUNG

A: The shadow at the root of the left lung consists of a local dense infiltration of the lung together with large hilar nodes. The broad streak extending to the axillary region is due to atelectasis of the anterior segment of the upper lobe. The bronchus was obstructed by the lymphomatous disease. *B:* The lesion underwent cavitation following radiotherapy. The tomogram shows the cavity to be extremely thick-walled and irregular. The roentgen appearance is indistinguishable from that of a broken down carcinoma.

roentgen picture which indicates the obstructive origin of the atelectasis.

In many cases the lesion responsible for the obstruction can be identified on the roentgen film. This is particularly true if it extends or is situated outside the bronchus as is often the case with neoplastic disease involving the bronchial wall (Figs. 76, 77 and 79). The shadow of a large mediastinal tumor or of an aneurysm that causes bronchial obstruction by external pressure, is always evident. Some purely intrabronchial lesions, such as foreign bodies or bronchial stones, are sufficiently dense so that they are visible.

Secondary infection of the atelectatic lung is common in bronchial obstruction and this alters the roentgen picture by producing areas of infiltration or cavitation. However, no matter what the cause of the obstruction or the secondary effects, the characteristics peculiar to obstructive

atelectasis usually remain if the obstructed bronchus is a large one (Fig. 70).

Atelectasis of an Entire Lung. When an entire lung is atelectatic, the pulmonary field is uniformly clouded, and its tone depends on the completeness of the atelectasis. When the atelectasis is slight, the pulmonary field is only slightly grayer than the opposite, normal lung, and when it is more complete, the shade is lighter. Usually, the color is not entirely white, because some air remains in most atelectatic lungs. The shadows of the blood vessels are often seen radiating from the hilum through the gray tone of the pulmonary field. The shadow of the partly collapsed lung has been described as "veil-like," since the vessels are seen through it, as if covered by a veil. In the cases in which the atelectasis is complete and there is no contrasting air within the lung, the vessels cannot be seen and the

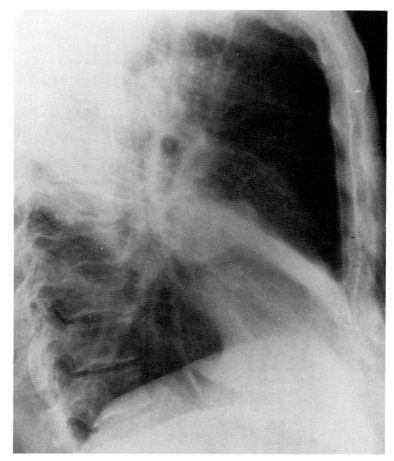

FIG. 77. OBSTRUCTION OF MIDDLE LOBE BRONCHUS BY BRONCHIAL CARCINOMA

The lateral view shows an oblique, band-like density extending to the anterior costophrenic sinus, representing a collapsed middle lobe. The nodular mass at the root of the lobe is caused by the carcinoma which has extended through the wall of the middle lobe bronchus to involve the surrounding lung and adjacent lymph nodes.

diffuse density of the pulmonary field suggests the presence of fluid in the pleural cavity (Fig. 78).

In lesser degrees of atelectasis, slight graying of the pulmonary field on the side of the obstruction in inspiration is comparable to the appearance of the normal lung in expiration. In such instances, the film made in expiration may show both lungs to be of the same density. However, in inspiration the difference between the two becomes apparent. This difference is more striking on fluoroscopy. The healthy side illuminates well on inspiration, while the diseased side shows no change in its tone. Whereas on expiration the mediastinum may be situated in its normal position, on inspiration it shifts sharply toward the side of the obstruction. When the atelectasis is more complete, the heart and mediastinal structures remain displaced to the side of the obstruction in expiration as well as inspiration. In addition, the chest wall is usually flattened and the diaphragm is considerably elevated. These evidences of contraction of the lung are usually present even when there is a complicating pleural effusion unless the latter is extremely large. One would ordinarily expect that an effusion would displace the mediastinum to the opposite side. If the mediastinum is displaced toward the side of the effusion one must consider that there is, in addition, atelectasis of the lung secondary to bronchial obstruction.

Lobar Atelectasis. The changes produced by atelectasis of a lobe of the lung depend on which lobe is involved and the presence or absence of pleural adhesions. Here again the picture is modified by the completeness of the atelectasis. In each case there is seen a homogeneous shadow which varies in intensity with the degree of airlessness of the involved lobe. The characteristics which differentiate lobar atelectasis from other causes of a similar roentgen shadow are to be found by observing the change in the position of the fissures, the lung roots, and the mediastinum, particularly the trachea.

RIGHT UPPER LOBE. Atelectasis of the right upper lobe characteristically results in elevation of its lower border (Fig. 73). This causes upward retraction of the short fissure and elevation of

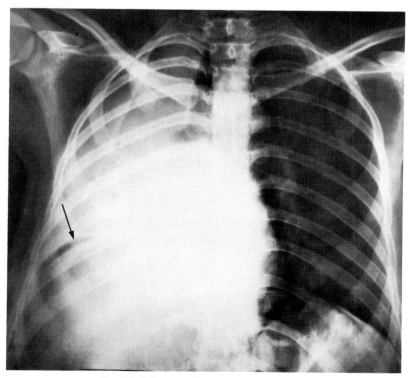

FIG. 78. MASSIVE COLLAPSE OF THE LUNG

The right hemithorax is completely opacified. The rib spaces are narrowed and the heart and trachea are markedly displaced to the right. The right diaphragm (arrow), which is outlined by air in the peritoneal cavity, is elevated. These findings indicate complete atelectasis of the right lung. This occurred immediately after an abdominal operation under general anesthesia. The lung reexpanded promptly after obstructing secretions were removed from the bronchi.

the lung root. In addition, the long fissure may be displaced anteriorly. The elevation of the short fissure is seen on the frontal view while the lateral view discloses the displacement of both fissures.

If there are extensive adhesions of the lung to the parietes, the outer border of the short fissure is fixed in its normal position while its midportion is raised. This causes the short fissure to assume a curved shape with an upward convexity (Fig. 79) in place of the straight line which is ordinarily seen when the short fissure is not bound down.

If there are adhesions on the mesial aspect of the upper lobe but not over its lateral surface, the mesial portion of the fissure remains fixed at its normal level at the upper border of the fourth rib near the mediastinum, while its lateral portion is free to move upward. The fissure is then represented by an oblique line that extends outward and upward on the frontal view (see Fig. 226). If the posterior portion of the upper lobe is free of adhesions, there will be considerable displacement of the upper part of the long fissure in a superior and anterior direction.

If the pleura is free of adhesions, atelectasis of the upper lobe usually produces no discernible displacement of the mediastinum (Fig. 80). The lower and middle lobes expand freely and take up the space relinquished by the collapsed upper lobe. However, in such a case one may note a sharp movement of the upper mediastinum to the right on sudden inspiration. This causes a

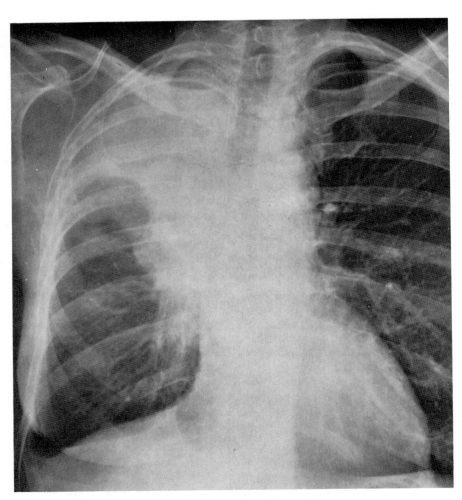

FIG. 79. ATELECTASIS RIGHT UPPER LOBE

The right upper lobe is completely collapsed. Because of pleural adhesions over the outer portion of the lobe, the lateral margin of the short fissure is fixed in place. The remainder of the fissure is bowed upward as a result of loss of volume of the upper lobe. Because of the pleural adhesions, the lobe is not free to collapse against the mediastinum and therefore the trachea is displaced to the right. The large mass at the right hilum represents a primary bronchogenic carcinoma.

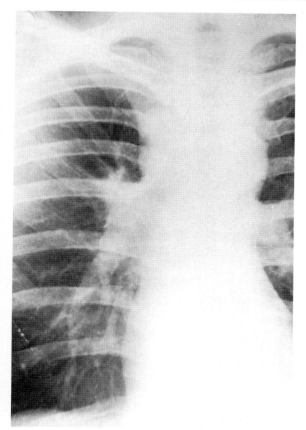

FIG. 80. ELEVATION OF LUNG ROOT IN ATELECTASIS

There is a triangular shadow over the mesial portion of the upper part of the right lung. This blends with the shadow of the mediastinum. The appearance suggests a mass in the superior mediastinum or consolidation in an azygos lobe. However, the right hilum is elevated, indicating loss of volume of the upper lobe. The patient had a carcinoma which obstructed the right upper lobe bronchus and produced complete atelectasis of the lobe. Because of the absence of adhesions, the upper lobe was able to retract mesially and its space was taken up by hyperexpansion of the middle and lower lobes. The trachea was therefore not displaced.

much more marked negative pressure in the pleural cavity than does a slow, prolonged inspiration, particularly in the presence of bronchial obstruction. The important factor which makes the mediastinal shift apparent is not the depth of inspiration but the suddenness with which the inspiration is performed. This is the reason for having the patient sniff when lateral movement of the mediastinum is being observed fluoroscopically.

If the atelectatic upper lobe is bound to the chest wall by adhesions, the middle and lower lobes cannot overexpand to compensate for the volume relinquished by the upper lobe. In this

event, a considerable shift of the mediastinum will occur (Fig. 73B). In the presence of such adhesions it is characteristic for the trachea to become more or less sharply angulated towards the side of the atelectatic lobe. In unusual cases, the trachea and the vessels in the superior mediastinum show only moderate displacement despite marked shrinkage of an adherent upper lobe. Instead, there is a marked displacement or herniation of the anterior portion of the left upper lobe into the mesial part of the right upper chest. This occurs in those instances in which the anterosuperior mediastinum is very thin and consists almost entirely of the two parietal pleural layers which are practically in contact with each other, and when the anterior mesial part of the chest is free of adhesions. The roentgen film then shows a curved, linear shadow, convex to the right, a short distance to the right of the sternum and extending from the clavicle to the level of the middle lobe. Mesial to this line the aerated appendage of the left upper lobe, which has crossed the midline, obliterates the shadow of the atelectatic right upper lobe in this region. Examination in the lateral view in these cases shows the upper anterior mediastinum to be abnormally well aerated (Fig. 81). The right lung root is elevated to a variable degree.

The shadow of an atelectatic right upper lobe merges with the shadow of the anterosuperior mediastinum. The right border of the mediastinum, which corresponds to the outer border of the superior vena cava, is then either poorly demarcated or not visible at all.

LEFT UPPER LOBE. The roentgen appearance of an atelectatic left upper lobe differs from that of atelectasis of the right upper lobe because of the absence of the short fissure and the presence of a lingular segment on the left side. A veil-like shadow is seen over the upper part of the chest, from the mediastinum to the upper axillary region. Often this shadow occupies only the mesial part of the chest adjacent to the upper border of the heart. When the lobe is not bound by adhesions, it collapses toward the root of the lung. The veil-like shadow of the lobe is then seen primarily in the perihilar region. The uppermost part of the chest is occupied by the superior segment of the hyperexpanded lower lobe. Blood vessels ascending from the lung root, seen in the shadow of the collapsed lobe, belong to the lower lobe behind it (Fig. 82).

Because the left upper lobe is situated adjacent to the mediastinum, when it becomes atelectatic its shadow merges with those of the main pulmonary artery and the upper part of the heart

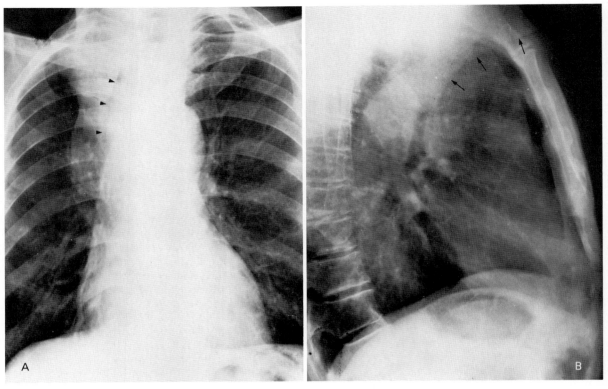

FIG. 81. ATELECTASIS OF RIGHT UPPER LOBE

A: Frontal view. The homogeneous, sharply circumscribed density adjacent to the right border of the mediastinum is associated with evidence of hyperinflation of the right lung and herniation of the anterior lappet of the left upper lobe (arrows) across the midline. These findings indicate atelectasis of the right upper lobe with compensatory hyperinflation of the remainder of the lung. The lobe was able to retract mesially toward the mediastinum because there were no adhesions to the lateral chest wall. The fact that the ascending aorta is seen within the shadow indicates that the lobe has also retracted posteriorly. The apex of the lobe is fixed by adhesions. *B:* Lateral view. The atelectasis of the upper lobe is not apparent. The anterior mediastinum is abnormally lucent because of herniation of the left upper lobe. The curvilinear shadow (arrows) extends beyond the chest and represents the lower border of the arm. Bronchoscopy revealed an obstructing carcinoma of the right upper lobe bronchus.

and obscures their borders (Fig. 83). If the long fissure is held in place by adhesions, the aortic knob is also obscured. However, when there are adhesions over only the anterior surface of the upper lobe and its mediastinal surface is free, the entire lobe may be displaced anterior to the aortic arch. The aortic knob is then outlined within the shadow of the contracted left upper lobe (see Fig. 420).

As with atelectasis of the right upper lobe, the lung root is somewhat elevated and, if there are adhesions immobilizing the outer portion of the lobe, the trachea becomes sharply angulated to the left. In the absence of such adhesions, the trachea may not be displaced although there is usually some bowing toward the left side.

In more highly penetrated films, the left main bronchus can be seen to pursue a more horizontal course than normal. This alteration in the course

of the left main bronchus is particularly apparent when the mediastinal structures are fixed by adhesions or neoplastic involvement. The tracheobronchial angle then becomes a sweeping curve as the distal portion of the left main bronchus is bent perpendicular to the trachea (Fig. 84).

If there are extensive adhesions over the lower part of the lobe, the lingular segment cannot retract upward and remains in its normal position in contact with the anterior portion of the diaphragm. This may create the impression on the frontal film that the left lower lobe is also involved. Examination in the lateral view will practically always clearly demonstrate that the abnormal shadow is due solely to atelectasis of the left upper lobe. If there are no adhesions over the anterior surface of the lobe, the anterior lappet of the right upper lobe can overexpand

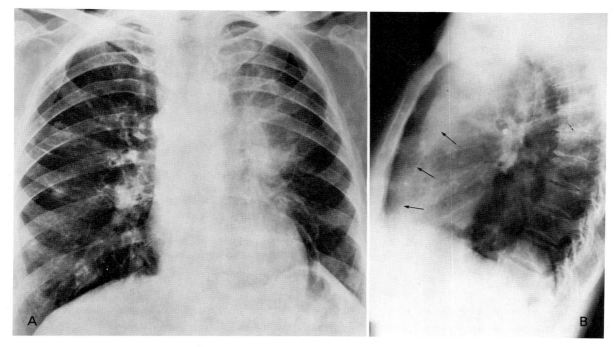

FIG. 82. ATELECTASIS OF LEFT UPPER LOBE

A: There is a veil-like shadow over the upper inner part of the left lung. The left hilum, which is seen through the shadow, is elevated. These changes are indicative of atelectasis of the left upper lobe in the absence of pleural adhesions. The aortic knob is visualized because the lobe had retracted anteriorly as it collapsed. The vessels visualized within the shadow belong to the overexpanded left lower lobe. Multiple small nodular densities are present in the right lung. The atelectasis was due to endobronchial metastasis from a carcinoma of the colon which also produced metastases in the right lung. *B*: Lateral view. The collapsed left upper lobe is represented by a tongue-like shadow in the upper part of the chest. Its posterior border is formed by the long fissure (arrows) which is bowed forward. Behind this the hyperinflated lower lobe can be seen extending to the dome of the thorax. The clear space between the collapsed lobe and the sternum is due to herniation of the anterior lappet of the right upper lobe. In this case the lingula was free of adhesions and retracted into the upper part of the chest.

and herniate across the anterior mediastinum. This creates a clear dark area just behind the sternum and in front of the white atelectatic left upper lobe which has become flattened from before backward in "pancake" fashion (Fig. 83). The collapsed left upper lobe then appears as a long, band-like shadow running downward and forward, sharply demarcated anteriorly by the overexpanded right lung and posteriorly by the long fissure and overexpanded left lower lobe.

If the anterior surface of the left upper lobe is adherent to the chest wall, herniation of the right upper lobe is prevented and the clear space in the upper anterior mediastinum, normally seen on the lateral view, is clouded by the airless left upper lobe. The long fissure is then displaced even more markedly forward and there is a corresponding anterior displacement of the trachea (see Fig. 186).

MIDDLE LOBE. The atelectatic middle lobe casts a characteristic shadow on the frontal view only when the short fissure, at its upper border,

is held in place by adhesions. The lobe then casts a triangular, rather homogeneous shadow which becomes fainter as it extends downward. Its upper border, represented by the short fissure, is sharply outlined and courses horizontally at the level of the anterior part of the fourth rib (Fig. 85). The base of the triangle is situated alongside the right cardiac border, usually reaching the diaphragm. The lower border extends upward and outward from the region of the cardiophrenic angle toward the axilla to meet the short fissure at a variable distance from the lateral chest wall, depending on the degree of contraction of the lobe and the presence of parietal adhesions. This lower border is poorly outlined on the frontal view.

A triangular right paracardiac shadow with a normal appearance of the lower outer portion of the pulmonary field is rather characteristic of middle lobe disease. The mesial border of the triangular shadow merges with the shadow of the heart and tends to obliterate this portion of the

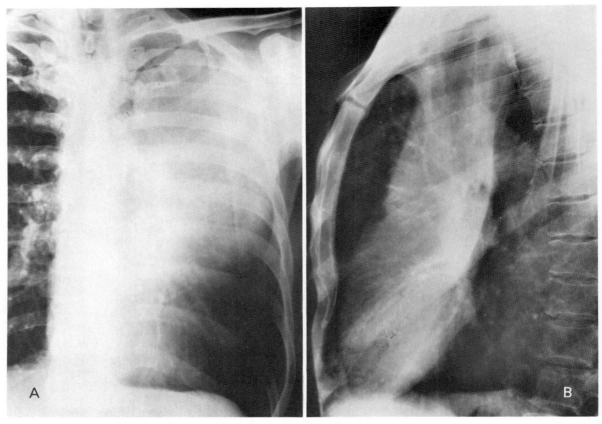

FIG. 83. LOBAR ATELECTASIS: PANCAKED LEFT UPPER LOBE

A: There is a homogeneous shadow over the upper part of the left chest through which the pulmonary vessels are faintly outlined. The heart is shifted slightly to the left and the left cardiac border is obliterated by the opacified lung. *B*: The oblique band-like density is characteristic of collapse of the left upper lobe when there are adhesions between the lingula and the diaphragm. The clear space behind the sternum is due to a herniation of the anterior lappet of the right upper lobe across the mediastinum. The upper portion of the long fissure is displaced forward so that the lower lobe, which has undergone compensatory emphysema, extends almost to the dome of the thoracic cavity. The patient had a carcinoma obstructing the left upper lobe bronchus.

cardiac silhouette. Disease of the lower lobe can cast a shadow in the same general region on the frontal film but the cardiac border remains sharply delineated by the contrasting air in the middle lobe.

If the short fissure is not held in place by adhesions, its anterior border is displaced downward and forward by contraction of the middle lobe, while the posterior part of the fissure is held in place by the pleural reflection at the root of the lobe. This causes the entire plane of the fissure to slant sharply downward (Fig. 12). On the ordinary posteroanterior view, the rays are no longer parallel to the fissure. They cross it from behind forward so that the upper part of the shadow cast by the atelectatic lobe represents only the thin, posterior upper portion of the lobe, and is not sharply outlined. The shadow

increases in density for a distance below the upper border and then gradually fades out again as the thin lower portion of the lobe is traversed. The shadow of the collapsed middle lobe, in the absence of fixation of the short fissure, is, therefore, faint and not so characteristic. However, it usually still maintains a roughly triangular shape with the base toward the poorly delineated right cardiac border. This appearance should always suggest the presence of atelectasis of the middle lobe. Occasionally, particularly when there is little active inflammation, the collapsed middle lobe becomes completely flattened and casts little or no shadow on the frontal projection. The only abnormality noted in this view may simply be poor delineation of the right cardiac border (silhouette sign of Felson). The fact that this is caused by atelectasis of the middle lobe can be

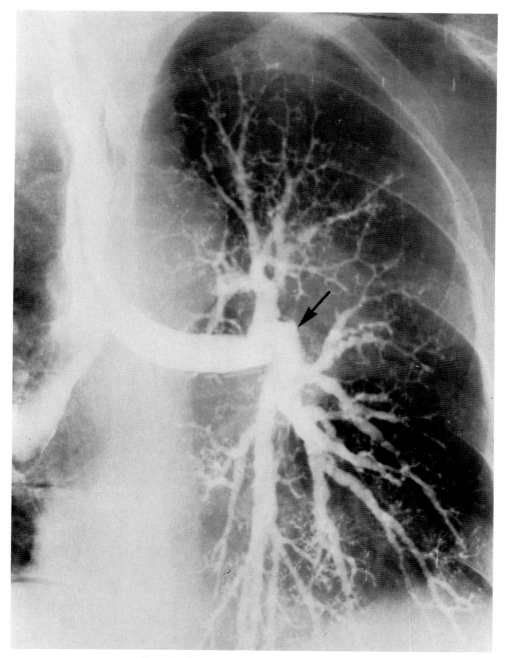

FIG. 84. ATELECTASIS OF LEFT UPPER LOBE

The bronchogram shows complete occlusion of the left upper lobe bronchus (arrow). The shadow at the hilum represents the completely collapsed lobe. This has resulted in elevation of the left main bronchus so that it pursues an almost horizontal course. The bronchial branches extending to the dome of the left hemithorax belong to the hyperexpanded superior segment of the left lower lobe.

demonstrated on other views. Obliteration of only the lower part of the cardiac contour can be caused by atelectasis of the mesial segment of the middle lobe while the upper portion of the cardiac contour is clearly delineated by the hy-perexpanded adjacent lateral segment.

The characteristic appearance of an atelectatic middle lobe may be obtained in the frontal projection if the lordotic position is used (Fig. 16). With the patient facing the cassette, his body is

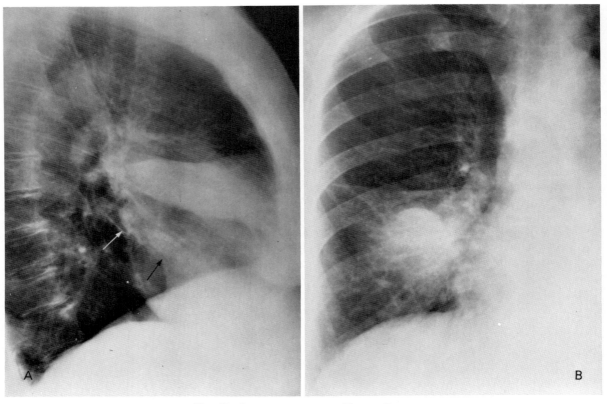

FIG. 85. ATELECTASIS OF THE MIDDLE LOBE

A: Lateral view. The triangular shadow represents the collapsed middle lobe. The density of the shadow is due to inflammation as well as atelectasis. Except for a slight downward bowing in its midportion, the short fissure maintains its normal position. The long fissure which forms the lower border of the shadow is considerably elevated. The long fissure on the left side (arrows) is seen in its normal position. B: Frontal view. The collapsed middle lobe is represented by a hazy shadow which obscures the right cardiac border and is sharply delimited by the short fissure. The normal position of the short fissure indicates that it is fixed to the chest wall both anteriorly and laterally. The area of increased density within the shadow was caused by an abscess.

inclined slightly backward thus separating the upper part of the chest from the film, and the tube is elevated. This directs the rays downward and forward, so that they are parallel to the short fissure which has been inclined in the same direction by the contraction of the middle lobe. The upper border of the shadow then becomes sharply outlined. In addition, since the rays are also more parallel to the long fissure in this projection, the lower border also becomes sharply demarcated. The roentgen appearance, then, of the collapsed middle lobe in the lordotic position, is that of a sharply outlined triangular density with a foreshortened base adjacent to the heart with its apex mesial to the axillary border of the chest.

The most characteristic representation of the atelectatic middle lobe is produced by examination in the lateral position. In this view, the rays are parallel to both the long and short fissures, regardless of any change in their inclination. A sharply outlined silhouette of the middle lobe is, therefore, obtained. This consists of a triangular shadow with the apex at the origin of the middle lobe bronchus from the intermediate bronchus, the two sides diverging from this point downward and forward to the anterior border of the chest (see Fig. 136). The width of the triangle varies with the degree of atelectasis. In complete atelectasis of the right middle lobe, the triangular shadow may measure only 1 cm in its widest portion adjacent to the lower part of the sternum (Fig. 12).

It may be difficult to differentiate the shadow of a collapsed middle lobe from an interlobar effusion even on the lateral view. Useful in the differentiation is the fact that an interlobar effusion, which represents an expanding lesion, widens either the long or the short fissure in a bulging manner. The bulging borders produce a

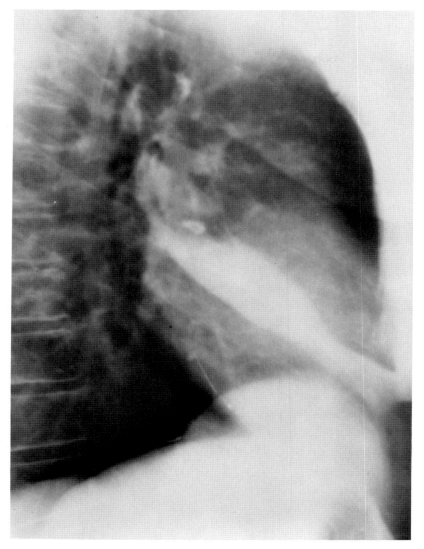

FIG. 86. INTERCALATED MIDDLE LOBE

The lateral view of the chest shows a spindle-shaped density in the region of the long fissure. The appearance suggests an interlobar effusion. However, there is no thickening of the upper portion of the long fissure or of the short fissure, making this diagnosis unlikely. The shadow was due to a completely collapsed middle lobe which had retracted from the anterior chest wall. The atelectasis was secondary to a broncholith which can be identified in the region of the orifice of the middle lobe bronchus.

more or less fusiform shadow. On the other hand, the shadow of a collapsed middle lobe has straight or concave borders which diverge in an anterior and downward direction. Extension of the shadow more posteriorly than the position of the root of the middle lobe is indicative of an interlobar effusion.

An additional aid in differentiation between an interlobar effusion and a collapsed middle lobe is the fact that a loculated interlobar effusion is necessarily associated with pleural adhesions.

These interlobar adhesions usually are visible at both the upper and lower borders of the middle lobe on the lateral view. The aerated middle lobe is well outlined by them and this permits the effusion, whether in the short or long fissure, to be easily recognized (see Fig. 534).

If the middle lobe collapses completely, in the absence of adhesions to any of the surrounding structures, the lobe may retract toward the lung root (Fig. 86). The collapsed lobe then becomes completely surrounded by the upper lobe in front and by the lower lobe behind. Below and anterior to it is the long pulmonary fissure which now connects the lower surface of the upper lobe with the anterior surface of the lower lobe. Because of the displacement of the middle lobe from its normal position adjacent to the heart, the cardiac border is no longer obscured as it generally is when the middle lobe or its mesial segment is collapsed.

This rare type of contracted middle lobe may be called an *intercalated lobe,* since it is hidden within the lung by the junction of the short and long fissures connecting the upper and lower lobes in front of it. The intercalated, collapsed middle lobe presents on the lateral view as a fusiform shadow which is indistinguishable from an interlobar effusion in the lower part of the long fissure. However, the absence of a demonstrable short fissure, ordinarily present with such an interlobar effusion, should lead one to suspect the possibility of collapse of the middle lobe. If there is no apparent cause for an interlobar effusion in such a case, an obstruction of the middle lobe bronchus should be suspected.

Middle Lobe Syndrome. This term was originated by Graham to indicate a vicious cycle characterized by atelectasis and infection of the middle lobe and adenitis of the regional nodes. He considered that there was compression of the middle lobe bronchus by large lymph nodes which were inflamed as a result of a pneumonia of this lobe. The obstruction of the bronchus led to persistence or recurrence of the middle lobe pneumonia which then perpetuated the lymphadenitis and middle lobe obstruction. He was able to relieve the obstruction and the atelectasis and infection by removal of the offending lymph nodes in one of his cases.

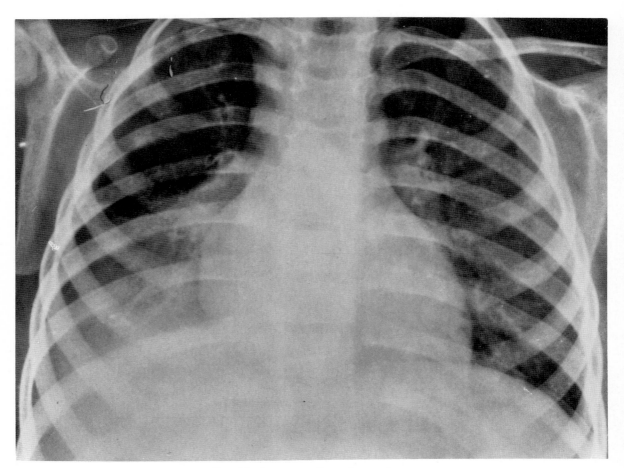

FIG. 87. COLLAPSED RIGHT LOWER LOBE

There is a veil-like shadow over the right lower lobe. This obscures the contour of the right hemidiaphragm but not the right cardiac border. The upper portion of the right lung is hyperlucent. These findings indicate atelectasis of the lower lobe. Obstruction of the lower lobe bronchus was due to aspiration of a pencil eraser.

The syndrome, as described by Graham, must be exceedingly rare. Cases presenting with atelectasis and recurring infection of the middle lobe, together with bronchial obstruction, have almost uniformly been associated with a permanent obstructive lesion. When due to inflammatory disease, the obstruction, in the cases we have observed, was caused by a stricture of the bronchus. While this was undoubtedly secondary to inflammation of the adjacent lymph nodes, the bronchial narrowing was the result of partial destruction of the bronchial wall with scarring, rather than simply extrinsic pressure of inflamed nodes. Under such circumstances it is more accurate to speak of bronchial stricture with secondary middle lobe atelectasis and pneumonia than to use the term "middle lobe syndrome," which should be confined to the rare condition described by Graham.

RIGHT LOWER LOBE. The appearance of an atelectatic right lower lobe depends largely on the completeness of its collapse. When the atelectasis is moderate, only a faint shadow is seen over the region of the lobe, more dense near the diaphragm (Fig. 87) and becoming imperceptible in the region of the apex of the lobe and inter-

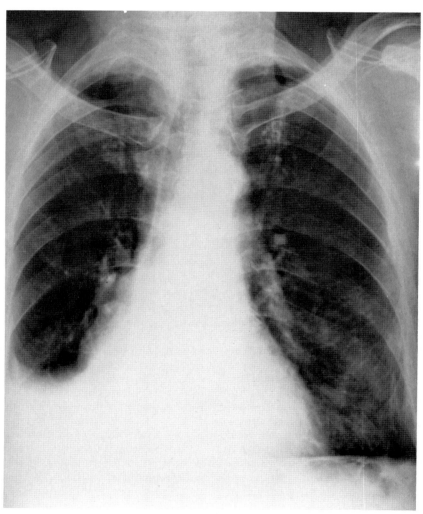

FIG. 88. STENOSING CARCINOMA OF RIGHT LOWER LOBE BRONCHUS

There is an effusion at the right base, largely obscuring the lower part of the right lung. However, the diagonal course of the trachea which is in line with the right lower lobe bronchus indicates atelectasis of the right lower lobe. Bronchoscopy showed the bronchus to be occluded by a small-cell carcinoma. At necropsy, this was found to have invaded the pleura and there was extensive involvement of the lymph nodes at the root of the right lung. The obliteration of the left costophrenic sinus and the shadows over the left lower lobe are due to pleural adhesions from previous inflammatory disease.

scapular region. The lack of density in this region is due to the thinness of this portion of the lobe and the overlying upper and middle lobes which are well aerated and hyperexpanded. A faint, veil-like shadow on the frontal view, and a slight posterior and downward displacement of the long fissure on the lateral view may be the only noticeable changes. A lowering of the right lung root makes the diagnosis of atelectasis clear.

As the atelectasis becomes more complete, the right lung root becomes more depressed and the course of the trachea and right main bronchus is altered. These structures become aligned along a continuous diagonal outward and downward course (Fig. 88). The heart may be displaced slightly or not at all, but on fluoroscopy it may be seen to shift to the right on inspiration, particularly on sniffing. The right leaf of the diaphragm is apt to be elevated only if there is complete atelectasis of the right lower lobe, but even then the elevation is only slight.

The elevation of the diaphragm and the displacement of the heart to the right are more marked when both the middle and lower lobes are collapsed. The right cardiac border is then poorly demarcated and the diaphragm is usually so obscured that no part of its border can be seen (Fig. 89).

The downward displacement of the posterior part of the long fissure, which occurs in the case of the more completely collapsed lower lobe, is sometimes evident in the frontal view, particularly if the x-ray tube is high. The fissure can be more sharply outlined by having the patient assume the lordotic position while he is facing the film.

The long fissure shifts in accordance with the degree of atelectasis and the presence or absence of pleural adhesions. If there is complete adhesion of the lower surface of the lobe to the diaphragm, the lobe becomes contracted from above downward. The long fissure then becomes more horizontal so that it can be seen on the frontal projection. The completely collapsed lower lobe has a sharply outlined upper border and the shadow of the dense, airless lobe beneath this border merges with that of the diaphragm and the liver. This produces an appearance which is easily confused with that of an elevated diaphragm or an infrapulmonary effusion. Often the collapsed lower lobe may be identified on the lateral view because of the relation of its shadow to the fissures.

If the outer part of the collapsed lower lobe is adherent to the chest wall, the lateral costophrenic sinus is obliterated, and the appearance on the frontal projection is easily confused with that of a pleural effusion. On the lateral view, however, the shadow of the collapsed lower lobe is seen to be bounded anteriorly by the sharp line of the long fissure which is frequently bowed backward. If the lobe is only partially atelectatic, there may be no increased density, and the only manifestation may be the posterior curve of the long fissure on the lateral projection.

In the absence of adhesions, the long fissure is free to change its position. When the lower lobe becomes collapsed, the fissure may be displaced directly backward, but more frequently it rotates posteriorly about the axis formed by the pulmonary ligament which fixes the mesial portion of the lobe. With complete collapse, the fissure rotates almost 90 degrees and the lobe flattens against the spine. The fissure is practically parallel to the x-ray beam on the frontal projection, and is seen in this view as an oblique line running from the root of the lung downward and outward to the diaphragm. The lobe then appears as a triangular density bounded mesially by the spine, below by the diaphragm, and laterally by the long fissure (Fig. 90). Since the plane of the fissure is now almost perpendicular to the rays on the lateral view, it is no longer visible on this projection. Moreover, since the lobe is pancaked against the spine, it casts very little shadow. The only evidence of atelectasis on the lateral view may be some increase in the density of the shadows of the lower dorsal vertebrae and loss of the silhouette of the posterior portion of the diaphragm (Figs. 91 and 194).

If there is only partial rotation of the fissure, it cannot be visualized on either the frontal or lateral projection, and all that is seen in these views is a hazy, poorly demarcated shadow, suggesting a pneumonia. That the shadow is due to a collapsed lower lobe can be determined by examination in the oblique view in which the x-ray beam is parallel to the partially rotated fissure. In the case of atelectasis of the right lower lobe, this will be the left anterior oblique or the right posterior oblique projection (Fig. 92).

If the fissure is not rotated, but simply displaced backward, possibly because of adhesions on the posterior surface of the lobe, or if the lobe is only slightly collapsed, the fissure remains sharply outlined on the lateral view. It maintains its oblique course parallel to and behind its normal position, extending from the root of the lung to about the midportion of the diaphragm (Fig. 69).

LEFT LOWER LOBE. Practically everything that has been said concerning atelectasis of the right lower lobe applies to the left lower lobe as well. However, the mesial basal triangular

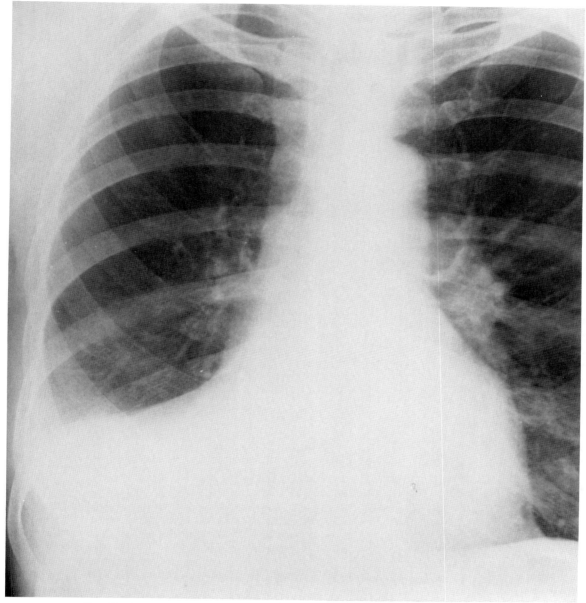

FIG. 89. ATELECTASIS OF RIGHT LOWER AND MIDDLE LOBES: BRONCHIAL CARCINOMA

The homogeneous density at the right base has a sharply outlined upper border which runs obliquely upward toward the mediastinum. The border of the diaphragm and the right side of the heart are obscured. The right lung root is depressed and is partly hidden by the heart, which is displaced to the right. The vessels in the upper part of the right lung are thinner than those on the left. The shadow at the right base is caused by atelectasis of the middle and lower lobes. The thinning of the vessels in the upper part of the right lung is due to obstructive emphysema of the right upper lobe. Bronchoscopy disclosed a carcinoma completely obstructing the intermediate bronchus and partly obstructing the bronchus to the right upper lobe.

shadow representing a completely atelectatic left lower lobe on the frontal view, may not be visible on insufficiently exposed films because it is hidden by the heart (Fig. 93). The typical triangular density is clearly visualized through the shadow of the heart on films made with proper exposure (See Fig. 209). If the fissure is partly rotated, the frontal projection will disclose only a faint increase in the density of the left side of the cardiac shadow together with obscuration of the blood vessels in this region. There is simply a condensation of the retrocardiac vascular shadows when

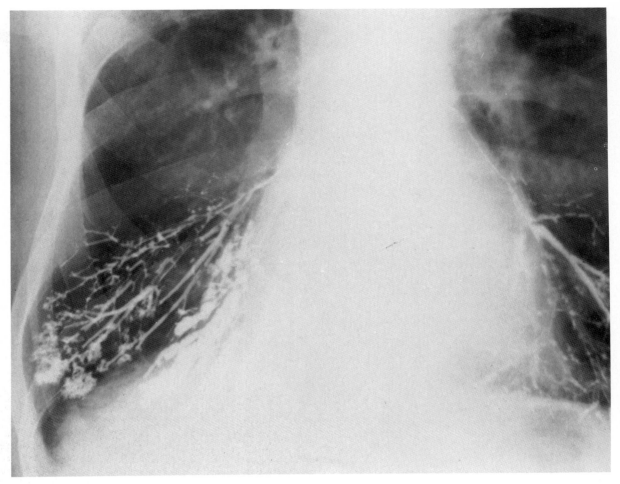

FIG. 90. BRONCHIECTASIS, RIGHT LOWER LOBE

The patient had an atelectatic, suppurative bronchopneumonia which produced a dense, triangular shadow in the right cardiophrenic angle. The shadow persisted after resolution of the pneumonia. Bronchography reveals cylindrical dilatation of the right lower lobe bronchi. Obliteration of their branches was responsible for the atelectasis of the lobe and the approximation of its bronchi. The normal bronchi in the region of the costophrenic sinus belong to the middle lobe which has shifted to fill in the space relinquished by the lower lobe.

the lobe is only partially collapsed. With partial rotation of the fissure, the triangular shadow of the lobe is visualized only on films made in the right anterior or left posterior oblique position.

COMBINED MIDDLE AND LOWER LOBE ATELECTASIS. When both lobes are collapsed, the appearance is quite similar to that of a pleural effusion. The right leaf of the diaphragm and the right cardiac border are obscured, but although the shadow reaches the lateral chest wall, it does not extend upward as in most cases of pleural effusion. The upper border of the shadow is fairly well demarcated, but usually is higher in its mesial than its lateral portion (Fig. 91). The short fissure, instead of being horizontal, slopes downward and outward. The heart and mediastinal structures are displaced to the right. The trachea pursues a straight, oblique, downward and outward course in contradistinction to the curve or angulation that occurs in atelectasis of the right upper lobe. The tracheal displacement is much more marked than that which occurs in atelectasis of the right lower lobe alone. The root of the lung, which is depressed, is hidden by the shadow of the collapsed lobes. Increased lucency of the upper lobe, which is due to compensatory emphysema, indicates that the shadow over the lower part of the chest is due to atelectasis.

Segmental Atelectasis. Complete obstruction of a main bronchus or a lobar bronchus almost always results in atelectasis, since the air in the lung distal to the obstruction is absorbed

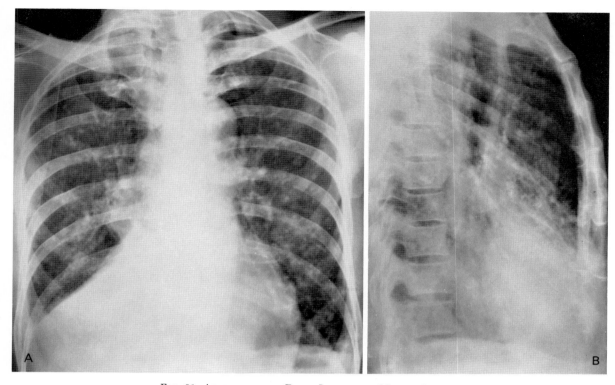

FIG. 91. ATELECTASIS OF RIGHT LOWER AND MIDDLE LOBES

A: Frontal view. The right leaf of the diaphragm and the right cardiac border are obscured by a homogeneous triangular density at the base of the lung. The right hilum is obscured by a mass. There are numerous small nodules throughout both lungs. These represent metastases from a hypernephroma. Metastasis to the intermediate bronchus was responsible for the atelectasis of the right middle and lower lobes. *B*: The lateral view shows relatively little compared to the frontal projection. However, only one diaphragmatic leaf can be identified and the lower vertebral bodies are denser than the ones immediately above them. These findings are indicative of disease of the lower lobe or an effusion.

and there is no way for air to bypass the occluded bronchus. Atelectasis does not occur, however, when the obstruction is in a segmental bronchus or one of its branches so long as the respiratory movements are free and the lung beyond the point of obstruction is not diseased. While the affected lung cannot receive air through its bronchus, it can be ventilated from the neighboring segments by way of the pores of Kohn through which the alveoli communicate with each other and, possibly, by way of small bronchiolar communications. If there is inflammation or congestion and edema of the lung distal to the obstruction, the alveolar communications become closed, the air in the obstructed segment is not renewed, and it then becomes atelectatic as the air within it is absorbed. The presence of segmental atelectasis, therefore, suggests some complicating factor in the affected portion of the lung.

Generally speaking, atelectasis of a pulmonary segment is recognized by a condensation of the shadows of the vessels within the segment. These are not spread out as far as they are under normal circumstances and do not fan out on inspiration (see Fig. 363). The density of the shadow cast by the affected area depends on the completeness of the atelectasis and the extent of infiltration or consolidation of the lung. When the segment is only partially atelectatic and the infiltration is not extensive, the shadow is faint.

The position and the shape of the shadow of an atelectatic segment depend on the particular segment that is involved. A thorough knowledge of the anatomy of the bronchopulmonary segments and their location on the films is essential for identification of the involved segment.

The segments of the lung are wedge-shaped, widening as they extend from the root to the periphery of the lobe. However, the roentgen projection does not correspond to this on all views. Thus, a segment whose bronchi are directed either anteriorly or posteriorly will not appear wedge-shaped on the frontal view but will

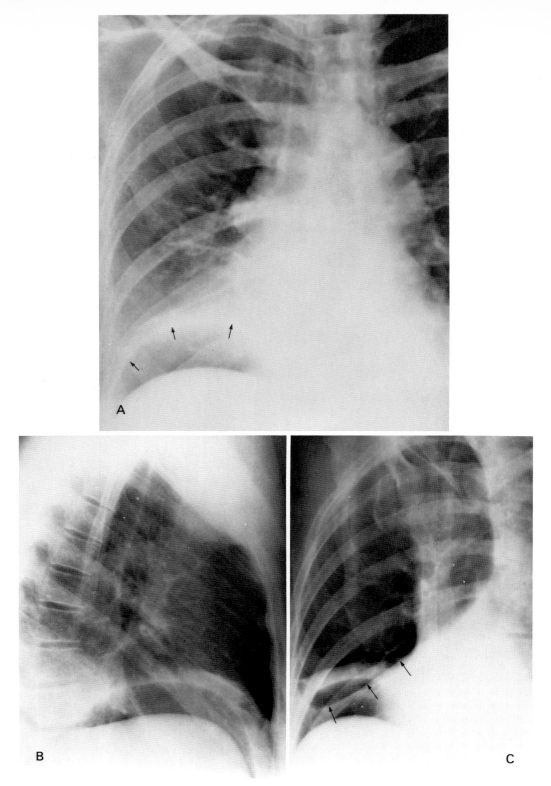

FIG. 92. ATELECTASIS OF THE RIGHT LOWER LOBE

The films were made following removal of a kidney for transplantation. Air is still present in the peritoneal cavity. *A*: Frontal view. There is a hazy density at the right base which obscures the upper border of the diaphragm. The border of the density is hazy. The appearance is most suggestive of a pneumonia. The undersurface of the diaphragm (arrows) and the upper border of the liver are outlined by the air in the peritoneal cavity. *B*: Lateral view. The disease in the lower lobe appears to be confined to the posterior basal portion. The density over the anterior portion of the diaphragm is caused by atelectasis of the adjacent portion of the middle lobe. *C*: Left oblique view. The true shape and extent of the lesion in the lower lobe is now evident. The picture is that of atelectasis of the entire lower lobe. The border of the shadow is sharply outlined and corresponds to the long fissure (arrows) which is displaced downward and backward. The anterior border of the right diaphragm is projected above the lower part of the fissure and is outlined by the atelectatic portion of the middle lobe. The atelectasis was due to a mucous plug which caused bronchial obstruction. The lung reexpanded promptly after bronchial suction.

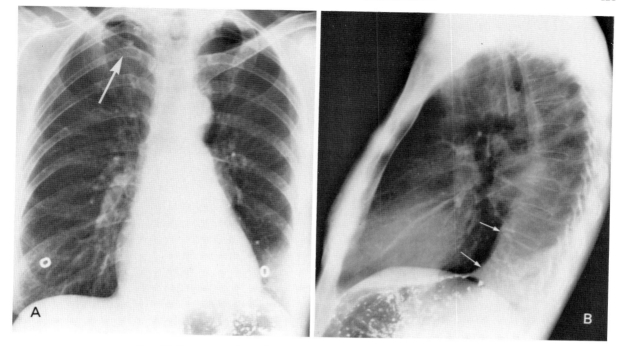

FIG. 93. SQUAMOUS CELL CARCINOMA OF LEFT LOWER LOBE BRONCHUS

A: On the frontal film, the cardiac shadow appears abnormally dense and the vascular markings of the left lower lobe cannot be visualized. The left lung root is displaced downward. These findings indicate atelectasis of the left lower lobe. The typical triangular shadow of an atelectatic lower lobe cannot be seen within the cardiac silhouette because it is not sufficiently penetrated. There is a pathologic fracture of the medial portion of the right clavicle (arrow). *B*: Lateral view. There is marked posterior displacement of the long fissure (arrow) and obscuration of the posterior portion of the left diaphragm due to the collapsed, airless lower lobe.

on the lateral projection. To demonstrate the triangular shape of any particular segment, it is necessary to position the patient so that the plane of the base of the segment is parallel to the rays. The long axis of the segment will then be aligned perpendicular to the rays and parallel to the plane of the x-ray film.

The views in which the narrow, wedge-shaped shadows of atelectasis in the various segments are demonstrated best are: the posteroanterior view for the apical segment and the axillary portion of the anterior segment of the upper lobes (Fig. 94), the lateral segment of the middle lobe and the anterior basal, posterior basal and mesial segments of the lower lobe. On the lateral view, the triangular shadow is best seen in atelectasis of the posterior segments and the pectoral portion of the anterior segment of the upper lobes, the lingular segments, the superior segment of the lower lobes, the anterior basal segment of the lower lobes (Fig. 69), and the posterior basal segment of the lower lobes. The triangular shadow of atelectasis of the mesial segment of the right lower lobe is also well depicted on the lateral view. The oblique views are best for disclosing the characteristic shape of atelectasis

of the lateral basal segment of the lower lobe and the subscapular portion of the posterior segment of the upper lobe. The right lateral basal segment, which has its parietal representation in the right posterior axillary line, is best observed in the right oblique view and the left lateral basal segment is best seen in the left oblique view. The anterior segments of the upper lobes are often more clearly demonstrated in the oblique views than on any other projection. The anterior segment of the right upper lobe is best seen in the left oblique and the anterior segment of the left upper lobe is best delineated in the right oblique projection.

The effect of segmental atelectasis on the pleural fissures and lung roots is often quite characteristic, especially when more than one adjacent segment is involved. Thus, in atelectasis of the posterior segment of the upper lobe, there usually is elevation of the posterior part of the long fissure, best seen on the lateral view. This is more marked when the apical segment is atelectatic as well. When both of these segments are shrunken, the vessels at the root of the lung are usually strikingly elevated. This occurs commonly in tuberculosis and it may be quite marked

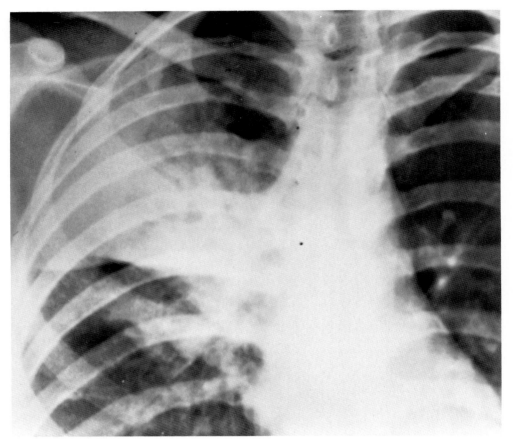

FIG. 94. ATELECTASIS IN CASEOUS PNEUMONIA

The dense, rather homogeneous shadow involving the lower two-thirds of the right upper lobe is due to a tuberculous pneumonia in the anterior segment and the outer, or subscapular, part of the posterior segment. The elevation of the short fissure indicates that the pneumonic lung is also partially atelectatic. Normally, this fissure, which separates the base of the anterior segment of the upper lobe from the middle lobe, is situated at the level of the anterolateral portion of the fourth rib. In this case it is projected at the level of the third rib. The density below the mesial part of the short fissure is due to consolidation of the superior segment of the right lower lobe.

even though the shadow of the lesion itself is hardly noticeable (Fig. 95).

In atelectasis of the pectoral portion of the anterior segment of the right upper lobe, the short fissure is almost always elevated. If the axillary part of this segment is involved as well, the outer portion of the fissure tends to become more elevated so that the fissure slants upward and outward (Figs. 96 and 226). If the lateral part of the short fissure is fixed to the chest wall by adhesions, the fissure becomes curved and bulges upward (Fig. 73B).

Considerable depression of the upper part of the long fissure occurs if the basal segments of the lower lobe are collapsed and the superior segment is not held in place by adhesions (see Fig. 237).

In atelectasis of the middle lobe, the short fissure is usually depressed, and on the lateral view it may be seen to course in a more downward and forward direction than under normal circumstances (Fig. 12). When the superior segment of the lower lobe is atelectatic, there is a depression of the upper part of the long fissure (Figs. 97 and 260). The entire long fissure may be displaced downward and backward if all of the basal segments are contracted, and this is usually accompanied by a depression of the lung root even though the apical and subapical segments are fully aerated (see Fig. 237).

Focal Atelectasis (Plate, Disc or Streak Atelectasis). As in the case of obstruction of the segmental bronchi, obstruction of their branches does not ordinarily cause atelectasis. The lung beyond the obstruction remains ventilated through communication with neighboring

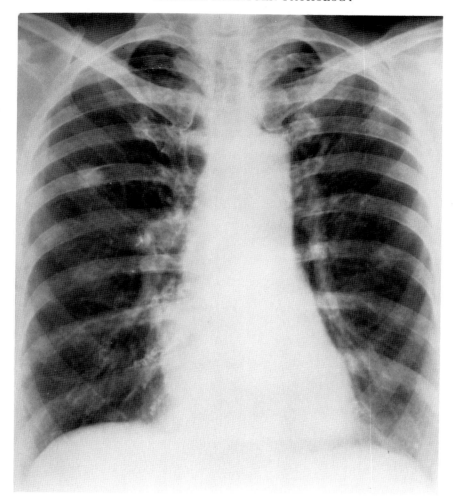

FIG. 95. ELEVATION OF LUNG ROOT

The left lung root is markedly elevated despite the lack of any significant density in the upper lobe. The displacement of the root is due to marked diminution in the volume of the apicoposterior segment, the result of an old tuberculous infection. The small, circumscribed nodule in the right upper lobe shows two crossing linear shadows. These are Fleischner lines and indicate that the nodule almost certainly represents a peripheral bronchogenic carcinoma. This diagnosis was confirmed at thoracotomy.

alveoli. However, when there is local interference with ventilation through these communications or a general diminution in the ventilation of the lungs, renewal of air in the involved region is prevented and a small focus of atelectasis results.

A focus of atelectasis in a portion of a segment is manifested radiologically by the presence of a horizontal or oblique, linear shadow (Figs. 98, 232 and 307). This has been referred to as streak, or discoid atelectasis. However, the term *focal atelectasis* is preferable as it indicates atelectasis of a small portion of a pulmonary segment. The streak-like shadows may be single or multiple, depending on the number of small bronchi that are occluded. They are most commonly situated in the lower lobes because obstructing secretion

is most apt to accumulate in the lower lobe bronchi. The edges of the lung are poorly aerated in patients whose breathing is limited. The atelectic streaks, therefore, are most frequently seen in the region of the costophrenic sinuses.

The significance of these streak-like shadows was first pointed out by Fleischner and they are therefore often called *Fleischner lines*. When a small portion of lung becomes atelectatic, it shrinks in length as well as in width and draws the overlying pleura inward (Fig. 99). The retraction of the pleura causes a puckering of the surface of the lung, clearly visible when the chest is first opened. It is apt to disappear when the lung is permitted to collapse but reappears when the lung is reinflated. The puckering consists of

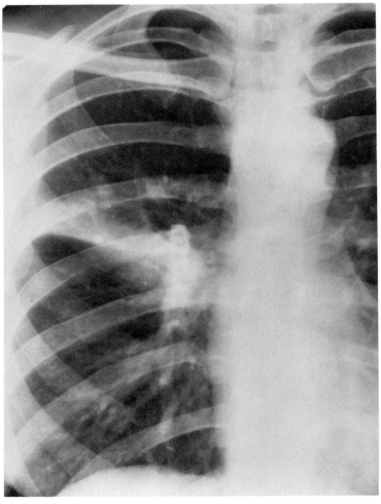

FIG. 96. BRONCHOLITHIASIS

The patient had recurrent attacks of fever and hemoptysis. The frontal film shows a narrow strip of homogeneous density abutting on the short fissure. This represents atelectasis and infection of the anterior segment of the right upper lobe. The short fissure is slightly elevated as a result of the collapse of the anterior segment. At the root of this segment there is an irregular calcific deposit representing a broncholith. Complete resolution took place after the stone was removed through the bronchoscope.

a groove or a combination of several crossing grooves dipping into the inflated lung. The grooves are lined by indrawn visceral pleura. When the newly formed fissure and the thin layer of condensed lung tissue adjacent to it lie parallel to the x-ray beam, they produce a sharply defined linear shadow, the Fleischner line. If the plane of the infolded pleura is at an angle to the rays, the lesion may not be visualized at all or may appear only as an extremely faint, poorly outlined density (see Fig. 402).

A tiny triangular shadow is occasionally visible at the distal extremity of a Fleischner line when the projection is such that the line extends to the border of the pulmonary field. This triangle is probably due to a small amount of exudate or fibrous tissue in the outer portion of the pleural groove (see Fig. 320). When there is an associated pleural effusion, a larger, well-demarcated triangular shadow may be formed by fluid which has entered into the newly formed fissure (Fig. 100). The shadow may disappear after the fluid has been aspirated or absorbed, leaving only the streak-like Fleischner line. In some cases, the triangular shadow may be visualized only in the recumbent position as the fluid shifts into the region of the atelectatic focus, disappearing when the fluid gravitates to the bottom of the chest as

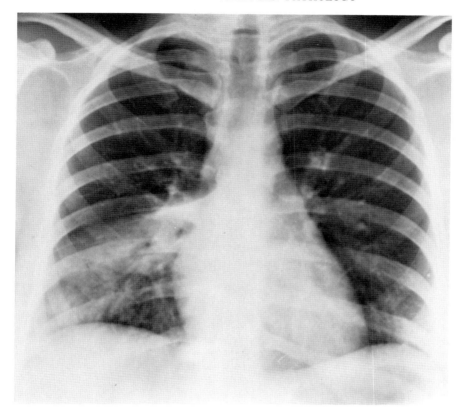

FIG. 97. LOWER LOBE TUBERCULOSIS

There is an area of dense consolidation involving the superior segment of the right lower lobe. The mesial portion of the long fissure which forms its upper border is depressed indicating that the segment is also atelectatic. There has been spread of the tuberculosis to the lateral basal segment which is stippled with acinar-nodose lesions.

the upright position is assumed.

Most focal atelectases are due to transitory obstruction of the bronchi or to obstruction associated with only a temporary disturbance in pulmonary ventilation. The streak-like shadows usually disappear within a comparatively short time (see Fig. 418), but in some cases they are permanent. The latter occurs particularly in destructive diseases such as suppurative bronchopneumonia, lung abscess, tuberculosis and bronchiectasis—conditions which are associated with destruction of bronchial branches and their occlusion by scar.

When there is an associated pleuritis, the indrawn pleural surfaces may become adherent and the streak-like shadow persists (Fig. 98). The permanent Fleischner line represents an adherent, newly formed fissure, together with an underlying atelectatic focus which cannot expand because of restriction by the fixed pleura. This is the cause of most of the permanent streaks at the base of the lung. Not infrequently this occurs as the result of pulmonary embolization or in-

farction (see Fig. 114). It is also the cause of many of the persistent streak-like shadows in the upper part of the lungs in tuberculosis. These may not be distinguishable from fibrosis of the tuberculous lung tissue.

If the area is only partly collapsed it is depicted on the film by a broader streak or by a small, wedge-shaped, faint shadow. Attention to the details within the shadow will show that the pulmonary vessels within it are closer together than they should be, and that they branch at a more acute angle than in corresponding parts of the normal lung.

Bilateral Diffuse Atelectasis. This occurs in stillbirths and in the newborn who has not drawn a breath, possibly because of an intracranial injury or some other abnormality resulting in respiratory paralysis. The same picture can result from obstruction of the trachea and main bronchi by meconium. Aside from these instances atelectasis of both lungs is never complete, because the patient dies of respiratory failure before this can take place.

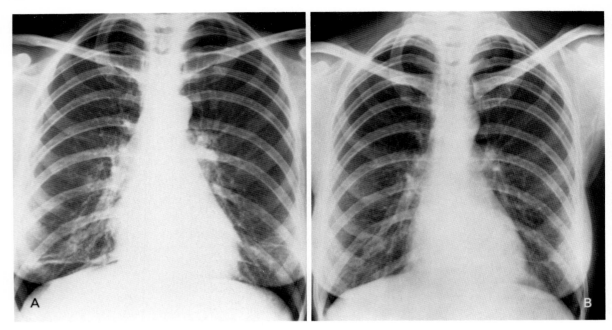

FIG. 98. FOCAL ATELECTASIS

A: The horizontal streaks at the base of each lung represent focal areas of atelectasis. The term "Fleischner lines" is commonly used to denote the atelectatic streaks. In this case, the atelectatic foci were due to plugging of small bronchi in the course of a bronchiolitis. *B*: A film made several years later shows all the streaks except one at the left base to have disappeared. The persistence of the streak indicates that fibrosis has taken place so that the atelectasis is permanent.

Incomplete atelectasis in both lungs may result from massive pulmonary or bronchial hemorrhage. In such cases asphyxia from obstruction of the main bronchi by blood clot is the usual cause of death rather than exsanguination. In the nonfatal cases, films made during the course of the hemoptysis often show poor aeration of the lungs with numerous focal areas of diminished lucency. The latter are due partly to extravasation of blood into the alveoli and partly to multiple areas of atelectasis.

A generalized diminution in the aeration of the lungs occurs in lymphangitic carcinosis. Here, the partial atelectasis of the lung is due to the interlacing cords of carcinoma tissue in the lymphatics (see Fig. 411), which prevent the lungs from expanding during inspiration. A similarly diffuse atelectasis, but of more focal distribution, is present in diffuse bronchiolitis. This is seen most frequently in association with tracheobronchitis, particularly in children. The lungs appear to be less lucent than normal. However, careful inspection of the film shows that the diffuse lessening of illumination is really due to the presence of innumerable, minute areas of clouding which represent tiny foci of atelectasis. Between these foci are areas of increased illumination due to emphysema. If the atelectasis predominates, then the pulmonary field appears grayer than normal, whereas if emphysematous areas dominate, the lung fields, on casual examination, appear hyperilluminated.

HYPERINFLATION

Hyperinflation of the lung denotes only overdistention of the alveoli. This is in contrast to the disease emphysema in which destruction of alveolar septa is a prominent feature. Rupture of alveolar septa rarely occurs in hyperinflation unless the overdistention is severe and then only scattered alveoli are affected.

Hyperinflation of the lung may be divided into three categories: that which occurs in the aged (usually called senile emphysema), the type secondary to atelectasis of a lung or part of a lung (compensatory emphysema), and finally, that which results from partial obstruction of the larger air passages (obstructive emphysema).

Senile Emphysema. In senile emphysema the lungs are moderately enlarged. The alveolar septa are atrophic and stretched. While the alveolar walls are ruptured in places, this change

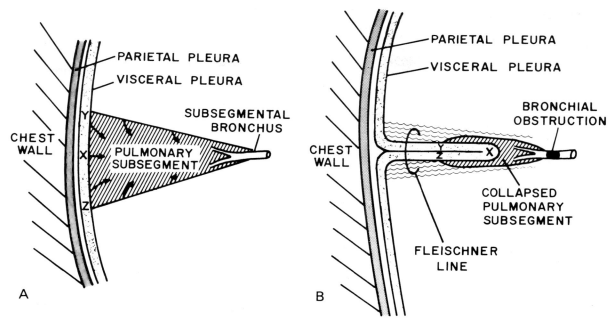

FIG. 99. MECHANISM OF FLEISCHNER LINE FORMATION

A: Normal pulmonary subsegment. The visceral pleura is intimately applied to a lung and cannot be separated from it without tearing pulmonary tissue. X, Y and Z are arbitrary reference points on the visceral pleura. The arrows indicate the directions in which the subsegment collapses as it becomes atelectatic. *B*: Atelectatic pulmonary subsegment following obstruction of its bronchus. The lung has collapsed toward the bronchus. The visceral pleura covering the subsegment has been pulled inward and now forms a double layer that extends to the chest wall. The shaded areas on either side on this pleural fissure represent alveoli in the adjacent pulmonary tissue where respiration is impaired, impeding collateral air drift. The Fleischner line represents the double layer of infolded pleura together with collapsed alveoli in the adjacent lung, projected on end. The atelectatic subsegment lies at the base of the pleural cleft. (Reprinted with permission from *Circulation, 45:* 171, 1972.)

is minor. Since there is no obstructive component, the large, irregular airspaces, characteristic of true emphysema, are absent. While the vital capacity of the lungs is diminished, the expiratory flow rate remains unchanged.

The hyperinflation is probably due to two factors: atrophy of the pulmonary septa, which interferes with the elastic recoil of the lung during expiration, and diminished mobility at the costovertebral junctions, so that the ribs tend to be fixed in the inspiratory position.

The enlargement of the lungs often cannot be recognized on films. Even when the process is quite advanced, the lungs usually appear normal in size or only slightly enlarged on the frontal projection because the diaphragms are not depressed and show little, if any, flattening in this view. Since there is no bronchial obstruction, diaphragmatic motion is not impeded. The lungs show little change in overall density, although there is frequently an area of increased lucency on either side of the upper part of the sternum because of the hyperinflation of the anterior lappet of each upper lobe. Since the condition is not associated with infection, there is no infiltra-

tion or consolidation of the lung in the absence of coincidental disease. The vascular markings sometimes appear accentuated and can result in confusion with interstitial disease of the lungs.

On the lateral view, the anteroposterior diameter of the chest is seen to be increased, the ribs course more horizontally than normal, causing widening of the rib spaces, especially in their anterior portion. In addition, there usually is kyphosis of the dorsal spine which further increases the anteroposterior diameter of the chest. In advanced cases, the upper part of the anterior portion of the chest is elevated, probably because of increased use of the accessory muscles of respiration. This causes an increase in the angulation between the manubrium and body of the sternum. The retrosternal space is deepened and abnormally lucent. The depth of the retrosternal space is greater in the presence of dorsal kyphosis. While the contour of the diaphragm is usually normal in the frontal projection, it is apt to appear flattened in the lateral view because of the increase in the anteroposterior diameter of the chest.

There is no evidence of obstruction to the flow

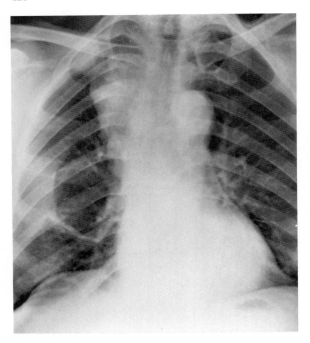

FIG. 100. FOCAL ATELECTASIS

The patient had a lymphosarcoma involving the right side of the mediastinum. An oblique Fleischner line is present in the right lower lobe. A small amount of fluid is collected over the atelectatic portion of lung and extends into the newly formed fissure.

of blood through the lungs. The peripheral vessels are of normal caliber, the hilar vessels are not prominent, and there is no enlargement of the heart secondary to the disease in the lungs.

Compensatory Hyperinflation. When a lung or part of a lung becomes atelectatic or is resected, there is an increase in the negative pressure in the pleura. This can result in elevation of the diaphragm, flattening of the thorax, shift of the mediastinum or hyperinflation of the remaining lung tissue. If the lung is normally distensible, compensatory hyperinflation, commonly referred to as compensatory emphysema, is the main mechanism whereby the relinquished space is occupied (see Fig. 186). The distention of the lung occurs in a passive manner and is no greater than that which is necessary to fill the space of the shrunken or missing portion. If the hyperinflated lung has not been the seat of previous disease, dilatation of the alveoli is more or less uniform so that the enlargement of individual alveoli is not so great as to cause rupture of their walls.

Compensatory hyperinflation of a portion of lung is recognized by an increase in its radiolucency compared with the corresponding area on

the opposite side (Fig. 70). Because the alveoli surrounding the arteries and veins are overdistended, the vessels tend to be more sharply demarcated than normal. Their course is abnormally straight and their bifurcations are splayed (Fig. 101). However, they are not narrowed as in the case of obstructive hyperinflation.

If one lung is atelectatic, the other becomes overinflated. The same changes take place after pneumonectomy (Fig. 102) unless the space previously occupied by the resected lung is filled by a large pleural effusion or pneumothorax, or is diminished by a thoracoplasty or phrenicotomy. The mediastinum shifts toward the side of the lung resection and the mesial border of the remaining lung usually herniates across the mediastinum into the opposite pulmonary field. This herniation most commonly occurs through the superior, anterior mediastinum. Less prominent herniation may occur through the posterior mediastinum, lower down, behind the heart (see Fig. 126). The herniation of the lung can be seen on standard chest films but is better demonstrated on overpenetrated Bucky or lordotic projections. Since the thoracic pressure in compensatory hyperinflation is not increased, there is no flaring out of the chest wall or depression of the diaphragm.

Obstructive Hyperinflation. Partial obstruction of the air passages can result in hyperinflation of the lungs and is most marked when the obstruction is of the check valve type. There is then little obstruction of air flow during inspiration but marked obstruction during expiration. This produces an increase in the volume of air in the alveoli together with an elevation of the intraalveolar pressure. The effect is accentuated by the fact that inspiration is an active process and is more forceful than expiration, which normally is passive. If the obstruction is marked, air accumulates in the alveoli with each breath, causing overinflation of the affected portion of lung during inspiration as well as expiration. The term obstructive hyperinflation is used when the lung is overdistended in expiration, even if it is incompletely or normally inflated in inspiration.

Because of its mobility, a polypoid tumor or a foreign body can act as a ball valve and cause obstructive hyperinflation. Simple stenosis of an air passage can act in a similar fashion even in the absence of a mobile tumor. Normally the bronchi expand during inspiration and contract during expiration. The lumen of a bronchus which is already considerably narrowed thus becomes narrower during expiration to the point of interference with the expulsion of air from the alveoli.

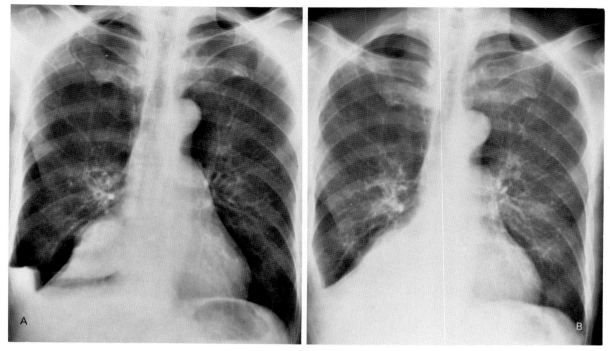

FIG. 101. COMPENSATORY HYPERINFLATION

A: The patient was admitted to the hospital with a large pleural effusion. The film made after aspiration of the fluid shows a small pneumothorax at the right base with a fluid level. In addition there is an unusual, sharply demarcated density that obliterates the right cardiac border. The vessels in the right lung are more clearly visible then those on the left and are spread apart. This is the picture of compensatory hyperinflation of the lung. The right lung root is markedly depressed. These findings indicate atelectasis of the lower lobe. The lucency between the collapsed lobe and the diaphragm is due to the pneumothorax. *B*: After absorption of the pneumothorax the typical appearance of a collapsed right lower and middle lobe is evident. A similar shadow can be caused by a paramediastinal collection of fluid. However this possibility is excluded because of the evidences of compensatory hyperinflation of the remainder of the lung and the extremely low position of the right lung root. Bronchoscopy revealed a carcinoma of the intermediate bronchus.

Obstructive hyperinflation differs from the compensatory type in that the pressure of the air in the lung is increased and the blood vessels are narrowed, especially during expiration (Fig. 17). It is also different from emphysema. Obstructive hyperinflation is usually reversible because there is little or no destruction of pulmonary tissue. In most instances, once the obstruction is relieved, the lung rapidly reverts to normal. If it is complicated by infection, expansion of the alveoli is interfered with and the degree of hyperinflation is lessened. If the obstruction becomes complete, atelectasis supervenes.

OBSTRUCTION OF THE LARYNX AND TRACHEA. Extreme narrowing of the larynx or trachea can act as a check valve. The valve-like effect is due to the resistance that the extremely narrow lumen offers to the passage of air, and the fact that the inspiratory effort is stronger than the force of expiration. The inspired air is not exhaled completely so that the residual volume of the lung increases slightly with each breath. This is

cumulative until a balance is reached.

The resulting gross overdistention of the lungs causes an increase in the size of the thoracic cavity. This is accomplished by a change in the course of the ribs, which become more horizontal, an increase in the width of the intercostal spaces, and depression of the leaves of the diaphragm. The retrosternal space is widened and there is an increased angulation between the manubrium and the body of the sternum.

On films made with standard exposure factors, the lungs appear abnormally dark and the retrosternal space appears hyperilluminated on the lateral view. The blood vessels are spread apart and appear thinner and straighter than normal. They are sharply outlined because of the contrast with the hyperinflated surrounding lung. The heart may be small. This is especially noticeable during expiration, an effect similar to that which occurs in the Valsalva maneuver.

The bilaterality of the roentgen changes and the absence of any shadows to indicate the pres-

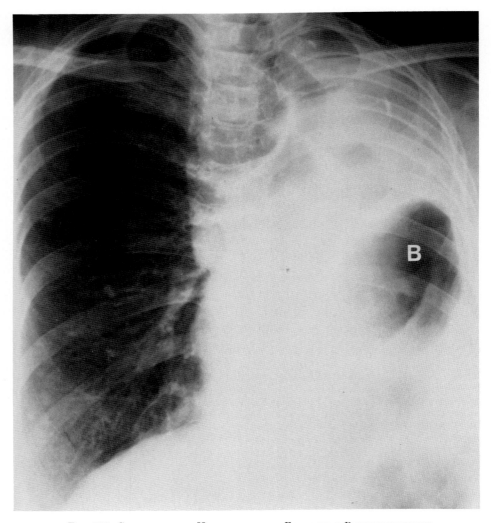

FIG. 102. COMPENSATORY HYPERINFLATION FOLLOWING PNEUMONECTOMY

The space previously occupied by the resected left lung has been diminished by an approximation of the ribs and by an extreme elevation of the left leaf of the diaphragm whose position is outlined by the large stomach bubble (B). The heart and mediastinal structures are displaced to the left side of the chest and the trachea is sharply angulated to the left. There probably is a small amount of gelatinous fluid in the left pleural cavity. Despite these changes, there still remains a considerable amount of space on the left side of the thorax. This is taken up by compensatory overexpansion of the right lung.

ence of diffuse disease of the smaller bronchi should suggest obstruction in the upper respiratory tract, although the same picture can be caused by acute bronchial asthma (see Fig. 192). When the obstruction is due to edema or inflammatory disease of the larynx, no abnormality aside from hyperinflation of the lungs may be seen. However, in severe laryngotracheobronchitis there is often evidence of bronchopneumonia.

A foreign body or tumor of the trachea, or a tracheal stricture is usually best seen on the lateral view. It can be visualized on frontal Bucky films but tomography is the method of choice. The shadow of a mediastinal mass or of a neo-

plasm of the main bronchus which obstructs the trachea, is usually visible on conventional films. However, additional studies are necessary to demonstrate involvement of the trachea.

OBSTRUCTION OF THE MAIN BRONCHUS. In most cases of check valve obstruction of a main bronchus, the hyperinflation of the lung is temporary because the obstruction tends to become complete and produce atelectasis. A striking example of this occurs in massive collapse of the lung following operations, particularly under general anesthesia. In the early stage, the patient may be severely ill with cyanosis and tachypnea. Films made at this time show hyperinflation of the lung rather than the collapse which occurs later. The obstruction is due to tenacious secretion. If this is expectorated or removed by suction, the symptoms clear rapidly and atelectasis does not take place. Transient hyperinflation of an entire lung can also result from obstructing malignant bronchial neoplasms or tuberculous lymph nodes.

More prolonged hyperinflation of the lung can occur when the check valve mechanism is due to a foreign body (Fig. 43) or a polypoid tumor. However, even here, atelectasis generally supervenes after a few months. In children, hyperinflation of a lobe or of an entire lung may result from incomplete development of the bronchial cartilages. This permits the bronchus to collapse during expiration from pressure of the adjacent lung tissue (see Fig. 315). In infants, the same picture may result from compression of the left bronchus by an enlarged heart.

Obstructive hyperinflation of one lung is easily overlooked on routine films. Since the standard examination is made in forced inspiration, the obstructed lung may appear no different than the healthy one. However, the diagnosis becomes obvious if the examination is repeated in expiration. The involved lung cannot expel its air and remains lucent, while the good lung becomes normally clouded (Fig. 17). The upward motion of the diaphragm on the involved side is limited. The heart and mediastinal structures are displaced toward the opposite side during expiration and return toward their normal position on inspiration. These changes are best noted on fluoroscopy.

OBSTRUCTION OF A LOBAR BRONCHUS. Partial obstruction of a lobar bronchus by malignant neoplasms is more common in the upper lobes. Secretions, bronchopneumonia, and foreign bodies affect the lower lobes more commonly, while bronchial narrowing from tuberculous bronchitis in adults occurs most frequently in the upper lobes.

In obstructive hyperinflation, the involved lobe appears more lucent than the remainder of the lung or its counterpart on the opposite side. This appearance is accentuated during expiration. The secondary effects of the overdistention, such as shift of the mediastinum, depend upon the lobe involved.

In obstructive hyperinflation of the right upper lobe, the mediastinal shift may be slight and is confined to its upper portion. In some cases there is herniation of the mesial lappet of the lobe through the anterior mediastinum to the opposite side. In the lateral view the retrosternal space then appears widened and more lucent

than normal. The short fissure is displaced downward during expiration and the upper part of the long fissure may be displaced backward as well as downward.

Partial obstruction of the left upper lobe bronchus produces more marked changes because of the greater volume of lung affected. The mediastinal shift is greater and involves the heart as well as the upper mediastinum. Motion of the diaphragm is usually not significantly affected.

Obstructive hyperinflation of the lower lobe causes pendular movement of the mediastinum, most marked in the region of the heart. Although the diaphragm is usually depressed, its upward movement during expiration may not be restricted to any considerable degree. However, restriction does occur when there are extensive adhesions over the upper lobe. Herniation through the posterior mediastinum is rare. If the overdistention is moderate, the chief signs are lack of clouding of the affected lobe during expiration and absence of the normal outward fanning of the vessels during inspiration. These changes are more easily discerned on fluoroscopy.

The pendular movement of the heart is more marked when the middle lobe is involved together with the lower lobe. A striking sign of obstructive emphysema in both lobes (Golden's sign) can be observed when the short fissure is visible. The fissure moves upward and downward together with the diaphragm because the diaphragmatic motion is transmitted through the middle and lower lobes whose air cannot be expelled during expiration.

When there is obstructive emphysema of only the lower lobe, the short fissure remains stationary during respiration. However, there is movement of the long fissure. This is detectable only on the lateral view. During expiration the fissure is pushed forward and upward and returns to its previous position during inspiration.

Hyperinflation of the lower lobe can also result from a lesion that partially obstructs the main bronchus and completely obstructs the upper lobe bronchus. Atelectasis of the upper lobe is then associated with hyperinflation of the lower lobe.

OBSTRUCTION OF SMALLER BRONCHI. Obstruction of a segmental bronchus rarely causes pulmonary hyperinflation. Communications between the alveoli permit collateral respiration with neighboring segments, preventing build-up of increased pressure and overinflation. If infection takes place beyond the obstruction, the small bronchi become completely occluded with exudate and the lung tissue becomes atelectatic rather than overinflated.

Tumors involving the subsegmental or smaller bronchi usually cause complete bronchial obstruction early in their development. Partial obstruction of these bronchi occurs frequently in bronchopneumonia, particularly in children. The appearance of the lungs at necropsy is often quite remarkable. Here and there, interspersed among areas of lobular atelectasis and pneumonia, are seen raised lobules of pink, hyperaerated lung, which do not collapse when the organ is removed. The small bronchi leading to these areas contain purulent secretion which interferes with the expulsion of air from the affected lobules while collateral respiration is prevented by blockage of the pores of Kohn by the inflammatory disease. The areas of hyperinflation are quite small and generally cannot be differentiated radiologically from normal lung between areas of lobular consolidation. Areas of increased aeration, large enough to be recognized on the films, probably result from rupture of alveolar walls and are therefore more properly considered in the section on emphysema.

INFILTRATION

The word infiltration is often used loosely in the description and interpretation of shadows on roentgen films of the chest. Not infrequently it is applied indiscriminately to mottled shadows caused by areas of consolidation or neoplastic masses without regard to the true meaning of the world. The term is adopted from pathology and when used in radiology it should be applied in the description of shadows caused by infiltration in the pathologic sense. It is useful in radiologic terminology because it describes a pathologic process which generally can be recognized by its roentgen characteristics.

Definition. Infiltration denotes the insinuation between the cells of the tissues of substances that are foreign to that location. Thus, tissues may be infiltrated with fluid, foreign solid materials, neoplastic cells or exudate from the blood. Properly speaking, when these substances have assumed their place in the tissues one should speak of an infiltrate rather than an infiltration. However, the word infiltration has been in common use for so long that it is now acceptable.

Infiltration should not be confused with consolidation of the lung. In the latter, the alveoli are the seat of the pathologic accumulation and it is not present between the cells of the lung tissues. In effect, the substances which cause consolidation of the lung are situated outside of the body proper. It is true that in most cases of infiltration of the lung there is also some consolidation. Conversely, with the exception of lobar pneumonia, pure consolidation is uncommon. It is impossible to determine the exact proportion of each of these two processes without microscopic study. However, it is usually possible roentgenologically to determine which of them is more prominent. Recognition that the lesion is solely or mostly infiltrative is useful in the roentgen interpretation of the nature of the disease.

Roentgen Appearance. In contrast to the process of consolidation, in which the pulmonary alveoli become filled, infiltration involves the interstitial tissues and, in the absence of complicating consolidation or atelectasis, the alveoli remain aerated. The tissues about the bronchi and blood vessels and within the interlobular septa and alveolar walls become thickened and cast shadows which are separated by the more or less lucent alveoli.

The roentgen manifestations of pulmonary infiltration depend upon the degree of thickening of the interstitial tissues and whether this occurs in an even fashion or in the form of localized nodular thickenings. In the absence of nodules, the thickened interstitial tissue produces a fine reticular pattern (see Fig. 369). When the infiltration is more intense, the shadows are coarser and appear as streaks which are either straight or irregular in outline (see Fig. 344). Nodular infiltrations produce miliary or submiliary shadows.

Infiltrations about the blood vessels tend to blur the outlines of these structures. Thickening of the interstitial tissues in the mesial portion of the lungs adjacent to the heart may impart a fuzzy appearance to the cardiac silhouette (Fig. 103). When there is infiltration of the pulmonary tissue bordering on a fissure, the latter is delineated by a line of variable thickness and density.

Fine, diffuse infiltrations are easily overlooked, especially if the film is overexposed even to a slight degree. The infiltrations are more prominent on films which are somewhat underexposed but this also causes an accentuation of the normal pulmonary markings which are then easily confused with infiltrations. The presence of pulmonary infiltration should be suspected if there is an unusual clouding of the lower third of the pulmonary field on films made in expiration. In addition, infiltrations which cannot be appreciated on conventional films can sometimes be

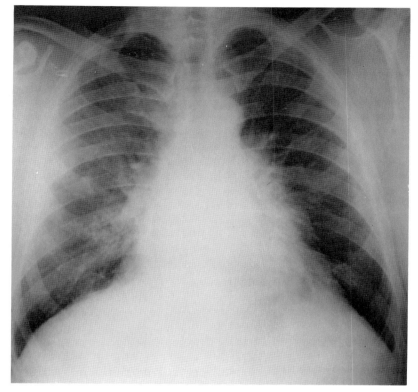

FIG. 103. PORCUPINE HEART IN ASBESTOSIS

There is a moderate degree of interstitial fibrosis involving mainly the lower half of the lungs. The shadows of the fibrotic interstitial tissues of the middle lobe and lingula overlap and blend with the cardiac silhouette, causing it to appear spiculated.

clearly seen through the superimposed liver on films made with increased exposure, particularly with the use of the Bucky grid and the patient supine. Not uncommonly, infiltrations in the lung bases are first detected within the liver shadow on films of the abdomen.

Inflammatory Infiltration. The most common *acute* inflammatory infiltrations of the lungs are those associated with acute interstitial pneumonia (see Fig. 236). This type of pneumonia is most often due to a viral infection, and occurs in a pure form in the early stages before it is complicated by pyogenic infection. The roentgen film shows fine, streak-like shadows which may be difficult to differentiate from blood vessels. On close inspection, however, the shadows can be seen to extend to the periphery of the lung and, in general, seem finer than the streaks produced by blood vessels. They do not diverge and, in many cases, the streaks are interspersed with fine, nodular shadows. The densities represent the interstitial tissues of the lungs thickened by inflammatory infiltration. The infiltrations are most frequently situated in the lower lobes where they are usually seen in the form of fine streaks

and miliary and submiliary nodules (Fig. 104). The process may be complicated by atelectasis resulting from obstruction of small bronchi by plugs of mucoid exudate. When these are expectorated, the lung reexpands and the characteristic pattern of the interstitial pneumonia again becomes visible. Lesions of this nature are not uncommon in the upper lobes. When they are mainly in the infraclavicular region it may be impossible, from a single examination, to differentiate them from tuberculosis. Acute interstitial infiltrations also occur in rickettsial infections, such as endemic typhus and Q fever.

Although pneumonia caused by pyogenic organisms is usually associated with consolidation, there are cases of streptococcus pneumonia which are predominantly interstitial in character. These generally follow streptococcus pharyngitis or cervical lymphadenitis, and may be associated with diffuse mediastinitis or mediastinal lymphadenitis together with purulent lymphangitis of the lungs (see Fig. 235). The infiltration extends along the lymphatics about the bronchi and the blood vessels and in the interlobar septa. When the alveolar walls become involved, a variable

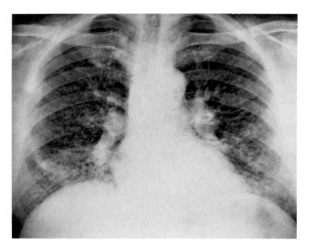

Fig. 104. Mycoplasma Pneumonia: Miliary
Infiltrations

The pulmonary fields on both sides are studded with fine
miliary and submiliary densities which are most numerous in
the lower part of the chest. The clinical picture was that of
a virus type of pneumonia. Focal areas of atelectasis developed later. All of the lesions resolved after a few weeks.

amount of exudation occurs.

Similar infiltrations, often more noticeable
near the roots of the lungs, occur in the acute
stages of measles and whooping cough. More
nodular lesions occur in chicken pox, especially
in the adult (see Fig. 249) and in tropical eosinophilia. An acute interstitial pneumonia sometimes complicates chronic bronchitis, particularly in asthmatics. In these cases, the lower
lobes are the site of predilection. Interstitial infiltrations occur in the pneumonia complicating
diffuse vascular disease. They are present in
periarteritis nodosa and in the eosinophilic pneumonia that often accompanies this disease or a
similar type of diffuse arteritis. In these cases the
infiltrations are usually bilateral and often simulate tuberculosis. However, they tend to be
fleeting and migratory.

The more chronic inflammatory infiltrative
diseases of the lungs are associated with fibrosis.
The fibrous tissue is deposited especially about
the bronchi and blood vessels and within the
interlobular septa. It is also present in the alveolar septa in association with infiltrations of lymphocytes, large mononuclear cells, and, occasionally, giant cells. The streak-like and fine nodular
shadows in tuberculosis are largely interstitial in
location. Similar interstitial infiltrations also occur in association with bronchiectasis and in the
neighborhood of chronic lung abscesses. Fungous
infections of the lungs, particularly in the chronic
state, are characterized by interstitial infiltrations of granulation tissue and white blood cells.

The tubercles in miliary tuberculosis form in
the alveolar septa in relation to the capillaries
and, therefore, the miliary shadows in this disease represent interstitial infiltrations. The
larger, tubercle-like shadows which characterize
the dust diseases and Boeck's sarcoid, together
with the streak-like shadows which occur in these
diseases, represent infiltrations of inflammatory
cells and granulation and fibrous tissue in the
pulmonary septa. The fine reticulation of the
lungs often present in the dust diseases represents an infiltration of the finer septa. These
finer septa are also involved in the fibrosis of the
lung of unknown etiology, described by Hamman
and Rich (Fig. 105). In this disease, fine nodules
may occur in addition to the more streak-like
infiltrations.

Neoplastic Infiltration. When the interstitial tissues of the lung are infiltrated by neoplastic cells in primary carcinoma of the lung, the
infiltrations usually extend outward from the
lung root into the involved lobe (see Figs. 390
and 411). The infiltrations are obscured if the
involved segment of the lung is atelectic. When
the infiltration is secondary to a carcinoma of a
large bronchus, it is more dense at the root (Fig.
106). The infiltrations spread outward into the
pulmonary fields in the form of linear densities
along the course of the lymphatic channels about
the bronchi and blood vessels, and in the interlobular septa. In some cases the carcinoma cells
grow within the lymphatic channels themselves.
The infiltrations then are fine, widespread and
extend throughout the lungs. However, here too,
there usually is a condensation of the shadows at
the root of the lung or of a lobe, indicating the
bronchial origin of the neoplasm.

In carcinomatous lymphangitis of the lungs
secondary to a neoplasm in the abdomen, the
shadows are more uniformly distributed despite
the fact that the lymphatic channels converge at
the lung roots (see Fig. 436). The metastatic
tumor is largely confined to the lymphatic channels which are very fine and there is little extension into the surrounding tissues and therefore
no coarse infiltrations at the hila. The roentgen
film simply shows a general accentuation of the
pulmonary markings by fine streaks and tiny
nodules. The interlobular septa above the costophrenic sinuses often become clearly outlined
when the lymphatics within them are permeated
by the spreading carcinoma. They appear on the
film as parallel, horizontal streaks just within the
lateral border of the chest, Kerley B lines (Fig.
107). Spread of the tumor cells in the subpleural
lymphatics causes demonstrable thickening of
the interlobar fissures.

Lymphangitic spread can also result in the

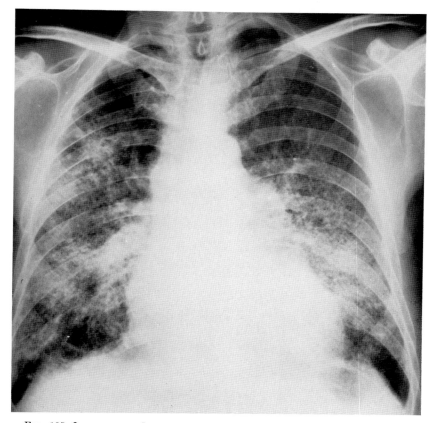

FIG. 105. INTERSTITIAL INFILTRATIONS AND FIBROSIS: HAMMAN-RICH DISEASE

Fine, sharply edged, interlacing and nodular shadows are present throughout the lower part of each lung except at the extreme bases. These portions are spared because they are the seat of bullous emphysema. The nonspecific interstitial fibrosis and infiltration of unknown etiology which characterize this disease were demonstrated by lung biopsy. The enlargement of the heart and of the main pulmonary arteries is indicative of pulmonary hypertension.

formation of larger nodules throughout the lungs by growth of the tumor tissue through the walls of the lymph channels. Despite their lymphatic origin, these simulate hematogenous metastases. The presence of streak-like infiltrations between the nodules indicates diffuse permeation of the lymphatics.

Miscellaneous Infiltrations. HODGKINS'S DISEASE. The lungs are involved in Hodgkin's disease with considerable frequency, particularly in the later stages (Fig. 76). Generally, the infiltrations are associated with rather massive involvement of the mediastinal nodes. The infiltrations are coarse and extend outward from the lung root about the larger bronchi and blood vessels. They are clearly visualized until the bronchi become so narrowed that atelectasis supervenes and obscures the underlying infiltrative pattern. Occasionally, Hodgkin's disease produces infiltrations in the lung without visible enlargement of the mediastinal lymph nodes. In rare instances this is seen in untreated cases (Fig.

108), but more commonly the absence of adenopathy is due to previous irradiation of the mediastinum. Again, the infiltrations are extremely coarse. They may be so extensive that they compress the alveoli and produce a dense shadow simulating the consolidation of pneumonia.

LEUKEMIA. Infiltration of the lung by leukemic cells is rare. The few instances we have observed have been in the lymphatic form of the disease. The infiltrations were generally dense and presented the appearance of a bronchopneumonia of the interstitial type. The infiltrations were coarser near the root and became finer as they extended into the lung. In two cases the infiltrations were in the form of fine nodules, distributed uniformly throughout the lungs.

HISTIOCYTOSIS X. Several types of pulmonary infiltrations have been observed in the histiocytoses. Fine infiltrations simulating miliary tuberculosis are probably the most frequent manifestations (Figs. 356 and 358). Some cases have shown coarse infiltrations extending out from the

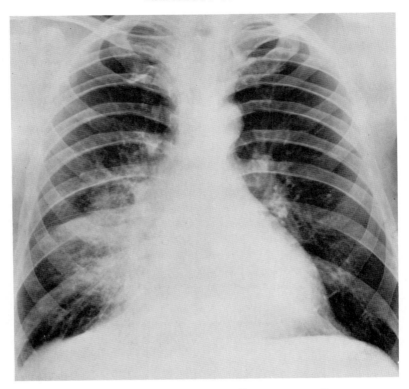

FIG. 106. INTERSTITIAL INFILTRATION BY BRONCHOGENIC CARCINOMA

The coarse infiltrations in the mesial portion of the right lower lobe are caused by carcinomatous invasion along the peribronchial, perivascular and interlobular lymphatic channels. The appearance simulates pneumonia from which it cannot be differentiated from the frontal film alone. However, the fact that the shadows were seen to radiate outward from the lung root on the lateral as well as on the frontal view indicates that they represent neoplastic disease. Unilateral lymphangitic spread points to a primary bronchogenic carcinoma rather than metastatic neoplasm.

lung roots, fine infiltrations in the periphery of the lungs, or irregularly rounded shadows with poorly demarcated borders from which fine infiltrations extend into the neighboring lung tissue. The latter appear more like areas of consolidation surrounded by fine, local infiltrations. In essence, these are granulomatous lesions and consist of a dense, focal type of infiltration in which the lung tissue is destroyed and replaced by the granuloma which sends out finer offshoots into the neighboring pulmonary septa.

CONSOLIDATION

Definition. Consolidation denotes solidification of the lung by material which replaces the air in the alveoli. The consolidated lung, therefore, is about the same size as the normal lung in mid or full inspiration. Consolidation should be differentiated from infiltration of the lung in which the pathologic process involves primarily the interstitial tissues rather than the alveolar spaces. In many instances of consolidation there may be some associated infiltration, but the solidification of the lung is due mainly to the material in the alveoli. In any case, the consolidated area appears more or less homogeneous on the cut section of the specimen because all the alveoli are filled with exudate. Similarly, the shadow of the lesion on the roentgen film appears homogeneous because of the absence of air in the involved area. It is this homogeneity of the shadow that characterizes the roentgen appearance of consolidation (Fig. 109).

Consolidation may involve the entire lung, one or more lobes, or a portion of a lobe. The consolidation may be confined to a bronchopulmonary segment, a number of lobules, or portions of the lobules, the pulmonary acini (Fig. 2). Uninvolved radiolucent lung may be present between areas of consolidation so that despite the homogeneity of the shadows of the consolidated

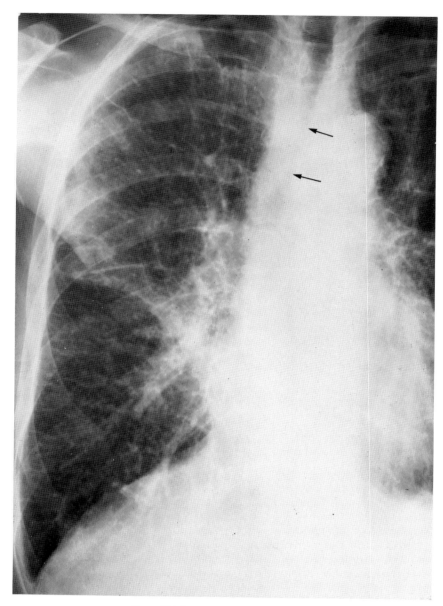

FIG. 107. LYMPHANGITIC CARCINOSIS

Extremely fine, linear shadows are scattered throughout the right lung, radiating from the hilum. The horizontal streaks in the periphery of the right lung above the costophrenic sinus are Kerley B lines and are due to infiltration of the interlobular septa. The left lung was similarly involved. The thoracic portion of the trachea (arrows) is diffusely narrowed. Postmortem examination revealed lymphagitic spread of a mucin-producing adenocarcinoma. The narrowing of the trachea was due to invasion of the mediastium.

areas, the overall pulmonary field may have a variegated appearance. The shadow of consolidation should be differentiated from that of pulmonary infiltration, atelectasis with or without infiltration, pleural effusion, a local neoplastic mass or a filled cavity.

Roentgen Recognition. The differentiation between consolidation and diffuse infiltration of the lung is usually a simple matter. However, where the infiltration is dense and localized, confusion may arise. This is especially true if the interstitial tissues are so thickened that they compress the alveoli and obliterate the alveolar spaces. The distinguishing feature of infiltration

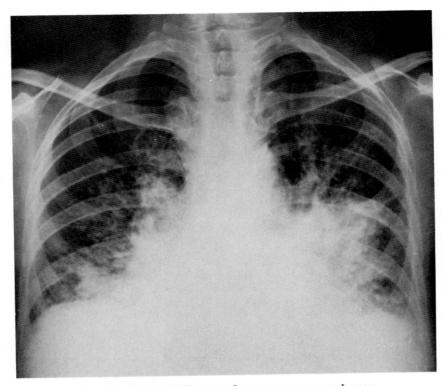

FIG. 108. HODGKIN'S DISEASE: INFILTRATION OF THE LUNGS

The manifestations in this case of Hodgkin's disease were essentially pulmonary. Dense infiltrations extend from the root of each lung, mainly to the lower lobes. The infiltrations become finer as they extend to the periphery. A faint shadow along the right border of the upper mediastinum is caused by enlarged paratracheal lymph nodes. Although pulmonary infiltration is not unusual in Hodgkin's disease, particularly in the later stages, it is rarely present without concomitant enlargement of the mediastinal nodes, provided the latter have not been treated by radiation.

is the lack of homogeneity of the shadow. This lack of uniformity in the roentgen image is due to the presence of air-containing alveoli within the lesion. The presence of a shadow in the region of the lung root, projecting with finger-like densities toward the periphery would indicate infiltration rather than consolidation (Fig. 108).

The pathognomonic roentgen sign of consolidation is the air bronchogram (Felson). Normally, the branch bronchi are not visible on the film because their walls are thin and there is little difference between the density of the air within their lumen and the surrounding air-containing lung. However, when the air in the alveoli is replaced by liquid or cellular material, there is a marked contrast between the lungs and the air in the bronchi. The latter then appear as branching linear lucencies within the consolidated, opacified lung (Fig. 110).

During the stage of resolution the roentgen appearance of the consolidated area may be indistinguishable from pulmonary infiltration be-cause of irregularity in the process of resolution and plugging of numerous small bronchi by fibrinous exudate originating from the alveoli. The resulting picture consists of numerous irregular areas of lucency representing aerated lung interspersed with small remaining areas of consolidation (see Figs. 227 and 231), together with atelectatic streaks.

In the absence of complicating infection, it is usually not difficult to differentiate consolidation from atelectasis. Atelectasis of a lung or a lobe produces sufficient displacement of the adjacent structures to indicate that there has been shrinkage of lung tissue. The shadow of atelectasis of individual pulmonary segments is much fainter than that of consolidation. Moreover, in the latter condition the pulmonary markings are completely obscured while they usually can be visualized within a partially collapsed area and appear drawn together. Atelectasis of still smaller portions of the lung is manifested by streak-like shadows which bear no resemblance to those of consolidation.

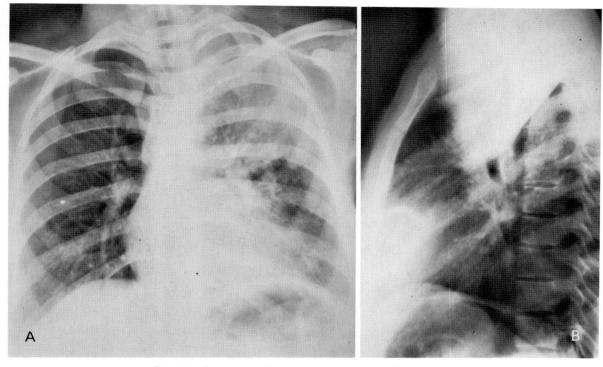

FIG. 109. SEGMENTAL CONSOLIDATION IN LOBAR PNEUMONIA

A: Frontal view. There is a homogeneous density over the upper part of the left upper lobe. The indistinctness of the left cardiac border indicates involvement of the lingula as well. The band-like density along the outer part of the left chest is caused by exudate on the pleura. The patient had high fever, and pneumococci were found in the sputum. *B:* Lateral view. The triangular area of homogeneous consolidation in the upper part of the left upper lobe corresponds to the apicoposterior segment of the lobe. The opacification above the anterior costophrenic sinus is due to the pneumonia in the lingula.

When infection and inflammation occur in the atelectatic lung, its shadow becomes denser and the contraction of the lung may no longer be so evident. As a rule, if the inflammatory process is mainly interstitial, sufficient evidence of atelectasis remains to allow its recognition, particularly when a large portion of the lung is involved. Lateral views are often required to demonstrate the displacement of the fissures and the approximation of the vascular markings indicative of atelectasis (see Fig. 237).

The bronchi within consolidated lung are frequently outlined by the radiolucent air within them (Fig. 110). This *air bronchogram* is usually not seen within the dense shadow of inflamed, atelectatic lung secondary to obstruction of a large bronchus. The bronchi distal to the obstruction are usually filled with secretion and exudate which have the same density as the adjacent collapsed lung, and are therefore not visible on the film. The air bronchogram of consolidation is not visible on films that are too lightly exposed. It is best demonstrated on to-mograms, but even the smaller bronchi are frequently seen on films made with increased penetration or with the aid of the Potter-Bucky diaghragm.

Pleural effusions also cast a homogeneous shadow which may be difficult to differentiate from the shadow of consolidation. Large effusions displace the mediastinum to the opposite side in both phases of respiration. In consolidation, the mediastinum may shift to the opposite side in expiration, but it returns to its normal position during inspiration. Smaller effusions are usually situated at the base and are apt to obliterate the outline of the diaphragm. They tend to spread upward along the border of the ribs, while the shadow of consolidation ends abruptly as it reaches the parietes. More laterally situated, partially loculated effusions simulate consolidation of the lung more closely. However, consolidation usually involves a definite anatomic division of the lung, whereas the shadow cast by a loculated effusion bears no relation to the distribution of the bronchi and blood vessels which

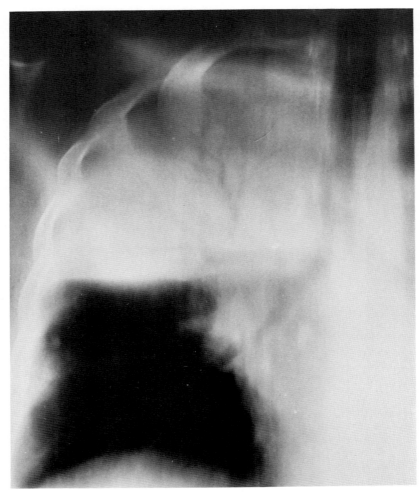

FIG. 110. LOBAR PNEUMONIA: AIR BRONCHOGRAM

The tomogram shows branching lucencies within the opacified right upper lobe. These represent bronchial air columns contrasting with the surrounding consolidated pulmonary parenchyma. The air bronchogram was also seen on the conventional film. The patient had pneumococcal pneumonia.

generally determine the boundaries of a consolidated area. Moreover, the air-containing bronchi are not delineated in the absence of consolidation of the lung about them. When the effusion is indistinguishable from consolidation of the lung in the frontal view, oblique or lateral views may disclose the characteristic pattern of fluid extending along the border of the chest wall.

An effusion in the long fissure may simulate consolidation of the lung in the frontal projection. However, on the lateral view, the sharp boundary of the shadow, its fusiform shape, and its relation to the fissure serve to identify an interlobar collection of fluid.

It is often impossible to differentiate between a cavity filled with exudate and an area of consolidation, for both may present identical shadows (see Fig. 270). If the possibility of a cavity is suspected, films should be made with increased penetration or with a Potter-Bucky diaphragm, or tomography should be utilized. These may disclose a fluid level or a small bubble of air within a cavity that is almost completely filled with fluid. If a dense, homogeneous shadow appears where a cavity was seen on previous films, it should be concluded that the opacity represents the cavity filled with exudate (see Fig. 131). If the original cavity had really closed, only a small linear streak or irregular infiltration would be visible. Differentiation between a filled cavity and an area of consolidation, can sometimes be accomplished by making another film after postural drainage or bronchoscopy. The removal of some of the exudate from the cavity and its replacement by air produces an air-fluid level where previously there existed a uniform shadow. Dense infiltration of the lung by a neoplasm in the periphery of the pulmonary field is easily confused with consolidation. Similarly, large inflammatory granulomas which, essentially, represent dense infiltrations of the lung, often cannot be differentiated from areas of consolidation (see Fig. 348). Fine finger-like projections about the border of the homogeneous density caused by the granuloma suggest the infiltrative nature of the disease.

Types of Consolidation. The types of consolidation may be classified as inflammatory, hemorrhagic, and neoplastic. More often than not it is impossible to differentiate these types from observation of a single film. But the serial changes noted on repeated examinations often disclose a more or less characteristic course from which the diagnosis of a specific disease may be made. In other cases, there are collateral changes which indicate the cause of the consolidation.

INFLAMMATORY CONSOLIDATION. With the possible exception of pneumococcal pneumonia, some infiltration of the interstitial tissues is present in addition to the exudate in the alveoli in practically all of the inflammatory diseases causing consolidation of the lung.

It may be said, in general, that consolidation is the prominent feature in those pneumonias which have an acute onset and in which the primary seat of the disease is in the lungs. Where the acuteness of the clinical picture is due to a generalized infection of the body, as in most viral diseases, the pathologic process in the lung, which is only one part of the disease, is largely interstitial, and manifests itself by infiltration rather than by consolidation. An acute inflammatory disease situated primarily in the lungs, therefore, is characterized by consolidation.

One or more local areas of consolidation may be superimposed upon more diffuse inflammatory infiltrative disease when there is secondary infection. This is the case in viral infections of the lungs in which a complicating bacterial infection takes place. Clearing of areas of consolidation in lungs involved by viral pneumonia is often observed during treatment with antibiotics. This effect is almost certainly due to the action of the drugs on secondary bacterial invaders which are responsible for the exudate in the alveoli, rather than to any effect on the underlying viral disease. The practical importance of recognizing the presence of consolidation is apparent if one accepts this as a clinical rule.

The occurrence of consolidation denotes a severe inflammatory response on the part of the lung but this reaction is not to be considered proportional to the severity of the injury that the pulmonary tissue has suffered. The reaction which produces consolidation is often said to be an hyperergic one, and in many cases has been shown to be caused by an undue sensitivity of the pulmonary tissues to the injurious agent. In this respect it is not unlike an allergic reaction.

Lobar Pneumonia. The consolidation that results from a sudden outpouring of exudate into the alveoli is best exemplified by lobar pneumonia. In this disease, the structure of the alveolar walls remains intact, while the infection spreads rapidly from alveolus to alveolus through the pores of Kohn, and from one small bronchial branch to another. In the early stages, the consolidation usually involves only a single portion of a segment. The consolidation spreads to involve the entire segment (see Fig. 226) and then rapidly extends to affect most, if not all, of the alveoli of an entire lobe (Fig. 51). Further spread of the infection and consolidation generally takes place later by way of the larger bronchi to other lobes of the lung (Fig. 230). These portions of the lung may be involved in a different manner than the initial site. Rather than a diffuse, homogeneous consolidation of entire lobes, there may appear simultaneously many smaller areas of consolidation such as characterize lobular bronchopneumonia.

Lobular Pneumonia. In lobular pneumonia, as in lobar pneumonia, consolidation is the dominant pathologic process and there is little infiltration or destruction of pulmonary tissue. However, the disease does not begin with a small area of consolidation that spreads diffusely through a lobe or an entire lung. Instead, it manifests itself by the more or less simultaneous appearance of several small areas of consolidation scattered in the lungs (Fig. 111). Radiologically, the consolidated areas appear as poorly defined, homogeneous shadows of variable size, some of which may be coalescent. They may be confined to one lobe or may be situated in several lobes. Usually both lower lobes are involved. The disease begins as a bronchial infection, as do the other forms of bronchopneumonia. In this way it differs from lobar pneumonia which appears to originate as an infection in the lung tissue. The lobular areas of consolidation which may be seen in lobar pneumonia, occur as the result of extension of the infection through the bronchi.

Tuberculosis. Consolidation of the lung is the predominant pathologic change in what has been termed the exudative type of pulmonary tuberculosis (Fig. 94). This is an expression of the hyperergic reaction which accompanies reinfec-

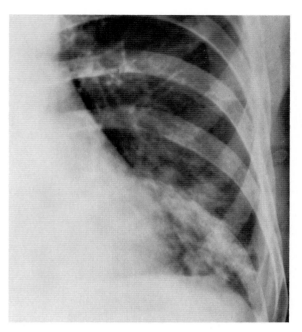

FIG. 111. LOBULAR CONSOLIDATION IN PNEUMONIA

Small, irregular, rather discrete, patchy shadows are seen above the left leaf of the diaphragm. These represent groups of consolidated lobules. The mesial portion of the left leaf of the diaphragm is straightened as the result of an adhesion to the undersurface of the lung.

tion with the tubercle bacilli in the adult form of tuberculosis. It also occurs when the infection is massive and tissue resistance low. Areas of tuberculous consolidation of considerable size may appear quite suddenly in individuals belonging to races which have little resistance to the disease, in diabetics, and in persons suffering from malnutrition. Large areas of consolidation are also encountered when there is massive infection from inhalation of caseous material extruded from cavities or ruptured tuberculous lymph nodes in patients with diminished resistance to the tubercle bacilli (see Figs. 286 and 295).

Lung Abscess. The early stage of a putrid lung abscess is characterized by a local area of consolidation confined to that part of the lung supplied by the bronchial branch into which the causative organisms have been aspirated (see Fig. 270). Although the infection of the bronchus is severe and extends through the bronchial wall, causing a certain amount of interstitial infiltration, there soon occurs extensive exudation into the alveoli, producing the picture of consolidation. The roentgen appearance at this time cannot be distinguished from that of the early stage of lobar pneumonia. However, the pneumonia

that initiates a putrid lung abscess is gangrenous in type and sooner or later exhibits its destructive character by the appearance of a cavity. It also differs from the consolidation of early lobar pneumonia by the fact that it tends to remain localized and stable for a much longer period of time. The lesion is apt to remain unchanged in size, appearance and distribution until cavitation becomes evident, even if this change is delayed for many weeks.

Suppurative Bronchopneumonia. Consolidation also occurs in suppurative bronchopneumonia (see Figs. 239 and 240). Since the pathologic process is primarily an interstitial one, pulmonary infiltrations are present in addition to the areas of consolidation. The consolidation can overshadow the infiltration in some instances so that it may be confused with lobar pneumonia for a time. However, films made early in the disease practically always show pulmonary infiltrations as the predominant change. In those cases with large areas of consolidation, cavitation usually develops (see Fig. 246). These changes suffice to differentiate suppurative bronchopneumonia from lobar pneumonia and simple bronchopneumonia.

The nonputrid abscesses which occasionally complicate suppurative bronchopneumonia can generally be differentiated from a putrid lung abscess because they tend to be multiple in the early stages of the disease. Occasionally, a single nonputrid abscess forms in suppurative bronchopneumonia and casts a shadow that is identical to that of a putrid lung abscess. The two can be differentiated from films made at the beginning of the disease. In the early stage of suppurative bronchopneumonia, the lesions are more widely distributed and consist mainly of areas of infiltration, indicating its interstitial nature.

Bronchial Obstruction. Consolidation can occur when a portion of lung distal to an obstructive lesion becomes infected. This takes place particularly beyond ulcerating bronchial carcinomas which not only serve to produce bronchial obstruction but also act as a nidus for infection. The lung distal to the obstruction need not be atelectatic. In fact, it is more likely to become infected if the obstruction is incomplete. In such a case, no evidence of the bronchial lesion may be noted on the film and an erroneous diagnosis of lobar pneumonia may be made. Only the persistence of the shadow, or its slow resolution with later evidence of atelectasis or recurrence of the pneumonia might indicate its obstructive cause. Instances such as these emphasize the necessity for repeated roentgen examinations until the consolidated area has entirely cleared before dismissing any case as one of simple pneumonia (see Fig. 416).

HEMORRHAGIC CONSOLIDATION. A portion of lung may become consolidated by filling of the alveoli with blood (Fig. 210). This may occur in inflammatory disease, either from the diapedesis of blood through intact capillaries or from actual rupture of these vessels. Injury to the pulmonary vessels by poison gases, by trauma, or as a result of infarction may also cause a filling of the aveoli with blood (Fig. 112).

Pneumonia. Hemorrhagic consolidation occurs in the early stage of lobar pneumonia when, as a result of the diapedesis of great numbers of red corpuscles into the alveoli, the affected portion undergoes the changes associated with red hepatization. The roentgen appearance is that which has been described in lobar pneumonia. The homogeneous shadow is generally confined to a lobe or to one of its segments and is well demarcated. Its segmental distribution is denoted by the involvement of a portion of the lung extending outward from the root and widening

as it approaches the chest wall. This may be visualized on films made in the positions that show the profiles of the segments involved.

Toxic or Hemorrhagic Diseases. More severe hemorrhage into the lung occurs from more marked disruption of the pulmonary capillaries either as a result of toxic or mechanical influences. This generally results in the production of multiple smaller areas of consolidation which, as a rule, do not conform to the boundaries of the segments. The shadows are also homogeneous in texture as in the case of all pulmonary consolidation, but they are not so well demarcated as the areas of consolidation in lobar pneumonia. Such areas of hemorrhage of varying size are present in the hemorrhagic stage of influenzal pneumonia and a similar appearance is present in poisoning by some of the more irritating gases. In these cases there is, in addition, edema of the surrounding lung which lessens the contrast of the shadows produced by the hemorrhagic foci and renders their borders less sharp. Multiple foci of hemorrhagic consolidation which are

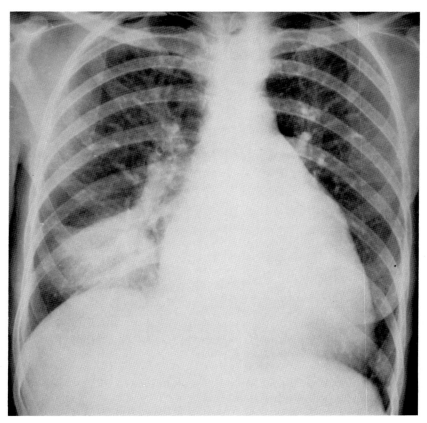

FIG. 112. HEMORRHAGIC CONSOLIDATION

The poorly outlined, homogeneous shadow at the base of the right lung represents an area of pulmonary consolidation. In this case, it was due to filling of the alveoli with blood as a result of an infarct. The heart has the typical mitral configuration. There is an increased incidence of pulmonary infarction in patients with mitral disease.

somewhat more sharply demarcated, occur in thrombocytopenia (Fig. 113), but, even in these, the borders of the consolidated areas are not well defined. Very small areas of hemorrhagic consolidation involving only portions of lobules, the pulmonary acini, occur together with larger, ill-defined areas of consolidation during the hemorrhagic phase of pulmonary hemosiderosis. Large areas of hemorrhagic consolidation, usually involving a considerable portion of the lungs, occur in Goodpasture's syndrome (see Fig. 374).

Contusions. A similar lack of sharp demarcation of the shadow is noted in mechanical injuries of the lung confined to a single area. A local area of hemorrhage may be the result of a contusion from a direct blow to the chest (see Fig. 380) with or without fracture of the ribs. Penetrating wounds or the excision of a portion of the lung may result in local hemorrhage into the pulmonary tissue. In these cases a single shadow of uniform density and of variable size is seen in the region of the injury. Because of the irregular seepage of blood into the alveoli and, perhaps

into the interstitial tissues, at the periphery of the hemorrhagic lesions, the borders are poorly demarcated at first. Later, as the blood in the tissues at the edges of the lesion is absorbed, the shadow becomes more sharply delineated. As clotting takes place within the center of the lesion, the shadow tends to become somewhat more dense. The persistence of the shadow, together with the sharpness of its outline, may suggest the presence of a round neoplasm.

Blast Injury. Multiple small areas of alveolar hemorrhage occur as a result of blast injuries, particularly when they are sustained under water. The hemorrhagic foci are quite small and their shadows blend with the surrounding edematous lung to produce a picture similar to that of acute hemorrhagic bronchopneumonia or severe gas poisoning. If anything, the pathologic process is even more diffuse. Roentgenologically, it is marked by the presence of numerous tiny foci of consolidation on an indistinct, gray background of edema.

Infarcts. The pulmonary infarct is an excellent

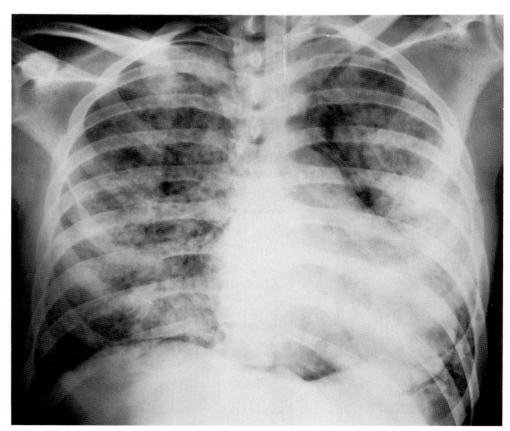

FIG. 113. PULMONARY HEMORRHAGE

The patient with terminal aplastic anemia developed massive hemoptysis. A portable film shows numerous, small, indistinct areas of consolidation throughout the right lung. The areas of consolidation on the left side are confluent. At autopsy, the alveoli were found to be distended with blood.

example of hemorrhagic consolidation (see Fig. 310). Although infarcts of the lung are generally found to be multiple at post mortem examination, most of those which are observed roentgenologically are single. This discrepancy is due to the fact that multiple infarcts generally occur as terminal events, particularly in patients with cardiac failure, and roentgen examinations are usually not performed at that time. Although pulmonary infarction secondary to embolization occurs most frequently in association with cardiac disease, particularly in the presence of heart failure, infarction is not so uncommon in embolization in the absence of heart disease.

The shadow of the infarct itself cannot be differentiated from that of consolidation in pneumonia. However, other changes associated with pulmonary embolization are often present, and they may be sufficiently characteristic to indicate the cause of the consolidation. These are the presence of associated areas of focal atelectasis, involvement of the other side, and the occurrence of effusions (Fig. 114).

The characteristic outline presented by the infarct at postmortem examination is rarely seen on films made in the frontal projection. The silhouette of the truncated conical lesion is not wedge-shaped in this position unless the base of the infarct happens to lie against the lateral border of the chest or against the short fissure. The sharply delineated shadow of uniform density which characterizes an infarct is sometimes seen on the lateral view. In this position, the much larger area represented by the anterior and the posterior surfaces of the lungs, a considerable portion of the base of the lung, and the fissural surfaces of the lobes, lie parallel to the rays and perpendicular to the film.

Multiple small areas of infarction occur in sickle cell anemia. In this disease, the smaller vessels of the lung may be occluded by tiny thrombi or agglutinated red cell sludge. The infarcts tend to be numerous. They are depicted as small, irregular, flocculent shadows throughout the pulmonary fields.

NEOPLASTIC CONSOLIDATION. Benign neoplasms of the lung and many of the metastatic tumors in this organ grow by expansion and, as they increase in size, push away the surrounding lung tissue. Primary carcinomas of the lung, however, as well as some metastatic growths extend not only by expansion of the tumor but also by infiltration into the adjacent pulmonary parenchyma. In addition, there are some tumors, both primary and metastatic, which appear to grow into the alveoli without invading or destroying the alveolar septa to any marked degree. The walls of the air sacs seem to act as a framework along which the tumor cells grow and proliferate to fill the alveoli. The filling of large numbers of contiguous alveoli with tumor cells produces, in effect, a consolidation of the lung. Because the framework of the lung is preserved, the cut section of such a neoplasm has the appearance of a pneumonia, so much so that this type of neoplastic involvement has been called *pneumonia carcinomatosa*.

The roentgen appearance of carcinomatous consolidation of the lung, as well as the characteristic pathologic appearance is best exemplified by cases of alveolar cell carcinoma. In this disease, the alveoli are lined by cuboidal cells whose arrangement suggests a benign growth of glandular origin. However, the tumor is not encapsulated and the consolidation of the lung proceeds actively at the border of the neoplasm. This tendency to contiguous spread indicates that it is malignant. It apparently grows not by expansion or infiltration of the surrounding tissue but by actual spread from alveolus to alveolus.

Since the tumor causes no symptoms for a long time, the first film often shows a farily large area of consolidation. This may present as a homogeneous shadow whose borders fade out into the surrounding lung in conformity with the manner of growth of the tumor. The appearance then cannot be differentiated from lobar pneumonia at a single examination (Fig. 115). However, the progressive growth of the shadow suggests its neoplastic nature. These growths may involve the adjacent lobe and, in most instances, they eventually produce additional lesions in the opposite lung. More often, the neoplasm is represented by multiple smaller foci of consolidation and infiltration. It is then impossible to differentiate the lesion from metastatic carcinoma.

Primary Carcinoma. A localized peripheral bronchogenic carcinoma may cause consolidation in the same way as pulmonary adenomatosis. This is most common with anaplastic growths but can also occur with adenocarcinoma. Squamous cell tumors usually expand and infiltrate and do not cause consolidation. The consolidating tumors are fairly well circumscribed. They show themselves as large masses of homogeneous density whose borders are relatively sharp because of their slow growth. They have a tendency to grow throughout the alveoli of an entire lobe (see Fig. 397). The border then becomes even more sharply outlined by the interlobar fissure. This eventually bulges in the direction of the adjacent healthy lobe because of the distension of the alveoli by the proliferating cells. This type of tumor is extremely rare. Because of its distribution, it has been termed lobar carcinoma. It

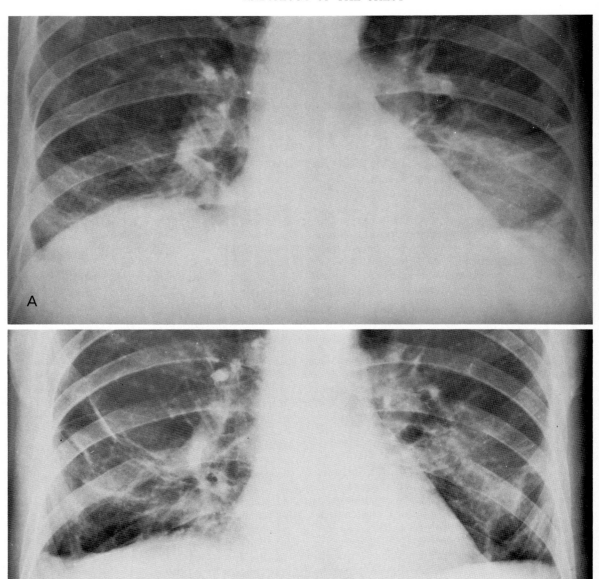

FIG. 114. PULMONARY INFARCTION

A: The shadow at the left base represents an area of hemorrhagic consolidation due to infarction of the posterior and lateral basal segments. There is a small effusion at the left base together with several linear streaks on both sides. Bilateral Fleischner lines are common manifestations of pulmonary embolization. *B:* Repeated embolization. Three weeks later, the infarct has almost completely resolved. Pleural adhesions now bind the outer part of the left leaf of the diaphragm to the lateral chest wall, obliterating the costophrenic sinus. Shortly before this film was made the patient developed sudden pain in the right chest. A small effusion has appeared in the right costophrenic sinus together with a number of new Fleischner lines, indicating recurrent embolization.

can be distinguished from lobar pneumonia on the film when it has attained large proportions and causes a bulging of the interlobar fissure.

Metastatic Carcinoma. Consolidation of the lung may be caused by a metastatic neoplasm. The most common site of origin is in the pancreas, but it has also been observed in carcinoma of the colon and stomach and, more rarely, from

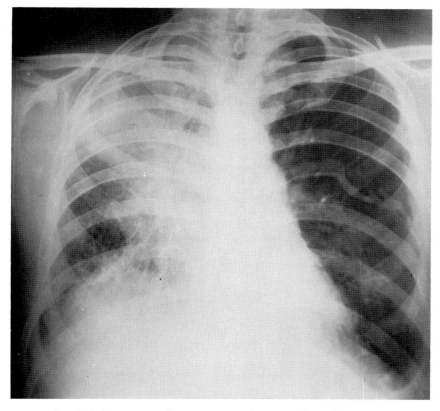

FIG. 115. NEOPLASTIC CONSOLIDATION: ALVEOLAR CELL CARCINOMA

The homogeneous shadow over the right upper lobe and the mesial part of the right middle lobe is due to consolidation of the alveoli by neoplastic cells. The obscuration of the contour of the right diaphragm indicates involvement of the right lower lobe as well. The neoplasm first appeared in the left lower lobe which was resected 2 years previously. The posterior portion of the left seventh rib was removed at that time and has undergone regeneration.

primary lesions in other organs. The pulmonary lesions are usually multiple and the individual areas of involvement smaller than in lobar carcinoma. The appearance is not unlike that of a lobular bronchopneumonia from which it can be differentiated roentgenographically only by the persistence of the shadows.

CIRCULATORY DISTURBANCES

Most of the individual shadows in the periphery of the lungs, the pulmonary markings, are cast by the blood in the pulmonary arteries and veins. The size of the vessels is determined largely by the volume of blood that flows through them. Alteration in the pattern of blood flow can be caused by abnormalities of the pulmonary parenchyma, disease of the heart, or lesions directly involving the pulmonary vessels.

Decreased Pulmonary Vasculature. A localized paucity of pulmonary vessels indicates diminished blood flow in the affected portions, or overexpansion of the lung. In compensatory hyperaeration, the vessels are intrinsically normal but are spread apart, thus giving the impression of hypovascularity. In obstructive hyperinflation or emphysema, the vessels are narrowed as well.

Decrease in blood flow to a portion of the lung results when one or more of the regional arteries are occluded or when there is an increase in the local vascular resistance so that blood is diverted to other areas where the impedance to flow is less. A localized elevation of vascular resistance is most often due to disease in the lung such as bullae, atelectasis, or obstructive emphysema, all of which compress the capillary bed. Occlusion of an arterial branch can be caused by invasion of the vessel by a pulmonary or mediastinal neoplasm or by thrombosis secondary to an adjacent inflammatory lesion in the lung. In most of these instances, the roentgen picture is dominated by the primary disease. When the arterial occlusion is due to an embolus, a localized oligemia is frequently the only roentgen sign of the disease (see Fig. 305).

Diffuse pulmonary hypovascularity can result from a generalized increase in intrapulmonary pressure as in emphysema, or from a cardiac abnormality that causes a right-to-left shunt. In the former case, the central arteries are enlarged because of the pulmonary hypertension that results from the high peripheral resistance. When there is a right-to-left shunt, some of the blood from the right side of the heart bypasses the pulmonary circuit and the hilar vessels are small. In both instances, peripheral pulmonary blood flow is decreased, the small vessels are narrow and the lungs appear more radiolucent than normal.

The appearance of the pulmonary vasculature in cyanotic congenital heart disease is modified by collateral circulation through the bronchial arteries. When this is well developed, it can create the impression of normal and even increased pulmonary blood flow. However, the pattern of the pulmonary vessels is distinctly abnormal. The hilar arteries are small and the peripheral vessels do not branch in an orderly fashion. Rather, the lung fields show a random, reticular pattern without radiation from the lung roots. The abnormal vascular shadows extend to the periphery of the lungs (Fig. 116).

Pulmonary Arterial Hypertension. The roentgen appearance of the vessels in pulmonary

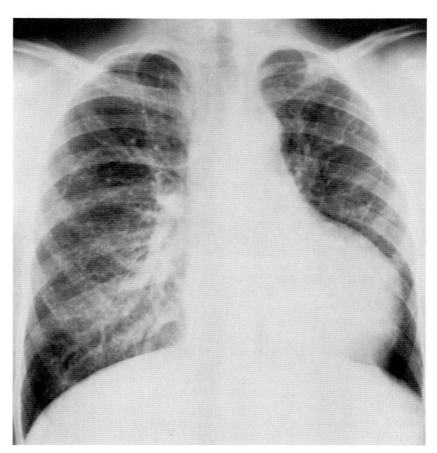

FIG. 116. BRONCHIAL COLLATERAL CIRCULATION

The patient had cyanotic congenital heart disease, characterized by pulmonary atresia and a ventricular septal defect. Despite the absence of major pulmonary arteries the lungs appear well vascularized. However, the pattern is distinctly abnormal. The central pulmonary vessels are small and do not branch in regular fashion from the hila. The peripheral vessels are disorderly and extend to the surface of the lung. The reticular appearance of the pulmonary vasculature is characteristic of collateral bronchial circulation. The heart is boot-shaped, its apex is elevated and rounded, and the normal bulge of the pulmonary artery segment is absent.

hypertension depends on whether the elevated arterial pressure is due to an increase in flow, as in a left-to-right shunt, or to an increase in pulmonary vascular resistance.

When there is a large left-to-right shunt, the pulmonary vascular bed is overloaded. Not only must the vessels transmit the volume of blood representing the systemic venous return to the heart, but they must also carry the additional blood shunted into the right heart chambers. Both the pulmonary arteries and veins dilate and give the picture of diffuse hypervascularity (Fig. 117). Once the cardiac defect is corrected, the increased blood flow ceases and the vessels rapidly return to normal caliber. A similar diffuse increase in vascularity can occur in any disease associated with an increased blood volume, such as polycythemia (Fig. 118).

Generalized increase in pulmonary vascular resistance can be caused by diffuse narrowing of the pulmonary arterioles and capillaries secondary to pulmonary disease such as emphysema or

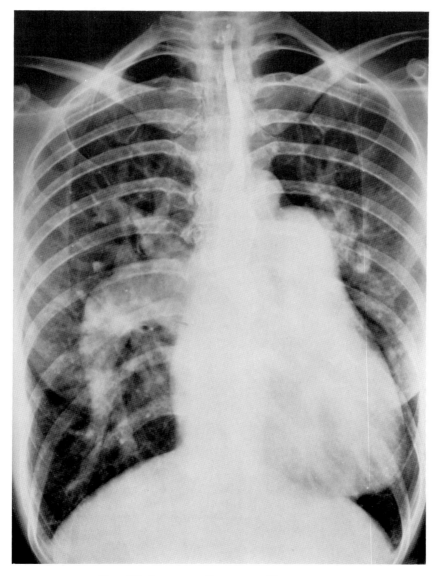

FIG. 117. INCREASED PULMONARY VASCULATURE

The arteries and veins throughout the lungs are dilated and there is inordinate enlargement of the main pulmonary artery and its major branches. The heart is moderately enlarged. The picture is typical of an atrial septal defect with a left-to-right shunt. In this case, however, the shunt was due to anomalous insertion of the right pulmonary veins into the right atrium.

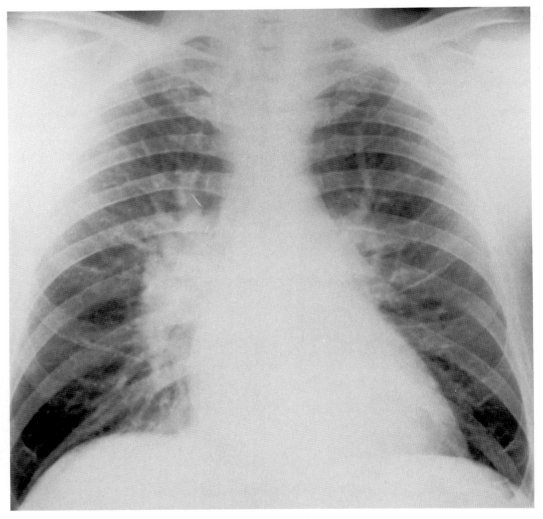

FIG. 118. PULMONARY VESSELS IN POLYCYTHEMIA

There is generalized widening of the pulmonary arteries and veins. Dilatation of the vessels is common in polycythemia because of the increased blood volume in this disease. The vessels revert to their normal size when the polycythemia is controlled. The elongation of the cardiac silhouette downward and to the left indicates dilatation of the left ventricle.

diffuse interstitial filbrosis, occlusion of substantially more than half of the peripheral vessels from repeated showers of pulmonary emboli, or proliferation of the intima of the pulmonary arterioles. Intimal hyperplasia can develop secondary to a prolonged increase in pulmonary blood flow as in a left-to-right shunt, or from chronic elevation of pulmonary venous pressure as in mitral stenosis. In some instances, no cause can be identified, and the condition is therefore referred to as primary pulmonary hypertension.

In severe resistive pulmonary hypertension, the central pulmonary arteries become considerably dilated. Their enlargement is rendered even more striking because of the diminished size of the peripheral vessels (Fig. 119). The dilatation involves the vessels down to the third or fourth order, after which they become abruptly narrowed. This may give the impression that the vessels are amputated. The prolonged elevation of pulmonary artery pressure is also reflected in the configuration of the heart. In chronic cor pulmonale the right ventricle is hypertrophied and may be somewhat dilated (see Fig. 268). This is usually difficult to detect. However, the outflow portion of the ventricle is abnormally prominent and produces a localized bulge on the left border of the heart when viewed in the right anterior oblique projection. The right atrium may be dilated and the superior vena cava and azygos vein unduly prominent, particularly when the right ventricle fails.

Pulmonary Venous Hypertension. In general, pulmonary venous pressure reflects left atrial pressure. The venous hypertension is most often caused by left ventricular failure, usually from coronary artery disease or systemic hypertension, or by obstruction of the left atrium as in mitral stenosis. The rare cases of total anomalous pulmonary venous drainage with stenosis of the common pulmonary vein, or stenosis of multiple pulmonary veins as in venoocclusive disease, have the same effect.

As the left atrial pressure increases, there is generalized dilatation of all the pulmonary veins, producing the picture of pulmonary congestion. This is a transitory stage and often difficult to detect from a single roentgen examination. The change in the caliber of the pulmonary veins may be quite evident if a film of similar technique made at a time when the patient was not in failure, is available for comparison.

The earliest roentgen manifestation of pulmonary venous hypertension that can be regularly identified is narrowing of the veins at the lung bases and widening of the vessels in the upper lobes. This reflects a redistribution of pulmonary blood flow, with an increased proportion of the right heart output going to the upper lungs (Fig. 120). Whether the narrowing of the veins is due to a reflex vasoconstrictive mechanism or to interstitial edema or some other cause is not certain. The roentgen picture may be quite striking. Normally, the vessels in the lower lung fields are appreciably larger than those in the upper. When the veins at the bases narrow, resistance to blood flow through them is increased and blood is diverted to the upper lobes. The arteries as well as the veins in the upper lobes dilate, while those in the lower lobes become smaller. This pattern is most commonly seen with mitral stenosis but can occur with any type of left heart failure.

If the cardiac condition is not corrected, the

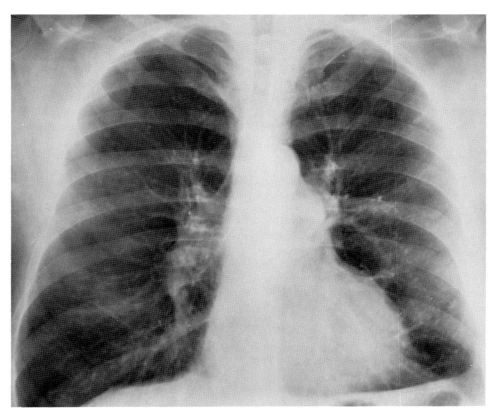

FIG. 119. PULMONARY HYPERTENSION

The central pulmonary arteries are abnormally prominent and the peripheral vessels are narrow and sparse. The change in the caliber of the vessels occurs abruptly a short distance from the hilum. This vascular pattern is characteristic of resistive pulmonary hypertension. In this case it was due to diffuse pulmonary emphysema. The outer portion of the left leaf of the diaphragm is elevated and fixed to the chest wall by adhesions as a result of previous inflammatory disease.

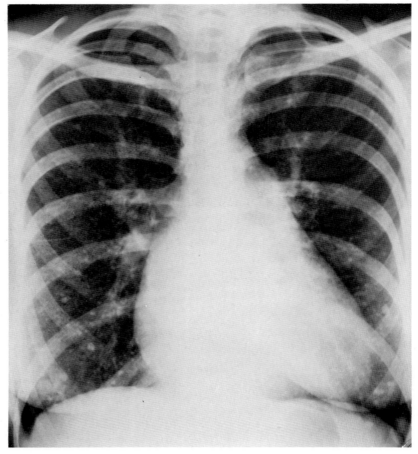

FIG. 120. PULMONARY OSSIFICATION IN MITRAL STENOSIS

Many small densities are scattered throughout both lungs, most numerous in the lower lobes. These represent deposits of calcium and bone which form as a result of intraalveolar hemorrhages in some cases of mitral stenosis. The irregularity and varying size of the calcific densities are characteristic of these lesions. The heart has a mitral configuration. The border of the enlarged left atrium is seen through the shadow of the right atrium. The central portion of the heart is abnormally dense, and the left cardiac border is straightened by the enlarged left atrial appendage. The vessels in the upper lobes are more prominent than those in the lower lobes because of redistribution of blood flow in the lungs as a result of pulmonary venous hypertension.

pulmonary venoconstriction eventually becomes generalized. This causes a diffuse increase in vascular resistance and eventually results in the roentgen picture of pulmonary arterial hypertension. Except when there are changes in the cardiac silhouette reflecting the underlying disease, the roentgen appearance of the lung is essentially the same as that of primary pulmonary arterial hypertension.

PULMONARY EDEMA

Under normal conditions, the intravascular and extravascular fluid compartments of the lungs are in balance. Small amounts of fluid from the blood constantly transude through the semipermeable capillary walls into the interstitial tissues. These are drained by the pulmonary lymphatics and the fluid is eventually returned to the blood stream. The major factors that control the volume of the transudate are the hydrostatic pressure within the vessels, which tends to force fluid out, the osmotic pressure of the blood plasma, which tends to hold it in, and the permeability of the capillary walls. A significant change in one or more of these factors can result in an outpouring of plasma fluid at a rate that exceeds the capacity of the lymphatics to clear it, so that the interstitial tissues become waterlogged—*interstitial pulmonary edema*. As fluid continues to accumulate in the interstitium, it begins to leak through the alveolar walls and fill the air spaces—*alveolar pulmonary edema*. At first, when the edema fluid is largely limited to the interstitial tissue, the patient is often tachypneic but there is little in the way of physical findings. The bubbly rales typical of pulmonary edema do not become evident until the fluid begins to displace the air in the alveoli.

Congestive Failure

Even moderate impairment of left ventricular contractility can result in a marked increase in pulmonary venous and capillary pressures. When the osmotic pressure of the plasma is exceeded, pulmonary edema ensues. Although the most common cause of pulmonary venous hypertension is failure of the ventricular myocardium, stenosis of the pulmonary veins or obstruction of the left atrium as in mitral stenosis, can produce the same effect.

Interstitial Edema. The interstitial tissues form a diffuse network throughout the lungs but the septa are too fine to cast individual shadows on the chest roentgenogram. However, they do contribute a faint, overall background density to the pulmonary fields which, because of its homogeneous character, does not interfere with visualization of the pulmonary vessels.

As fluid accumulates in the interstitial tissues, they become increasingly prominent and some of the thickened septa, when projected on end, cast moderately well-defined linear shadows. The majority of the septa still are not seen as individual structures, but the summation of their shadows now imparts an irregular, crisscross pattern to the pulmonary fields. This increase in "background noise" presents so many confusing shadows that the pulmonary vessels, although still outlined by air-containing alveoli, are no longer clearly visualized (Fig. 121). Because the interstitial tissues converge toward the lung roots, this portion of the pulmonary field becomes denser than the periphery, creating a perihilar haze (Fig. 122).

The interlobular septa at the lung bases are the ones most commonly oriented parallel to the

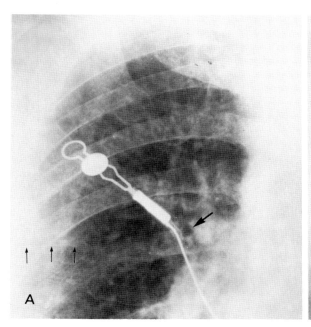 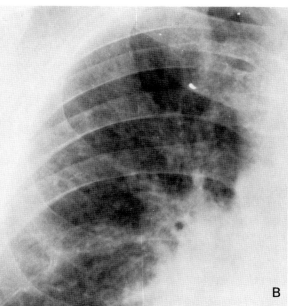

FIG. 121. INTERSTITIAL PULMONARY EDEMA

A: Portable film made shortly after myocardial infarction when the patient was not in congestive failure. The blood vessels in the upper part of the right lung are clearly outlined. The thin, circular shadow (arrow) represents the bronchus to the anterior segment of the upper lobe, which courses directly forward and is projected on end. The outer part of the short fissure (arrows) is visualized at this time. *B:* Several days later the patient developed incipient cardiac failure. The only overt symptom was tachypnea. The pulmonary vessels are now poorly outlined because of thickening of the interstitial tissues by edema fluid. The wall of the anterior segmental bronchus is thick and hazy as a result of peribronchial edema. The short fissure is not well outlined even though the patient is in failure. The "disappearance" of the fissure is due to a change in the angulation of the x-ray tube.

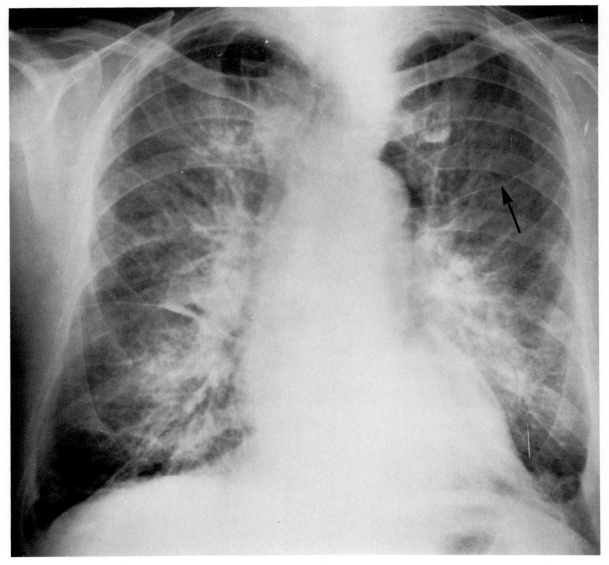

Fig. 122. Interstitial Pulmonary Edema

Patient with acute myocardial infarction. Numerous indistinct, streak-like densities are present throughout both lungs, most marked at the lung roots. These represent edematous interstitial tissues of the lung which converge at the hila. The short fissure on the right side is thickened because of subpleural edema. The angular, linear streak in the upper part of the left lung (arrow) is a Kerley A line. Kerley B lines are present at the lung bases.

x-ray beam on standard projections and are therefore viewed on end. They cast short, horizontal lines which always extend to the pleural surface. These are the B lines first described by Kerley (Fig. 123). They are best seen in the lateral and posterolateral costophrenic sulci, especially in the oblique projections. Kerley lines caused by interstitial edema are identical to those from other causes, such as lymphangitic carcinosis or pulmonary fibrosis, but they disap-

pear rapidly once the congestive failure is controlled.

Kerley A lines are longer, measuring as much as 6 cm in length. They are straight or angled, linear shadows that course obliquely across the upper lung fields, often not extending to the pleura. Superficially, they may be confused with blood vessels but the A lines are thinner and denser and do not branch (Fig. 122). The pathogenesis of these lines is not certain. Some believe they represent thickened interlobular septa like the B lines, but Trapnell has produced evidence indicating that they can be caused by dilated lymphatic channels together with the edematous tissues surrounding them.

Edema of the subpleural connective tissue causes broadening of the shadows of the visceral pleura. This cannot be appreciated over the surface of the lung because the shadow of the visceral pleura merges imperceptibly with that of

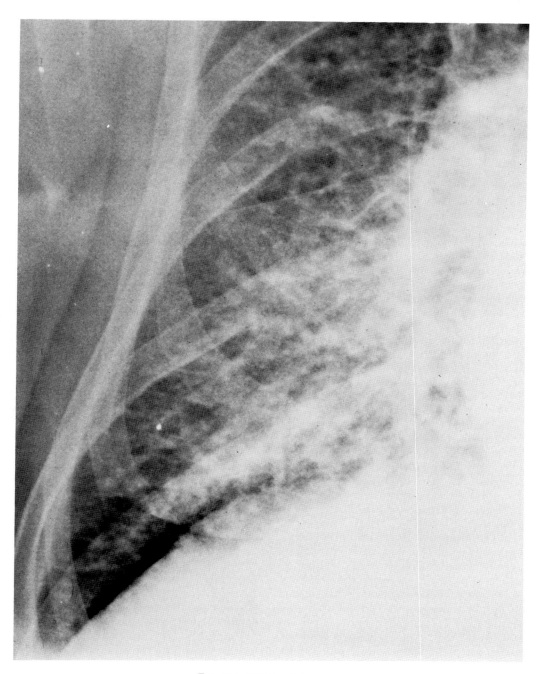

FIG. 123. KERLEY B LINES

A 65 year old man in congestive failure following myocardial infarction. The outlines of the pulmonary vessels are obscured by edema of the interstitial tissues. The parallel, horizontal linear shadows above the right costophrenic sulcus are Kerley B lines. They represent edematous interlobular septa seen on end.

the parietal pleura and chest wall. However, the double layer of visceral pleura lining the interlobar fissures is outlined on both sides by air-containing lung. The normal fissures cast too fine a shadow to be visualized on standard films. However, the additional density contributed by the edematous subpleural tissue is usually sufficient to outline the fissures clearly when they are projected on end although not when viewed obliquely or *en face*. The short fissure, which lies in a cross-sectional plane, is usually the only one that can be identified on a frontal chest film. However, if the x-ray beam is not aligned perpendicular to the long axis of the patient, the fissure will not be visible even though it is thickened (Fig. 121). Films in a cardiac intensive care unit are usually made with portable equipment and the angulation of the tube can vary from examination to examination. Because of this lack of standardization, the appearance or disappearance of the short fissure is of limited usefulness in the evaluation of congestive failure.

Interstitial edema also causes thickening of the bronchial and peribronchial tissues. This is most easily appreciated in the anterior segmental bronchus of the upper lobe since this bronchus is usually projected on end on the frontal film. Normally, the bronchus is seen as a smooth-walled, sharply outlined ring shadow just lateral to the upper part of the hilum (Fig. 33). It is always accompanied by a branch of the pulmonary artery which appears as a round, homogeneous density. When the tissues are edematous, the shadow of the bronchial wall thickens and becomes denser and somewhat indistinct—peribronchial cuffing (Fig. 121). Since pulmonary edema on a cardiac basis is always accompanied by congestion of the vessels, the artery next to the bronchus is dilated. However, because of the variation in size of blood vessels from one patient to the next, the vascular engorgement often cannot be appreciated except by comparison with previous films.

The roentgen picture of interstitial pulmonary edema is not a specific one and can be produced by a variety of diseases that cause thickening of the interstitial tissues. In general, the shadows cast by edematous tissues are more hazy than the sharply etched, linear pattern seen with pulmonary fibrosis.

Obscuration of the pulmonary vessels is one of the earliest signs of interstitial pulmonary edema. In many cases, it is difficult to appreciate this from a single roentgen study. However, when a series of films are available, the changes are usually quite obvious. Since sequential films are routinely obtained in patients with myocardial infarction, it is usually possible to detect developing congestive failure radiologically before it becomes apparent clinically.

Alveolar Edema. The basic roentgen picture of alveolar edema is simply one of pulmonary consolidation. However, the picture differs from that of most other causes of consolidation because the shadows do not have a segmental distribution and because they are relatively unstable, tending to clear rapidly in one place while new ones appear elsewhere. It is rare for all of the alveoli in any area to be completely filled with fluid. The shadow of alveolar edema, therefore, is not as dense or homogeneous as that of lobar or lobular pneumonia. The pulmonary vessels in the area of edema are obscured because the fluid-filled alveoli have the same radiodensity as the arteries and veins so that their shadows merge with each other. However, the opacification of the alveoli sets off the air columns within the bronchi to produce an air bronchogram.

The most characteristic picture of alveolar edema is a hazy, poorly defined opacification of the central portion of each lung, radiating out from the hila in a butterfly pattern (Fig. 124). Rarely, a reverse pattern occurs, the perihilar regions remaining clear while the outer third of the lungs is clouded. More often, pulmonary edema appears as scattered, patchy areas of consolidation. Occasionally the edema is unilateral (Fig. 125), but this is generally transient and is soon followed by involvement of the opposite lung.

The shadows of pulmonary edema can be distinguished from other lesions because they tend to be evanescent and often show considerable change from day to day as the severity of the congestive failure varies. Their fleeting nature resembles that of the shadows in Löffler's pneumonia, but pulmonary edema is not associated with eosinophilia. In almost all cases of edema on a cardiac basis, the heart is enlarged. However, in acute congestive failure following a myocardial infarction, pulmonary edema may appear almost immediately while dilatation of the heart does not become manifest for 24 to 48 hours. Although both pulmonary edema and pleural effusion are related to left heart failure, either can occur in the absence of the other.

Pulmonary edema without cardiomegaly can also be caused by the administration of excessive intravenous fluids, certain central nervous system disorders, azotemia, shock or by exposure to high altitudes.

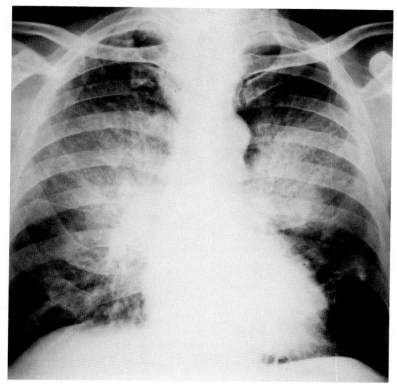

FIG. 124. BUTTERFLY SHADOWS IN PULMONARY EDEMA

The distribution of the shadows extending from the lung roots into the middle of each pulmonary field is characteristic of pulmonary edema. The shadows are not homogeneous because some alveoli are filled with fluid while others are partly or completely aerated. The streaks within the shadows are cast by the edematous interstitial tissues. The film was made soon after a massive myocardial infarction.

CAVITATION

Because of its elastic structure, its relation to the airways and the negative pressure in the pleural space around it, the lung is prone to cavity formation in many diseases of widely diverse nature. These include a variety of inflammatory diseases, neoplasms, infarcts, traumatic injuries, and disturbances in pressure relationships in which bronchial obstruction due to various causes plays a part.

Pulmonary cavities are usually detected by roentgen examination and only rarely can their presence be determined from the findings at physical examination. The ability to recognize the presence of a cavity is essential for the diagnosis of several of the diseases. It is important in estimating their prognosis and in the choice of proper treatment. Although the diseases in which cavities form are diversified, there are common factors which operate in their production.

Factors in the Production of Cavities. Pulmonary cavities may be either congenital in origin or acquired. Although congenital cavities may occur in relation to cystic disease, this seems to be quite rare. Such cavities will be discussed with other congenital malformations of the lung.

Several factors operate in the production of acquired pulmonary cavities. Foremost is the disruption of pulmonary tissue in relation to a bronchus, second is the tension under which the elastic tissue is held, and third is the degree of patency of the entering bronchus.

DESTRUCTION OF LUNG. Disruption of pulmonary tissue certainly occurs in mechanical trauma to the lung. This may produce a contusion or laceration which occasionally is associated with cavitation. In the case of pulmonary infarcts, cavitation is more common but it appears to occur practically only in the presence of secondary infection. The reason for the absence of cavitation despite the destruction of lung tissue in the majority of contusions and infarcts of the lung apparently is the absence of any well-

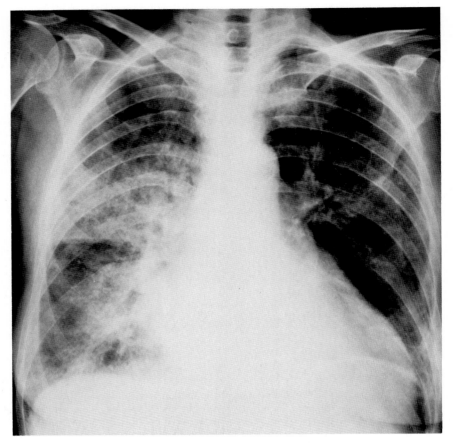

FIG. 125. UNILATERAL PULMONARY EDEMA

The shadows in the right lung are due to patchy alveolar filling of acinar distribution. The heart is markedly enlarged. The association of an enlarged heart with this type of consolidation, even though unilateral, is most suggestive of pulmonary edema. A film made the following day showed evidence of edema of the left lung as well.

marked communication between a bronchus and the injured area. In addition, in these cases, the dead tissue does not have a tendency to become liquefied.

Cavitation occurs rather frequently within bronchogenic carcinomas (Fig. 404). Several factors enter into the production of these cavities. The bronchial tumor grows largely by invasion as well as by expansion, and its growth causes obstruction of major blood vessels which lie in close relationship to the bronchus. This produces necrosis of the tumor. There is a tendency to infection of the necrotic material by bacteria entering through the involved bronchus. Finally, necrotic infected tissue is expectorated through the bronchus which is the primary site of the neoplasm, leaving a cavity within the growth.

The factors that favor cavitation in primary bronchogenic carcinoma rarely come into play in the case of metastatic neoplasms of the lung. These grow largely by expansion rather than

invasion, and do not tend to involve important blood vessels. They rarely involve bronchi of any considerable size so that infection of the tumor and extrusion of necrotic infected material through the bronchus is a most unusual occurrence. Cavitation, therefore, occurs rarely in the case of metastatic neoplasms of the lung. However, cavitation does occur occasionally in metastatic neoplasms or in Hodgkin's disease of the lungs following radiotherapy. This causes extensive necrosis of the tumor and, if a bronchus is involved, a cavity can form (Fig. 76).

Cavitation takes place in infections of the lung, when there is considerable destruction of tissue together with liquefaction of the exudate. The diseases most often associated with cavitation are the destructive forms of bronchopneumonia, either suppurative, caseous or gangrenous.

A bronchopneumonia associated with necrosis of pulmonary parenchyma is also accompanied by necrosis of bronchial walls. As the necrotic tissue separates, a communication is established between the bronchus and the destroyed portion of lung. If the suppurative or caseous focus is small, it is not apt to communicate with a bronchus of any consequential size. However, if the destroyed portion of lung is large, the necrosis will generally involve a sizeable bronchus. As the partly liquefied, necrotic tissue is eliminated through the bronchus, it is replaced by air which enters through the same bronchial communication. In this way a cavity containing air and a variable amount of detritus and fluid exudate is formed within the lung (Fig. 126).

In the case of an infarct or contusion which has become secondarily infected, liquefaction of the dead tissue takes place through the action of the exudate that forms in response to the infection. This produces an abscess in the contused or infarcted area. As the abscess expands it ruptures into one of the bronchi. Similarly, a metastatic abscess of the lung whose pathogenesis does not involve the bronchi, may perforate into the bronchus in the course of its invasion of the neighboring structures and empty its contents

through that bronchus. In all of these instances, a cavity forms because of destruction of lung tissue and communication with a patent bronchus through which the exudate is eliminated and air can enter (see Fig. 309).

Destruction of lung tissue in infections may be hastened by secondary infarction of the inflamed portion of lung. The severe infection of the bronchi present in the destructive types of bronchopneumonia often spreads through the bronchial wall to the adjacent pulmonary artery. As this becomes thrombosed, the blood supply is cut off from the most severely affected portion of the lung. Two factors are then active in the destruction of lung tissue, namely infection and infarction.

Uncomplicated lobar pneumonia is not a destructive disease. It is manifested almost entirely by an inflammatory reaction with only a minimum of necrosis of the pulmonary parenchyma. However, if complicated by arteritis, infarction of a portion of the consolidated lung may result. The leukocytic exudate causes liquefaction of the dead tissue which may be expelled through a

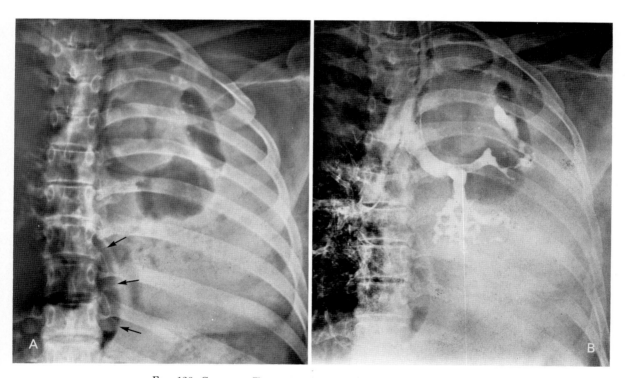

FIG. 126. CAVITARY TUBERCULOSIS: BRONCHIAL COMMUNICATION

A: Bucky film. The left lung is completely atelectatic, and the right lung has herniated across the lower part of the mediastinum (arrows). There are two large cavities in the left upper lobe. Since they contain air, a bronchial communication must be present. *B:* Bronchography. Most of the branches of the left upper lobe bronchus have been cut off as the result of tuberculous bronchitis. The contrast material reaches the cavities through a communication with an irregularly narrowed branch bronchus. The lower lobe bronchi are crowded together and irregularly widened. The terminal branches are amputated.

bronchus. The cavity which forms is the result of the aputrid necrosis caused by the arteritis (Figs. 127 and 233).

TENSION OF ELASTIC TISSUE. The elastic tissue which forms a network throughout the lung is under tension at all times in expiration as well as in inspiration. A tear in the lung inevitably interrupts elastic fibers. Retraction of these torn fibers in an otherwise normal lung causes the formation of a cavity which is many times the size of the tear. In the absence of any limiting factors, the cavity tends to be round in shape, even though the tear in the lung is linear or irregular. This is due to the pull of the elastic tissue in all directions from the point of injury.

The formation of fairly large, round or oval cavities from injury to a small portion of lung was beautifully demonstrated by Moolten. He made a small, irregular tear in the lung by means of a bronchoscopic forceps. The lung was then inserted in a negative pressure chamber with the bronchus free to communicate with the outside air. This put the elastic tissue of the lung under tension. As the lung inflated, a round or oval cavity appeared which was many times the size of the tissue torn by the forceps. An analogous experiment may be performed by producing a slit in a piece of cheesecloth and then exerting tension on all sides of the material. A round hole appears where the slit was made. How much

larger this cavity would be if the cloth were made of more elastic material!

PATENCY OF THE ENTERING BRONCHUS. An air-containing cavity will not develop in the absence of a communication between the destroyed lung and a bronchus. Once a cavity has formed, if the bronchial communication is occluded, the air within it is gradually absorbed and cannot be renewed. If the cavity does not contain fluid, its walls become approximated and the cavity disappears. Should the bronchus reopen before the walls of the cavity fuse, the cavity reappears.

Exudate within the cavity may be expectorated or absorbed if the infecting organisms are destroyed. On the other hand, if the organisms cause more destruction of tissue and more exudate, the collection of pus grows and either drains through the entering bronchus or perforates through the cavity wall into a neighboring bronchus or into the pleural space. Caseous material within a blocked cavity may be only partly absorbed while the remainder becomes calcified.

If there is a check valve obstruction of the bronchus leading to a cavity, the bronchial lumen is open only during inspiration. Air is then permitted to enter the cavity but cannot exit. In this way a positive pressure is built up within the cavity and pushes its walls outward. The increase in the size of the cavity may be considerable, especially when the wall is thin (Fig. 128). When

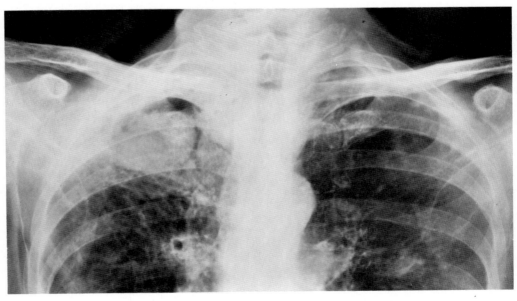

FIG. 127. APUTRID NECROSIS IN LOBAR PNEUMONIA: PULMONARY SEQUESTRUM

The round density in the right upper lobe represents a portion of necrotic lung which has sequestrated and lies within a cavity. The film was made in the erect position and the mass of dense, consolidated tissue has dropped to the base of the cavity. It is sharply outlined by a crescentic area of radiolucency which represents air in the upper part of the cavity. The patient had lobar pneumonia, pneumococcus type VIII.

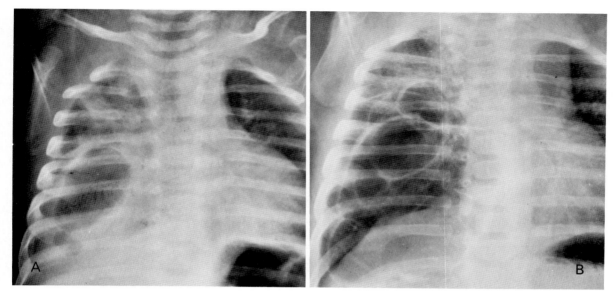

FIG. 128. PNEUMATOCELE IN SUPPURATIVE BRONCHOPNEUMONIA

A: Two weeks before this film was made, there was only a small area of atelectatic pneumonia involving the right upper lobe. The infection then spread to the lower lobe which now shows a large, oval cavity and, beneath it, a smaller round cavity. An area of atelectatic pneumonia remains in the upper lobe and there is a triangular area of emphysema in the axillary portion of this lobe. *B:* Two weeks later, the pneumonia has almost completely resolved. However, the cavities have enlarged enormously. They are characterized by extremely thin walls and the appearance is that of air cysts. These cysts can remain permanently and, if first discovered in later years, may be confused with congenital cysts of the lung. Fortunately, even large cystic cavities of this type usually disappear spontaneously within a relatively short time, leaving no residual abnormality.

the wall is thick, the weakened portion may give way, leading to the formation of a second cavity communicating with the first. It is in this manner that cavities become multiloculated.

Appearance of Cavities in General. The roentgen appearance of a pulmonary cavity depends on its contents and the nature of its wall. The appearance is also determined, in part, by the type of bronchial communication.

The cavity may be located anywhere within the lung, but the site of predilection varies with the nature of the underlying disease. Most cavities are situated in the periphery of the lung adjacent to the parieties. Some of them are more deeply located, but even these are generally in the periphery of a lobe adjacent to an interlobar fissure. Cavities which appear to be situated at the root of the lung on the frontal film are almost always really located at a considerable distance from the hilum, either posteriorly or anteriorly. This may be determined from lateral or oblique views. The oblique view is also helpful in differentiating an annular shadow produced by crossing blood vessels from the wall of a cavity.

The *empty cavity* is depicted as an area of radiolucency surrounded by a density of varying thickness which separates it from the normal lung tissue. The cavity may be round, oval or

somewhat flattened on one side. It may be multiloculated, it may have a crenated or clover-leaf shape, or it may be totally irregular. The character of the cavity wall is important. It varies from a finely etched, thin, smooth line as in an air cyst, or a denser annular shadow consisting of condensed and partly atelectatic lung, as in certain cases of tuberculosis, to a dense, diffuse shadow representing consolidated lung.

The pulmonary markings extending from the root of the lung toward the cavity often stop abruptly as they reach its mesial border (Fig. 129). When this is the case, the diagnosis of cavitation is certain. However, the shadows of blood vessels anterior or posterior to the cavity frequently traverse the area of radiolucency. Tomograms at the proper level show only the structures within the plane of the cavity and eliminate the overlapping shadows. The cavity is then seen to be free of pulmonary markings.

Because overlapping shadows of branching blood vessels can create the impression of a cavity wall, certain precautions are required in the interpretation of tomograms before deciding that a cavity is really present. The entire wall of the suspected cavity should be carefully followed to make certain that it is continuous throughout its entire circumference. A gap in the border which does not communicate with a bronchus or lead into an adjacent loculation excludes a cavity from consideration. It is also important to study tomograms made in adjacent planes. Even small cavities should be delineated on two or three sections made a centimeter apart.

A more characteristic picture is obtained when there is *fluid as well as air* in the cavity. The fluid, naturally, accumulates in the dependent portion of the cavity. It produces a sharply demarcated, horizontal interface with the air above it. On films made with a horizontal beam the surface of the fluid is projected as an absolutely straight, horizontal line. This level is pathognomonic of a cavity containing fluid and air (Fig. 129). Shadows of blood vessels and infiltrations

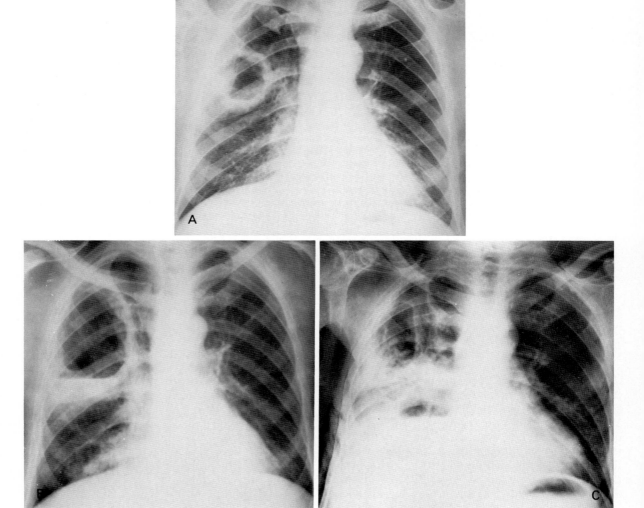

FIG. 129. PUTRID LUNG ABSCESS

A: There is a large, irregular cavity in the anterior segment of the right upper lobe. Despite the fact that the cavity had been draining rather freely, as evidenced by the small amount of fluid at its base, it contains a large quantity of air. *B:* A few days later. The cavity has enlarged rapidly because of incomplete obstruction of the entering bronchus, producing a check valve mechanism. The abscess has perforated into the pleura in the axillary portion of the chest. The irregularity of the mesial portion of the cavity indicates that this part, at least, is situated in the lung. An area of consolidation has appeared in the posterior basal segment of the right lower lobe. This represents a gangrenous bronchopneumonia caused by spread of the infection from the abscess, by way of the bronchi. *C:* A few days later. There is now definite evidence of perforation of the abscess into the pleura. It has become smaller and a loculated pyopneumothorax is present at the right base. Adhesions formed during the earlier stages have prevented general invasion of the pleural cavity.

in the lung or straightening of the diaphragm may cause a shadow easily confused with a fluid level (Fig. 111). Even a slight deviation of the line from the horizontal excludes the possibility that it is caused by fluid and air.

In almost all cases, the air-fluid level is demonstrable by roentgen means. When the amount of fluid is small, the level may not be obvious and appears only as a flattening of the base of the cavity (Fig. 130). When the cavity is obscured by other shadows, such as a markedly thickened

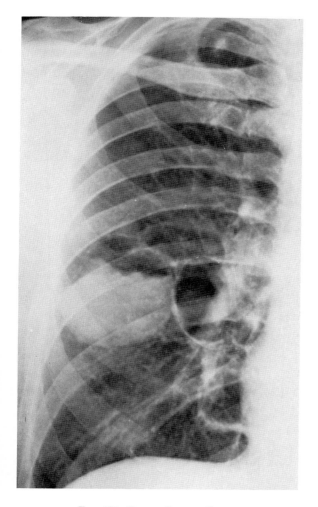

FIG. 130. BLOOD CLOT IN CAVITY

The cavities in the right lower lobe are thin-walled and resemble cysts. They are probably pneumatoceles, the result of a previous suppurative bronchopneumonia, although congenital cystic disease of the lung cannot be excluded. The film was made following a hemoptysis. The lower two-thirds of the outer cavity is occupied by a dense, homogeneous shadow with a sharply outlined, irregular, upper border. The unusual conformation is caused by blood clot projecting above the fluid within the cavity. The base of the lowermost cavity is flattened, indicating a small quantity of fluid.

pleura, a pleural effusion, or consolidated, infiltrated or fibrotic lung, the level can be demonstrated on Bucky films. It is important to remember that the fluid level is visible only if the direction of the rays is horizontal and, therefore, parallel to the surface of the fluid. Obviously, it is impossible to demonstrate the fluid level when the patient is recumbent with the tube above him, a position in which the rays are directed perpendicular to the plane of the air-fluid interface.

In the presence of air, the fluid is freely mobile within the cavity. Even though it is thick or grumous, the upper border of the fluid remains horizontal regardless of the position of the patient. This is often spoken of as a shifting fluid level, although, in reality, it is not the level which shifts, but rather the patient whose position is changed. Absolute proof of the presence of fluid and air is obtained if the level remains horizontal when the patient is tilted. This can be done under fluoroscopic observation or by making another film with the patient in the tilted or the lateral decubitus position, using a horizontal beam.

A small amount of fluid which produces only a slight flattening at the base of a cavity (Fig. 131C) can be recognized by reexamining the patient in a tilted or decubitus position. The flattening then shifts to the most dependent portion of the cavity.

After hemorrhage into a cavity, clotted blood as well as fluid may be present. This causes an irregularity in the straight line of the fluid level and may prove confusing (Fig. 130). The fact that clotted blood is responsible for the irregularity is determined from the history of hemoptysis and by the demonstration of fluid within the cavity. This is done by reexamination after tilting the patient.

An irregularity of the fluid level may also occur if, in addition to fluid, the cavity contains sequestrated, necrotic lung that has not been liquefied. Such material may often be present without accompanying fluid. The necrotic lung or inspissated material usually is free in the cavity and therefore lies in the most dependent portion regardless of the position of the patient. It is usually rounded in shape and when a horizontal x-ray beam is used, the air above it is represented by a crescentic area of radiolucency (Fig. 127). A similar appearance may be caused by an echinococcus cyst which has ruptured into the surrounding lung (see Fig. 266). When a vertical beam is used, as when the patient is x-rayed in the recumbent position, the round mass of the necrotic lung appears to lie within the center of the cavity, surrounded by a circular zone of lu-

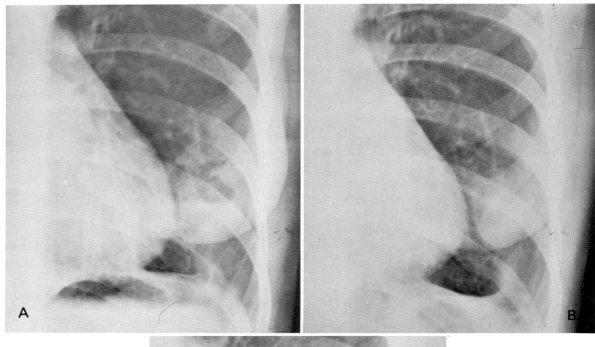

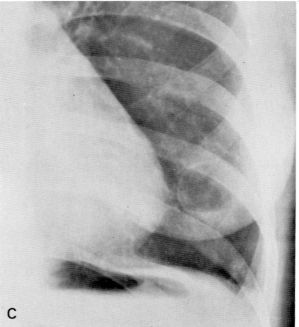

FIG. 131. DEVELOPMENT OF CHRONIC LUNG ABSCESS

A: There is an irregular cavity in the left lower lobe with a small collection of fluid at its base. The lung about the abscess is inflamed. *B:* The cavity became filled with exudate when its entering bronchus was obstructed. The patient stopped expectorating sputum at this time. The abscess is now represented by an irregular solid shadow. *C:* The abscess emptied itself after a communication was reestablished with the entering bronchus. However, because the abscess had become chronic, the cavity persisted. This is undoubtedly due to epithelialization of the bronchial entrance, resulting in a permanent bronchial communication. Air is then always free to enter the cavity, preventing its closure. A small fluid level is present within the cavity, indicating that infection is still present.

cency. The echinococcus cyst will appear the same, regardless whether the x-ray beam is horizontal or vertical because its wall is fixed within the lung.

When the cavity is *completely filled* with fluid, it exhibits a dense, homogeneous shadow on the roentgen film and neither air nor a fluid level is demonstrable. If the surrounding lung is aerated, the filled cavity presents the appearance of a round neoplasm. If the lung is consolidated, infiltrated or fibrotic, the borders of the cavity may be obscured. Thus, it may be impossible to determine whether a cavity is present from a single observation. The diagnosis can be made if a cavity had been previously demonstrated in the same location (Figs. 131 and 294).

Occasionally, a cavity contains a small amount of air which is not demonstrable in the ordinary frontal projection. It casts a dense, homogeneous shadow and is, therefore, unrecognizable as a cavity. Films made with increased exposure or oblique or lateral views may demonstrate a small air-fluid level near the summit of the shadow (Fig. 54). In some instances the air within the shadow can be demonstrated only by tomography. If the tomograms are made with the patient supine, the air appears as a radiolucent globule within the shadow. No matter how small the lucency is, so long as it is perfectly round and sharply demarcated, it unequivocally indicates the presence of a cavity.

It is sometimes difficult to determine whether a cavity, with or without a fluid level, is situated within the lung or within the pleura. A small or moderate-sized cavity within the lung rarely presents a problem because only a small part of its circumference touches the chest wall. On the other hand, a very large cavity which is broad-based against the chest wall, may simulate a loculated pneumothorax or pyopneumothorax. What appears to be a large circular cavity within the lung on one view, may be demonstrated to be flat against the chest wall when viewed tangentially. However, the upper border of a loculated pyopneumothorax is sharply outlined and forms a smooth, regular, arc-like curve (Fig. 132). Films in several projections may be required to demonstrate this. The presence of a scalloped upper border is indicative of a cavity within the lung even though it has a broad pleural representation.

An interlobar pyopneumothorax may present a roentgen apprerance identical with that of an abscess of the lung on the frontal projection, particularly if it is situated in the long fissure. Its relation to the interlobar fissure may be demonstrated clearly on the lateral view (see Fig. 528).

Pseudocavity. Shadows simulating cavities in the lung may be due to several causes. The most common is overlapping shadows of blood vessels, usually near the root of the lung. The vascular components which make up the annular shadow can be separated by turning the patient to the proper oblique position. Irregular calcification of the cartilage of the first rib can result in an annular shadow, easily confused with a tuberculous cavity (Fig. 1). Here again, oblique views resolve the problem. The appearance of a tuberculous cavity may also be simulated by synostosis of the first two ribs or by bifid ribs, particularly on films made with insufficient penetration. Careful attention to the ribs will obviate this difficulty (Fig. 47). Annular shadows can be produced by localized thickening of the pleura, particularly if calcified (Fig. 133). The fact that the lesion lies in the plane of the pleura can be demonstrated in either the lateral or oblique views.

Modification of Appearance by Causative Factors. The roentgen appearance of a cavity in the lung is determined by the factors which enter into its formation. These cause variations in the thickness and density of the cavity wall, in the size and shape of the cavity, and in its fluid and air content.

CAVITY WALL. The thickness and density of the cavity wall are largely determined by the disease responsible for the production of the cavity. A comparatively thick wall of homogenous density is usually present in infarcts which have undergone cavitation and in broken down, peripheral neoplasms. Especially with a carcinoma, the cavity can remain unchanged for a considerable period of time (see Fig. 403). A similar persistence of a thick wall may occur in tuberculosis, particularly in a broken down tuberculoma, and in old chronic cavities whose walls are markedly indurated by fibrous tissue. The wall of a putrid lung abscess is generally rather thin, although its lower portion may appear thick because of an accumulation of grumous fluid at its base. In suppurative bronchopneumonia, the thickness of the wall varies with the extent of the consolidation. Usually, in the early stages, the cavities are small and the infiltration about them is extensive.

In the inflammatory diseases, particularly the pyogenic infections, the wall of the cavity is apt to grow thinner as immunity develops. The organisms in the lung tissue about the cavity are destroyed and resolution of the inflammatory process takes place. As this occurs, the amount of exudate in the cavity diminishes and, if the entering bronchus permits good drainage, the

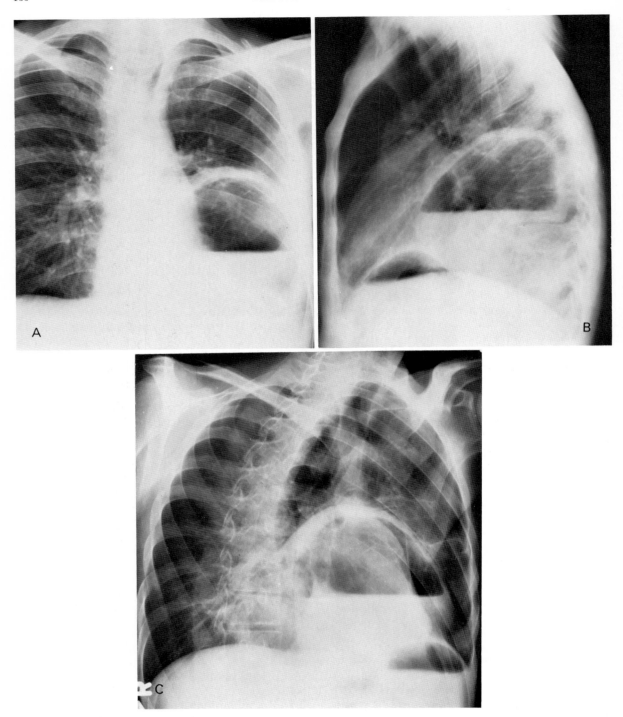

FIG. 132. PYOPNEUMOTHORAX

A: The frontal view shows a loculated collection of fluid and air in the lower half of the left chest. The upper border is thick and smooth indicating that the lesion is a pyopneumothorax rather than a cavity within the lung. *B:* The lateral view shows the lesion to be broad-based against the posterior chest wall. *C:* In the right oblique view, separate fluid levels are seen in the stomach and in the lesion. In the absence of symptoms referable to strangulation this excludes a diaphragmatic hernia from consideration. The patient proved to have a perforated lung abscess.

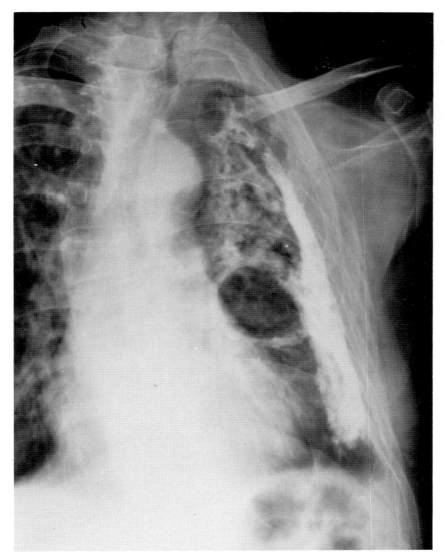

FIG. 133. PLEURAL CALCIFICATION: PSEUDOCAVITIES

The extensive pleural calcification followed a tuberculous pleurisy many years previously. Shrinkage of the left chest is responsible for the shingling of the ribs and the scoliosis. Where the calcified pleura is tangential to the x-ray beam, it appears as a band-like density paralleling the chest wall. The thick, fibrous portion of the pleura lies between the calcific layer and the rib cage. Where the pleural calcifications are viewed obliquely or *en face,* they cast a geographic type of shadow. Irregularities in the distribution of the calcium are responsible for the lucent areas resembling cavities in the lung. Pulmonary cavities were excluded because they could not be visualized on any other view. The thickness of the layer of calcium and the obliteration of the costophrenic sinus helped to differentiate this type of calcification from that which occurs in asbestosis.

cavity becomes empty. If this happens early in the disease, before epithelialization of the bronchocavitary junction, the cavity can heal. This occurs most frequently when the communicating bronchus is small. The bronchus becomes strictured at its point of entry so that no air can pass into the cavity. The latter then diminishes progressively in size as its air is absorbed until its walls become agglutinated and finally grow together.

SIZE AND SHAPE. The size and shape of the cavity depend on the amount of tissue destroyed, the density of the infiltration about the lung, and the mechanics of the entering bronchus. Destruction of a large portion of the lung naturally results in the formation of a large cavity. However, as has been pointed out, destruction of even a small amount of pulmonary tissue may result in the formation of a large cavity because of retraction of the disrupted elastic tissue. But if the region where destruction has taken place is surrounded by densely infiltrated lung, the elastic tissue may not be able to retract. The size of the cavity would then represent the amount of tissue destroyed. At this time the cavity is usually irregular in shape. Later, as resolution of the infection takes place, the pull of the elastic tissue may cause the cavity to become round. The round shape of an early cavity unaccompanied by any considerable infiltration in the surrounding lung suggests that the size of the cavity is largely due to the retraction of elastic tissue rather than extensive tissue destruction.

BALLOON CAVITIES. Rapid enlargement of a cavity in all directions, producing a sharply outlined annular shadow is usually due to a valve-like obstruction in the entering bronchus (Figs. 129 and 134). Ballooning of the cavity is sometimes followed by its rapid disappearance as complete obstruction of the bronchus takes place. If, however, active infection is still present during the stage of valve-like obstruction, as is usually the case with tuberculosis, the disease becomes more extensive. The cavity accumulates exudate and bacteria and the wall becomes caseous. When the entering bronchus reopens, the contents of the cavity are discharged into the bronchial tree. This can result in spread of the infection to other parts of the lung while the cavity may remain unchanged in size. Similar spread of infection can occur from the sudden drainage of a lung abscess into the bronchi.

When the lung about the cavity is densely indurated, a valve-like obstruction in the bronchus may not produce a uniform ballooning of the cavity. A portion of the cavity wall which offers less resistance may give way, causing loculation of the cavity.

Balloon cavities are common in children during the course of a suppurative bronchopneumonia (Fig. 128). The small size of their bronchi and the elasticity of their lungs make valve-like obstruction and retraction of the elastic tissue important factors in the production of extremely large cavities. Although most of these cavities eventually disappear by closure of the entering bronchi, occasionally they persist without producing any symptoms and may be detected in later life as incidental findings. Because of the thinness of the walls of the cavities and the absence of any surrounding disease, they are then often called air cysts and, if a history of the previous disease is not obtained and previous films are not available, they are wrongly considered to be of congenital origin (see Fig. 240).

Kinking of small bronchi by scar tissue, or strictures of tiny bronchi resulting from severe bronchial disease may produce a valve-like obstruction causing severe local emphysema of the lung. The overdistention may be so great that the walls of many of the alveoli rupture to produce a large air space, called a *pneumatocele*. The adjacent lung condenses about this area, forming a smooth wall. When the lung is removed at operation or autopsy, the pneumatocele does not deflate because its bronchus is obstructed and it projects above the surface of the excised, collapsed lung.

In essence, a bulla is similar to a pneumatocele in that it represents an area of emphysematous lung whose alveolar walls have been torn (Fig. 135). Bullae occur frequently at the apex of the lung in association with tuberculosis. It is important to differentiate them from true tuberculous cavities, which are caused primarily by destruction of lung tissue by the tubercle bacilli. In the absence of specific treatment, the infection in the tuberculous cavity persists, while the bulla, which is the result of mechanical factors, is not infected.

Large terminal sacculations in bronchiectasis really begin as cavities in the lung during the course of a bronchopneumonia. The bronchi that enter these sacculations are dilated during the early stages of the disease because of destruction of elastic tissue in their walls. The cavities at the ends of these bronchi are very small and represent the areas of destroyed lung tissue. There is no ballooning because the communicating bronchi are widened and do not permit air trapping. With time, the epithelium of the entering bronchi proliferates and extends into the cavities. The fact that the sacculations eventually are found to be lined by bronchial epithelium does not signify that they represent dilated bronchi. Serial roentgenograms of the suppurative bronchopneumonia that precedes the bronchiectasis demonstrate their origin as cavities in the lung tissue. If the infection becomes completely controlled, the roentgen appearance may suggest numerous air cysts. However, this is not an accurate term because bronchography will demonstrate the dilatation of the entering bronchi. The entire process is more clearly comprehended if it is called *cystic bronchiectasis* (see Fig. 200).

CAVITY CONTENTS. The contents of a cavity depend on the pathologic process in its wall and the patency of the entering bronchus. If there is no active infection in the wall, there can be no collection of exudate within the cavity. The fate

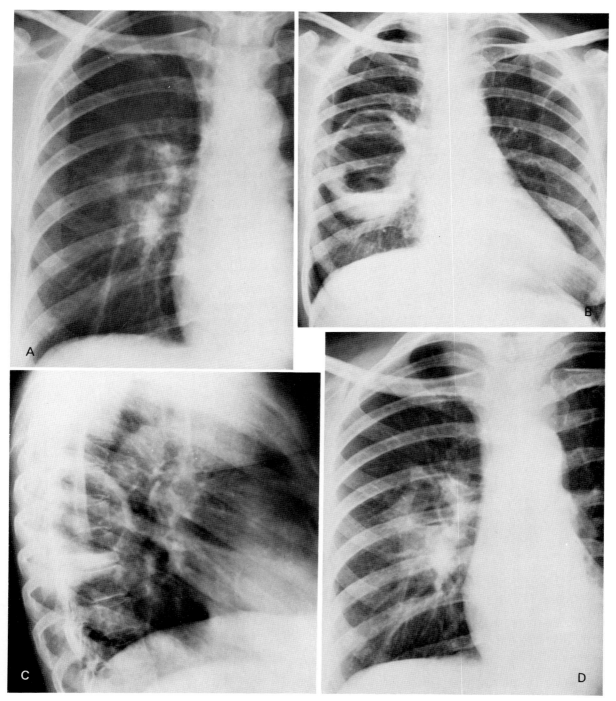

FIG. 134. PUTRID LUNG ABSCESS

A: There is a small cavity near the root of the right lung. It is irregular in shape and almost empty. The crenation of its wall and the fact that it is practically empty suggests that the abscess has been draining well and has diminished in size. *B:* Two weeks later, the patient stopped bringing up sputum and his temperature rose. There was a sudden increase in the size of the cavity and in the amount of exudate within it. Ballooning of the cavity was due to a valve-like obstruction by exudate at the bronchocavitary junction. This permitted air to enter the abscess but interfered with its egress. *C:* The cavity, which appeared to be at the root of the lung on the frontal projection, is seen to lie posteriorly in the superior segment of the lower lobe, abutting on the posterior chest wall. *D:* Eleven days later the patient again began to expectorate foul sputum as a free bronchial communication was reestablished. The remaining fluid level indicates that drainage is not complete.

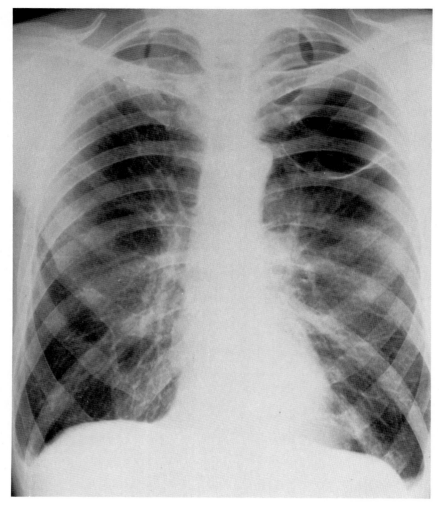

FIG. 135. BULLA

The large air space in the apex of the left lung represents a bulla. This was formed by coalescence of many overdistended alveoli due to rupture of their walls. The fine linear shadows within the bulla represent residual septae, some of which may contain blood vessels. The remainder of the lungs appears normal without evidence of diffuse emphysema.

and appearance of the cavity then depends on whether or not the bronchus leading to it is patent. If the bronchus is closed and remains closed, the cavity disappears. If it is open, the cavity contains only air and is represented by a thin-walled, annular shadow (see Fig. 275).

A persistent, thin-walled, empty cavity may suddenly fill with blood if one of the vessels in its walls should rupture. If the bronchus is plugged by a clot, the cavity becomes completely filled and then appears as a homogeneous, sharply demarcated, dense, round shadow. If the bronchus is not completely occluded, some of the blood is expectorated and air enters the cavity. The air-fluid level due to bleeding within a cavity does not always present as a straight line. Often,

clots project above the fluid blood and produce irregularities in the fluid level (Fig. 130). A similar appearance may be produced by necrotic material in a draining lung abscess.

Even though there is active infection in the wall of the cavity, comparatively little exudate may be present. The exudate is usually eliminated immediately if there is a wide bronchial communication in the dependent portion of the cavity. Such empty cavities are seen in indolent infections, particularly in tuberculosis. They also occur in lung abscess and in suppurative bronchopneumonia in the healing stage, when the infection is largely controlled. Persistence of a relatively large amount of fluid in the cavity indicates that drainage is poor.

A cavity may contain material other than exudate. When a necrotic bronchogenic carcinoma becomes excavated, there is often a persistent, irregular projection on the mesial wall of the cavity, representing the primary tumor (see Fig. 387). In cavitation secondary to broncholithiasis, one or more stones may drop into the cavity from the mouth of the entering bronchus. Larger deposits of calcium may be present in a cavity when the latter is due to infection about a calcific focus in the lung.

Occasionally a mass is seen within a cavity that contains little or no fluid. Most commonly it consists of a collection of hyphae (mycetoma), but, in rare instances, it represents an old blood clot, a sequestrum of necrotic lung (Fig. 127), or hardened, inspissated pus in a lung abscess from which the fluid exudate had been draining well. The cavity may be almost completely filled with this material which gravitates into its most dependent portion. Above the mass there remains a sharply outlined, crescentic area of radiolucency whose convex upper border represents the wall of the cavity and whose lower, concave border corresponds to the filling defect produced by the mass. An identical crescentic radiolucent shadow may also occur in a perforating echinococcus cyst. Here, the picture is produced by the insinuation of air between the cyst and its surrounding capsule (see Fig. 266).

The round mass is usually free to move and fall to the most dependent portion of the cavity as the patient changes his position. When the patient is supine, the mass settles against the posterior wall of the cavity. If the x-ray beam is then directed vertically, the mass will appear in the center of the cavity, encircled by a ring of lucency (see Fig. 251). This does not occur in the case of an echinococcus cyst because the air is trapped between the cyst wall and the capsule. Therefore, when viewed in the supine position, the perforating echinococcus cyst shows the same crescentic area of lucency as it does in the erect position.

CALCIFICATION

The recognition of calcification on roentgen films of the chest is extremely important in the diagnosis of thoracic diseases. The presence of calcium in a tumor usually indicates that it is benign. In inflammatory processes, calcification indicates that the disease is of long duration and probably healed. In addition, it may suggest the cause of the disease.

The main roentgen feature of calcification is the extreme density of its shadow. Usually the deposition of calcium occurs in an uneven fashion so that the shadow has an irregular, although sharply demarcated contour. This characteristic is useful in distinguishing calcification from other causes of dense shadows. Sometimes it is necessary to make a second exposure, with the patient twisted a few degrees, in order to differentiate calcified lymph nodes from blood vessels viewed on end (Fig. 33). In cases in which the detection of calcification is important for diagnosis, films made with a Potter-Bucky grid or tomograms may be required. Accurate localization of the calcific deposit is required for the diagnosis of broncholithiasis and in the differentiation of pleural calcification from a lesion in the underlying lung.

Bronchi. Calcification of the *bronchial cartilages* occurs frequently in elderly persons and is associated with ossification of the cartilages. It is rarely encountered in young individuals. The process is most marked in the trachea and the larger bronchi whose rings are demonstrated on the film as parallel white stripes. This abnormality is of no known clinical significance.

A much more important form of calcification associated with the bronchi occurs in *broncholithiasis*. In this disease, the calcific deposits lie within the bronchial lumen or in the bronchial wall. The stones originate as calcific deposits within caseous foci in the hilar lymph nodes, resulting from tuberculosis or histoplasmosis. If the disease extends into the wall of an adjacent bronchus, a stone can form within the bronchial wall—*intramural broncholithiasis*. If the mucosa over the calcific deposit becomes ulcerated, the stone may be extruded into the lumen— *endobronchial lithiasis* (see Fig. 190).

The stones lie at, or near, the root of the lung, most frequently in relation to the middle lobe bronchus or the anterior division of the upper lobe bronchus. They usually measure 2 to 8 mm in diameter and are recognized by the density and irregularity of their shadows. They are differentiated from calcifications within lymph nodes that are in their normal locations and from pulmonary calcific deposits by their relationship to the area of atelectasis and infection in the lung supplied by the involved bronchus. The characteristic roentgen picture of broncholithiasis consists of a dense, triangular shadow, representing the atelectatic, infiltrated pulmonary segment, and a small calcific density at its apex, representing the stone within the bronchus (Fig. 96). Especially when the middle lobe is involved, the triangular shape of the atelectatic lung may not be evident in the frontal projection and a lateral or oblique view is needed to demonstrate the characteristic shadow with the stone at its apex (Fig. 136).

It is important to differentiate the shadow of a stone from that of a blood vessel viewed on end. The latter casts a sharply demarcated, homogeneous, round shadow with a regular outline. It is usually adjacent to a small, annular shadow which represents the accompanying bronchus (Fig. 33). If there is any doubt as to whether a small, dense shadow at the apex of an area of atelectasis is due to a calcific deposit or to a blood vessel, a second film should be made with the patient slightly rotated. The density caused by a vessel will either disappear or become elongated, while that of a stone remains unchanged. The characteristic mottled density and irregularity of the outline of the stone may be brought out more clearly by Bucky films or tomography.

Lung. The most common cause of a calcific

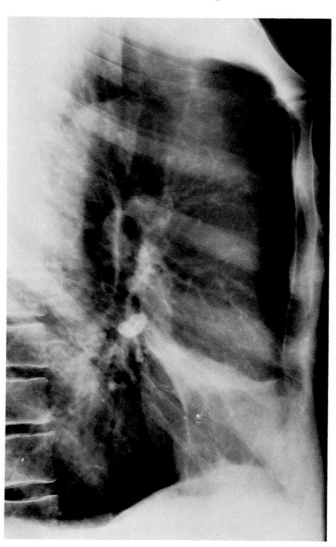

Fig. 136. Broncholithiasis

The right lateral view shows a triangular shadow extending downward and forward from the root of the lung. This represents the lateral segment of the middle lobe which has become atelectatic. Its superior margin is formed by the short fissure which is displaced downward. The mesial segment, which occupies the anterior costophrenic angle, remains aerated. The irregular density at the apex of the collapsed segment is cast by a calcified lymph node. This has eroded through the bronchial mucosa and is responsible for the atelectasis.

deposit within the lung is a healed primary tuberculous infection (Ghon tubercle). The size of the calcific deposit that remains as a result of this infection usually varies from 2 to 5 mm, although occasionally it is larger. Smaller ones are generally not visible. They may be situated anywhere within the pulmonary field, but are usually seen near the surface of a lobe if the film is made in the proper projection. The calcified tubercle is rarely of any clinical significance except as an indication that the patient was at one time infected with tubercle bacilli. Sometimes this is important in deciding that another lesion of the lung represents a reinfection type of tuberculosis rather than a primary infection.

In areas where histoplasmosis is endemic, a calcific deposit identical to that of a Ghon tubercle often represents the healed primary lesion of histoplasmosis.

In rare cases, mild reactivation of the tuberculous infection occurs about the calcified area and may produce a dense, fibrous nodule surrounding the calcific deposit. The calcified core may not be detected on ordinary roentgen films and the fibrous nodule can them be mistaken for a neoplasm. It is important in the examination of all solitary nodules of small or moderate size to look carefully for evidences of such a central calcific core, for its presence excludes the possibility of a malignant neoplasm. If a calcific deposit is not apparent on the standard films, Bucky films or tomograms should be obtained. Sometimes, in addition to the calcified core, there are concentric rings of calcification, caused by recurrent reactivations of the primary tuberculosis with subsequent calcification (see Fig. 257). These lesions, often called *tuberculomas*, are rarely of any clinical significance and almost never require resection (Fig. 137).

A most unusual complication of the calcified primary tuberculous infection in the lung results from secondary infection of the surrounding tissues by pyogenic organisms. This produces an abscess within which the calcified material may lie free. The latter is known as a *pneumolith*. However, most stones that lie within a cavity in the lung do not originate in the lung but represent hilar lymph nodes that have perforated into a bronchus (Fig. 20). As the lung tissue distal to the obstructing stone becomes infected and undergoes suppuration, one or more of the broncholiths may drop into the pulmonary cavity.

Calcium is also frequently deposited in the tubercles which result from hematogenous dissemination of tuberculosis. These calcific foci are most usually situated in the apices of the lungs. In rare instances they are scattered more or less diffusely throughout the lungs although they tend to be more numerous in the upper lobes. The calcifications are usually similar in size. Characteristically, the lung surrounding the multiple, small, well-demarcated densities appears normal. These lesions are practically always bilateral.

Considerably more common are the calcifications that occur within healed lesions of the reinfection type of tuberculosis. These vary in size and configuration. They usually occur in groups, particularly in the infraclavicular and supraclavicular regions, and are associated with fibrosis of the surrounding lung (see Fig. 289). Occasionally, a single, comparatively large, calcified nodule, measuring 1 to 2 cm or more in diameter, is found beneath the clavicle with few, if any, fibrous changes about it. This represents either the healed stage of a caseous tuberculous lesion that has never emptied itself through a bronchus, or calcified, inspissated material within a cavity whose bronchus became blocked.

Calcific deposits at the periphery of a dense, homogeneous shadow beneath the clavicle are also suggestive of a *blocked cavity* with calcification in its wall. In such cases, the remainder of the shadow is caused by caseous, uncalcified material. This may be extruded through the bronchus at any time and cause the cavity to reappear. Such circumscribed lesions are often wrongly considered to represent tuberculomas. The blocked cavity is more dangerous than the tuberculoma because its contents can be discharged into a bronchus and spread the infection to other parts of the lung. All medium and large nodular shadows beneath the clavicle should be studied by tomography. Calcifications along a portion of the periphery of the lesion strongly suggest a blocked tuberculous cavity.

Calcific deposits in the lung also occur in histoplasmosis and coccidioidomycosis. These are apt to simulate a healed primary tuberculous focus becuase they often consist of only a single, small area of calcification. Multiple calcific deposits scattered throughout the lungs not uncommonly result from histoplasmosis (Fig. 138). Miliary calcifications are rarely due to other mycotic infections. Similar small calcific deposits throughout the lungs sometimes follow in the wake of varicella pneumonia (see Fig. 249).

Multiple, rather small calcific densities, 2 to 4 mm in diameter, are occasionally found in the lungs of patients with mitral stenosis (Fig. 120). Characteristically, these vary in size and are most numerous in the lower portions of the lungs. They result from the deposition of calcium and the formation of bone within small areas of hem-

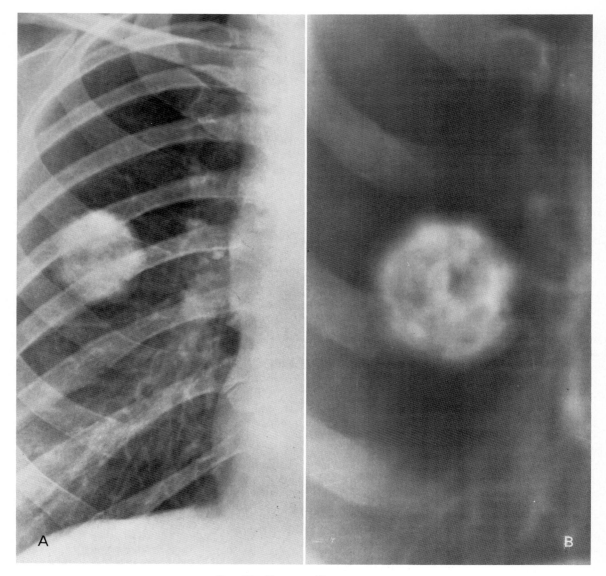

FIG. 137. NODULAR TUBERCULOSIS

A: The nodular shadow in the right upper lobe is unevenly dense. This suggests the possibility of calcification within the lesion. *B:* Tomography revealed irregular calcification throughout the lesion. The calcific deposits show a tendency to be arranged in lamellae. At operation, the mass proved to be a tuberculoma.

orrhage into alveoli. Why some patients with mitral stenosis develop these calcifications while the overwhelming majority do not, is unknown.

Occasionally calcium is deposited in the submiliary nodules of silicosis. In the early stages the nodules simply show a slight increase in density but as the calcification progresses, the nodules become quite dense and sharply demarcated so that the presence of calcium is unmistakable. Some of the nodules exhibit a central lucency, presumably because their core contains little or no calcium (see Fig. 321). The density of

these shadows is not as great as that cast by deposits of heavy metals, such as occurs in stannosis and baritosis.

In alveolar microlithiasis, calcium is deposited in proteinaceous material in groups of alveoli throughout the lungs. This causes the pulmonary fields to have a stippled appearance (see Fig. 376). As more and more alveoli become involved, the shadow of the lungs becomes more homogeneous and their density may become greater than that of the heart.

Diffuse calcification of the interstitial tissues

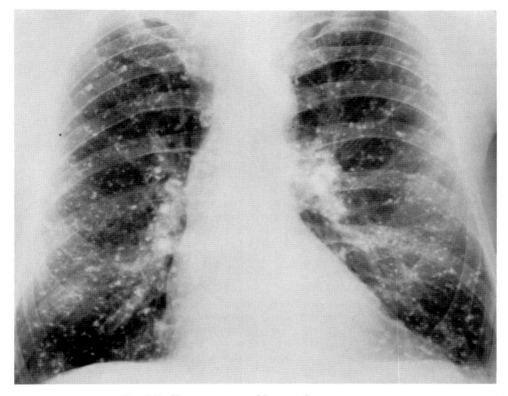

FIG. 138. HISTOPLASMOSIS: MILIARY CALCIFICATIONS

Both lungs are studded with tiny calcific densities. The patient was one of a group of people who contracted histoplasmosis in a cave in Oklahoma 20 years previously.

of the lungs is a rare accompaniment of hyperparathyroidism, vitamin D intoxication, and scleroderma. However, the calcific deposits are so fine that it is extremely rare for them to be visible on the film.

The tendency to deposition of calcium within hemorrhagic areas is exemplified by the occasional occurrence of calcification in old infarcts (Fig. 139). Broken down blood pigment remains within these areas for long periods, and occasionally calcium and iron are deposited along the connective tissues and elastic fibers in the infarcted area. Such encrustation with calcium and iron may also occur in diffuse hemosiderosis of the lung in patients who have suffered extensive hemolysis. The calcium and iron then form a fine reticular network throughout the lung. Calcification of benign pulmonary tumors of developmental origin is not uncommon (Fig. 140). These tumors are usually chondromas, in which there are areas of bone formation. They are classified as hamartomas because of the absence of a capsule and the presence of epithelial cells in the periphery. The calcium is usually distributed irregularly throughout the nodule. This pattern clearly differentiates them from malignant neoplasms. Their appearance is different from that of a tuberculoma as there is no well-defined central core of calcium nor is the calcium arranged in concentric rings. As with other lesions, the calcium is often not demonstrable on ordinary films and must be searched for with Bucky films or tomograms.

Malignant tumors of the lung rarely undergo calcification. Occasionally a bronchial adenoma (bronchial carcinoid), a tumor of relatively low grade malignancy, contains calcium or even bone. This is probably the result of hemorrhage within the growth. A large portion of the tumor may appear very dense as a result of the calcium content. Metastases from an osteogenic sarcoma usually do not contain calcium in sufficient quantity to be demonstrated radiologically. However, occasionally there is a sufficient amount of well-developed bone tissue within the tumors to produce dense mottling (see Fig. 434).

We have never observed development of calcific deposits within a bronchogenic carcinoma. However, the growth of a carcinoma about calcified lymph nodes at the lung roots is a common

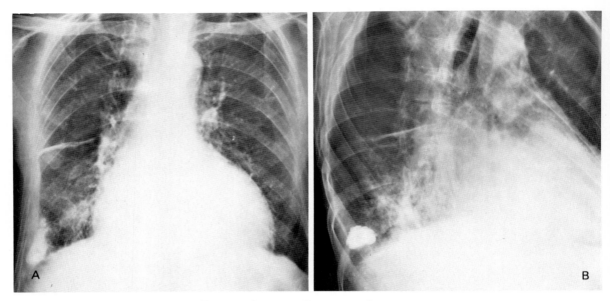

FIG. 139. CALCIFIED PULMONARY INFARCT

A: Frontal projection. The irregular calcific density in the region of the right costophrenic sinus is associated with marked thickening of the pleura over the right lower lobe and the short fissure. The heart is enlarged as a result of dilatation of the left ventricle. *B:* Right oblique projection. The calcified lesion lies within the lateral basal segment of the right lower lobe. Many years ago the patient had a pulmonary infarct in this portion of the lung and calcium was deposited within the hemorrhagic necrotic tissue.

occurrence. In addition, we have observed several instances in which a nodular carcinoma in the periphery of the lung has grown about a previously existing calcific deposit. The finding of a calcific focus within a round shadow may therefore lead to an erroneous diagnosis of a benign lesion. In this connection it is important to observe the exact location of the calcific deposit in relation to the nodule. If it is seen to be exactly in the center of the round shadow on the lateral or oblique projections as well as on the frontal view, it is fair to dismiss the lesion as benign. Otherwise, the possibility of a bronchogenic carcinoma which has grown around a previously existing calcific lesion is not excluded (see Fig. 410). Of course, examination in more than one position is always necessary before deciding that the calcific deposit is really within the lesion and not simply superimposed on it in one projection.

Calcium may be deposited in the wall of an echinoccocus cyst. Calcium appears as a dense, thin, regularly curved line, outlining a portion of the cyst. This local accentuation of a portion of the outline of the shadow is quite striking even on films made with standard exposure. It may involve a considerable portion of the circumference but even when small, it indicates that the sharply demarcated, round shadow most likely

represents an echinococcus cyst of the lung. Occasionally the entire circumference is calcified (Fig. 141) and in some cases the entire shadow of the cyst shows an irregular density because of extensive deposition of calcium. Rarely calcium is deposited in the wall of a bronchogenic cyst.

Chest Wall. Abnormal calcific densities of the chest wall occur most frequently within the ribs. These represent areas of bone condensation, called *bone islands* (see Fig. 163). They are not clinically significant but may be mistaken for nodules in the lungs. The problem of identification of these areas arises particularly when pulmonary metastases are suspected. The problem also presents itself when the density is seen in the infraclavicular region in which case the nodule may simulate a small tuberculous focus. The constant relationship between the density and the ribs on films made after lowering or raising the roentgen tube, or with a slight change in the position of the patient, proves that the lesion is located in the bone and not in the underlying lung.

Occasionally, irregular calcification of the costal cartilages simulates an infiltration in the lung. Often the calcific deposits are small and scattered within the cartilage and do not make a dense shadow. They can be recognized by their alignment, which corresponds to the course of the

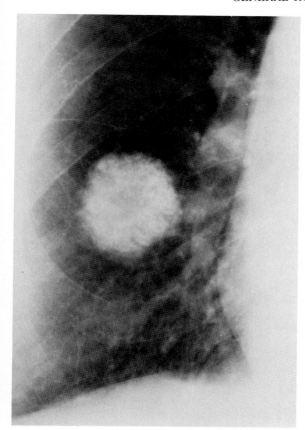

FIG. 140. HAMARTOMA OF THE LUNG

The nodule in the midportion of the right lung contains numerous calcific deposits. These are distributed throughout the lesion. The appearance is typical of an osteochondromatous hamartoma.

cartilages. Calcification in an *osteochondroma* also tends to occur in irregular fashion, but generally its relation to the shadow of the rib is easily demonstrated (see Fig. 158).

Round, calcified *phleboliths* in the chest wall may be confused with lesions in the lungs. The phleboliths are practically always situated within dilated veins of the breasts, and careful inspection of the films will show that they extend beyond the pulmonary field. Here the phleboliths may not be so clearly visualized because they are not contrasted with the air-containing lung. They are more clearly visualized and their location in the breast more definitely determined by examination in the oblique projections. Rarely, the phlebolith is a manifestation of a hemangioma in the chest wall. The characteristics of the shadow of the phlebolith are its homogeneity and the regularity of its round outline. Often the periphery of the phlebolith is denser than the center.

An unusual manifestation of a parasitic infestation of the chest wall is the presence of a wavy or coiled linear shadow in the soft tissues, representing calcification of the worm *Filaria medinensis*.

Mediastinum. The most common location of calcification in the mediastinum is within the lymph nodes. Calcification of the nodes usually represents the healed stage of the lymph node component of the primary complex of tuberculosis. However, even though calcification has taken place, viable tubercle bacilli may still be present within the nodes. The organisms may cause a reactivation of the infection and spread through the local lymphatics, thoracic duct and blood stream to cause distant hematogenous tuberculous foci.

The calcific deposits in the lymph nodes are generally larger than the calcified primary focus in the lung. A single group of regional nodes may

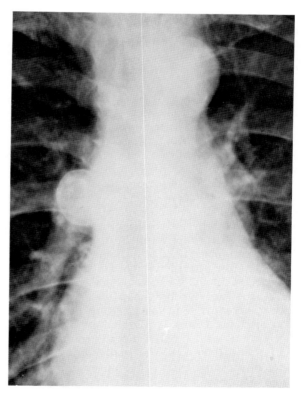

FIG. 141. CALCIFIED ECHINOCOCCUS CYST

A round, sharply demarcated mass with a completely calcified rim is present in the mesial part of the superior segment of the right lower lobe. This is quite characteristic of an echinococcus cyst but a similar appearance can occur in a bronchogenic cyst. The patient was a 47 year old Israeli sheep rancher. The lesion had not changed in size or appearance over a period of 9 years.

be involved, or there may be extensive calcification of many of the nodes throughout the mediastinum. In rare instances, a large calcific deposit of perhaps 4 or 5 cm in diameter occurs. This probably represents a calcified cold abscess originating in a node. Such large lesions in the paratracheal region or at the tracheal bifurcation may penetrate the trachea or one of the main or lobar bronchi. In a few instances, huge calcified nodes at the tracheal bifurcation have been known to cause obstruction of the esophagus.

The calcified lymph nodes are characterized roentgenologically by dense shadows. Their borders are sharp and irregular and, particularly in the larger calcified nodes, the density varies in different portions of the shadow. An unusual distribution of the calcium in the lymph nodes occurs at times in silicosis. In this disease the calcium may be deposited along the periphery of the node, forming a shell of calcification about it. On the roentgen film this appears as a ring-like shadow. These annular shadows which have been called *eggshell calcifications*, usually appear in multiple nodes throughout the mediastinum (see Fig. 320). The eggshell calcifications in silicosis occasionally are associated with tuberculosis of the lymph nodes but cases have been observed in which no pathologic evidence of tuberculosis could be found and in which the Mantoux reaction was negative. The explanation for the ring-like calcifications in these cases is not clear. Conversely, there are rare cases in which eggshell calcifications occur in the absence of silicosis (Fig. 142).

The finding of calcification in the lymph nodes was considered, at one time, to be an indication of previous primary tuberculosis. However, extensive surveys in the Mississippi Valley and the central part of the United States have shown that large numbers of persons living in this region have negative tuberculin reactions despite the presence of calcific mediastinal nodes. These patients were found to have positive skin tests for histoplasmosis. The primary complex of this disease is similar to that of tuberculosis, both in its distribution within the lung and regional nodes and its tendency to calcification (Fig. 143). Similar findings occur in coccidioidomycosis which is endemic in the San Jóaquin Valley.

Calcification sometimes occurs in the capsules of benign tumors of the mediastinum. It occurs particularly in the capsule of a dermoid cyst (see Fig. 454), but we have also observed it in the capsule of benign thymomas. The calcification may involve the entire circumference of the tumor which is then outlined by a sharply defined, dense, annular shadow. In most cases only a short segment of the capsule is calcified.

Calcification occurs particularly in adenomas of the thyroid gland both at the root of the neck and within the mediastinum. Here also there is a tendency for the calcium to be situated mainly in the capsule. However, in the case of a thyroid adenoma, as well as a thymoma, the lime tends to extend into the tumor. The calcification, then, is characterized not only by a thin layer of calcium on the surface of the growth, but also by an irregular deposition of lime within it. In some cases the calcium is deposited in multiple areas of necrosis and hemorrhage, causing a rather characteristic flocculated type of density.

The differentiation between an aneurysm and a malignant neoplasm in the mediastinum may be dependent on the finding of calcification. A thin rim of calcium is not uncommon in the wall of an aneurysm and serves to differentiate its shadow from that of a malignant growth (see Fig. 506).

Calcification of the ascending aorta, in the absence of calcification of any other part of the

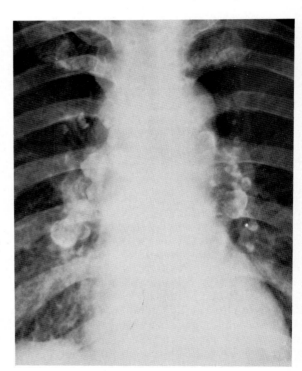

FIG. 142. EGGSHELL CALCIFICATION ON MEDIASTINAL
NODES: TUBERCULOUS LYMPHADENITIS

The hilar lymph nodes are enlarged and cast ring-like shadows because of a shell of subcapsular calcification. This pattern of calcification is practically always associated with silicosis. However, the patient had no exposure to siliceous dust. He had Addison's disease and autopsy showed caseous adrenals and tuberculosis of the mediastinal nodes.

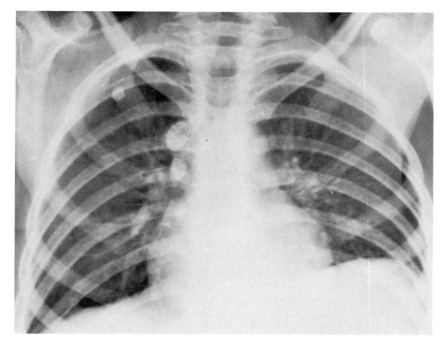

FIG. 143. CALCIFIED PRIMARY COMPLEX IN HISTOPLASMOSIS

The small calcific nodule beneath the outer part of the right clavicle is the residuum of a pneumonic focus in the right upper lobe. The calcific densities at the root represent calcified regional lymph nodes. The child was 7 years of age. The tuberculin test was negative and the histoplasmin test was positive. The left leaf of the diaphragm was elevated because of hemorrhage in the subphrenic space from traumatic rupture of the spleen.

aorta, is common in syphilitic aortitis. This finding is also useful in the diagnosis of an aneurysm. If the ascending aorta is found to be calcified, the shadow of a mass anywhere along the course of the aorta should suggest the possibility of aneurysm rather than a neoplasm. The exact diagnosis can be made by aortography.

From the facts outlined above, it is evident that the finding of calcification in relation to a mediastinal mass is useful in determining whether the mass is of a benign or a malignant nature. However, it should be borne in mind that malignant neoplasms in the mediastinum may grow around calcified nodes. The finding of calcified nodes in the midst of a mediastinal mass tends to indicate that it is malignant rather than benign. It is necessary, however, to take the precaution of making films in several projections to prove that the calcified node is situated within the mass rather than in front of or behind it.

Calcium deposits within malignant tumors in the anterior mediastinum represent calcification of the tumor itself and not engulfed lymph nodes. There are relatively few nodes in the anterior mediastinum and calcification of them from any cause is distinctly rare. On the other hand, calcification is not uncommon in malignant thy-

momas (see Fig. 487). It may take the form of several irregular deposits within the mass or appear as one or more ring-like densities. The latter configuration results when calcium is deposited in the periphery of an area of hemorrhage and necrosis in the tumor. A similar ring-like shadow may be present within a carcinoma of a substernal thyroid, the calcification having developed on the surface of an underlying thyroid adenoma. Calcification may also occur in Hodgkin's disease involving the anterior mediastinum, following radiotherapy or chemotherapy (see Fig. 475). We have seen one instance where calcification followed a biopsy of the lesion but have never seen it to develop spontaneously in the anterior mediastinum in this disease. It appears likely that the calcium is deposited in necrotic material resulting from treatment, or in an area of hemorrhage following biopsy. In all these instances, the calcification involved a rather small area, about 2 or 3 cm in diameter. The density was irregular in outline and appeared somewhat flocculant.

Pleura. Calcium is deposited in the pleura in tuberculous pleurisy, hemothorax, asbestosis and rare cases of chronic empyema.

Calcification of the pleura complicating pleural

tuberculosis or an old hemothorax usually occurs after the exudate has absorbed so that only the calcification and fibrous thickening of the pleura remain. The calcium is deposited irregularly in the thick plaque of fibrous tissue over the involved area and casts a large, bizarre, mottled shadow. This is easily confused with the shadow of an infiltration in the lung unless it is viewed tangentially (see Fig. 331). If the calcified plaque involves the axillary portion of the pleura, its edge will be projected as a sharp, straight line parallel to the chest wall in the frontal projection. The mottled continuation of this shadow over the pulmonary field is caused by extension of the calcific plaque onto the anterior or posterior pleura. When the plaque does not lie in the axillary part of the chest, it casts only a bizarre geographic pattern in the frontal projection. Films made in the proper oblique position or in the lateral view will project the plaque on end and make the diagnosis of pleural calcification quite clear.

In rare cases of nonspecific empyema of long duration, as well as in a persistent tuberculous effusion or persistent hemothorax, the pleura bordering on the collection of fluid may become calcified. Because of the density of the shadow of the fluid, the calcified material may not be visible on ordinary films but can be demonstrated on films made with the Potter-Bucky diaphragm.

A short, curvilinear shadow of calcification occurs occasionally in a portion of the capsule of a benign tumor of the visceral pleura. We have also seen an extremely thin shell of calcification in the border of a scalloped density representing an extrapleural lipoma bulging into the thoracic field.

Calcification can occur within a fibrin body in the pleural cavity. In the cases we have observed the calcium was irregularly distributed throughout the round, tumor-like nodule which was formed either during the course of pneumothorax treatment or as a result of hemothorax following an injury. These foreign bodies are usually situated in the region of the costophrenic sinus.

Calcific plaques at the apices of the lungs are usually bilateral and they probably result from hematogenous dissemination of tuberculosis. They appear on the film as small plaques viewed on end or as thin, arch-like structures bounding the extreme apex of each lung (see Fig. 518). Short, linear shadows of calcification, measuring 0.2 to 3 cm in length are visible at the boundary of the pulmonary field in many cases of silicatosis and are quite characteristic of this condition. They are seen most frequently in asbestosis and talcosis. Occasionally they occur in persons who have been exposed to mica dust or to diatomaceous earth. The calcification is usually situated on the diaphragm or over the lower part of the lung. It is an extremely important and reliable sign of occupational disease, and should be searched for carefully in all patients with fine infiltrations of the lungs, for it is easily overlooked. The line of calcification may be difficult to visualize on films made with insufficient exposure since the plaques are thin and rarely can be seen unless viewed on end. They may, therefore, be visible only in the lateral or oblique views (see Fig. 331) unless situated over the axillary or diaphragmatic surface of the lung. In rare instances the plaques are extensive and numerous and are visible over the upper portion of the lung as well as in the more typical locations.

Part III

Regional Roentgen Pathology: Roentgenologic Manifestations of Diseases

The roentgen manifestations that result from individual pathologic processes in the chest are limited in number. On the other hand, the spectrum of x-ray pictures produced by specific diseases is quite extensive because they represent various combinations of pathologic processes with differences in location and distribution of the lesions in the course of the illness. The effect of time and the response to treatment is helpful in the diagnostic evaluation of many diseases. For example, if a lesion in a lung is seen to diminish in size on serial films, the chances of its being malignant are quite small. The same is true if the lesion appears unchanged on a film made a number of years previously.

Comparison of films can be misleading unless the effects of differences in technique are taken into account. As a rule, a lesion appears larger on a light film than on a darker one. This pitfall is avoided if the shadow is actually measured with a ruler or calipers rather than relying on visual estimates for the comparison. Because the rays in an x-ray beam are not parallel but diverge slightly, a real difference in the size of the shadow cast by a lesion will be created if the patient is facing the x-ray tube for one exposure and has his back to it for the other, or if the tube-film distance is not the same for both examinations. If a lesion abuts on the anterior chest wall, it appears larger on an anteroposterior projection since it is further from the film than on the posteroanterior view. It will also become larger

as the tube-film distance is shortened. Allowance for the magnification factor can be made by noting the difference in the size of the rib adjacent to the lesion, or the width of the chest from film to film.

Differences in the appearance of the lesion may also be due to variation in the positioning of the patient, rotation into a slight oblique projection or tilting of the chest forward or backward. It is important to recognize these differences which can be responsible for an apparent change in the size or shape of a lesion. The relationship between the bony structures of the front and back of the chest are used to determine the tilt or rotation of the patient. On a true frontal projection, a line connecting the spinous processes of the upper thoracic vertebrae will be projected midway between the heads of the clavicles. In the absence of scoliosis, any variation from this indicates obliquity of the projection. Forward or backward angulation of the chest, or a change in the height of the x-ray tube can be evaluated from the position of the clavicles in relation to the posterior ribs. If the patient is leaning backward on a posteroanterior film, the clavicle will be projected over a higher rib than if the patient is bent forward.

Differences in degree of inspiration usually do not affect the size of a shadow unless the lesion is vascular in nature. However, the heart appears larger and the lungs appear less lucent on an expiratory film. A pleural effusion or pneumothorax will also appear larger. The degree of inspiration can be evaluated by determining the level of the diaphragm, using both the posterior and anterior ribs as markers.

The images on a roentgenogram represent a summation of the shadows of all structures within the path of the x-ray beam. A density projected over a pulmonary field may represent a lesion on the skin surface, or one involving a rib or the soft tissues of the chest wall. It may arise from the pleura or lie entirely within the lung. Determination of the structure that is involved is a necessary first step in the diagnostic process. More precise localization to a specific area is often required for the diagnosis of lesions in the lung or mediastinum. For example, tuberculosis is a primary consideration in lesions situated in the outer part of the posterior segment of the upper lobe but other diseases must be considered first if the lesion is situated elsewhere. Localization usually presents no great problem if there are multiple views of the chest or if the patient can be studied fluoroscopically. However, in many instances, only frontal films are available for review. Nevertheless, even with this limitation it is often possible to determine the exact location of the lesion.

Delineation of the entire circumference of a noncalcific lesion indicates that it is surrounded by air. This practically always signifies that the lesion is within the lung although a similar appearance can be produced by a mass on the skin surface or within an interlobar fissure. A lesion of the pleura viewed *en face* usually shows about half of its circumference sharply outlined while the remainder is poorly defined and fades off into the surrounding shadows. Indistinctness of the entire margin of the lesion has no localizing significance.

Obscuration of the normal vascular markings indicates that a lesion is within the lung. Normally the pulmonary arteries and veins are seen because they cast denser shadows than does the air in the adjacent alveoli. If the alveoli are collapsed or if the air within them is replaced by fluid or cells, the vessels are no longer delineated. Although a lesion of the chest wall or pleura casts a shadow over the pulmonary field, because the vessels are still outlined by air-containing lung, they are visible through the shadow. There are exceptions to this rule. If an intrapulmonary lesion is small or if it is situated against the chest wall, shadows of the vessels in the normal lung in front or behind are superimposed over the shadow of the lesion and create the impression of undisturbed vascular markings. Conversely, a lesion of the pleura or chest wall may be mis-

taken for one in the lung if the film is too light and penetration is inadequate to reveal the normal vessels through the shadow.

The air bronchogram sign unequivocally identifies a lesion as intrapulmonary. Normally the peripheral bronchi are not visualized on a chest film because their walls cast too fine a shadow to be detected between the radiolucent air within the bronchial lumen and the adjacent alveoli. However, when the surrounding lung is airless, regardless of whether this is due to consolidation or to compression of the alveoli by thickening of the interstitial tissues, the air columns within the bronchi stand out as dark, branching streaks against the opacified pulmonary parenchyma (Fig. 110). No lesion outside the lung can create this appearance.

The silhouette sign, first elucidated by Dr. Benjamin Felson, is an invaluable aid for localizing a lesion to a specific region of the lung or mediastinum. Normally, the heart, aorta, hilar structures and diaphragm are sharply outlined because of the contrast between their radiodensity and that of the air-containing lung bordering on them. Opacification of the lung or pleura contiguous to any of these structures will obscure its border in the area of contact. If a pulmonary lesion obliterates part of the right heart border, it can be assumed to be within the middle lobe because that is the only part of the lung in contact with this portion of the heart (Fig. 19). A density that merges with and obliterates the outline of the aortic knob must lie within the posterior mediastinum (see Fig. 168) or the posterior subsegment of the left upper lobe. A lesion in the posterior segment of the right upper lobe will not affect the silhouette of the ascending aorta because this is a more anteriorly placed structure. This silhouette will be obscured by disease in the anterior segment of the right upper lobe (see Fig. 416) or by a mass in the anterior mediastinum. A false positive silhouette sign can be obtained if the film is insufficiently penetrated (Fig. 26).

Obviously, the silhouette sign can be applied only to those lesions whose shadows contact or are projected over the mediastinum or the diaphragm. A nodule in the midlung cannot be localized in this manner. However, if more than one frontal film is available, the position of such a nodule can often be determined from parallax, utilizing the anterior and posterior ribs as landmarks. Even though a patient is carefully positioned in the frontal projection each time a film is made, it is not uncommon for the tube to be centered at different heights or for the patient to be tilted slightly forward or backward. As a result, the anterior and posterior ribs are projected at relatively different positions from film to film. The shadow of a nodule in the lung will also shift with a change in the angle between the x-ray beam and the patient. If the nodule is in a posterior pulmonary segment, its shadow maintains a constant relationship to the posterior ribs but shifts appreciably in relation to the anterior ones. The shadow of a nodule in the midchest will shift in relation to both the anterior and posterior ribs.

In certain specific instances, a lesion can be localized rather accurately on a single frontal film solely from the configuration of the shadow. For example, a density within the lung that is projected in the upper right parahilar region could represent disease within the upper lobe or in the superior segment of the lower lobe. However, if its inferior margin is sharply outlined and straight or concave, it must border on the short fissure and therefore lie within the anterior seg-

ment of the upper lobe, or possibly the subscapular portion of the posterior segment. If the upper border of a lesion in the right midlung field is outlined by the short fissure, then it must be within the middle lobe.

A mass in the superior mediastinum also can be localized from the frontal film if it reaches to the level of the clavicles, because of the tilt of the thoracic inlet. The inlet is delimited by the first ribs which lie on an oblique plane extending downward and forward from the spine. A mass in the posterior portion of the superior mediastinum can extend above the clavicle and still be within the thorax so that its upper and lower borders are outlined by air-containing lung. A mass at the same level but situated anteriorly, extends into the neck. Its lower border is still outlined by lung but its upper border fades off as it becomes lost in the shadow of the cervical soft tissues.

DISEASES OF THE CHEST WALL

Many abnormalities of the chest wall can be well evaluated by physical examination. However, it may be difficult to recognize lesions in the deeper tissues of the chest by external examination alone and these are often best studied by roentgen techniques.

The shadows of the structures of the chest wall are superimposed on those of the lungs and are especially prominent if the film is made with soft technique. The appearance of the breasts, nipples, subcutaneous fat and muscles of the chest wall vary considerably in different individuals. These variations must be appreciated if confusion with disease of the lungs is to be avoided (Figs. 4 and 144).

The Soft Tissues

The Breast. The roentgen appearance of the breast varies in accordance with its size and shape and the radiologic technique employed. On the frontal projection, the shadow of the small breast often lies completely within the pulmonary field. Large breasts cause bulging shadows extending laterally beyond the rib cage. If pendulous, the lower border is situated well below the diaphragm. The pendulous breast casts only a faint, rather homogeneous shadow over the lower, outer part of the lung, most dense over the costophrenic sulcus.

The opacity of the shadow of the breast is related to its thickness. If the patient does not

press firmly against the cassette so that the breast is flattened, its shadow is more dense and can simulate a pneumonia. The same effect is produced when the film is underexposed or made with low voltage. In most cases, the characteristic uniformity of the shadow, the gradual increase in its density as it approaches the diaphragm and chest wall, and the absence of any disturbance in the architecture of the vascular markings of the lung, indicate that the shadow is caused by the breast rather than a pulmonary lesion. Observing the continuity of the breast shadow with that of the axillary folds aids in this differentiation.

More difficulty is experienced in the interpretation of the shadow of the virginal breast where the typical, sharply defined, rounded border of the breast is not present and the organ is represented by an ill-defined shadow which does not extend to the diaphragm (Fig. 4). This shadow is easily confused with that of consolidated lung. In cases where the border is better delineated, the shadow may suggest a neoplasm. A similar difficulty in recognition of the breast shadow is encountered in gynecomastia (see Fig. 204) or mastitis in the male, especially when unilateral. In patients who have had a mastectomy, the shadow cast by the remaining breast may be mistaken for a lesion of the lung because of the difference in radiolucency of the two sides. This is also true when there is hypoplasia of one breast.

After a simple mastectomy, the only changes

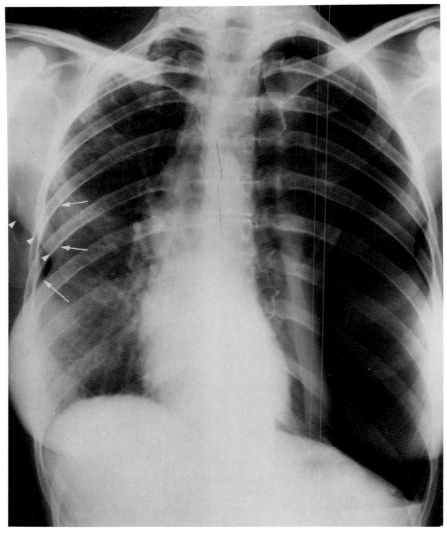

FIG. 144. PECTORAL MUSCLES

The patient has a tension pneumothorax on the left side. The curvilinear shadow (arrows) in the right axillary region represents the anterior axillary fold formed by the skin over the border of the pectoralis major muscle. This is continuous with the outline of the breast. The diagonal line crossing the pectoral muscle (arrow heads) represents the latissimus dorsi which forms the posterior axillary fold. The lucency lateral to the border of the pectoral muscle could be mistaken for a loculated pneumothorax.

noted on the film are absence of a breast shadow and an increased lucency of the lower part of the pulmonary field on that side. After a radical mastectomy, the lucency is more pronounced and extends almost to the clavicle. The axillary fold is absent. Instead, there is usually a narrow zone of density beneath the clavicle sharply demarcated from the hyperlucent pulmonary field below it. The line of demarcation is horizontal or slopes slightly downward and outward. It extends beyond the chest, is continuous with the inner border of the arm and corresponds to the line of

resection of the pectoral muscles and the fold in the skin which now forms the anterior border of the axilla (Fig. 145). It is important to recognize that a radical mastectomy has been performed because of the lead it gives in the detection and interpretation of other abnormalities on the chest film when no clinical information is available. An identical appearance is created by congenital absence of the pectoral muscles (Fig. 146).

The difficulties imposed by the breast shadows may be resolved by repeating the examination with increased exposure or using greater penetra-

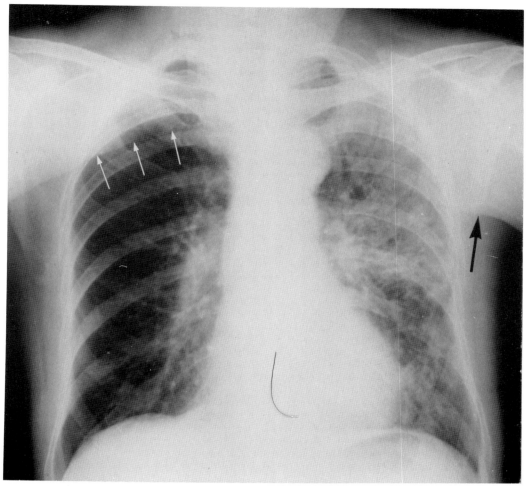

FIG. 145. BILATERAL MASTECTOMY

A radical mastectomy was performed on the right side and a simple mastectomy on the left. The axillary fold (arrow) is visible on the left side but not on the right. In its place is a long diagonal line of demarcation extending from the axilla across the infraclavicular portion of the thorax (arrows). This line represents the edge of the excised pectoral muscles together with the overlying skin fold. The patchy and streak-like shadows noted in the left lung are due to radiation reaction.

tion. In some cases it is also necessary to displace the breasts laterally in order to differentiate the shadow from that of a lesion in the lung. This is done by having the patient press more firmly against the cassette, or by displacing the breast either manually or by means of a bandage or adhesive tape.

A large breast frequently obscures the mediastinum on the oblique projection. In addition, it can cause a density with a sharply demarcated bulging border overlying the mesial portion of the opposite lung. In positioning the patient with large breasts for the oblique view, it is advisable to displace the breast which is in apposition to the cassette as far laterally as possible and to have the patient press firmly against it (Fig. 7).

Pressure of a flaccid or obese breast against the screen may produce a crease which appears as an indentation on the contour of the breast shadow. A similar indentation can result from excision of a portion of the breast.

On rare occasions, numerous small, round or oval shadows are seen over the region of the breasts, simulating shadows in the lungs. These shadows practically always represent phleboliths within dilated veins in the breast. Although frequently calcified, they are usually of moderate density, and close examination of the film may be required to recognize that they extend outside the border of the lungs. Their relationship to the breast is easily determined by oblique views or fluoroscopy.

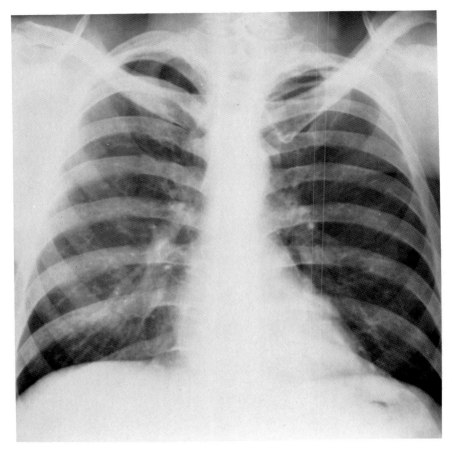

FIG. 146. CONGENITAL ABSENCE OF PECTORAL MUSCLES

A routine film of a 45 year old male shows an oblique line crossing the upper outer part of the left lung. The line is continuous with the inner border of the arm, and is the same as that seen after radical mastectomy. It also occurs in congenital absence of the pectoral muscles. The relative lucency of the left lung is due to associated hypoplasia of the breast as well as the deficiency of the chest wall musculature. (Courtesy of Dr. G. Genkins, New York City.)

A large, irregular shadow in the pulmonary field can be caused by a carcinoma of the breast. A dense fibroadenoma can cast a well-demarcated round shadow, simulating a neoplasm in the lung. Fainter, more irregular and poorly demarcated densities can, on rare occasions, be observed in cystic mastitis. We have seen a case in which the calcified rim of a cyst of the breast mimicked a cavity within the lung (Fig. 147).

Except in rare instances, details of breast structure are not visualized on films of the chest. Special mammographic techniques are required for this purpose.

NIPPLES. Not infrequently, a large nipple casts a round, sharply demarcated, dense shadow which, by itself, is indistinguishable on the frontal view from that of a small neoplasm in the lung. The position of the shadow in relation to the lower, outer border of the breast and the presence of a similar shadow on the opposite side serve to identify it as nipple. Interpretation is more difficult when the shadow is seen on only one side, particularly when the breasts are small and their lower borders poorly demarcated, or when the nipple is situated at an unusual level.

The nipple of the male, when bulbous, may also cast a small round shadow, easily mistaken for a nodule within the lung. The nature of the shadow is obvious if bilateral and symmetrical. However, it is possible for the shadow of only one nipple to be visualized even though both are prominent. This occurs when the patient flattens one nipple by pressing his chest unevenly against the cassette.

The shadow of the nipple poses a problem especially when the possibility of a metastatic neoplasm is considered. As in the case of other confusing shadows of soft tissues of the chest wall, the easiest method of differentiating the nipple shadow from that of a tumor in the lung

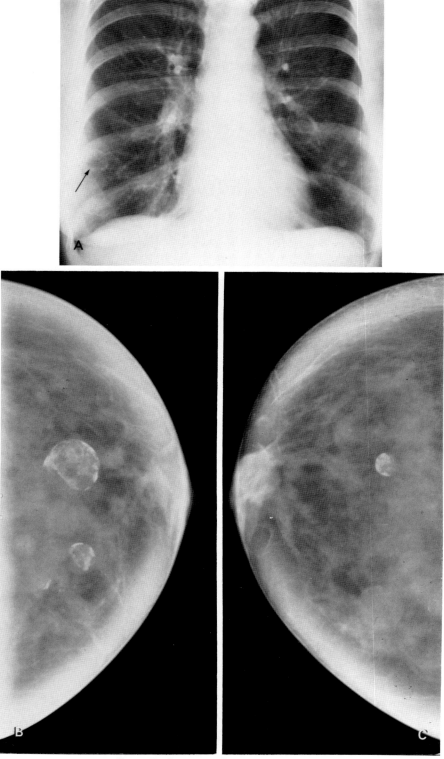

FIG. 147. CALCIFIED CYSTS OF THE BREAST

A: Routine film of the chest shows several lesions in the lower part of the pulmonary fields. The annular shadow (arrow) was thought to represent a pulmonary cavity. A poorly outlined density is present beneath this and a sharply circumscribed small calcific deposit is seen on the left side. *B:* Mammogram of right breast. Multiple round densities are seen throughout the breast. Two of them have calcified rims. *C:* A film of the left breast shows similar changes with one small densely calcified cyst. It is this lesion that accounts for the nodular shadow projected over the left lung.

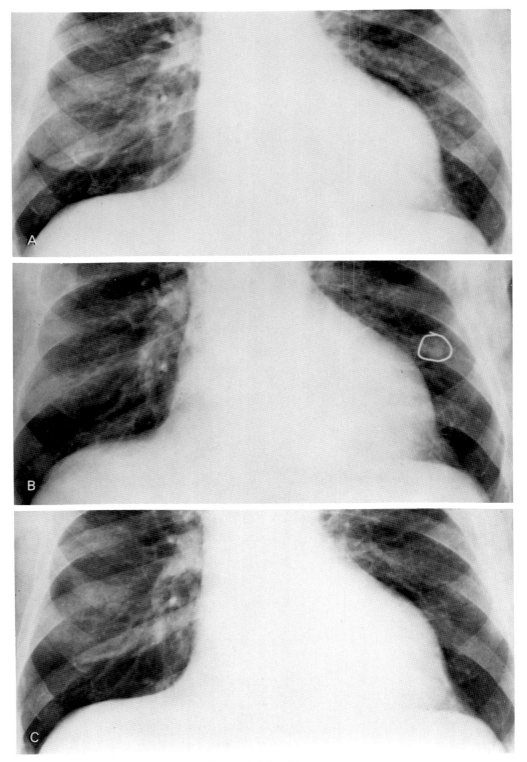

FIG. 148. MALE NIPPLE

A: A routine film of the chest shows a small nodule to the left of the heart. *B:* The examination was repeated after placing a wire around the nipple. The nodular shadow is seen within the center of the circular wire. *C:* After the nipple has been flattened by a firmly applied strip of adhesive tape, its shadow is no longer visible.

is by manipulation during fluoroscopy. This can also be accomplished by making an additional film after placing a metal marker around the nipple. The shadow may be obliterated by flattening the nipple with a tight band of adhesive tape (Fig. 148).

Skin and Subcutaneous Tissues. SKIN TUMORS. Especially when pedunculated, tumors of the skin can cast round shadows of considerable density simulating nodules in the lung. Subcutaneous tumors, such as lipomas or sebaceous cysts, cast shadows over the pulmonary field only when they are large. Their borders are indistinct in contrast to the pedunculated lesions which are sharply demarcated and clearly visualized (Fig. 149) even though quite small. Unless the shadows are demonstrated to be situated within the chest on films made in various projections, the skin should be examined clinically before deciding that a small or moderate-sized, sharply demarcated density represents a nodule within the lung.

Tumors arising from either the skin or the subcutaneous tissues may be recognized as such if they are seen to project beyond the boundary of the chest wall. Frequently the protuberance casts only a faint shadow which is not easily recognized in the black part of the film surrounding the chest unless the film is examined under bright illumination. However, pedunculated tumors of the skin, such as neurofibromas, are usually clearly visualized when they are projected over the axilla.

FOREIGN BODIES. Foreign bodies in the subcutaneous tissues are easily detectable if they are radiopaque. It is important to localize them accurately if an attempt at removal is to be made. In the case of needles which are broken off during aspiration of the chest, it is wise to take every possible precaution in localization for not infrequently they are missed in spite of prolonged search by the best of surgeons. If not readily found, it is advisable to perform the operation under fluoroscopic control. Bullets are usually situated at a considerable distance from the point of entrance. If they are not palpable in the soft tissues, they can be localized by special roentgen methods before attempting to remove them surgically (see p. 342). In these cases, roentgenographic examination is important not only to localize the bullet but also to determine the presence and extent of deeper injuries.

CALCIFICATIONS. Calcific deposits are rarely encountered in the soft tissues of the chest wall.

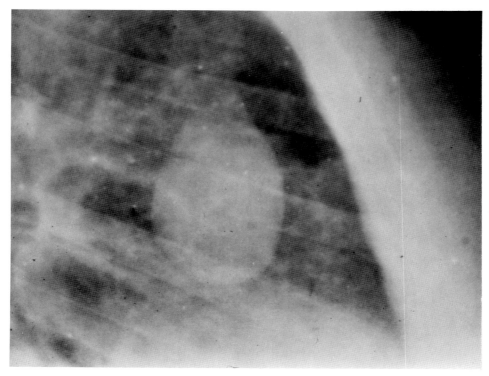

FIG. 149. CUTANEOUS NEUROFIBROMA

The steep oblique view shows a large teardrop shadow over the anterior chest. It is extremely well demarcated except at its uppermost border. This appearance is characteristic of a pedunculated lesion, which in this case was hanging from the skin.

Phleboliths which cause small, round shadows, usually with a more lucent center, may be seen outside the breast shadow. They are then usually situated within a cavernous hemangioma. Sheet-like densities of irregular shape, often having a streaky quality, occur in *myositis ossificans* and *calcinosis universalis*. That these shadows represent calcification is suggested by their density and characteristic conformation. This is confirmed by examination in different projections which show the calcified plaques on end.

Calcified *lymph nodes* in the cervical region or in the axillae are almost always easily recognizable because of their appearance and location. However, calcified nodes above the mesial portion of the clavicle may be confused with calcific deposits at the apex of the lung. Differentiation can be made from the apical lordotic view, in which the nodes are projected above the lung, or by manipulating the nodes during fluoroscopic observation.

Calcified *parasites*, such as the guinea worm (*Filaria medinensis*) can produce long, undulant or coiled shadows in the chest wall. Tiny, oval, calcific foci in the soft tissues may represent calcified *cysticerci*.

Extremely dense, often bizarre shadows, simulating calcific deposits, may represent radiopaque injected material. Contrast material injected during myelography may infiltrate along the nerve roots and present as densities in the intercostal spaces on both sides (Fig. 150). Many years ago it was common to inject bismuth into the lumbar muscles in the treatment of syphilis. The bismuth often migrated upward along the muscle and fascial planes to the lower portion of the chest where it remained for many years. Occasionally such cases are encountered today, and the roentgen picture of the chest presents great difficulty in interpretation if the history of previous bismuth injections is not provided.

INFECTIONS. Inflammatory diseases of the soft

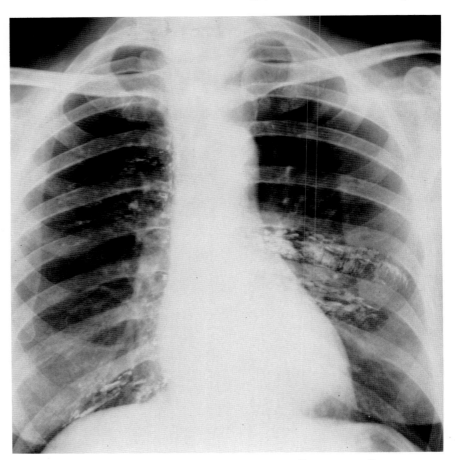

FIG. 150. MYELOGRAPHIC CONTRAST MATERIAL IN INTERCOSTAL SPACES

Radiopaque material is seen within the fifth, sixth and tenth posterior intercostal spaces on the right side and the seventh and eighth spaces on the left. This occurred as a complication of myelography, at which time the contrast material extended along the intercostal nerve roots. The linear density beneath the left clavicle is an artifact.

tissues occur in the form of acute phlegmons, abscesses or chronic inflammatory processes. They may originate in the subcutaneous tissues, lateral thoracic lymph nodes, ribs, costochondral junctions, pleura or lungs. The swelling of the soft tissues causes a localized intensification of the shadows of the chest wall and tends to obliterate the demarcation of the muscular planes. It produces a bulging shadow on the contour of the chest.

Phlegmons of the chest wall are usually caused by external infections. However, large abscesses in the soft tissues can result from suppuration of acutely inflamed thoracic lymph nodes, from osteomyelitis of the ribs or from an osteochondritis. An empyema may perforate between the ribs to produce a collection of pus within the chest wall (*empyema necessitatis*). In rare instances, a subcutaneous collection of fluid and air results from perforation of a lung abscess without an intervening empyema. If a chest wall abscess with an air-fluid level is projected over the pulmonary field, it may be confused with an abscess in the lung. This error can be avoided by fluoroscopy or examination in oblique and lateral views.

Cold abscesses of the chest wall secondary to tuberculous osteochondritis may be associated with erosions of the ribs at the costochondral junction (Fig. 18), but often they are not visible on the film. The same is true of pyogenic abscesses secondary to suppurative osteochondritis. Marked induration and thickening of a portion of the chest wall of a chronic nature is characteristic of mycotic infections of the lung (see Fig. 263), particularly actinomycosis. These changes are due to extension of the disease directly through the pleura into the superficial tissues. It is usually associated with a more or less diffuse widening of the shadow of the soft tissues, occasionally with a localized bulge on the contour of the chest wall. The ribs may or may not be involved.

NEOPLASMS. The lipoma is the most common neoplasm of the subcutaneous tissues. If it is situated in the lateral portion of the chest, its relation to the soft tissues is easily recognized on the frontal film. However, if it is in the anterior or posterior chest wall, it can cast a faint, homogeneous density which may seem to be within the lung (Fig. 151). Its true location, outside the thoracic cavity, can be determined from oblique or lateral films or by fluoroscopy with manipulation of the chest wall in the region of the shadow.

SUBCUTANEOUS EMPHYSEMA. Air may infiltrate into the soft tissues of the chest wall following an injury or surgery to the chest. This is not always recognized clinically but is usually demonstrable on films. The air appears as dark, linear streaks between the denser muscle bundles. On the frontal film the lucent streaks are seen most distinctly in the lateral portion of the chest, parallel to the chest wall. When the emphysema is confined to the anterior or posterior aspect of the chest, it can produce a confusing picture. The lung fields appear mottled, with irregular areas of increased lucency, particularly over the ribs. If the subcutaneous air is an extension from emphysema of the mediastinum, the dark, irregular areas of increased lucency are most prominent in the supraclavicular regions and the root of the neck. The presence of air in the mediastinum indicates the origin of the subcutaneous emphysema (see Fig. 356).

A localized collection of air in the axilla or immediately above the clavicle may be seen following biopsy in these regions (see Fig. 453). If exudate or blood is also present, an air-fluid level will be visible. The appearance can be confused with a cavity at the apex of the lung or a pulmonary abscess which has perforated into the chest wall in the region of the axilla.

Neck. Attention should always be paid to the shadows of the structures of the neck. Inflammatory, cystic or neoplastic diseases may cause a localized protuberance on the cervical contour. Large, supraclavicular lymph nodes frequently distort or obliterate the normal triangular lucency in the supraclavicular fossa.

The position of the trachea should be noted on both frontal and lateral projections. Displacement of the cervical trachea to one side in the absence of any demonstrable lesion in the upper lobe of the lung, is caused by an enlarged thyroid gland. This can extend beneath the sternum without producing a recognizable shadow on the film. Anterior displacement of the trachea with a corresponding increase in the width of the prevertebral space occurs in retropharyngeal or mediastinal abscess (Fig. 46) and in cardiospasm. In these cases, an air-fluid level may be seen crossing the trachea above the sternum on the frontal projection. The horizontal fluid level must be carefully watched for since it is easily mistaken for the upper border of a vertebra.

Occasionally, the pyriform fossae are visualized as oval-shaped areas of lucency. They are recognized from their position and characteristic pear shape, and because they are seen on both sides of the neck. This picture is usually caused by overdistention of the pyriform fossae with air when the patient strains after taking a deep breath. Laryngeal ventricles are occasionally seen about an inch above the sternum. Asym-

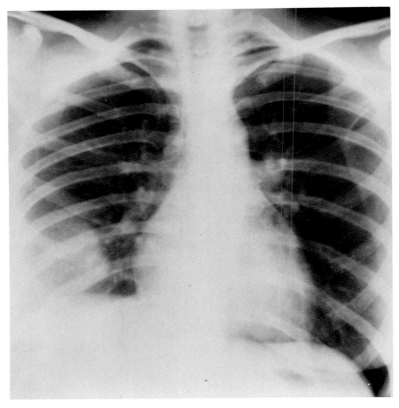

FIG. 151. SUBCUTANEOUS LIPOMA

The density over the lower part of the right chest has a well-defined inner border but fades out superiorly and laterally. This configuration suggests that the lesion is outside the lung. The shadow was due to a large lipoma on the patient's back. On fluoroscopy the shadow could be displaced by manipulation of the mass.

metry of the shadows of the ventricles may be due to laryngeal tumor or paralysis of a vocal cord.

The Bony Thorax

Sternum. Abnormalities of the sternum that can be recognized roentgenologically are neoplasms, osteomyelitis, fractures and erosions from adjacent lesions. The most common primary tumor of the sternum is the myeloma, and involvement of the sternum is not uncommon in this disease. Hodgkin's disease of the sternum is not particularly rare but in our experience this has always been associated with involvement of the anterior mediastinum and it appears most probable that is represents a direct extension of the mediastinal lesion. In rare instances other malignant tumors of the mediastinum and even tumors arising in the mediastinal lappet of the adjacent lung involve the sternum directly. Erosion of the sternum can result from pressure of an aneurysm of the ascending aorta. At first this

erodes only the posterior table of the bone but later the full thickness of the sternum may be destroyed. Osteomyelitis of the sternum is rare. Erosion of the lateral border occurs in either suppurative or tuberculous osteochondritis involving the junction of the sternum and the cartilage of the adjacent ribs and the junction between the manubrium and the clavicle. The bone may be extensively destroyed in fungal infections, particularly in the case of South American blastomycosis.

An abnormality of the sternum is difficult to visualize on the conventional frontal view of the chest because it is obscured by the spine and mediastinal structures. In some cases, destruction of the upper portion of the manubrium, particularly in the region of the sternoclavicular junction, can be recognized. A fairly good view of the sternum is provided by the lateral projection, but the patient must be carefully positioned to produce a true lateral view. This position is best for detecting fractures of the sternum and erosions of the posterior table alone, as well as for more complete destructive lesions of the bone (Fig. 152). The use of a grid is advisable. Examination in the anterior oblique position with the patient prone provides particularly good detail of the sternum (Fig. 153). A long exposure is used and the patient is instructed to breathe while it is being made. This blurs the shadows of the posterior ribs and the blood vessels while the sternum, which is relatively immobile and closer to the film is sharply defined.

Tomograms in the frontal plane yield particularly good detail of the manubrium but do not show the body of the sternum very well. Lateral and oblique tomograms are necessary when lesions of the sternum are suspected and not clearly visualized otherwise.

Posterior bowing of the sternum occurs in pectus excavatum (*funnel breast*). This is not clearly evident on the lateral view at first glance since the depressed sternum is covered by the ribs which extend further anteriorly. The presence of pectus excavatum may be suspected from the appearance of the chest on the frontal projection. The posterior ribs are more horizontally placed than in the average chest and the anterior ribs assume a more oblique downward course. Because of the change in the position of the ribs, the dome of the thorax loses its usual curve and becomes squared off (Fig. 154). The heart can be compressed between the sunken sternum and the vertebral column resulting in an increase in its transverse diameter. In many cases, pressure of the sternum results in cardiac displacement to the left, suggesting enlargement of the left ventricle. The heart may also be rotated somewhat toward the right oblique view, producing a conformation suggesting mitral disease. That these changes are due to narrowing of the anteropos-

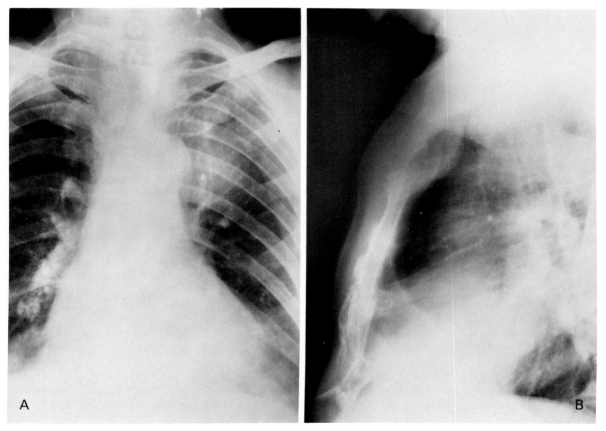

FIG. 152. METASTATIC NEOPLASM OF STERNUM

The patient had a carcinoma of the colon resected 14 months previously and presented with a mass on the anterior chest wall. *A:* The hazy density projected over the left hilum is associated with destruction of the anterior portion of the second rib. However, since blood vessels can be seen through the shadow, the latter cannot represent consolidation of the lung. The shadow did not correspond to the position of the chest wall mass which was situated in the midline. *B:* Lateral view. The lower half of the manubrium is destroyed and there is a large, soft tissue mass extending both in front and behind it. Biopsy revealed mucin-producing adenocarcinoma.

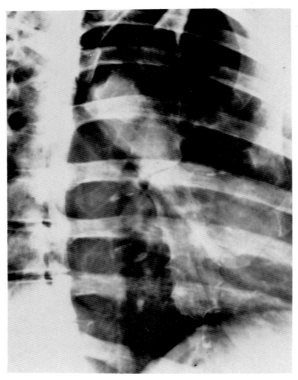

FIG. 153. USE OF THE ANTERIOR OBLIQUE PROJECTION
FOR VISUALIZATION OF THE STERNUM

terior diameter of the chest is suggested by the rather clear visualization of the spine and the ribs through the cardiac shadow on a film which is not obviously overexposed.

Forward bowing of the sternum occurs in the *pigeon breast* deformity. This increases the anteroposterior diameter of the chest and is therefore associated with an increase in the width and lucency of the retrosternal and retrocardiac spaces, changes ordinarily associated with emphysema. However, on the frontal projection the chest is usually seen to be narrow and the diaphragmatic curve is normal.

Spine. The spine is poorly visualized on ordinary films of the chest. Abnormalities in this structure often cast shadows which may be confused with lesions of the mediastinum. In scoliosis, the distorted spine can simulate a widened mediastinum, a dilated aorta or an enlarged heart, particularly if the film is insufficiently exposed (see Fig. 204). When the vertebral bodies are not clearly discernible, flaring of the ribs on the side of the bulging shadow and the closer approximation of the ribs on the opposite side would indicate the presence of scoliosis. This can be confirmed by films of the spine.

A cold abscess of the spine projects into the mediastinum and often extends laterally into the pulmonary field. It usually appears as a fusiform paravertebral shadow, often simulating an aneurysm of the thoracic aorta. Not infrequently the sharply demarcated shadow of the lesion can be seen through the heart. The diagnosis can usually be suspected when examining the ordinary films of the chest because of the position of the shadow in relation to the spine, its fusiform shape and the continuation of the shadow along the sides of the spine. Films of the spine will usually show evidence of erosion of the vertebral bodies, narrowing of one or more of the intervertebral spaces, or collapse of the vertebrae in the region of the shadow of the Pott's abscess.

Collapse of the vertebral bodies causes an approximation of the paraspinal portions of the ribs. The convergence of the ribs produces a spider-like arrangement which is characteristic of vertebral collapse (Fig. 155).

A similar appearance can be produced by pyogenic osteomyelitis with an associated paravertebral abscess, but calcification in the wall of the abscess suggests a tuberculous etiology. In either case the paraspinal abscess may be well formed before roentgen evidence of bone destruction appears, but narrowing of the intervertebral space is almost always present.

A neoplasm arising in a vertebral body may project outward from the bone and give the appearance of a mediastinal tumor. Chordomas which usually occur in the suboccipital or lumbosacral region may also involve the dorsal spine.

Occasionally, on the lateral chest film, one or more vertebrae appear abnormally dense. This is characteristic of involvement of those bones by Paget's disease or Hodgkin's disease. It may also result from osteoplastic metastasis from prostatic, breast, thyroid or lung carcinomas. It is a rare manifestation of urticaria pigmentosa.

Spinal deformities are frequently present in association with other lesions that are evident on the chest film, such as neurofibroma, ganglioneuroma, intrathoracic meningocele and neurenteric cyst. The neural tumors and the meningoceles are situated paravertebrally in the region of the intervertebral foramina. Not infrequently they cause enlargement of the foramina with erosion of the adjacent vertebral pedicles and the lateral wall of the vertebral bodies, and occasionally cause splaying of the ribs. The neurenteric cyst is located more anteriorly and is situated in the posterior mediastinum even though it has a connection with the spine. This, as well as the meningocele, is often associated with an anomaly of vertebral segmentation. Scoliosis is particularly common in association with meningoceles.

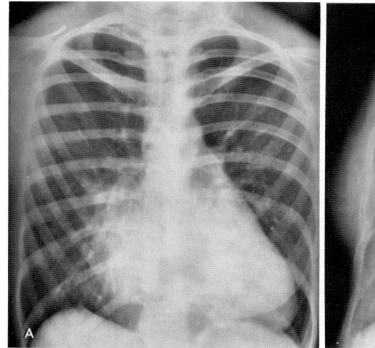
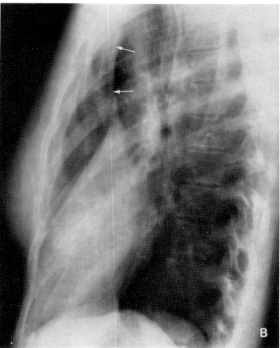

FIG. 154. PECTUS EXCAVATUM

A: In the frontal view the dome of the thorax is squared off and the sides of the chest are straightened. The posterior portions of the ribs are more horizontal than normal while anteriorly they course steeply downward. The apex of the heart is displaced to the left. The right cardiac border cannot be identified because of consolidation of the middle lobe. *B:* On the lateral view the depressed sternum is projected within the thorax (arrows). The entire middle lobe is consolidated.

Ribs. On the frontal projection of the chest the posterior portion of each rib is seen to course from its articulation with the upper part of the corresponding vertebra downward and outward to the axillary part of the chest, and then downward and inward to the costochondral junction. There is frequently some condensation of bone at the junction with the cartilage. The cartilage itself does not cast a shadow on the roentgen film unless it is calcified.

COSTAL CARTILAGES. Calcification in the rib cartilage is not clinically significant. However, the presence of calcium or bone formation in the cartilage may cause difficulty in roentgen interpretation. Occasionally there is overgrowth of bone at the costochondral junction of the first rib which may produce a shadow simulating a lesion in the lung, particularly on underexposed films (Fig. 1). Any unusual shadow in this region that may possibly be related to ossification of the first rib cartilage should be carefully investigated by additional films made with increased exposure, a grid or by a film made in a partial lordotic position. Calcification of the cartilages of the lower ribs may also cause confusion, particularly when the calcium is not deposited throughout the entire course of the cartilage. Sometimes the calcium deposit occurs in the form of small islands and may be confused with nodules in the lungs. In other cases, the calcium and bone formation occur along the lower border of the cartilage to produce a sharply defined linear shadow. This can be mistaken for the horizontal line of an air-fluid level. If the line follows the curve of the cartilage and crosses the shadow of a blood vessel, it may produce an annular shadow suggesting a cavity in the lung. Errors will be avoided if these possibilities are kept in mind.

COSTAL PATTERN. The course of the ribs is altered by a variety of conditions. An increased obliquity of the ribs with consequent narrowing of the intercostal spaces occurs when the chest is flattened for any reason. This change takes place in fibrosis of the parietal pleura and chest wall and in atelectasis secondary to bronchial obstruction. The ribs also become more oblique and approximated on the concave side of a scoliosis.

In emphysema the anterior part of the chest wall is elevated. This causes the ribs to pursue a more horizontal direction. Consequently there is

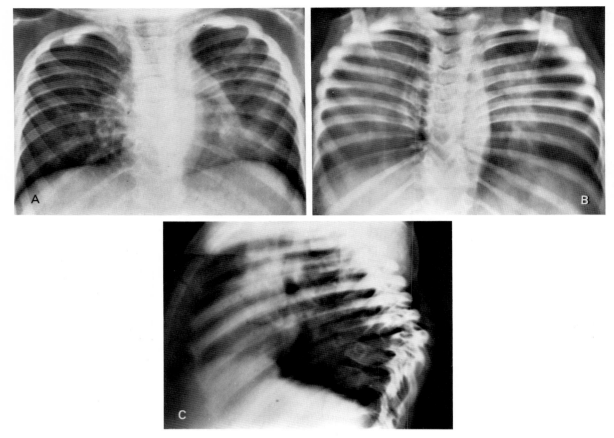

FIG. 155. POTT'S ABSCESS

A: The frontal film of a young child with infiltrations in both lungs shows the ribs to radiate from the spine in spider-like fashion. This is always due to collapse of one or more vertebral bodies. *B:* A Bucky film confirms the abnormal course of the ribs and shows a circumscribed fusiform density in the left paravertebral region. This appearance is characteristic of a tuberculous abscess. *C:* The lateral view shows destruction of several of the thoracic vertebrae and a sharp angulation of the spine forming a gibbus.

a corresponding increase in the anteroposterior diameter of the chest and an increase in the width of the intercostal spaces as seen on the frontal projection. A diminution of the obliquity of the posterior ribs with increased angulation of the anterior ribs occurs in persons with long flat chests. These are frequently associated with either saucer or funnel-shaped depression of the sternum. On the frontal projection the chest usually has a characteristic contour. The dome of the chest appears squared off and the lateral borders of the chest do not show the usual bulging curve. Rather, the lateral borders appear straightened. This change in the contour of the chest on the posteroanterior film is sufficiently characteristic of the flat chest to permit its recognition even in the absence of a lateral view (Fig. 154). Not infrequently the heart is compressed from before backward and its shadow

spreads out, increasing its transverse diameter. The heart may remain in its normal position. However, it is more frequently displaced to the left side and is rotated somewhat toward the right oblique view. The diminution in the anteroposterior diameter of the heart decreases its density and permits visualization of the ribs and spine more clearly than in the normal.

The ribs diverge as the spaces become increased in width on the convex side of a scoliosis. Similar divergence of the ribs occurs on both sides when one or more vertebral bodies are collapsed (Fig. 155).

ANOMALIES. Malformations of the ribs are common. One of the more usual is the cervical rib, which often occurs bilaterally (see Fig. 540). Ordinarily these are short and rudimentary but frequently they are more fully developed. A cervical rib can be the cause of a thoracic outlet syndrome. Most cervical ribs are clinically insignificant and symptoms ascribed to them may be the result of some other lesion, even though a cervical rib is present.

Rarely two ribs are seen to arise from a single costovertebral articulation. More often supernumerary ribs are the result of bifurcation of one of the ribs in more or less close proximity to the costochondral junction. The bifid portion of the rib is less dense than the remainder of the bone. The fourth rib is affected more often than any other. Bifid ribs are sometimes joined to the adjacent rib, either above or below, and thus cause the formation of a shadow over the underlying lung between the ribs. This shadow may be confused with a lesion in the lung if its connection with the ribs is not recognized (Fig. 47).

Sometimes two adjacent ribs are fused (see Fig. 448). While this is usually due to a congenital anomaly, bridging of two ribs can also occur after thoracotomy, particularly in childhood. It can take place simply following intercostal drainage of an empyema without rib resection, probably as a result of periosteal reaction from injury to the ribs by the intercostal tube.

Where there is a well-developed supernumerary rib, the adjacent rib may be missing or rudimentary. An underdeveloped rib can also be an isolated finding. The first rib is the one which is most apt to be rudimentary (Fig. 465). The incompletely developed rib is thin and may not extend as far as the normal costochondral junction. When a number of ribs are underdeveloped, the corresponding part of the chest wall is flattened. Occasionally one or more ribs are entirely absent.

FRACTURES. Fractures of the ribs are easily overlooked unless there is considerable displacement of the fragments or if there is well-marked callus formation. In the absence of a history of trauma, the pain caused by the fracture may be considered to be due to pleurisy or myositis. Strain during cough is a common cause of spontaneous rib fractures. Cough fractures occur either at the anterior or posterior bend of the ribs in the lower thoracic cage. Usually the anterior portion of the fifth or sixth rib, or the posterior of the seventh or eighth rib is the site of the fracture. Occasionally the same rib is fractured in two places. As in the case of other rib

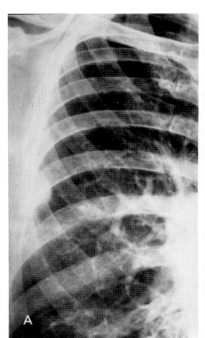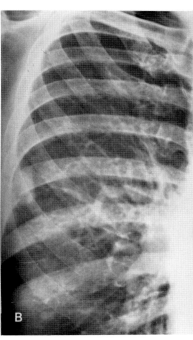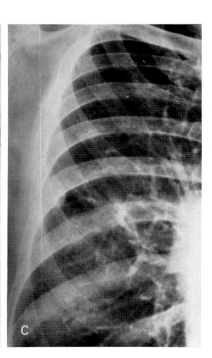

FIG. 156. COUGH FRACTURE

A: The patient was referred because of a nodule in the lateral portion of the right chest which was thought to represent a neoplasm of the lung. The lesion is sharply demarcated and based against the pleura. The appearance is identical with that of a tumor of the pleura. *B:* Because the patient had a chronic cough and had experienced sudden chest pain 2 months previously, an earlier film was sought for. This shows the shadow to have been hazy and associated with a fracture of the eighth rib at the posterior axillary bend. This portion of the rib is the most common site for a cough fracture. *C:* A year later the fracture is completely healed. The nodule has shrunken and obviously represents mature callus.

fractures with little or no displacement of the fragments, the only roentgen change may be a hairline lucency across the rib. This is frequently visible only in the oblique views. Even then there may be a question as to whether or not the lucency represents a fracture. Attention should be directed to the border of the ribs. Even the slightest lack of continuity of the cortex proves that a fracture is present.

It is a common experience, even in the case of severe trauma to the chest, to miss a good many of the multiple fractures on films made immediately after the accident. However, within a few days the pull of the intercostal muscles tends to draw the fragments out of alignment so that the fractures become evident. When there is no displacement of the fragments, the first roentgen manifestation of the fracture may be the presence of callus formation. The so-called "barracks-bag fracture" caused by the pressure of the

strap of the bag on the posterior part of the first rib, is often first evidenced by callus on this rib, noted on a film made because of pain in the region of the trapezius.

The callus may be confused with a nodular lesion in the lung, a primary tumor if it is single (Fig. 156) and metastases when the calluses are multiple. In osteoporotic ribs, the relationship of the density of the callus to the faint outline of the ribs, particularly in their anterior portions, is not clearly evident and makes for difficulty in diagnosis. Proof that we are dealing with a callus rather than a neoplasm of the lung is afforded by films in the oblique view which show that the lesion is extrapulmonary. Careful examination with proper illumination may disclose a hairline lucency within the density to indicate an underlying fracture.

Nontraumatic rib fractures are often due to underlying disease of the bone. Most frequently

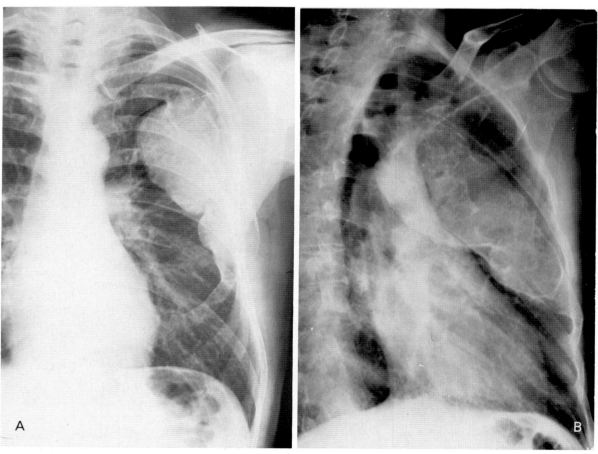

FIG. 157. FIBROUS DYSPLASIA OF RIB

A: The frontal film shows an elongated, lobulated mass which appears to be in continuity with the fifth rib. *B:* An overpenetrated right oblique view shows the mass to represent an expansile lesion of the rib. Fine bony septa are visible within the lesion.

they are due to destruction of the rib by metastatic neoplasm. Occasionally they result from osteoporosis, particularly in patients under prolonged steroid therapy. These fractures are associated with calcium deposition in the bone adjacent to the fracture but with little extension beyond the border of the bone as in the case of ordinary callus formation. The appearance is bizarre and may suggest metastatic tumors of the lung, particularly when they are multiple and if the hairline lucency running across the rib is overlooked.

PRIMARY NEOPLASMS: *Benign Tumors.* The most common benign tumors of the ribs are chondromas and osteochondromas. The *chondroma* presents as a well-demarcated radiolucent defect within the rib. Almost always the tumor is associated with a local widening of the bone. Not infrequently small densities representing calcific deposits are present within the lucent cartilagenous neoplasm. The *osteochondroma* produces a larger swelling of the rib, most often at the anterior extremity of the bone adjacent to the costal cartilage. Occasionally the tumor is situated at the head of the rib near the spine. Usually the border of the tumor is rather irregular. Because of the presence of bone within the growth, the shadow is denser than that of the

simple chondroma, and it may be mistaken for a tumor of the lung or mediastinum on the ordinary chest film. However, on overpenetrated or Bucky films, irregular bony septa are visible within the density, indicating its origin in the bone. Fibrous dysplasia, although not considered a tumor of bone, can cause marked local expansion of a rib and thinning of its cortex. The lesion consists mostly of fibrous tissue and, therefore, is relatively radiolucent although it often contains scattered foci of calcification and new bone formation (Fig. 157).

Malignant Tumors. The most common primary malignant rib neoplasm is the chondrosarcoma (Fig. 158). This is characterized by a noncircumscribed density associated with destruction of the bony cortex and irregular extension of the tumor mass into the soft tissues of the chest wall. The bony trabeculae crossing through the lucent cartilage are more irregular and have a more bizarre distribution than in a benign osteochondroma.

Less common are malignant tumors arising from the bone marrow, such as *Ewing's tumor* and *myeloma* or *plasmacytoma.* These are characterized by a homogeneous soft tissue density and the origin in the rib is easily overlooked,

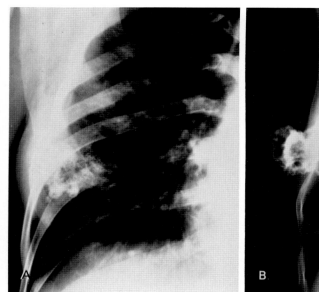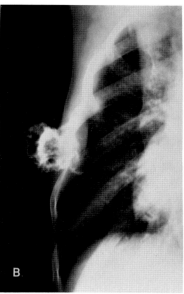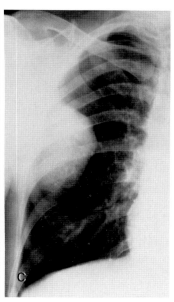

FIG. 158. OSTEOCHONDROSARCOMA OF THE RIB

A: Frontal view. An irregular area of calcification is seen in the outer part of the right pulmonary field. This might be considered to be within the lung except for the soft tissue swelling of the chest wall lateral to the calcific deposit. *B:* Left oblique view. The shadow of the bony tumor is now projected away from the pulmonary field and its connection with the anterior rib is demonstrated. The soft, circumscribed, homogeneous density mesial to the calcified area, represents the soft sarcomatous part of the growth. *C:* Recurrence 2 years after resection of the tumor. A frontal film shows a sharply demarcated, soft tissue mass with a fine tracery of calcification within it. This appearance is quite characteristic of osteosarcoma.

particularly if the tumor is large and obscures the rib from which it arises (Fig. 159). If the shadow is projected within the pulmonary field, it may be confused with a lesion in the lung. Overpenetrated or Bucky films will show an area of rib destruction usually extending throughout the entire length of the shadow. The rib at the periphery of the density is usually expanded. Ewing's tumor occurs more frequently in young persons and often grows to huge proportions. Multiple myelomas usually appear as small, sharply punched out, lytic defects, simulating metastatic carcinoma. Myelomas involving several bones in other portions of the body may show only a single mass on the chest film, similar to that of the Ewing tumor. Although a myeloma of the rib can be a solitary lesion, it usually proves, on bone survey, to be one of many. Even if the remainder of the bones appear to be free, repeated examination at a later date, generally shows the disease to be widespread.

METASTATIC NEOPLASMS. These may be secondary to vascular spread from a primary tumor of almost any organ. The most common origin is a neoplasm of the lung, breast, kidney, prostate or thyroid gland. When the metastatic lesions are small, they are represented simply by localized areas of rarefaction in the ribs, often difficult to recognize. They are more clearly defined in the outer portion of the chest where they are free from the shadows of the lungs.

Pathologic fractures make the metastases more evident. As the metastases become larger they may project into the pulmonary field as demarcated scalloped shadows of varying size. These are easily confused with neoplasms within

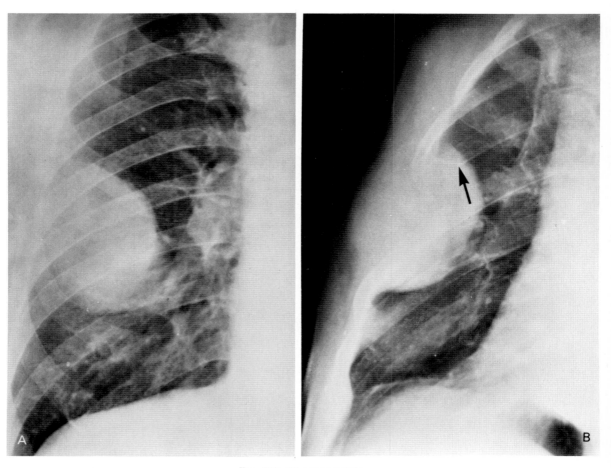

FIG. 159. PLASMACYTOMA

A: Frontal view. The large mass in the right side of the chest obscures the anterior portion of the fifth rib. It is difficult to determine from this film whether the lesion lies within the lung, the pleura or the chest wall. B: Left oblique view. The tumor, which is now projected tangentially, is seen to involve the chest wall. The anterolateral portion of the fifth rib (arrow) is destroyed throughout the length of the tumor. There is no sclerosis of the adjacent bony markings. Biopsy showed the lesion to be a plasmacytoma. No other lesions were present.

the lung. Close observation of the ribs within the shadows, or examination with a grid, will disclose areas of rarefaction or complete destruction of a portion of the rib. In contradistinction to most rib tumors, metastatic neoplasms rarely cause expansion of the rib.

If the lesions are multiple, it is safe to assume that they are metastatic. However, in the case of a single lesion, the possibility remains that we may be dealing with a primary carcinoma of the lung that has invaded the rib by direct extension (see Fig. 406). In general, the metastatic tumor causes destruction of the rib throughout the entire length of the mass, while a lung carcinoma causes destruction of the bone over only a part of the tumor. The metastatic tumor of the rib does not extend to destroy an adjacent rib. On the other hand, a primary neoplasm of the lung may cause destruction of two or even three adjacent ribs by direct invasion (Figs. 160 and 404).

It is possible to differentiate between the nodular mass representing a metastatic tumor of the rib and that of a carcinoma of the lung which has secondarily invaded the rib by inducing a pneumothorax. In the case of a primary carcinoma, the lung cannot be separated from the chest wall in the region of the tumor. On the other hand, it is possible to separate a metastatic tumor of the rib from the lung by a pneumothorax since these tumors do not invade the lung or produce pleural adhesions (Fig. 161).

Rib metastases are not always characterized by lytic changes. In most cases of carcinoma of the prostate and in many cases of carcinoma of the breast or thyroid, *osteoplastic* changes occur in the rib metastases. Similar changes occur in Hodgkin's disease. Osteoplastic metastases from bronchogenic carcinoma are rare. As a rule, in the case of osteoplastic rib metastases, some areas of bone destruction can also be found. The occurence of such associated *osteoclastic* lesions will indicate that the osteoplastic ones are due to bone metastases. In carcinoma of the prostate, only the osteoplastic changes may be present. These may be so diffuse that the shadows of the ribs appear almost uniform, and on casual inspection the entire process may be overlooked. However, if attention is directed to the shadows where the ribs cross each other, the increased density of the ribs becomes more noticable, and in addition, a haziness of the rib borders is apparent (Fig. 162). This is due to the irregular ossification of the metastases and constitutes an important sign of osteoplastic metastasis.

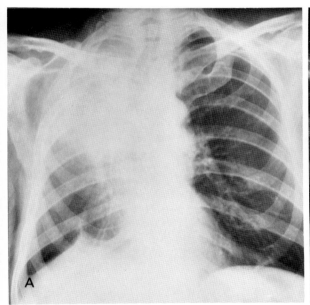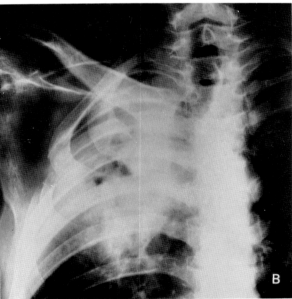

FIG. 160. CARCINOMA OF THE LUNG INVADING CHEST WALL

A: The dense shadow over the right upper lobe is associated with increased obliquity of the ribs, elevation of the right diaphragm and deviation of the trachea. These findings indicate atelectasis of the upper lobe together with an inability of the remainder of the lung to undergo compensatory hyperinflation because of pleural thickening and adhesions. *B:* A Bucky film shows destruction of the lateral portions of the third and fourth ribs. The irregular lucency within the shadow is due to cavitation within the lesion. The disruption of the ribs without periosteal reaction or other evidences of peripleuritis is indicative of an underlying carcinoma rather than actinomycosis. The involvement of two contiguous ribs excludes a metastatic lesion.

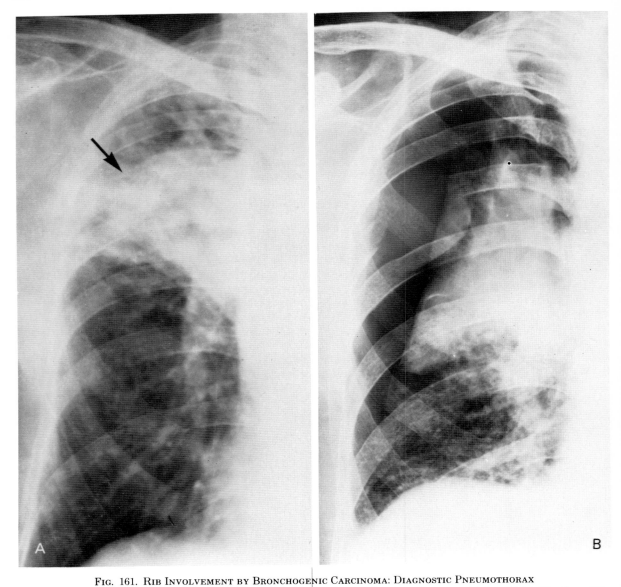

FIG. 161. RIB INVOLVEMENT BY BRONCHOGENIC CARCINOMA: DIAGNOSTIC PNEUMOTHORAX

A: There is a dense shadow in the right upper lobe with elevation of the short fissure, and interstitial infiltration of the peripheral portion of the lobe. The posterior part of the sixth rib (arrow) is destroyed, indicating the neoplastic nature of the disease. Continuity of the shadow of the neoplasm with that of the destroyed rib almost always indicates direct invasion of the chest wall. *B:* Reexamination after induced pneumothorax. The air has displaced the right upper lobe away from the destroyed rib. This excludes extension of the tumor into the chest wall and indicates that the lesion in the rib represents a distant metastasis. This contraindicated surgery which would have been undertaken if the rib had been involved simply by direct extension.

OSTEOPLASIA. In addition to neoplastic disease, increased density of the ribs resulting from bone formation occurs in Paget's disease and fibrous dysplasia. Irregular proliferation of osteoid tissue and of calcium in Paget's disease produces widened, irregular rib shadows. In fibrous dysplasia there may simply be a uniform increase in the density and some widening of a part of one or more of the ribs, or a soap-bubble appearance caused by cystic widening of the bone together with bony trabeculae.

More diffuse and regular density of the ribs occurs in osteopetrosis (Albers-Schönberg disease), myelofibrosis, or fluoride or vitamin A intoxication. In these conditions the borders of the shadows at the rib crossings are perfectly sharp and regular.

A local area of bone condensation in one of the

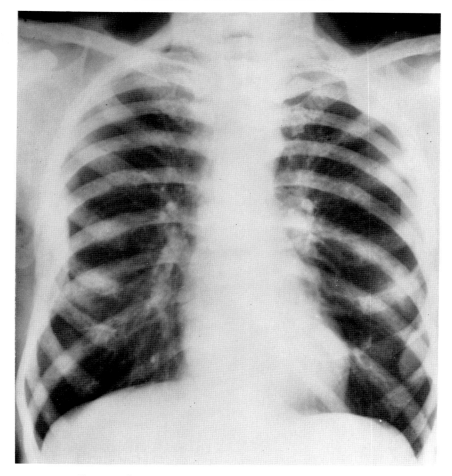

FIG. 162. OSTEOPLASTIC METASTASES: PROSTATIC CARCINOMA

The shadows of the ribs are abnormally dense. This is most apparent where the ribs cross each other. In many places the rib margins appear fuzzy because the metastases are osteoclastic as well as osteoblastic. There is marked thickening of the extrapleural tissues of the right lateral chest wall. It is not certain whether the scalloped shadows on the left side represent pleural or extrapleural metastases.

ribs, the so-called *bone island*, produces a small round or oval density easily mistaken for a nodule in the lung (Fig. 163). Whenever such a density is seen within the shadow of a rib, additional films should be made altering the position of the patient or the x-ray tube. If the density maintains its position in relation to the border of the rib on all films, the possibility of a nodule in the lung may be excluded.

RAREFACTION OF RIBS. In histiocytosis X, areas of rarefaction of the ribs are not uncommon. They are usually sharply punched out, either round or oval in shape, and without sclerosis of the adjacent bony tissue. Occasionally the rib is expanded in the region of the lesion. The areas of rarefaction are usually associated with infiltrations in the lungs in Letterer-Siwe's disease and in eosinophilic granulomatosis. The

lesions are less frequently seen in the Hand-Schüller-Christian type of histiocytosis. Generalized rarefaction and expansion of the ribs occurs in severe cases of thalassemia (Fig. 164).

OSTEOMYELITIS AND OSTEOCHONDRITIS. The infection in osteomyelitis of the ribs is either exogenous or endogenous. The external cause is usually an operation for suppurative disease within the chest. Occasionally osteomyelitis complicates a fracture of the rib. In these cases there is an irregularity of the end of the rib, not only of the broken edge but also of the upper and lower borders adjacent to the operative site or the site of fracture. The body of the rib in this region may also be demineralized and have a mottled appearance. Later, this portion may show evidence of periosteal proliferation and new bone formation.

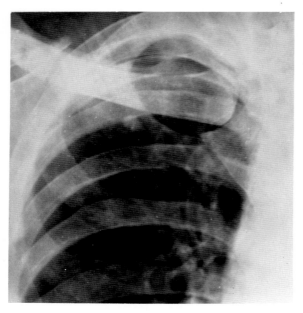

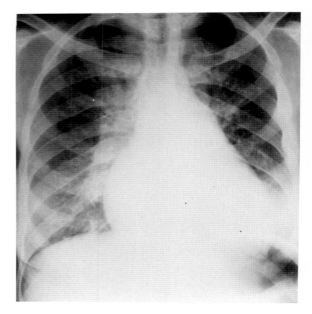

FIG. 163. BONE ISLAND

The sharply circumscribed oval density beneath the right clavicle resembles a calcified focus in the lung. However, since it lies within the shadow of the first rib the possibility of a bone island must be considered. A film was therefore made in the oblique projection. This showed the density to maintain its exact position in relation to the border of the rib confirming the fact that it lies within the bone.

FIG. 164. THALASSEMIA

The ribs and clavicles are widened and their cortices are thinned. This appearance is characteristic of extensive hyperplasia of the bone marrow. The prominence along the lateral end of the fourth rib on the left side represents callus from a fracture. The heart is enlarged and the pulmonary vasculature appears increased because of the increased cardiac output associated with the anemia.

The most common internal cause for osteomyelitis of the rib is disease of the underlying lung. Mycotic infections as well as nonspecific suppurative disease of the lungs can involve the adjacent ribs by direct extension. Metastatic osteomyelitis results from blood stream invasion by pyogenic organisms, tubercle bacilli or fungi. The affected portion of the rib may show only absorption of bone, but it can also exhibit evidences of bone proliferation. Tuberculous osteomyelitis of the ribs characteristically shows thickening of the bone in association with areas of destruction. It occurs most frequently as a result of direct extension of the infection from tuberculosis of the spine. When the rib is involved in association with tuberculous osteochondritis, the diseased bone usually becomes rarefied and sometimes the part adjacent to the cartilage is completely destroyed (Fig. 18).

Infections of the costochondral junctions are not rare. They may be due to tuberculosis, syphilis, or pyogenic organisms. Often the infection in this region causes no visible change on the film, but not infrequently there is an irregularity of the adjacent portion of the rib. When the disease is associated with abscess formation, the appearance may be that of a loculated empyema.

RADIATION OSTEITIS. With the increasing use of supervoltage radiotherapy, radiation injury to the ribs has become relatively uncommon. Irradiation with a beam of lesser voltage is more likely to result in damage to the ribs because the absorption of x-rays in the lower energy range is much greater in bone than in soft tissue.

A slight degree of osteoporosis may be the only change in the ribs following radiation injury. With more severe damage, there is increased destruction of the bone which undergoes patchy sclerosis and casts an irregularly dense shadow. In either case, the rib is weakened and is subject to fracture from minimal trauma. The fractures are frequently multiple, and, as in the case of cough fracture, are most apt to occur at the anterior and posterior bend of the ribs. Usually these fractures do not heal well.

Since radiotherapy is usually administered to patients with neoplastic disease, the possibility of radiation osteitis should be considered before assuming that the roentgen changes are due to metastases (Fig. 165). Such damage is especially

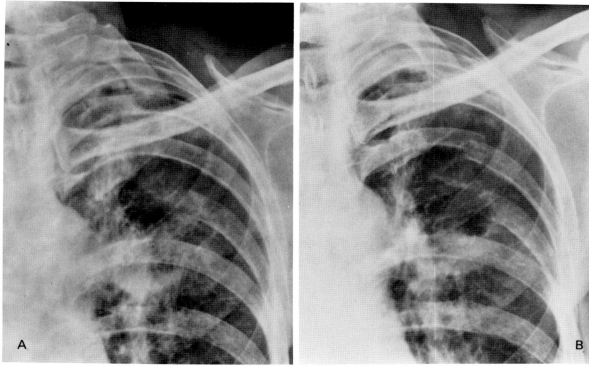

FIG. 165. RADIATION OSTEITIS

A: The patient has a peripheral carcinoma of the lung with destruction of the overlying portion of the sixth rib. The left hilar shadow is enlarged because of lymph node metastasis. *B:* Three weeks after completion of radiotherapy the primary tumor has almost completely disappeared and the hilar shadow has reverted to normal. However, there is now a fracture of the posterior portion of the fifth rib but no evidence of bone destruction to indicate that it was involved by the neoplasm. The fracture was due to radiation osteitis and eventually healed.

common when tangential fields are used in the treatment of breast carcinoma.

RIB NOTCHING. Notching of the ribs is almost always the result of localized bone atrophy from chronic pressure on the undersurface of the bones due to dilatation and tortuosity of the intercostal vessels or tumors of the intercostal nerves. These structures lie in the costal groove in approximation with the undersurface of the rib. Since they are separated from the ribs in the anterior portion of the chest, notching occurs only posteriorly. The notches appear as a series of scalloped defects in the lower border of the ribs, usually with some bone condensation at the margins (Fig. 166).

The most common cause of rib notching is coarctation of the aorta. The site of coarctation is usually distal to the origin of the left subclavian artery. A considerable portion of the blood reaches the distal aorta by way of a collateral circulation from the subclavian to the intercostal arteries. The intercostals become elongated and tortuous, as well as dilated, and are responsible

for the pressure atrophy. The first two intercostal arteries do not communicate with the descending aorta and the last three do not communicate with the subclavian. Therefore, rib notching in coarctation of the aorta involves only the third through the ninth ribs. Most commonly the notching is bilateral. However, when the right subclavian artery arises from the descending aorta distal to the coarctation, the rib notching is limited to the left side. In the absence of this anomaly, notching is confined to the ribs on the right side when the coarctation is situated proximal to the left subclavian artery. In rare instances no cause is known for unilateral rib notching in coarctation of the aorta.

When there is interruption of the flow of blood through the subclavian artery following the Blalock-Taussig operation or in Takayasu's disease (pulseless disease), a collateral pathway develops between the descending aorta and the axillary artery via the thoracic and intercostal arteries. The latter can then produce notching of the ribs on one or both sides, depending upon whether

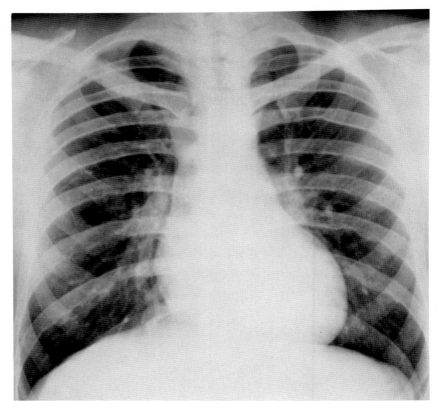

FIG. 166. COARCTATION OF THE AORTA

The heart is normal in size, but the curve of the left ventricle is accentuated suggesting hypertrophy of this chamber. The aortic knob is obscured and the left border of the superior mediastinum is straightened. This appearance is typical of coarctation of the aorta. The diagnosis is confirmed by the presence of notching on the undersurfaces of the fourth, fifth, seventh and eighth ribs on the left side. Notching of the right ribs is less prominent.

one or both subclavian arteries are interrupted. It is also possible for rib notching to occur when the abdominal aorta is occluded. The lowermost ribs are then involved.

In the case of diminished pulmonary arterial supply, additional blood can reach the lungs from the aorta by way of the intercostal and bronchial arteries. In rare instances, the dilatation of the intercostal arteries may be sufficient to produce notching of the ribs. This can be seen with many types of cyanotic congenital heart disease. In extremely rare instances it has been observed in severe pulmonary emphysema.

Dilatation of the intercostal veins, sufficient to cause rib notching, can occur in chronic obstruction of the superior vena cava involving the mouth of the azygos vein. The intercostal veins then form a collateral pathway for blood from the head and upper extremities to the patent portion of the azygos vein.

Rib notching also occurs when there is an arteriovenous fistula in the chest wall (Fig. 167). The arterial communication results in a marked increase in blood flow in the intercostal veins, which become markedly dilated and tortuous. This can also occur in the case of an arteriovenous fistula within the lung if there are overlying pleural adhesions so that vascular communication is established with the chest wall.

Tumors of the intercostal nerves often produce pressure atrophy on the undersurface of the ribs. When these tumors are multiple, as in neurofibromatosis, rib notching, similar to that seen in coarctation of the aorta, can occur (Fig. 168). The diagnosis is clear when the tumors themselves are visible.

Pressure atrophy of the upper margins of the ribs is not uncommon in paralytic poliomyelitis when the patient has been bedridden and lying on his back for some time. The third rib is the one most commonly involved, but any rib from the second to the eighth may be affected. The

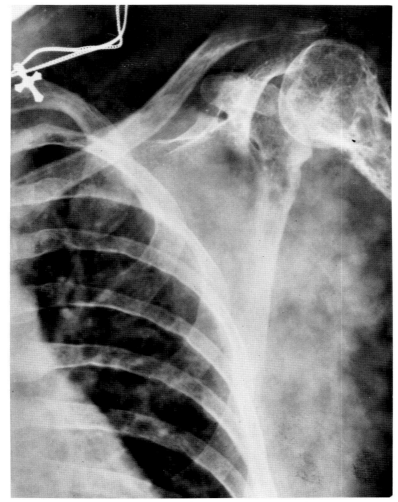

FIG. 167. UNILATERAL RIB NOTCHING: ARTERIOVENOUS MALFORMATION

The notching of the lower borders of the ribs is identical to that caused by coarctation of the aorta. In this case, the rib changes were secondary to an arteriovenous malformation involving the upper extremity and chest wall. Because of the marked shunting of blood, the intercostal veins draining the lesion are tortuous and dilated. Pressure of these vessels causes atrophy and sclerosis of the ribs. The racemose vessels are visible in the soft tissues of the chest wall and axilla. The bones of the shoulder girdle are also involved.

condition is apparently due to continued pressure of the medial border of the scapula against the rib.

The Shoulder Girdle

The clavicles, scapulae and upper portions of the humeri are included on the chest film and should not be overlooked. Evidence of a neoplasm, primary or metastatic, osteomyelitis, arthritis and calcific deposits about the shoulders, as well as a cyst of the head or neck of the humerus, may be found on the films and indicate the need for more detailed examination.

Diseases of the clavicle itself are quite rare. They usually involve the ends of the bone, either in relation to the acromioclavicular junction or the sternoclavicular joint. The clavicle is rarely the seat of neoplastic disease. Even when there is generalized involvement of the bones of the body by metastases or multiple myeloma, the clavicle is usually spared. However, the clavicle is not infrequently involved by Paget's disease which produces general widening and increased density of the bone with thickening of the cortex and coarsening of the trabecular pattern.

Demineralization of the outer ends of the clavicle, producing a frayed appearance of the bone

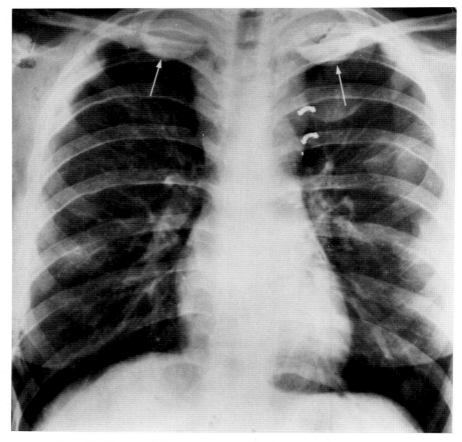

FIG. 168. MULTIPLE NEUROFIBROMAS (VON RECKLINGHAUSEN'S DISEASE)

Numerous neurofibromas involving the intercostal nerves are visible as scalloped shadows along the periphery of the pulmonary fields. A large circumscribed mass is present at each apex (arrows). In addition, there is a large mass in the superior mediastinum representing a neurofibroma of the vagus nerve. The lower borders of the posterior parts of the fifth and seventh ribs on the right side and of the sixth rib on the left side are notched by the tumors which proved to be neurofibromas. The metallic densities to the left of the mediastinum represent skin clips.

in the region of the acromioclavicular joint, may be the first roentgen sign of hyperparathyroidism. Destruction of this portion of the clavicle also occurs occasionally in rheumatoid arthritis. Less often the mesial ends of the clavicle are involved in this disease leading to partial absorption of the clavicular heads which become tapered mesially to a blunt, pointed end. The "pencil clavicle" is rather typical of rheumatoid arthritis. A more destructive process at the mesial ends of the clavicle occurs in syphilis and in South American blastomycosis. In these diseases the adjacent portion of the sternum and first rib may also be destroyed.

Occasionally there is a broad notch on the undersurface of the clavicle near its mesial end. This is a normal variant of the bone at the site of attachment of the rhomboid muscle. The notch can be differentiated from neoplastic dis-

ease because it is almost always bilateral and symmetrical and is bordered by an intact rim of dense cortical bone (see Fig. 473).

The shadows of the scapulae often obscure the upper part of the chest, particularly on underexposed films and in obese persons. Small tuberculous lesions, so common in this region, are easily hidden unless the scapulae are withdrawn from the pulmonary fields at the time of the examination. In rare cases of winged scapula, such as occur with damage to the spinal accessory nerve, the scapula may cover a large part of the upper chest and the shadow can simulate disease in the underlying lung (Fig. 169).

The vertebral border of the scapula varies in appearance. It may be irregular in outline or concave in shape. In the latter instance, the angle of the scapula can present as a rounded shadow over the middle outer part of the lung, while that

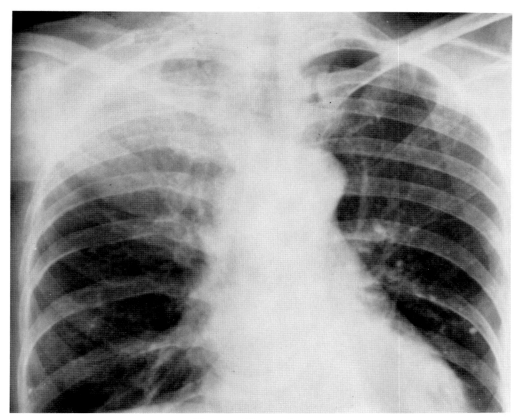

FIG. 169. WINGED SCAPULA

The shadow over the right upper lobe is due entirely to the density of the scapula which is in an abnormal position. The shift of the scapula was due to muscular imbalance from previous poliomyelitis. The blood vessels in the upper lobe appear normal, suggesting the extrapulmonary origin of the shadow. Close observation of its borders show them to correspond to the distorted image of the scapula.

part of the border of the scapula above it remains outside the pulmonary field. If the connection with the upper part of the scapula is not obvious, the shadow of the angle of the scapula may be wrongly considered to represent a lesion in the lung, pleura or ribs. This deformity is almost always bilateral.

Each scapula should be inspected carefully in examining the roentgen film of the chest. A well-defined area of rarefaction within the body of the bone or along one of its borders, may be indicative of a primary or metastatic neoplasm. The discovery of such an area of rarefaction in a patient with an indeterminate shadow in the lung would indicate that the patient has a primary pulmonary carcinoma with bone metastasis (Fig. 170).

The Extrapleural Tissues

Peripleuritis. Infections of the extrapleural tissues (the tissues between the parietal pleura and the ribs) are most often due to mycotic disease of the lungs, particularly actinomycosis, or to osteomyelitis of the ribs. The induration of the extrapleural tissues causes a homogeneous shadow in the periphery of the chest. This is usually most dense in the axillary region and fades gradually in its mesial portion. An extremely dense, band-like shadow is often present, running up and down the periphery of the chest adjacent to the ribs, representing exudate together with fibrosis of the pleura and extrapleural tissues seen on end. When the entire lesion is very dense, this band-like shadow may be obscured except in its upper and lower portions where it extends above and below the main density. The ribs are usually drawn together, suggesting atelectasis. Displacement of the mediastinal structures to the affected side is absent, however, and this helps to exclude bronchial obstruction from consideration (see Fig. 250). In addition, the ribs are frequently widened and their borders irregular as a result of periosteal

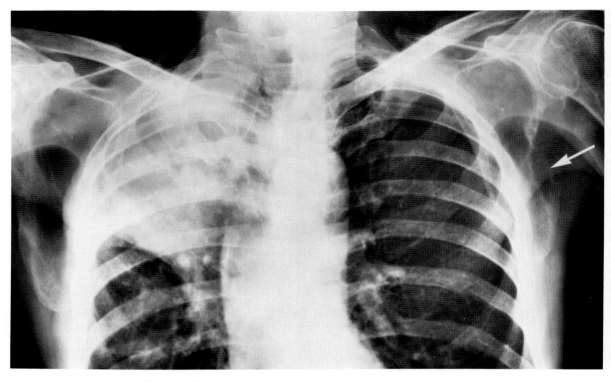

FIG. 170. METASTASIS TO SCAPULA FROM CARCINOMA OF THE LUNG

The shadow over the upper portion of the right pulmonary field has a sharply defined, concave inferior margin. This represents an elevated short fissure and indicates atelectasis of the upper lobe. The marked density of the shadow is due to infiltration of the lung in addition to the atelectasis. This appearance could be caused by pneumonia, or any lesion causing obstruction in the upper lobe bronchus. The area of destruction in the outer border of the left scapula (arrow) is characteristic of metastatic neoplasm, indicating that the atelectasis of the right upper lobe is due to carcinoma.

proliferation. A bulge of the soft tissues of the chest wall may also be evident.

Extrapleural Tumors: CONNECTIVE TISSUE TUMORS. Tumors which arise from connective tissue between the parietal pleura and the remainder of the chest wall are mostly in the nature of fibromas or fibrosarcomas. Occasionally lipomas are encountered in this region. Because these neoplasms may present the roentgen picture of tumors arising from the pleura itself, they are discussed in the section on Pleural Neoplasms (see p. 703).

NEUROGENIC TUMORS. Neurofibromas and ganglioneuromas, tumors which arise from the intercostal nerves and sympathetic ganglia, are often classed with mediastinal tumors because they appear to be situated in the mediastinum on the frontal projection. However, these tumors are actually within the chest wall, since the posterior mediastinum extends only to the anterior borders of the vertebral bodies. The tumors are located adjacent to the vertebral foramina which are at a considerable distance behind the mediastinum. They lie in the vertebral gutter formed by the posterior part of the lateral surface of the spine and the mesial, posterior portions of the ribs.

The tumors are usually single and benign. Those that are malignant or multiple are generally associated with neurofibromas elsewhere or with skin lesions which are part of von Recklinghausen's disease (Fig. 168).

The neurofibroma or ganglioneuroma is most often situated in the upper part of the chest, in the region from the second to the fifth ribs. It is represented by a homogenous, semicircular density with the base adjacent to the spine. It is characterized by an extremely sharp outer border (Fig. 171). Its location in the paravertebral gutter is depicted on the lateral view. Here, the semicircular shape of the shadow with its diameter along the posterior chest wall, differentiates it from most of the nodular lesions in the lung or mediastinum, which appear either oval or circular in shape. Occasionally, a few calcific deposits are visible within the shadow of the neoplasm. These are due to calcification of hemorrhagic or necrotic areas within the tumor. In some cases,

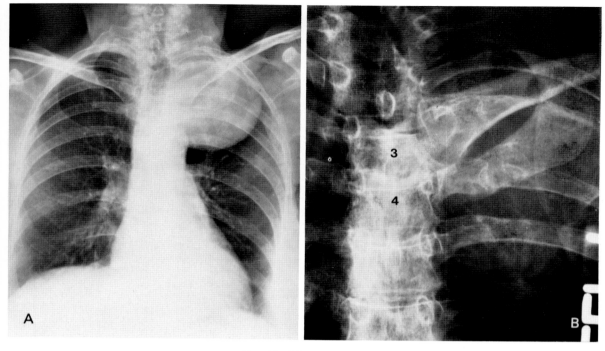

FIG. 171. NEUROFIBROMA

A: The sharp demarcation and the smooth round border of the mass in the upper part of the left chest are indicative of a benign tumor. The outline of the aortic knob is obliterated because the mass is situated posteriorly. Its location, adjacent to the spine, and the spreading of the third and fourth ribs are characteristic of a neurogenic tumor. *B:* Bucky film of the spine. The undersurface of the third rib is partially destroyed because of pressure atrophy. The pedicle on the left side of D_3 is missing because of erosion by the expanding tumor in the intervertebral foramen. These findings confirm the neurogenic origin of the tumor. It proved to be a neurofibroma.

the capsule of the growth shows small, thin, calcific plaques.

In rare instances, a neurofibroma arises from an intercostal nerve some distance from the spine. Its shadow then may be round or oval, but if it is located in the axillary region, it appears semicircular. It cannot be differentiated from a tumor of the pleura, a peripheral carcinoma of the lung or some other neoplasm of the chest wall unless it spreads the ribs apart or causes atrophy of the adjacent ribs (Fig. 172).

Large neurofibromas spread the ribs apart and cause atrophy or erosion of the ribs adjacent to the growth. If the tumor arises in the intervertebral foramen, it may grow in dumbbell fashion (Fig. 173). Part of the growth projects into the pulmonary field while the remainder grows into the vertebral canal. Because of this possibility, a special examination of the spine should be made in all cases where neurofibroma is suspected to determine whether there is any erosion of the spine or enlargement of the interverterbral foramen.

A roentgen appearance identical with that of the neurofibroma occurs in rare cases of pheochromocytoma, a tumor that can develop anywhere along the course of the paravertebral sympathetic chain as well as in the adrenal medulla. Additional information concerning these tumors is provided in the section on the Mediastinum (see p. 564).

DISEASES OF THE TRACHEOBRONCHIAL TREE

The Trachea

The trachea is visualized as a vertical radiolucent band representing the air in its lumen contrasted against the soft tissues of the neck and mediastinum. The entire wall of the trachea is usually not visible on the frontal projection but it is often seen on the lateral or oblique views as a linear density bordering the air column. In the position usually used for the lateral view, part of the trachea is obscured by the arms and shoulders. More complete visualization is best ob-

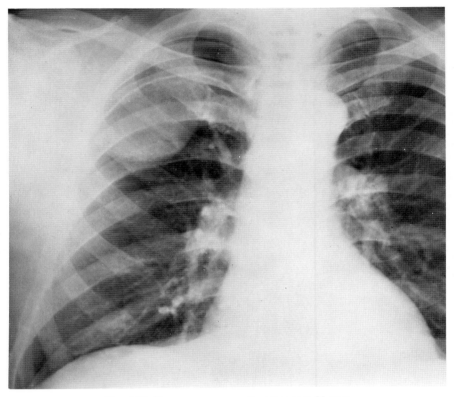

FIG. 172. NEUROFIBROMA OF INTERCOSTAL NERVE

The mass over the outer part of the right upper lobe has a sharply defined lower border without a distinguishable upper margin. This appearance is characteristic of a pleural or extrapleural lesion. The fifth and sixth ribs are somewhat spread apart. The fifth rib is markedly narrowed and shows sclerosis of its lower border, indicating pressure atrophy. These findings are characteristic of an intercostal neurofibroma.

tained in this projection by having the arms folded behind the back, the shoulders retracted and the head extended.

While displacement of the trachea is usually obvious on conventional films, intrinsic diseases of the trachea are not so easily recognized. They are frequently overlooked because the possibility of disease of the tracheal wall is usually not borne in mind at the routine examination. However, the abnormalities are often recognized in conventional, oblique and lateral projections if the attention is directed to the trachea.

Calcification of the tracheal cartilages, which is not abnormal in older people, is recognizable in all views. The calcified cartilages appear as transverse, parallel, dense, stripe-like shadows crossing the air column. At the margins of the trachea where the cartilaginous rings are projected tangentially there is a local increase in the density of the shadows, producing a beaded appearance.

Lautkin has noted an increase in the width and density of the wall of the trachea in cases of severe tracheitis and other conditions causing diffuse thickening of the trachea (Fig. 174). Lesions intruding into the tracheal lumen can often be recognized on lateral or oblique views when they cannot be seen on ordinary frontal films. Overpenetrated or Bucky films disclose the tracheal air column more clearly and are more apt to reveal the intratracheal lesions. However, tomograms are required whenever a thorough study of the trachea is indicated. The trachea is outlined exceptionally well by coating the mucosa with a contrast medium. The technique is essentially the same as that used in laryngography. It is useful in revealing fine details of abnormalities of the tracheal mucosa and for ciné recordings to demonstrate tracheal dynamics. The movements of the trachea can also be observed by fluoroscopy without the aid of contrast material. This is best performed in the oblique position.

Normally there is little change in the caliber of the trachea during respiration, but a slight increase in width may sometimes be seen during

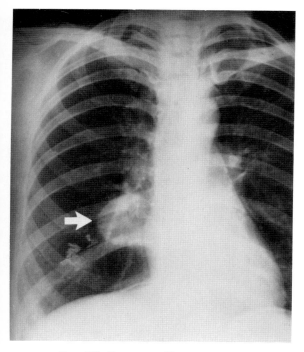

FIG. 173. DUMBBELL NEUROFIBROMA

The mass (arrow) does not obliterate the right cardiac border and therefore lies posteriorly. It is round and sharply demarcated. A lateral view showed it to be situated in the paravertebral gutter. The adjacent intervertebral foramen was enlarged. At operation the neurofibroma was found to lie partly outside the parietal pleura adjacent to the spine and partly within the spinal canal. The irregular opacity lateral to the growth represents iodized oil and methylene blue injected within the intercostal muscles for localization.

the inspiratory phase. In asthma and in severe emphysema the trachea frequently becomes markedly narrowed during *expiration*. This is due to the increase in intrathoracic pressure resulting from the force required to expel the air through the bronchi which are narrowed during this phase. The high pressure causes an invagination of the posterior wall of the trachea, which is not protected by cartilage. Since the transverse diameter of the trachea remains relatively unchanged, the narrowing of the organ is visible mainly in the oblique and lateral views. A similar narrowing of the trachea occurs normally during the act of coughing. In tracheomalacia there is a marked increase in the caliber of the trachea during *inspiration* because the normal negative intrathoracic pressure is sufficient to draw the relatively flaccid tracheal walls outward. This is visible on the frontal as well as on the lateral views.

Tracheal Displacement and Compression.
With few exceptions the trachea is normally sit-

uated in the midline. The lateral borders of the trachea should be equidistant from the mesial ends of the clavicles. The clavicles rather than the spine are used as points of reference because the trachea is situated anteriorly. A slight deviation from the true frontal projection will cause a considerable shift of the shadow of the trachea in relation to the spine but will cause little change in its relationship to the clavicles. Moreover, even a slight scoliosis will separate the shadow of the spinous processes from that of the trachea which maintains its position between the heads of the clavicles even if the curvature of the spine is extreme (see Fig. 568). Displacement of the trachea below the level of the thoracic inlet must be judged by its position in relation to the spine. However, the possibility of apparent displacement resulting from poor positioning of the patient or the presence of spinal curvature must be taken into consideration.

The trachea is frequently situated somewhat to the right of the midline in infants. In older people with arteriosclerosis of the aorta the trachea is frequently displaced to the right at the level of the aortic knob. If the displacement continues for a significant distance above the knob, an additional cause for the tracheal deviation should be considered.

With the exceptions mentioned above, displacement of the trachea demands explanation because it may signify the presence of important disease not immediately apparent on examination of the films. Displacement of the trachea may result from pressure of an adjacent mass or from an imbalance of the pressures in the lungs or pleura on the two sides.

The trachea is not easily compressed because of the support afforded by its cartilaginous rings and the fact that it is quite mobile. However, its mobility is limited at the thoracic inlet so that a relatively small mass in this location can compress the organ. Within the thoracic cavity only large masses can cause compression of the trachea, unless it is surrounded by the mass, or the mediastinum is fixed by inflammatory or neoplastic disease.

Compression of the trachea with little or no displacement can be caused by a vascular ring, most commonly a persistent double aortic arch. The vascular ring encircles the esophagus as well as the trachea and causes characteristic indentations on both sides and the back of the esophagus. When the left pulmonary artery arises from the right pulmonary artery it swings around the right main bronchus and courses behind the trachea and in front of the esophagus to reach the left lung. It can then cause compression of the

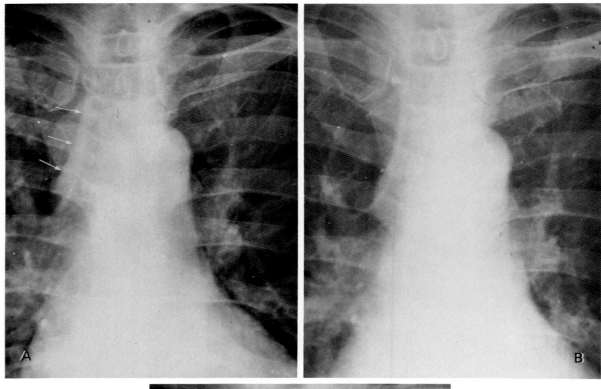

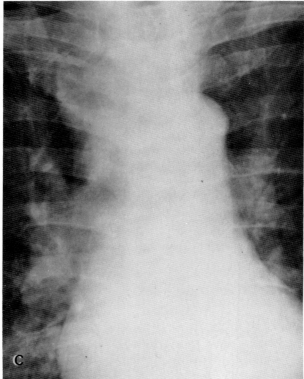

FIG. 174. THICKENING OF TRACHEAL STRIPE

A: June 14, 1971. A routine film of the chest revealed thickening of the tracheal stripe (arrows). This is indicative of an infiltrative process in the mediastinum. B: November 1, 1969. At this time, the tracheal stripe was normal. The stripe represents the wall of the trachea, the adjacent mediastinal tissues and the pleura, outlined by air in the tracheal lumen on one side and the right upper lobe on the other. C: November 3, 1971. A mediastinal tumor is now obvious. Biopsy revealed anaplastic carcinoma. (Courtesy of Dr. Arthur Lautkin, New York, N.Y.)

air passages. The anomalous vessel can be seen in the lateral projection as an oval density between the trachea and esophagus, producing an indentation on the anterior esophageal border.

Displacement of the trachea to either side may be limited to the neck. Most frequently this is due to a large thyroid (see Fig. 519), but the deviation may be caused by a cyst, neoplasm or inflammatory disease in the adjacent tissues. The same holds true for lateral displacement of the trachea at the thoracic inlet (see Fig. 234).

Lateral displacement of the trachea within the chest is more commonly due to disease of the lung or pleura and is usually associated with displacement of the other mediastinal structures. A pleural effusion or a pneumothorax may displace the trachea for a considerable distance to the opposite side. Such displacement also occurs in emphysema resulting from obstruction of a large bronchus. In any case, the displacement is more marked during expiration and may not be present on films made during inspiration.

Displacement to the side of a pulmonary lesion occurs when one lung, or a considerable portion of a lung, is contracted from any cause (Figs. 175 and 296). The traction on the trachea may also cause it to become widened. When the entire lung or the right middle and lower lobes are shrunken, the trachea pursues an oblique course, downward and outward to the carina which is also displaced to the right (see Fig. 241). The long axis of the trachea now forms a single, continuous line with that of the lower lobe bronchus. When the upper lobe alone is contracted

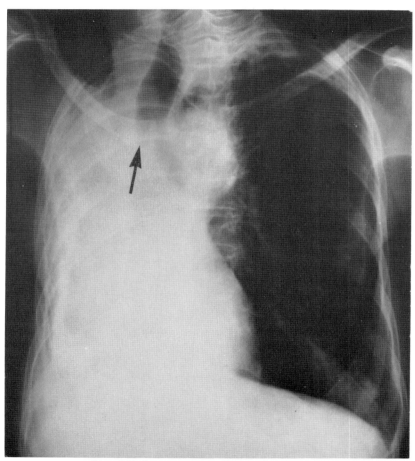

FIG. 175. ATELECTASIS OF ENTIRE RIGHT LUNG

The right hemithorax is opaque. The heart and mediastinal structures are displaced markedly to the right. The right chest is much smaller than the left. The ribs are drawn together and the dome of the thorax is flattened. The dense streak along the lateral border is due to extensive calcification of the pleura, the result of tuberculous pleurisy following pneumothorax treatment. However, this is insufficient to explain the marked shift of the mediastinum which must be due to complete atelectasis of the lung. The sharp cutoff of the air column of the right main bronchus (arrow) indicates complete obstruction just beyond the carina. This was due to a bronchogenic carcinoma.

there is only slight displacement of the trachea or possibly no displacement at all if pleural adhesions are absent and the lower lobe can shift to take up the space relinquished by the shrunken upper lobe. On the other hand, if the upper lobe is fixed to the lateral chest wall before it becomes shrunken, the trachea is more markedly deviated to the side of the pulmonary lesion (Fig. 73). Because the carina tends to maintain its normal position, the trachea becomes bowed or even sharply angulated.

Occasionally, tracheal displacement occurs in the absence of shadows in the lung to indicate the presence of atelectasis. Displacement of the lung root upward or downward, displacement of the fissures or herniation of the opposite lung, will indicate that the deviation of the trachea is due to atelectasis. In unilateral hyperlucent lung, the trachea may be displaced to the side of the lesion because the lung is often decreased in volume despite the fact that it is emphysematous.

Lateral displacement of the trachea to the opposite side by purely intrathoracic disease also occurs in the case of large mediastinal lymph nodes, mediastinal cysts, aneurysms of the aorta and very large pleural tumors. However, even a relatively small carcinoma of the lung can cause local displacement if it is situated, adjacent to the mediastinum. This can occur in the absence of mediastinal involvement by the growth.

Paradoxical displacement of the trachea away from the side of an atelectatic lung is an indication of massive involvement of the mediastinal lymph nodes by the neoplasm responsible for the bronchial obstruction (see Fig. 421). A similar shift of the trachea can occur in primary tuberculosis associated with extremely large mediastinal nodes together with bronchial obstruction (see Fig. 279).

Paradoxical displacement of the trachea can also occur in cases of pneumothorax. This happened rather frequently when pneumothorax treatment was employed for pulmonary tuberculosis. Often, when the lung had been collapsed for a considerable period of time the pleura would become thickened and prevent full reexpansion of the lung. As the pneumothorax space became smaller during the course of treatment, the lung would be unable to expand sufficiently to take up the space relinquished by the pneumothorax, and the trachea and mediastinal structures would consequently be drawn toward the side of the pneumothorax. Displacement of the trachea toward the side of a pneumothorax in the absence of evidence of fibrosis of the lung indicates that the lung is imprisoned by thickened pleura (Fig. 75).

The presence of anterior or posterior displacement of the trachea is determined from the lateral projection. It is frequently difficult to decide whether the trachea is displaced because of variations of its normal position in relation to the spine and the sternum. In patients with loss of the normal kyphotic curve of the dorsal spine (straight back syndrome), the space between the trachea and the vertebral column is diminished. In the presence of an accentuated angulation at the sterno-manubrial junction there is an increase in the space between the trachea and the sternum. In these instances the trachea maintains its straight course. Bowing of the trachea, either forward or backward, is an absolute indication of tracheal displacement.

The width of the space between the vertebral column and the trachea at the root of the neck is relatively constant and serves as an excellent guide for its position. Lateral films of the neck are therefore useful when there is any question concerning anterior displacement of the trachea (Fig. 46). Widening of the retrotracheal space is a constant finding in retropharyngeal abscess and in perforation of the upper part of the esophagus. In the latter condition, one or more air bubbles are frequently seen in the widened prevertebral space. Anterior displacement of the trachea by a Zenker's diverticulum (see Fig. 499) or by the dilated esophagus in cardiospasm or above an obstructing esophageal carcinoma may be associated with a fluid level behind the trachea. A posteriorly situated goiter, a paraesophageal cyst, a Pott's abscess, a neuroenteric cyst or an anterior meningocele may also cause anterior displacement of the trachea.

Posterior displacement of the trachea is most commonly caused by a substernal (cervicomediastinal) thyroid. Such displacement of the trachea can also be caused by a large dermoid cyst, thymic neoplasm, malignant teratoma of the mediastinum or an aneurysm of the ascending arch of the aorta.

Tracheobronchomegaly (Mounier-Kuhn Syndrome). This condition is characterized by a marked widening of the trachea and the main bronchi associated with outpouchings of the muscular walls between the rings of the affected airways. There is also an increase in the width of the posterior wall of the trachea which is not protected by cartilage. A chronic tracheobronchitis is present in most cases. This is usually associated with emphysema, occasionally with bronchiectasis (Fig. 176). The condition is frequently first noted during childhood, and appears to be associated with a deficiency of elastic tissue in the walls of the trachea and the main bronchi. In fact, it has been described in association with

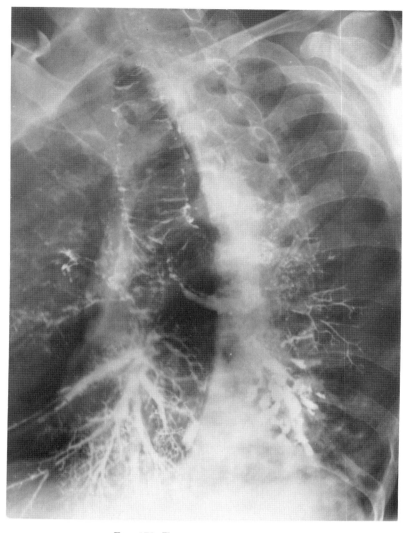

FIG. 176. TRACHEOBRONCHOMEGALY

Bronchogram, left oblique view. The trachea and the right and left main bronchi are markedly dilated. However, the bronchial branches are of normal caliber with the exception of the basal divisions of the left lower lobe. These are bronchiectatic as a result of a previous suppurative bronchopneumonia. The coarse striations in the trachea and main bronchi represent contrast material puddled in the outpouchings of the wall between the cartilaginous rings.

the Ehlers-Danlos syndrome which is caused by a congenital defect in the elastic tissue throughout the body. The association with chronic infection is probably due to stagnation of secretions in the outpouchings between the cartilages which may be large enough to have the appearance of diverticula. Tracheomegaly may also be secondary to chronic bronchitis and emphysema. Here the widening is probably due to disruption of elastic tissues secondary to inflammatory disease together with the increased pressure caused by coughing. However, the changes are moderate in comparison to the striking abnormalities encountered in what appears to be a primary form of tracheobronchomegaly. Moderate widening of

the trachea can also occur when it is drawn to one side in association with shrinkage of an entire lung or of an upper lobe.

The widened trachea which may measure from 3 to 5 cm in width can be visualized on the conventional film but is better seen on the oblique views which also disclose the widened main bronchi. Transverse strips of increased lucency are often seen crossing the trachea. These dark bands represent air in the horizontal troughs produced by outward bulging of the tracheal wall between the cartilaginous rings. A considerable change in the caliber of the trachea is noted during respiration, with widening during inspiration and narrowing during expiration.

This change is particularly notable during the Müller and Valsalva maneuvers. It indicates poor support of the trachea by its cartilages. Extreme narrowing of the tracheal lumen, seen on the lateral view during expiration, is due to infolding of the wide posterior wall which has no cartilaginous support.

The characteristic outpouchings between the cartilaginous rings can be seen on Bucky films or tomograms but are more clearly visualized by bronchography. The contrast material puddles in the recesses and produces a series of broad transverse opaque stripes alternating with lucent bands, representing the cartilages (Fig. 176). Often there are scattered, localized puddles outlining small diverticula and dilated ducts of the mucous glands. The border of the trachea has a characteristic corrugated appearance, caused by the uniform outward bulges of the mucosa between the cartilages. These changes are also visible in the widened main bronchi.

Tracheomalacia. Since this term denotes softening of the tracheal wall, tracheomegaly, which is caused by a weakening of the wall, is to be considered as a manifestation of diffuse tracheomalacia. A more localized form of tracheomalacia is due to incomplete development of one or more of the tracheal cartilages. The trachea in the affected region is apt to collapse during expiration, producing expiratory stridor. The collapse during expiration can be visualized on fluoroscopy or cinébronchography. A diverticulum of considerable size may result from a local outpouching of the weakened tracheal wall. While this may be visible on conventional films or tomograms, it is best demonstrated by tracheography.

Tracheoesophageal Fistulae. Fistulous communications between the trachea and esophagus may be congenital or acquired. In either case, ingested material or secretions enter the air passages and cause respiratory difficulties, particularly during feeding, and frequently cause aspiration bronchopneumonia. In most cases of *congenital* tracheoesophageal fistula there is an associated atresia of the esophagus, and in these cases the infants survive only a few days if the condition is not corrected. In the absence of esophageal atresia, the infant with a congenital tracheoesophageal fistula can survive for months and even years, but the course is marked by recurrent episodes of pneumonia which causes increasing respiratory disability. *Acquired* fistulae occur at any age, depending upon the nature of their cause. They occur most frequently in adults. The onset is frequently insidious. The symptoms may not appear to be related to the ingestion of liquids or solids but simply to the chronic lung infection and the presence of a fistula not suspected.

Congenital Tracheoesophageal Fistula. The roentgen manifestations of congenital tracheoesophageal fistula depend upon the presence or absence of atresia of the esophagus and the relation of the fistula to the site of the atresia. In all instances there is a tendency for the development of patchy areas of pneumonia, frequently associated with atelectasis resulting from the aspiration of food and secretions. The upper lobes are most commonly involved because the infants are usually recumbent.

In most cases associated with esophageal atresia, the upper esophagus consists of a blind pouch while the lower portion, below the atresia, communicates with the trachea a short distance above the carina. The upper portion, which is cut off from the rest of the esophagus, is usually distended by air and secretion. Since the films are practically always made with the infant in the supine position, this portion of the esophagus appears as a sharply defined lucency overlying the spine extending from the neck usually to the level of the second or third dorsal vertebra. On the lateral view the lucent, distended esophagus is seen to occupy the space in front of the vertebral bodies and displaces the trachea forward. An air-fluid level may be seen in the esophagus if the films are made with the patient suspended in the erect position. Since there is a free communication between the lower portion of the esophagus and the trachea, air passes from the lungs through the esophagus into the stomach and intestines. The roentgen films, therefore, usually show these organs to be distended with air (Fig. 177). The diagnosis of this anomaly is confirmed by passing a soft catheter into the esophagus as far as it will go and injecting an oily or water-soluble contrast substance. A sterilized, thin barium water mixture may also be used. The radiopaque material provides a perfect outline of the blind esophageal pouch (Fig. 178). The presence of the fistula is inferred because of the air in the stomach. Frequently the contrast material spills over from the blind esophageal pouch into the larynx to enter the trachea and bronchi. Spillover of ingested material in this way predisposes to aspiration pneumonia. However, pneumonia may also occur as the result of regurgitation of gastric secretions into the air passages through the esophagotracheal communication.

In rare instances the portion of the esophagus proximal to the atresia communicates with the trachea while the lower portion opens only into

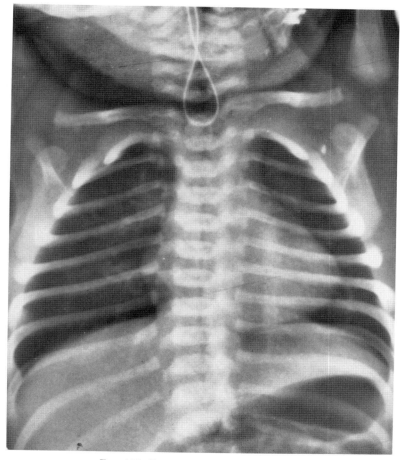

FIG. 177. TRACHEOESOPHAGEAL FISTULA

Because the infant regurgitated all of his feedings, a soft rubber nasogastric tube was inserted. It could be advanced only to the level of the jugular notch. At this point it doubled back on itself, outlining a blind esophageal pouch. The air in the stomach indicates a fistulous communication between the distal esophagus and the trachea or a bronchus.

the stomach. Contrast material injected into the esophagus flows directly into the trachea. The upper portion of the esophagus usually is not distended and the stomach and intestines which have no communication either with the pharynx or the trachea are free of air. An exception to this occurs in the extremely rare instances in which there is a second fistula connecting the trachea with the distal portion of the esophagus.

In the absence of esophageal atresia, aspiration pneumonia and its complications may be the only abnormalities to be seen on conventional films. The diagnosis then can be made only with the aid of contrast material. It may be quite difficult to demonstrate the fistula because the tract is often narrow and the contrast substance passes through it in short, rapid spurts. It is therefore necessary to monitor the examination fluoroscopically and to make spot films or preferably a ciné recording. Because the fistula usu-

ally courses upward and forward from the anterior wall of the esophagus to the trachea, the child is best examined in the oblique prone position with the head of the table tilted downward. A satisfactory examination can generally be obtained by having the patient drink the contrast material, making it unnecessary to pass a catheter into the esophagus. Even if the fistula itself is not clearly visualized, opacification of the lower trachea and bronchi without opacification of the larynx may be considered diagnostic. However, the oropharynx and larynx must be watched carefully during the act of swallowing to exclude the possibility of spillover through the larynx as the source of the contrast material in the air passages.

ACQUIRED TRACHEOESOPHAGEAL FISTULAS. Acquired fistulas are most commonly secondary to perforation of an ulcerating carcinoma of the esophagus into the trachea. Frequently the fis-

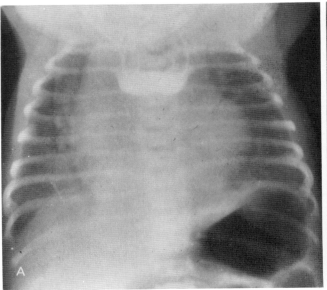
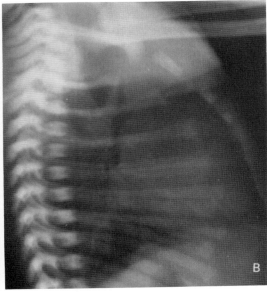

FIG. 178. TRACHEOESOPHAGEAL FISTULA

A: The diagnosis of a tracheoesophageal fistula is confirmed by injection of contrast material through a soft rubber catheter into the esophagus. The opaque material outlines the blind upper pouch of the atretic esophagus. There is considerable air in the stomach and intestines indicating that the lower portion of the esophagus communicates with the trachea. *B:* A lateral film made before the instillation of contrast material. The blind esophageal pouch is distended with air and is easily identified behind the trachea.

tula follows destruction by irradiation of an esophageal carcinoma that has invaded through the tracheal wall. A fistula may also result from perforation into the trachea and esophagus of necrotic lymph nodes in tuberculosis or histoplasmosis. A mediastinal abscess secondary to a tear in the esophagus during esophagoscopy or from a foreign body may also perforate into the trachea and establish a persistent communication between the two organs.

The roentgen picture is dominated by infection of the lung, manifested by one or more areas of bronchopneumonia which have a tendency to undergo suppuration and cavitation. However, pneumonia may be absent, particularly in recent fistulas. The presence of a fistula is often first suspected when the air passages are outlined during a barium meal. Since the fistula itself is rarely visualized, it is necessary to exclude the possibility of aspiration of the contrast material into the trachea or bronchi through the glottis. This occurs particularly in patients who are very ill and in those with laryngeal paralysis. Spillover aspiration can be excluded with certainty only by fluoroscopy or ciné filming of the pharynx and larynx while the contrast material is being swallowed.

Rupture of the Trachea. Rupture of the thoracic trachea occurs as a result of a severe crushing injury to the chest. The x-ray examination soon discloses evidence of mediastinal emphysema which extends to the neck. Almost always there is a pneumothorax involving the right side. This may be accompanied by a hemothorax. Not infrequently the pneumothorax is bilateral. A common complication is a tracheoesophageal fistula, evidence of which may first appear some time after the accident. In patients who survive without operation, a tracheal stricture may form.

In a considerable number of the cases of tracheal rupture there is concomitant rupture of a bronchus. This usually involves one of the main bronchi or the bronchus to the right upper lobe. The x-ray manifestations will then include those of the ruptured bronchus (see p. 241).

Tracheal Strictures. Significant strictures of the trachea are extremely rare. They may be congenital, follow tracheostomy or trauma, or result from inflammatory diseases. Those which follow tracheostomy occur either at the level of the stoma from an overgrowth of granulation tissue, or below this region as a result of pressure necrosis from the cuff of the tracheostomy tube. Inflammatory strictures are encountered in rare instances in the course of specific infections, such as tuberculosis, histoplasmosis or syphilis. In these diseases the trachea may be involved locally by direct extension of the disease from adjacent lymph nodes or may be more widely affected as a result of diffuse involvement of the mucous membrane. In the former instance the stricture usually involves the lower part of the trachea while in the case of generalized endotracheal disease the narrowing is more diffuse and irregular and occurs at any level. Diffuse narrowing of the trachea also occurs in Wegener's granulomatosis (see Fig. 368) or lethal midline granulomatosis (noninfectious necrotizing granulomatosis).

On conventional films the narrowing is best seen in the oblique or lateral projections. In addition to the stricture, the films may also show thickening of the wall of the trachea, particularly when it is diffusely involved. Both the stricture and the thickening of the tracheal wall are better seen on tomograms. Demonstration of mucosal detail is afforded by tracheography.

In the case of strictures following trauma or tracheostomy, the stenosis is localized and the tracheal wall in the narrowed area is sharply defined and smooth. A similar narrowing can occur either from rupture of an infected lymph node or a gumma into the trachea. In specific endotracheal infections or noninfectious necrotizing granulomatosis, the tracheogram shows an elongated area of narrowing, often with wavy or irregular borders.

Benign Tumors. Almost all primary tracheal tumors in children and in about half of those in adults are benign. A wide variety of histological types are represented, such as the osteochondroma, hemangioma, fibroma, leiomyoma and papilloma. Of these, the papilloma in the adult may become malignant.

The tumors vary in size from those which can be visualized only by tracheography to those which cause complete obstruction of the trachea. With the exception of papillomas, the benign tumors originate submucosally and are covered by mucous membrane. The margin of the tumor projecting into the lumen is therefore rounded and sharply demarcated with a smooth border which can frequently be seen on conventional films. Most of the lesions are sessile but occasionally there is a well-developed pedicle which permits the tumor to change its position with respiration or coughing. This can be observed fluoroscopically, using image intensification or during tracheography. Radiologic evidence of calcification is exceedingly rare, except in the case of osteomas.

Tracheal scleromas and some amyloid tumors may also be single. They cannot be differentiated radiologically from true neoplasms. The scleroma, a specific infectious granuloma, is almost always associated with similar lesions in the larynx and the nasal mucous membrane. Aberrant thyroid tissue may develop beneath the mucosa of the trachea and project within the lumen in the same manner as a benign neoplasm. It may be recognized by scanning after the administration of radioactive iodine.

TRACHEOPATHIA OSTEOPLASTICA. This term has been applied to multiple tumors containing cartilage and bony tissue. The tumors arise in relation to the cartilages and therefore are situated at the anterior and lateral walls of the trachea. They involve a considerable portion of the trachea and often the major bronchi as well. They produce rather flat nodular intrusions into the lumen which narrow the airway. The topography of the lesions is best demonstrated on tomograms which show a narrowing of the trachea whose border exhibits a wavy appearance. Although bone is present in the tumors, there is usually insufficient calcium deposited for recognition on the films.

TRACHEAL AMYLOIDOSIS. Amyloid deposition in the trachea occurs in the *primary* form of amyloidosis, in which there is no known underlying cause. It is usually associated with a diffuse thickening of the tracheal wall with tumor-like masses projecting into the lumen, causing a picture similar to that of tracheopathia osteoplastica or that of Wegener's granulomatosis. Most commonly the bronchi are also involved. The condition therefore is described more completely in the section on diseases of the bronchi (see p. 239).

PAPILLOMATOSIS. Papillomas are the most common tracheal tumors in children and are almost always multiple in this age group. Solitary papillomas of the trachea are more common in adults although multiple papillomas are occasionally encountered.

The papillomatous tumors most frequently involve the larynx as well as the trachea, particularly in children. They are sessile, and while they usually involve the cervical trachea just beneath the larynx, they often extend throughout the entire length of the trachea and the larger bronchi. Rarely the papillomas are distributed down to the smallest bronchi. Spontaneous regression of the tumors has been observed in children.

In contrast to other benign tumors, the papillomas arise from the mucous membrane itself, producing wart-like conglomerations. They therefore appear as irregular masses projecting from the wall of the trachea into the lumen. Those situated in the upper part of the trachea are best seen on lateral views of the neck. When

there are numberous small papillomas the entire
length of the tracheal air column is diffusely
narrowed with an irregular undulating border.
Larger papillomas or groups of papillomas produce more localized densities. The border of
these opacities is irregular, corresponding to the
cauliflower appearance of the growths. The irregularity of the masses and their extent may be
demonstrated by tomography. Tomograms made
in more than one projection are particularly useful in evaluating the extent of involvement. The
characteristic irregularity of the tumors is best
depicted by instilling contrast material which
coats the papillomas and fills the clefts between
their excrescences.

Primary Malignant Neoplasms. Of the primary malignant neoplasms of the trachea, *carcinoma* is the most common. It is most frequently situated in the lower third of the trachea
and is largely endotracheal. Extension into the
mediastinum is due mainly to involvement of the
paratracheal lymph nodes. The *cylindroma* occurs next in the order of frequency. Unlike most
of the carcinomas it arises from the depths of the
mucous membrane which covers the tumor forming a smooth surface (Fig. 179). The neoplasm is
often of the "iceberg" type with its major portion
growing outward into the surrounding tissues. It
is more apt to involve the upper part of the
trachea. *Carcinoid* tumors of the trachea are
extremely rare. They grow like the cylindromas
but metastasize less frequently. Those we have
observed have been situated in the lower portion
of the trachea. *Sarcomas* are also rare. Like the
cylindroma, the sarcomas have a tendency to
extend through the tracheal wall into the mediastinum. Both tumors can give rise to hematogenous metastases studding the lungs. This
type of metastasis occurs less frequently with
carcinomas of the trachea.

If the malignant tumor does not extend for any
considerable distance beyond the tracheal wall,
the roentgen appearance is often similar to that
of benign tumors. This is especially true of the
cylindroma, sarcoma and carcinoid, for these
present a sharply outlined density protruding
into the air column which, although lobulated, is
characterized by a smooth border. On the other
hand, the tracheal carcinoma tends to ulcerate
and produce a more irregular mass. When it is
localized and mostly endotracheal, it may be
indistinguishable from a solitary benign papilloma. In some instances the carcinoma is relatively flat, infiltrating the trachea more diffusely
and appears as an irregular thickening of the
tracheal wall. If the carcinoma involves a considerable portion of the circumference of the tra-

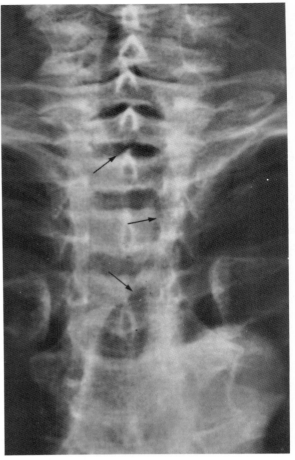

FIG. 179. CYLINDROMA OF THE TRACHEA

The tracheal lumen is narrowed by a smooth mass (arrows) projecting in from the right side. The fact that the
trachea is not displaced indicates that the lesion is within its
wall and that the narrowing is not due to pressure from an
extrinsic mass.

chea, it can produce a napkin-ring type of narrowing of the lumen. However, this appearance
is not entirely pathognomonic of carcinoma since
we have observed it in a case of tracheal cylindroma.

The extratracheal portion of a tracheal neoplasm can be recognized only when it is quite
large. When situated at the thoracic inlet it may
be manifested only by local increase in density
without a discernible border, but like an enlarged
thyroid, the mass can displace the trachea to the
opposite side. When the neoplasm is situated at
a lower level, the extratracheal portion of the
tumor may produce a localized bulge on the
superior mediastinal border. More diffuse mediastinal widening is produced by spread of the
carcinoma.

It should be emphasized that most of the carcinomas that involve the lower end of the trachea represent upward spread of a carcinoma originating in a main bronchus. The only roentgen evidence may be a mass projecting into the trachea, best seen on oblique views or tomograms (Fig. 180). More commonly, however, the roentgen examination discloses evidence of stenosis of the main bronchus or infiltration of the lung.

Extrinsic Neoplasms. Hematogenous metastases to the trachea are extremely rare. Secondary involvement of the trachea by neoplastic disease is practically always due to direct extension from an adjacent organ. Most commonly this is due to the upward spread of a carcinoma of a main bronchus. Direct extension to the trachea from an adjacent carcinoma of the esophagus is not unusual. In either instance it may be difficult, if not impossible, to determine whether the carcinoma has originated in the trachea. Ulceration of a carcinoma involving both the esophagus and trachea may result in a tracheoesophageal fistula. This occurs much more frequently when the primary lesion is situated in

the esophagus. Other causes of secondary neoplastic involvement of the trachea are extension from a metastatic carcinoma of the subcarinal lymph nodes, a primary carcinoma of the thyroid or in extremely rare instances, direct invasion of the trachea from a peripheral carcinoma of the mesial surface of the upper lobe immediately adjacent to the trachea.

Pulmonary Complications of Tracheal Obstruction. The most common abnormality secondary to obstruction of the trachea is bronchopneumonia. This is due not only to spread of infection into the lung from an infected ulcerative lesion in the trachea, but also to impairment of drainage of secretions from the tracheobronchial tree. The pneumonia occurs more frequently in the lower lobes and may take the form of a single area of consolidation or multiple patchy areas involving both lungs. Persistent or recurrent pneumonias are not uncommon and may result in chronic changes. Atelectasis or obstructive emphysema of one lung or of the right upper lobe occur when the tumor extends downward to cause either complete or partial

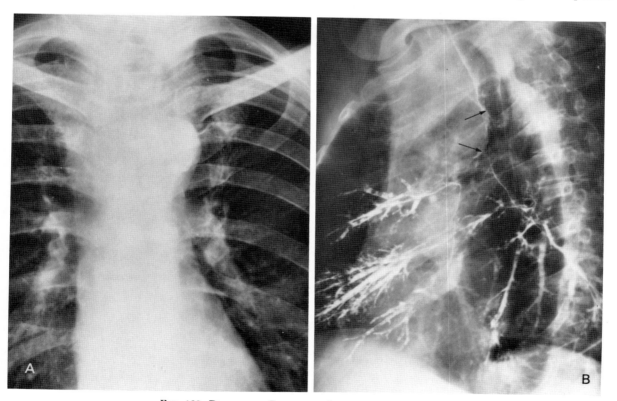

FIG. 180. BRONCHIAL CARCINOMA INVOLVING THE TRACHEA
A: The right side of the mediastinum is widened and the root of the right lung is elevated as a result of atelectasis of the right upper lobe. *B:* Bronchogram, left oblique view. The right upper lobe bronchus is completely occluded by a large mass which also extends through the tracheal wall (arrows). The triangular shadow above this represents the atelectatic right upper lobe. Bronchoscopy disclosed a squamous cell carcinoma infiltrating the trachea.

obstruction of a large bronchus. Obstructive emphysema of both lungs occurs when the tracheal lumen is severely compromised. Bilateral bronchopneumonia is then an early additional complication.

Since the obstructive lesion in the trachea is usually not obvious on the conventional frontal film, the roentgen picture is dominated by the pulmonary complications. It is important to bear in mind the possibility of tracheal obstruction in all cases of pneumonia, obstructive emphysema or of atelectasis of an upper lobe in association with wheezing or stridor. In all of these instances the trachea should be observed on oblique or lateral views.

Adherent Mucus. A gob of mucoid secretion resting on the mucous membrane of the trachea can simulate a neoplasm. In rare instances it may be observed on a conventional oblique or lateral view of the chest but it is more frequently seen on tomograms (Fig. 181). On the sections it appears as a semioval or semicircular intrusion on the lumen with a sharp, regular border, which in some instances even appears lobulated. In the absence of clinical evidences of a neoplasm or of additional roentgen findings to indicate the presence of a tumor, the possibility of an adherent collection of mucus must always be considered whenever such a shadow is seen. In these instances the tomogram should be repeated after coughing to make certain that the shadow persists. Disappearance of the shadow would indicate that it is due to mucus. Even in patients presenting other evidences suggesting the possibility of tracheal obstruction, all of the tomograms should be studied carefully to determine whether the shadow has shifted its position on one or more of the sections. A change in the

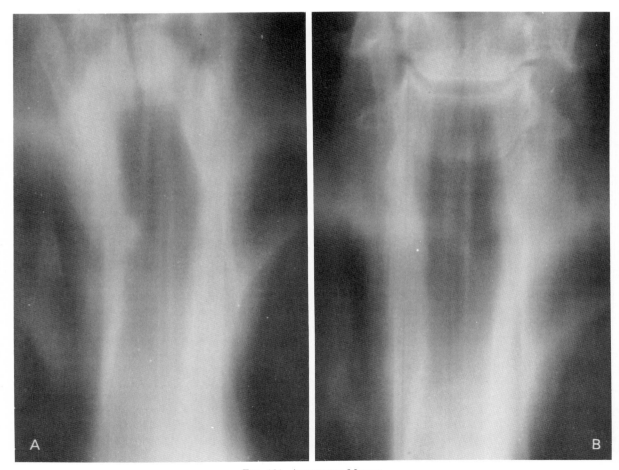

FIG. 181. ADHERENT MUCUS

A: The patient had been considered to have a neoplasm of the trachea because of a mass seen on the right tracheal wall on tomograms. Because such a shadow can be caused by a gob of mucus, tomograms were repeated before subjecting the patient to bronchoscopy. *B:* Tomograms made several days later show the shadow to have disappeared.

position of the shadow may be seen with a pedunculated neoplasm but it is more likely to occur in the case of tenacious mucus. The tomograms should then be repeated after coughing to determine whether the shadow disappears before making a final diagnosis. Repetition of tomography of the trachea is also advisable when bronchoscopy fails to disclose a tumor of the trachea suspected from a previous radiologic examination. Observation of the lesion on the second set of films is an indication for repeat bronchoscopy.

The Bronchi

On most films, only the main bronchi are visualized with any degree of clarity. They are seen because of the contrast between the radiolucent air within them and the density of the mediastinal structures around them. Under normal conditions, the small bronchi are not outlined because their walls are thin and they are surrounded by radiolucent lung. However, if their walls are thickened, as in chronic bronchitis, they may be recognizable on ordinary films. If the adjacent lung is consolidated, even the more peripheral bronchi may be seen quite clearly because the air within their lumen stands out against the opaque, solidified lung (Fig. 110).

The walls of the normal upper and lower lobar bronchi are sufficiently thick to be delineated, particularly on oblique views. The anterior division of the upper lobe bronchus is projected on end on the frontal view and is often seen as a small, ring-like shadow adjacent to the round, homogenous density of its accompanying blood vessel (Fig. 33). The small bronchial branches are accompanied by blood vessels which can usually be seen on the films, even though the bronchi themselves cannot be identified. Displacement or distortion of these structures can be inferred from the distribution of the vessels.

The bronchi are better seen on high contrast films, especially when made with a Bucky grid (Fig. 175). Still better visualization is afforded by tomography. However, caution must be exercised in interpreting funnel-shaped narrowing of the bronchi on the tomograms. Such a narrowing can be produced when the bronchus does not lie parallel to the plane of the section and is cut obliquely. It is justifiable to conclude that a stenosis is present only if the sections demonstrate a distinct shadow within the bronchial lumen (see Fig. 389), or if they show an irregularity of the bronchial wall (Fig. 22). Tomograms are also useful in demonstrating widening of the bronchi and the entrance of bronchi into cavities.

Bronchography is required for detailed studies of the bronchi. The bronchogram clearly demonstrates displacement and distortion of the bronchi, the degree and type of bronchial dilatation, and irregularities and stenosis of the lumen. In many cases, the nature of an obstructive lesion can be inferred from the brochogram (Fig. 182). Bronchography has proved useful in the study of the pathogenesis of bronchiectasis and is indispensable for mapping out the distribution of the dilated bronchi prior to resective surgery. It can also be employed to demonstrate obstructive lesions beyond the range of the rigid bronchoscope (see Fig. 190). It is helpful in the localization of abscesses within the lung and for the demonstration of cavities which communicate with the bronchi (see Fig. 240).

The movements of the bronchi may be studied fluoroscopically at the time of bronchography by ciné techniques and on films made during inspiration and expiration. Bronchography may also disclose the presence and location of bronchopleural or bronchoperitoneal fistulas.

Bronchial Displacement

Displacement of the main bronchi may be the only obvious sign of disease in the adjacent lung or mediastinum. Widening of the angle at the tracheal bifurcation is most often produced by an enlarged left atrium which elevates the left main bronchus and displaces the right main bronchus laterally. This occurs most frequently in patients with mitral valve disease or atrial fibrillation. A large pericardial effusion produces the same effect. Widening of the angle is usually not evident on ordinary films because the bronchi are obscured by the increased density of the cardiac shadow. However, the obtuse angle formed by the main bronchi can be seen on more highly penetrated films.

Splaying of the tracheal bifurcation can also be caused by a mass in the subcarinal region. This almost always represents large lymph nodes involved by neoplasm, tuberculosis or sarcoidosis. Rarely a bronchogenic cyst occurs in this location and produces the same effect (Fig. 446).

The left main bronchus may be displaced upward when the left upper lobe is atelectatic. Even when the lobe is completely collapsed, it may produce only a faint density in the frontal projection. This is easily overlooked. However, elevation of the left main bronchus should suggest the possibility of atelectasis and indicate the need for a lateral film. This will clearly disclose the outline of the shrunken upper lobe (Fig. 186). The presence of bronchial obstruction can be

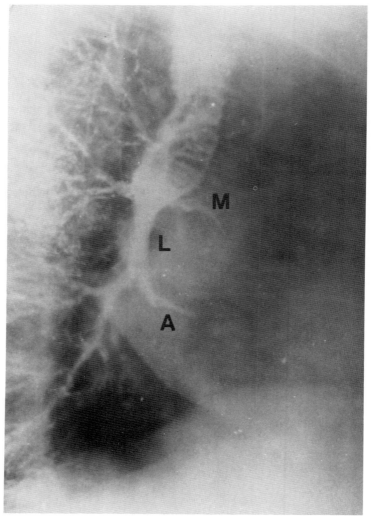

FIG. 182. RAT TAIL STENOSIS OF THE BRONCHUS

Bronchogram of the right lung, lateral view. The longitudinal narrowing of the lower lobe bronchus (L) is caused by carcinomatous infiltration of its wall. The neoplasm has also extended into the anterior basal division (A) of the lower lobe bronchus and into the middle lobe bronchus (M). These bronchi taper to a fine point a short distance from their origin. This appearance, which has been likened to a rat's tail, is characteristic of bronchogenic carcinoma.

confirmed by fluoroscopy which discloses a swing of the mediastinum to the left on inspiration.

Large nodes in the tracheobronchial angle may depress the main bronchus and narrow the angle of the tracheal bifurcation. When such nodes are associated with an obstructing carcinoma of the upper lobe, they produce a rather characteristic alteration in the course of the bronchi. The downward displacement of the mesial portion of the main bronchus by the nodes and the upward displacement of the upper lobe bronchus resulting from the atelectasis, produce a hook-like deformity which is quite striking (Fig. 421).

The tracheal bifurcation may also be narrowed when there is atelectasis of a lower lobe. As this portion of lung collapses, the main bronchus tends to assume a more vertical position.

Bronchial Obstruction

The presence of bronchial obstruction is usually recognized roentgenologically by its effect on the lung, particularly the occurrence of atelectasis and emphysema. However, the roentgen picture is often modified by infection which so frequently occurs beyond the obstruction. This may be manifested by recurrent pneumonias confined to one area, or by a pneumonia that fails to resolve promptly. Bronchiectasis or suppuration with the formation of one or more cavities may further complicate the picture of bronchial obstruction. In some cases, the process is entirely overshadowed by a pleural effusion or a pyopneumothorax.

Because of the possibility of an underlying obstructing bronchial lesion, bronchoscopy should be performed in all cases of unilateral bronchiectasis or chronic lung abscess. Bronchography may also be required. However, bronchography cannot be relied on as a primary procedure because it is possible to overlook a partially obstructing lesion, such as an adenoma, even when it is situated within a large bronchus.

The presence of atelectasis is indicated by a drawing together of the bronchial branches which is easily recognized on bronchography if the branches can be filled (Fig. 90). On ordinary films, one may infer that the bronchi are drawn together from the fact that the vessels appear approximated.

In emphysema, the bronchi are separated from each other to an appreciable degree. Widening of the angles formed by the branches is most marked in compensatory emphysema. The overexpansion and shift of the rest of the lung are most striking when one or more lobes are completely collapsed. The compensatory emphysema may be so effective that no shrinkage of the hemithorax takes place and the fact that a major bronchial branch is obstructed is easily overlooked. In order to avoid this error, it is necessary to identify and trace the course of each bronchus on the bronchogram.

When the emphysema is due to obstruction of a large bronchus, the film made in inspiration may be entirely negative because both lungs can be equally expanded. During expiration, however, the obstructed lung does not show normal clouding and the mediastinum may shift toward the opposite side (Fig. 17). Therefore, whenever the history suggests inhalation of a foreign body or if there are wheezing respirations of unknown cause or unilateral diminution in breath sounds, the patient should be observed in both phases of respiration by fluoroscopy or with films made in inspiration and expiration.

Bronchial Strictures. The most common cause of bronchial strictures are tuberculous bronchitis and perforation of diseased lymph nodes into or through the bronchial wall. A stricture of a large bronchus can also result from damage caused by a foreign body and may persist even after this has been removed. Slight narrowing of the larger bronchi sometimes occurs in association with bronchiectasis. It results from

severe ulcerative bronchitis that is part of the suppurative bronchopneumonia responsible for the bronchiectasis. While slight narrowing of the main bronchi can also occur in sarcoidosis, this is rare. Significant strictures are not uncommon in bronchi of medium size, such as the middle lobe or segmental bronchi. Stricturing of small bronchial branches occurs frequently in sarcoidosis, as well as in all destructive, inflammatory diseases of the lung.

A bronchial stricture is rarely visible on conventional films. The manifestations on these films are referable to complications of the obstruction rather than to the stricture itself, i.e., atelectasis, persistent or recurrent pneumonia, or bronchiectasis. Bucky films may disclose the point of narrowing in some instances but the strictures are more frequently demonstrated by tomography. In the case of the middle lobe bronchus, which is the most frequent site of stricture, the narrowing is best demonstrated on the tomograms made in the lateral or the right posterior oblique position. Of course, the best method of demonstrating the stricture is by bronchography which discloses its exact position, shape and extent.

The bronchial narrowing caused by tuberculous bronchitis in the *reinfection* type of the disease extends characteristically over a considerable length of the bronchus, producing an elongated irregular stricture. This differs from that which occurs from direct extension of the disease from an adjacent lymph node in *primary* tuberculosis. Bronchography in the latter usually discloses the narrowing of the bronchus to be localized to a point in the region of the lung root directly adjacent to the diseased nodes. Similar changes occur in histoplasmosis.

In tuberculous bronchitis, other, more characteristic, evidence of tuberculosis is usually visible at the time of the examination. In some cases, collapse of the upper lobe obscures the underlying disease. In these instances, however, additional evidence of tuberculosis is usually present on previous films or in the opposite lung. In the case of an old stricture resulting from perforation of a tuberculous node, there may be a history referable to childhood tuberculosis. If the disease is still active, large nodes may be seen at the lung root (see Fig. 279).

Anthracotic lymph nodes which are the seat of nonspecific infection may perforate into a bronchus and cause a stricture in the absence of tuberculosis or histoplasmosis. Such strictures are practically always situated at the origin of the segmental bronchi, and usually involve the anterior division of the upper lobes although they may affect the middle lobe bronchus or one of its segmental divisions.

Congenital strictures are extremely rare. Those which are recognized occur in the large bronchi. The ones that we have seen have been long and tapering, ending in a cord which represents the anlage of the malformed bronchus.

Bronchial Compression. Benign tumors of the mediastinum rarely cause significant compression of the bronchi unless they are very large. We have seen one case in which a bronchogenic cyst, the size of a walnut, caused obstruction of a main bronchus. In this instance there was an associated chondromalacia of the bronchial wall so that the cyst was able to compress the bronchus. Radiologically, this presented the picture of obstructive emphysema of the left lung.

Bronchial obstruction by a malignant neoplasm of the mediastinum is almost always due to infiltration of the bronchial wall rather than compression. Obstruction of one or both main bronchi does occur, on occasion, from the pressure of large subcarinal nodes involved by metastatic neoplasm. Most often this is due to a bronchogenic carcinoma but it can be secondary to metastasis from a distant organ, such as the breast.

In the past, the sudden appearance of a homogeneous shadow in the lung of a child with primary tuberculosis was considered to represent consolidation caused by reaction to the toxins of the tubercle bacilli. This was known as *epituberculosis*. It is now quite clear that the picture is due to atelectasis resulting from obstruction of a bronchus by large tuberculous nodes in the mediastinum or lung root. The atelectasis usually disappears quite promptly when the disease in the nodes regresses, but it may persist if a bronchial stricture forms.

Graham described compression of the middle lobe bronchus by lymph nodes which were enlarged as the result of a nonspecific pneumonia involving the middle lobe. He concluded that the pressure of the inflamed nodes resulted in obstruction of the middle lobe bronchus. This prevented resolution of the middle lobe pneumonia which, in turn, caused persistence of the lymphadenitis. He called this vicious cycle the *middle lobe syndrome*. The sequence of events described by Graham must be extremely rare. Our experience has been that inflammatory obstruction of the middle lobe bronchus is due to a stricture rather than to compression by a large node. The most common cause of this stricture is involvement of the bronchial wall by infection that has spread from a contiguous lymph node. This is usually due to tuberculosis or histoplasmosis. In

some cases the stricture follows perforation of the diseased node into the bronchus. Rarely this is due to nonspecific suppurative lymphadenitis. In any case, the persistent obstruction is caused by a stricture of the bronchus rather than pressure by a large node.

An aneurysm of the aorta can compress the left main bronchus or the bronchus to the left upper lobe. It does not cause obstruction of the left lower lobe bronchus alone or the bronchi on the right side. Compression of the right main bronchus can be due to a *vascular sling*. In this anomaly the left pulmonary artery arises from the right pulmonary artery and courses behind the bifurcation of the trachea to reach the left lung. The right bronchus is compressed between the right pulmonary artery which lies anterior to it, and the left pulmonary artery behind. Aneurysmal dilatation of either pulmonary artery can also result in compression of a major bronchus.

The left atrium lies immediately beneath the carina. In rare instances, when this chamber is markedly enlarged, it can compress the left main bronchus and cause atelectasis of the lung. It may also partially obstruct the right main bronchus. In adults, this complication is practically always associated with disease of the mitral valve. In infants and young children it is more often produced by generalized enlargement of the heart. In these cases, the left lower lobe bronchus is the one most commonly obstructed, but it is possible for the left main bronchus to be compressed (Fig. 183).

Bronchial Neoplasms. The most common bronchial neoplasm, the carcinoma, is discussed in the section on Carcinoma of the Lung, since this tumor practically always involves the lung as well as the bronchus. Other neoplasms that arise in the bronchus are generally less malignant. The most common of these is the bronchial carcinoid. The cylindroma is considerably less common, while the mucoepidermoid tumor of the bronchus is very rare. These three tumors had previously been grouped under the single heading of bronchial adenoma, the bronchial carcinoid being designated as the carcinoid type of adenoma, and the cylindroma as the mixed tumor type. However, observations in recent years indicate that these tumors differ in their clinical course as well as in their pathologic picture and therefore should be considered as separate entities.

BRONCHIAL CARCINOID. The tumor is properly called a carcinoid because of its similarity in cell type and behavior to the carcinoid tumor of the bowel and because it tends to produce serotonin and the carcinoid syndrome when it metasta-

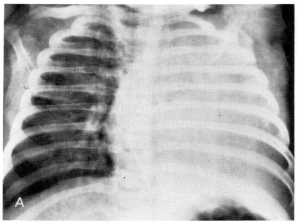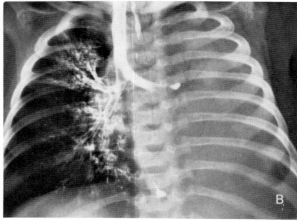

FIG. 183. BRONCHIAL COMPRESSION BY LARGE HEART

A: An 11 month old child with endocardial fibroelastosis and marked enlargement of the left atrium and left ventricle, presented with complete atelectasis of the left lung. The left cardiac border cannot be visualized at this time because of the opacity of the lung. *B:* The bronchogram shows the bronchial obstruction to be situated where the left bronchus lies in relation to the left atrium. There was no endobronchial lesion.

sizes. The tumor arises from the bronchial mucous membrane beneath the epithelial layer. Most commonly, the tumor originates in a large bronchus. In about 10% of the cases the carcinoid is situated in the periphery of the lung and its bronchial origin may be difficult to demonstrate because it arises from a very small bronchus.

With the exception of the peripheral carcinoids, the neoplasms project into the bronchial lumen, forming a polypoid mass which has a smooth surface because it is covered with intact bronchial epithelium. In most cases the tumor infiltrates the depths of the bronchial wall and grows between the cartilages into the peribronchial tissues. Here it may form a mass much larger than the intrabronchial component. However, there is only local invasion of the lung. Regional lymh nodes are involved in about 10% of the cases almost always by direct invasion of the tumor (Fig. 184). In about 5%, there are distant metastases, particularly in the liver, rarely in the bones. We have not observed metastases in the lungs in our series of 140 cases.

A carcinoid of a large bronchus is rarely detected before it produces bronchial obstruction. The roentgen picture is usually dominated by atelectasis which, in turn, is often complicated by secondary infection. In rare instances, the only manifestations are those of obstructive emphysema (Fig. 17) or dilated bronchi filled with mucus (See Fig. 193). When the extrabronchial component is large, the tumor itself may be visible on ordinary films (Fig. 185). This occurs in about one-fifth of cases. In the remainder, secondary infection usually obscures the tumor.

The roentgen picture then is that of pneumonia, bronchiectasis or lung abscess. Occasionally, despite the complications, the mass is clearly outlined at the root of the infected lobe. In some instances the entire picture is overshadowed by a pleural effusion secondary to the inflammation of the lung.

The polypoid tumor can sometimes be recognized within a main or lobar bronchus on overpenetrated films. More often it is clearly demonstrable on tomograms (Fig. 186). Practically all these tumors when first recognized have already produced bronchial obstruction. Only the proximal free border of the mass can be identified. It presents as a sharply demarcated convexity projecting into the bronchial air column. Because the tumor tends to produce local dilatation of the bronchus, the air column may be splayed about the proximal portion of the mass. Bronchogenic carcinomas in the same region are more irregular and flatter, and usually produce an irregular narrowing of the bronchial lumen proximal to the growth.

The smooth globular or polypoid outline of a carcinoid and the splaying of the bronchus are clearly outlined by bronchography (Fig. 187). As a rule, the column of contrast material ends abruptly with a sharply outlined, concave border where it meets the endobronchial component of the tumor. When the bronchus is not completely occluded, the radiopaque dye may trickle past the obstruction to outline the entire mass. In rare instances, the tumor cannot be identified and the only visible abnormality is dilatation of the bronchi beyond it.

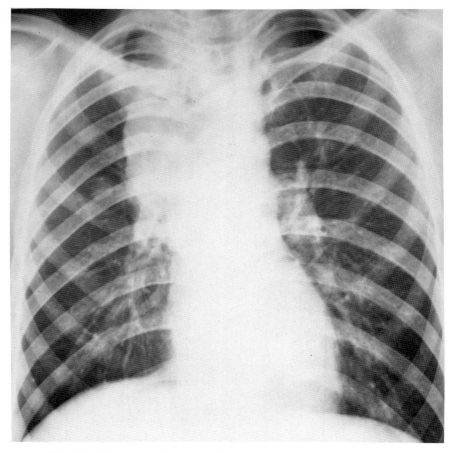

FIG. 184. BRONCHIAL CARCINOID, INVOLVEMENT OF MEDIASTINAL NODES

The patient was 15 years old at the time of examination. The same shadow along the right side of the mediastinum had been present since the age of 6. Bronchoscopy disclosed a smooth, polypoid neoplasm projecting from the right upper lobe into the right main bronchus. At operation, the right upper lobe was found to be completely collapsed and the neoplasm invaded the adjacent lymph nodes which were greatly enlarged. All of the aerated lung on the right side, extending to the apex of the right pulmonary field represents the hyperexpanded right lower and middle lobes. These were able to fill the space relinquished by the collapsed upper lobe since there were no pleural adhesions. The trachea, therefore, remains in the midline.

The peripheral carcinoid completely obstructs the small bronchus from which it arises while it is still very small. Because collateral respiration is not interfered with, distal atelectasis is uncommon and infection beyond the tumor is rare. The adenoma appears radiologically as a round, well-demarcated pulmonary nodule with a smooth border, indistinguishable from a benign tumor. Since the tumor completely occludes the bronchus, only the obstruction can be demonstrated by bronchography.

Rarely, calcific deposits and bone formation occur within a bronchial carcinoid. This may lead to error because calcification within a peripheral nodule is considered to be a sign of benignancy. However, if such a mass is observed to grow, the possibility of a carcinoid should be considered. Calcification within a tumor situated in a major bronchus does not cause any difficulty because the carcinoid is readily recognized when viewed through a bronchoscope.

The roentgen picture of bronchial carcinoid is usually nonspecific, consisting of atelectasis and the results of secondary infection. These changes, when associated with a tumor at the lung root, suggest carcinoma. However, certain facts in the clinical history taken together with the roentgen findings aid greatly in the diagnosis. A long history, beginning before the age of 40, particularly in a female, a story of recurrent pulmonary infections over a long period of time and the expectoration of pure red blood in a patient with

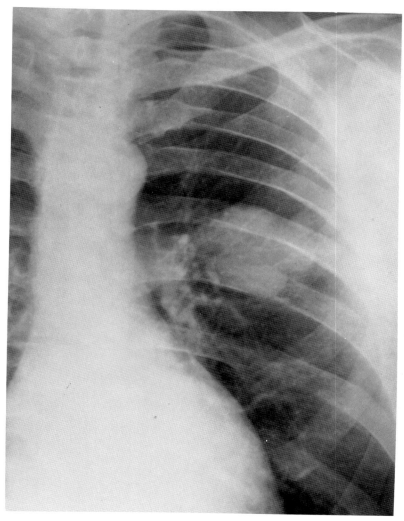

FIG. 185. PERIPHERAL BRONCHIAL CARCINOID
Ordinarily, bronchial carcinoids develop in large bronchi and are obscured on the roentgenogram by the shadow of the atelectatic inflamed lung which the bronchus supplies. In this case, the neoplasm originated in a small bronchus and the lobulated, sharply circumscribed density represents the tumor itself. It was resected at thoracotomy.

evidence of bronchostenosis, should always arouse the suspicion of a carcinoid or some other type of bronchial tumor rather than carcinoma.

OTHER PRIMARY BRONCHIAL TUMORS. *Cylindromas* are grossly similar to bronchial carcinoids, presenting as smooth, polypoid protrusions into the bronchus. The bronchographic appearance of the two tumors is the same. However, the cylindroma is a much more malignant tumor and has a tendency to cause considerable infiltration of the lung. Thus the pulmonary component of the tumor is apt to be more evident on the films. In addition, there is a tendency for growth into the large pulmonary vessels, producing hematogenous metastases. When the pulmonary artery is involved, numerous, well-demarcated, round nodules may form in the portion of lung supplied by the artery that is invaded. In rare instances, both lungs are the seat of numerous round metastases.

We have had the opportunity to observe two examples of true *bronchial adenomas*. These are benign tumors arising from the mucous glands, consisting of large acini widely distended with mucus and lined by columnar and cuboidal cells. There was no infiltration of the bronchial wall in these instances nor in the few similar cases that have been described. Radiologically, there were

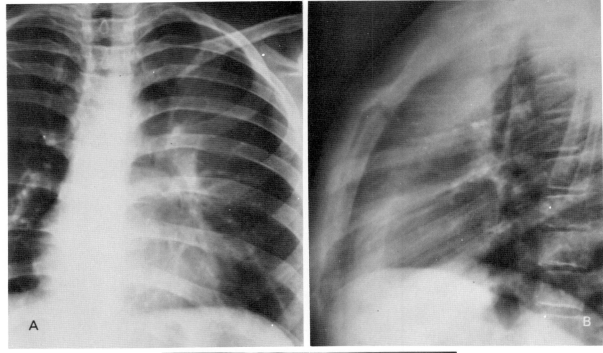

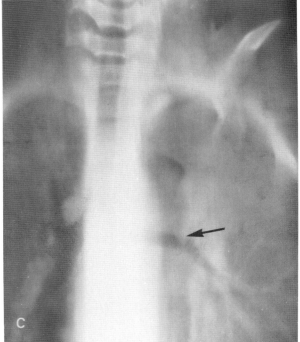

FIG. 186. BRONCHIAL CARCINOID

A: The frontal film shows a hazy density over the upper part of the left lung through which blood vessels are visible. The left cardiac border is obscured and the left main bronchus is elevated. These findings indicate atelectasis of the left upper lobe. *B:* In the lateral view the collapsed upper lobe is seen as a band of density behind the sternum with extreme anterior displacement of the long fissure. The lower lobe is hyperexpanded and reaches the dome of the thorax. Its vessels are projected through the shadow of the collapsed upper lobe on the frontal film. *C:* The frontal tomogram shows a smoothly outlined filling defect (arrow) on the superior border of the left main bronchus. This represents a bronchial carcinoid protruding from the orifice of the left upper lobe bronchus. The trachea remains in the midline because of the compensatory hyperexpansion of the lower lobe.

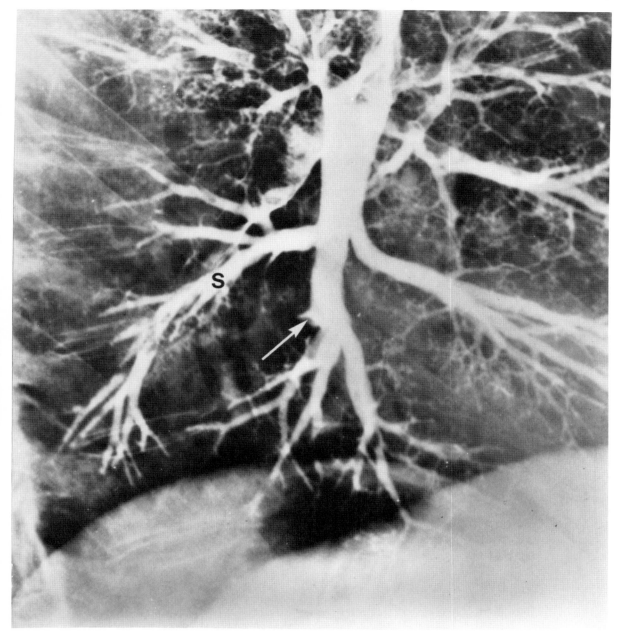

FIG. 187. BRONCHIAL CARCINOID

A bronchogram shows complete occlusion of the posterior basal bronchus of the right lower lobe. The bronchus just proximal to the obstruction is splayed (arrow). This is a rather characteristic finding of a bronchial carcinoid. The diagnosis was confirmed by bronchoscopy. The bronchi to the superior segment of the lower lobe (S) are displaced downward, filling the space relinquished by the collapsed posterior basal segment.

only manifestations of an obstructing polypoid bronchial tumor, without evidence of growth outside the confines of the bronchus.

Other benign tumors of the bronchi are the chondroma and osteochondroma, usually considered *hamartomas,* the lipoma and the granular cell myoblastoma. These also do not infiltrate

beyond the bronchial wall. In three of the chondromas that we have seen, the intrabronchial polypoid mass appeared somewhat irregular with a knurled surface similar to that of some intrapulmonary cartilaginous hamartomas. In one of these the filling defect seen on the bronchongram had a raspberry-like contour (Fig. 188). Calcifi-

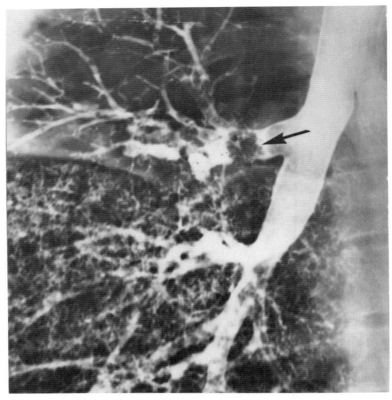

FIG. 188. ENDOBRONCHIAL HAMARTOMA

The hamartoma in the right upper lobe bronchus is seen on the bronchogram as a round defect with an irregular border (arrow). Several of the anterior segmental branches show cylindrical dilatation. There is some loss of volume of the anterior segment which appears clouded. The short fissure is bowed upward.

cation may be visible in the rare cases of osteochondroma.

METASTATIC NEOPLASMS OF THE BRONCHUS. Although microscopic metastases to the bronchi are not uncommon in widely disseminated neoplasms, it is unusual for the metastases to be large enough to cause obstruction of the larger bronchi. The renal hypernephroma tends to metastasize to large bronchi more commonly than any other tumor (Fig. 91). Such metastases may become clinically evident many years after the primary lesion has been removed. Metastases from breast carcinoma to a large bronchus are not very rare. We have also seen endobronchial deposits from carcinoma of the colon and one instance from a carcinoma of the prostate. In some cases, the metastases lodged in the bronchial wall itself. In others, they undoubtedly occurred in the lung or in lymph nodes adjacent to the bronchus and involved the bronchial wall secondarily. In either case they produced atelectasis of a segment or a lobe of the lung. In some this was the only roentgen manifestation. In others, additional lesions were present either in the

mediastinum or in other parts of the lung (Figs. 82 and 189).

When evidence of bronchial obstruction is found in a patient with a primary cancer somewhere else in the body, it cannot be assumed that an endobronchial metastasis is responsible for the atelectasis in every case. We have seen several such patients in whom it was proved that an additional primary carcinoma of the bronchus was responsible for the pulmonary lesion. One must always bear in mind the possibility of multiple primary malignant neoplasms in this situation.

Broncholithiasis. It used to be thought that bronchial stones form within the bronchial lumen. However, available evidence indicates that this is not the case, and it is generally agreed that the stones originate in calcified lymph nodes which perforate into the bronchi. The calcific deposits in the nodes are usually the result of healed primary tuberculosis but may also be caused by histoplasmosis. During the active stage of the disease the infection spreads from the nodes to the adjacent bronchus and partially

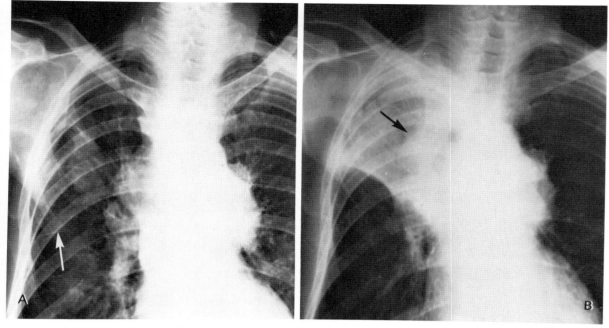

FIG. 189. METASTATIC NEOPLASM OF THE BRONCHUS

A: The patient had a primary carcinoma of the rectum. The lymph nodes on each side of the mediastinum are enlarged and there are several indistinct nodular densities in the right upper lobe. The appearance is due to metastases to the lung and mediastinal nodes. The short fissure (arrow) is in its normal position. *B:* Several weeks later. The short fissure is bowed upward because of partial atelectasis of the right upper lobe due to obstruction of its bronchus by extension of the neoplasm from the adjacent nodes. The mass (arrow), seen within the shadow of the upper lobe, represents the enlarged tracheobronchial nodes which have been displaced laterally together with the right main bronchus, because of collapse of the lobe.

destroys its wall. In this manner the caseous node becomes incorporated into the bronchial wall. The stone then forms in the bronchial wall and may remain there or may be extruded into the lumen.

Roentgenologically, it is impossible to differentiate between intraluminal and intramural stones. Although the latter are entirely within the bronchial wall and covered by intact mucous membrane, they bulge into the lumen and can obstruct the bronchus. In other cases, the broncholith is associated with a stricture which develops during the healing of the original infection. In any of these instances, the term broncholithiasis is applicable.

The typical roentgen picture of broncholithiasis consists of a calcific deposit at the root of an atelectatic portion of the lung. In about half of the cases the stone is situated at the root of the right middle lobe bronchus, and the roentgen film shows the classic picture of atelectasis of the middle lobe (Fig. 136). In about 25%, the anterior segmental bronchus of either upper lobe or the lingular bronchus is the site of the stone (Fig. 96). The posterior division of the upper lobe bronchus and the superior segmental division of

the lower lobe are the next most frequently involved (Fig. 190). It is rare for the stone to be situated in the basal divisions of the lower lobe. Involvement of the main bronchi and lobar bronchi other than that of the middle lobe is unusual but not rare.

Infection of the lung distal to the obstructed bronchus is common and frequently results in bronchiectasis and abscess formation. Infection of the pleura and the formation of an empyema from rupture of one of the suppurative foci may obscure the underlying disease.

The possibility of broncholithiasis should be considered whenever the roentgen film shows calcification near the root of the lung in association with segmental or lobar atelectasis or pneumonia. Films should be made in those projections which outline the silhouette of the diseased segment to demonstrate the relationship of the calcific deposit to the entering bronchus. The presumptive diagnosis of broncholithiasis is justified if the calcific deposit is situated at the apex of the involved area. This relationship must be confirmed by films made in at least one additional projection before a final diagnosis can be made. When the stone is not well visualized on

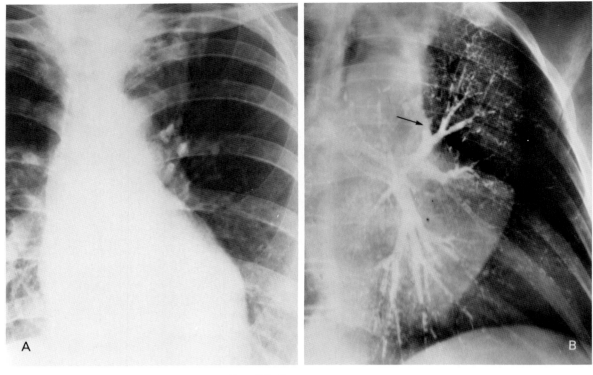

FIG. 190. BRONCHOLITHIASIS

A: Bucky film. The ordinary frontal film showed a triangular shadow in the left upper lobe adjacent to the mediastinum.
The apex of the shadow was situated at the root of the lobe where there was a suggestion of small calcific deposits. The Bucky
film clearly outlines three calcific deposits at the root of the left upper lobe. The atelectatic apicoposterior segment is visible
as a faint shadow. *B:* Bronchography. All of the bronchi of the left lung are well outlined with the exception of the apicoposterior
branch. This is completely obstructed by a stone immediately beyond its origin (arrow). A short distance above, two more
stones are visible. At operation, these were found immediately beyond the bifurcation of the bronchus into its apical and
posterior branches. A stone was present in each branch.

conventional films, Bucky films (Fig. 19) or tomograms (Fig. 20) are required. These are essential when the pulmonary field is obscured by a
pleural effusion or complicating pulmonary infection.

The diagnosis of broncholithiasis can be made
with a high degree of accuracy from the roentgen
studies, but it should always be confirmed by
bronchoscopy. The finding of a stricture at the
site of the calcific deposit, proved to be inflammatory through biopsy, confirms the diagnosis of
broncholithiasis almost as certainly as direct visualization of the stone. If the obstruction is beyond the view of the bronchoscopist, bronchography should be done. The demonstration of
bronchial obstruction at the point where the
calcific deposit is located, also confirms the diagnosis (Fig. 190).

Because of the frequency of calcification of the
hilar nodes close to the main bronchi and the
comparative rarity of obstruction of these bronchi by stones, relatively little significance can be

attached to calcific deposits found in association
with atelectasis of an entire lung or any lobe
other than the middle lobe (Fig. 191). However,
attention should be paid to the relationship of
the calcified nodes to the bronchi in these cases
even though it is likely that the disease of the
lung is due to a cause other than broncholithiasis.

The x-ray examination of the chest should be
repeated periodically even after one or more
stones have been expectorated or removed at
bronchoscopy. Some calcific deposits may remain, but these are insignificant if they are not
related to the bronchial tree. On the other hand,
one or more residual calculi may still be present
within the lumen or in the bronchial wall.

Abnormal shadows in the lung distal to the
bronchial obstruction can clear completely after
the stones have been eliminated. However, the
affected lung tissue may remain altelectatic. Abscess cavities may disappear, but bronchiectases
practically always remain unchanged. The importance of these residual shadows in the lung

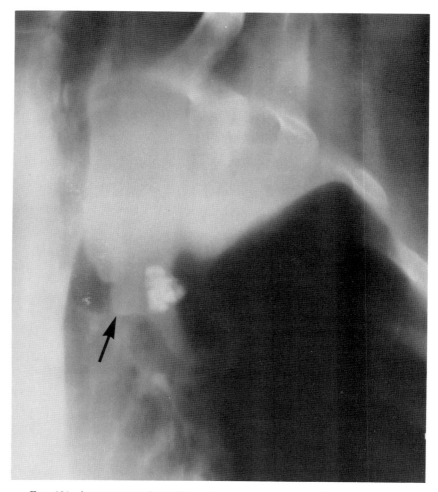

FIG. 191. ATELECTASIS, LEFT UPPER LOBE: CARCINOMA VS. BRONCHOLITHIASIS

The conventional films showed an atelectatic left upper lobe with a calcific density near its root. The tomogram, made in the frontal projection, shows the calcified node to be situated somewhat lateral to the origin of the left upper lobe bronchus. Mesial to this is a mass (arrow) occluding the left upper lobe bronchus and projecting into the main bronchus. This proved to be a squamous cell carcinoma.

should not be overestimated. Fibrotic, atelectatic lung tissue, even if associated with bronchiectasis, does not necessarily cause clinically significant disease. The indication for resection of such diseased lung tissue cannot be drawn from the roentgen findings. It will depend entirely upon the clinical course.

Bronchial Asthma. In an acute asthmatic attack, many bronchial branches are occluded by spasm and by mucoid secretion. The spasm is most severe in the smallest bronchi while the mucus obstructs those of medium size. During the severe paroxysms of asthma, both lungs become markedly hyperaerated (Fig. 192). The diaphragms are displaced downward and their upward movement during expiration is greatly limited. In some cases, the mucus plugs are fairly large and cast well defined, branching shadows, usually without evidence of atelectasis. These have been observed particularly in the allergic form of aspergillosis.

Bronchography may show obstruction of many of the medium-sized bronchi. These are sharply cut off and there is an absence of filling of their smaller branches. Here and there globules of secretion within the bronchi appear as radiolucent bubbles within the contrast-filled bronchi. Even after the acute attack, the fine bronchial branches may not fill well because of spasm.

Bronchial Obstruction by Mucus. MUCUS PLUGS. Mucoid secretion which is not cleared promptly, can obstruct a lobar bronchus or a main bronchus. This happens more often in children whose bronchi are small and easily oc-

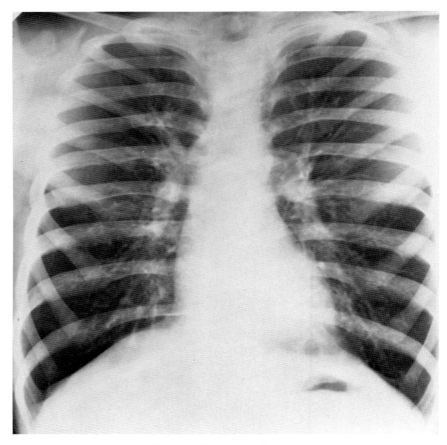

FIG. 192. BRONCHIAL ASTHMA

The film was made during an acute attack of bronchial asthma. There is hyperaeration of both lungs, particularly of the lower lobes. Both leaves of the diaphragm are markedly depressed and flattened. In addition, elevation of the anterior part of the chest has caused the ribs to run transversely. The intercostal spaces are widened. The branches of the pulmonary vessels are abnormally straight and spread apart.

cluded. In adults, it occurs particularly when the cough reflex has been abolished by narcotics, so frequently administered in large doses after operations (Fig. 78). Otherwise, the obstruction by mucus tends to occur in patents with pulmonary as well as bronchial infections, although the pneumonia is generally overshadowed by the effects of the obstruction.

In the postoperative state, the lower lobe bronchi are the ones most frequently obstructed. Occasionally, the stagnant secretion extends to the main bronchus, producing more striking symptoms. In children, obstruction of the middle and lower lobes is not an uncommon complication of measles, whooping cough or suppurative bronchopneumonia. The middle lobe bronchus is occasionally occluded during the course of bronchopneumonia in adults (Fig. 12).

Plugging of a lobar or main bronchus at first causes obstructive emphysema which can result in severe dyspnea and cyanosis. This stage is transitory and by the time the roentgen examination is made, atelectasis has usually supervened (Fig. 92). The underlying bronchopneumonia is usually obscured at this time and is not recognized until the lung reexpands after the secretion is expelled by the patient or removed by suction. Occasionally, the pulmonary field clears completely immediately after the obstruction is relieved. In these cases it must be assumed that the obstructive bronchitis existed without a concomitant pneumonia.

MUCOID IMPACTION OF THE BRONCHI. This condition differs from the type of mucus plugging described above in that segmental or subsegmental bronchi are involved rather than the major bronchi, and there is no association with pulmonary or bronchial infection. It occurs most commonly in asthmatic patients or in patients with allergic aspergillosis. It also has been reported in association with chronic bronchitis or mucoviscidosis. In about 15% of reported cases, no underlying disease has been identified.

Because the involved bronchi are situated beyond the hilar shadows, the mucus plugs themselves often can be seen. They cast round or oval, well-demarcated, homogeneous shadows when viewed on end. Otherwise, the shadows appear more elongated and serpentine. If they occur at a bronchial bifurcation, they are V shaped with the apex pointing towards the hilum (Fig. 193). Involvement of multiple adjacent bronchi produces an appearance that has been likened to a cluster of grapes.

In general, although the mucus plugs completely obstruct the bronchus, they do not cause atelectasis because of collateral ventilation between the segments. They are most common in the upper lobes but can occur anywhere in the lung. Involvement of a lower lobe as the sole site is distinctly uncommon. If the plug is expectorated, the shadow disappears but new ones can form elsewhere.

Amyloid Disease. Amyloid may be deposited within the walls of the bronchi as well as the trachea without involvement of the lungs. The amyloid accumulates beneath the intact mucosa and causes diffuse thickening of the wall with narrowing of the lumen. Generally, the amyloid is not evenly distributed and local accumulations can produce mound-like elevations that protrude into the lumen.

Involvement of the trachea and main bronchi can be recognized on ordinary films, particularly on oblique views, because of the increased thickness, density, and irregularity of their walls. The accumulation of amyloid imparts a rather characteristic wavy or scalloped contour to the lu-

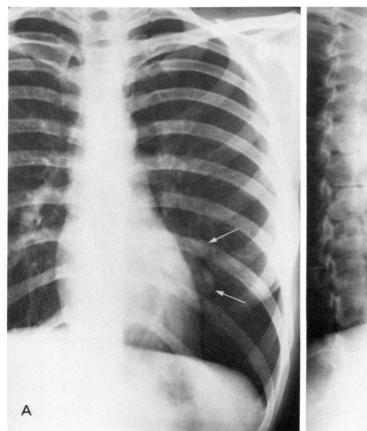
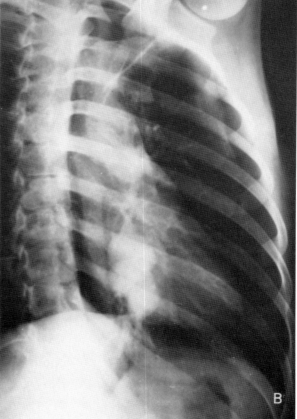

FIG. 193. MUCOID IMPACTION

A: The frontal film of a 26 year old female shows two elongated, oval shadows (arrows) converging toward the root of the left lower lobe. The shadows are sharply circumscribed and smooth and form two arms of a V. This appearance is characteristic of impaction of mucus in the bronchi. *B:* In the right oblique view the distended bronchi are superimposed on each other and form a serpentine shadow. The lung beyond the shadows is not collapsed. Bronchoscopy disclosed a carcinoid tumor of the left lower lobe bronchus. At operation, the bronchi beyond the carcinoid were distended by tenacious mucus.

men. Often the amyloid is heaped up at the carina, rounding off its normal sharp angle and narrowing the origin of both main bronchi.

The changes are more clearly visualized on tomograms or bronchograms. However, bronchography is deemed inadvisable because the viscid contrast material can cause asphyxia from obstruction of the bronchi, many of which are already narrowed by the disease. When the deposition of amyloid is sufficient to occlude a bronchus, the roentgen picture is dominated by the effects of the bronchial obstruction and its complications—obstructive emphysema, atelectasis and secondary infection. The changes produced by amyloidosis of the tracheobronchial tree cannot be distinguished roentgenologically from those associated with Wegener's granulomatosis.

In rare instances, amyloidosis occurs in the form of one or more localized nodules in the trachea or bronchi. The nodules are covered by smooth mucous membrane and project into the lumen in precisely the same manner as a bronchial carcinoid. In the trachea, the localized amyloid tumor is seen as a smooth, well-demarcated, round or semicircular density within the lumen. Similar localized tumors within the bronchi are generally overshadowed by the complications of bronchial obstruction.

Foreign Bodies. The diagnosis of a foreign body in a bronchus is usually quite simple when the aspirated substance is radiopaque. If the foreign body is radiolucent, it cannot be detected on films and only the effects of the bronchial obstruction may be visible (Fig. 43). This is particularly true of foreign bodies composed of organic material. The fact that the roentgen changes are due to aspiration of a foreign body can then be determined only from the history.

Most visible foreign bodies are metallic or contain metal. The metal casts an extremely dense shadow whose contour is so clearly outlined that the nature of the foreign body can usually be identified (Fig. 194). Aspirated teeth are also quite radiopaque and can usually be differentiated from other shadows in the lung. However, fragments of bone may cast a faint shadow and are easily overlooked. Whenever there is a suspicion of an aspirated bone, Bucky films and even tomograms may be necessary for its detection. Some fish bones, however, are so fine and contain so little calcium, that they cannot be visualized even by these methods.

It may be difficult to differentiate the shadow of a dense foreign body from that of calcified hilar lymph nodes on the frontal film alone. Oblique and lateral projections, exposed to demonstrate the bronchial air column, will generally show whether the density is within the bronchus or outside of it. In some cases, tomography is necessary for this purpose.

Foreign bodies are almost always located in the main or lower lobe bronchi. It is extremely rare for one to be lodged in the bronchus to the middle lobe or one of the upper lobes. A foreign

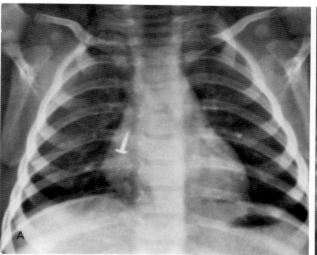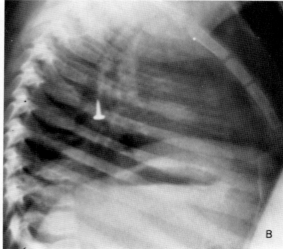

FIG. 194. BRONCHIAL FOREIGN BODY

A: The child aspirated a tack which is seen in the position of the right lower lobe bronchus. No other abnormality is evident on the frontal film. *B:* The lateral view shows evidence of atelectasis and possibly pneumonia of the posterior segment of the right lower lobe. The density of this portion of the lung is only slightly increased, but the striking finding is the obliteration of the posterior portion of the right diaphragmatic contour.

body in a main bronchus can cause complete obstruction with atelectasis of the lower lobe and incomplete obstruction with emphysema of the upper lobe.

Bronchial Rupture. Rupture of a bronchus results from a severe type of crushing injury involving the upper part of the chest. In children and in young adults it may occur without associated fractures of the ribs. However, over the age of 30, there is almost invariably a fracture of one or more of the first three ribs. In most cases there is evidence of pneumomediastinum or pneumothorax or both. One would rather expect to find either of these complications in every case, but in 10% no abnormality has been noted on the early films other than the rib fractures.

The rupture of the bronchus may be complete or incomplete. In either case, the connective tissue about the bronchus frequently remains intact. The ends of the severed bronchus may retract for a distance as great as 3 cm while the peribronchial tissues maintain continuity of the airway through the affected lung. This makes for great difficulty in the diagnosis of bronchial rupture in the early stages. Even though the peribronchial tissues are intact, air becomes insinuated between the bronchus and the surrounding sheath. This can be demonstrated as a fine linear lucency alongside the bronchus. It is best seen on tomograms or on films made with high kilovoltage technique. Dislocation of the severed ends of the bronchus may produce a bayonet-shaped deformity of the column of air.

Collapse of the lung can occur soon after the accident as the result of a large pneumothorax or from obstruction of the airway by blood or thick secretion. When the airway is preserved by the peribronchial tissues, obstructive emphysema can result from collapse of the connecting fibrous, tubular channel during expiration. The late stage of bronchial rupture is characterized by a bronchial stricture. Evidence of this appears within a month after the accident. A partial tear of the bronchial wall may result in stenosis of the bronchus, but complete rupture eventually causes total obstruction by fibrous scar at the site of the injury. In the latter instance, there is complete atelectasis of the portion of lung supplied by the ruptured bronchus.

The occurrence of atelectasis of a lobe or of an entire lung, 2, 3 or 4 weeks after a crushing injury to the chest, should suggest the possibility of rupture of a bronchus (Fig. 195). This should also be strongly suspected if there is a pneumothorax following an injury and the lung cannot be expanded despite adequate suction drainage. The diagnosis is much more difficult in the earlier stages because the airway can be well maintained despite the bronchial rupture. Therefore, whenever there is a fracture of one or more of the first three ribs, tomograms or films made with high voltage technique should be made in a search for a mantle of air about one of the main bronchi. All patients who have sustained a severe crushing injury to the chest should be reexamined a month after the injury, even though the original films were negative, to determine whether atelectasis has developed.

Bronchitis

Acute Bronchitis. Conventional films of the chest are of little value in the diagnosis of acute bronchitis. In the majority of cases the lungs appear normal while in the remainder there may be evidence of hyperinflation due to bronchial spasm. This is particularly common in children with laryngotracheobronchitis. Although in this disease the hyperinflation is due largely to laryngeal edema, congestion of the bronchial mucosa and bronchospasm are contributing factors. Densities in the lung fields associated with acute bronchitis almost always represent a complicating pneumonia.

Chronic Bronchitis. This disease is generally conceived of as a clinical rather than a pathologic entity. It has been defined as a chronic disorder characterized by excessive mucus secretion in the bronchi, manifested by chronic or recurrent productive cough for periods of at least 3 months in 2 or more consecutive years. The diagnosis cannot be made until other diseases which can produce similar clinical findings, such as neoplasm, bronchiectasis, or heart disease are excluded. The main pathologic change of chronic bronchitis is hypertrophy and hyperplasia of the bronchial mucous glands. Impairment of pulmonary function is due to increased air flow resistance because of bronchial spasm or stricturing of bronchioles. In addition, chronic bronchitis is often complicated by emphysema.

Radiologic abnormalities have been reported in 20 to 50 % of patients with a clinical diagnosis of chronic bronchitis. The roentgen findings include overinflation of the lungs, tubular shadows extending beyond the hila, an increase in the interstitial pulmonary markings with decrease in the peripheral pulmonary vasculature and characteristic changes on the bronchogram.

Hyperinflation of the lungs is related to bronchospasm which impedes the outflow of air during expiration. It is rarely striking in chronic bronchitis unless associated with emphysema.

The walls of second or third order bronchi and

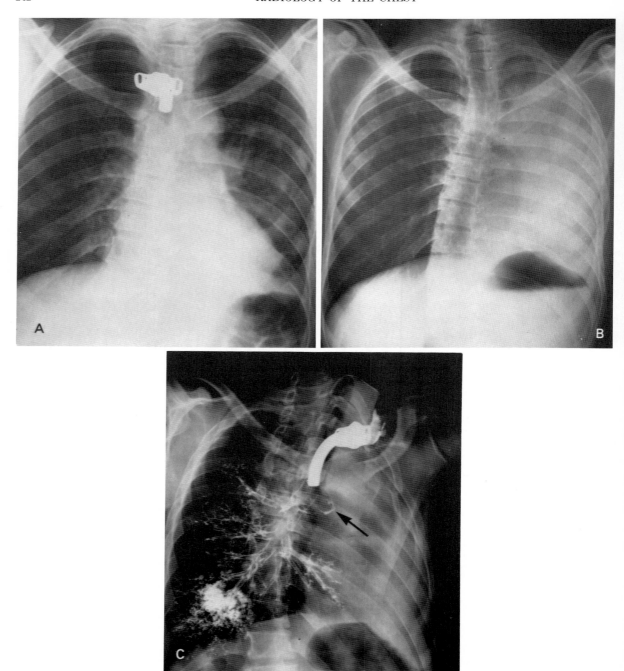

FIG. 195. BRONCHIAL RUPTURE

A: The patient sustained a crushing injury of the chest and a fractured leg in an automobile accident. The second, third and fourth ribs on the left side were fractured and there was a large pneumothorax and pneumomediastinum. This film made five days after the institution of drainage shows reexpansion of the left lung. *B:* Six weeks later, when the patient was ambulated, he exhibited considerable dyspnea. The film made at this time shows opacification of the left hemithorax with shift of the mediastinum into the left chest and herniation of the right lung across the midline, indicating complete atelectasis of the left lung. *C:* The bronchogram shows occlusion of the left main bronchus (arrow) which was responsible for the atelectasis of the left lung. The fractures of the upper ribs on the involved side are visualized. Operation disclosed complete rupture of the left main bronchus. The ends were anastomosed, the lung reexpanded, and normal pulmonic function was restored. (Case, courtesy of Dr. J. W. Comer, New York, N. Y., reported in JAMA 196:194, April 11, 1966).

their branches are relatively thin and cannot be identified on routine chest films when normal. However, as they become thickened in chronic bronchitis, they can be visualized in the lung fields in a moderate percentage of patients with this disease. The bronchial walls are then seen as two parallel or slightly converging linear shadows. Their appearance has been likened to that of railroad tracks. The visualized bronchi do not appear distended and are situated more centrally than the affected bronchi in bronchiectasis (Fig. 196).

Accentuation of the pulmonary markings producing a picture that has been described as "the dirty chest" is quite common in chronic bronchitis. In most cases this is caused by infiltration of the peribronchial tissues and interstitial fibrosis secondary to repeated bronchial infections. The vessels seem prominent and are often irregular as a result of distortion of the pulmonary architecture by small areas of partial atelectasis together with localized zones of hyperinflation. These result from varying degrees of obstruction of small bronchi. Diminished vascularity in the periphery of the lungs is indicative of complicating emphysema.

Bronchography often shows a sharp cutoff of bronchi of the fifth to the eighth order. This is usually due to obstructing mucus but can also be caused by bronchial spasm. The changes are not evenly distributed throughout the lung but tend to occur in scattered patchy areas. The contrast material often fills the widened neck of hypertrophied bronchial glands which appear like small diverticula communicating with the lumen of the larger bronchi (Fig. 197). Small, smoothly outlined, round or oval pools of opaque material are occasionally seen at the ends of small bronchi.

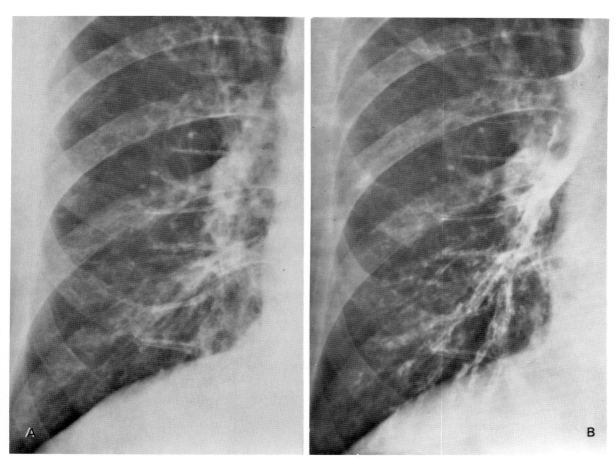

FIG. 196. CHRONIC BRONCHITIS

A: The diffuse accentuation of the pulmonary markings is due to the thickening of the bronchial walls and interstitial tissues rather than to widening of the blood vessels. This creates the appearance of "dirty lung." The thickening of the bronchial walls is best noted in the cardiophrenic region where they appear as pairs of parallel lines. *B:* Posttussive bronchogram. The bronchial walls are coated with radiopaque oil. This confirms the origin of railroad track shadows seen on the plain film.

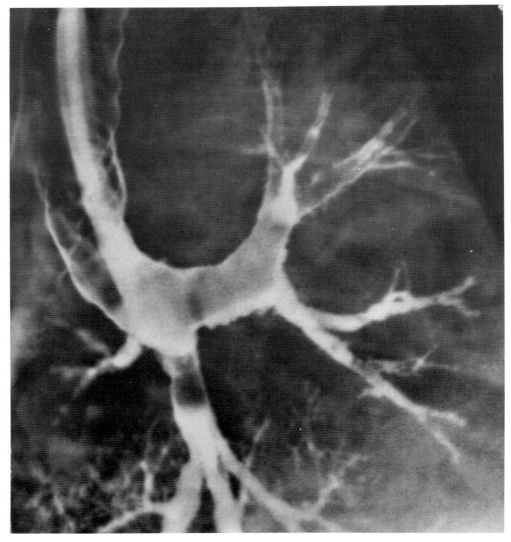

FIG. 197. CHRONIC BRONCHITIS

A bronchogram of the left lung shows multiple projections of the radiopaque material from the lower border of the left upper lobe bronchus. These represent widened mouths of hypertrophic bronchial glands. Similar changes are present in several of the segmental bronchi.

These have been shown to represent dilated bronchioles. Spider-like extensions from these pools are seen when there is filling of the tiny branches of the dilated bronchioles.

In some cases the medium-sized bronchi do not taper normally and may, in fact, show some degree of varicose dilatation (Fig. 198). This is caused by weakening of the bronchial wall by the chronic inflammatory disease and the repeated periods of increased intrabronchial pressure produced by spasms of coughing. The caliber of the lumen is often normal in the region of the cartilages which support the bronchi, but between the cartilages the weakened bronchial wall bulges

outward. Although the bronchi are dilated, this condition must be differentiated from the disease bronchiectasis. The changes of chronic bronchitis have a more widespread distribution throughout the lungs and the dilatation of the bronchi is not associated with pruning of their branches. True bronchiectasis is a more local or focal disease.

A rather striking bronchographic finding is caused by puddling of the radiopaque material in the areas where the bronchial wall bulges outward between the cartilages. This creates the appearance of a series of transverse stripes. Similar findings are seen in the trachea in tracheo-

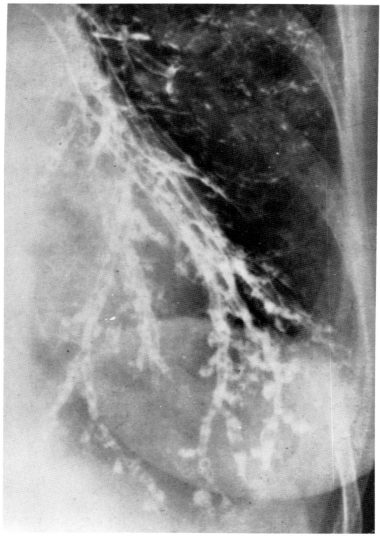

FIG. 198. VARICOSE BRONCHIECTASIS

The branches of the left lower lobe bronchus show irregular localized dilatations resembling varicosities. This pattern occurs in chronic bronchitis and emphysema and also in the severe bronchitis which accompanies suppurative bronchopneumonia. It should not be confused with the *disease* bronchiectasis. The radiolucent defects within the opacified bronchi are caused by bubbles of air and secretion.

megaly. In some cases, local outpouching of the bronchial musculature is more marked and true diverticula are formed.

Membranous Bronchitis. Bronchi can be obstructed by the exfoliated diphtheritic membrane which forms in diseases associated with extensive necrosis of the bronchial mucosa. This occurs in diphtheria, influenza and following the inhalation or aspiration of caustic agents. The roentgen appearance is overshadowed by the pneumonia that is almost always present in these conditions. The atelectatic nature of the pneumonia is due to the plugging of the bronchi.

Fibrinous Bronchitis. This is a rare allergic condition involving the bronchi in which there is outpouring of an exudate containing large amounts of fibrin. This forms fibrinous casts which obstruct the bronchial lumen. The casts may be quite large, and in children may occlude a main or lobar bronchus. In adults, segmental or subsegmental bronchi are usually obstructed although, on occasion, a lobar bronchus is occluded. The roentgen appearance is characterized by the sudden development of atelectasis of a segment, a lobe or an entire lung. When only a segment is collapsed, the fibrin casts may be presumed to extend into the main bronchus of the lobe, for otherwise, collateral respiration would keep the lung aerated despite the bronchial obstruction.

Numerous eosinophils are intermingled with the fibrin in the bronchial plug. This is associated with a high eosinophil count in the peripheral blood. The diagnosis of fibrinous bronchitis is justified when atelectasis appears suddenly in a patient who has a high peripheral eosinophilia.

BRONCHIOLITIS. Bronchiolitis is practically always associated with interstitial pneumonia or consolidation of pulmonary acini. The latter changes may not be recognizable roentgenologically. The picture then is only one of emphysema or acute bronchial asthma. When the infiltrations are visible the bronchiolitis is manifested by the presence of irregular, streak-like markings and of minute nodules in the lungs (see Fig. 337). Characteristically, the nodular lesions are seen following bronchial dissemination of tuberculosis. Since these nodules represent consolidation of acini, they have been termed *acinar-nodose* lesions by Aschoff. However, similar lesions occur in bronchiolitis from other causes, e.g., viral infections, acute infections in the course of bronchial asthma, and in fungus and dust diseases.

A special form of bronchiolitis is that called *bronchiolitis obliterans*. The essential lesion consists of an obliteration of small bronchi by endobronchial protuberances of granulation and fibrous tissue. The condition occurs particularly after the inhalation of irritating gases, but similar bronchial lesions are found in nonspecific infections. The roentgen films may show numerous tiny nodular shadows throughout the lungs, similar to those which occur in other types of bronchiolitis. In the chronic stage, the roentgen picture is often dominated by fine interstitial fibrosis and emphysema.

Bronchiectasis

Definition of Terms. The word bronchiectasis signifies nothing more than dilatation of the bronchi. It occurs in a variety of conditions. Often the bronchial widening is unimportant and the term is used simply for purposes of description. Thus, widening of the bronchi is commonly noted at necropsy in association with pneumonia but it is in itself of no significance. Some widening of the bronchi is extremely common in chronic bronchitis. Here again, the bronchial dilatation is generally of little or no importance in relation either to the symptoms or the course of the disease. On the other hand, the *disease bronchiectasis* is a separate and distinct entity in which

the widened bronchi are responsible for important clinical manifestations. Bronchial function is impaired, secretions tend to stagnate in their lumen and many of the bronchial branches are destroyed, interfering with transmission of air into the lungs.

Bronchiectases can be divided into three morphologic types: cylindrical, saccular and varicose. *Cylindrical* bronchiectasis refers to a generalized, more or less regular widening of the larger bronchi. In *saccular* bronchiectasis, the bronchi terminate in sac-like cavities. These are usually associated with cylindrical widening of the entering bronchi (see Fig. 274). When the saccules are large and thin-walled, the term *cystic* bronchiectasis is often used. In these cases the bronchi communicating with the cysts frequently show little widening. *Varicose* bronchiectasis refers to irregular dilatation of the bronchial wall between intact cartilages (Fig. 198). This is characteristic of suppurative or chronic bronchitis rather than the disease bronchiectasis. However, there are cases in which there is destruction of the bronchial wall in scattered areas with herniation between the cartilages of the larger bronchi, producing sacculations measuring up to a centimeter in diameter. These may be responsible for symptoms in addition to those referable to the chronic bronchitis itself.

From a clinical standpoint, bronchiectasis may be divided into reversible, suppurative and dry forms. *Reversible* bronchiectasis occurs during the course of bronchopneumonia, as a result of relaxation of the bronchial walls rather than a destructive process (Fig. 199). As the name implies, the bronchi revert to their normal caliber after the acute disease resolves. Most cases of the disease bronchiectasis are associated with chronic or recurrent bronchial infections associated with purulent sputum and are clinically considered as *suppurative* bronchiectasis. *Dry* bronchiectasis refers to the end stage of bronchopulmonary disease in which the active infection has completely subsided, leaving in its wake dilated bronchi which produce little or no secretion.

Pathology. Bronchiectasis may be congenital or acquired. The former is extremely rare. In most instances it is impossible to differentiate it from the acquired form except in the newborn. Most cases which are thought, clinically, to be congenital are probably acquired, resulting from an acute infection during infancy.

Acquired bronchiectasis comes about as a result of the interplay of several factors. Most important of these is weakening of the bronchial wall from destruction of muscle and elastic tissue

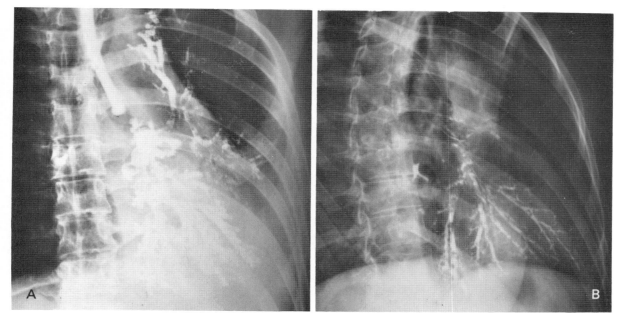

FIG. 199. REVERSIBLE BRONCHIECTASIS

A: The right oblique view of the bronchogram made during the course of an atelectatic suppurative bronchopneumonia, shows irregular, cylindric dilatation and some sacculation involving all of the branches of the left lower lobe. The lingular segment of the left upper lobe is also affected. *B:* The bronchogram made several weeks later, after resorption of the pulmonary infiltrations, shows the bronchi to have returned to their normal caliber.

fibers in the course of the severe bronchial infection that accompanies suppurative bronchopneumonia (see Fig. 238). Additional factors are an increase in the intrabronchial pressure resulting from cough or partial bronchial obstruction which tends to distend the bronchi, and a diminution in the extrabronchial pressure which exerts an outward pull on the bronchial wall. The diminished extrabronchial pressure is caused by atelectasis of the surrounding lung, and this in turn is due to obstruction or destruction of many small bronchial branches during the course of the suppurative bronchopneumonia. The bronchial branches that are destroyed are replaced by fibrous tissue, resulting in permanent atelectasis. Others are temporarily occluded by swelling of their walls and by exudate within their lumina, and reopen as the pneumonia resolves, permitting the lung to reexpand. However, pulmonary fibrosis frequently occurs during the atelectatic phase and the fibrous tissue prevents reexpansion of the lung even after patency of the bronchi is reestablished.

Destruction of pulmonary parenchyma and terminal bronchi by suppurative disease of the lung results in the formation of numerous small cavities. These communicate with the weakened bronchi which have become widened. As the acute infection is controlled, the bronchial epi-

thelium proliferates distally and lines the cavities, producing the final picture of sacculated bronchiectasis. Larger sacculations which have the appearance of air cysts and which simulate congenital bronchiectasis, probably result from persistent pneumatoceles whose bronchial openings have never closed off. The cyst-like cavities differ from sacculated bronchiectases in that they do not correspond in size to the area of lung that was destroyed. Rather, they are the result of ballooning of small areas of destroyed parenchyma and communicate with bronchi that show little widening.

There is a tendency for the bronchiectatic lung to remain chronically inflamed because of retention of infected secretions. This is due to diminution of ciliary action resulting from destructive changes in the epithelium and to impairment of bronchial motility. This is especially true when the lingula or the lower lobes are involved, because drainage from these portions of the lung is poor. An inflammatory process in the upper lobes, with the exception of the lingula, can subside completely despite the presence of extensive bronchiectasis, because bronchial drainage from these portions of the lung is favored by gravity. The term, *dry bronchiectasis,* is usually applied to such cases in which active infection is absent (Fig. 200). The mucosa lining the bronchiectases

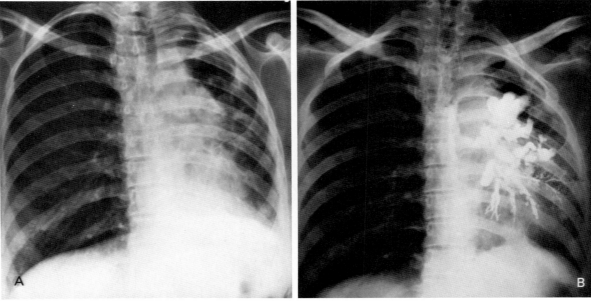

FIG. 200. DRY BRONCHIECTASIS: HEMOPTOIC FORM

A: The left chest is markedly shrunken and the heart and mediastinum are displaced into the left hemithorax. There are many small, round, thin-walled cavities throughout the left lung. The appearance is characteristic of cystic bronchiectasis. *B:* The bronchogram shows large sacculated cavities which communicate with the main bronchus through dilated bronchi. Most of the cavities are in the upper lobe. The patient was 31 years old and developed the disease when she was 4 years of age. However, there was no cough for many years before this examination and bronchoscopy disclosed no secretion. Severe hemoptysis was the only symptom.

is generally atrophic and associated with marked dilatation of the bronchial vessels. Rupture of these vessels is not uncommon because of lack of support by the atrophic mucosa and results in expectoration of bright red blood without admixture of sputum.

Roentgen Features. The roentgen appearance of the lungs in bronchiectasis is usually dominated by the presence of dense pulmonary infiltrations and fibrosis, often with changes due to atelectasis. Most commonly the lower lobes are affected and frequently the disease is unilateral. The superior segment of the lower lobe is often spared. Not infrequently there is involvement of the lingula when the left lower lobe is diseased. Similarly, the middle lobe is frequently involved together with the right lower lobe.

The degree of atelectasis associated with bronchiectasis varies considerably. A dense trianglular shadow, representing a collapsed and infiltrated bronchiectatic lower lobe or its basal segments, may be manifest when the atelectasis is fairly complete. The triangular shadow is situated adjacent to the spine with its base extending for a variable distance along the mesial portion of the diaphragm. On the right side it obliterates the cardiophrenic angle (Fig. 90). On the left side it is often hidden by the heart unless sufficient

exposure is used to penetrate this organ (Fig. 201).

When there is less infiltration and fibrosis, the shadows are less dense and condensation of the vascular markings is more clearly evident. In addition, the dilated bronchi may be visible with ordinary exposures. If the dilated bronchi are free of secretions, they appear on the film as dark strips of radiolucency converging in the direction of the lung root. If the bronchi are filled, they may be depicted as elongated, gray shadows arranged in the manner of finger-like projections extending from the root of the lung into the lower lobe. Occasionally small fluid levels are seen within these shadows. The rather broad, stripe-like densities, representing secretion in the dilated bronchi, disappear after effective postural drainage (Fig. 202). In their place radiolucent, empty, dilated bronchi may now be visible. Such changes are seen in *cylindrical* bronchiectasis with or without terminal sacculations.

Saccular bronchiectases, when visible on the ordinary film, are represented by more or less irregular areas of radiolucency within the shadow of the inflamed lung (Figs. 203 and 241). If large, they may show fluid levels. When the inflammation in the lung is mild, the sacculations have the appearance of multiple, thin-walled cavities

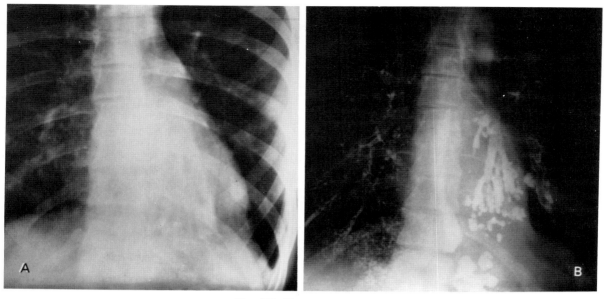

FIG. 201. BRONCHIECTASIS

A: A triangular density containing air-filled dilated bronchi is seen through the cardiac silhouette. The heart is displaced to the left and partially rotated into the right oblique position. This was due to a suppurative bronchopneumonia which resulted in bronchiectasis. *B:* Bronchography. The triangular shadow behind the heart is more clearly outlined on a Bucky film. The bronchi which are filled with contrast material are cylindrically dilated and have club-shaped extremities. The bronchi are crowded together as a result of the atelectasis. There is also marked widening of the branches of the lingular division of the left upper lobe. The right lower lobe bronchi are of normal calibre.

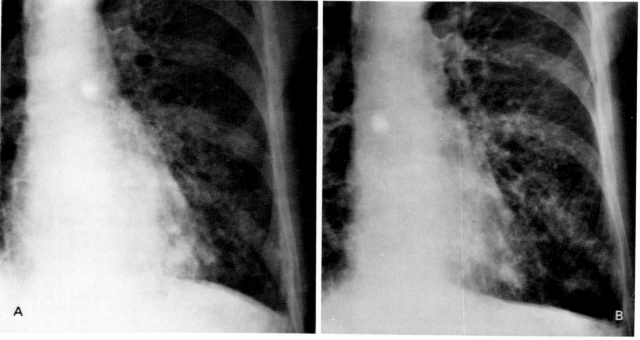

FIG. 202. CYLINDRICAL BRONCHIECTASIS

A: The finger-like shadows extending downward from the left lung root behind the heart represent dilated bronchi filled with secretion. The generalized infiltrations are due largely to interstitial fibrosis resulting from chronic inflammatory disease. *B:* Reexamination after postural drainage shows that most of the tubular shadows have cleared. The small density at the cardiac apex represents a collection of retained secretion. The oval, white area over the spine is identical on both films. It represents a "kissing" artifact.

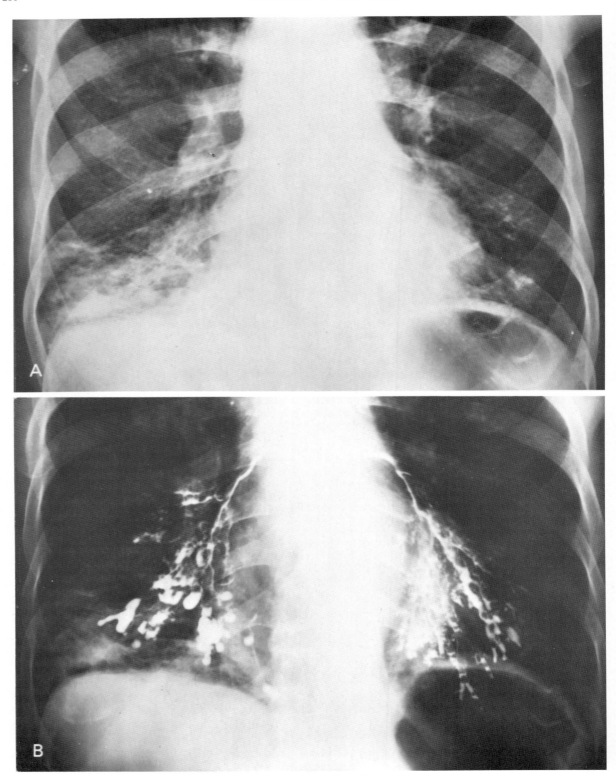

FIG. 203. BRONCHIECTASIS OF BOTH LOWER LOBES

A: There is dense infiltration of the right lower lobe. Within the infiltrated area are a number of small, irregular lucencies which represent air in dilated bronchi. The density seen through the cardiac shadow represents a partially collapsed infiltrated left lower lobe. *B:* The bronchogram shows cylindric dilatation of the branches of the left lower lobe. These are drawn together because of the associated atelectasis. The basal divisions of the right lower lobe bronchus show sacculated dilatations. The bronchi have club-shaped extremities and the small bronchial branches are absent. Presumably they have been destroyed in the suppurative bronchopneumonia that initiated the bronchiectasis.

(Fig. 204). If they are small, they produce a picture not unlike that of a honeycomb. When the thin-walled cavities are large, they simulate multiple air cysts. These differ from multiple bullae in that they have a tendency to be round and the classical angular shape of bullae is lacking (Fig. 205).

When there is little active infection or when the bronchiectases are dry, the conventional film may be entirely negative. In some cases there is simply some distortion of the pulmonary markings. The blood vessels in one area of the lung may be drawn together or show an irregular course. The possibility of dry bronchiectasis should be considered when such milder changes are found in patients with a history of hemoptysis. Immediately after an hemoptysis the x-ray film may show one or more nodular shadows representing saccular bronchiectases filled with blood. The ring-like shadows representing the bronchiectases may be evident on previous films or on ones made a few days after the hemoptysis.

Bronchography. Bronchography is required for the definitive diagnosis of bronchiectasis and for precise delineation of the type and extent of the disease. It is advisable to perform bronchography when there is a chronic productive cough the cause of which is not clear despite complete investigation, particularly when there is a persistent infiltration in the lung (Fig. 11). It is also required in cases in which the diagnosis of bronchiectasis is obvious, in order to determine the distribution of the disease as a guide to possible surgical management. In this connection it is advisable to map out the entire bronchial tree in order to avoid overlooking important bronchiectases in portions of the lung which otherwise appear normal. Bronchography is also indicated

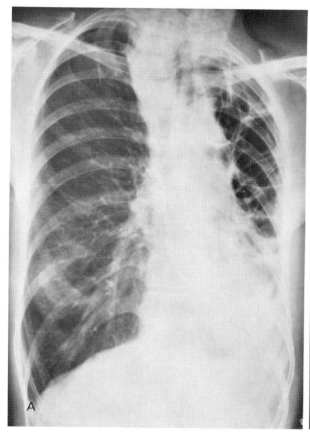
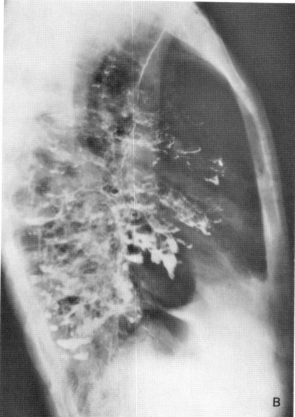

FIG. 204. CYSTIC BRONCHIECTASIS

A: This is an acquired lesion, often confused with congenital cystic disease of the lung. The left lung is small and is replaced by numerous large, thin-walled, cyst-like cavities. The dome of the left chest is flattened, the left side of the thorax is narrowed, and the heart is displaced far to the left, exposing the vertebral bodies. The lower part of the left lung is obscured by dense fibrosis and infiltration. There is a scoliosis of the upper dorsal spine, convex to the right, causing a density which may be confused with a mediastinal tumor. *B:* A bronchogram in the lateral view shows cylindric and sacculated dilatations of almost all the bronchi of the left lung. The lower lobe branches show fluid levels within the large bronchiectatic cavities.

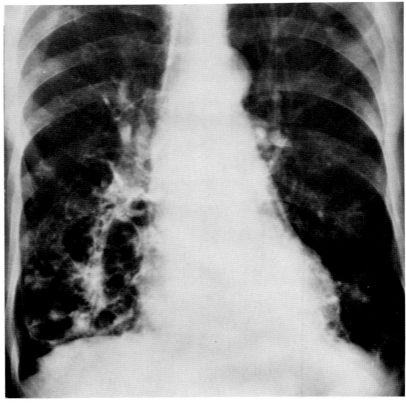

FIG. 205. BILATERAL BRONCHIECTASIS

The numerous honeycomb shadows throughout the right lower lobe together with the larger thin-walled cavities impart a cystic appearance to the lobe. These cavities are due to cystic dilatations of the terminal bronchi. The triangular shadow seen through the cardiac silhouette represents an atelectatic, bronchiectatic left lower lobe.

in hemoptysis of obscure origin even when the conventional films are entirely negative. In such a case, bronchography may disclose an underlying obstructive lesion which is beyond the reach of the bronchoscope.

Normally the bronchi have relatively smooth walls and branch in an orderly fashion, tapering gradually as they extend to the periphery. In bronchiectasis, widening is noted in branch bronchi, frequently beginning in those of the third order and increasing in the smaller branches. Many of the smaller bronchi are obliterated and the remaining widened bronchial branches are drawn together and distorted (Fig. 90). In some cases of cylindrical bronchiectasis, the larger bronchi are uniformly dilated while the peripheral branches show little change from their normal caliber and distribution. Most frequently, however, the branches are widened and end abruptly, producing a club-shaped contour.

In saccular bronchiectasis, the contrast material accumulates in puddles at the ends of the bronchi. These puddles usually are in the form of clusters and are best seen in recumbent films. On films made in the upright position the contrast material layers at the base of the sacculations which are then incompletely outlined. In this form of bronchiectasis there is considerable destruction of bronchial branches so that there is little normal lung between the saccules. Well-marked cylindrical widening is usually observed in the bronchi that lead to the sacculations. In cystic bronchiectasis, the bronchi entering the air cysts may be of normal caliber so that only a small quantity of the rather viscous contrast material can enter the cavity. The small collections of radiopaque material at the base of the cavities then show only short air-fluid levels.

In dry bronchiectasis the dilated bronchi are particularly well outlined because of the absence of secretion. There is an especially sharp, smooth definition of the contrast material because of the atrophy of the bronchial mucous membrane (Fig. 200). Bronchograms in dry bronchiectasis may show either sacculations or cylindrical bronchiectases with club-shaped terminations.

Usually it is possible to differentiate between the widening of the bronchi that occurs in association with chronic bronchitis from that of true bronchiectasis. In the former there may be slight cylindrical dilatation of the bronchi with diminished tapering of the branches. The changes are diffusely distributed throughout the bronchial tree and there is no obliteration of bronchial branches and therefore no atelectasis. Furthermore, the bronchi are seen to contract well during expiration. Bronchial cartilages are not destroyed so that the larger bronchial branches show outpouching of the wall between the cartilages rather than regular, diffuse cylindrical dilatation.

Most important from the standpoint of surgical treatment of bronchiectasis is the determination of the distribution of the disease. Ideally, all of the bronchi in both lungs should be outlined for this purpose. This may be done in either one or two sittings. In this connection, it should be borne in mind that complete outlining of the bronchi with the contrast material is not always attained because of the presence of retained secretions. It is therefore advisable to perform postural drainage before the examination is begun.

In bronchiectasis of the lower lobe it is necessary to obtain a good view of the superior segmental branches for, if these are free of disease, the resection may be confined to the basal segments. In bronchiectasis of the left lower lobe it is necessary to examine the lingular branches of the left upper lobe with particular care. Because of the contraction of the left lower lobe which is so common in this disease, the lingular branches are often displaced downward so that they are easily mistaken for branches of the lower lobes (Fig. 201). Overlooking these bronchiectases may result in serious consequences in the postoperative period if the diseased lingular segment is not resected together with the lower lobe. This error may be avoided by studying the branches of the lingular division in the right oblique and lateral views.

Special efforts should be made to prevent alveolar filling during bronchography because retained contrast material tends to cause an inflammatory reaction which may interfere with expansion of the remaining lung after lobectomy. In general, it is advisable to delay the operation for several weeks if there has been a significant degree of alveolar filling in an area of lung which is not to be resected.

To avoid alveolar filling, the following precautions should be taken:

1. Sufficient sedation and anesthesia should be given to minimize cough during the procedure, for the sudden inspiration that follows a coughing spell tends to draw the contrast material into the alveoli.

2. The minimum amount of material necessary to outline the bronchi should be used.

3. The examination should be concluded as quickly as possible and postural drainage should be carried out immediately after termination of the procedure to help the patient eliminate the contrast substance.

Complications of Bronchiectasis. As a result of the suppurative bronchopneumonia, which is the cause of most cases of bronchiectasis, and persistence or recurrence of infection with involvement of the lymphatics, there is usually an associated chronic pleuritis. This may be evidenced simply by obliteration of the costophrenic or cardiophrenic angles, but frequently there is, in addition, thickening of the pleura above these regions. The pleural thickening may be visible only as a band along the chest wall in the oblique or lateral views, but occasionally the pleura becomes so thick that it produces a generalized haze over the diseased portion of lung on the frontal projection.

The course of suppurative bronchiectasis is usually punctuated by acute pulmonary infections. Most frequently these involve the lung in the region of the bronchiectases. Spread often occurs through neighboring bronchi to adjacent pulmonary segments. Sometimes the infection extends to more distant portions of the lung. In the case of bronchiectasis of the left lower lobe, infection may spread to the lingular segment of the left upper lobe; and in bronchiectasis of the right lower lobe, the middle lobe frequently becomes secondarily involved. More rarely the disease extends to the opposite lung.

The complicating infection takes the form of a suppurative bronchopneumonia. Although this may resolve fairly promptly, there is a tendency for the development of bronchiectasis in the newly involved portion of the lung. In other cases there eventually occurs a diffuse chronic bronchitis throughout the lungs with accompanying interstitial fibrosis and emphysema. All of these changes are manifestations of the progressive nature of the disease.

Special Types of Bronchiectasis. CONGENITAL. This is extremely rare. Most cases thought to be congenital in origin are really acquired, resulting from suppurative bronchopneumonia early in life. True congenital bronchiectasis is of the sacculated variety with little or no functional pulmonary tissue in the involved area. The bronchiectatic lung often appears cystic as in congenital cystic adenomatoid malformation of the lung.

Widening of the smaller bronchi and bronchioles also occurs in absent or incomplete development of a main pulmonary artery. This produces the picture of unilateral hyperlucent lung, indistinguishable on plain films from the atrophic lung resulting from a bronchopulmonary infection during early childhood. Bronchography discloses bulbous dilatation of the ends of the small bronchi without alveolar filling. The differentiation from the acquired type of the disease can be made only by *selective* pulmonary arteriography.

Kartagener described a syndrome consisting of bronchiectasis in association with situs inversus, incomplete development of the frontal sinus, and sinusitis (Fig. 206). The relationship of the bronchiectasis to the associated anomalies is not clear. However, the relation between the sinusitis and the bronchial infection is probably no different in Kartagener's syndrome than in other forms of bronchiectasis.

TUBERCULOSIS. Some degree of bronchiectasis is regularly seen about tuberculous cavities. As in the case of suppurative bronchopneumonia caused by pyogenic organisms, destruction of bronchial walls and pulmonary parenchyma occurs regularly in the caseous bronchopneumonia caused by tubercle bacilli. This may result in bronchiectasis with or without persistence of the tuberculous infection.

The process practically always occurs in an upper lobe. Because of the extensive destruction of bronchial branches, the lobe becomes markedly shrunken and fibrotic. If the tuberculous process is controlled and nonspecific infection does not supervene, the bronchiectasis is dry and, despite the presence of atelectasis, the shadow of the contracted lobe is not very dense. If, on the other hand, secondary pyogenic infection occurs and persists, the affected upper lobe becomes quite opaque. In general, it may be concluded that atelectatic bronchiectasis confined to an upper lobe, in the absence of bronchial obstruction, is tuberculous in origin. The bronchiectases may appear as ring-like cavities or as irregular or longitudinal areas of lucency within the shrunken upper lobe (see Fig. 296).

A similar situation occurs in the case of chronic lung abscess. Severe destructive disease in the adjacent lung tissue results in bronchiectases about the cavity. Where there has been spillover infection causing extensive gangrenous bronchopneumonia, the resulting bronchiectases may be widespread. As the infection resolves and the cavity diminishes in size, the end stage of chronic putrid lung abscess may not be distinguishable

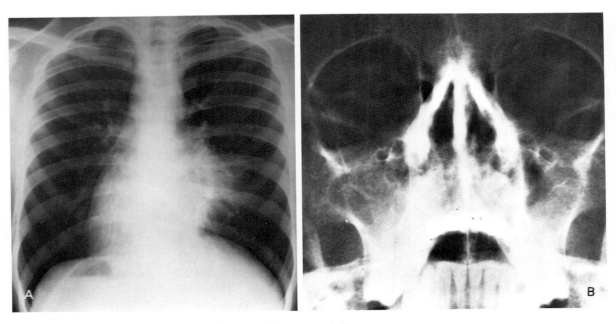

FIG. 206. KARTAGENER'S SYNDROME

A: The aortic knob, the cardiac apex and the gastric air bubble are all on the right side indicating situs inversus. The left border of the heart is obliterated by an infiltration of the adjacent middle lobe. The patient had been expectorating purulent sputum for several years suggesting underlying bronchiectasis. *B:* A Water's view of the skull shows opacification of the maxillary antra. The triad of situs inversus, bronchiectasis and sinusitis comprises Kartagener's syndrome.

from that of ordinary suppurative bronchiectasis unless films are available to depict the original lesion.

SECONDARY TO OBSTRUCTION. Bronchiectasis often occurs distal to bronchial obstruction. It results either from weakening of the bronchial wall secondary to complicating infection, from distention of the bronchi by accumulating bronchial secretions or from a combination of the two.

Bronchiectasis localized to the middle lobe or to the lingular or anterior segmental bronchi, is most frequently due to a bronchial stricture resulting from disease of adjacent lymph nodes. If the bronchi are completely obstructed, either as a result of the stricture itself or impaction of thick secretion in the strictured area, there is only a homogeneous shadow representing the atelectatic portion of the lung together with the bronchi filled with secretion. In rare instances, when there is no pulmonary infection, the filled widened bronchi themselves are visible within the atelectatic lung which casts only a faint shadow. Under these circumstances, cylindrically dilated bronchi may appear like wide blood vessels (Fig. 386). A lobulated, racemose or cloverleaf density may represent a cluster of sacculated bronchiectases distal to obstruction of a small bronchus, filled with either secretion or blood.

Bronchial Fistulas

Fistulous tracts may form a communication between a bronchus and the esophagus, the pleural space, the peritoneal cavity or one of the abdominal organs. They may also extend from a bronchus to the surface of the skin.

Bronchoesophageal Fistula. The causes of bronchoesophageal communications are generally the same as those of tracheoesophageal fistulas. However, congenital bronchoesophageal fistulas are rare and carcinomatous fistulas of the esophagus tend to involve a bronchus rather than the trachea. Such a fistula can also be caused by perforation of a carcinoma of a bronchus into the esophagus but this is distinctly less common than the reverse. In any instance, the manifestations are the same as those of a tracheoesophageal fistula with the exception that complicating pulmonary infection is usually confined to one side. Similarly, ingested contrast material outlines the bronchial tree primarily on the side of the lesion. As a result of coughing, however, the contrast material may enter the bronchi on the opposite side. The picture then mimics that of a tracheoesophageal fistula (Fig. 207).

Fluoroscopy or ciné filming during the barium swallow is then required to identify the location of the fistula.

Bronchopleural Fistula. Bronchopleural fistulas result from a disruptive lesion involving the lung as well as the bronchi and pleura. The fistulas may result from destructive bronchopulmonary disease extending through the pleura or from rupture of a bulla or air cyst in the lung even though the bronchial communciation is extremely small. The fistulas may also form as a complication of partial or complete resection of the lung. Rarely they are traumatic in origin.

In the absence of infection, the fistulous communication tends to close spontaneously unless the bronchial opening is large. Thus, the fistulas that result from ruptured bullae, local resection of lung, and many of those caused by trauma usually heal within a relatively short time. When the fistula is infectious in origin or when there is complicating pleural infection it will not close spontaneously. However, even in the presence of infectious disease in the lung, the bronchopleural fistula is not necessarily due to perforation of an infective focus. It may result simply from rupture of a bulla or pneumatocele associated with the underlying disease. Such noninfected bullae are common in chronic tuberculosis. These, as well as pneumatoceles occurring during the course of staphylococcal pneumonia, can rupture into the pleura without causing an empyema.

The characteristic roentgen manifestation of a bronchopleural fistula is the presence of air in the pleural cavity. The pneumothorax may be extremely small or it may be large enough to cause complete collapse of the lung and displacement of the mediastinum to the opposite side. The size of the pneumothorax is not necessarily related to the diameter of the fistula. The largest pneumothoraces are more commonly associated with small fistulas which act as a trap valve, permitting air to flow only in the direction of the pleural space.

Fluid is present whenever the fistula is caused directly by infection of the lung. However, fluid also occurs in association with traumatic fistulas and may be present in small amounts following rupture of a bulla or a pneumatocele. A large collection of fluid in the case of a ruptured bulla is usually due to hemorrhage into the pleural cavity.

The fluid and air in the pleural cavity may be free or loculated (Fig. 208). In the case of a small loculation the air which indicates the presence of a fistula may not be visible on conventional films because of marked thickening of the pleura. Overexposed upright Bucky films or tomograms

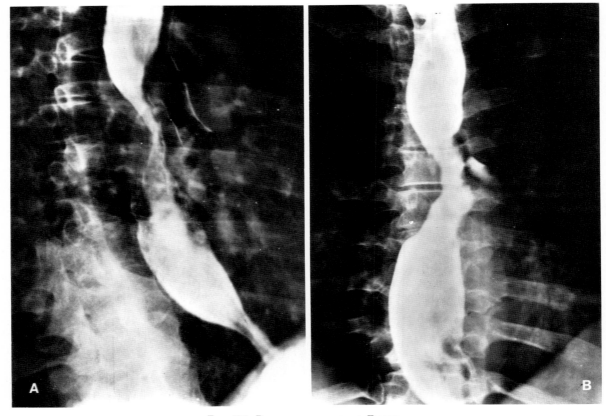

FIG. 207. BRONCHOESOPHAGEAL FISTULA

A: A film of a barium study of the esophagus shows a large, irregular carcinoma of the esophagus encroaching on the lumen. The trachea and left main bronchus are outlined by barium. On this film, it is impossible to determine whether the barium entered the airway by aspiration from the pharynx or through a tracheal or bronchial fistula. *B:* A spot film made at the beginning of the examination shows a small fistulous connection between the involved portion of the esophagus and the left main bronchus. The barium reached the trachea when the patient coughed.

will usually disclose even very small amounts of air.

The presence of air in the pleural cavity, not introduced from the outside or from a rupture of the esophagus, is pathognomonic of a bronchopleural fistula. It is not necessary to demonstrate the fistulous tract to make the diagnosis. In most instances, the bronchial openings are too small to allow the viscid contrast material used in bronchography to pass into the fistula. However, fistulous tracts connected with the stump of a large bronchus following lobectomy or pneumonectomy are usually well outlined on bronchograms.

Bronchocutaneous Fistulas. A communication between a bronchus and the surface of the body may occur with or without an intervening empyema. Bronchocutaneous fistulas most frequently follow surgical drainage of a pyopneumothorax or of a suppurative focus in the lung that communicates with the bronchus. Infected,

penetrating chest wounds may also result in such a fistula.

Rarely, suppurative infections of the lung extend spontaneously through the chest wall (*empyema necessitatis*). This also occurs with certain fungous infections of the lung, notably actinomycosis and nocardiosis. Characteristically, these diseases produce an extensive productive pleuritis which obliterates the pleural cavity over the lesion. The infection usually extends through the area of pleurodesis and forms one or more fistulous tracts through the chest wall without producing an empyema. In rare instances, a putrid lung abscess, which is always connected with a bronchus, behaves in a smiliar manner.

On occasion, an abscess of the chest wall burrows into the lung through adherent pleura and empties part of its contents into a bronchus. When the abscess opens onto the surface of the chest wall, either surgically or spontaneously, a bronchocutaneous fistula results. Such abscesses

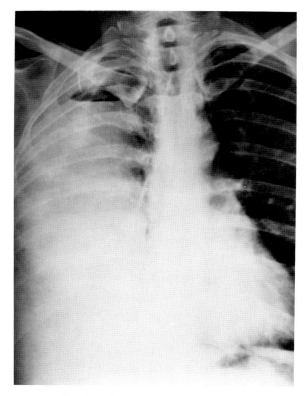

FIG. 208. BRONCHOPLEURAL FISTULA

Eighteen years previously the patient received pneumothorax treatment for cavitary tuberculosis. This was complicated by a pleural effusion which has persisted to the present time. Shortly before this film was made he began to cough up purulent material. The shadow in the right hemithorax which had been homogeneous throughout all the years now shows an air-fluid level. Operation disclosed a chronic tuberculous empyema which had not been recognized until it ruptured into the lung and established communication with a bronchus.

practically always originate in an osteomyelitis of a rib or costochondral junction and are frequently tuberculous. In rare instances a mediastinal abscess can drain externally as well as into a bronchus.

Radiologically, the picture is dominated by a dense shadow caused by the diseased pleura. Disease of the underlying lung may be apparent, and one or more air-fluid levels may be seen in the lung or pleural cavity. Frequently the ribs are drawn together as a result of peripleuritis. Swelling of the chest wall may be evident together with obliteration of the soft tissue planes. Thickening and increased density of the ribs occurs frequently as the result of periosteal reaction. Destructive or productive changes within the ribs indicate the presence of an osteomyelitis which may be the cause of the bronchocutaneous fistula.

The possibility of a fistula should be considered whenever a sinus tract in the chest wall fails to heal within a reasonable period. The diagnosis is made by the injection of radiopaque material into the sinus. A portion of the bronchial tree will almost always be outlined if a bronchocutaneous fistula is present. The study must be performed carefully, preferably with fluoroscopic control, as the sinus tract may be extremely tortuous and have a number of side branches which end blindly. The opening in the skin may be some distance from the bronchial communication. This occurs particularly when the cause is a mediastinal abscess, which can burrow as far as the lumbar region before it breaks through the skin.

Other Bronchial Fistulas. Fistulous tracts connecting a bronchus with a subphrenic abscess practically always result from rupture of the abscess into the base of the lung which has become adherent to the diaphragm. Where the subphrenic abscess is secondary to perforation of the stomach or intestine, a communication is established between the bronchus and the alimentary canal. The bronchial fistula may then be visualized on barium examination of the gastrointestinal tract. It is difficult to demonstrate the fistula by means of bronchography in such cases.

A biliary fistula can be produced by rupture of a liver abscess through the diaphragm into the lung. An air-fluid level may then appear within the liver. Perforation of a lung abscess into the pericardium results in a pneumopericardium.

Benign Bronchial Bleeding

Hemoptysis occurs occasionally in persons who do not appear to have any significant pulmonary or bronchial disease, and is referred to as benign bronchial bleeding. The bleeding originates in vessels in the bronchial mucous membrane and occurs especially when they are dilated or under increased pressure as in mitral stenosis, hypertension, congestive heart failure, and polycythemia. It may also be a manifestation of hemorrhagic disease. The roentgen films show no evidence of pulmonary disease to account for the hemorrhage although they may show widening of the pulmonary vessels and enlargement of the heart.

There is also a tendency to hemorrhage from the atrophic mucous membrane that lines the bronchi in dry bronchiectasis. The ordinary roentgen film may be entirely negative in this condition. In some cases the film shows only slight changes resulting from old, healed tuberculosis which has left in its wake a few small dilated bronchi whose mucous membrane is atrophic.

One must guard against the error of considering hemoptysis to be related to tuberculosis when the film shows only fine fibrous strands in the upper lobe. Furthermore, the possibility of the hemoptoic form of bronchiectasis should not be excluded because the film of the chest appears to be negative. All of the bronchi in both lungs should be studied bronchographically before this condition is eliminated from consideration.

In cases of benign bronchial bleeding, clotted blood may obstruct one of the bronchi and produce atelectasis (Fig. 209). If a lobe of the lung is found to be collapsed in a patient with hemoptysis, the error will usually be made of considering that both the bleeding and the atelectasis are due to the same obstructing bronchial lesion. This error can be avoided only by bronchoscopy or by further observation which shows a normal lung after the expectoration of firm, dark blood clot.

Occasionally a faint, rather homogeneous shadow is present in a segment of the lung after a hemoptysis (Fig. 210). This may be due to inundation of alveoli by aspirated blood or to obstruction of a small bronchus by clot. If the shadow is situated under the clavicle, particularly if there is a small scar of a healed tuberculous lesion, the patient may be considered to have active tuberculosis. Repetition of the roentgen examination after an interval may show complete clearing of the shadow to indicate that it was simply the result of the hemoptysis.

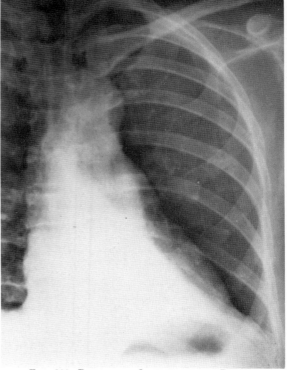

FIG. 209. BRONCHIAL OBSTRUCTION IN BENIGN BRONCHIAL BLEEDING

The triangular shadow behind the heart represents a completely collapsed left lower lobe whose bronchus was obstructed by clotted blood. The heart is displaced to the left, exposing the right border of the vertebral column. The vessels seen on the left side are spread apart as a result of compensatory hyperinflation of the upper lobe. After removal of the clot at bronchoscopy, the lung returned to normal.

DISEASES OF THE LUNGS

Anomalies

The anomalies of the lung consist essentially of absence of a lung (agenesis), malformation of a portion of a lung (hamartoma and bronchogenic cyst), abnormalities of bronchial distribution, abnormalities of lobulation, development of an accessory lung (Nebenlunge), and malformations of the pulmonary arteries and veins.

Agenesis and Aplasia of the Lung. When one lung fails to develop, the space on that side of the chest is taken up by the heart and mediastinal structures which are markedly displaced, by the diaphragm which is elevated and by compensatory overexpansion of the opposite lung. Because of the extreme mobility of the mediastinum in the newborn, the normal lung herniates across the midline and fills the chest on the affected side. The intrathoracic pressure

tends to be equal on both sides because so little resistance is offered by the mediastinal barrier. The chest wall on the abnormal side, therefore, is not drawn inward. Only one lung root is visible on conventional films. No large blood vessels are seen within the hilar region on the affected side because this contains only the peripheral portion of the hyperexpanded lung from the opposite side. The same general appearance is noted in both agenesis and aplasia of the lung. However, in the latter, the stump of the main bronchus is present and may be seen, particularly on overexposed Bucky films.

Agenesis and aplasia of the lung are asymptomatic and often are not discovered until unrelated symptoms lead to an x-ray examination of the chest. The problem is then one of differentiation from atelectasis of the lung. Atelectasis of an entire lung is associated with contraction of

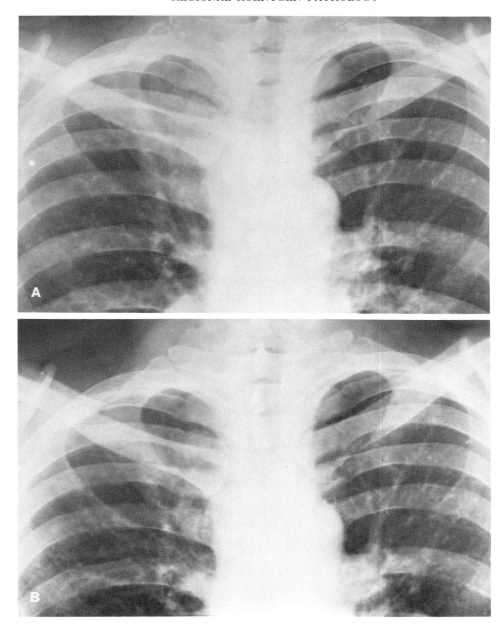

FIG. 210. HEMORRHAGIC CONSOLIDATION IN BENIGN BRONCHIAL BLEEDING

A: The film made at the time when the patient was expectorating bright red blood shows an irregular area of consolidation in the paravertebral portion of the right upper lobe. Bleeding stopped abruptly after a few days. *B:* A film made a few weeks later shows complete clearing. Later studies showed no evidence of an underlying lesion.

the chest wall. Marked displacement of the mediastinum without diminution in the size of the hemithorax constitutes a cardinal sign of agenesis of the lung (Fig. 211). In those cases of agenesis in which the chest is contracted, absence of large blood vessels and a main bronchus leading to the affected side should suggest the diagnosis. A picture simulating agenesis can occur following pneumonectomy, particularly if done early in life (Fig. 212).

In agenesis or aplasia of one lobe of the lung, the remaining lobe or lobes on that side tend to enlarge and fill the entire hemithorax. The diaphragm may remain in its normal position, there is little or no displacement of the mediastinum and the chest wall has a normal contour. Roent-

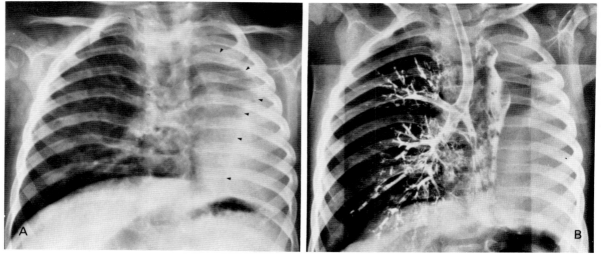

FIG. 211. AGENESIS OF THE LUNG

A: The left hemithorax is clouded. The heart is shifted entirely into the left chest and the trachea is displaced markedly to the left. There is compensatory emphysema of the right lung which has herniated across the mediastinum and almost reaches the left lateral chest wall (arrows). There is very little contraction of the left hemithorax. This favors the diagnosis of agenesis rather than atelectasis of the left lung. *B:* The bronchogram shows total absence of bronchi to the left lung. The vertical shadow to the left of the spine represents contrast material in the esophagus.

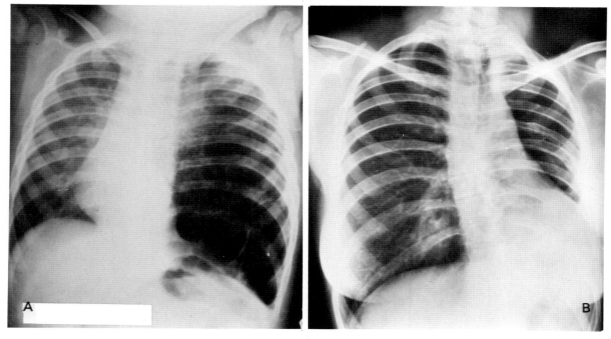

FIG. 212. PNEUMONECTOMY IN INFANCY: CYSTIC ADENOMATOID MALFORMATION

A: Age 16 months. The infant was in severe respiratory distress. The left lung is enlarged and cystic and displaces the diaphragm downward and the heart into the right chest. Pneumonectomy was performed at this time. *B:* Age 24 years. Although the left lung is absent, air-containing lung showing pulmonary vascular markings is present on that side. This is due to herniation of the right lung across the mediastinum. The patient is asymptomatic and her activity is not limited. (Courtesy of Dr. I. A. Sarot, New York, N. Y.)

genologically, the chest appears normal and the anomaly is discovered only by bronchography. In aplasia of the upper lobe, there may be mediastinal herniation to that side as in upper lobe atelectasis. However, in atelectasis of the upper lobe, the lateral view discloses the characteristic shadow of the collapsed lobe.

Pulmonary Hypoplasia. In hypoplasia of the lung, all of the component parts are smaller than normal. As the small lung expands to fill the hemithorax, it becomes emphysematous and it is impossible, in most cases, to differentiate between this condition and acquired unilateral hyperlucent lung. The diagnosis of congenital hypoplasia may be made with certainty only under special circumstances. If unilateral lucency is noted in an infant who has not had a severe respiratory infection, one may assume that the abnormality represents a congenital defect. Even then there is a possibility of error. The increased lucency may simply be due to compensatory hyperexpansion secondary to agenesis of a single lobe. This can be determined only by bronchography. The congenital, as well as the acquired hyperlucent lung often shows cystic changes which represent small, sacculated, terminal bronchiectases.

Congenital hypoplasia of a lung may be associated with complete absence of the pulmonary artery. It must be borne in mind, however, that inability to demonstrate the pulmonary artery on the diseased side by means of venous angiography does not mean that it is absent. Lack of opacification of the pulmonary artery may be due simply to diminished blood flow through the diseased lung. Selective pulmonary arteriography is required for confirmation in these cases.

Anomalies of Lobulation. Anomalous lobulation of the lungs is of clinical as well as anatomic significance and can affect the roentgen appearance of pulmonary disease. Thus, a pneumonia, a lung abscess, or tuberculosis may not be delimited by the border of a lobe if the fissure is absent. On the other hand, the inflammatory process may be sharply limited by an anomalous fissure, producing an unusual conformation to the shadow of the lesion. Absence of a fissure may cause difficulty in resective surgery while the presence of a supernumerary fissure may simplify segmental resection.

Many of the anomalies of lobulation are not visible on the roentgenogram. However, two of the most common malformations, the azygos lobe and the inferior accessory lobe, can almost always be recognized on the ordinary frontal projection. The anomalous fissure separating the superior segment from the basal segments of the lower lobe is best identified on the lateral view.

AZYGOS LOBE. In the embryo, the azygos vein courses upward in the posterior chest wall outside the parietal pleura, then arches over the apex of the right lung and runs downward, forward and mesially to empty into the superior vena cava. As the chest grows, the vein does not elongate proportionately. It slides off the apex of the lung to assume its normal position in the mediastinum just above the lung root.

If the mesial migration of the vein is arrested before it reaches the mediastinum, it will hold down a double fold of parietal pleura. This fold is called the azygos membrane and the azygos vein lies within its free border. The membrane forms a cleft in the right upper lobe. The portion mesial to the membrane is known as the azygos lobe.

The azygos lobe is part of the right upper lobe. Its size and bronchial supply depend upon the point at which migration of the azygos vein was arrested. It is not supplied by a segmental bronchus of its own.

The azygos membrane and the layers of visceral pleura which lie on either side of it are in a plane parallel to the roentgen beam in the frontal projection. They are represented on the film by a sharp, thin, curved line extending from the apex of the lung toward the hilum. At the lower end of this line there is a small oval or pear-shaped shadow which represents the azygos vein, seen on end (Fig. 213).

In rare instances, the bronchus to the azygos lobe is partly or completely compressed by the azygos vein. This may result in atelectasis, bronchiectasis, and chronic inflammation of the lobe. When the azygos lobe is collapsed or consolidated, its shadow merges with that of the mediastinum and simulates a mediastinal tumor. An azygos lobe should be suspected whenever the shadow is bounded by an extremely sharp, smoothly curved outer border. The presence of the characteristic shadow of an azygos vein at its base confirms the diagnosis. In doubtful cases, azygos venography may be required.

The azygos lobe may be separated from the rest of the lung by fluid if there is a pleural effusion, or by air in the case of a pneumothorax.

INFERIOR ACCESSORY LOBE (CARDIAC LOBE). The mesial basal segment of the right lower lobe is regularly supplied by a bronchus of its own. Not uncommonly there is a distinct fibrous septum separating this segment from the remainder of the lobe. When the lung is inflated, an indentation may be seen on its diaphragmatic surface,

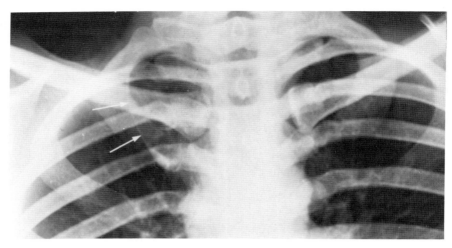

FIG. 213. AZYGOS LOBE

The sharply defined, curvilinear shadow (arrows) in the right upper lobe represents the azygos membrane, composed of a double layer of infolded parietal pleura, together with a double layer of visceral pleura. The teardrop shadow at its base is cast by the azygos vein as it curves forward to empty into the superior vena cava.

corresponding to the lower border of the septum. In rare instances the pleural indentation is so deep that it forms a complete fissure bounding the entire mesial basal segment. This anomaly is often spoken of as a mesial or cardiac lobe.

A fairly well-developed septum separating the mesial segment from the remainder of the lobe may present radiologically on the frontal view as a fine, oblique line, extending from the lower portion of the lung root downward and outward to the midportion of the diaphragm (Fig. 214). Whether this line represents a septum or a complete fissure cannot be determined roentgenologically in the absence of a pneumothorax. In either event, there is no collateral respiration between the segment and the adjacent lung. The segment then acts as a separate lobe. Radiologically, the isolated mesial segment is generally referred to as the inferior accessory lobe even when it is bounded by a septum rather than a fissure.

ADDITIONAL FISSURES. Fissures have been described in anatomic specimens separating every segment from the remainder of the lung. Most of these are extremely rare. One of the more common is an accessory fissure separating the superior segment of the right lower lobe from the basal segments. Usually this fissure is incomplete. It lies in a horizontal plane at about the same level as the normal short fissure and can be seen in all conventional projections. In the lateral view, the anomalous fissure is seen to extend backward from the long fissure, more or less as a continuation of the line of the short fissure (Fig. 51).

Anatomically, an incomplete fissure between the anterior segment of the left upper lobe and

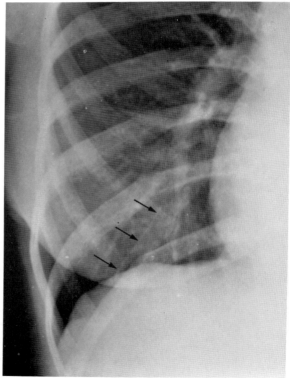

FIG. 214. INFERIOR ACCESSORY LOBE

The thin, sharply demarcated, oblique line (arrows) represents a fibrous septum which separates the mesial basal segment from the remainder of the lower lobe. This is sometimes referred to as a cardiac lobe.

lingula is rather common. Occasionally the fissure is complete. Because the plane of the fissure slopes downward and forward, it is rarely visible on the frontal projection but can be recognized on the lateral view.

ABSENCE OF FISSURES. An interlobar fissure may be absent without any change in the bronchial or vascular pattern of the lung. Absence or incomplete development of the short fissure is common, while incomplete development of the long fissure is rare. This abnormality cannot be recognized roentgenologically since, in most instances, fissures which are not thickened cannot be identified (Fig. 215). Absence of the fissure may affect the roentgen appearance of pneumonia or a neoplasm which will no longer be confined to the usual limits of a lobe (see Fig. 426). It is also of importance to the surgeon in the performance of a lobectomy.

Anomalies of Bronchial Distribution. Variations in the pattern of division and distribution of the subsegmental bronchi are relatively common but are of little clinical significance. The pattern of the major or segmental bronchi is fairly constant. One of the more frequent variants is a separate bronchus to the subapical segment of either lower lobe. It arises from the posterior wall of the lower lobe bronchus, distal to the origin of the superior segmental division. In such instances, the superior segmental bronchus may originate at a higher level than usual. The most common variation in the upper lobes is a separate axillary segmental bronchus in place of the axillary branch of the anterior segmental bronchus.

Of particular significance is the more unusual anomaly consisting of a second upper lobe bronchus arising either from the trachea (Fig. 216) or from the main bronchus. In most cases it occurs on the right side and supplies the apical or the apical and posterior segments. The corresponding branches of the normal upper lobe bronchus are usually absent and the segments of lung supplied by the anomalous bronchus are normal. In other instances, the anomalous bronchus is truly supernumerary, the right upper lobe bronchus having all its normal branches. The lung supplied by the accessory bronchus then represents a second upper lobe. However, in most instances, it is not separated by a fissure. The pulmonary tissue of this lobe is often malformed and may be the seat of chronic inflammatory disease.

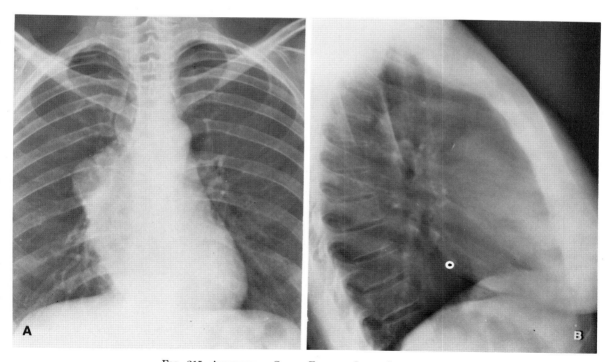

FIG. 215. ABSENCE OF SHORT FISSURE: LUNG CARCINOMA

A: The frontal projection shows a sharply demarcated lobulated mass to the right of the mediastinum. The border of the heart and ascending aorta is obscured indicating that the lesion is situated anteriorly. The appearance cannot be distinguished from that of a tumor of the anterior mediastinum. *B:* The lateral view confirms the anterior location of the mass which has the appearance of a thymoma. However, because the patient was coughing up blood the possibility of a carcinoma was considered more likely. The mass involves the middle lobe and the contiguous portion of the upper lobe. Extension of a carcinoma across a fissure causes thickening of the fissure. In this case the short fissure is not visualized. At operation a primary carcinoma of the lung was found involving both lobes with absence of the fissure between them.

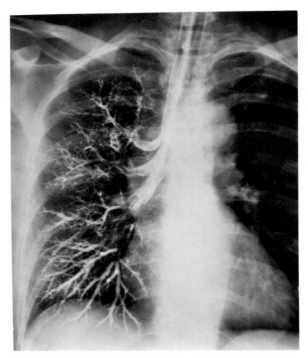

FIG. 216. SUPERNUMERARY BRONCHUS

The bronchogram shows an anomalous bronchus (arrow) arising from the lower trachea. It supplies the apical and posterior segments of the right upper lobe. The normal right upper lobe bronchus arises in its usual position.

Abnormalities of bronchial distribution and lobulation of the lungs may occur as part of a developmental disturbance involving several organs. In the *asplenia syndrome,* the body develops symmetrically. Each lung has three lobes and the bronchial pattern on both sides is that of a right lung. Multiple cardiac abnormalities, including transposition of the great vessels and anomalous pulmonary venous drainage together with abnormalities in the position of the abdominal viscera are almost always associated with absence of the spleen.

Abnormalities of pulmonary lobulation also occur in the *scimitar syndrome* (see p. 266), in which there is anomalous venous drainage of the right lung into the inferior vena cava. In this condition the right lung usually has only two lobes with a hyparterial bronchial pattern like that of a normal left lung. Bilateral left lungs have also been encountered in *polysplenia.*

Anomalies of Pulmonary Arteries. Almost all anomalies of the main pulmonary artery are associated with anomalies of the heart and aorta. Idiopathic dilatation of the pulmonary artery can occur as an isolated malformation. In most cases, dilatation of the pulmonary artery is secondary to increased blood flow resulting from a left-to-right shunt or to stenosis of the pulmonic valve. When both major pulmonary arteries are dilated, the increased size of the hila may mimic large lymph nodes.

The shadow of the main pulmonary artery may be small or absent when the vessel is underdeveloped, as in tricuspid or pulmonary atresia, or tetralogy of Fallot. In these anomalies, there is usually a sizable right-to-left intracardiac shunt, pulmonary blood flow is diminished, and the peripheral pulmonary vessels are small. A pulmonary artery of normal size may not be visible on the frontal chest film in transposition of the great vessels because the artery is mesially placed and largely hidden by the aorta and the heart.

The hilar shadows are generally elevated when both pulmonary arteries arise from the ascending aorta in persistent truncus arteriosus. The right lung root may be elevated in corrected transposition of the great vessels.

Coarctation of a major pulmonary artery usually produces no significant change in the appearance of the hilar shadows. Rarely, poststenotic dilatation causes undue prominence of the hilum. The root shadow may be small when the stenotic segment is long.

Absence of one pulmonary artery almost always occurs on the side opposite the aortic arch. While it can represent an isolated anomaly, it is often associated with tetralogy of Fallot. In contrast to agenesis of a lung, when a central pulmonary artery is missing, fairly well developed bronchial and pulmonary tissue is present on the involved side. The lung and hemithorax are small, the mediastinum is displaced toward the abnormal side, and the diaphragm is elevated (Fig. 217). Ventilation of the involved lung may be normal so that there is no significant shift of the mediastinum with respiration. The lung is commonly hyperlucent and presents a reticular appearance because its blood supply is derived entirely from the bronchial arteries.

The diagnosis of absence of one pulmonary artery can be established with certainty only by selective pulmonary arteriography. On a venous angiogram, it may not be possible to distinguish between an absent pulmonary artery and acquired unilateral hyperlucent lung. In this condition, the pulmonary vascular resistance in the involved lung is increased. As a result, most of the blood pumped by the right ventricle tends to flow to the opposite lung. Because of the decreased flow, the pulmonary artery on the involved side is quite small and often cannot be identified on a venous study.

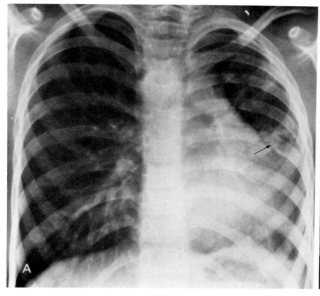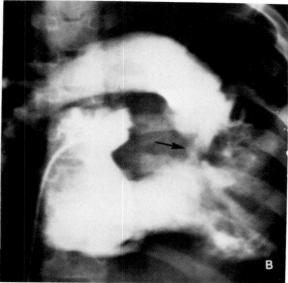

FIG. 217. ABSENCE OF LEFT PULMONARY ARTERY: TETRALOGY OF FALLOT

A: A 5 year old cyanotic boy was admitted with massive hemoptysis. The left lung is small and the heart is shifted into the left hemithorax. There are several patchy areas of consolidation in the left lung and a cavity (arrow) in the lingula. These lesions were subsequently proven to be caused by active tuberculosis. The trachea is deviated to the left by a right aortic arch.
B: Angiocardiogram. Contrast material injected into the right atrium outlines a marked stenosis (arrow) of the infundibular portion of the right ventricle. The right pulmonary artery appears normal. The left pulmonary artery is absent. Subsequent films showed a sizable right-to-left shunt at the ventricular level.

In a *congenital arteriovenous fistula,* a branch of a pulmonary artery and vein communicate directly, bypassing the capillary plexus that normally intervenes between them. Since the vascular resistance offered by the fistula is less than that in the remainder of the lung, blood flow through the fistula is relatively great. Both the involved pulmonary artery and vein may become aneurysmally dilated.

Not uncommonly, arteriovenous fistulas are multiple and involve both lungs. In some cases they are part of the generalized vascular anomaly of hereditary hemorrhagic telangiectasia (Osler-Weber-Rendu disease).

An arteriovenous fistula usually presents as a nodular density within the lung (Fig. 30). It is homogeneous, often has a lobulated contour, and is easily confused with a peripheral pulmonary neoplasm. Dilated vessels between the mass and the hilum are usually recognizable on routine films of the chest but are more clearly visualized by tomography. In some cases, instead of presenting as a mass, the arteriovenous fistula is characterized by a collection of dilated, racemose vessels radiating from the hilum. In either instance, fluoroscopy may disclose pulsation of the lesion and diminution of its size during the Valsalva maneuver. The diagnosis can always be established by angiocardiography.

Small fistulas, clearly demonstrable by angiography, may not cast a shadow on the film. Because arteriovenous fistulas are often multiple, pulmonary arteriography should always be performed before resection of what is presumed to be an isolated lesion.

Anomalies of Pulmonary Veins. Early in embryonic life, the four pulmonary veins join to form a single common pulmonary venous trunk. This establishes communication with the left atrium. As the heart grows, it is absorbed into the atrium so that the four pulmonary veins eventually open independently into the chamber. Anomalous development can result in communication of one or more of the pulmonary veins with the right atrium, the superior or inferior vena cava, or the portal vein. The roentgen picture associated with these anomalies is determined by the number of veins that are involved, their course and termination, and whether or not there is obstruction to venous blood flow.

PARTIAL ANOMALOUS VENOUS DRAINAGE. Return of pulmonary venous blood to the right side of the heart represents a left-to-right shunt. When only one vein drains anomalously, the chest film is usually completely normal. However, involvement of two or more veins often causes overloading of the pulmonary circulation sufficient to produce dilatation of the main pulmonary artery and a recognizable increase in the vascularity of the lungs. Not uncommonly, the picture is indistinguishable from that associated with an atrial septal defect.

A characteristic roentgen picture is often associated with anomalous venous drainage of the right lung or the right lower lobe into the inferior vena cava. This forms one part of a complex of malformations popularly known as the *scimitar syndrome*. The right lung is usually hypoplastic and often has only two lobes. A part of this lung may receive its arterial supply from the abdominal aorta.

Commonly, the right hemithorax is smaller than the left and the heart and mediastinum are shifted to the right. There is increased pulmonary vascularity and the anomalous vein appears as a crescent-shaped shadow along the right heart border, resembling a scimitar (Fig. 218).

SUPRADIAPHRAGMATIC TOTAL ANOMALOUS PULMONARY VENOUS DRAINAGE. Total anomalous pulmonary venous drainage is almost always associated with persistence of the embryonic common pulmonary vein. Most often this communicates with the upper remnant of the left superior vena cava and drains into the innominate vein. The left superior vena cava forms a prominence along the left side of the mediastinum. The normal right superior vena cava is dilated because it carries the venous return from the lungs as well as from the upper extremities and head. This causes a widening of the right side of the mediastinum. The appearance caused by the bilateral bulge of the superior mediastinum above the cardiac silhouette has been likened to that of a snowman or a figure-of-eight (Fig. 219). In the frontal view, this may be confused with a thymic tumor. The lateral projection easily differentiates the two conditions because both vena cavae lie in the middle mediastinum so that with anomalous venous drainage, the anterior mediastinum remains clear. When the common pulmonary vein drains into the coronary sinus, it usually cannot be identified on films. In either case, the diagnosis is easily made by angiocardiography.

INFRADIAPHRAGMATIC TOTAL ANOMALOUS PULMONARY VENOUS DRAINAGE. When all the pulmonary veins drain into the portal vein, the common venous channel leading through the diaphragm cannot be identified because it lies within the mediastinum. The venous structure is usually narrowed, either as it passes through the diaphragm or at its junction with the portal vein. This stenosis results in pulmonary venous hypertension and pulmonary congestion. Although the appearance of the lung is typical of congestive failure, the heart is normal in size because of the obstruction to venous return. This anomaly, if uncorrected, is almost universally fatal and

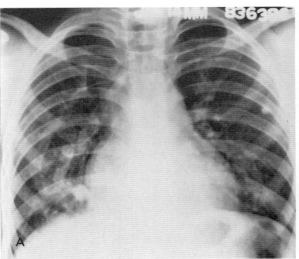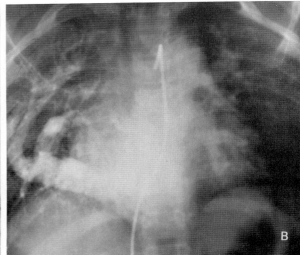

FIG. 218. SCIMITAR SYNDROME

A: Two broad curvilinear shadows converge toward the right cardiophrenic angle. This appearance is characteristic of drainage of the veins of the right lung into the inferior vena cava. A sharply circumscribed round density at the right cardiac border represents a large vein seen on end. There is an increase in the pulmonary vasculature as a result of the left-to-right shunt. In this case the right lung is normal in size. *B:* A late film of a selective pulmonary angiogram shows the pulmonary veins from the left lung draining into the left atrium while all the veins from the right lung join to form one large common vein which empties into the inferior vena cava immediately below its entrance into the right atrium.

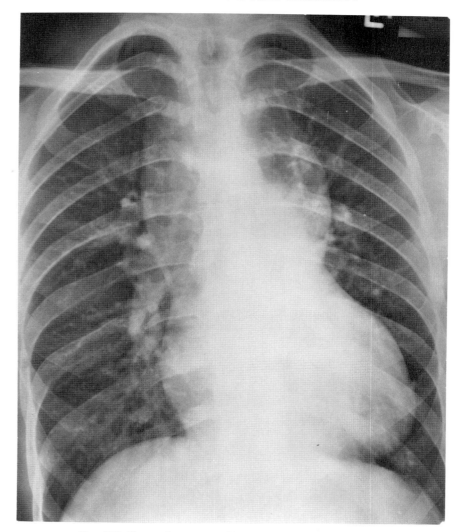

FIG. 219. TOTAL ANOMALOUS PULMONARY VENOUS DRAINAGE

The superior mediastinum bulges to both sides. The density of the mediastinal shadow is less than would be expected with a tumor of this size. The heart is moderately enlarged and the pulmonary vasculature is increased. The appearance of the superior mediastinum and heart, which is characteristic of anomalous pulmonary venous drainage into the left innominate vein, has been likened to that of a snowman.

therefore is seen only in infants. The combination of pulmonary edema with a normal-sized heart in these children strongly suggests the diagnosis of anomalous pulmonary venous drainage below the diaphragm.

VARICOSE PULMONARY VEINS. Localized dilatation of the pulmonary veins usually occurs near their junction with the left atrium. It rarely is an isolated congenital abnormality. Most often, dilatation of the pulmonary veins results from increased pulmonary blood flow when there is a left-to-right shunt or as a manifestation of pulmonary venous hypertension. The dilated vein may be seen on end in the frontal projection and

resembles a tumor in the lung. Distinction is not difficult in the oblique views in which the vein is not foreshortened and the smaller veins entering it can be identified. Tomography in the oblique projections makes this even more obvious. Angiocardiography is rarely required.

Malformation of a Portion of the Lung. The malformations most commonly met with are bronchogenic cysts, hamartomas, and pulmonary cysts.

BRONCHOGENIC CYST. A bronchogenic cyst is the result of improper development of a bronchial bud. Since these buds originate near the root of the lung, congenital bronchial cysts are generally seen in that region. The cyst is usually unilocular. In most cases it is lined by ciliated epithelium and its wall contains smooth muscle and cartilage. Generally, there is no bronchial communication, although a fibrous attachment to one of the larger bronchi at the root of the lung can usually be found. Occasionally there is a free bronchial communication, either congenital, or acquired from rupture of an infected cyst into a bronchus.

When there is no communication with a bronchus, the cyst is represented by a sharply demarcated, homogeneous, round or oval density. If there is a bronchial communication, the fluid contents of the cyst are partly expelled and the film shows a fluid level. When the cyst empties completely, only an annular shadow, representing the cyst wall, remains. The bronchial communication may be demonstrated by bronchography.

Of paramount importance in the diagnosis of bronchogenic cysts is the situation of the lesion adjacent to or near the root of the lung on all views (Fig. 220). It is rare for any other sharply demarcated, round or oval lesion, or a thin-walled, smoothly outlined cavity to be situated in this location. Cavities due to inflammatory disease are rarely located centrally, and neoplasms which have undergone cavitation rarely have a smooth outline. It is most unusual for a bronchogenic cyst to be situated in the anterior or posterior mediastinum. When the cyst lies in the subcarinal region it tends to splay the main bronchi. Cysts in the paratracheal region are fixed to the trachea and therefore rise on swallowing.

PULMONARY CYSTS. Multiple cysts, usually limited to one lobe, but sometimes involving the entire lung, can be manifestations of congenital cystic adenomatoid malformation of the lung. This condition appears to be due to an overgrowth of the terminal respiratory structures without an orderly bronchial pattern. The interstitial tissues of the lung between the cystic areas are markedly thickened. The cysts are of varying size and usually communicate with each other.

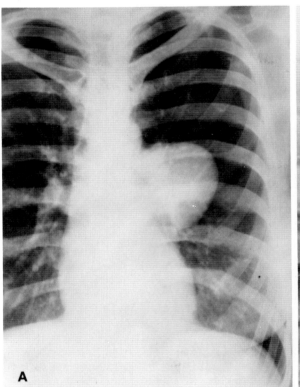
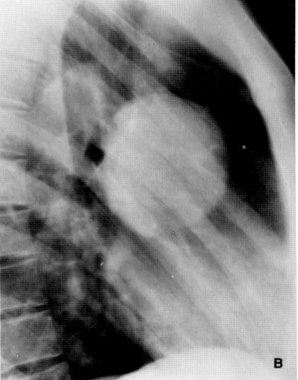

FIG. 220. BRONCHOGENIC CYST

A: Frontal projection. The extremely sharp demarcation of the mass near the root of the left lung is indicative of a benign tumor. Since the outline of the left pulmonary artery is not obliterated, the mass must lie in a different plane, in front of or behind the hilum. *B:* Lateral projection. The round mass is situated immediately in front of the root of the lung. The anterior mediastinum is clear. This excludes a teratoma or thymic tumor from consideration. Paraesophageal cysts and neurofibromas occur more posteriorly. This case illustrates the site of predilection or bronchogenic cysts.

They may be filled with fluid but often they contain air because of the presence of bronchial communications.

The involved portion of the lung is usually larger than normal. It compresses the adjacent pulmonary tissue and may displace the mediastinum to the opposite side (Fig. 212). The malformation appears on the films as an area of soft tissue density containing multiple lucencies. The roentgen picture can simulate consolidation of the lung with multiple pneumatoceles as in staphylococcal pneumonia. Congenital cystic adenomatoid malformation involving a lower lobe can be confused with a diaphragmatic hernia. An incomplete outline of the left diaphragm together with a relative lack of gas-filled bowel in the abdomen, favors the diagnosis of hernia.

Multiple cysts without adenomatoid malformation of the lung may result from defective development of the pulmonary tissue in relation to the bronchioles. If there is free communication between the bronchi and the lung, the cysts contain air and form numerous thin-walled cavities. Otherwise, the cysts are filled with fluid and cast round, solid shadows. If a communication develops, multiple air-fluid levels may appear. Unless the cystic lesions are seen in infants soon after birth, their congenital origin cannot be inferred from the roentgen examination (Fig. 221). In the great majority of cases, cystic disease of

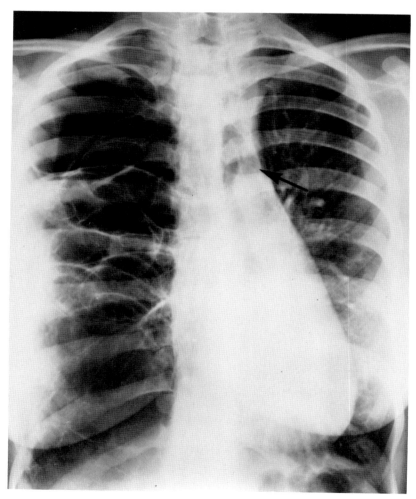

FIG. 221. CYSTIC DISEASE OF THE LUNG

The right lung is composed of numerous large, thin-walled cavities whose annular shadows overlap each other. No vessels can be seen on this side. The heart and trachea are displaced to the left. The right diaphragm is depressed and there is herniation of the right lung through the superior mediastinum (arrow). These changes indicate increased pressure within the cysts in the right lung. The marked thickening of the right pleura suggests that the cavities may have been acquired during a pneumonia in childhood. However, in the absence of any history of such infection, the possibility of congenital cystic disease of the lung cannot be denied.

the lung is an acquired lesion, the result of bronchopulmonary infection (Figs. 128, 204 and 240).

HAMARTOMA. A hamartoma is a tumor resulting from maldevelopment of certain tissues in embryonal life, producing an overgrowth or an abnormal arrangement of these tissues. Commonly the hamartoma presents as a localized nodule within the parenchyma of the lung. Since the hamartoma represents tissue indigenous to the body it is not encapsulated. Nevertheless, it remains localized and does not infiltrate the surrounding tissues. Despite its congenital origin, the localized form of hamartoma is rarely seen in children. It is most commonly discovered in the third and fourth decades. We have observed a number of cases in which the hamartomas were not visible on films made between 2 and 7 years previous to their discovery. These observations would indicate that the tumors developed from tiny, quiescent embryonal rests.

The most common form of localized pulmonary hamartoma is the chondroma or chondroadenoma. This is composed mainly of cartilage together with connective tissue and epithelial elements, mostly in acinar formation. Bone may be admixed with the cartilage. Rarely, hamartomas are hemangiomatous or consist largely of muscle or fatty tissue. In any case, there may be considerable variation in the degree of maturity of the tissues.

Radiologically, the hamartoma usually appears as a sharply circumscribed, round or slightly lobulated homogeneous density within the lung (Fig. 222). It is almost always separated from the pleura and is usually situated within the depths of the lobe. Most hamartomas are quite small when first discovered, usually measuring 1 to 3 cm in size. While observation over a period of years may show no growth, usually there is a gradual and constant increase in the size of the nodule. On the average the tumors seem to grow about one millimeter in diameter

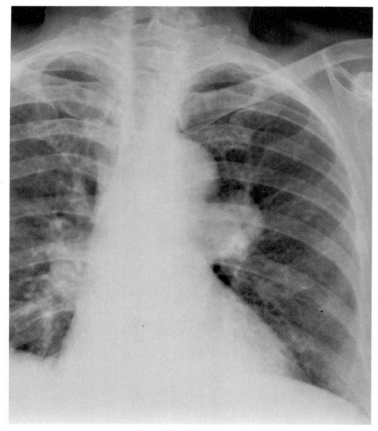

FIG. 222. HAMARTOMA

The smoothly outlined, round mass projected over the left hilum proved to be a hamartoma in the superior segment of the left lower lobe. Despite its size, no calcium could be demonstrated histologically. Visualization of the outline of the pulmonary artery within the shadow of the mass indicates that the lesion is not situated at the lung root.

per year. Rarely growth is quite rapid. Nodules over 5 to 6 cm in diameter are unusual. In any case, malignant change in the hamartoma is so rare that it does not merit serious consideration.

Calcium can be demonstrated radiologically in a considerable portion of the chondromatous hamartomas, particularly in the ones over 3 or 4 cm in diameter. The demonstration of calcium is particularly important in differentiating the hamartoma from a malignant tumor. If, as is usually the case, calcium is not demonstrable on ordinary films, tomograms should be made whenever the possibility of a hamartoma is considered.

The pattern of calcification within a hamartoma can vary considerably and often is nonspecific. However, when the calcium is deposited in small nodules scattered irregularly throughout the tumor, or when arranged in "popcorn" or "mulberry" fashion, a hamartoma can be diagnosed with a considerable degree of certainty (Fig. 140). This pattern of calcification differs from that of a tuberculoma or a blocked tuberculous cavity (Fig. 137). A tuberculoma or histoplasmoma usually has a dense central deposit of calcium or the lime may be deposited in concentric rings (Fig. 257). Concentric arrangement of the calcium does not occur in a hamartoma but a central focus of calcium may be present in a hamartoma as well as in a tuberculoma. Calcification of a blocked tuberculous cavity appears radiologically as a thick, irregular, shell-like density in one portion of the periphery of the shadow. This appearance is not seen with a hamartoma.

Hamartomas other than those which consist largely of cartilage, do not show evidence of calcification. Their borders are exquisitely demarcated on ordinary films as well as on tomography. The possibility of a hamartoma rather than a granuloma should be considered whenever the lesion is situated at a distance from the surface of the lobe. Inflammatory nodules, such as the tuberculoma, histoplasmoma and coccidioidoma are regularly situated immediately beneath the pleura.

In the absence of calcification, it is usually impossible to differentiate the hamartoma from some cases of peripheral bronchial adenoma, a cavity filled with fluid, or a solitary metastatic neoplasm. If the border of the nodule is not smooth and sharply demarcated, the possibility of a primary bronchogenic carcinoma cannot be excluded. Moreover, a primary bronchogenic carcinoma cannot be excluded if a small calcific deposit is noted in the outer part of the tumor. We have seen several cases of nodular carcinoma in which the tumor grew about and enveloped a preexisting calcific focus in the lung.

Endobronchial hamartomas are encountered rarely. Most of them are chondromatous, but others contain a considerable amount of myxomatous and fatty tissue as well as epithelial elements. In any case, the radiologic picture is that of bronchial obstruction and its complications, and the nature of the obstructing lesion can rarely be determined without bronchoscopy or surgical exploration (Fig. 188) even if calcium is present within the tumor. The lesion is easily confused with a calcified lymph node because the tumor is located near the lung root.

In contrast to most localized hamartomas, which occur in adults, the diffuse type is almost always seen in infants. This maldevelopment involves a fairly large portion of the lung, usually a lobe, or even the entire lung, but is sometimes confined to only one or more segments. In some cases, the involved lung appears solid, while in others there are cystic spaces. When the cysts predominate, the term *congenital cystic adenomatoid malformation* of the lung is applicable.

Radiologically, the anomaly appears as a dense shadow containing one or more lucent areas. The malformed lung may be so large that it displaces the mediastinal structures to the opposite side (Fig. 212).

TUBEROUS SCLEROSIS. Tuberous sclerosis is a generalized condition with hamartomatous changes in several organs. The lungs are only occasionally involved, much less frequently than the brain, skin and kidneys. The pulmonary abnormality is generally diffuse and affects both lungs. There is an overgrowth of the pulmonary interstitial tissue involving smooth muscle and vascular elements, as well as the connective tissue. This produces a thickening of the interstitium of the lung. Tiny, scattered nodules, representing leiomyomas and capillary angiomas may be present (Fig. 223).

Tuberous sclerosis is one of the causes of the roentgen picture described as honeycomb lung. In addition to reticular shadows throughout the lungs due to thickening of the interstitial tissues, there are innumerable tiny cystic areas. These may be poorly defined and easily overlooked. They are best seen at the edge of the pulmonary field, especially on lateral and oblique films. Often the honeycomb pattern is most evident within the shadow of the liver on films of the abdomen. In addition, the tiny leiomyomas may cause miliary stippling of the lung fields. Spontaneous pneumothorax from rupture of one of the cysts is relatively common.

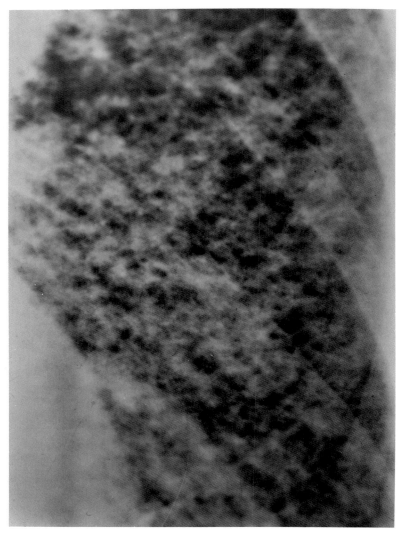

FIG. 223. TUBEROUS SCLEROSIS
A close-up view of the left lung shows diffuse, irregular thickening of the interstitial tissues with many small nodules. Innumerable cystic areas are interspersed throughout the lung. The pulmonary changes are more pronounced than in most cases of tuberous sclerosis.

A diagnosis of tuberous sclerosis cannot be made from the chest film alone since it cannot be distinguished from other varieties of honeycomb lung. The diagnosis can be made when roentgen or clinical examination discloses the presence of hamartomas in other organs, such as tuberosclerotic lesions of the brain, retinal phakoma, adenoma sebaceum, and hamartomatous tumors of the kidneys.

PULMONARY SEQUESTRATION (NEBENLUNGE). An accessory or sequestrated lung developing apart from the normal bronchial tree or normal pulmonary arterial circulation probably arises from a supernumerary lung bud of the primitive foregut in early embryonic life. The major arterial supply to the sequestrated lung is from the systemic circulation, most commonly by means of one or more arteries arising from the aorta at about the level of the diaphragm. The venous drainage is generally into the normal pulmonary veins although in some instances, the drainage is into the azygos system.

The anomalous lung is most commonly incorporated within the normal lung and is then designated as an *intralobar* pulmonary sequestration. Almost always it is situated within the posterior basal segment of the lower lobe, more commonly on the left side than on the right.

Rarely the sequestered lung is found within one of the upper lobes. Sometimes it is independent of the normal lung and lies on the diaphragm, within the abdomen, or within the pericardial cavity. This accessory lung is frequently associated with diaphragmatic and other thoracic anomalies and is referred to as *extralobar* pulmonary sequestration. Rarely there is a persistent connection between the anomalous lung and the gastrointestinal tract.

The anomalous lung is generally rudimentary and composed of a mass of poorly differentiated tissue containing mesenchymal elements, epithelial tissue, bronchi, fetal alveoli and cartilage. In rare instances, the abnormal lung is composed largely of irregularly dilated arteriovenous malformations.

The mass of tissue may be solid or it may contain multiple fluid-filled cysts. The sequestered lung is prone to recurrent and chronic infections which are probably originally hematogenous. If the infection spreads to the adjacent normal lung, a bronchial communication may be established. The sequestered lung may evacuate some or all of its contents and assume the appearance of a lung abscess or air cyst.

The roentgen appearance of the sequestered lung depends largely on whether or not it communicates with a bronchus. In the absence of such communication its shadow is more or less homogeneous. The density of the sequestered lung can vary considerably. It may cast only a faint, hazy shadow which can be overlooked. More often the shadow is dense enough to simulate a pulmonary neoplasm (Fig. 224). The shadow usually has a rather poorly demarcated border. It may be roughly round or curvilinear in shape but its contour tends to be irregular.

If there is a bronchial communication, multiple cystic spaces containing air and fluid may be seen. It can then mimic a localized area of bronchiectasis. When the mass is largely cystic and empty, it can appear as an annular shadow. If there is a check-valve obstruction in the communicating bronchus, the cyst can balloon out (Fig. 225). When the cyst is infected, an air-fluid level appears and it then simulates an abscess.

Bronchography shows the normal bronchial branches of the lower lobe to be spread apart or simply displaced by the mass of the sequestered lung. If there is a bronchial communication, the contrast material may enter and puddle within the diseased anomalous lung. Pulmonary arteriography will demonstrate the lack of a pulmonary arterial supply to the nebenlunge. Aortography, however, is the diagnostic procedure of choice as this reveals the abnormal branches of the aorta which supply the sequestered lung.

The diagnosis of pulmonary sequestration should be suspected whenever there is a localized density situated in the region of the lower lobe adjacent to the spine and posterior mediastinum and lateral to the aorta, particularly when it does not extend backward as far as the posterior chest wall. Consideration of this possibility is especially important when surgical treatment is planned for a mass in this region as considerable bleeding may be encountered from the anomalous systemic vessels if their presence is not suspected.

The Pneumonias

Conventionally, the pneumonias have been divided into three types: lobar pneumonia, bronchopneumonia, and interstitial pneumonia. This division was made largely from the appearance of the lungs at postmortem examination and had little to do with the etiology of the disease or with the pathologic changes occurring during its course. It was recognized that most of the cases of lobar pneumonia were due to the pneumococcus and that the bronchopneumonias consisted of a group of diseases caused by various agents and presenting a variety of pathologic characteristics. Caseous bronchopneumonia was known to be caused by tubercle bacilli, suppurative and gangrenous pneumonias were generally due to pyogenic organisms and hemorrhagic bronchopneumonia was often associated with influenza. However, little of the pathogenesis and life history of the pneumonic diseases could be determined from pathologic examination. It was appreciated that the bronchopneumonias begin essentially as bronchial infections and that the involvement of the lung occurs secondarily to the disease in the bronchi. The disease in the lungs, therefore, consists of multiple foci. In some, the reaction in the lung takes the form of multiple localized areas of consolidation, each of which is similar to lobar pneumonia, and if these are confluent the gross appearance could simulate that disease. In others, the infection and the inflammatory reaction occur mainly in the interstitial tissues so that the pathologic picture is mainly that of an interstitial pneumonia.

Today much more is known about the natural history of the pneumonias because of serial roentgenographic examinations during the course of the disease, the use of bronchography and tomography and the study of specimens removed at operation. This has helped us in

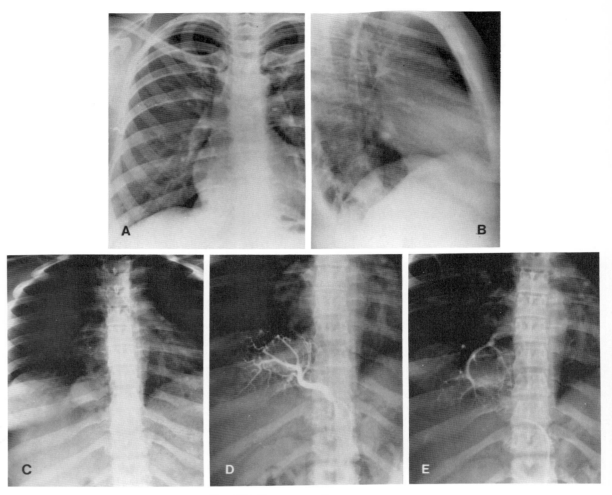

FIG. 224. PULMONARY SEQUESTRATION

A: The shadow in the right cardiophrenic angle does not obliterate the cardiac border, indicating that it is situated behind the heart. The appearance is suggestive of a neoplasm. A tumor arising from a nerve root can be excluded because the mass is separated from the spine. *B:* Lateral view. The mass is projected over the lower dorsal spine but does not extend to the posterior chest wall. *C:* Supine Bucky film. The mass is now more clearly visualized. It is round and well demarcated. Because of its appearance and location, it was considered necessary to exclude the possibility of pulmonary sequestration before subjecting the patient to thoracotomy. *D:* Selective arteriogram. A flush aortogram revealed an anomalous artery arising from the abdominal aorta. Selective opacification of this vessel shows that it supplies the mass in the lower part of the right lung. *E:* Selective arteriogram, venous phase. The veins from the mass drain by way of the normal inferior pulmonary vein into the left atrium. This vascular pattern is typical of intralobar sequestration.

recognizing the different diseases which more or less conform to the pathologic pictures of lobar, bronchial and interstitial pneumonia. It has been found that several of the diseases are characterized by the presence of all three pathologic processes, by the presence of lobar consolidation, bronchopneumonic patches, and infiltrations of the interstitial tissue, either concomitantly or in different stages of their course. Although the division of pneumonias into three categories is helpful in diagnosis, the mere ascertainment that the pneumonia in question falls into one of the groups is not adequate for a final diagnosis. However, the roentgen findings, particularly those which pertain to the changes occurring during the course of the disease, are extremely helpful in placing the disease in its proper, specific category.

The clinical manifestations of pneumonia are often nonspecific and there may be no signs to indicate that the disease is situated in the lungs. Not uncommonly, the diagnosis of pneumonia

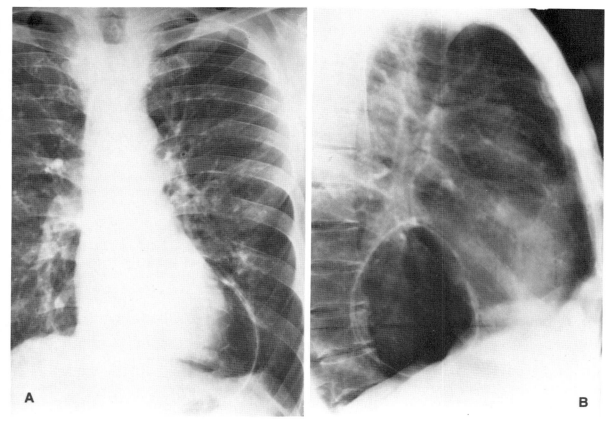

FIG. 225. INTRALOBAR SEQUESTRATION

A: A large cyst is present just lateral to the apex of the heart. The differential diagnosis on this film should include a large pneumatocele, a diaphragmatic hernia and a cystic sequestrated lobe. *B:* The cyst, which is situated adjacent to the descending aorta, is projected over the posterior mediastinum. This is the characteristic location for a pulmonary sequestration. At operation, the cystic lung was supplied by a large artery that arose from the abdominal aorta. An anomalous bronchus connected the cyst to the left lower lobe. The wall of the cyst showed evidence of embryonal pulmonary malformation.

can be made only from roentgen films of the chest. This examination may disclose a pneumonia as the cause of fever of unexplained origin or of abdominal pain, vomiting and rigidity which seem to be characteristic of an acute abdominal disease. In other instances, a pneumonia associated with a generalized disease may present characteristic pulmonary changes which are helpful in making a specific diagnosis. Conversely, the roentgen examination of the chest can exclude the possibility of pneumonia and may lead to a correct diagnosis by directing the attention to other parts of the body.

Since the routine roentgen examination of the chest often includes only a frontal view, this film should be made with sufficient penetration to show the vessels through the cardiac shadow. Otherwise, a pneumonia involving the left lower lobe will be overlooked. Oblique and lateral views are useful in disclosing not only the retrocardiac region but also the portions of the lungs obscured by the diaphragm on the frontal projection. These additional views also help to demonstrate the exact extent of the disease in relation to the lobes and their segments.

All cases of pneumonia should be documented radiologically and followed with serial films until the lungs are entirely clear. It is extremely rare for a pneumonia caused by pyogenic bacteria not to undergo complete resolution if the infection is controlled. Resolution may be delayed if antibiotic treatment is inadequate, but eventually no sign of the disease remains unless a complicating factor is present. A diagnosis of unresolved pneumonia should be made with extreme caution since it almost always proves to be incorrect. Lack of resolution is usually due to bronchial obstruction, neoplastic disease, bronchiectasis, or infection by other organisms, such as tubercle bacilli or fungi, or to one of the granulomatous diseases.

Lobar Pneumonia

Lobar penumonia represents a type of inflammation of the lung characterized by outpouring of exudate into the alveoli with little change in the bronchi or interstitial tissues. In essence, this is a purely consolidative pneumonia. The most characteristic roentgen appearance of lobar pneumonia is produced when there is diffuse consolidation of an entire lobe of the lung. Before the x-ray era, when only postmortem material was available for study, this was thought to occur soon after the onset of the disease. This is not correct. The disease begins with filling of a group of pulmonary lobules with edema fluid and bacteria and relatively few inflammatory cells. The outpouring of fluid is generally considered to result from a local sensitivity reaction to the polysaccharides in the capsule of the pneumococcus. The bacteria are rapidly carried by the edema fluid from alveolus to alveolus through the pores of Kohn and the bronchioles, so that by the time the patient's symptoms indicate the need for x-ray examination, one or more segments of the lobe are involved.

Early Stage. INFLAMMATORY EDEMA. Pathologically, the early stage of lobar pneumonia consists of inflammatory edema associated with pleuritis. The latter is manifested clinically by chest pain and occurs quite early. At the time of the first roentgen examination, the infection and edema have usually spread throughout a segment of the lung. Nevertheless, the film may show only a faint shadow which does not completely obscure the pulmonary vessels in the area because many of the alveoli are still aerated. At this stage, the lesion may be overlooked unless films of good technical quality are available. This is especially true of examinations made at the bedside.

Even under the best of circumstances, the area of congestive edema may not be apparent. However, the possibility of early pneumonia should be considered if one leaf of the diaphragm is elevated or its motion restricted. Diaphragmatic motion can be evaluated by fluoroscopy or from films made at the end of inspiration and expiration. Limitation of motion can also be inferred from a single film if the patient breathes during the exposure. The diaphragm on the normal side appears blurred because of its motion, while that on the involved side tends to be sharply outlined because it remains stationary.

Stage of Consolidation. *The Blood Vessels.* The appearance of the consolidated portion of the lung is characterized by a rather dense shadow of uniform opacity. The shadows of the blood vessels in the affected segments are lost because their density is the same as that of the consolidated lung and there is no air in the adjacent alveoli to set them off. The absence of clear visualization of the blood vessels is particularly important in the detection of consolidation of the left lower lobe behind the heart. Normally, films made with proper exposure disclose these vessels clearly. If they cannot be seen on a film which is sufficiently penetrated to disclose the shadows of the ribs through the cardiac silhouette, the presence of consolidation of that portion of the lung should be suspected.

Often the shadows of blood vessels may seem to course through an area of consolidation. Almost invariably, these are situated within the more or less normal lung in front of or behind the consolidated segment. This can be determined by following the direction and distribution of the vessels. The presence of consolidation is confirmed on films made in the oblique or lateral projections.

The Air Bronchogram. Ordinarily, the smaller bronchi are not well visualized on roentgen films because their walls are thin and there is no contrast between the density of the air within the bronchi and that of the surrounding, aerated lung. When the air in the alveoli is replaced by exudate, the radiodensity of the involved lung increases. If the bronchi remain patent, the air columns within them stand out as dark, linear bands against the surrounding, homogeneously gray lung (Fig. 110). The presence of an air bronchogram within a shadow in the pulmonary field indicates that the density is due to consolidation of lung.

Borders of the Shadow. Most frequently, the area of consolidation is poorly delimited from the adjacent lung except where it abuts on a fissure lying in a plane parallel to the rays (Fig. 109). On the frontal view, the lower border of a consolidated anterior segment of the right upper lobe, which is limited by the short fissure, appears as a sharp, straight, horizontal line (Fig. 226). Similarly, this fissure will sharply limit the upper boundary of the shadow of a consolidated middle lobe.

On occasion, the entire border of the lesion is fairly well circumscribed, and if only one portion of a segment is involved, the shadow may be round and simulate a neoplasm. In these cases, the clinical history and the rapid change in the size and appearance of the shadow within a few

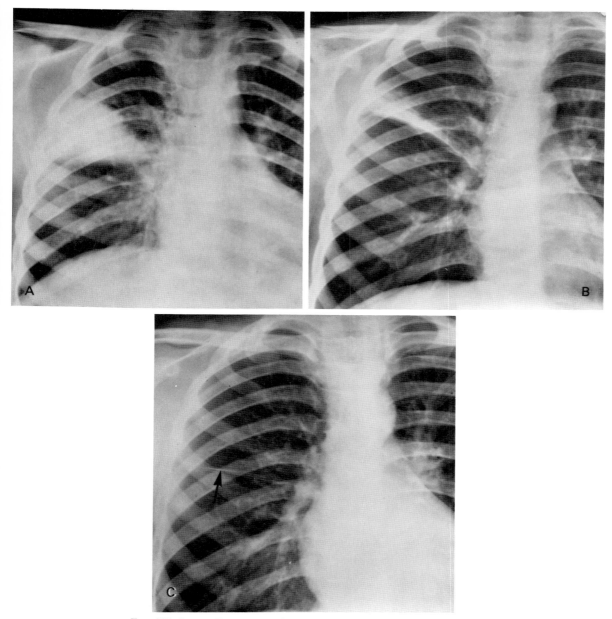

FIG. 226. LOBAR PNEUMONIA: ANTERIOR SEGMENT, RIGHT UPPER LOBE

A: The consolidation involves most of the axillary portion of the anterior segment of the right upper lobe. The inferior border of the consolidated lung is bounded by the short fissure which extends from the third space in the mesial portion of the chest to the fourth rib in the anterior axillary region. *B:* During resolution, the anterior segment has become partially atelectatic because of plugging of many of the small bronchi by exudate. The short fissure is elevated and now follows the course of the anterior part of the third rib. The fissure was able to shift because of the absence of parietal adhesions. *C:* After complete resolution, the right upper lobe appears normal. The short fissure (arrow), which is outlined by pleural adhesions, has returned to its normal position, indicating that the lobe has completely reexpanded.

days make the diagnosis quite clear (Figs. 227 and 232).

For complete delineation of the distribution of the disease, the lateral view is required as well as the frontal. This projection will show the rela-

tionship of the area of consolidation to the long fissure which delimits the posterior segment of the upper lobe, the middle lobe or lingula, and the anterobasal and medial basal segments of the lower lobe. Usually, in one of these views, the

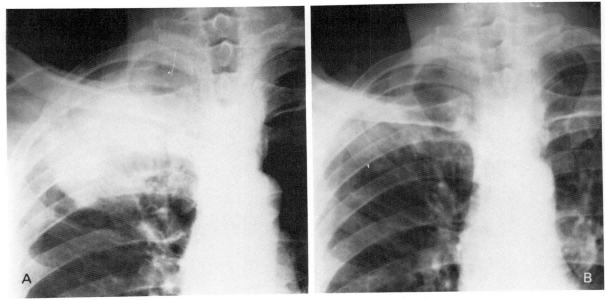

FIG. 227. LOBAR PNEUMONIA: RIGHT UPPER LOBE

A: The homogeneous shadow in the right upper lobe simulates that of a neoplasm because of its round, circumscribed border. It represents consolidation of the apical and posterior segments of the lobe. This is an unusual distribution of lobar pneumonia because the anterior segment is spared. *B:* Eight days later, there has been partial resolution and the remaining disease is confined to the outer part of the posterior segment of the upper lobe. The shadow is mottled because of irregular resolution and the appearance suggests tuberculosis. Subsequent films showed complete clearing. Although a film made at any one stage of the disease can mimic other conditions, the correct diagnosis of lobar pneumonia becomes obvious when serial films are available.

consolidated area shows a triangular shape with its apex directed toward the lung root and its base along the chest wall or diaphragm (Fig. 51).

Segmental Distribution. In most cases, the roentgen examination of the chest in lobar pneumonia is first made when only one or two segments of a lobe are consolidated. If adequate antibiotic treatment is given, no further spread takes place. Most often, the basal segments of the lower lobes are the ones involved at the onset (Fig. 228), but it is not uncommon for the disease to begin in the superior segment of the lower lobe (Fig. 229). When the disease originates in the upper lobe, the anterior segment is usually first involved. Primary involvement of the posterior segment is less common (Fig. 109) but it is the next segment to be affected if the disease is permitted to progress. The apical segment is usually spared, even when the remainder of the upper lobe is entirely consolidated and the disease has progressed to involve other lobes of the lung. It is unusual for the middle lobe to be consolidated if the lower lobe is not already involved. As a rule, when the anterior segment of the left upper lobe is consolidated, the lingular segment is also affected.

Lobar Consolidation. In untreated cases, the disease extends rapidly to neighboring segments so that soon most or all of an entire lobe is consolidated. In the lower lobes, usually all of the basal segments are involved but the superior segment may be spared for a time. The apical portion of the upper lobe is usually free of consolidation.

It has often been stated that the completely consolidated lobe is larger than a normal lobe. This impression is gained from the following observations: (1) The fact that the diseased lobe appears larger at postmortem examination than the rest of the lung; (2) on microscopic examination the alveoli, containing exudate, are widely distended while the remaining alveoli, containing air, appear small, and (3) because on roentgen examination a consolidated lobe appears to occupy more of the chest than it should.

There is a fallacy in the conclusion that is drawn from each of these observations. At postmortem examination, the consolidated lobe remains distended and therefore appears to be enlarged because it is compared with the smaller, normal lobes which are largely collapsed. If the remainder of the lung is inflated, the consolidated lobe no longer appears abnormal in size. This is also the cause of the disparity between

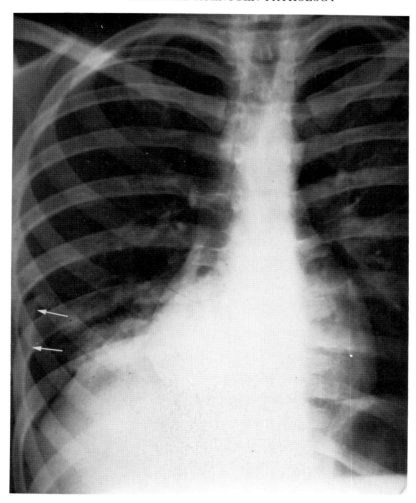

FIG. 228. LOBAR PNEUMONIA: BASAL SEGMENTS, RIGHT LOWER LOBE

The posterior and lateral basal segments of the right lower lobe are consolidated. The right cardiac border is clearly visible. The right leaf of the diaphragm is elevated and there is a small collection of exudate over the right lower lobe. This appears as a narrow density running upward over the outer portion of the lobe and extending into the long fissure (arrows).

the size of the alveoli as seen on microscopic examination. The involved alveoli are distended by exudate while the air-containing alveoli are partly collapsed. If sections are made after the lungs have been fixed in the inflated state, there does not appear to be much difference in size. The impression of an abnormally large, consolidated lobe gained from the roentgen film is due to comparison with the remaining aerated lobe on the same side. This comparison does not take into account the fact that the diaphragm on the affected side is usually elevated to a considerable degree so that the remaining air-containing lobe is not fully distended in inspiration.

A more reliable indication of the size of an affected lobe is the contour of its fissural surface. If the lobe were actually enlarged, its borders would be rounded and its fissural surface would bulge. However, at necropsy, the fissural surface appears flat and the edges of the involved lung adjacent to the fissure are not blunted. Likewise, on the roentgen film, there is no evidence of bulging of the fissure toward the adjacent normal lobe. In fact, when the upper lobe is consolidated, the short fissure is apt to be somewhat elevated above its normal position at the level of the fourth rib (Fig. 226). In consolidation of the lower lobe, the lateral film usually shows the long fissure displaced backward. In other words, the involved lobe, if anything, is somewhat smaller in size than the normally aerated lobes.

Spread to Other Lobes. In rapidly progressing cases of lobar pneumonia and in those where treatment has not been instituted promptly, the

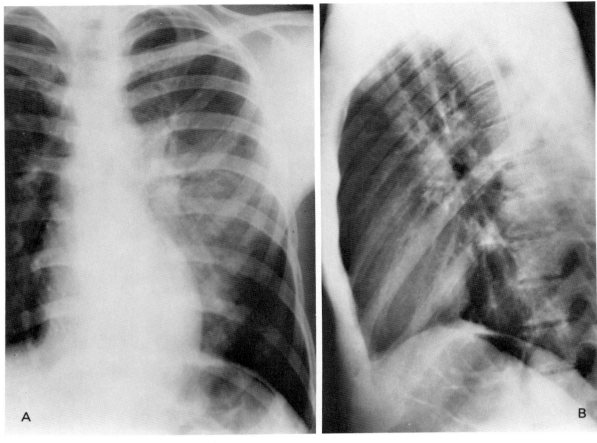

FIG. 229. LOBAR PNEUMONIA: SUPERIOR AND SUBAPICAL SEGMENTS, LEFT LOWER LOBE

A: Frontal view. The distribution of the consolidation in the left lung seems to correspond to the anterior and lingular segments of the upper lobe. However, the clear demarcation of the left cardiac border indicates that the upper lobe, which lies adjacent to the heart, is well aerated. It must be concluded, therefore, that the consolidation involves the superior and subapical segments of the lower lobe. The clear area at the outer part of the left base corresponds to the aerated anterior and lateral basal segments of the lobe. *B:* Lateral view. The abnormality is easily overlooked on the lateral projection. However, the increased density of the midthoracic vertebrae is indicative of an overlying lesion. The remainder of the consolidated area is projected behind the spine.

consolidation often extends into a neighboring lobe. The usual spread of pneumonia from the upper lobe is to the superior segment of the lower lobe. The roentgen appearance in the frontal projection is rather characteristic when the right lung is involved in this manner. A uniform density is projected over the right upper lobe or its lower two-thirds. The lower portion of this shadow is delineated by a sharp border, representing the lateral portion of the short fissure. Mesially, this sharp demarcation is lost. Here the shadow of the consolidation continues downward from the lower mesial portion of the right upper lobe to the region of the lung root. This part of the shadow, caused by consolidation of the apex of the right lower lobe, is poorly demarcated from the remainder of the lower lobe. On the left

side, involvement of the apex of the lower lobe is usually not recognizable on the frontal view because there is no short fissure and the uppermost portion of the lower lobe is hidden by the consolidated lingular segment.

When an area of consolidation is situated in the mesial portion of the lower chest, it may be difficult to determine its exact location from the frontal film alone. The shadow may represent consolidation either in the lower lobe or in the right middle lobe or lingular segment of the left upper lobe. This is easily resolved by making an additional film in the lateral projection.

In many cases, this determination is possible from the frontal projection alone. The borders of the heart are normally sharply outlined on the frontal film because of the contrast between the density of the heart and the adjacent air-filled lung. In the absence of a pleural effusion, obscuration of even a small part of a cardiac border indicates an absence of air in the adjacent lung. Obliteration of the right cardiac border is caused by involvement of the middle lobe, obliteration of the left cardiac border, by the lingular segment. If the cardiac borders can be seen through the shadow of the consolidated lung, the disease must be limited to a lower lobe (Fig. 229). The dome of the diaphragm is clearly outlined when the consolidation involves only the right middle lobe. The lingular portion of the left upper lobe has a fairly broad base on the diaphragm and in some cases of consolidation of this segment, the diaphragmatic contour is lost. Conversely, it is possible for the silhouette of the diaphragm to remain well outlined when the consolidation is limited to a lower lobe. On the left side, this is due to the aeration of the lingular segment, while on the right side, the long fissure may be displaced backward, thus increasing the area of contact between the aerated middle lobe and the diaphragm.

If the middle lobe or the lingular segment of the left upper lobe is consolidated together with the corresponding lower lobe, a dense, homogeneous shadow is produced, which merges imperceptibly with the diaphragm as well as with the heart. This shadow can simulate a pleural effusion. Differentiation usually can be accomplished by examination in the oblique and lateral projections. If these fail to show the characteristic ascending course of the shadow of fluid along the posterior outer portion of the chest, an effusion is unlikely. Lateral decubitus films which do not show any significant change in appearance of the shadow in the lung, serve further to exclude the possibility of pleural effusion.

Spread of the infection may result in consolidation of an entire lung, although the apex is usually spared. This produces a picture simulating a large pleural effusion. Although an effusion of this size almost always displaces the mediastinum to the opposite side, this is not a conclusive differential feature because the mediastinum can remain in the midline if the effusion is associated with underlying atelectasis of the lung, as in bronchial obstruction due to a carcinoma. If one of the basal segments of the lung is spared, the diagnosis of consolidation is usually clear (Fig. 230), but if the entire hemithorax is opacified, the correct roentgen diagnosis may not be apparent until resolution begins to set in. Differentiation from a large pleural effusion is simpler when the disease is situated on the left side, particularly if the colon or stomach is distended

with gas. This serves to localize the undersurface of the diaphragm. In the case of a large effusion, these organs should be depressed. If not, it may be concluded that the homogeneous shadow in the left chest is caused by consolidation rather than fluid (see Fig. 286).

Most often, when an entire lung is opacified the diagnosis of pneumonia is indicated by the fact that the opposite lung shows one or more areas of consolidation. This frequently does not take the form of a segmental or lobar consolidation, the disease more often being *lobular* in distribution. The shadows, therefore, are usually multiple and small in size, and represent collections of contiguous lobules filled with exudate. The borders of these consolidated areas are generally ill-defined.

Stage of Resolution. The time of the crisis in lobar pneumonia does not usher in so dramatic a change in the roentgen appearance as it does in the condition of the patient. Resolution does begin at this time, whether the crisis is a natural one or induced by drugs, but it occurs gradually. Although resolution may be complete within a few days if only a small area of lung was involved, some evidence of consolidation usually remains for a week, and two or three weeks may elapse after the temperature drops before the lung returns to normal.

During the stage of resolution, the homogeneity of the shadow of consolidation is lost and it becomes mottled as the exudate in various portions of the affected lung is absorbed and alveoli here and there are filled with air. Although the alveolar exudate is absorbed through the lymphatics, many small bronchi remain plugged by cellular and fibrinous exudate and the corresponding portions of the lung become atelectatic. The pathologic picture, then, consists of intermingled areas of consolidation of varying degree, aeration of the alveoli and areas of atelectasis. The latter are often represented on the film by streak-like shadows (Fig. 231). These shadows disappear as the lung reexpands and resolution is completed (Fig. 226).

The roentgen appearance during the stage of resolution has little to identify it with lobar pneumonia (Fig. 232). It is not difficult to make the correct diagnosis if previous films made during the stage of consolidation are available, or if the clinical history is taken into consideration. In the absence of this information, the roentgen appearance is confusing. The only aid in the diagnosis of lobar pneumonia may be the tendency to lobar distribution of the disease and the progressive resolution of the process as determined from later examinations.

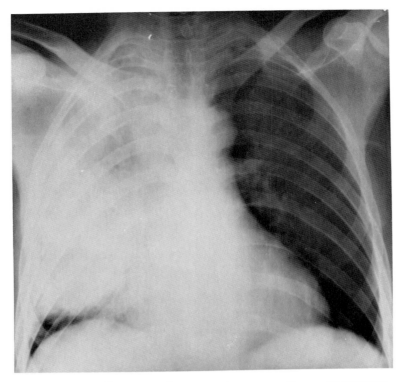

FIG. 230. LOBAR PNEUMONIA INVOLVING ALMOST THE ENTIRE RIGHT LUNG

The entire right lung is consolidated with the exception of a small portion at the base. The patient was observed before antibiotics were available. Today, the disease is almost always checked before it causes such extensive consolidation. A film made 12 days later showed complete restitution to normal.

When the lower lobes are the seat of the disease, the roentgen picture during this stage suggests bronchial rather than lobar pneumonia. The shadows are mottled and the blood vessels are usually drawn together because of the atelectasis due to obstruction of many of the smaller bronchi. When the disease is situated in the anterior segment of the upper lobe, this problem does not arise because bronchial pneumonia is rarely confined to this segment unless there is an underlying obstructive lesion in a large bronchus.

When only the posterior segment of an upper lobe is involved, it is impossible, from the single examination, to exclude tuberculosis from consideration (Fig. 231). A positive diagnosis of lobar pneumonia can be made only when subsequent films show rapid resolution. An additional problem in the diagnosis of resolving lobar penumonia results from the presence of localized areas of aeration within the consolidated region, suggesting cavitation. This may lead to a mistaken diagnosis of suppurative bronchopneumonia or tuberculosis. The diagnosis of a cavity should not be made unless the border surrounding an area of lucency is complete, or if there is a well-defined

fluid level. When there is question of cavitation, it is advisable to repeat the roentgen examination after a few days. By that time the appearance of the lungs will have changed and the suggestion of cavitation disappeared if the case is one of resolving lobar pneumonia.

The process of resolution continues until the lung returns to normal. At this time, the chest films should show no residual changes except for evidence of pleural adhesions. Resolution may be delayed for a considerable interval if treatment has been inadequate, but eventually all shadows disappear if the diagnosis of lobar pneumonia was correct. If an error is to be avoided, the x-ray examination should be repeated until the lungs are completely clear.

Complications. The three complications of lobar pneumonia that are manifested radiologically are pleuritis, pericarditis and aputrid necrosis.

PLEURITIS. Pleurisy occurs early in the disease and the pain it causes is usually one of the first symptoms. In the beginning, only a thin layer of fibrinous exudate covers the pleura and this may not be recognizable radiologically. However, the

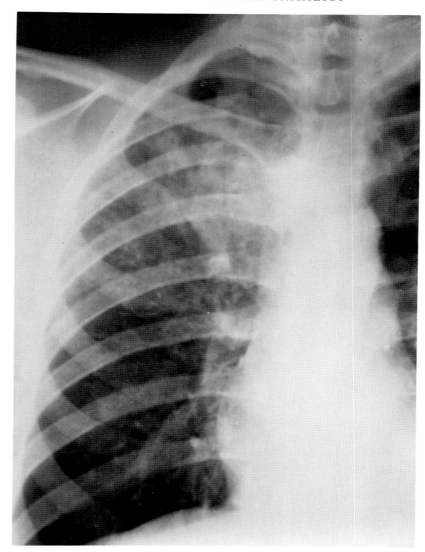

FIG. 231. LOBAR PNEUMONIA: STAGE OF RESOLUTION

The irregular shadows in the right upper lobe suggest a tuberculous lesion. Although the diagnosis of resolving pneumonia may be quite evident clinically, it cannot be made roentgenologically without serial films.

irritation of the pleura limits respiratory excursion. The diaphragm tends to be elevated and its range of movement is decreased.

As the fibrinous layer becomes thicker, it outlines the interlobar fissures. The short fissure appears as a sharp, horizontal line on both the frontal and lateral views, while the long fissure is visualized as an oblique line on the lateral projection. Frequently, the fibrinoplastic exudate forms a dense coat on the surface of the lung. This is manifested on the chest film by a long, narrow strip of increased density along the lateral border of the pulmonary field, adjacent to the chest wall and sharply demarcated from the lung.

It is best seen on the frontal view, particularly when the lower lobe is involved. The density often extends upward from the diaphragm along the outer surface of the consolidated lower lobe into the long fissure. In the frontal projection, the exudate in the fissure casts a faint shadow which usually has a characteristic shape. The density over the lateral portion of the lobe arches upward and mesially and gradually narrows as it progresses toward the apex of the lobe (Fig. 228).

The strip of fibrinoplastic exudate becomes wider as the pleurisy progresses, and an effusion may form. This first obliterates the costophrenic sinus and then merges with the shadow of the

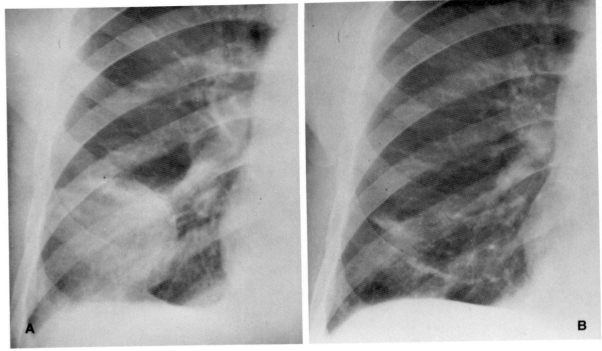

FIG. 232. LOBAR PNEUMONIA

A: The sharply demarcated, round shadow in the lateral basal segment of the right lower lobe resembles a peripheral bronchogenic carcinoma. However, the clinical picture was that of a lobar pneumonia which proved to be pneumococcal in origin. *B:* A week later all that remains of the lesion are several areas of discoid atelectasis.

consolidated lower lobe. The fluid may remain clear and finally disappear, even in untreated cases. In patients who receive antibiotics early in the course of the disease, fluid forms rather infrequently, and even when it does, it is usually absorbed rapidly. In cases which have not been treated, the fluid tends to increase and become purulent. However, a free collection of purulent fluid in the pleura (pyothorax) is rare in lobar pneumonia, because by the time pus is formed the effusion is loculated by fibrinous adhesions. The loculated collection of fluid is often poorly demarcated on the roentgen film because its shadow merges with that of the consolidated lung adjacent to it. The sharp border of the empyema becomes clearly outlined as the pneumonia resolves.

The empyema is usually situated in the posterolateral portion of the pleural cavity, immediately above the diaphragm. However, it may be located between the undersurface of the lung and the diaphragm (infrapulmonary empyema), in the mediastinal pleural space, in the subscapular region or even over the apex of the lung.

We have never observed an empyema in lobar pneumonia that was confined to an interlobar fissure. In every case, it has represented an extension of an empyema involving the parietal portion of the pleural cavity. The interlobar component of the empyema is often obscured by the parietal portion, even though the pneumonia in the underlying lung has resolved completely. However, there is always one view, usually the oblique or lateral, in which the interlobar collection is demonstrable.

PERICARDITIS. Since the advent of antibiotics, pericarditis has become an extremely rare complication of lobar pneumonia. Suppurative pericarditis is often associated with only a small effusion that is difficult to detect. When the effusion measures less than 250 cc, it causes little or no enlargement of the cardiac shadow. However, it does tend to produce a straightening of the cardiac border by obliterating the angles between the cardiac chambers, those delineating the pulmonary artery segment, and the angle formed by the root of the aorta and the right border of the heart.

APUTRID NECROSIS. Pneumococcal lobar pneumonia is not a destructive disease. However, cavitation occasionally does occur within the consolidated lung as the result of an arteritis of one of the branches of the pulmonary artery. Thrombosis of the vessel results in infarction of the portion of lung it supplies. Because of the presence of great numbers of leukocytes which form lytic enzymes in the stage of resolution, the necrotic tissue is liquefied. Ordinarily, the necrotic infart does not communicate with an open bronchus. Air cannot enter the lesion and the cavity is not visualized. With time the liquefied material is absorbed. However, if a bronchial communication is established, the material expectorated is replaced by air, and a cavity, often with an air-fluid level, becomes evident. This condition has been termed aputrid necrosis (Figs. 127 and 233). It should not be confused with a true lung abscess. The cavity of aputrid necrosis is generally not important clinically except when it perforates into the pleura, producing either an empyema or a pyopneumothorax. If perforation does not occur, the cavity will close spontaneously within a short time after resolution of

the underlying pneumonia and does not lead to chronic disease. However, if the diagnosis of pneumococcal pneumonia is not certain, the importance of the cavity cannot be ignored because it may be a manifestation of tuberculosis, putrid lung abscess, suppurative bronchopneumonia or even a broken down neoplasm.

Bronchopneumonia

In contradistinction to lobar pneumonia, which begins as a focal area of infection and spreads from alveolus to alveolus and from one pulmonary segment to an adjacent one, bronchopneumonia begins primarily as a bronchial infection and has a tendency to involve separate parts of the lung. In most cases, the pulmonary component of a bronchopneumonia consists largely of areas of consolidation. However, in some forms

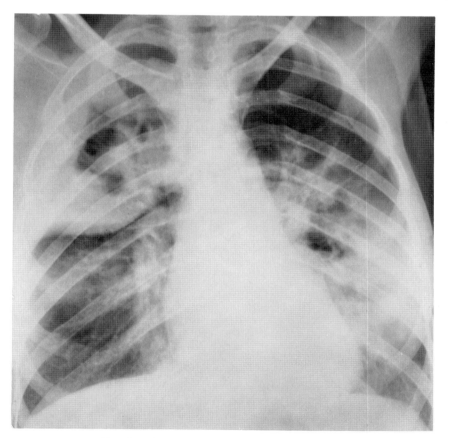

FIG. 233. APUTRID NECROSIS IN LOBAR PNEUMONIA

The pneumonia was due to pneumococcus type III. The films shows a large cavity within the right upper lobe with consolidation of the surrounding lung. The downward bulge of the short fissure is due to ballooning of the cavity. The superior, subapical and posterior basal segments of the left lower lobe are consolidated and there is an irregular cavity in this region. In addition, there is consolidation of the posterior basal segment of the right lower lobe. The fact that the middle lobe and the lingula are free of disease is evidenced by the clear delineation of the outline of the heart. Resolution took place slowly. The cavities disappeared and the lungs appeared normal on a film made 5 weeks later.

of bronchopneumonia, the infection spreads along and through the bronchial walls, and results in infiltration of the interstitial tissues with little involvement of the alveolar air spaces. In most cases, both consolidation and interstitial infiltration are present. In addition, there is often plugging of the smaller bronchi by secretion and exudate resulting from the bronchial inflammation. Frequently, this causes atelectasis which complicates the roentgen picture (Fig. 234). If the pneumonia is caused by destructive organisms, foci of suppuration or even a true abscess may result.

Lobular Bronchopneumonia. This form of bronchopneumonia is characterized by consolidation of collections of lobules in the lungs, with or without changes due to bronchial inflammation. Because the bronchial changes are often slight, there is little, if any, interstitial infiltration or atelectasis. In effect, the process is similar to that of lobar pneumonia, except that the areas of consolidation are scattered and generally small. In some cases, the lobular areas of consolidation become confluent.

Lobular pneumonia is usually due to the pneumococcus or other pyogenic organisms but can be caused by other agents. The roentgen picture consists of irregular, patchy shadows (Figs. 111 and 245). These are of uniform density and fade out at the edges. They involve groups of lobules rather than entire segments. During the course of the disease, the patches may become confluent and produce large areas of consolidation that can simulate lobar pneumonia. Nevertheless, it is often possible to differentiate the two diseases, because in lobular pneumonia the density of the shadow is not completely uniform and there is an absence of characteristic segmental or lobar distribution. Lobular patches of pneumonia may appear during the spread of infection in lobar

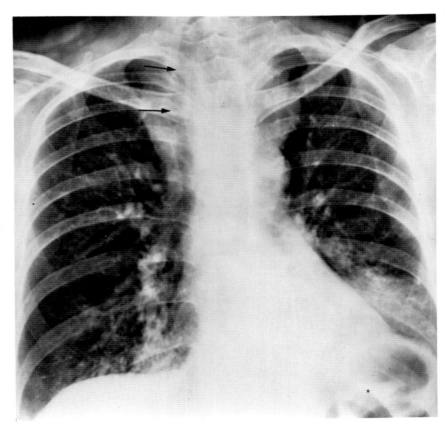

FIG. 234. BRONCHOPNEUMONIA

There is an irregular infiltration which is largely interstitial, involving the mesial part of the right lower lobe, and a rather homogeneous density in the left lower lobe. The left leaf of the diaphragm is elevated. Although the process in the left lower lobe represents a bronchopneumonia similar to that on the right, the shadow is homogeneous because of atelectasis secondary to bronchial obstruction by secretion. Incidentally, there is a mass in the superior mediastinum displacing the trachea to the right (arrows). This is characteristic of a cervicomediastinal goiter.

pneumonia. Most often, the lobular patches are associated with the more characteristic changes of bronchopneumonia, namely, interstitial infiltration and areas of atelectasis in other portions of the lung.

Interstitial Pneumonia. This form of bronchopneumonia involves mainly the tissues around the bronchi and blood vessels and those which compose the interlobular and interalveolar septa. In rare instances, the interstitial tissues are involved in the absence of any bronchial inflammation. This occurs in some cases of mediastinitis in which the infection spreads from the mediastinum by way of the lymphatics and causes an acute lymphangitis of the lung (Fig. 235). We have seen a similar purulent lymphangitis of the lungs as the result of extension from a phlegmonous gastritis. In congenital syphilis, interstitial pneumonia also occurs without a preceding bronchitis. Here, the interstitial pneumonia assumes a chronic form. These are the exceptional cases. In general, interstitial pneumonia is secondary to a bronchial inflammation which involves the depths of the bronchial wall and extends directly to the peribronchial tissues and from here to the remaining interstitial tissues.

Pure interstitial pulmonary inflammation without some lobular consolidation is rare. Frequently, however, the interstitial pneumonia is predominant and little lobular consolidation is seen (Figs. 104 and 236). Acute interstitial pneumonia is most commonly due to a viral infection of the lung. It also occurs in association with lobular consolidation in suppurative bronchopneumonia and in exacerbations of purulent infections complicating bronchiectasis or lung abscess. Chronic interstitial pneumonia is most often associated with chronic bronchial infection, particularly in persons with asthmatic bronchitis. In these cases it is usually associated with emphysema. Chronic interstitial infiltrations are also one of the main features of the dust diseases and of suppurative bronchiectasis in the quiescent stage. Interstitial pneumonia together with more or less extensive lobular consolidation also occurs as a rather characteristic feature of fungous infections.

The roentgen appearance of interstitial pneumonia is characterized by fine, streak-like, or nodular shadows in the lungs. Often, both types of shadows coexist. The fine, linear densities, which are usually rather closely approximated, are easily confused with prominent vascular markings. However, interstitial infiltrations do not show branching, which typifies blood vessels. Rather, they lie between the vessels as well as being superimposed on them. Most often, the streaks are confined to the lower lobes, but the lower lateral portions of the upper lobes are not

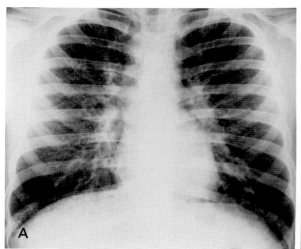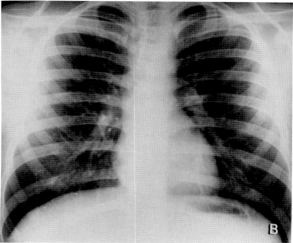

FIG. 235. PURULENT PULMONARY LYMPHANGITIS

A: The film of an acutely ill, 17 year old boy with high fever and acute pharyngitis, shows a generalized increase of the interstitial markings. This is responsible for the increased density of the lung roots and the indistinctness of the vascular shadows in the periphery. Kerley lines are present at the right base. The hilar and right paratracheal lymph nodes are enlarged. In this case the changes were due to a purulent lymphangitis caused by a beta hemolytic streptococcus. A similar picture can occur in sarcoidosis or lymphangitic carcinosis. Viral pneumonia rarely produces sufficient enlargement of the lymph nodes to be detected roentgenologically. *B:* After 9 days of antibiotic treatment the nodes have regressed considerably. The pulmonary vessels are now clearly outlined, indicating that the interstitial lesions have resolved.

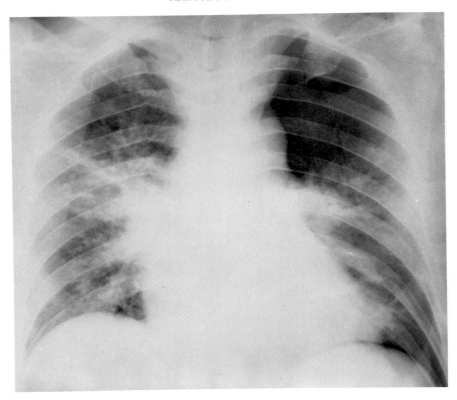

FIG. 236. INTERSTITIAL INFILTRATIONS IN VIRAL PNEUMONIA

Fine and coarse interstitial infiltrations extend outward from the lung roots. In the lower part of the right upper lobe there is an oblique linear streak, representing a focal area of atelectasis due to plugging of a bronchus by secretion. The area of radiolucency in the left upper lobe is caused by a large bulla which antedated the pneumonia. No infiltration is present in this area because of the absence of pulmonary tissue.

infrequently involved. In some cases, the streaks are largely limited to a single segment, while in others several scattered segments of the lung are involved. Both lungs are usually affected in a diffuse manner in the interstitial pneumonia that complicates chronic bronchitis and emphysema.

The nodular infiltrations of interstitial pneumonia represent small localized inflammatory thickenings of the interstitial tissue. The shadows are quite small. Most of them are miliary in size, but they can be as large as a pea.

The more chronic forms of interstitial pneumonia are associated with fibrosis of the interstitial tissues. This produces a roentgen appearance similar to that of acute inflammatory infiltration except that the fibrotic streaks tend to be more sharply outlined.

Small fibrotic areas in the upper lobes due to interstitial pneumonia are easily confused with tuberculosis. The presence of additional similar lesions in the lower lobes and the association with emphysema are generally sufficient to exclude tuberculosis from consideration. It is often

difficult to differentiate between the diffuse form of chronic interstitial pneumonia and lymphangitic carcinosis. This is especially true when the fibrotic pneumonia is associated with contraction of the lung. In most cases of chronic interstitial pneumonia, however, there is hyperinflation of the lung, as evidenced by depression of the diaphragm and limitation of its mobility, and the presence of emphysematous bullae. In addition, there is usually obliteration of the costophrenic sinuses together with other signs of pleural adhesions. In the absence of these changes, diffuse, fine, linear infiltrations with tiny nodules in the lungs, more pronounced toward the roots, are suggestive of lymphangitic carcinosis.

Atelectatic Bronchopneumonia. In many cases of bronchopneumonia, the small bronchi in the inflamed lung become plugged by secretions and by swelling of the bronchial mucous membrane. The segments or portions of the segments supplied by these bronchi may become atelectatic (Fig. 234). The shadow cast by the inflamed atelectatic portion of lung appears homogeneous and simulates consolidation as in lobar or lobular pneumonia. However, the extremely sharp definition of the collapsed and inflamed portion of the lung and its triangular shape, with the apex directed toward the lung root, are indicative of atelectasis (Fig. 237). If the atelectasis is incomplete and some air remains in the affected portion of the lung, the blood vessels within it can be visualized. Their close approximation indicates the loss of lung volume. That there is atelectasis associated with the pneumonia is also indicated by displacement of the pleural fissures or a portion of a fissure toward the lesion. Streak-like shadows (Fleischner lines) within the shadow of the pneumonia indicate atelectasis of small portions of the lung. That the atelectasis is related to a bronchopneumonia is clear when evidences of this disease are found in other parts of the lung.

Special Pathologic Types of Bronchopneumonia. In general, the bronchopneumonias are caused by single, specific organisms and undergo resolution quite promptly, leaving little or no evidence of infection. In certain cases, however, resolution occurs slowly and there is a tendency to complications. These can be caused by a variety of bacteria, many of which are not virulent by themselves but which act in symbiosis to produce serious disease. The rather distinctive pathologic entities that result from this type of infection are suppurative bronchopneumonia, gangrenous bronchopneumonia, and the pneumonia that occurs beyond a bronchial obstruction. Occasionally such a chronic pneumonia is associated with deposition of cholesterol crystals in the lung.

SUPPURATIVE BRONCHOPNEUMONIA. This type of bronchopneumonia is associated with the formation of multiple, purulent foci within the lungs. These may be large or small, but in either case the destruction of pulmonary tissue occurs within a more or less diffusely inflamed portion of lung. The disease is associated with a purulent bronchitis and, in contradistinction to gangrenous bronchopneumonia, the exudate is not foul. The bronchitis is usually quite severe and it frequently is associated with weakening of the musculature of the bronchial wall. This can result in varicose bronchiectasis (Fig. 198). Serial bronchograms in the course of suppurative bronchopneumonia have shown reversion of the bronchi to their normal caliber after recovery from the disease (Fig. 199).

The suppurative disease may be due to a spe-

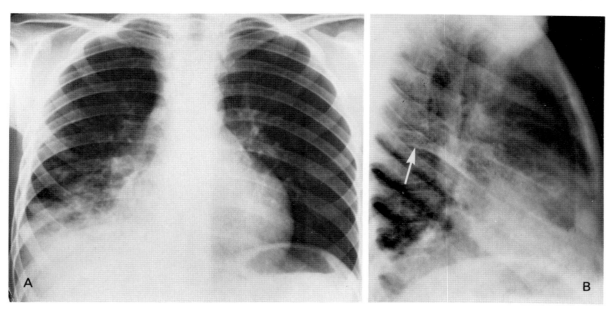

FIG. 237. ATELECTATIC BRONCHOPNEUMONIA

A: Frontal view. The irregular infiltration of the right lower and middle lobes is due to bronchopneumonia. The increase in the density of the triangular area adjacent to the right border of the heart is caused by complete collapse of the basal segments of the right lower lobe. The root of the right lung is depressed because of the atelectasis. *B:* Lateral view. The inflamed, collapsed basal segments of the right lower lobe cast a triangular shadow at the base, obscuring the right leaf of the diaphragm. The long fissure (arrow) is depressed and the well-aerated superior segment of the lower lobe extends downward almost to the diaphragm because of the shrinkage of the basal segments. Faint infiltrations above the anterior part of the long fissure indicate that the bronchopneumonia also involves the middle lobe.

cific organism. In children in whom suppurative bronchopneumonia is particularly common, it is usually caused by the staphylococcus, and in some adults it may be due solely to the Friedländer bacillus. But in general, suppurative bronchopneumonia is due to a mixture of bacteria which singly may be nonpathogenic. It can occur from spread of infection from bronchiectatic cavities, the inhalation of organisms from an esophageal diverticulum, from an esophagotracheal or bronchial fistula, from the inhalation of bacteria from the mouth during anesthesia or submersion, or in diseases that interfere with the normal process of deglutition. Many cases of suppurative bronchopneumonia follow in the wake of a viral infection of the lung, while others occur distal to an obstruction.

Suppurative bronchopneumonia is characterized by interstitial infiltration, lobular consolidation, and a tendency to atelectasis, cavity formation, and pleural complications. In the simplest form, where the suppurative foci are minute, only fine, streak-like and nodular infiltrations may be seen, similar to other acute interstitial pneumonias. The pulmonary markings in the affected region are generally drawn together

to some degree because of small areas of atelectasis, caused by plugging of bronchi with thick exudate. The presence of atelectasis is further manifested by longer, sharply outlined, linear streaks within the lesion. The disease may progress no further than this but resolution of the small purulent foci is generally slow, requiring a few weeks for complete restitution to normal. Usually the atelectatic streaks are the last to disappear.

In more severe cases, areas of lobular consolidation appear (Fig. 238). These often become confluent, especially in children, and may involve an entire lobe in what appears to be uniform consolidation. When an entire lobe is involved, well-marked signs of atelectasis are generally present. The mediastinum is usually shifted toward the lesion and the fissures are displaced in a similar fashion.

In many of the cases showing extensive lobular consolidation, necrosis of a variable degree takes place in one or more segments of the lung and, as the necrotic, purulent material is expectorated, cavities form (Fig. 239). The presence of extensive necrosis of pulmonary tissue in these cases has given rise to the term *necrosuppurative*

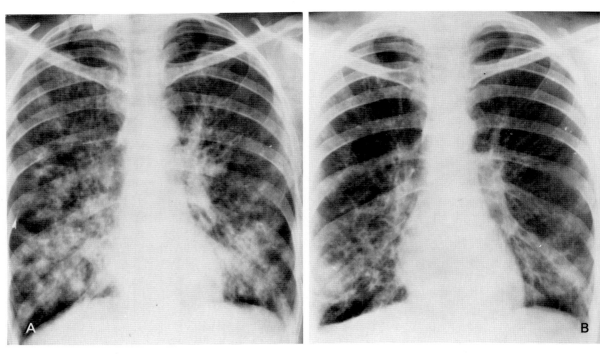

FIG. 238. SUPPURATIVE BRONCHOPNEUMONIA

A: The poorly demarcated nodular shadows in the lower half of each lung represent areas of lobular consolidation. The patient was acutely ill and expectorating purulent sputum. There is coalescence of the lesions on the left side. The patient improved but the lesions never resolved completely. *B:* Four years later. There are chronic infiltrations in the lower part of each lung. On the right side, small round lucencies are visible. These represent sacculated bronchiectases. The right leaf of the diaphragm is flattened and the extreme lung bases are hyperlucent as a result of local bullous emphysema.

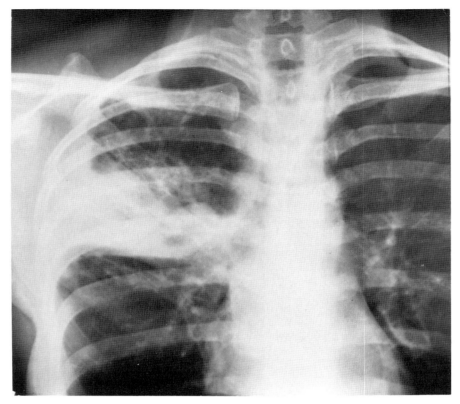

FIG. 239. SUPPURATIVE BRONCHOPNEUMONIA

There is a confluent lobular consolidation of the anterior segment of the right upper lobe. Within the shadow are several areas of increased radiolucency, representing cavities within the consolidated lung. The short fissure, which sharply delimits the lower border of the inflamed segment, is slightly elevated, indicating that the lesion is associated with some degree of atelectasis.

bronchopneumonia. The first manifestation of cavitation is the appearance of irregular areas of increased aeration within the consolidated region. In contradistinction to a putrid lung abscess, the cavities are multiple, even in the early stages of the disease, and lie within areas of diffuse bronchopneumonia (Fig. 240). They should not be considered abscesses. True abscesses are characterized by localization of the inflammatory process to the wall surrounding the purulent collection, while in suppurative bronchopneumonia, the cavities represent purulent foci within the diffusely inflamed lung.

Many of the small cavities disappear quite promptly. Others may increase rapidly in size as they become ballooned out by the accumulation of air within them. This occurs when the exudate in the communicating bronchus acts as a check-valve (Fig. 240). As the pneumonia about these ballooning cavities resolves, the retraction of the torn elastic tissue of the lung enlarges them even more (Fig. 128). The cavities then present as thin-walled annular shadows, appearing like large air cysts. These usually disappear spontaneously when the entering bronchus becomes strictured at its junction with the cavity. If the bronchi remain open, the air cysts persist indefinitely (Fig. 130).

Not infrequently a subpleural suppurative focus causes pleurisy with effusion. The pleural fluid is clear or only slightly cloudy if the infection does not extend into the pleural cavity *(sympathetic effusion)*. If the suppurative focus perforates into the pleura, it is usually walled off by adhesions and an empyema results. If a patent bronchus communicates with the suppurative focus, a pyopneumothorax usually develops. Any of these pleural complications can occur early in the disease and overshadow the pulmonary lesion completely. However, it is important that the underlying focus be recognized because it frequently determines the course of the disease and the manner in which the empyema should be handled.

Occasionally the pneumonia and the smaller suppurative foci resolve, leaving a single, sizeable

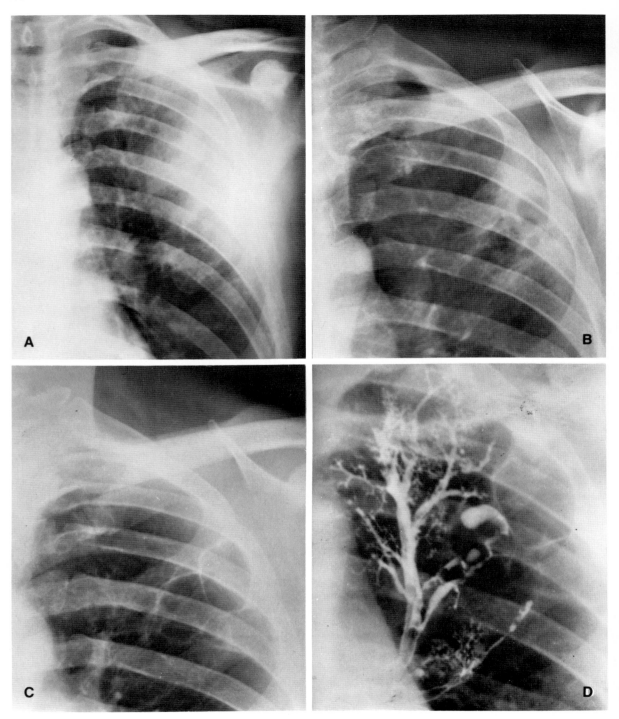

FIG. 240. SUPPURATIVE BRONCHOPNEUMONIA IN ASTHMA

A: The patient developed the typical picture of suppurative bronchopneumonia following an acute attack of bronchial asthma. The subscapular part of the posterior segment of the left upper lobe is consolidated. The homogeneity of the shadow is due to confluence of lobular areas of consolidation. *B:* Considerable resolution of the pneumonia has taken place. At least two cavities can now be seen within the lesion. *C:* Five weeks later. The pneumonia has completely cleared, leaving behind only a series of pneumatoceles. These form because of check valve obstruction of the tiny bronchi entering the area of necrosis. They are characteristically thin-walled and empty, identical to air cysts considered to be congenital. *D:* The bronchogram of the left upper lobe shows filling of one cavity by way of the posterior segmental bronchus. The thin-walled cavities lateral to this are not outlined because their bronchial communications are too small for passage of the oil. The size of the cavities is due to ballooning which occurred because of the small caliber of the entering bronchi, rather than to extensive destruction of lung tissue.

cavity, which has not drained its contents through the bronchi. This produces a rather round, homogeneous shadow with a fairly well demarcated border. Since the lesion consists of a localized collection of pus surrounded by a limited wall of inflammation, it now represents a true lung abscess. Such a nonputrid abscess of the lung is uncommon.

When host resistance is low or treatment is inadequate, a suppurative bronchopneumonia can become chronic. The disease is most apt to persist in the lower lobes and in the lingular segment, from which bronchial drainage is poor. Persistence of the infection results in a weakening of the walls and permits them to become overstretched. The diseased, widened bronchi communicate with the suppurative foci in the lung, giving rise to the formation of sacculated bronchiectases.

During the course of the suppurative bronchopneumonia, while the bronchiectases are forming, many small bronchi are destroyed. Simultaneously, fibrous tissue is laid down in the interstitial tissues of the lung. Because of the obliteration of the small bronchi, the affected portion of the lung becomes atelectatic. The fibrous tissue deposited in the atelectatic lung prevents it from reexpanding even when the acute inflammation resolves. It is for this reason that bronchiectasis is often associated with permanent atelectasis of the lung (Fig. 241).

Despite the rather extensive changes caused by suppurative bronchopneumonia, it is usually not a prolonged or disabling disease and serious complications are infrequent. In most of the cases, even in those that are complicated by extensive cavitation early in the disease, restitution to normal takes place. Even when fairly extensive bronchiectasis has occurred, the lung may clear completely and the dilated bronchi return to their normal caliber (Fig. 199).

After complete resolution of the inflammation, there usually is no abnormality discernible on the films. In some cases there remains simply a drawing together of the pulmonary markings or one or more fine scars in a portion of the lung. In others, there is some bronchial dilatation but this cannot be discovered without bronchography. Finally, there may be some reduction of lung volume which causes permanent displacement of the mediastinum or interlobar fissure toward the lesion, particularly in patients who have developed a moderate degree of pleural thickening which imprisons the lung.

GANGRENOUS BRONCHOPNEUMONIA. Gangrenous bronchopneumonia occurs in two forms, localized and diffuse. The localized form is the precursor of a putrid lung abscess. It is due to the inhalation of particulate matter contaminated with a mixture of anaerobic organisms. If the aspirated material becomes impacted in a segmental bronchus or one of its branches, a localized area of consolidation occurs in that portion of the lung. Within a week after the onset, practically the entire consolidated area forms a gangrenous slough. This later becomes liquefied and is expectorated, leaving a foul abscess cavity surrounded by a limited wall of inflammatory tissue.

Diffuse gangrenous bronchopneumonia results from the simultaneous infection of many portions of the lung by material containing anaerobic organisms. Numerous gangrenous foci develop, some of which liquefy to form cavities. The diffuse involvement of the bronchi is due to massive inhalation of liquid material, most commonly from a putrid abscess of the lung. It may also be caused by submersion or by perforation of the esophagus into the trachea or one of the main bronchi. A diffuse gangrenous bronchopneumonia sometimes occurs in alcoholics. Here it is due to the inhalation of vomitus in a patient with a foul infection of the gums during a period of drunken stupor. Gangrenous bronchopneumonia that is limited to one of the lower lobes can be caused by perforation of a subphrenic abscess which communicates with either the stomach or the intestine.

While gangrenous bronchopneumonia is really lobular in distribution, the consolidated foci may be confluent by the time the roentgen examination is made. In this case there may be nothing to distinguish the shadow of the localized form of the disease from that of lobar pneumonia (see Fig. 270). A helpful feature may be the location of the lesion which, in gangrenous bronchopneumonia, is most often situated in either the apex of the lower lobe or the outer portion of the anterior or posterior segment of the upper lobe. When there is uniform consolidation of either of these segments and a history suggesting the possibility of aspiration, or when the clinical picture does not suggest lobar pneumonia, a gangrenous pneumonia, which will develop into a putrid abscess unless treated, must be considered.

Generally, the area of consolidation remains unchanged in size for a week or so after the onset. Then, within a short time, a fluid level usually appears within the diseased segment, indicating the presence of a lung abscess.

The diffuse form of gangrenous bronchopneumonia cannot be differentiated from suppurative bronchopneumonia by the roentgen findings alone. The diagnosis of gangrenous broncho-

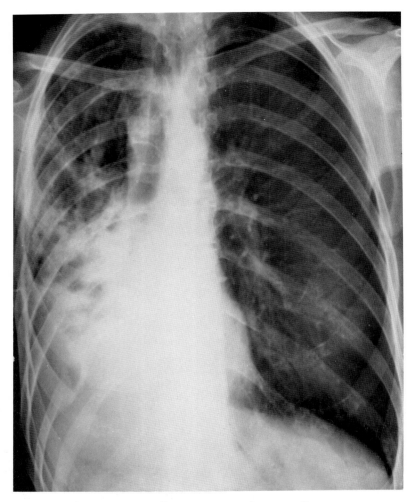

FIG. 241. ATELECTASIS IN BRONCHIECTASIS: ACQUIRED DEXTROCARDIA

This 20 year old patient had a suppurative bronchopneumonia and empyema in childhood. There is dense infiltration of the right lower and middle lobes and the lower part of the upper lobe. The irregular areas of radiolucency within the diseased lung represent large sacculated bronchiectases. The heart and mediastinal structures are displaced to the right, the right chest is diminished in volume, and the trachea pursues a straight downward course. These are characteristic signs of atelectasis of the lower lobe when its outer portion is adherent to the chest wall. The atelectasis and bronchiectasis undoubtedly date back to the time of the original suppurative bronchopneumonia.

pneumonia is clear if areas of consolidation with or without cavitation occur during the course of a subacute or chronic lung abscess. It should also be suspected if such shadows appear in a patient with carcinoma of the esophagus or a subphrenic abscess.

PNEUMONIAS SECONDARY TO BRONCHIAL OBSTRUCTION (OBSTRUCTIVE PNEUMONIA). It has been mentioned that suppurative bronchopneumonia is often complicated by atelectasis because of the obstruction of bronchi by thick secretion. Conversely, obstruction of bronchi from any cause frequently leads to secondary infection and pneumonia which is often suppurative in type. It would appear difficult to differentiate radiologically between a pneumonia complicated by secondary obstruction and obstructive disease complicated by pneumonia. However, the differentiation can usually be made.

In obstructive pneumonia, the pulmonary infection is confined to that portion of the lung supplied by the obstructed bronchus. If additional pneumonic foci are present, it is most likely that the disease process is a bronchopneumonia complicated by atelectasis rather than a primary obstructive lesion. The possibility of a pneumonia beyond a bronchial obstruction must be considered whenever the area of atelectatic pneumonia is confined to a single bronchopulmonary segment, adjacent segments, or a lobe of the lung. However, the final diagnosis can be made only if the obstructive cause is visualized. Thus, a large mediastinal tumor or aneurysm compressing a bronchus, a dense, persistent infiltration about the lung root representing a bronchogenic carcinoma, or a radiopaque foreign body or broncholith within a bronchus would indicate that the atelectatic, inflamed area is secondary to the obstruction.

Bronchial obstruction as the cause of a pneumonia rather than the reverse, may be inferred with some degree of reliability if the pneumonia persists despite adequate treatment or if it recurs in exactly the same area (see Fig. 416). However, persistence of an atelectatic pneumonia or recurrence of the lesion may be due to chronic inflammation associated with bronchiectasis. This possibility merits serious consideration only if the localized inflammatory lesion is situated at the base of a lower lobe. In any event, persistence or recurrence of the pneumonia warrants further investigation. If bronchoscopy fails to disclose an obstructive lesion, bronchography is indicated (Fig. 190).

Abscess formation and bronchiectasis are common complications in pneumonia secondary to bronchial obstruction (Figs. 20 and 70). The possibility of an underlying bronchial obstruction must therefore always be considered in cases of chronic lung abscess and bronchiectasis. However, a distortion of the bronchi in these conditions may cause some difficulty in interpretation and it is possible to overlook an obstruction of one of the larger bronchi unless the bronchograms show all of the bronchi clearly.

If bronchiectases have been present for any considerable length of time distal to an obstructive lesion, they remain permanently. They may persist even though the cause of the obstruction, whether it be a foreign body, a broncholith or benign tumor, is removed. While the roentgen shadow may then become less dense, it usually persists because of a complicating fibrosis and atelectasis. Nevertheless, the active infection usually clears and cough and expectoration generally disappear even though the infection behind the obstruction has been present for a long time. On the other hand, the infection of nonobstructive suppurative bronchiectasis is apt to persist unless antibiotics are given, and even then it has a tendency to recur at intervals. This difference in behavior between the infection that occurs in simple suppurative bronchiectasis and that which is associated with bronchial obstruction, is noteworthy. Apparently the defenses of the patient against infection in simple suppurative bronchiectasis are insufficient to eliminate the infectious agents while the important factor in maintaining the infection in the lung distal to an obstruction is the obstruction itself.

CHOLESTEROL PNEUMONIA. The pathologic examination of the specimens in chronic forms of pneumonia sometimes discloses cholesterol deposits in the inflamed lung. Grossly, these are manifested by the presence of typical bright yellow, refractile areas in the indurated, fibrotic pulmonary tissue. The lipoid deposits occur particularly in cases of bronchial obstruction, bronchiectasis and chronic lung abscess. The occurrence of extensive cholesterol deposition in only some of these cases suggests that there may be an underlying disturbance in cholesterol metabolism. Beyond this, however, the presence of the cholesterol in the tissues simply suggests that the patient has a chronic form of pneumonia associated with destruction of pulmonary tissue or bronchial obstruction. There is no roentgen characteristic by which the presence of cholesterol deposits can be recognized.

Recurrent Pneumonias. Mention has been made of recurrences of pneumonia distal to bronchial obstruction. Similar recurrences of pneumonia in the same place frequently occur in bronchiectasis. However, here, as well as in chronic lung abscess, pneumonias may occur in other portions of the lung as the result of spillover infections. Recurrent pneumonias in various parts of the lungs are common in a variety of conditions. They are apt to occur in the case of excessive or thick bronchial secretions which cause obstruction in the small bronchi. Such pneumonias are usually associated with areas of atelectasis or emphysema and frequently lead to chronic infection and interstitial fibrosis. Cystic fibrosis of the pancreas is classically associated with this type of recurrent pneumonia. Thickened bronchial secretions also occur in Sjögren's syndrome. Increased secretions that are not properly expectorated are the cause of obstruction in the small bronchi in the Riley-Day syndrome. This is characterized by a disorder of autonomic function, excessive perspiration and salivation and hyporeflexia. The x-ray films show evidences of lobar, segmental or focal atelectasis or emphysema. These may be due simply to complete or partial bronchial obstruction, or recurrent areas of consolidation which vary from submiliary nodules representing consolidation of acini to larger, patchy areas of consolidation, representing disease of groups of lobules or portions of bronchopulmonary segments. Atelectatic foci may persist for several weeks. Recurrent infections may result in chronic interstitial fibrosis similar to that which takes place in cystic fibrosis (Fig. 242).

Recurrent infections of the lung occur as the result of aspiration from the esophagus in achalasia, esophageal diverticula, tracheoesophageal fistula or abnormalities in the swallowing mechanism, such as occur in a variety of neurological and muscular disorders.

Defects in the immune mechanism also predispose to recurrent pneumonias. The most common examples of these are hypo- or agammaglobulinemia, dysgammaglobulinemia and the Wiskott-Aldrich syndrome. The latter is a congenital

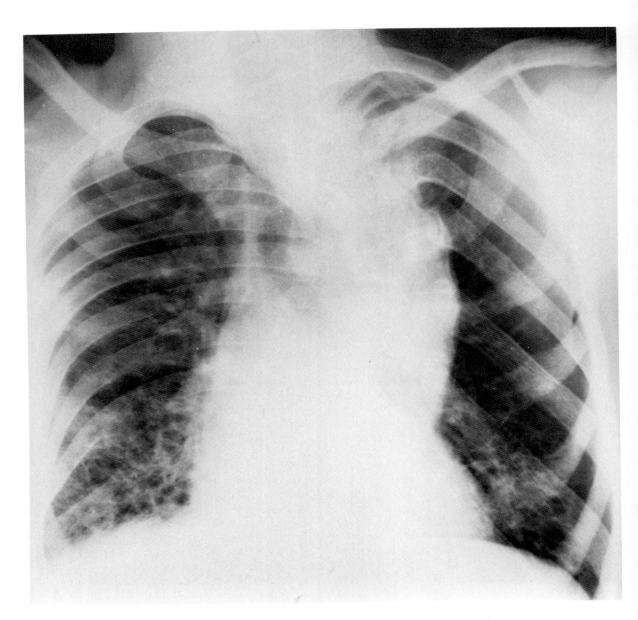

FIG. 242. RILEY-DAY SYNDROME

The patient was a 23 year old male with a history of multiple pulmonary infections. The fibrosis of the lower lobes is the result of repeated bronchopulmonary infections with inflammatory thickening of the interstitial tissues. The honeycomb appearance on the right side is caused by foci of emphysema interspersed with areas of atelectasis and fibrosis. There is marked scoliosis of the dorsal spine with the convexity to the left.

immunologic defect with a tendency to other infections as well as recurrent pneumonia together with thrombocytopenia.

Specific Infections of the Lungs

In the foregoing section, the result of infection on the lung was considered from the standpoint of roentgen changes in the different pathologic types of pneumonia without consideration of the etiology. The pathologic manifestations of inflammatory disease of the lung depend on several factors. Among them are the immunity or susceptibility of the patient and the agent that causes the infection. From the clinical standpoint, the etiology of the disease is extremely important. In many instances, the roentgen changes are sufficiently characteristic to suggest a specific etiologic agent. This is especially true if these findings are correlated with the clinical manifestations.

Infections of the lungs will be discussed according to the nature of the infecting agents: (1) infections caused by bacteria, (2) spirochetal, viral and rickettsial infections, (3) the fungous diseases, protozoan infections and parasitic infestations.

Bacterial Infections. Some bacteria tend to cause a more or less characteristic response when they infect the lung. Thus, the pneumococcus regularly produces consolidation rather than infiltration and is the common cause of lobar pneumonia, although it may also cause lobular consolidation. The tubercle bacillus produces characteristic pathologic alterations in the lung which are represented by corresponding roentgen manifestations from which the disease can usally be recognized. Tuberculous infections of the lung will be discussed in a separate section. The remaining specific bacterial infections will be discussed under the headings of the individual organisms.

STAPHYLOCOCCUS AUREUS. The *Staphylococcus aureus* may cause infection in the lungs either through the bronchi or the blood stream. Bronchogenic infection is the more common and causes the typical picture of suppurative bronchopneumonia, while hematogenous infection results in the formation of one or more abscesses in the lungs.

The *bronchogenic* infection occurs most commonly in infants and children, usually without evidence of any preceding illness. In adults, however, staphylococcal infection of the lungs is generally superimposed upon a viral infection, or it occurs in patients who have diabetes or a debi-litating disease. It may also appear as a postoperative complication or in patients with a tracheostomy.

In general, the pathologic process is that described in the section on Suppurative Bronchopneumonia (p. 289) and the roentgen picture is characterized by areas of consolidation, infiltration, cavitation and atelectasis, often with secondary involvement of the pleura. While the pneumonia usually begins in one portion of the lung, it tends to spread through the bronchi to involve other lobes, but frequently remains localized to one lung. In infants and young children the disease is apt to be more extensive than in adults. Cavities appear early in the course, producing multiple areas of lucency in the consolidated lung. The small bronchi entering the cavities are often partially obstructed, producing a check valve mechanism, resulting in balloon cavities (pneumatoceles). These are common in staphylococcal pneumonia and frequently become quite large. In infants, since the lungs are small, the pneumatocele is relatively large and is easily mistaken for a pneumothorax. The course of staphylococcal pneumonia is usually prolonged and when the infection is inadequately treated the disease may persist for many weeks and even months.

The pleural complications of staphylococcal bronchopneumonia occur predominantly in infants. In adults they have been encountered particularly during epidemics of influenza, when complicating suppurative foci in the periphery of the lungs tend to produce pleural irritation and effusions. These may be clear and sterile (sympathetic effusion). If treatment is inadequate, the pleural cavity is invaded by the staphylococci and becomes the seat of a purulent effusion. This is usually rich in fibrin and therefore tends to become loculated. Often, in infants, one of the suppurative foci in the lung connected with a bronchus ruptures into the pleura and produces a pyopneumothorax.

In unusual instances an uninfected pneumatocele ruptures into the pleura and produces a simple pneumothorax. Occasionally, however, an extremely large intact pneumatocele simulates a pneumothorax. The differentiation between the two is sometimes difficult, but it usually can be made if the smooth, regular border of the collapsed lung is seen. This is indicative of a pneumothorax rather than a pulmonary cavity.

It is especially important to differentiate between a pyopneumothorax and a large, infected pneumatocele. An infected pneumatocele practically always disappears on medical treatment while a pyopneumothorax almost always requires drainage. Moreover, aspiration of the infected pneumatocele can result in the formation of a complicating pyopneumothorax. A large pneumatocele containing a fluid level can be differentiated from a pyopneumothorax by observing the border of the cavity above the fluid level and the angle that this border forms with the chest wall. A scalloped border indicates that the lesion is within the lung rather than within the pleura. When the border of the pneumatocele is regular and smooth, it is more difficult to differentiate it from a pyopneumothorax. It is then necessary to make films in a projection in which the area of contact between the lesion and the chest wall is projected tangentially. In a pyopneumothorax, the upper border of the cavity makes an obtuse angle with the chest wall, while in the infected pneumatocele this angle is acute and appears rounded because of the presence of

a shell of lung adjacent to the pleura (Fig. 243).

Hematogenous infection of the lung occurs as a secondary spread from a focus elsewhere in the body. Usually it comes about during the course of a bacteremia complicating a serious infection such as acute osteomyelitis, suppurative thrombophlebitis or acute bacterial endocarditis. However, on occasion, hematogenous infection of the lung results from a relatively insignificant lesion, such as a furuncle, a paronychia or a small, infected abrasion which is easily overlooked. Such infections are not uncommon in addicts who administer their narcotics intravenously.

Blood-borne staphylococcal infections of the lung produce one or more pulmonary furuncles. Roentgenologically, they appear as poorly circumscribed, scattered areas of consolidation measuring from 1 to 5 cm in diameter (Fig. 244). When these increase in size they often empty into a bronchus and then exhibit an air-fluid

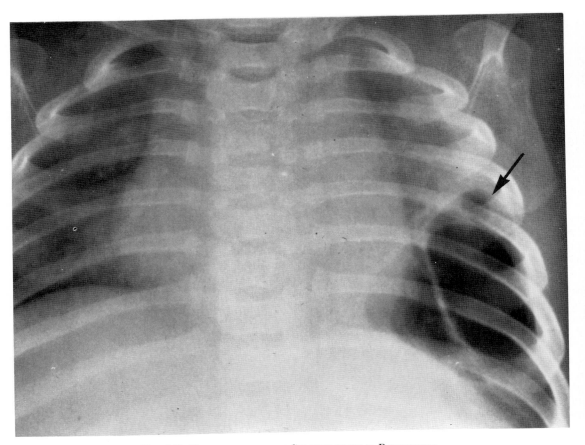

FIG. 243. PNEUMATOCOELE IN STAPHYLOCOCCAL PNEUMONIA

During the course of the pneumonia, the infant developed a localized area of lucency in the lower left chest. The acute angle (arrow) where the air space meets the chest wall indicates that it represents a pneumatocele rather than a loculated collection of air in the pleura. Areas of pneumonic consolidation are present in both lungs. The pneumatocele disappeared after complete resolution of the pneumonia.

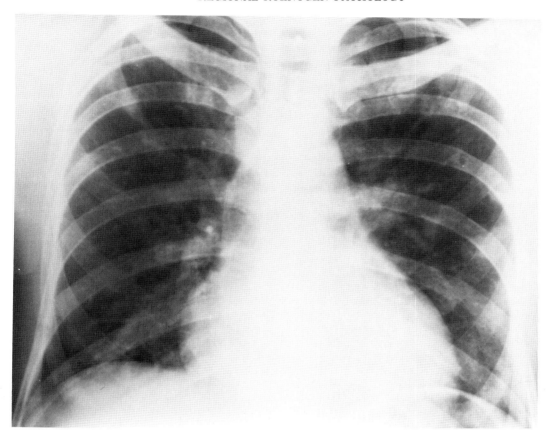

FIG. 244. HEMATOGENOUS STAPHYLOCOCCUS INFECTION

The patient, a heroin addict, was admitted to the hospital with high fever and thrombophlebitis of an antecubital vein. There are several, poorly defined, nodular densities in both lungs. The lesions in the upper lobes have the appearance of irregular areas of consolidation suggesting inflammatory rather than neoplastic disease. Blood cultures were positive for *Staphylococcus aureus*.

level. A pleural effusion and occasionally a pyopneumothorax may occur at any stage of the disease.

Local, less extensive involvement of the lung is the result of a transient bacteremia. Often only a single, poorly defined, rather round area of consolidation is produced, resembling a small focus of pneumonia, an infarct or a neoplasm. The presence of a skin infection may be the only clue to suggest the diagnosis of metastatic abscess. The lesion may resolve completely or it may break down to form a single cavity. If this drains well and the infection is controlled, the cavity empties and the surrounding inflammatory disease clears, leaving a sharply defined, smooth, thin-walled cavity which eventually disappears.

In some cases the infection extends through the pleura to produce an empyema. Most often the patient is not seen in the early stages, and

pain in the chest refereable to the empyema is the first indication of the disease. The empyema is almost always well loculated but may be associated with a sympathetic effusion. Our experience has been that staphylococcal empyema in the adult is usually due to hematogenous infection, whereas in infants and children it is generally secondary to suppurative bronchopneumonia.

STREPTOCOCCUS HEMOLYTICUS. This organism is found in association with others in many of the suppurative diseases of the lung. However, as a specific infection, streptococcal pneumonia occurs particularly in children. The lungs are usually involved secondary to an infection in the nasopharynx. The infection then follows lymphatic pathways to the mediastinum where it produces a phlegmon and suppurative lymphadenitis. Extension of the infection along the lymphatics from the root of the lung results in an infiltration of the perivascular, peribronchial, and interlobular connective tissues. The purulent lymphangitis often spreads to the pleura. The roentgen picture is essentially that of fine interstitial infiltrations extending from the root toward the periphery of the lung (Fig. 235). These are manifested by poorly defined, streak-like shadows, together with tiny, miliary or submiliary densities, most often involving both lungs. In some cases, the mediastinal shadow is diffusely widened because of the phlegmonous involvement. In addition, there may be small protuberances from the mediastinum in the paratracheal regions and at the lung roots, representing inflamed lymph nodes. Not infrequently, the pulmonary changes are associated with a pleural effusion which may be bilateral.

FRIEDLÄNDER'S BACILLUS (*KLEBSIELLA PNEUMONIAE*). Friedländer's pneumonia is primarily a disease of the old and debilitated and of the alcoholic. It is uncommon in healthy adults and is extremely rare in children. By far the majority of cases result from aspiration of material from the mouth or pharynx, although in isolated instances the pulmonary infection results from hematogenous spread from a focus elsewhere in the body. Essentially, the infection takes the form of a suppurative bronchopneumonia. Although interstitial infiltrations are present, they are usually overshadowed in the early stages of the disease by consolidation of the lung. The lesions are lobar or lobular in distribution. In the latter instance there is a tendency for extensive confluence of the individual areas of consolidation. The disease most often begins in an upper lobe or the superior segment of a lower lobe. This is probably due to the fact that aspiration of the material containing the bacilli usually occurs when the patient is in the recumbent position.

Areas of suppuration develop rapidly in the consolidated lung and lead to the formation of multiple small cavities. These may collect to form a well-defined lung abscess which not infrequently becomes chronic.

When the consolidation occurs in a lobular pattern, Friedländer's pneumonia presents a roentgen appearance similar to other forms of suppurative bronchopneumonia. In general, the disease progresses to produce large, confluent areas of consolidation within which cavitation takes place. Plugging of the bronchi by the thick and tenacious secretion characteristic of the disease, produces areas of atelectasis. The infection tends to spread to other segments of the same lung and to the opposite lung to produce additional areas of consolidation and possibly cavitation. This tendency for migration of the infection is rather characteristic of Friedländer's pneumonia. When one area begins to resolve, other portions of the same or opposite lung may become involved (Fig. 245). Despite the suppurative nature of the disease and its tendency to spread, important pleural complications are rare. A plastic pleuritis is common, and results in the early formation of adhesions. Obliteration of the pleural space soon after the onset of the infection probably prevents the development of pleural effusion, empyema or pyopneumothorax.

In many cases, the disease takes the form of a lobar pneumonia. This differs from pneumococcal lobar pneumonia in several ways. In the Friedländer infection, multiple suppurative foci soon form in the consolidated lung in contradistinction to the single cavity that characterizes the aputrid necrosis complicating some cases of pneumococcal pneumonia. The cavities in Friedländer's pneumonia drain poorly because the exudate within them is thick and tenacious. The accumulated exudate often causes the lobe to become enlarged, despite the presence of foci of atelectasis. In the case of consolidation of the right upper lobe, this frequently causes a downward bulge of the short fissure (Fig. 246). The appearance then differs sharply from that of lobar pneumonia in which the lower border of the consolidated area is either straight or bowed upwards. A similar bulge of the fissure occurs in a shutoff lung abscess or a large round neoplasm. The demonstration of multiple areas of cavitation within the shadow, however, suggests Friedländer's pneumonia. The multiple cavities which occur in staphylococcal pneumonia are not associated with a bulging of the fissure. Moreover, unlike Friedländer's pneumonia, the staphylococcus infection of the lung occurs most frequently in children and is often associated with fluid in the pleural cavity.

Unlike pneumococcal pneumonia, the Friedländer infection undergoes very slow resolution and has a tendency to become chronic. In the chronic form, there is considerable interstitial fibrosis and contraction of the lung together with marked thickening of the pleura. One or more persistent cavities may be present and there is a variable amount of associated bronchiectasis. When this occurs in the upper lobe, it is impossible to differentiate the disease roentgenologically from cavitary tuberculosis or a chronic fungous infection. Rarely, hematogenous infection by the Friedländer bacillus involves the lungs and produces one or more abscesses. In the early

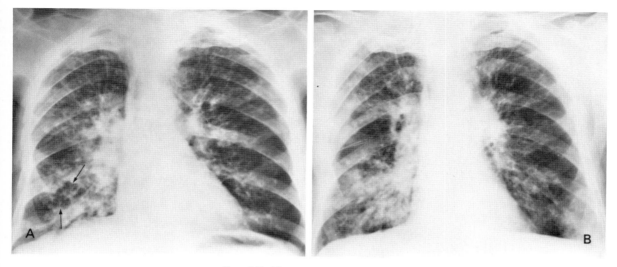

FIG. 245. KLEBSIELLA PNEUMONIA

A: Focal emphysema. Lobular areas of consolidation are present at the right base and near the root of the right lower lobe. There are interstitial infiltrations in both lungs. A cluster of small, irregular areas of increased lucency (arrows) is seen a short distance above the diaphragm. These represent collections of emphysematous lobules which are overdistended because of partial obstruction of small bronchi by secretion. *B:* Spread of infection. Sixteen days later, the lobules which were previously emphysematous, are now consolidated. A homogeneous shadow has appeared above the outer portion of the left leaf of the diaphragm. This represents consolidation of the anterior basal segment of the left lower lobe. A prolonged course and migration of the disease to other parts of the lung are rather characteristic of Friedländer's pneumonia.

stage, these form round, poorly demarcated, homogeneous shadows. Cavities with or without a fluid level become evident later. Extremely thin-walled cavities may persist for a considerable length of time before they close.

HEMOPHILUS PERTUSSIS (WHOOPING COUGH). Although the ordinary case of whooping cough is characterized particularly by a severe tracheitis and bronchitis, pulmonary involvement by the causative organism, and complications secondary to obstruction of small bronchi are not uncommon. The changes in the lungs often produce no abnormal physical signs and therefore are unrecognized unless roentgen films are made during the course of the disease.

Frequently there is infiltration of the interstitial tissues by inflammatory exudate containing mainly round cells. This produces the characteristic roentgen picture of interstitial pneumonia, varying in severity from faint infiltrations near one lung root to extensive infiltrations occurring throughout both lungs. Small areas of atelectasis in the form of linear shadows or broader, faint streaks are common as a result of obstruction of small bronchi by tenacious exudate. Atelectasis of an entire lobe is rarely encountered.

In some instances there is a patchy, lobular form of bronchopneumonia but lobar consolidation is rare. An appearance suggesting lobar

pneumonia may occur when there is a combination of atelectasis of a lobe due to obstruction of its bronchus together with underlying patchy consolidation.

Because of the rather diffuse distribution of the pulmonary lesions, either in the form of infiltrations or atelectasis, the lung adjacent to the heart is often involved in irregular fashion. This causes the cardiac border to be indistinct and irregular, an appearance that has been described as "shaggy heart." The same appearance may be produced by any disease in which there are foci of infiltration or atelectasis adjacent to the heart.

Examination at autopsy practically always discloses considerable enlargement of the lymph nodes at the lung roots and in the mediastinum. However, the nodes are rarely large enough to be detected radiologically.

In some instances, the pneumonia is caused by secondary invaders. In such cases pulmonary suppuration may occur and can lead to bronchiectasis.

PASTEURELLA TULARENSIS. The lungs become infected in almost half of the cases of tularemia. This usually results from dissemination of the infecting organism through the blood stream. A purely pneumonic form of the disease occurs from inhalation of large numbers of the orga-

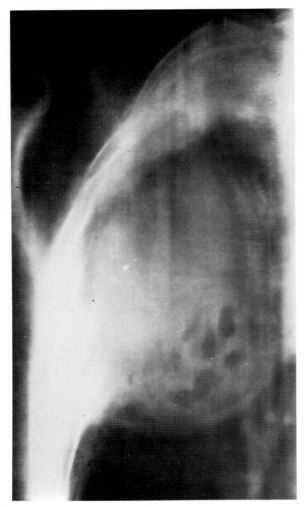

FIG. 246. KLEBSIELLA PNEUMONIA

The conventional film showed a large, homogeneous density with a sharply demarcated, convex lower border, occupying most of the right upper lobe, suggesting a neoplasm. The tomogram, however, shows several areas of radiolucency in the lower half of the shadow. The downward bowing of the short fissure and the presence of multiple cavities within the area of consolidation are quite characteristic of Klebsiella pneumonia.

nisms and is encountered particularly in laboratory workers.

The bacillus usually produces a lobular form of bronchopneumonia, characterized by ill-defined foci of consolidation scattered throughout both lungs. Occasionally the disease is more limited and produces only a single area of consolidation which may be quite large and even involve most of a lobe. There is no tendency to cavitation. Often there is enlargement of the lymph nodes at the lung roots or the paratracheal region. Occasionally, lymph node involvement is most extensive and produces considerable widening of the mediastinal shadow. A small pleural effusion may be present.

The roentgen appearance is nonspecific and the diagnosis depends upon the demonstration of the causative organisms on culture of the sputum, the blood or the skin lesions. The occurrence of an unusual pneumonia, particularly one associated with enlargement of the lymph nodes in a butcher or a hunter who has had contact with rabbits, or in a laboratory worker who has been dealing with the organism, should suggest the possibility of tularemia.

MELIOIDOSIS. This disease, caused by *Pseudomonas pseudomallei* is endemic in Southeast Asia. The great majority of cases observed in this country have been in soldiers returning from Vietnam. Infections in patients who have not been in the endemic area have been extremely rare.

Most of the original reports of this disease were of the acute form with widely disseminated lesions. More recently an increasing number of subacute and chronic cases have been detected. In addition, the results of serologic testing have disclosed a considerable incidence of healed subclinical infections.

In the acute form of the disease the most common roentgen pattern consists of numerous poorly defined, irregular nodules, 4 to 10 mm in diameter, disseminated throughout the lungs. If suitable antibiotic treatment is not instituted, the lesions become larger and coalesce and may produce a picture resembling pulmonary edema. There is a tendency for one or more of the lesions to form cavities which may be thin-walled. Less commonly the acute form of the disease is associated with a large area of consolidation, most frequently in an upper lobe, usually together with multiple smaller lesions scattered throughout the lungs. The large lesions are prone to break down and exhibit one or more cavities if the patient does not succumb in the early stage. Pleural reactions are rare. In the cases we have reviewed the films have not revealed evidence of lymph node enlargement. Many of the severe, acute cases are complicated by a septicemia resulting in suppurative lesions in the subcutaneous tissues, viscera and bones.

The subacute and chronic forms of melioidosis are radiologically quite similar to tuberculosis. In the large majority of cases an upper lobe or the apical segment of the lower lobe is affected. At first there is an area of consolidation and infiltration which usually undergoes cavitation. As in tuberculosis, the cavity is most commonly seen in the infraclavicular region. There is a tendency for the disease to spread to other portions of the lung if treatment is not adequate or sufficiently prolonged. Under treatment the infiltrations subside, the cavity becomes thin-walled and eventually closes in most of the cases. At any time during the course of the disease evidences of infection may appear in other parts of the body. Osteomyelitis may occur with minimal pulmonary symptoms.

The disease may have a long latent period and it may first appear years after the patient has left the endemic area. Not infrequently there are no pulmonary symptoms and the disease is discovered on a routine x-ray examination of the chest or at an examination made because of fever or weight loss. The differentiation of the latent or chronic form of the disease from tuberculosis is most difficult and depends upon demonstration of *P. pseudomallei* in the sputum or a positive serological test.

SALMONELLA. Salmonella infections of the lung are not common. Perhaps the most frequent is the pneumonia that occurs in the early stage of typhoid fever. There is nothing specific roentgenologically about this pneumonia. However, its occurrence as part of the typhoid infection must be appreciated if the general disease is not to be overlooked because it is overshadowed by the pneumonia.

Other salmonella infections can also cause pneumonia and suppurative disease. We have seen one case of segmental consolidation of the lung resulting in the formation of a salmonella abscess. Two cases of salmonella empyema have come under our observation; one showed a moderate-sized free effusion in the acute stage, later followed by the formation of a well-loculated small empyema; the other was a small, chronic empyema which had been overlooked for many years and whose walls were extensively calcified.

CORYNEBACTERIUM DIPHTHERIAE. Pneumonia occurs in diphtheria particularly when the larynx is involved. The diphtheritic membrane not infrequently extends into the trachea and may involve the bronchial tree. It then produces roentgen evidence of bronchial obstruction. Where the lung is not atelectatic, areas of lobular consolidation may be seen.

Spirochetal Infections. Syphilis of the lung may take various forms. Congenital syphilis in the newborn most frequently causes a diffuse, dense infiltration of the lung. The infiltrations are generally so extensive and the interstitial tissues so swollen that the alveoli are compressed and may be obliterated. The cut section of the lung is white and homogeneous, suggesting con-

solidation. This pathologic appearance has given rise to the term *pneumonia alba*. The roentgen picture is characterized by a dense uniform opacity which may involve an entire lung. Congenital syphilis also occurs in a nodular form which is seen in both infancy and childhood. The lungs show multiple irregular, persistent nodular shadows interspersed with coarse interstitial infiltrations and fibrosis. Bullae may be present. The appearance cannot be differentiated from the large granulomas of histiocytosis X.

The characteristic lesion of tertiary syphilis is the *gumma*. This produces a circumscribed, round shadow which cannot be differentiated from that of a neoplasm at a single examination (Fig. 247). The diagnosis can be made only by observing the effects of antiluetic therapy. However, it must be emphasized that gummas of the lung are extremely rare. Almost all syphilitic patients of cancer age whose film shows a nodular shadow will prove to have a carcinoma.

Gummas of the trachea are usually small and tend to produce a stricture of the organ. They are rarely large enough to project beyond the mediastinum.

Diffuse interstitial fibrosis of the lung is rarely due to the syphilitic infection itself. Rather, there appears to be a tendency for delayed resolution of ordinary pneumonias and residual fibrosis in these individuals.

Spirochetosis of the lung is a rare infection. While it is true that spirilla and fusiform bacilli are present in the gangrenous infections such as putrid lung abscess and gangrenous bronchopneumonia, these organisms are not the important cause of the infection, which is due to a mixture of anaerobic and aerobic bacteria. The few cases of spirochetal infection of the lungs that have come under our observation have shown interstitial infiltrations and patchy areas of consolidation in various parts of both lungs. They were associated with a tendency to the formation of small cavities within the consolidated areas. We have seen one case of *Spirillum minus* infection which showed persistent interstitial infiltrations and partial atelectasis, together with fibrosis of the lower lobes.

Viral, Rickettsial and Similar Infections. This group of infections is caused by a variety of agents which have been classified rather recently. Some organisms, previously regarded as viruses, are now classified as rickettsia. In others the classification remains uncertain. Because of this and the fact that the pulmonary infection caused by the different organisms have certain features in common, they are grouped together. In general, the pathologic picture in the lungs is

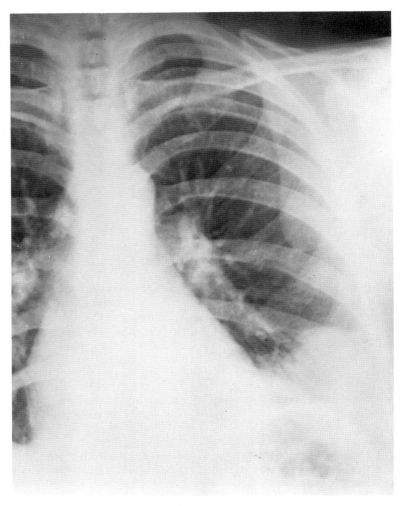

FIG. 247. GUMMA OF THE LUNG

The fairly well circumscribed mass in the left lower lobe was thought to represent a carcinoma. The positive Wassermann reaction was disregarded because gummas of the lung are extremely rare and the lesion did not regress during the administration of bismuth. The mass was resected and proved to be a gumma.

predominantly that of inflammation of the interstitial tissues. Most often there is very little evidence of pulmonary consolidation. On occasion, however, the gross appearance of the lung is mainly that of lobular or confluent lobular consolidation even though extensive interstitial disease is seen on microscopic examination.

While the infection is often primarily one of the respiratory tract, in many instances, particularly in the rickettsial infections, the involvement of the lung is only one part of a generalized infection. In fact, the pulmonary component may be so insignificant clinically that it is not associated with any respiratory symptoms or abnormal physical signs. However, the roentgen changes can be quite distinct and well marked despite the paucity of clinical signs.

The infections are frequently complicated by secondary invasion by other organisms. While the latter may be virulent enough to produce serious disease of the lungs by themselves, there is reason to believe that other, less virulent organisms may cause serious pulmonary complications when they are implanted on a lung already infected by a virus, rickettsia, or similar type of organism.

INFLUENZA. The pulmonary lesions of influenza vary in accordance with the severity of the disease. Sporadic cases are practically always mild. This is also true of the infections which occur in mild epidemics. Most of the severe or fulminating types of influenza are encountered during severe, recurrent pandemics.

The mild cases, which may be characterized

clinically only by fever without any respiratory symptoms, are usually associated with fine interstitial infiltrations in one or more portions of the lung. In association with these infiltrations, there may be an area of lobular or of confluent lobular consolidation of small or moderate size. In the more severe form, the interstitial infiltrations are often quite marked throughout both lungs. In addition, there may be a large, irregular area of lobular consolidation in one or more lobes. Bilateral patches of consolidation are frequent. In the fulminating form of the disease, the earliest change is that of a diffuse, hemorrhagic edema involving both lungs. The roentgen picture cannot be differentiated from pulmonary edema due to other causes. As a matter of fact, even the pathologic picture may be identical with that produced by the inhalation of irritating gases. Death may occur in this stage. If the patient survives, the generalized edema subsides but large patchy areas of consolidation occur and produce large, irregular, more or less homogeneous shadows on the film.

In the more serious cases of influenza, there is usually a severe bronchitis which may be hemorrhagic or necrotizing. Destruction of small bronchi as a result of the severe bronchial disease often produces foci of atelectasis. These may appear either in the form of streak-like shadows or in the form of atelectatic pneumonia.

There is a great tendency to secondary infection by pyogenic organisms, resulting in a suppurative bronchopneumonia. In the early stages, the suppurative bronchopneumonia cannot be differentiated on the roentgen film from the consolidation caused by the influenza itself. A definite roentgen diagnosis of secondary infection can be made only later, when cavitation or pleural effusion occurs. It may then be impossible to differentiate the disease roentgenologically from cavitary tuberculosis or a chronic fungous infection.

MEASLES. Cough is a prominent symptom in the early stage of measles. Although the physical examination is usually negative at this time, the roentgen films often show interstitial infiltrations in the lungs (Fig. 248). Usually the interstitial infiltrations are very fine and easily overlooked. They tend to be more evident at the lung root, but in some cases the bases are more extensively involved. Miliary infiltrations, such as occur in atypical pneumonia, are also seen in measles. Enlargement of the hilar lymph nodes is notable on the roentgen film in a relatively small percentage of the cases.

Although the measles virus alone can produce extensive infiltration of the lung, the severe pneumonias associated with measles are usually due to secondary infection by pyogenic organisms which produce a purulent bronchitis and a pneumonia of the suppurative type. Segmental areas of atelectasis are not uncommon but more extensive atelectasis also occurs, especially of the middle lobe. The frequency of atelectasis of the middle lobe is undoubtedly due to the fact that this is a small lobar bronchus, and therefore the one most easily obstructed by secretions. As in all suppurative bronchopneumonias, the course tends to be prolonged and may be further complicated by the development of an empyema or bronchiectasis.

CHICKEN POX PNEUMONIA. Although chicken pox is mainly a disease of childhood, involvement of the lungs by the varicella virus occurs almost exclusively in adults. The pulmonary lesions appear within a few days after the onset of the skin eruption and occur in two forms. The one which causes the most serious clinical manifestations is the pneumonic form. This consists of patchy areas of consolidation in various parts of the lungs. The nodular form may cause little in the way of symptoms if the lesions are few. When the lungs are studded with nodules dyspnea may be quite severe.

The nodules in varicella pneumonia vary from about 1 to 3 mm in size. They are quite well demarcated as a rule. When few and scattered they tend to be easily overlooked. If the nodules are localized to the upper part of each lung, the appearance suggests the hematogenous form of tuberculosis. When there are many nodules diffusely distributed throughout the lungs, the roentgen appearance is indistinguishable from metastatic carcinoma and the diagnosis depends on the clinical picture. Usually the lesions resolve completely, but in some cases they undergo calcification (Fig. 249). Varicella pneumonia is one of the more common causes for calcific nodules scattered diffusely throughout both lungs.

MISCELLANEOUS VIRAL INFECTIONS. A number of viruses, such as the adenovirus, the ECHO virus, and others which are as yet not specifically identified, are responsible mainly for upper respiratory disease, but, on occasion, do involve the lungs. In addition, the viruses responsible for infectious mononucleosis, smallpox, and the Stevens-Johnson syndrome can affect the lungs. The usual roentgen picture is that of interstitial pulmonary infiltrations of moderate extent. In the case of infectious mononucleosis, the infiltrations are associated with enlarged mediastinal and hilar lymph nodes. The Coxsackie virus appears to cause disease of the pleura and pericardium rather than pneumonia. It is responsible for epi-

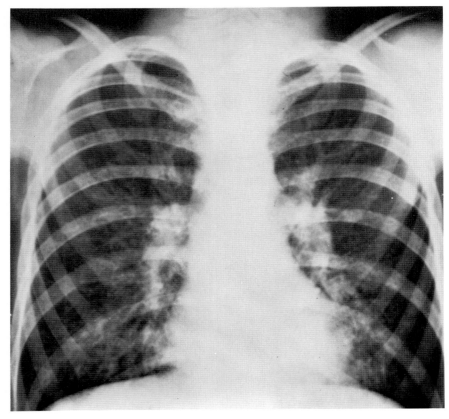

FIG. 248. MEASLES PNEUMONIA

A 6 year old boy developed high fever and cough 1 week after onset of the typical rash of measles. The chest film shows diffuse interstitial infiltration of both lungs. The hilar nodes are moderately enlarged. (Courtesy of Dr. T. F. VanZandt, Rochester, N. Y.)

demic pleurodynia and relapsing pleuropericarditis.

ATYPICAL PNEUMONIA. The term, "atypical pneumonia" was first applied to a group of pulmonary infections that occurred in the form of small epidemics prevalent in army camps in the United States during World War II. Clinically, these resembled grippe or virus infections in their course and in their roentgen appearance. Quite specific for this disease was the finding of a high titre of cold agglutinins in the blood. Eventually it was discovered that this disease was caused by the Eaton agent, a pleuropneumonia-like organism, the *Mycoplasma pneumoniae*.

In most cases, there are interstitial infiltrations which appear as irregular, streak-like shadows either in one or both lower lobes. There is often atelectasis of a segment or part of a segment of the involved lung, producing homogeneous densities suggesting consolidation. In a day or two this portion of lung may reexpand, again revealing the interstitial infiltrations. If the atelectatic portion of the lung is small, it appears on the film as a streak-like shadow which may be broad or thin. Frequently, in addition to the irregular, fine, streak-like infiltrations in the lower lobes, there are fine miliary infiltrations in the outer parts of the upper lobes. In some cases the entire process takes the form of miliary or submiliary shadows scattered throughout the lungs (Fig. 104). A small collection of fluid is sometimes present in the pleural cavity in association with the pneumonic infiltrations.

Most often dense shadows of lobular consolidation appear when a suppurative bronchopneumonia is produced by secondary pyogenic invaders.

Prolongation of the pulmonary disease is usually due to secondary infection. However, there are some cases in which the interstitial infiltrations are widespread and the primary infection itself persists for a long period (Fig. 236). The infiltrations may recede, but recurrences can take place over a period of several months.

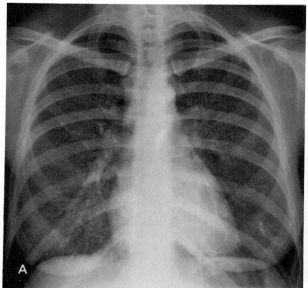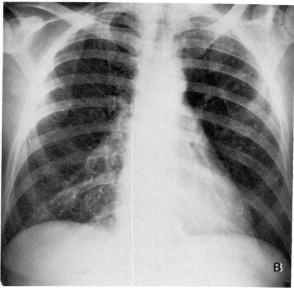

FIG. 249. CHICKENPOX PNEUMONIA

A: 7-18-60. The chest film of a 28 year old woman with cough and fever and the typical rash of chickenpox shows numerous tiny, nodular densities throughout both lungs. *B:* 10-12-70. Although many of the lesions of chickenpox pneumonia have cleared, others have become calcified. Characteristically, the calcifications following varicella pneumonia are of uniform size.

The disease is milder than influenza pneumonia and is less apt to produce lobular consolidation. Nevertheless, in severe cases, areas of confluent lobular consolidation do occur and simulate those seen in epidemic influenza.

ORNITHOTIC PNEUMONIAS. These infections, produced by what appear to be large viruses, are transmitted by parrots and parakeets (psittacosis), pigeons, ducks, grouse and other birds. The ornithotic pneumonias are primarily of the interstitial type. Infiltrations and focal areas of atelectasis may be scattered throughout the lungs. They are most prominent in the region of the lung roots and the basal segments of the lower lobes where the shadows may appear confluent. Rarely, a large area of homogeneous consolidation is present, simulating lobar pneumonia. The course of the disease is prolonged and may be characterized by spread to other areas while the original one clears.

RICKETTSIAL DISEASES. Of the rickettsial diseases, Q fever is the one in which the lungs are most likely to be involved since the disease appears to be contracted principally by inhalation. The lesions are characterized by interstitial infiltrations, but scattered areas of consolidation are not uncommon.

Pulmonary infiltrations are rarely seen in endemic typhus. Those that we have observed appeared as small, faint, poorly defined shadows, representing small, localized interstitial infiltrations. Denser patches of consolidation sometimes occur in severe cases of typhus, particularly if there is secondary infection with pyogenic organisms. Patchy consolidation also occurs in Rocky Mountain spotted fever.

Fungous Diseases of the Lung. The diagnosis of fungous disease of the lungs can rarely be made from the roentgen films alone because the appearance is usually identical to that of a variety of other conditions. Where the fungous infection is merely bronchial, the picture may be that of chronic bronchitis and emphysema. Localized fungous infections of the lungs usually simulate neoplasm or abscess. More diffuse infections resemble disseminated lobular pneumonia and, if associated with cavity formation, the appearance is identical to suppurative bronchopneumonia. When the disease is confined to the lymph nodes, the roentgen picture simulates Hodgkin's disease. If, in addition, there is a lesion in the lung, the condition may be confused with primary tuberculosis or a pulmonary neoplasm with mediastinal metastases. Disseminated nodular lesions produce a roentgenographic appearance like that of miliary tuberculosis, pneumoconiosis or metastatic neoplasm. Perhaps the only specific picture of a fungous infection is that which occurs in actinomycosis and, less frequently, in nocardiosis or North American blastomycosis, when the disease is associated with a chronic peripleuritis and changes in the overlying ribs. A round mass within a pulmonary cavity is most suggestive of a fungus ball but this also occurs in other conditions.

Despite the absence of characteristic shadows, the roentgen appearance, if taken together with the clinical information, is helpful in the diagnosis. A fungous disease of the lung should be suspected in chronic pulmonary lesions of insidious onset when the clinical findings tend to exclude the usual diseases suggested by the roentgen appearance. Thus, the failure to find tubercle bacilli in the sputum or a negative skin test in a patient whose films suggest active tuberculosis, leads to a suspicion of a fungous infection. The presence of chronic suppurative disease of the lung in the absence of an obstructive lesion, a foul infection, or bronchiectasis should likewise suggest this possibility.

One of the fungous diseases must be considered in the differential diagnosis of all slowly resolving pneumonias and especially when the roentgen film shows a localized, persistent, dense shadow with or without enlargement of the regional nodes. This applies particularly to patients under prolonged steroid therapy, those being treated with antimetabolites, and patients suffering from leukemia or a lymphomatous disease. The possibility of a specific fungous infection should be considered in patients who have been in regions where these are endemic, i.e., coccidioidomycosis in the southwestern United States, and histoplasmosis in the Mississippi Valley.

The roentgen diagnosis of a fungous infection of the lungs is justified if a patient with a fungous infection of the skin or mucous membrane develops pulmonary lesions, particularly if these are in the form of disseminated nodules. Similarly, the diagnosis may be made if a patient with a chronic pulmonary lesion develops multiple subcutaneous or cutaneous nodules in which the fungus can be found.

It is important to bear in mind that the finding of certain fungi in the sputum is insufficient to warrant a conclusion that a pulmonary lesion is due to infection by these organisms, even though they are of proven pathogenicity. *Candida albicans* commonly contaminates sputum on exposure to the air and this organism, as well as the *Geotrichum*, is frequently present in the mouth and thus contaminates the sputum. Even secretions removed through the bronchoscope may be thus contaminated. In addition to these organisms, *Streptothrix, Sporotrichum, Aspergillus* and *Actinomyces* may grow in a saprophytic manner within bronchiectases or abscess cavities where the infection is really due to other pyogenic organisms. The fungi may also implant themselves on ulcerating neoplasms without causing any invasion of the lungs. The mere fact, therefore, that these fungi can be grown consistently from the sputum does not prove that they are important in the pathogenesis of the disease depicted on the film.

In addition to the demonstration of the fungus, it is necessary to exclude the presence of tuberculosis, putrid lung abscess and neoplasm before deciding that the roentgen abnormality is due to a fungous infection. The diagnosis is tenable when the fungus is recognized invading the tissues on a biopsy specimen or when there are associated characteristic lesions in other organs.

Exposure to *spores* of fungi may produce disease without infection by the fungi themselves. Here the clinical manifestations are due to a sensitivity reaction to the spores. Examples of this are bagassosis, farmer's lung and similar conditions which will be discussed in the section on Sensitivity Diseases.

ACTINOMYCOSIS. *Actinomyces israeli*, the anaerobic fungus which causes actinomycosis, forms part of the normal flora of the mouth. It flourishes in carious teeth, gingival pockets and tonsilar crypts as a saprophyte. It may also occur as a saprophyte in exudates resulting from infection by other, more virulent mouth organisms. The diagnosis of actinomycosis, therefore, should not be made simply from the finding of these organisms in the sputum or in pus from the lung or pleura.

The lung usually becomes infected by aspiration into a bronchus of material containing the fungus. A local area of bronchopneumonia results, and is characterized by both consolidation and infiltration of the interstitial tissues. This is persistent and is complicated by the production of small areas of suppuration, but large cavities such as in lung abscess, are rarely formed.

The infection is situated in the periphery of the lobe and has a tendency to invade the pleura, which becomes covered with exudate. This results in dense adhesions and obliteration of the pleural space. In some instances, the disease extends directly through the adherent pleura to involve the chest wall. This is characteristic of actinomycotic infections which are of a burrowing nature, not limited by anatomic boundaries. Empyemas are uncommon.

In the early stages, there is nothing specific about the roentgen appearance of actinomycosis to differentiate it from a segmental pneumonia or an early lung abscess. Later the more characteristic picture of actinomycosis usually develops. This consists of a fairly large area of chronic consolidation and infiltration together with evidences of peripleuritis. The shadow in the lung usually appears more or less homogeneous, and increases in density as it extends to the periphery of the lobe where there is marked thickening of the pleura. The ribs are drawn together over the lesion, flattening the chest wall. Often they appear thickened as a result of periostitis. New bone formation is often manifested by fine lines of increased density paralleling the long axis of the ribs. The ribs themselves may show ill-defined lucencies representing areas of bone destruction.

In some cases there is swelling of the superficial tissues of the chest wall. The infection may extend further, involving the skin with the production of one or more sinuses. Injection of radiopaque material into a sinus tract may demonstrate communication with small, irregular cavities within the lung.

When the actinomycotic infection is extensive, a considerable portion of one hemithorax may appear opaque. This suggests atelectasis secondary to bronchial obstruction because the ribs are drawn together (Fig. 250). However, despite the extent of the actinomycosis, the mediastinal structures are usually not displaced to the affected side. The approximation of the ribs, which is due to a fibrosing peripleuritis, also occurs in other conditions, such as empyema necessitatis or osteomyelitis of a rib due to other organisms.

Less commonly, actinomycosis of the lung results from extension of the disease from the abdomen, usually from a subphrenic or hepatic abscess. The infection generally spreads directly through the diaphragm and pleura into the lung. If the pleura is not adherent an empyema can develop. The infection may also extend through the upper abdominal or chest wall to produce swelling and induration of the soft tissues (see Fig. 263).

Actinomycosis of the mediastinum may result from direct extension of the infection from the mesial portion of the lung. Not uncommonly, however, the mediastinum is involved by spread of an infection of the jaw down through the fascial planes of the neck. The actinomyces may also enter the mediastinum through a perforated esophagus to cause diffuse mediastinitis. In either case, the infection can then extend from the mediastinum into the lung. It may also spread downward in the posterior mediastinum to the retroperitoneal tissues and produce swelling and fistulas in the lumbar region.

In extremely rare cases, actinomycosis produces a fairly well circumscribed nodular shadow in the lung, simulating a well-demarcated peripheral pulmonary neoplasm. Multiple patches of lobular consolidation throughout the lungs may occur as a result of bronchogenic spread late in the disease. Numerous poorly defined nodules may also result from hematogenous dissemination. An unusual roentgen manifestion which simulates bronchogenic carcinoma, is a hilar density, either triangular in shape or associated with faint shadows radiating outward from the hilum. The root shadow may be mistaken for large lymph nodes. However, enlargement of the lymph nodes is extremely rare in actinomycosis. The hilar mass is usually due to granulomatous reaction in the wall of a large bronchus and in the peribronchial tissue.

ASPERGILLOSIS. *Aspergillus fumigatus*, the causative organism of aspergillosis, is a ubiquitous organism which almost always acts as a saprophyte. It rarely causes pulmonary disease in healthy people. Most frequently it is found in the sputum simply as a contaminating organism. In certain instances it implants itself on a preexisting lesion. It may then give rise to clinical symptoms, and even produce an abnormal shadow on the film, but still not be responsible for important disease. Colonies of aspergilli may grow upon a necrotic bronchial carcinoma, the mycelia may form masses within preexisting cavities in the lung, and they may be present in mucous plugs in patients with asthma. Significant infections with *A. fumigatus* generally occur in patients with lowered resistance, particularly in leukemia and in persons undergoing a prolonged course of treatment with corticosteroids.

The most common roentgen manifestation of aspergillosis is caused by a fungus ball (mycetoma) made up of a mass of mycelia within a pulmonary cavity. Any preformed cavity within the lung, whether the result of old tuberculosis, a healed lung abscess, a broken-down infarct, or even a large bulla, can be the site of implantation of the aspergilli. The mass of mycelia is depicted as a more or less well-demarcated, round density within the cavity. The mycetoma is almost never attached to the wall and, since it rarely fills the entire cavity, it is freely movable and gravitates to the most dependent portion as the patient changes his position (Fig. 251). The shift of the mycetoma is well demonstrated when films are made in the lateral recumbent as well as the erect position. The air within the cavity appears on the film as a crescentic area of lucency between the fungus ball and the uppermost portion of the cavity wall. When the patient is supine, the mycetoma lies against the posterior wall of the cavity so that in the frontal projection the air is seen as a circular band of lucency around the mass. This is the usual appearance on to-

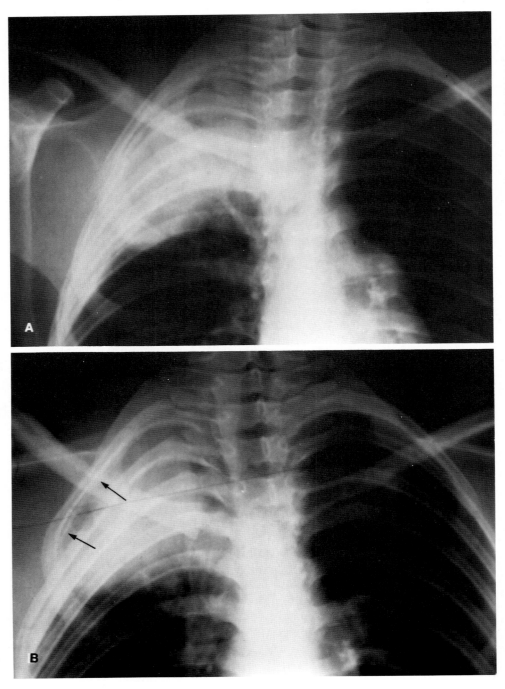

FIG. 250. ACTINOMYCOSIS

A: The right upper lobe is opacified. The overlying ribs are drawn together suggesting atelectasis. However, neither the hilum nor the short fissure is elevated and the trachea remains in its normal position. This indicates that the narrowing of the rib spaces is due to disease involving the chest wall. *B:* A Bucky film was made to show better rib detail. The periosteum at the lower border of the outer portion of the second rib is thickened (arrows). The combination of the consolidation of the lung with periostitis and peripleuritis is characteristic of actinomycosis or nocardiosis. The small area of lucency beneath the second rib represents air in relation to a sinus tract in the chest wall.

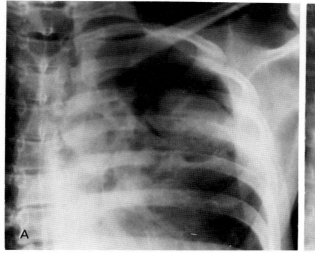 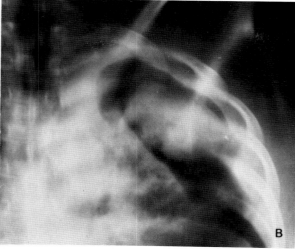

FIG. 251. ASPERGILLOMA

A: The patient had cavitary tuberculosis several years ago. The tuberculous infection cleared completely but the cavity persisted because its entering bronchus became epithelialized (open healing). The upright film shows a large lobulated mass at the base of the cavity. There is marked thickening of the pleura over the lesion. *B:* A film made with the patient supine shows the mass to be completely encircled by air. This indicates that it lies free within the cavity and has shifted to its posterior wall which is now the most dependent portion. Movement of an intracavitary mass with change in the position of the patient is characteristic of a mycetoma.

mograms because the sections are made with the patient in the prone or supine position. When the mycelial mass has been present for a long time, calcium may be deposited within it. The calcific deposits are usually seen only on tomograms.

The symptom which frequently calls attention to the pulmonary disease is hemoptysis. The question then arises as to whether a mass within a cavity represents a blood clot or a mycetoma. This question can usually be settled by observation over a relatively short period of time. A blood clot will soon diminish in size or disappear completely, while the shadow of a mycetoma remains unchanged.

The cavity wall outside the mycetoma varies in appearance, depending upon the nature of the underlying disease. Cavities resulting from healed tuberculosis or a healed lung abscess generally have extremely thin walls and lateral decubitus films or tomography may be required for their recognition. Thick-walled cavities are often present in bronchiectasis and broken down carcinomas or infarcts. The fungus ball may be poorly visualized if the wall is extremely thick or associated with considerable induration of the surrounding lung or pleura. Well-penetrated Bucky films or tomograms may be necessary to demonstrate the lucency about the mycetoma.

Because mycetomas are most often formed within tuberculous cavities or bullae, they are usually situated in the upper lobes. Not infrequently the surrounding lung is infected by the aspergilli or by secondary invaders. This produces marked thickening of the overlying pleura, sometimes with peripleuritis and flattening of the dome of the thorax (see Fig. 350).

Primary aspergillosis of the lung is extremely rare. Confluent, lobular areas of consolidation have been described and have a tendency to persist. Suppuration and cavitation may occur within the lesions.

Atelectatic foci are occasionally seen in cases of asthma in which the sputum is persistently positive for aspergilli. The atelectasis appears to be due to bronchial mucous plugs rather than to disease of the bronchial wall itself. Sensitivity to the aspergilli is probably responsible for the asthma as well as the mucous plugs.

NORTH AMERICAN BLASTOMYCOSIS. This form of blastomycosis is caused by *Blastomyces dermatitidis* and occurs mainly in the United States and Canada. While a considerable number of cases are associated with skin lesions, in most instances the pulmonary disease is predominant.

The most common roentgen manifestation in the early stage of the disease, is a rather homogeneous density in a pulmonary segment, representing consolidation and infiltration. Local spread of the infection causes enlargement of the area of consolidation. Further spread through the bronchi results in patchy areas of lobular consolidation (Fig. 252) which may be distributed throughout both lungs. Interstitial infiltrations are usually present about the areas of consolidation. Cavities can form, but are often hidden by the indurated lung. Localized thickening of the pleura over the pneumonic area is common, but pleural effusions are rare.

As in other fungal diseases, the pulmonary lesions are persistent. When there is only a single, rather well-demarcated area of consolidation, the roentgen picture is easily confused with that of a bronchogenic carcinoma. If, as is frequently the case, the lesions are confined to the upper lobes, they simulate tuberculosis. When the disease presents as a small, sharply demarcated, round focus, the diagnosis of blastomycosis can be determined only by biopsy. In rare instances, the disease spreads directly from the pleura to the overlying ribs where it causes periosteal thickening and an appearance which may be identical with that of actinomycosis. Enlargement of the hilar lymph nodes occurs occasionally.

In some instances, miliary or submiliary infiltrations are seen throughout the lungs. These probably result from hematogenous dissemination of the infection. Extension of the disease through the blood stream may cause destructive lesions in the ribs, manifested by lytic areas which are often surrounded by sclerotic bone.

SOUTH AMERICAN BLASTOMYCOSIS. This disease is particularly prevalent in Brazil and is caused by *Blastomyces brasiliensis* (*Coccidioides brasiliensis*). Most commonly it begins with ulceration of one of the mucous membranes. When it occurs in the mouth there is usually marked enlargement of the submandibular and cervical lymph nodes. The visceral form of the disease begins with infection of the intestine. In any case, the lungs are apparently involved secondarily, either as the result of aspiration or hematogenous spread.

When the pulmonary infection results from aspiration, the first manifestation is usually a segmental area of consolidation. The disease tends to spread through the bronchi to produce diffusely scattered infiltrations throughout one or both lungs. Hematogenous involvement of the lungs is characterized by multiple small, ill-de-

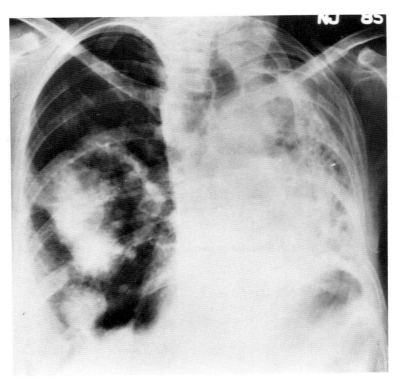

FIG. 252. NORTH AMERICAN BLASTOMYCOSIS

The left lung is shrunken and its pleura extensively calcified because of previous pneumothorax treatment for tuberculosis. At this time the patient presented with hemoptysis and persistent low grade fever. The large, irregular areas of consolidation in the right lung are unlike the lesions resulting from spread of tuberculosis. There is no evidence of a cavity in either lung and the sputum was negative for tubercle bacilli. The diagnosis of blastomycosis was made by open biopsy of the lung.

fined, nodular densities diffusely distributed throughout both lungs.

COCCIDIOIDOMYCOSIS. The causative organism, *Coccidioides immitis*, is endemic to the southwest desert regions of the United States, particularly the San Joaquin Valley in California. Occasional cases of coccidioidomycosis have been contracted elsewhere in North America.

The disease usually begins with a poorly demarcated area of pulmonary consolidation with indistinct borders. This may be quite small, involving only a small portion of a pulmonary segment, but it may be of segmental distribution or even involve a large portion of a lobe in a confluent lobular pneumonia. In most cases, the initial lesion is very small and because it is asymptomatic it passes by unnoticed. In others, there is more extensive involvement of a lobe of the lung early in the disease with considerable enlargement of the hilar or paratracheal lymph nodes (Fig. 253). All grades of severity between these extremes occur. There is a tendency to spontaneous resolution of the disease. When resolution is incomplete, the pulmonary lesions become smaller and more sharply defined, forming

a round nodule. This may represent a solid granuloma, *coccidioidoma* (Fig. 254), or a blocked cavity filled with pus and caseous material. Either type of nodule may remain unchanged in size for years and resemble a benign tumor. It may gradually diminish in size and eventually undergo calcification. A blocked cavity can rupture into a small bronchus and discharge its contents leaving only an empty cavity or one with a fluid level (see Fig. 510). Most often the wall of the residual cavity is extremely thin. If the bronchial communication closes, the cavity may rapidly disappear but it can refill and once more appear as a solid nodule. If the bronchial communication remains open, the cavity can persist indefinitely (Fig. 255).

A persistent cavity often changes in size and appearance as a result of temporary, complete or partial obstruction of the entering bronchus. It may become quite small and almost disappear, only suddenly to balloon out and become larger than ever. The fluid level may appear and disappear, depending upon the occurrence of secondary infection or reestablishment of good bronchial drainage. Although it has been stated

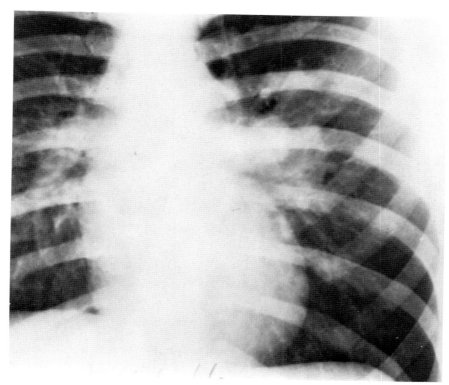

FIG. 253. COCCIDIOIDOMYCOSIS

The area of consolidation in the superior segment of the left lower lobe is associated with enlargement of the left hilar lymph nodes. The patient developed fever while in an area in which coccidioidomycosis is endemic. Skin and serological tests were positive.

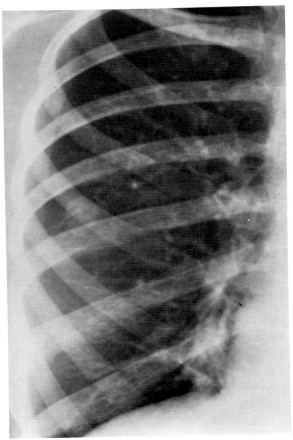

During the acute phase of the disease, the infection may extend directly into adjacent portions of the lung, or spread through the bronchi to produce disseminated, patchy areas of consolidation. Spread of the disease is sometimes complicated by pleural effusion or an empyema.

In both the acute and chronic forms of coccidioidomycosis, there is a tendency to hematogenous or lymph-hematogenous dissemination throughout the body. This may result in the formation of innumerable miliary and submiliary lesions in the lungs. Hematogenous spread to the bones may then appear as predominantly lytic lesions in the ribs, spine or shoulder girdle.

CRYPTOCOCCOSIS (TORULOSIS). This disease, caused by *Cryptococcus neoformans*, often presents clinically as a subacute meningitis. In most cases, however, the primary infection is in the lung. The pulmonary lesion may be so small that it is not detected, either clinically or radiologically, and the primary focus is found only at necropsy. However, the pulmonary disease is apparent clinically in about two-thirds of the cases.

Usually the pulmonary lesion appears as a dense, homogeneous shadow representing an area of consolidation. This is often quite large and poorly demarcated. The density tends to persist for a relatively long time and simulates a

FIG. 254. COCCIDIOIDOMYCOSIS: NODULAR FORM

The patient went to the desert region because of bilateral lower lobe bronchiectasis. On her return, the small nodular shadow at the level of the fourth anterior intercostal space, was found. The nodule remained unchanged during 1 year's observation. The coccidioidin skin test gave a positive reaction. The tuberculin test was negative.

that the residual cavities do not give rise to spread of coccidioidomycosis to adjacent or distant parts of the lung, this is not always true. We have observed several cases of such bronchogenic spread of the disease and others have recently been reported. In rare instances, residual cavities result in pleural complications.

When the disease is extensive, necrotic foci within the area of confluent lobular pneumonia may result in the formation of multiple cavities. These may be thin-walled and resemble the pneumatoceles of staphylococcal pneumonia. They may disappear rapidly when the pneumonic process resolves, but more commonly, a round, caseous or suppurative focus remains. In at least 10% of the cases multiple nodular shadows persist. These undergo the same course as the solitary nodular lesions described above.

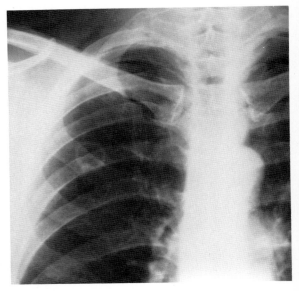

FIG. 255. COCCIDIOIDOMYCOSIS: RING CAVITY

A sharply demarcated annular shadow without any surrounding reaction is rather characteristic of coccidioidomycosis. It follows the expectoration of necrotic material from a circumscribed nodular focus. This sequence of events occurred in this patient who contracted the disease while in the San Joaquin Valley.

neoplasm. A smaller granulomatous lesion presents as a solitary nodule in the lung, usually without pulmonary symptoms, fever or other clinical manifestations for a long period. Occasionally, there are patchy areas of consolidation in one or more lobes of the lung. Many of these eventually resolve completely. In some, the lesions shrink to small size and then persist indefinitely in what may prove to be a healed stage of the disease. Rarely is calcium deposited in the lesions. Cavitation is most unusual and pleural complications are rare.

While in many of the cases the first symptoms are referable to involvement of the brain and meninges, in others they are referable to the lungs. The pulmonary disease may be active for years before cerebral or meningeal symptoms appear. In fact, the pulmonary lesions may appear to have resolved when the central nervous system complications first become manifest.

Hematogenous spread of the disease may also produce lesions in the bones. These are predominantly destructive in character and may lead to the formation of sinus tracts from which the causative organisms can be isolated. Hematogenous dissemination can result in studding of the lungs with numerous small nodules (Fig. 256). Spread from the primary focus in the lung to the regional lymph nodes is probably common, for the organisms can be found in the nodes at postmortem, but the nodes are seldom large enough to be detected on the films.

GEOTRICHOSIS. *Geotrichum candidum* is frequently found as a normal inhabitant of the mouth. A true infection of the respiratory tract by this organism is extremely rare. The diagnosis of geotrichosis, therefore, must be made with great caution when the organism is found in the sputum of a patient with pulmonary disease. The geotrichum should be demonstrated in the sputum repeatedly and all other causes of the condition in question carefully excluded before the possibility of geotrichosis is considered. Even then, a final diagnosis of geotrichosis should be

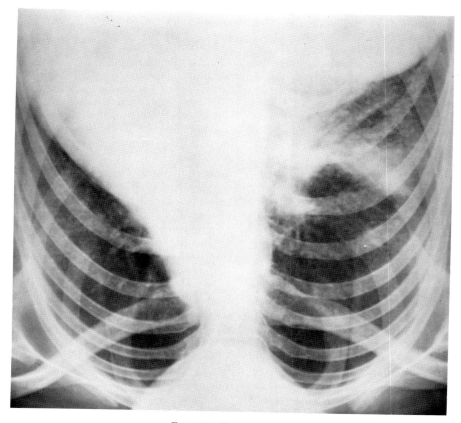

FIG. 256. CRYPTOCOCCOSIS

A young female under steroid treatment for lupus erythematosus developed fever and eventually died of meningitis. The film shows consolidation of the lower part of the right lung together with numerous, tiny, nodular shadows throughout both lungs. Autopsy disclosed *Cryptococcus neoformans*. The tiny nodules were the result of hematogenous dissemination from the pneumonic focus in the right lung.

made with some reservation unless the organism can be demonstrated in the tissues or evidence of dissemination of the infection is found elsewhere.

Two forms of the disease have been described, the bronchial and the pulmonary. The bronchial form is manifested by a bronchitis and peribronchitis which is characterized roentgenologically by accentuation of the pulmonary markings and interstitial infiltration of the lungs. It seems likely that most of the cases that have been presented as bronchial infection with the geotrichum really represent cases of nonspecific bronchitis in which the geotrichum has been found in the sputum. The diagnosis of geotrichosis is presumptive if the organisms are found on direct smears from the bronchi and is definite if they are found within the tissue on bronchial biopsy.

The pulmonary form of the disease is characterized by dense patches of consolidation which may undergo cavitation. These are exceedingly rare. We have observed one such case in which the diagnosis was proved by demonstration of the organisms within the pulmonary tissue at postmortem examination. In another case, patchy areas of consolidation had become localized and sharply demarcated to form nodules in the lungs varying up to 3 or 4 mm in size. A small calcified focus was demonstrable in the center of several of the nodules. Biopsy of one of them revealed geotrica within the lesion.

HISTOPLASMOSIS. This disease, caused by inhalation of the spores of *Histoplasma capsulatum*, is most prevalent in the Mississippi valley. A large percentage of the population in this region shows evidence of having had the infection. The disease is also fairly common in the Middle Atlantic States and as far west as the western parts of Nebraska, Kansas, Oklahoma and Texas. A recent survey has also shown widespread infection of the population in the Panama Canal Zone. Apparently it is contracted easily; only a short exposure is required to produce the disease. It is, therefore, not surprising that sporadic cases of histoplasmosis have been found throughout the United States.

In many respects histoplasmosis is quite similar to tuberculosis. Both diseases exist in a primary and a reinfection form. Like tuberculosis, the primary infection in histoplasmosis is usually asymptomatic unless there has been massive exposure to the organism. The primary infection in the lung is associated with involvement of the regional lymph nodes, and there is a tendency for both the pulmonary lesion and the involved nodes to undergo calcification (Fig. 143). In the more severe cases, the infection may be dissem-

inated through the bloodstream to produce lesions in the liver, spleen and other organs, as well as miliary foci in the lungs. The reinfection type of disease, as in tuberculosis, is often associated with cavitation and fibrosis. Because of the high incidence of histoplasmosis, it is not surprising that this disease should exist together with tuberculosis in certain individuals. The danger then exists of overlooking one of the two diseases.

Primary Histoplasmosis. As a rule, the primary infection is manifested by one or more small areas of consolidation in the lung, together with enlargement of the regional lymph nodes. Multiplicity of the primary lesions is unusual in tuberculosis. As in tuberculosis, however, the pulmonary lesion in histoplasmosis may not be evident on the x-ray film, the roentgen picture being dominated by enlargement of the paratracheal or hilar lymph nodes on one side. In other cases, the pulmonary lesion is visible while the lymph nodes are not large enough to produce an abnormal shadow.

The area of consolidation representing the primary lesion is usually small, but it may involve an entire bronchopulmonary segment. In any case, the lesion tends to resolve spontaneously, becoming smaller and more circumscribed to form a round nodule. This usually undergoes calcification but the calcium may not be detected radiologically. Often the calcium is deposited in concentric rings presenting the roentgen appearance of a target, with or without a central calcific core (Fig. 257). The entire lesion may become more or less uniformly calcified or there may simply be a calcific center surrounded by a circumscribed round, faint density, giving the appearance of a halo (Fig. 258). In other cases, no calcification can be seen within the lesion, even on tomography. The lesion appears as a round, homogeneous density, 1 to 2 cm in diameter, situated in the periphery of a lobe, indistinguishable from a neoplasm (Fig. 259). Whether calcified or not, the nodule may persist indefinitely and even increase in size over a period of years.

When the disease is contracted by inhalation of dust containing a high concentration of spores, it is characterized by numerous lesions throughout the lungs. The chest film shows the pulmonary fields to be studded with small, poorly demarcated densities, an appearance that has been likened to that of snowflakes. The shadows represent groups of consolidated acini. Occasionally, the pulmonary disease is complicated by a small pleural effusion.

The lesions become circumscribed and appear more nodular during the process of resolution.

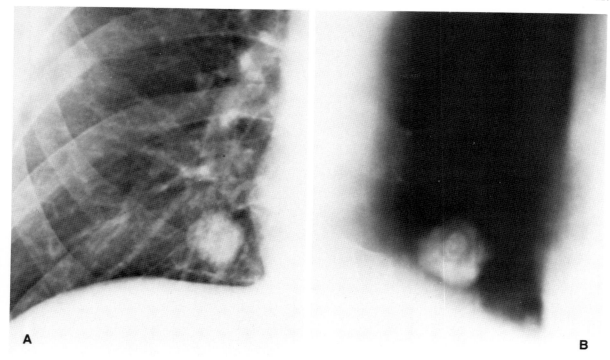

FIG. 257. HISTOPLASMOMA

A: The lobulated nodule in the right cardiophrenic angle cannot be differentiated from a peripheral bronchogenic carcinoma. *B*: The tomogram shows a central core of calcification surrounded by alternating dense and lucent rings. This is pathognomonic for a chronic granuloma, most often due to tuberculosis or histoplasmosis.

They may disappear entirely over a period of months or years, but often the centers of many of the nodules undergo calcification. Eventually, the inflammatory component disappears and only the calcific deposits remain. These are scattered rather uniformly throughout the lungs (Fig. 138), although the apices are usually least involved. Such calcific foci, all of uniform size, scattered throughout the lungs, are quite characteristic of a previous massive infection with the spores of *Histoplasma capsulatum*. They differ from the calcifications that follow in the course of a bronchial dissemination of tuberculosis in that the latter are more apt to be clustered rather than uniformly distributed, and are more variable in size. In the rare cases of calcified miliary tuberculosis, the lesions are uniform in size and distribution but are more numerous and closely packed. The calcific deposits in mitral stenosis vary in size, and are more numerous in the lower portions of the lungs (Fig. 120). The calcifications that occur following varicella pneumonia are indistinguishable from those of histoplasmosis (Fig. 249).

Enlargement of the lymph nodes is usually evident during the acute stage of the disease. In severe infections both lungs are often involved and are associated with bilateral enlargement of the hilar nodes. This is in contradistinction to the common form of primary infection which is mild and in which the lymphadenopathy is confined to the regional nodes draining a single focus in the lung.

As in tuberculosis, the diseased lymph nodes may cause obstruction of a bronchus by direct spread of the infection into the adjacent bronchial wall. Granulation tissue forms and, together with edema of the mucosa, can result in complete obstruction of the bronchus with collapse of the corresponding portion of the lung (Fig. 260). This phase may be temporary. As the inflammatory process subsides, the obstruction may be partially or completely relieved. However, in some cases a permanent stricture results and leads to recurrent episodes of secondary infection and bronchiectasis.

Calcification of diseased lymph nodes involving the bronchial wall can result in broncholithiasis. The stones may be situated within the bronchial wall and cause narrowing of the bronchus, or they may erode through the wall to form intraluminal stones. They are indistinguishable

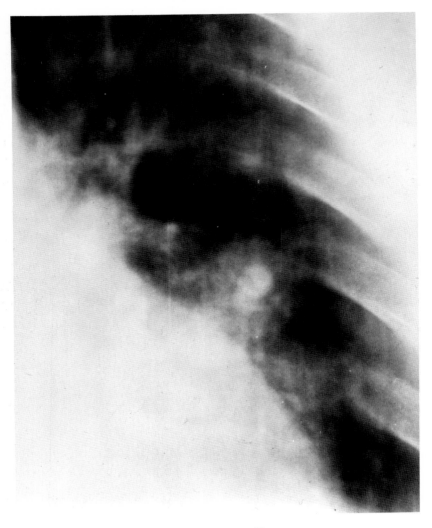

FIG. 258. CALCIFICATION IN A HISTOPLASMOMA

A tomogram shows a faint, round, soft tissue density with a central calcific core in the superior segment of the left lower lobe. The central location of the calcification is indicative of a granuloma. In this case it was due to histoplasmosis.

from those which originate in tuberculous nodes. Perforation of a diseased lymph node into the esophagus can lead to the formation of a small traction diverticulum (see Fig. 467). This occurs in the region of the subcarinal nodes. The traction diverticula are therefore always situated on the anterior wall of the esophagus at this level.

The course of resolution of the pulmonary lesion may be interrupted by local spread of the disease, causing enlargement of the roentgen shadow, before the lesions finally shrink. In some cases, hematogenous dissemination of the disease occurs, resulting in the formation of scattered caseous foci in various organs. These frequently undergo calcification. Calcified foci in the spleen may be visible on the chest film.

Miliary involvement of the lungs occurs as a result of more extensive invasion of the blood stream. The shadows differ from the "snowflake" type of involvement that follows inhalation of the organisms in that they are extremely small and much more numerous than the bronchogenic lesions. The miliary nodules represent tiny granulomas in the interstitial tissues of the lung rather than the acinar nodose areas of consolidation that characterize the inhalation form of the disease. As in miliary tuberculosis, the lesions may not be visible for 2 or 3 weeks after the invasion of the blood stream.

Reinfection Histoplasmosis. The reinfection form runs a chronic course with a tendency to cavitation and fibrosis. It generally occurs in older people and commonly involves the upper lobes, presenting an appearance similar to chronic tuberculosis.

The cavities are usually thick-walled and multiple, and not infrequently involve both upper lobes. They tend to be multiloculated and irregular, and most often do not show a fluid level. In rare instances, the cavity ruptures to produce a bronchopleural fistula. There is usually extensive fibrosis and shrinkage of the lung, causing elevation of the lung root, displacement of the trachea to the affected side and flattening of the chest wall.

Areas of dense infiltration and fibrosis without evidence of cavitation may persist unchanged for years. This is comparable to the arrested form of tuberculosis. However, reactivation of the infection is common. The lesions then increase in extent and cavities may appear. Other portions of the lungs can be involved as a result of bronchogenic spread of the infection. Hematogenous dissemination can occur at any time from direct involvement of a pulmonary vein.

MONILIASIS (CANDIDIASIS). While large numbers of *Candida albicans* can be isolated from the mouth, gums or tooth sockets of a great

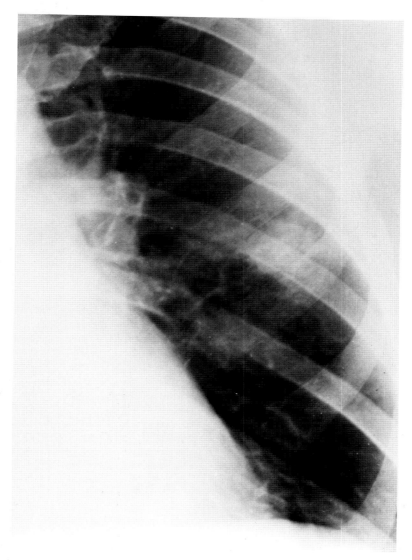

FIG. 259. HISTOPLASMOMA

The poorly demarcated nodule in the left lung showed no calcification on tomograms and could not be distinguished from a bronchogenic carcinoma. The lesion was resected and showed actively budding forms of histoplasma within it.

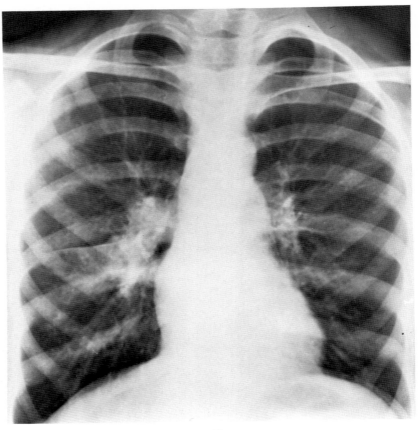

FIG. 260. PRIMARY HISTOPLASMOSIS

The round shadow at the right root represents a large lymph node. Below this there is a homogeneous density caused by disease of the superior segment of the right lower lobe. The upper margin of the shadow represents the long fissure which has been displaced downward as a result of atelectasis of the involved segment. The appearance is identical to that of the primary complex of tuberculosis.

many persons, and from the sputum of patients, especially those who have received antibiotics, this organism rarely causes disease of the lungs. The incidence of monilial infestation is so great in patients being treated for nonfungal respiratory disease, that the finding of monilia in the sputum is of little diagnostic significance. The diagnosis of moniliasis, therefore, cannot be made with certainty unless the organism is demonstrated in excised tissue or in cultures of the blood. Positive cultures of the urine may be significant in the male, but they are without diagnostic value in the female because of the high incidence of monilia in vaginal secretions.

In the majority of reported cases of moniliasis, the infection has been in the kidney, on a heart valve, or at the site of an indwelling venous catheter. There are few authenticated cases of bronchopulmonary moniliasis. These have occurred almost exclusively in patients on long term steroid treatment, or in those with a debi-litating disease, most commonly leukemia or one of the lymphomas.

Because of the small number of verified cases of moniliasis, it is difficult to draw the roentgen picture. It is generally stated that the disease occurs in the lungs in two forms: the bronchial, which is associated with fine peribronchial infiltrations producing a hazy appearance to the pulmonary field, and the pulmonary, which is characterized by consolidation of the lung. The pulmonary lesions consist of a single area of consolidation or infiltration or multiple lesions (Fig. 261), some of which may clear while new ones develop during the course of the disease. A review of the reported cases suggests that true moniliasis is characterized by involvement of the pulmonary parenchyma. It is doubtful that fine, peribronchial infiltrations alone are really due to this disease. It seems more likely that the roentgen changes in such cases are due to a nonspecific bronchial infection in a patient who has monilia

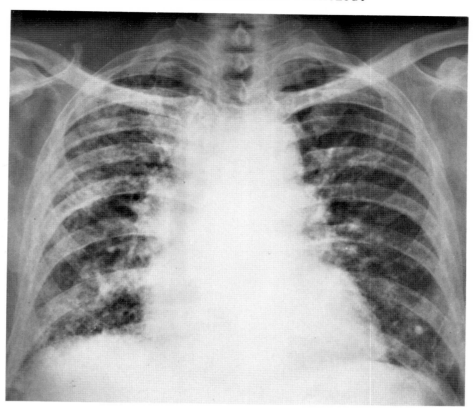

FIG. 261. MONILIASIS

The diffuse, streak-like shadows represent interstitial infiltrations throughout the lungs. They cannot be differentiated radiologically from lymphangitic carcinosis. In this man, monilia were found in the urine as well as in the sputum, indicating that the organisms were pathogenic.

in the sputum. Several instances of pleural effusion and of empyema, caused by monilia, have been described. There is nothing specific about the roentgen picture in these cases.

The diagnosis of moniliasis may be justified in a patient with longstanding, debilitating disease associated with one or more persistent patches of consolidation, in whom neoplastic disease can be excluded, and when no specific organisms are found in the sputum aside from monilia.

MUCORMYCOSIS. This is an infection caused by a fungus belonging to the family *Mucoraceae*. The organisms are generally saprophytic, but in rare instances they cause serious and fatal disease in man. The cases reported have occurred mostly in patients with an underlying debilitating disease, such as diabetes or leukemia, and in patients treated with cancerocidal drugs and corticosteroids. Most often the infection appears to involve the paranasal sinuses, the central nervous system and the intracranial veins. The lungs may be affected by inhalation, or by embolization from a thrombophlebitic focus.

The films show one or more areas of consolidation. These may be large or small, and can undergo cavitation. The appearance cannot be differentiated from bacterial pneumonia or pulmonary infarction (Fig. 262). As a matter of fact, when the pulmonary lesion is due to embolization from an infected venous focus it represents an infarct together with infection. Like other infected infarcts, cavitation may occur. The wall of the cavity may be quite thick and suggest a broken down neoplasm.

NOCARDIOSIS. Nocardiosis is caused by *Nocardia asteroides*, an aerobic acid-fast organism which lives free in nature as a saprophyte, but can cause disease in humans. The pulmonary disease apparently occurs as the result of inhalation of the organism. It is frequently associated with lesions in the skin and brain from hematogeneous dissemination of the pulmonary infection.

The pulmonary lesions are characterized by consolidation and interstitial infiltration. Not infrequently, the process begins in the upper por-

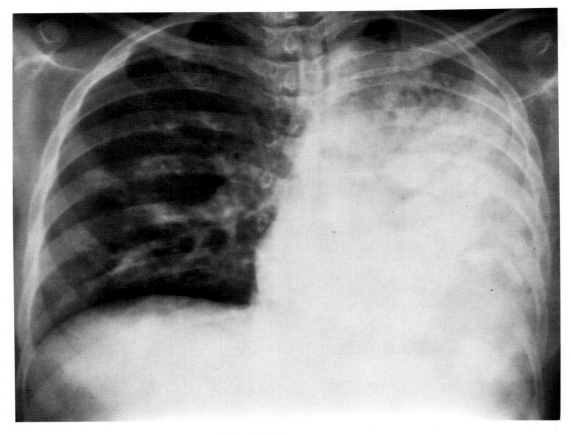

FIG. 262. MUCORMYCOSIS

A 16 year old female diabetic presented with high fever, hemoptysis and dyspnea. The entire left lower lobe and the lingular and anterior segments of the upper lobe are opacified. An air bronchogram is seen indicating consolidation of the lung. The heart is shifted slightly to the left because of loss of lung volume secondary to plugging of small bronchi. The organisms of mucormycosis were found in necrotic tissue removed from the left main bronchus at bronchoscopy. The patient was treated with amphotericin B followed by left pneumonectomy. (Courtesy of Dr. T. F. VanZandt, Rochester, N. Y.)

tion of an upper lobe. The roentgen picture is then indistinguishable from tuberculosis, particularly when interstitial infiltration is the prominent feature. In other cases the disease begins with a patch of dense consolidation situated anywhere in the lung. This usually increases in size as a result of local spread of the infection and often involves more than one segment. It may affect an entire lobe or the entire lung. There is little tendency to spontaneous resolution.

Although areas of suppuration are regularly found within the lesions at postmortem examination, roentgen evidence of cavitation is not so common. When cavities are visible, they appear to be part of a diffuse inflammatory process, as in suppurative bronchopneumonia, rather than in the form of a distinct abscess with a well-defined wall. A pleural effusion may occur during the acute stage of the disease and an empyema can result from perforation of a superficial sup-

purative focus at any stage. As in actinomycosis, the infection may spread directly through the parietal pleura to produce a peripleuritis, osteomyelitis of the overlying ribs, suppuration in the soft tissues and the formation of draining sinuses (Fig. 263).

Nocardiosis, like other fungous infections, has a tendency to occur in debilitated individuals. Recently, a number of cases have been found in association with pulmonary alveolar proteinosis. The rather characteristic picture of diffuse clouding of the lungs by the proteinaceous material in the alveoli then becomes complicated by the presence of one or more areas of dense inflammatory consolidation.

SPOROTRICHOSIS. This is caused by *Sporotrichum schenckii*, an organism growing either as a saprophyte or parasite on certain plants. In humans, the infection occurs particularly in those who handle contaminated plants or soil,

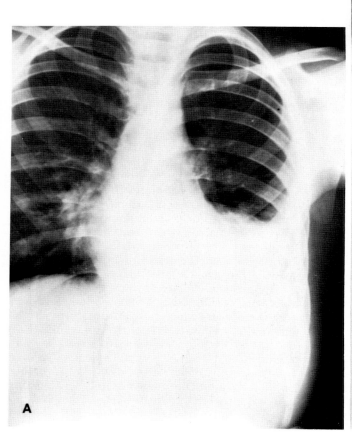
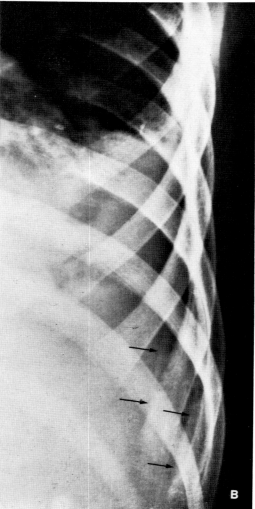

FIG. 263. NOCARDIOSIS

A: The film shows a homogeneous opacification of the lower part of the left hemithorax. In addition, there is thickening of the soft tissues of the left chest wall extending down the left flank. An area of infiltration is also present in the mesial portion of the right lower lobe. *B*: Close-up of a Bucky film of the lower left ribs shows linear streaks (arrows) paralleling the upper borders of the anterior ribs, representing periosteal new bone formation. Several lucencies are present in the lower part of the left lung, indicating a suppurative process. The combination of the findings in the lung and chest wall is indicative of actinomycosis or nocardiosis.

and most commonly affects the skin and lymph nodes. Pulmonary infection is unusual and rarely occurs in the absence of skin lesions.

The pulmonary lesion begins as an area of consolidation and infiltration which has a tendency to undergo cavitation. The wall of the cavity may be thick and irregular at first but as drainage takes place it becomes thin. Patchy areas of consolidation and additional cavities result from bronchogenic spread of the infection. A blocked cavity, filled with exudate, can simulate a round pulmonary neoplasm. Numerous

small nodules, scattered throughout the lungs, suggesting metastatic neoplasm, can result from hematogenous spread. These may be associated with lesions in the skin or bones. Enlargement of the hilar lymph nodes has been described.

Protozoan Infections. Protozoan diseases of the lungs are unusual. The most important are amebiasis, *Pneumocystis carinii* pneumonia and toxoplasmosis.

AMEBIASIS. Infection with *Entamoeba histolytica* begins in the intestines. Often the amebae travel through the portal system to the liver and produce one or more hepatic abscesses. Perforation of one of these beneath the diaphragm results in a subphrenic abscess. As with any subphrenic abscess, a sterile, sympathetic effusion may form in the pleural cavity. An empyema forms if the amebae traverse the diaphragm, either by rupture of the subphrenic abscess or spread through the lymphatic channels of the diaphragm into the pleura. The liver abscess itself may rupture through the diaphragm to produce an empyema without an intervening subphrenic abscess.

If the undersurface of the lung becomes adherent to the diaphragm, either the subphrenic abscess or the liver abscess can perforate directly into the lung. This usually occurs in the anterior basal or mesial basal segment of the right lower lobe. The involved portion of lung becomes consolidated and soon undergoes suppuration. Not infrequently the suppurative focus drains through a bronchus, producing a bronchial fistula which communicates with the abscess in the liver either directly or through a subphrenic abscess. Further spread of the amebic infection may then occur through the bronchi to neighboring portions of the lung, producing additional suppurative foci.

The lungs can also be infected by hematogenous spread of the amebae, resulting in the formation of one or more pulmonary abscesses. Most commonly the hematogenous dissemination occurs from infection of a hepatic vein from an adjacent liver abscess. However, it is possible for hematogenous infection of the lungs to occur without an intervening liver abscess. The infection can reach the lungs from the rectum or sigmoid colon by way of the inferior hemorrhoidal vein and inferior vena cava.

The thoracic manifestations of amebiasis are elevation of the right leaf of the diaphragm with or without evidences of pleurisy, pneumonia of the contiguous portion of the right lung often associated with suppuration or a bronchial fistula extending through the diaphragm, and metastatic pulmonary abscesses.

Not infrequently the diaphragm is markedly elevated simply as a result of extreme enlargement of the liver by one or more abscesses. There may be little impairment of the motion of the diaphragm which can retain its smooth, regular contour. Marked limitation or absence of diaphragmatic movement is more characteristic of a subphrenic abscess. This is often associated with obliteration of the costophrenic sinus as a result of diaphragmatic pleurisy. A collection of free fluid, usually of moderate extent, may be present in the right pleural cavity, and may signify nothing more than a reactive pleurisy without invasion by the amebae. Large collections of fluid or loculated effusions are generally due to actual infection of the pleura. The diaphragm may be obscured if the effusion is large and its elevation not recognizable on films made in the erect position.

Since infection of the lung is usually secondary to an abscess in the liver, the amebic pneumonia is characteristically situated immediately above an elevated right diaphragm (Fig. 264). The pneumonia may be overshadowed by an effusion in the pleural cavity and not recognized until the effusion has been aspirated.

There is a tendency for early suppuration of the pneumonia. This is manifested by one or more lucent areas within the shadow of the consolidated lung. In some instances, there is only a single cavity with a fluid level. However, unlike a putrid lung abscess, in which the surrounding inflammatory process is minimal, in amebic disease an extensive area of consolidation remains about the cavity. In addition, there is a tendency to early local spread of the infection with enlargement of the area of consolidation.

The presence of one or more lucencies or of a fluid level within the consolidated lung indicates that the abscess which has ruptured through the diaphragm communicates with a bronchus. However, these changes may be absent if the communication is small or blocked by exudate. Even bronchography may fail to disclose the fistula, but it can often be demonstrated by injecting contrast material into the sinus tract which forms following drainage of the abdominal abscess. Bronchography may show only separation of the branches of the middle lobe bronchi from those of the lower lobe. This is due to displacement of the two lobes by the elevated diaphragm and to lack of filling of the bronchi of the anterior basal segment which is the portion of lung that is usually involved.

Metastatic amebic abscesses are situated anywhere in the lungs. They may be single as well as multiple. They may appear as more or less well defined, discrete, homogeneous opacities or show fluid levels. In this respect, they do not differ from other types of pulmonary abscess. The wall is generally quite thin with little surrounding inflammation. When the metastatic abscess is secondary to an abscess in the liver, the right leaf of the diaphragm is usually elevated. This may be associated with a pleural reaction at the right base or an area of consolidation in the lower part of the right lung. These changes

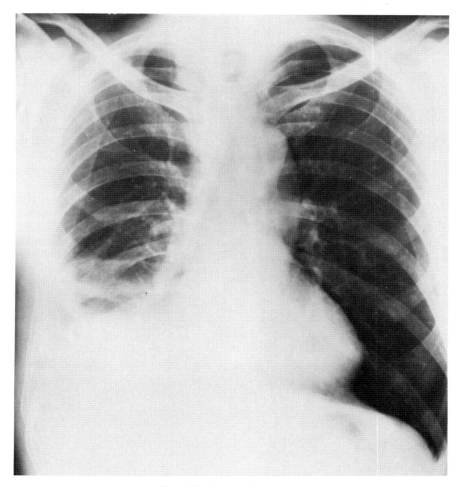

FIG. 264. AMEBIC PNEUMONIA

There is infiltration of the right lower lobe in association with elevation of the right leaf of the diaphragm and thickening of the pleura. The patient had an amebic abscess of the liver which had perforated into the lung.

are absent when the metastatic abscess results from infection of the lower portion of the intestinal tract without an intervening liver abscess.

PNEUMOCYSTIS CARINII PNEUMONIA. This disease, previously called interstitial plasma cell pneumonia, occurs most frequently in infants between the ages of 6 weeks and 6 months. In almost all of the reported cases the infants have been born prematurely or were suffering from a debilitating disease. In some instances, there was an underlying hypo- or agammaglobulinemia. In adults also there is practically always an underlying debilitating condition, such as leukemia or Hodgkin's disease, particularly during treatment with cytotoxic agents.

On pathologic examination, the lungs are large and heavy and do not collapse. Sections show confluent foci of consolidation, interspersed with areas of emphysema. The interlobular septa are thickened. Microscopically, the alveoli are seen to be filled with eosinophilic material which contains numerous vacuoles which impart a foamy appearance to the section. Within these, the pneumocystis can be demonstrated. The interstitial tissues are infiltrated with round cells, causing marked thickening of the alveolar septa. The interlobar septa are also thickened by edema fluid.

In general, the roentgen appearance is that of a rather diffuse bronchopneumonia which is almost always bilateral. In the early stage, the involved portions of lung appear diffusely clouded, and on close inspection present a fine granular appearance. Later, denser patchy areas of consolidation appear. These have a tendency to coalesce and become confluent during the course of the disease. Emphysematous areas become manifest between the patches of consolidation. Interstitial emphysema, resulting from alveolar rupture, may lead to mediastinal emphysema or pneumothorax.

The roentgen appearance is not unlike that of hyaline membrane disease. However, the latter condition occurs exclusively in the newborn while the pneumonia caused by the *Pneumocystis carinii* does not become manifest until the infant is at least 6 weeks of age. The diffuse cloudiness of the lungs and the granular appearance are not unlike the changes that occur in pulmonary edema and alveolar proteinosis. Extremely rapid respiration and cyanosis, which are characteristic of pneumocystis pneumonia, also suggest pulmonary edema. However, the physical examination discloses surprisingly few abnormal signs in the chest and the crackling and bubbling rales, characteristic of pulmonary edema, are absent. The acuteness of the disease and the age incidence of the great majority of the cases serves to exclude alveolar proteinosis. In an adult with a debilitating disease, the sudden onset of clouding of the pulmonary fields in the presence of a normal-sized heart should suggest the possibility of pneumocystis pneumonia (Fig. 265).

TOXOPLASMOSIS. Infection by *Toxoplasma gondii* is common in humans as evidenced by serological tests. Clinical disease, when it occurs, usually involves the eyes or central nervous system. Pulmonary infection is extremely rare. Most of the reported cases have been in the newborn, associated with generalized infection. In the pulmonary disease of the adult, the roentgen picture is that of an interstitial pneumonia. In the early stage, clouding of the lungs, particularly at the roots, has been described. The later picture is more like that of atypical pneumonia with spotty or coalescent densities.

Parasitic Infestations. Parasitic diseases of the lungs are rare in this country. The most common is that caused by the echinococcus and is characterized by the formation of one or more cysts in the lungs, mediastinum and pleura. More

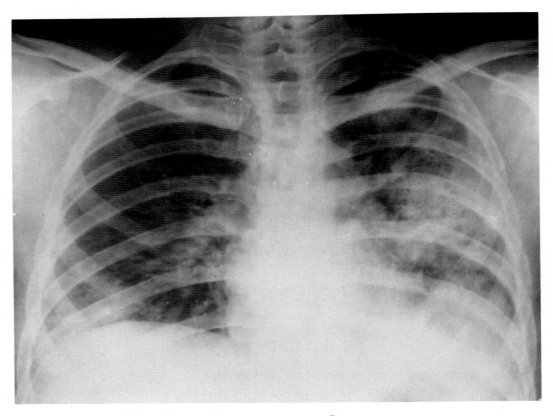

FIG. 265. *PNEUMOCYSTIS CARINII* PNEUMONIA

This 32 year old female, who was receiving chemotherapy for Hodgkin's disease, became acutely ill with shortness of breath and fever. The film shows bilateral pulmonary infiltrations, more marked on the left side. The involved areas have a granular appearance as a result of filling of many of the alveoli with exudate. The disease cleared rapidly on treatment with pentamidine.

or less diffuse eosinophilic infiltrations in the lungs occur in paragonimiasis and *Ascaris* infestations. Miliary nodules are characteristic of tropical eosinophilia, and interstitial fibrosis occurs in some cases of schistosomiasis.

ECHINOCOCCUS DISEASE (HYDATID CYST). Echinococcus disease is caused by a small tapeworm, *Echinococcus granulosus*, which is found in the intestines of dogs and related animals. The dog develops the tapeworm after the ingestion of infected organs, particularly the liver, of sheep or cattle which contain the parasite in its encysted form. These animals represent the intermediate or secondary host, contracting the disease by ingesting the echinococcus ova from the stool of the dog. Man contracts the disease from the dog in the same way as do sheep and cattle. The ova hatch in the bowel and release embryos which burrow into the intestinal wall. From here, some are carried by the portal circulation to the liver where they develop into hydatid cysts. One or more of the embryos may pass through the capillaries of the liver and reach the lungs where they form cysts.

The echinococcus cyst is a fluid-filled sac with a complex wall. The inner layer consists of a germinal epithelium which produces a brood capsule containing scolices that form the adult tapeworm when ingested by a dog. The brood capsules can form daughter cysts. These, as well as many of the scolices, float freely in the hydatid fluid and are liberated when the cyst ruptures. The middle layer of the cyst is formed by laminated elastic material elaborated by the cyst, while the outer layer is composed of fibrous tissue produced by the host. Occasionally calcium is deposited in the cyst wall. There is little inflammatory reaction about the intact cyst. However, if the cyst ruptures, the hydatid fluid causes an inflammatory reaction in the surrounding tissues.

Radiologically, the intact hydatid cyst appears as an extremely sharply outlined, round or oval, homogeneous density which may be somewhat lobulated. The cysts are either single or multiple and may be tiny or huge. As a rule, when multiple cysts are present, they vary greatly in size. Growth of the cysts can often be demonstrated by periodic examination. The density of the cyst depends on its size, the smaller ones casting a faint shadow while the larger ones appear quite dense. When the wall of the cyst is calcified, the lesion usually appears mottled because of irregular deposition of the lime.

The shadow of an uncomplicated echinococcus cyst differs from that of a primary bronchogenic carcinoma in the remarkable homogeneity of its density and the extreme sharpness and smoothness of its border. However, sarcoma of the lung, either primary or metastatic, or a benign tumor of the pleura, can produce a shadow indistinguishable from that of an echinococcus cyst. The presence of a calcific border is characteristic of hydatid disease (Fig. 141). Marked elevation of the right leaf of the diaphragm in association with one or more round shadows in the lungs, should suggest the possibility of echinococcus disease with involvement of the liver by large cysts. Obviously, similar findings may occur in patients with metastatic neoplasm.

When a tear develops in the wall of the cyst, some of its fluid seeps into the adjacent lung. The ensuing inflammatory reaction obscures the characteristically sharp outline of the cyst and the appearance is then the same as that of a neoplasm. If the cyst ruptures into a small bronchus, air may enter between the outer fibrous layer of the cyst wall and the middle elastic layer. The localized collection of air appears as a crescentic zone of radiolucency within the border of the cyst. This *crescent sign* has been considered pathognomonic of echinococcus cyst (Fig. 266). However, it can also be present in a variety of conditions in which a pulmonary cavity is partly filled with solid material. In these instances, when the patient assumes the decubitus position, the location of the area of lucency usually changes as the contents of the cavity shift to the most dependent portion. The lucent crescent remains unchanged in the case of an echinococcus cyst regardless of the position of the patient, because the air is trapped in the cyst wall.

Rupture of a hydatid cyst into a larger bronchus may result in complete evacuation of its contents and disappearance of the cyst. In other instances, an empty, smooth-walled cavity persists, leaving a thin, ring-like shadow like that of a tuberculous cavity or the residual cavity of a healed lung abscess. When the cyst is only partially evacuated, an air-fluid level appears. The level may be perfectly straight and regular, as in other cavities containing air and fluid. However, in some cases crumpled remnants of the inner germinal membrane of the cyst float on the fluid and cause an irregularity of the fluid level. This has been described as the *sign of the water lily*. A pulmonary cavity partly filled with fluid and blood clot can present a similar appearance. After draining its contents, the ruptured cyst may become small and unrecognizable on conventional films, presenting simply as a localized inflammatory process. However, the underlying cavity may be demonstrable by tomography or bronchography.

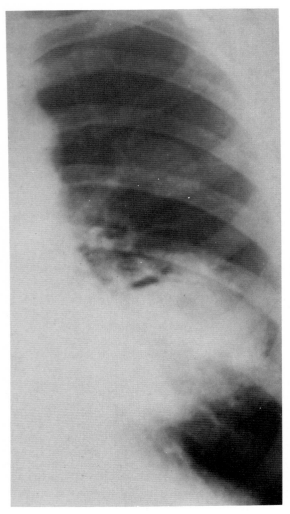

FIG. 266. PERFORATING ECHINOCOCCUS CYST: CRESCENT
SIGN

The round, dense shadow in the left lower lobe represents
an echinococcus cyst. The crescentic lucency near its upper
border is caused by air that has insinuated itself between the
layers of the cyst wall. This is a characteristic sign of the
early stage of rupture. The oval shadow in the upper lobe is
a second cyst.

Not infrequently a ruptured cyst becomes secondarily infected. It then cannot be differentiated from a lung abscess unless previous films
showing the intact cyst are available. Infection
of the surrounding lung can obscure the entire
picture.

Rupture of a cyst, spontaneously, at operation,
or as the result of needle aspiration, releases the
daughter cysts together with the fluid. Intrathoracic spread of the disease may also follow rupture of a hydatid cyst of the liver through the
diaphragm. If the cyst ruptures into a bronchus,

the daughter cysts may be disseminated throughout the lungs and develop into large cysts (Fig.
267). These may be uniform in size. Rupture into
the mediastinum may result in the formation of
large masses in the mediastinum.

Rupture into the pleura produces a pleural
effusion. The daughter cysts can sometimes be
recognized on the pleura after the fluid is aspirated, particularly if a pneumothorax is induced.
Spread into the pleura also results in the formation of one or more localized cysts on the surface
of the lungs surrounded by dense, granulomatous, thickened pleura.

PARAGONIMIASIS. This disease is caused by the
lung fluke, *Paragonimus westermani*. The adult
worm develops and ovulates in the human lung.
The ova are expectorated in the sputum and are
picked up by the intermediate host, the crayfish
or crab, which carries the encysted parasites in
its liver and muscle tissue. When these are ingested by the human, the cysts liberate their
larvae in the small intestine. The larvae penetrate through the intestinal wall into the peritoneal cavity, and then make their way through
the diaphragm, finally piercing the visceral
pleura to enter the lung. Usually several larvae
find their way into the lungs and often burrow
for considerable distances before developing into
adult worms. These cause a rather localized inflammation of the lung with central areas of
necrosis in which the ova are deposited. The
disease is most prevalent in the Far East, although cases have been observed in certain parts
of Africa and South America.

The roentgen appearance of the chest in paragonimiasis varies in accordance with the stage
of the disease. Each stage of the development of
the worm has its counterpart in special pathologic alterations which are reflected on the roentgen film. The three stages are the larval, the
adult and the healing stage.

Penetration of the pleura occurs at least a
month after the encysted parasites are ingested.
It may be associated with a pleurisy evidenced
by plastic exudate or a small effusion, or a complicating pneumothorax. The pleurisy is often
bilateral. As the larvae enter and wander through
the lung, they produce ill-defined, more or less
irregular areas of consolidation. These vary in
size and can occur anywhere in the lungs. They
are usually bilateral and are not limited by the
boundaries of any segment. Many of the densities
are evanescent, clearing while new ones appear
in other portions of the lung. In this respect they
resemble the shadows seen in eosinophilic pneumonia due to other causes. These changes may
continue for a number of months before the

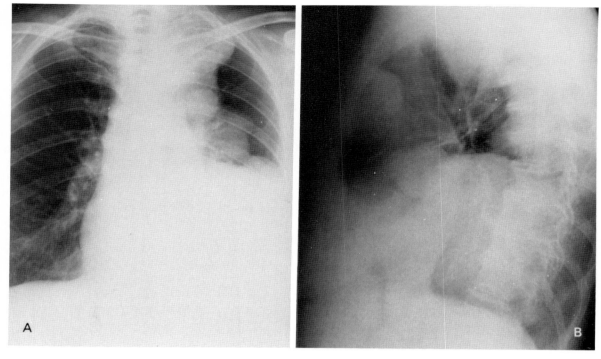

FIG. 267. ECHINOCOCCUS CYSTS

A: Ten years previously the patient had a single hydatid cyst in the left lung. This ruptured into a bronchus and the patient expectorated scolices at that time. This examination shows multiple cysts of varying size. The opacification at the left base simulates a pleural effusion. *B*: The lateral view shows the opacification at the left base to be due to a large cyst. Smaller cysts are seen above it. The trachea is bowed forward by a cyst in the posterior superior mediastinum. The patient also had cysts of the liver and spleen.

appearance of the lesions caused by the adult worm. A pericardial effusion has been noted during this period in rare instances.

The stage of the mature worm is characterized by bilateral, moderately well defined densities, varying from 1 to 4 cm in diameter. However, only a single lesion may be present. Cavitation can occur in one or more of the lesions. As the cavity develops, the shadow of the lesion becomes round and sharply marginated, and presents the appearance of a cyst. Characteristically, it is free of fluid. It may be thin-walled but more commonly, the wall is rather thick, at least in one portion of its circumference. Perforation into the pleura may produce an empyema or a pyopneumothorax. The active, adult stage of the disease, during which changes occur in the shadows, lasts anywhere from 6 to 10 years. In the later phases, bronchography may disclose local areas of bronchiectasis.

When the worms die, the lesions either disappear completely or become stabilized. Residual lesions are represented simply by small areas of fibrosis, sometimes associated with calcification. Small, localized bronchiectases may remain.

SCHISTOSOMIASIS (BILHARZIASIS). Schistosomiasis is caused by one of the blood flukes. S. *japonicum* is endemic in the Far East, while S. *mansoni* and S. *haematobium* are prevalent in Africa and the Middle East. S. *mansoni* is also the cause of schistosomiasis in South America and the Caribbean.

In all instances, the disease is contracted by man from water containing the young forms of the schistosome (cercariae), which emerge from infected snails. The cercariae penetrate the skin or mucous membranes, from which they are carried by the lymphatics, through the venous system, into the lungs. The larvae are small enough to pass through the pulmonary capillaries into the systemic circulation. Those which enter the mesenteric artery pass through the capillaries of the small intestine, into venules of the portal system. Here the S. *mansoni* and S. *japonicum* complete their development into the mature worm, while S. *hematobium* migrates retrograde into the venous system about the urinary bladder. The ova of the mature S. *hematobium* either perforate the bladder, to be excreted in the urine, or enter the inferior vena cava by way of the iliac veins to be transported to the lungs, where they become impacted in the arterioles. The ova of *S. mansoni* and *S. japonicum* are either deposited in the bowel or are carried by the portal vein into the capillaries of the liver, where they become impacted and cause hepatic cirrhosis. When collateral circulation develops, many of the ova bypass the liver and lodge in the pulmonary arterioles.

The ova of all three types of blood fluke produce a necrotizing arteriolitis in the lungs. They pass through the walls of the necrotic arterioles and cause a granulomatous reaction. Many of the arterioles eventually become obliterated by fibrous tissue, leading to pulmonary hypertension. In some instances, adult worms also reach the lungs in similar fashion and lodge in small branches of the pulmonary arteries. Here the worms die and produce a severe inflammatory reaction complicated by thrombosis.

Only a small percentage of cases of schistosomiasis develop pulmonary complications. The earliest changes occur when the larval form enters the pulmonary capillaries. At this time they may cause transient shadows associated with eosinophilia as in Löffler's syndrome. The more permanent manifestations result from impaction of the ova in the arterioles. This may produce miliary shadows which then develop into diffuse, more or less fine, fibrotic infiltrations throughout the lungs. The pulmonary hypertension which occurs in this phase of the disease may overshadow the picture by producing marked enlargement of the major pulmonary arteries at the lung roots (Fig. 268). When the pulmonary involvement is mostly confined to the arterioles and the granulomatous reaction is minimal, the outer two-thirds of the lungs appear clear. The roentgen picture is then identical with that of primary pulmonary hypertension.

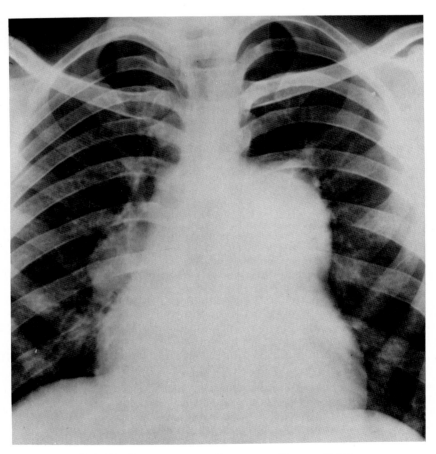

FIG. 268. SCHISTOSOMIASIS: PULMONARY HYPERTENSION

The main and right pulmonary arteries are markedly dilated while the vessels in the outer portions of the lungs are extremely small. Disparity in the size of the central and peripheral vessels is indicative of severe pulmonary hypertension. The cardiac silhouette is enlarged as a result of hypertrophy and dilatation of the right heart chambers and obscures the left pulmonary artery. The patient had schistosomiasis of long standing. (Courtesy of Dr. Ali Rida Henedi, Alexandria, Egypt).

TROPICAL EOSINOPHILIA. The name, tropical eosinophilia, is applied to a disease occurring in the tropics, characterized by low grade fever, severe paroxysmal cough and shortness of breath often associated with wheezing, a high blood eosinophilia, and a strongly positive filarial complement fixation test. In almost all cases, pulmonary lesions can be demonstrated on the films. The clinical manifestations of the disease, including the eosinophilia, respond quickly to treatment with arsenicals or diethylcarbamazine. The disease is most prevalent in India and Malaya, but a large number of cases have been observed in Africa and in Puerto Rico.

The finding of microfilaria in the lungs in a few of the reported cases, the positive complement fixation test against the filarial antigen, and the response to specific treatment indicate that some form of filaria is probably responsible for the disease.

The roentgen changes most frequently observed are caused by inflammatory infiltration in the interstitial, peribronchial and perivascular tissue. The lower two-thirds of the lungs are most involved. There is a generalized grayness of the pulmonary fields, with obscuration of the peripheral vessels and blurring of the borders of the larger vessels at the lung roots. The infiltrations also tend to form a reticular pattern throughout the lungs although, in many places, they appear as more streak-like, linear densities. In about a third of the cases, usually in addition to the above, there are tiny nodular densities throughout the lungs, representing small granulomas. These are 1 to 3 mm in size, somewhat larger than miliary tubercles, and unlike hematogenous tuberculous lesions, they are more numerous in the lower portions of the lungs. Occasionally, larger nodular lesions occur, measuring up to 0.5 cm in diameter. These are irregular and poorly demarcated and in places, may be confluent. Areas of lobular or subsegmental consolidation occasionally occur in conjunction with the other lesions. Thickening of the pleura, as manifested by accentuation of the fissures, occurs quite frequently. Pleural effusions are extremely rare.

Response of the lesions to specific therapy is important in the diagnosis. Resolution has been observed to begin within 3 days after the onset of treatment, but there is a tendency to chronicity and interstitial fibrosis so that complete resolution does not occur in all cases. However, the nodular infiltrations and the diffuse grayness of the pulmonary fields usually clear, leaving the linear or reticular pattern of interstitial fibrosis. Relapse of the disease is not uncommon within a year or two after cessation of treatment, and this is usually associated with a return of the original picture of the disease.

Tropical eosinophilia should not be confused with other conditions characterized by pulmonary infiltrations and eosinophilia, such as Löffler's syndrome, eosinophilic pneumonia and periarteritis nodosa. In contrast to tropical eosinophilia, these diseases are manifested by the presence of either single areas of consolidation which are transient, disappearing in one place and appearing in another, or multiple such areas, irregularly scattered throughout the lungs. On the other hand, the picture may be indistinguishable from the diseases associated with an allergic response to certain organic dusts, such as farmer's lung.

MISCELLANEOUS PARASITIC DISEASES. A variety of parasites can infest the lungs and produce lesions visible on the films. These may be in the form of small nodular foci or larger patches of consolidation which may be evanescent, clearing in one place and appearing in another. The inflammatory reaction is associated with an outpouring of eosinophils in the blood as well as the pulmonary exudate.

The parasite most frequently responsible for transient eosinophilic infiltrations of the lung is the roundworm *Ascaris lumbricoides*. The adult worm lives in the human intestine, and its ova are excreted with the stool. The disease is contracted when the ova are ingested with contaminated food or soil, and develop into larvae in the small intestine. The larvae burrow into the wall of the bowel and are carried by the blood to the lungs. Here they penetrate the capillary wall to enter the alveoli where they call forth an eosinophilic pneumonic reaction. The larvae are then coughed up and some are swallowed, returning to the small bowel where they complete their cycle by developing into adult worms.

Two cases of infestation of the lung by *Strongyloides stercoralis* have been reported by Berk, Woodruff and Frediani. One showed transient nodular infiltrations in the lungs, while the other showed only increased markings in the lower lobes, wrongly attributed to bronchiectasis. Eosinophilia was present in each case.

Small, nodular infiltrations of the lungs, associated with eosinophilia, have been described in patients in whose sputum mites have been found (*acariasis*). A search should be made for these parasites, as well as for evidence of helminthic infestation in all patients with pulmonary infiltrations and eosinophilia of unknown cause.

A solitary nodule can be formed in the lung as a result of infestation by the dog heartworm, *Dirofilaria immitis*. The human is an accidental host, the microfilaria entering the blood stream through a mosquito bite. The worm matures in the right side of the heart or pulmonary artery. It is carried into a small pulmonary vessel where it causes a local inflammatory reaction. The inflammatory nodule that is formed is persistent and fibrotic and may undergo necrosis and calcification. In the absence of calcification the appearance suggests a circumscribed neoplasm of the lung.

Multiple, small, discrete, calcific deposits in the lungs sometimes occur in *pentastomiasis*. The lesions are caused by the encysted larval form (tongue worm) of the arachnids *Linguatula serrata* and *Armillifer armillatus*. The pulmonary lesions are rare in this country but are not uncommon in Europe and parts of Africa and South America. They are about 0.5 cm in diameter and the calcium may be deposited in an annular form.

Putrid Abscess of the Lung

An abscess can be defined as a collection of pus surrounded by a limited, localizing wall of inflammation. An abscess of the lung, therefore, is to be differentiated pathologically from foci of suppuration within a diffuse inflammatory lesion such as that of suppurative bronchopneumonia. The true abscesses that occur occasionally in the course of suppurative bronchopneumonia are nonputrid. They are not so common as putrid lung abscesses and almost all of them heal spontaneously. They rarely reach a chronic stage unless they are secondary to an obstructive lesion in the bronchus.

Metastatic abscesses are usually multiple. Since many of them do not communicate with a bronchus, they often appear as solid shadows without fluid levels. The clinical picture associated with metastatic abscesses is dominated by the general sepsis of which they are one part and, unless they perforate into the pleural cavity to produce an empyema, they do not cause any characteristic symptoms or present a therapeutic problem in themselves. In extremely rare instances, a metastatic abscess may be single and produce either a small nodular shadow or one which is poorly delineated and suggestive of an area of consolidation. It may be situated anywhere in the lungs. If it perforates into the pleura and produces an empyema, the underlying lesion will be obscured. Otherwise the metastatic abscess undergoes slow, progressive resolution.

The problem of the putrid lung abscess is a different and more important one because the disease is bronchogenic and has a tendency to progress and requires active treatment which may entail surgery. The type and manner of treatment depends on the evolution of the abscess, requiring careful and repeated roentgen examinations during the course of the disease. These will disclose whether the abscess is draining well or whether it is increasing in size, or resolving. The films will also demonstrate spread of the disease to adjacent portions of the lung and complicating infections of the pleura. The roentgen examination is indispensable for the determination of the extent of the disease and its localization. This information is essential in cases requiring surgical treatment.

The roentgen appearance of a putrid lung abscess varies considerably, being influenced by many factors. Among these are the stage of the disease, the patency of the entering bronchus and the presence of pleural complications. Occasionally, the findings on a single roentgen examination may be sufficiently characteristic to permit a diagnosis of putrid lung abscess. More commonly, however, the roentgen appearance simulates that of pneumonia, tuberculosis or a neoplasm.

The diagnosis usually becomes more evident if serial examinations are made during the course of the disease. A localized area of consolidation which remains unchanged for a number of days and then undergoes cavitation, is generally satisfactory evidence of an abscess. Similarly, the occurrence of a pleural effusion a short time after the appearance of a localized area of consolidation suggests an abscess of the lung. Although either of these patterns may be seen with a pulmonary infarct, the differentiation is not difficult if the clinical picture is taken into consideration.

When the patient presents with a chronic lesion, the nature of which cannot be determined from the roentgen examination at that time, every effort should be made to obtain previous films for review. These will unfold the entire course of the disease and are invaluable for establishing the diagnosis. In addition, study of the early films is useful for localization of abscesses that are obscured by complicating shadows in the later stages of the disease.

Acute Stage. The putrid lung abscess begins as an area of gangrenous bronchopneumonia which is practically always due to aspiration of particulate material from the mouth or throat, containing a mixture of organisms capable of producing putrefaction. The diseased area almost always consists of a single focus and its location depends on the bronchus into which the material has been aspirated. The involved bronchus is usually of the order of a branch of a segmental bronchus and the inflamed area of the lung corresponds to the distribution of this branch.

Since by far the most common source lies in an infection of the gums in relation to a tooth socket, putrid lung abscess is extremely rare in the edentulous person. In some cases the abscess results from inhalation of an infected plug from a tonsillar crypt. This accounts for the frequency of putrid abscess of the lung as a complication of tonsillectomy. Comatose states also predispose towards aspiration of material from the mouth and throat. Putrid lung abscess is, therefore, prone to occur after operations under general anesthesia or following alcoholic stupor or convulsive seizures.

Although any of the segments of the lung may be the seat of the disease, the fact that the aspiration usually takes place when the patient is recumbent predisposes to infection of certain of the segments. When the patient lies on his back, aspiration is most apt to occur into the superior segment of the lower lobe, and when he lies on his side, the aspirated material tends to lodge in the outer portion of the anterior or posterior segment of the upper lobe.

The area of consolidation and inflammation extends in wedge-shaped fashion from the impacted, aspirated material in the bronchus to the periphery of the lobe. It usually extends to the costal surface of the lung because almost all the medium sized bronchi, in which the disease originates, have branches distributed toward the surface. The only branch of considerable size that does not supply the lung adjacent to the costal parietes is the medial basal division of the right lower lobe (Fig. 54). The segment that it supplies faces only the diaphragmatic and mediastinal surfaces of the lung. In rare instances, an abscess which originates in a small bronchus faces only an interlobar fissure and does not extend to the periphery of the chest.

The area of gangrenous pneumonia can be identified on the chest film within a few days after the aspiration. The roentgen picture is essentially that of segmental or subsegmental consolidation of the lung. In the frontal projection, it most frequently appears as a poorly defined, more or less round, homogeneous density. The typical wedge-shaped shadow of segmental consolidation is more often demonstrable in the lateral or one of the oblique views. In at least one of the projections, the shadow can be demon-

strated to extend to the periphery of the lung in almost all of the cases (Fig. 269). About 2% of abscesses abut only on a pleural fissure and fail to extend to the boundary of the thoracic cavity.

The pleura over the lesion becomes intensely inflamed and covered by fibrinous exudate at the onset of the disease. This soon becomes organized, producing firm adhesions between the lesion and the chest wall. The presence of adhesions is demonstrated fluoroscopically by absence of motion between the lesion and the overlying ribs during respiration. Of course, this is not the case in the rare instance in which the abscess faces only the interlobar fissure or when it lies in the mesial segment of the lower lobe and faces only the diaphragm.

Within a week after the aspiration, liquefaction of the necrotic tissue within the area of gangrenous pneumonia occurs. It usually takes 10 days to 2 weeks for the tissue about the bronchus leading to the lesion to become sufficiently liquefied and separated to permit drainage. During this period, the shadow remains unchanged and cannot be distinguished from the consolidation of pneumonia (Fig. 270). If it is situated beneath the outer part of the clavicle, the appearance is similar to that of caseous tuberculosis.

Once bronchial drainage has been established, the diagnosis is suggested by the appearance of a cavity with a fluid level. The air enters the cavity by way of the bronchus through which the pus and necrotic material are extruded (Figs. 269 and 271). At this time the diagnosis usually becomes obvious clinically because the sputum is foul.

If the abscess continues to drain freely, all of the necrotic material is gradually expelled from the cavity. The inflammatory process about the abscess gradually resolves, no further exudate is formed, and the fluid level disappears. Usually the entering bronchus heals by stricture, the remaining air in the cavity is absorbed and the lung assumes a normal appearance. The only residual change may be some local distortion of the vascular markings and, possibly, a thin, linear, fibrous strand. Complete healing generally occurs in 6 to 10 weeks after the onset of the disease. In about 20% of the cases, the abscess heals without any specific treatment. With adequate antibiotic and chemotherapy, begun early in the disease, at least 85 to 90% of the cases go on to recovery.

The x-ray examination of the chest is the only way of determining when complete healing has taken place. If any shadow remains other than a thin, fibrous streak, it must be concluded that

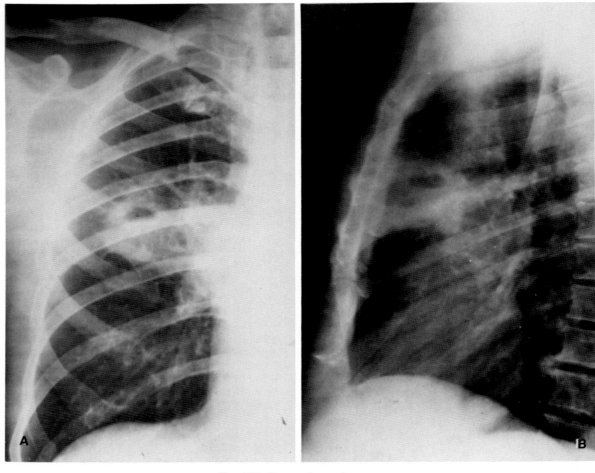

FIG. 269. PUTRID LUNG ABSCESS

A: The shadow overlying the anterior portion of the fourth rib contains an air-fluid level, indicating that it represents a cavity. It is impossible from this view to determine whether the lesion is in the lowermost part of the right upper lobe or the superior segment of the lower lobe. *B*: The lateral view shows the cavity within the anterior segment of the upper lobe. As in practically all cases of putrid lung abscess, the lesion extends to the pleura.

active infection is still present and that the lesion may recur if treatment is stopped. The only exception to this is the persistence of a *residual cavity* (p. 336).

When drainage of the necrotic material in the abscess is incomplete because of blockage of the entering bronchus, the air-fluid level reappears. If the bronchus remains completely obstructed, the air in the abscess cavity is absorbed and replaced with exudate. The film again shows a solid, homogeneous shadow (Fig. 131). Increasing tension within the abscess may force pus through its wall with consequent spread of the disease to the adjacent lung tissue (Fig. 272).

If the entering bronchus is only partially obstructed, a check-valve mechanism may occur, so that air can enter the cavity readily but re-

mains trapped within it. This causes a striking enlargement (ballooning) of the abscess cavity. The increased pressure within the abscess predisposes to local spread of the infection and may lead to perforation into the pleura.

Subacute Stage. This is a stage in the natural history of putrid lung abscess which was important in the preantibiotic era when surgical drainage was generally necessary for cure. It was found that drainage procedures were almost uniformly successful if performed within 6 weeks of the onset of clinical manifestations. After this time, the mortality and morbidity of the disease gradually increased. The subacute stage was arbitrarily defined as the period between 6 weeks and 3 months after the onset of infection. After 3 months the abscess was considered to be chronic.

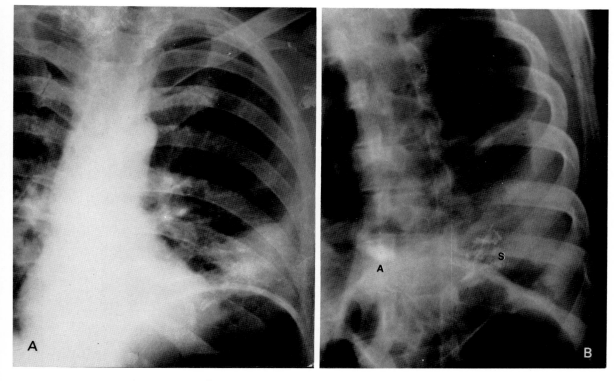

FIG. 270. SHUT-OFF PUTRID LUNG ABSCESS

A: The homogeneous shadow in the left lower lobe, appearing as an area of consolidation, actually represents an abscess in the anterior basal segment, which had not been draining. The patient did not cough or bring up any sputum. An abscess was suspected because of pain in the chest and fever without the cough that is usually associated with a pneumonia. There was severe foul infection of the gums. A foul odor was detected during coughing when the patient was positioned for postural drainage. *B*: A few days later, the patient developed a clear sympathetic effusion, best demonstrated in the left anterior oblique projection. The position of the underlying abscess, obscured by the fluid, is marked by a mixture of iodized oil and methylene blue which was injected into the muscle of the fifth intercostal space in the anterior axillary region (S). The shadow marked (A) is an artifact.

The subacute stage of lung abscess presents a variable roentgen picture. During this period fibrosis of the wall becomes established and there is a greater tendency for the infection to spread to the adjacent pulmonary parenchyma. In many cases the shadow of the abscess is quite small. An air-fluid level or other evidences of a distinct cavity may be lacking when the bronchus is blocked and the cavity completely filled with inspissated necrotic material. When the tension within the cavity increases and the pus extrudes through one or more weak points in the abscess wall, additional densities appear adjacent to the original lesion. As air enters these foci, one or more may show fluid levels. This type of spread is always in contiguity with the original abscess even though an adjacent segment of the lung is involved. The infection can spread in this way through an interlobar fissure to produce a cavity in an adjacent lobe.

In occasional cases, an acute abscess does not establish an adequate bronchial communication. It remains as a solid round shadow of uniform density which may be unchanged in size and shape for many weeks. The pus-filled abscess then has the appearance of a pulmonary neoplasm.

Chronic Stage. Although a chronic lung abscess may consist of a single lesion with a roentgen appearance similar to that of an abscess in an earlier stage, the lesion is generally a more complicated one. In the interval between the acute and chronic stage, as a rule, several changes have occurred which alter the roentgen appearance of the abscess. During the course of the disease, the draining bronchus is usually obstructed intermittently, causing an extension of the abscess in an irregular fashion into the neighboring pulmonary tissue. The abscess which originally was represented by a single round cavity,

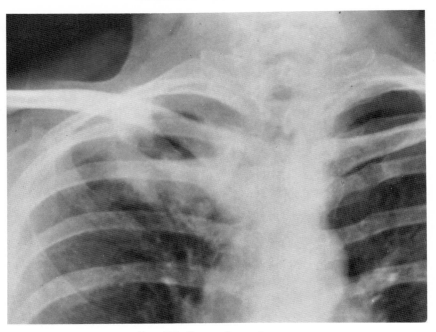

FIG. 271. PUTRID LUNG ABSCESS

There is a cavity with a fluid level in the upper part of the right upper lobe. The differential diagnosis lies between a lung abscess and tuberculosis. The location of the cavity in the paravertebral part of the posterior segment rather than in the subscapular portion where tuberculous cavities are more common, suggests a lung abscess. Expectoration of foul pus made the diagnosis clear.

now is loculated. The loculations often communicate with each other by narrow channels. Frequently, spread of the infection into neighboring bronchi produces a gangrenous or suppurative bronchopneumonia in the adjacent lung (Figs. 129 and 273). This often causes the formation of additional cavities and bronchiectasis. The involved portion of lung, in the meantime, has undergone some degree of contraction because of the closing off of many small bronchial branches by secretion in their lumen and by destruction of their walls. At the same time, fibrous tissue is deposited throughout the lesions.

The roentgen picture of chronic lung abscess, therefore, is characterized by evidence of fibrosis and contraction of a chronically inflamed and indurated lung, often involving more than one segment. Not infrequently, the adjacent portion of a neighboring lobe is also involved. Within the chronically inflamed area, there are one or more cavities but often these are hidden on routine films by the dense shadow cast by the surrounding, inflamed, fibrotic and atelectatic lung. The entire picture is complicated by the presence of associated bronchiectasis (Fig. 274). Because of these changes, it is often difficult to differentiate a chronic lung abscess from advanced pulmonary tuberculosis, bronchiectasis, or bronchial carcinoma.

Diffuse spread of the infection throughout both lungs is not uncommon in the chronic stage of the disease, when the patient's resistance is low. The spread occurs by way of the bronchi and results in a gangrenous bronchopneumonia which, if extensive, may result in death. The chest film in this stage shows scattered patches of lobular consolidation, several of which may be confluent. Extension of the infection from any of the areas of gangrenous bronchopneumonia may lead to the formation of an empyema or a pyopneumothorax on the side of the original lesion or on the opposite side. A diffuse gangrenous pneumonia may also occur at any stage of the disease if the patient's resistance is diminished by a pleural infection.

Residual Cavities. Occasionally, when a lung abscess heals, a thin-walled cavity remains (Fig. 131). The persistence of the cavity is due to the fact that the bronchial opening into the cavity has become epithelialized before becoming obliterated by fibrous tissue. The epithelialization at the bronchocavitary junction prevents further stricturing at this point so that the bronchial communication is permanent.

The residual cavities are usually quite round and the wall is extremely thin, producing a fine, annular shadow at the site of the previous abscess. This may be so faint as to be unnoticed on

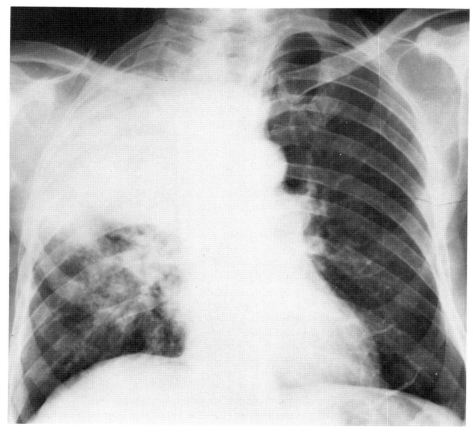

FIG. 272. GANGRENOUS BRONCHOPNEUMONIA

There is a dense, homogeneous consolidation of the entire right upper lobe and lobular consolidation of the superior segment of the right lower lobe. Previous films showed a putrid lung abscess in the outer part of the posterior segment of the right upper lobe. Spread of the infection occurred through the bronchi in the first few weeks of the disease. The changing roentgen appearance of a lung abscess is exemplified by the fact that a fluid level was visualized within the outer part of the dense shadow both on the day before and the day after this film was made.

casual examination. There is a tendency for the cavity to remain unchanged over a long period— in some cases throughout life. Frequently, however, a fluid level develops within it either from new infection, or as a result of accumulation of blood from rupture of a vessel in the cavity wall. In the latter instance, the fluid level may appear irregular because of projection of blood clots above the fluid (Fig. 130). Sometimes the cavity becomes completely filled with clotted blood and then appears as a solid, round, circumscribed shadow. This is more apt to take place when the cavity is small.

Pleural Complications. The pleura directly over a putrid lung abscess becomes inflamed at the onset of the disease. The pleurisy is intense and is characterized by a thick, fibrinous exudate which soon becomes organized into fibrous tissue. This effectively seals off and obliterates the pleural cavity over the abscess by the time that

clinical evidence of the disease becomes manifest. Pleurisy with effusion, or an empyema, which represents spread from the lung abscess, occurs only from a recent lesion. It is most common within the first 2 or 3 weeks after the onset of the abscess. Important infection of the pleura in the later stage of the disease does not result directly from the original lung abscess. Rather, it complicates new pulmonary lesions which follow intrapulmonary or bronchial spread of the infection.

FISSURAL PERFORATION. Abscesses located adjacent to a pleural fissure cause adhesions to form within the fissure. If the bronchus draining the abscess is blocked, the pus may work its way through the area of pleurodesis into an adjacent lobe. The pus then drains through a bronchus in this lobe. The fibrous adhesions which seal off the fissure prevent perforation into the free pleural space in that region. Perforation of a

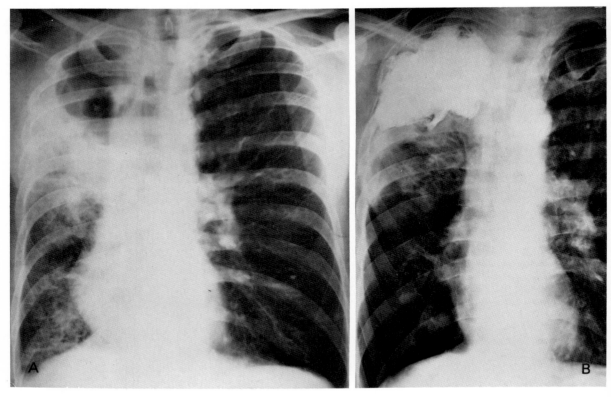

FIG. 273. LUNG ABSCESS IN UNILATERAL HYPERLUCENT LUNG

A: There is a huge abscess with a fluid level in the right upper lobe. The consolidation immediately beneath the abscess and the interstitial infiltrations in the right lower lobe are the result of spread of the infection. The right chest is considerably smaller than the left because of atrophy of the lung despite the presence of emphysema (Swyer-James syndrome). An abscess in an emphysematous lung is apt to assume large proportions. *B*: Following surgical drainage, the abscess was packed with radiopaque gauze. Persistence of a shadow beneath the packing indicates a residual area of suppuration that has not been drained. The pneumonia in the right lower lobe has resolved.

fissure occurs most commonly during the chronic stage of a lung abscess. The most common site for perforation is the upper portion of the long fissure. An abscess of the posterior segment of the upper lobe may perforate in this region into the apical segment of the lower lobe or vice versa. Similarly, an abscess in the anterior segment of the upper lobe may penetrate the short fissure and discharge its pus through the middle lobe bronchus.

It is important to bear in mind that fissural perforation almost always signifies blockage of the normal drainage of the abscess. Otherwise it would be impossible to explain the discrepancy between the findings of the bronchoscopist who notes pus issuing from a segmental bronchus of one lobe, while the main roentgen shadow is situated in an adjacent lobe.

PYOPNEUMOTHORAX. Perforation of a putrid abscess into the pleura usually produces a pyopneumothorax. This may be quite small and

localized or it may involve a large part of the pleural cavity. In the former instance, the patient often does not appear extremely ill and the pleural complication is first identified from the roentgenogram.

A small, loculated pyopneumothorax is often difficult to differentiate from a large lung abscess (Fig. 129). The fact that perforation into the pleura has occurred can be suspected from the appearance of the border of the shadow. The upper border of a large lung abscess is usually irregular and appears scalloped as the air within it bulges between the pulmonary septa (Fig. 275). On the other hand, the upper wall of a pyopneumothorax presents as a single, sharply outlined, sweeping curve (see Fig. 545). The fluid level in the perforated abscess appears to touch the chest wall if the film is made with the x-ray beam tangential to the parieties over the lesion, while the fluid level of an unperforated abscess is usually separated from the chest wall by a thin shell

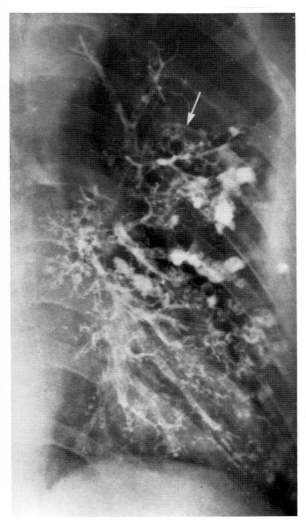

FIG. 274. BRONCHIECTASIS IN CHRONIC LUNG ABSCESS

Following drainage of a chronic lung abscess, a fistulous tract remained in the anterior chest wall. Iodized oil injected into the tract outlined an irregular cavity in the axillary part of the anterior segment of the left upper lobe (arrow). The oil then entered the bronchus communicating with the cavity and outlined the bronchi throughout the left lung. Sacculated bronchiectases are visualized in the remainder of the anterior segment and in the lingular segment of the upper lobe.

of indurated lung. In the tangential projection, the localized pyopneumothorax has a semicircular shape based against the chest wall.

Recognition of a localized pyopneumothorax is important because it usually does not remain localized for any length of time. Perforation into the free pleural cavity can occur at any time. The toxic effects of this are great and the patient may soon become moribund. The extensive pyopneumothorax is easily recognized by its large

air-fluid level. The pleural disease tends to obscure the exact location of the underlying pulmonary lesion.

EMPYEMA. A collection of pus in the pleura without air is not very common in putrid lung abscess. It results from perforation of a small abscess that does not have a well-established bronchial communication. Because of this, the patient may not cough or expectorate any sputum and an empyema or an underlying abscess is not suspected clinically. Usually the patient is thought to have pneumonia because of the sudden onset of pain in the chest, dyspnea and fever. The empyema is generally first recognized when the roentgen examination discloses a pleural effusion. The fact that this is due to perforation of an abscess of the lung is often not appreciated until aspiration of the chest reveals foul pus. Frequently, however, air enters the pleura as a freer communication between the abscess and its bronchus is established. The empyema cavity then enlarges and may perforate into the free pleural space.

An empyema confined to an interlobar fissure is practically always due to a lung abscess or suppurative pneumonia. On the other hand, an interlobar pyopneumothorax is uncommon in these conditions because the bronchi supplying the interlobar surfaces of the lobes are relatively small. The interlobar collection of pus that complicates lobar pneumonia is always part of a more generalized empyema that involves the costal pleura as well.

Localization of an empyema or pyopneumothorax within an interlobar fissure may not be suspected from the frontal projection (see Fig. 528). It is usually clearly represented on the lateral view. One must be careful not to confuse the normal fusiform shadows caused by the overlapping of the heart and liver with that of an interlobar effusion (Fig. 59).

SYMPATHETIC EFFUSIONS. A pleural effusion may occur even though the lung abscess has not perforated the pleura and can form even though bacteria have not wandered into the pleural space. Such a collection of fluid is known as a *sympathetic effusion*. It is serous in character and results simply from irritation of the pleura by toxins of the bacteria which are still confined to the lung. Such effusions in unperforated lung abscesses are most often small and usually disappear if the abscess is drained or the patient receives antibiotic treatment. In untreated cases, the sympathetic effusion soon becomes infected and is converted into an empyema.

More often, sympathetic effusions occur adjacent to a loculated collection of pus and air in

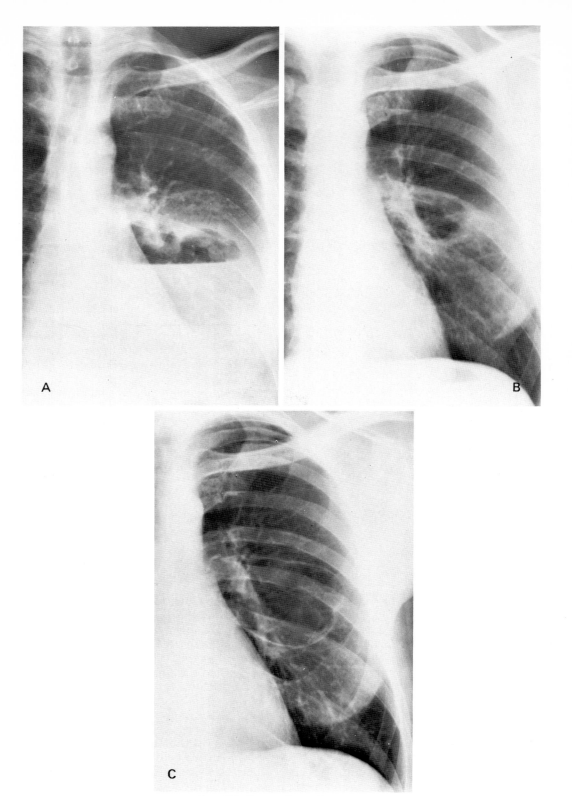

FIG. 275. PUTRID LUNG ABSCESS

A: 7-6-76. The patient developed fever and coughed up foul sputum after an epileptic attack. The huge cavity with an air-fluid level in the left lower lobe suggests a pyopneumothorax. However, the irregularity of the cavity wall indicates that it lies within the lung rather than in the pleura. *B*: 8-3-76. On antibiotic therapy, the cavity has become much smaller and there is no longer an air-fluid level. *C*: 9-20-76. Although the patient was clinically well, the cavity has increased in size. Its wall is thin and smooth and there are no infiltrations in the lung around the cavity. The ballooning of the cavity was noted after an attack of asthma. The increase in size was due entirely to air trapping because of the bronchospasm and does not indicate reactivation of the infection.

the pleura that follows perforation of a lung abscess. These sympathetic effusions are usually quite large and tend to obscure the underlying disease in the lung as well as the loculation of pus, or pus and air, in the pleura. The recognition that a clear effusion in the pleural cavity is sympathetic and is related to an underlying lung abscess is quite difficult, and often requires special methods of roentgen examination.

Special Diagnostic Procedures. The roentgen diagnosis of lung abscess often depends on the demonstration of a cavity within a shadow which otherwise has the appearance of a pneumonia or a neoplasm. The cavity may not be visualized on ordinary films if it contains very little air or if the lung about it is extensively inflamed. Moreover, the entire process in the lung may be obscured by a pleural effusion. These difficulties can be resolved by positioning the patient so that the abscess is projected clear of overlying shadows or by increasing the penetration so that the cavity can be seen through these shadows.

Occasionally, a cavity with a fluid level can be demonstrated in the lateral or the oblique view when it cannot be seen on the ordinary frontal projection (Fig. 54). Overexposed or Bucky films may disclose a fluid level which cannot be seen with the usual exposures. If there is a question concerning the presence of a fluid level, films should be made either in the lateral decubitus position or in the erect position with the patient tilted toward one side. If the line noted on the original examination remains horizontal despite the shift in the position of the patient, the presence of air and fluid within the cavity is confirmed (p. 163).

Tomography may disclose cavities where other methods fail. The tomograms aid not only in the demonstration of the original cavity but also in the detection of additional loculations. Since tomography is usually performed with the patient in the supine position and the beam directed more or less vertically, a fluid level is not demonstrated. However, even small collections of air not visible by other techniques, can be clearly demonstrated on the sections. Only a tiny, well defined lucency within a large, fairly well demarcated density is sufficient to indicate the presence of an abscess. Tomography may also aid in differentiating a broken down neoplasm or a cavity secondary to broncholithiasis (Fig. 20) from an ordinary putrid lung abscess.

None of these methods can disclose the cavity if it is completely filled with fluid or necrotic material. Therefore, if an abscess is suspected despite the inability to demonstrate the cavity radiologically, the examination should be repeated after an attempt is made to empty the abscess cavity of some of its content. This may be done by bronchoscopy or by postural drainage. A knowledge of the approximate location of the lesions is necessary to facilitate drainage by these procedures.

Bronchography is of limited value in the diagnosis of putrid lung abscess. The radiopaque material rarely reaches the cavity during the acute phase because the entering bronchus is markedly inflamed and narrowed. On the other hand, the contrast substance usually will enter the diseased area in other localized inflammatory conditions. It is evident that bronchography is of no value in differentiating the shadow of an acute putrid lung abscess from that of an obstructing bronchial neoplasm.

In chronic lung abscess the entering bronchus is frequently wide and permits the passage of the contrast material into the cavity. Bronchiectases are usually present in the lung about a chronic lung abscess. In those cases in which the cavity cannot be filled, the demonstration of bronchiectases surrounding a dense shadow in the lungs strongly suggests the diagnosis of chronic lung abscess.

Localization of Lung Abscess. In some cases of lung abscess, special methods of treatment may be necessary. These include selective instillation of antibiotics into the segmental bronchus leading to the abscess, segmental resection of the lung, and drainage of the abscess through the chest wall. All of these require accurate localization of the abscess. This is best accomplished when the abscess first becomes manifest.

In the early stage, a lung abscess is confined to a small portion of the lung and its precise localization is a relatively simple matter. However, if the disease does not respond satisfactorily to antibiotic treatment, it may become complicated by local spread of the infection or by occurrence of a pleural effusion or pyopneumothorax. These obscure the original lesion and make localization quite difficult.

Where the proposed treatment consists of instillation of antibiotics through the bronchoscope, or where segmental resection is contemplated, it is necessary to determine only the bronchopulmonary segment in which the abscess lies. The methods outlined in the section on Fluoroscopic Localization (p. 63) usually suffice for this purpose. In chronic lung abscess, where the cavity is obscured by the shadow of the secondary infection and in cases of perforated lung abscess in which the cavity is not visible, bronchography may be required to identify the involved segment.

More precise localization is required if the cavity is to be drained through the chest wall. Ninety-five per cent of the abscesses are situated immediately beneath the chest wall and the pleural space over the lesion is obliterated by dense adhesions. If drainage is accomplished through the area of pleurodesis, the operation can be completed in a single stage without contamination of the pleural cavity.

Once the involved segment has been identified, localization of an abscess in the mesial half of the chest can be made from the frontal projection alone. The rib crossing the middle of the abscess is identified and the distance from the center of the abscess to a bony landmark in the mesial portion of the chest is measured. If the abscess is situated anteriorly, the costochondral junction or the edge of the sternum is used as the point of reference for this measurement. For posterior lesions, the distance between the abscess and the nearest transverse process or spinous process is determined. An abscess in the mesial part of the posterior segment of the upper lobe poses a special problem. Because of the obliquity of the long fissure which bounds the lower part of the abscess posteriorly, only the upper portion of the shadow seen on the frontal view, makes contact with the chest wall. The superior segment of the lower lobe is interposed between the chest wall and the lower part of the abscess. A lateral view is essential (Fig. 276) to demonstrate the actual area of contact between the abscess and the chest wall.

If the abscess lies in the outer half of the lung, it is impossible to localize it adequately from the frontal projection because the ribs in the axillary region are foreshortened and cross each other in this view. Localization must be performed in the projection in which the ribs over the abscess are the least distorted. If the abscess is situated approximately midway between the front and back of the chest, the lateral view is used for localization. A point along the rib or interspace overlying the center of the shadow will prove to be situated directly over the central part of the lesion where the adhesions are most dense. This point must be marked on the patient's chest for there is no natural landmark to which it can be related.

When the abscess is located in the anterior or posterior part of the outer portion of the lung, oblique views are required for localization (Fig. 14). On one oblique view the abscess will be seen to extend to the border of the chest wall. This will be the right oblique in the case of lesions situated in the anterolateral portion of the left lung and the posterolateral portion of the right lung. However, in this projection, the ribs overlying the lesion are markedly foreshortened and cross each other, so that it is impossible to locate the lesion in relation to them or to the intercostal spaces. The opposite oblique projection will show the ribs over the abscess in their true length. It is on this view, then, that the ribs and rib spaces are counted and the chest wall marked over the center of the lesion for its precise localization. In a similar way, lesions in the posterior outer portion of the left lung and the anterior outer portion of the right lung are located. The left oblique view shows their proximity to the chest wall, while the right oblique view is used to mark the location of the lesion.

SPOT METHOD. Because of the free movement of the skin in relation to the chest wall, and because of difficulty in accurately counting ribs, the *spot method* was devised to guide the surgeon to the abscess (Figs. 14 and 270). The abscess is localized exactly as described above. However, instead of marking the skin as a point of reference for the surgeon, a mixture of 0.25 cc of iodized oil and 0.25 cc of a solution of methylene blue is injected into the intercostal muscles. This is done under fluoroscopic control and the injection is made as closely as possible to the center of the abscess with the patient in the position in which the ribs show the least distortion. Films are then made in this position and the relationship of the center of the abscess to the patch of iodized oil is determined. Since the patch is visible to the surgeon because of its blue stain, he can easily follow the directions of the roentgenologist to the point where the abscess abuts on the chest wall.

The spot method is not useful in the rare cases where the abscess faces the diaphragm or an interlobar fissure instead of the chest wall. These cases can be recognized radiologically by the fact that the abscess is separated from the chest wall in all views.

POSTOPERATIVE RADIOPAQUE PACKING. After drainage of an abscess of the lung we have found it useful to reexamine the patient radiologically following the insertion of a radiopaque packing within the drained cavity. Either iodoform gauze or plain gauze saturated with iodized oil may be used (Fig. 273). The precaution should be taken to fill only the abscess cavity with the radiopaque packing and not pack the wound itself with this material. The remainder of the wound may be packed with plain gauze as this will not cause a confusing roentgen shadow.

Within a few days after the drainage of an abscess, there should be little or no density beyond the drained area. The radiopaque packing will serve to delineate the cavity. Any dense

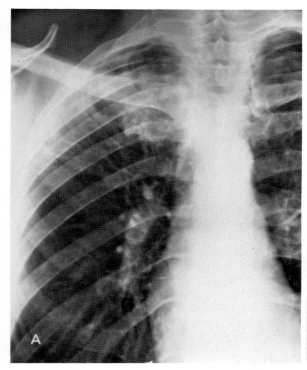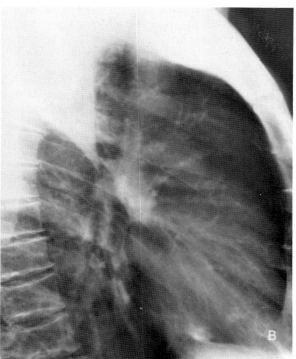

FIG. 276. LUNG ABSCESS: POSTERIOR SEGMENT, RIGHT UPPER LOBE

A: The shadow in the mesial portion of the right upper lobe was due to a poorly draining abscess. The frontal projection alone is not adequate for proper localization of the lesion. *B*: The lateral view demonstrates the lesion to be situated in the posterior segment of the right upper lobe. The involved segment is represented by a sharply outlined, triangular shadow whose apex is directed toward the root of the lobe. Its lower border is bounded by the long fissure and its anterior border corresponds to the anterior limits of the segment. Although the lower border of the lesion is projected at the level of the sixth intercostal space posteriorly on the frontal projection, its area of contact with the chest wall actually extends no lower than the fourth space. Below this, the apex of the lower lobe is interposed between the involved segment and the chest wall. Drainage, therefore, was carried out through the bed of the posterior part of the third rib.

shadow or area of increased aeration persisting about the cavity indicates the presence of an additional focus. The exact location of the undrained focus can be determined by using the iodoform packing as seen on the roentgen film for a guide. Films made in the frontal, lateral and oblique views will disclose its relationship to the drained cavity and aid the surgeon in the location of the residual purulent collection.

Pulmonary Tuberculosis

Before the roentgen era, the diagnosis of tuberculosis in its early stages was most difficult and uncertain. Today, by means of the roentgen examination, not only is the diagnosis made clear in most instances, but even slight changes occurring in the lungs during the course of the disease are visible if the examinations are made frequently enough. Little reliance can be placed on the results of physical examination in this disease, and determination of the stage of its development and the indications for treatment depend largely on roentgenographic findings.

Incipient tuberculosis is usually asymptomatic. By the time symptoms appear, the disease is often quite far advanced. Since treatment in the more advanced stages can be complicated and difficult, and because the results are uncertain, it is essential that the disease be discovered early. This can be done only by reasonably frequent roentgen examination of apparently normal people.

Classification of Tuberculosis. Basically, pulmonary tuberculosis exists in two forms. The first occurs in the individual who has never had the disease before, *primary tuberculosis*. Since it occurred almost exclusively in childhood in previous years when tuberculosis was more common, it was also called the *childhood form* of tuberculosis. Today, the primary infection with tuberculosis occurs with considerable frequency in adults. The term, "childhood tuberculosis" has thus lost its significance and the term, *primary* or *first-infection* tuberculosis, is used to denote the first infection in either the child or the adult. Pulmonary tuberculosis that occurs in a person who has previously had a primary infection with tubercle bacilli is designated the *reinfection* type of tuberculosis. It is essential to be acquainted with these two types of tuberculosis because they run a different course and often present different problems from the standpoint of roentgen diagnosis.

The primary, or first-infection, type of tuberculosis, usually produces only a small lesion within the lung. This is apt to stay small and has little tendency to spread through the bronchial tree to infect other portions of the lung. However, it does spread by the lymphatics to the regional lymph nodes, and from them to the lymph channels and vascular system, to other parts of the body. Lymphatic or lymphhematogenous spread is inhibited in the secondary or reinfection type of tuberculosis. Here the spread of the disease is predominantly bronchogenic.

The roentgen picture following hematogenous dissemination of tuberculosis to the lungs usually differs from the local lesion of primary tuberculosis and from that resulting from bronchial dissemination. Furthermore, the hematogenous lesions are of special pathologic and clinical significance and, therefore, they will be considered separately.

Allergy and Immunity in Tuberculosis. The person who has never had a tuberculous infection displays no allergic reaction to tuberculoprotein. The inflammatory reaction to the first infection with tuberculosis is, therefore, limited to the area of infection. Since immunity has not as yet been established, the toxins of the tubercle bacilli cause destruction of the involved lung tissue. Thus, a local area of caseation necrosis appears soon after the development of the infection. Manifestations of an allergic response do not appear until a period of about six to eight weeks has elapsed. By this time a certain degree of immunity has developed which tends to limit the spread of the infection. Whether the lesion will increase in size or not will depend upon the severity of the infection and the intensity of the immune reaction.

The immune reaction, acquired as a result of the primary tuberculous infection, is a permanent one and modifies the response of any further infections by the tubercle bacillus. Because of the prior sensitization to tuberculoprotein, when reinfection occurs the inflammatory reaction extends far beyond the area of bacterial invasion. Destruction of tissue, however, is limited to the infected area and bears no direct relationship to the size of the lesion. On the other hand, a severe allergic reaction results in an outpouring of exudate which can carry the bacilli throughout the inflamed area, thus spreading the disease. The extent of tissue destruction may then be quite great despite a considerable degree of immunity.

Exudative and Productive Lesions. The earliest stage of tuberculosis in both the primary and the reinfection type is characterized by a bronchopneumonia associated with outpouring of exudate into the alveoli as well as into the interstitial tissues. This is the *exudative* stage of the disease. If the disease is arrested before significant destruction of pulmonary tissue takes place, the exudate absorbs and the lung may return to a practically normal state. The extent of the exudative process depends upon the severity of the infection and the allergic response. If the latter factor is predominant, the area involved in the exudative process may be most extensive and yet a remarkable degree of resolution can take place.

The term, *productive* tuberculosis, is used when there is a predominance of tuberculous granulation and fibrous tissue. In addition to the connective tissue reaction, there is extensive infiltration of the interstitial tissues of the lung with small and large round cells and epithelioid cells. The smallest unit of the productive type of tuberculosis is the tubercle and this, as well as the other productive lesions, involves the interstitial tissue rather than the alveolar spaces. Numerous tubercles conglomerate to form large tubercles which are often surrounded or connected by tuberculous granulation tissue. Where the inflammatory reaction is not intense, the productive type of inflammation may be a rather early manifestation of the disease. In other cases, where there is an extensive exudative reaction, the latter may undergo resolution, leaving areas of productive inflammation which persist for a considerable length of time. However, despite the fact that these productive lesions contain numerous fibroblastic elements and cause dense induration, they may disappear almost completely, leaving only thin, fibrous strands. This marked involution of the lesion is due to breakdown and absorption of the lymphocytes and large round cells, and atrophy of the fibroblastic elements.

Caseation, Cavitation and Calcification. Characteristic of the destructive effect of the tuberculosis toxin is necrosis of lung tissue and of the inflammatory exudate and granulation tissue, to form a crumbly, caseous mass. If the caseous area is large, it may be evacuated through a bronchus, leaving a cavity within the lung. If it is small, it may become encapsulated by fibrous tissue. The caseous area can remain unchanged for a considerable length of time. As a rule, calcium is deposited within it after a period of several months. However, it usually takes a number of years for the deposition of sufficient calcium to be recognizable on the roentgen film. In occasional instances of larger caseous foci, the presence of calcification can be recognized comparatively early. The shortest interval between the onset of infection and recognizable calcific deposits in our experience has been 7 months. Tubercle bacilli may remain viable within the caseous foci for a great many years and may even be cultured from lesions which contain a considerable amount of calcium. The organisms, however, are effectively sealed off by the surrounding, dense, fibrous capsule so that the disease may be considered to be inactive from a clinical standpoint.

Primary Tuberculosis

The tuberculosis of childhood practically always represents a primary infection. Reinfection with tuberculosis is rare before puberty even if the primary infection occurred during infancy. It may, therefore, be stated *a priori* that tuberculous lesions in the lungs discovered before puberty, represent the first infection with the disease.

In previous years, when tuberculous infection was far more common than it is today, particularly in cities, most of the population became infected by tubercle bacilli before the 20th year. Tuberculous infection of the lung occurring after that time could safely be considered a reinfection. Today, better standards of living and hygiene have sharply reduced the incidence of primary infection so that in many cases the first infection not infrequently takes place during adult life. The basic pathologic form of the disease remains the same, whether this first infection is contracted during childhood or later in life. However, the course of the primary lesions in the adult tends to differ from that in the child.

The Primary Complex. Most cases of primary tuberculosis are due to the inhalation of tubercle bacilli. The organisms provoke an inflammatory reaction, producing a small area of tuberculous bronchopneumonia. At the outset, the infection spreads from the intial focus in the lung to the regional and mediastinal lymph nodes by way of the lymphatic channels. The constant association of tuberculous adenitis with the pulmonary lesion is characteristic of the primary infection with tubercle bacilli. The combination

of these two lesions is known as the *primary (Ghon) complex* (Figs. 2 and 277). There is no relationship between the size of the pulmonary lesion and of the diseased lymph nodes. Neither may be especially prominent. Enlargement of the nodes, far out of proportion to the pulmonary lesion, occurs particularly in children. In most adults with primary tuberculosis only the parenchymal lesion is visible although the lymph nodes are always the seat of a more or less extensive caseous tuberculosis.

THE PRIMARY PULMONARY FOCUS. In the majority of children who have developed a primary tuberculous infection, evidenced by a positive tuberculin reaction, the pulmonary lesion is not visible at the time when the roentgen film is made. The lesions that are seen are usually less than 2 cm in diameter. They are poorly demarcated and are always situated in the periphery of the lobe. Usually the primary focus is single. In

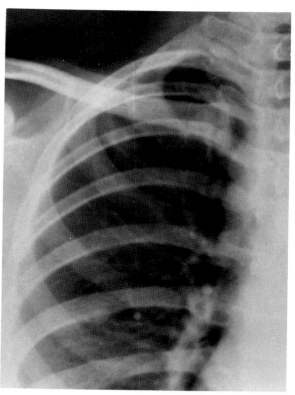

FIG. 277. PRIMARY TUBERCULOSIS: ACTIVE PRIMARY COMPLEX

The patient, who is 12 years old, had been exposed to tuberculosis and the tuberculin test was positive. There is a small area of infiltration beneath the outer part of the right clavicle and enlargement of the right paratracheal lymph nodes. Together these lesions constitute the primary complex.

children it occurs without specific predilection for any lobe or segment of the lung. However, in adults, the primary pulmonary infection is usually situated in the upper lobe (Fig. 417) and is seen beneath the clavicle in the frontal projection.

The inflamed area soon becomes caseous and is surrounded by a dense capsule of connective tissue. As this occurs, the lesion becomes more sharply defined. Within a period varying from a number of months to a few years, calcium is deposited and, in a considerable percentage of cases, bone is eventually formed in the lesion (Fig. 137). The shadow of the calcified pulmonary lesion of primary tuberculosis is identical with that of histoplasmosis and occurs in several different forms. It may appear simply as a small calcific deposit or one surrounded by a halo of lesser density. In some cases there are, in addition, one or more concentric rings of calcium about the halo, presenting an appearance similar to that of a target. In others, there is a central lucency surrounded by one or more calcific rings.

THE REGIONAL LYMPH NODES. The inflamed lymph nodes regularly undergo caseation as does the primary lesion in the lung. Most commonly the regional lymph nodes at the root of the involved segment become diseased. In addition, the neighboring nodes in the mediastinum are usually involved. Most often, however, only the enlarged nodes at the root of the diseased lobe are recognizable on the film. In upper lobe tuberculosis, the nodes at the tracheobronchial angle and the paratracheal chain are the ones that appear prominent.

Probably the most frequent type of shadow caused by the caseous mediastinal lymph nodes is a small, nodular protuberance in the paratracheal region, more prominent on the right side than on the left (Figs. 277 and 278). On the left, the protuberance sometimes overlies the shadow of the aortic knob and produces an irregular density in this region. When it is situated lower down on the left side, the appearance may suggest an abnormally prominent pulmonary artery. A double shadow in the region of the aortic arch or pulmonary conus is indicative of an abnormality in the mediastinum, and one of the conditions to be considered is tuberculosis of the lymph nodes. A large bronchopulmonary lymph node, situated at the root of the lung, must be differentiated from branches of the pulmonary artery.

Frequently all the groups of lymph nodes on

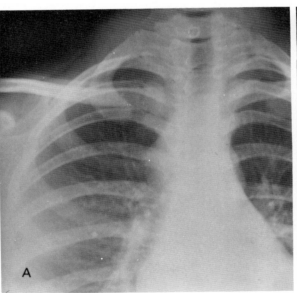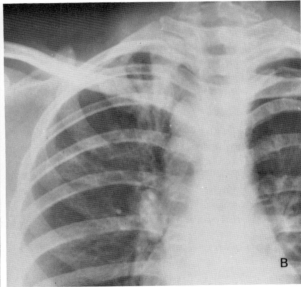

FIG. 278. PROGRESSIVE PRIMARY TUBERCULOSIS

A: The bulging shadow at the right of the superior mediastinum is due to a mass of tuberculous paratracheal lymph nodes. A less well-defined bulge on the left side of the mediastinum is caused by involvement of the tracheobronchial nodes. The tuberculin test was positive. *B*: Ten months later. The tuberculous lesion in the lung is now visible. It appears as a wedge-shaped shadow at the right apex, due to atelectasis as well as infiltration of the lung. This indicates the presence of tuberculous bronchitis. A second area of atelectatic pneumonia is present in the outer part of the anterior segment, causing upward retraction of the short fissure. The disease in the mediastinal nodes has progressed. The tracheobronchial and hilar nodes are now also enlarged.

the side of the pulmonary lesion are enlarged and project from the mediastinum for a considerable distance into the pulmonary field. Sometimes the mediastinal outline is not distorted, but appears simply to be widened on that side. More commonly, the matted masses of enlarged lymph nodes impart an irregular, sharply demarcated, scalloped outline to the mediastinum. When the disease is extensive, the appearance may be identical with that of a mediastinal neoplasm because the outlines of the individual nodes are obscured. If the mediastinum is involved more diffusely, it becomes generally widened. The borders may then be straight and regular, producing an appearance like that of an enlarged thymus. The trachea may be displaced to the opposite side by the large nodes. If the subcarinal nodes are markedly enlarged, they tend to displace the main bronchi upward, widening the angle of the tracheal bifurcation. A large group of tracheobronchial lymph nodes often depresses the main bronchus on that side, close to its origin. This causes an increase of the normally obtuse tracheobronchial angle.

The nodes gradually diminish in size as the infection is controlled, and the areas of caseous necrosis within them eventually become calcified. The calcific foci usually vary from 1 or 2 mm to 1 cm in size. Occasionally, however, a group of lymph nodes remains enlarged and when they calcify, produce an irregular, dense mass. Such a group of nodes may displace the esophagus backwards or produce permanent widening of the carinal angle. In rare instances, the entire superior mediastinal shadow is the seat of calcific deposits. These may not be easily recognizable on conventional films so that the appearance suggests a mediastinal neoplasm.

The healing and calcification of the lesions in the lung and the lymph nodes proceed independently of each other. The pulmonary lesion usually undergoes more rapid and complete resolution than the nodes. Thus, at one stage during the course of primary tuberculosis, enlarged mediastinal nodes may be the only abnormality noted on the chest film. Since enlargement of the lymph nodes without extensive infiltration in the lungs is extremely rare in childhood from any cause other than tuberculosis, such nodes should be considered as tuberculous even though there is no visible pulmonary lesion.

PROGRESSION OF THE PULMONARY LESION. As caseation takes place, there is destruction not only of the pulmonary parenchyma but also of the bronchi within the lesion. Since the focus is generally small and the peripheral bronchi in children are of fine caliber, there is usually little tendency for the disease to spread to other parts of the lung. When the primary lesion is more extensive and involves larger bronchi, or in the adult, in whom the peripheral bronchi are sizable, there is more tendency to spread of the disease, particularly in the neighborhood of the original focus. The lesion may then involve a large portion of a pulmonary segment (Fig. 94). Under these circumstances, caseous material can be extruded from the lung into a bronchus, resulting in formation of a cavity. Before the days of chemotherapy, the presence of a cavity in primary pulmonary tuberculosis was an ominous sign because it was almost always associated with widespread bronchial dissemination and usually resulted in death. Apparently, children who develop lesions large enough to result in cavitation have little resistance to the disease. With chemotherapy, however, the course has changed. If treatment with antituberculosis drugs is begun while the lesion is small, progression is halted and resolution takes place quite rapidly.

In the adult with primary tuberculosis, the disease often runs a different course. Cavitation takes place much more frequently, and occurs even in relatively small primary tuberculous foci. Apparently the resistance of the adult is greater than that of the child because there is much less tendency to extensive spread of the disease from the cavity, and the outlook, even without chemotherapy, is not so grave. Whereas the wall of the tuberculous cavity in the child is apt to be quite thick, in the adult it is often thin. Because the cavity in the adult is most often situated in an upper lobe, the bronchial communication is located in its lowermost portion. This facilitates free drainage so that a fluid level is generally absent.

Local spread of tuberculosis in the region of a cavity is common, and takes the form of small, nodular areas of consolidation of acinar distribution. However, larger areas of consolidation may appear at any time. Except for the fact that hematogenous dissemination of the disease to other organs is more common, the further course of primary cavitary tuberculosis in the adult is not unlike that of reinfection tuberculosis.

In most instances of primary tuberculosis without cavitation, the caseous focus shrinks in size, becomes encapsulated, undergoes calcification and does not present a clinical problem. When calcification is absent or incomplete, the encapsulated lesion contains a considerable amount of granulation and fibrous tissue, infiltrated to a variable extent with inflammatory elements, and forms a well circumscribed nodule which is termed a *tuberculoma*. Occasionally the encapsulated lesion is large and remains large for an indefinite period. It then may be confused with a neoplasm.

In some instances, especially in adults with a large primary infection, local spread of the disease occurs despite the presence of calcification (*progressive primary tuberculosis*). The infection apparently extends here and there through the capsule resulting in concentric inflammation about the lesion, causing it to increase in size. This change may occur from time to time over a period of years. The tuberculoma then gradually increases in size like a benign neoplasm of the lung. Occasionally small, tubercle-like foci appear about the tuberculous nodule. These satellite foci usually disappear under chemotherapy. They may clear spontaneously if untreated but, not uncommonly, they persist indefinitely and undergo calcification.

In rare instances the nodule which has remained unchanged in size for a long time, discharges its content into a bronchus and thus undergoes cavitation. In such cases the wall of the cavity remains quite thick, and the lesion is not likely to undergo complete resolution. It may shrink considerably under the influence of chemotherapy but a small nodular focus usually remains.

PROGRESSION OF LYMPHADENITIS. In primary tuberculosis, extensive involvement of the mediastinal lymph nodes is more common in children than in adults. Progression of the lymphadenitis occurs as the infection spreads from the regional lymph nodes to the paratracheal and subcarinal nodes. In some instances, the lymph nodes on the opposite side of the mediastinum also become involved (Fig. 278) but this is usually not recognizable on the roentgen films. The diseased lymph nodes may cause bronchial obstruction by spread of the infection into the bronchial wall (Fig. 279) or by perforation of the bronchus by a caseous node resulting in permanent stricture. Perforation of the node into the esophagus produces a so-called traction diverticulum. Suppuration of the diseased nodes in the mediastinum can produce a cold abscess (Fig. 280).

The disease in the lymph nodes may become reactivated many years after the primary infection. In fact, nodes which have become calcified and in which there is every reason to believe that the disease has been controlled, may show evidence of reactivation of the infection. Autopsies at institutions for the aged have shown an appreciable incidence of recent caseation in the mediastinal lymph nodes, sometimes with spread of the infection throughout the body, in patients who had contracted primary tuberculosis in childhood. While the association of calcified lymph nodes with bronchial obstruction suggests broncholithiasis without active tuberculosis, there are occasional cases in which the bronchial obstruction is due to reactivation of the disease in the adjacent nodes.

BRONCHIAL OBSTRUCTION. In previous years, radiologists and pediatricians interested in tuberculosis were impressed by the occasional appearance of a faint, homogeneous shadow which occurred suddenly during the course of a childhood tuberculous infection. The shadow had a tendency to disappear almost as suddenly as it appeared. Many thought that it was due to a nonspecific inflammatory reaction which was a manifestation of an allergic state, and that the lesion was akin to a gelatinous bronchopneumonia which resolved rapidly. The name *epituberculosis* was given to this lesion. However, not many years after the introduction of the term epituberculosis, it was found that the shadow really represented an area of atelectasis secondary to pressure or erosion of the bronchus by involved lymph nodes.

Bronchial obstruction from diseased lymph nodes occurs mainly in children because their bronchi are small and the walls are easily compressed. The obstruction may be due simply to pressure of the enlarged nodes. However, in addition, there generally is extension of the infection beyond the capsule of the nodes into the adjacent bronchial wall. Although the obstruction is usually incomplete and may produce no roentgen signs, it may be sufficient to interfere with the flow of air through the bronchus. Since, as a rule, the force of inspiration is greater than that of expiration, the lung supplied by the narrowed bronchus becomes overdistended, and the roentgen picture of obstructive emphysema develops.

If the obstruction is complete, atelectasis occurs. This usually involves an entire lobe. In rare instances, a main bronchus is obstructed, resulting in atelectasis of a lung. In some cases only a single portion of a lobe is involved—most commonly the anterior segment of the upper lobe or the superior segment of the lower lobe.

Atelectasis may supervene after a short period of obstructive emphysema when the obstruction becomes complete. It disappears when the bronchial obstruction is relieved as the tuberculous lymphadenitis resolves. During the stage of reexpansion, streak-like shadows are often seen within the newly aerated lung. These represent focal areas of atelectasis which remain because some of the small bronchi are still obstructed by secretion and exudate.

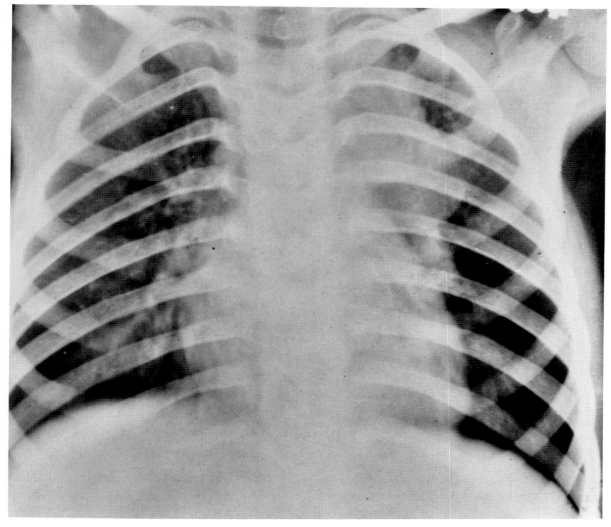

FIG. 279. PRIMARY TUBERCULOSIS: BRONCHIAL OBSTRUCTION

The frontal film of a 5 year old child shows a lobulated mass along the left side of the mediastinum, representing enlarged tuberculous lymph nodes. The sharply outlined lower border of the left upper lobe is raised to the level of the second anterior intercostal space, indicating atelectasis of the lobe. The pulmonary markings in the lower lobe are sparse because this portion of the lung has undergone compensatory emphysema. Despite the atelectasis of the left upper lobe, the trachea is displaced to the right by the large nodes.

It is possible for the nodes to cause complete obstruction of one bronchus and incomplete obstruction of a neighboring bronchus. This results in atelectasis of one lobe and emphysema of the other. In the cases we have seen, the upper lobe was atelectatic and the lower was emphysematous. There was a uniform density over the contracted upper lobe and marked upward displacement of the interlobar fissure, together with elevation of the lung root. The lower lobe appeared hyperaerated, it displaced the heart toward the opposite side and depressed the diaphragm. There was bulging of the posterior mediastinum

for a considerable distance into the opposite chest behind the heart. Such displacement of the lower posterior mediastinum occurs more easily in children because the structures are loosely bound by thin connective tissue which allows free mediastinal movement.

The obstructing node may be extruded into the lumen and coughed up, relieving the obstruction. In rare instances the node lodges in the trachea, causing a ball-valve obstruction which produces severe bilateral emphysema. It has caused death from suffocation.

It is surprising that the extrusion of a tuber-

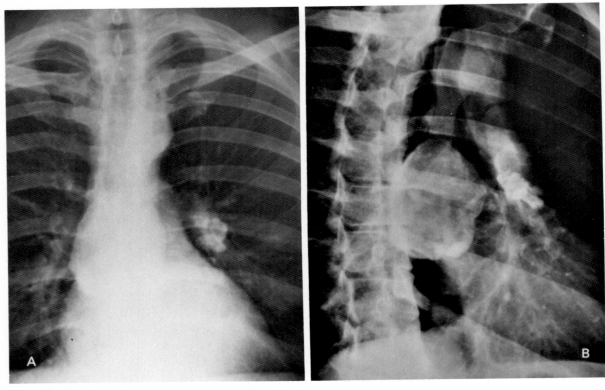

FIG. 280. SUBCARINAL COLD ABSCESS

A: Frontal projection. The oval shadow in the midline below the carina represents a cold abscess. Its density is due to calcium within its wall. A group of calcified lymph nodes is present at the left hilum. *B*: Right oblique projection. The main bronchi are spread apart by the mass of caseous nodes. The shadow differs from that of a bronchogenic cyst in that its border is irregular and there is a patchy distribution of the calcium.

culous node into a bronchus does not always produce extensive bronchial dissemination of the disease. One would expect this at least in the affected lobe or lung. It has been our experience that such dissemination is not the rule and that more often the lobe eventually reexpands without showing evidence of any important extension of the tuberculosis. Occasionally the destruction of tissue causes a bronchial stricture with scarring of most of the circumference of the ulcerated bronchus. The stricture results in either permanent atelectasis or bronchiectasis.

The diagnosis of obstruction by tuberculous nodes can usually be made from the roentgen findings because the nodes often are large enough to be seen on the films. In a child, atelectasis of a pulmonary segment, a lobe, or of an entire lung with large nodes at its root, justifies a presumptive diagnosis of primary tuberculosis.

Caseation of the lymph node is followed by deposition of calcium. If the infection extends beyond the capsule of the node to involve the adjacent bronchial wall, the calcification may involve the bronchus as well. In this way a stone is formed within the wall of the bronchus (*intramural broncholith*) and causes narrowing of the bronchial lumen. In some cases this erodes through the mucosa and becomes a true *intraluminal broncholith*.

INVOLVEMENT OF MEDIASTINAL STRUCTURES. Tuberculous lymphadenitis may progress to abscess formation. A cold abscess of the mediastinum can form in the early stage of the infection or much later, as a result of reactivation of the infection in the lymph nodes. The roentgen film shows a sharply defined, semicircular protuberance in the paratracheal or tracheobronchial region. This may have the appearance of a paratracheal cyst.

A similar abscess involving the subcarinal nodes causes a widening of the tracheal bifurcation. In the frontal projection this portion of the mediastinum appears abnormally dense, while in the lateral and oblique views the cold abscess is seen to project backwards over the posterior mediastinum, displacing the esophagus (Fig.

280). If the inflammatory process extends beyond the bounds of the paratracheal nodes, it can result in superior vena caval obstruction.

The pus within a cold abscess may become inspissated and undergo extensive calcification. The finding of irregular, calcific deposits in the paratracheal or subcarinal regions suggests an old tuberculous lymphadenitis. If, in addition, there is widening of the mediastinum and superior vena caval obstruction, it is almost certain that a cold abscess was the cause. This can result from either tuberculosis or histoplasmosis. A cold abscess or caseous nodes in the subcarinal region can perforate into the esophagus and lead to the formation of a traction diverticulum on its anterior wall.

Involvement of the Pleura. In a considerable percentage of early cases of primary tuberculosis there is roentgenologic evidence of pleuritis. The pleurisy is due either to the pulmonary lesion, which is practically always situated immediately beneath the visceral pleura, or to disease in the lymph nodes directly under the mediastinal pleura. The pleuritis may be fibrinous and localized to the region of the pulmonary lesion or it may be serous and gravitate to the base. The only roentgen evidence of the pleurisy may be a slight thickening of the short fissure, seen on the frontal projection or a similar accentuation of the long fissure on the lateral view. In some cases there is a small amount of fluid in the costophrenic sinus, best seen in the oblique and lateral projections. Some observers have been able to demonstrate a small quantity of fluid in the pleural cavity in a great majority of cases of primary tuberculosis by employing the lateral decubitus position, using a horizontal beam. Usually the effusions are small in young children, but moderately large collections of fluid may accompany the primary infection in adults. The larger tuberculous effusions are more characteristic of a later stage of the disease, and will be discussed separately.

Reinfection or Postprimary Tuberculosis

The pathogenesis of pulmonary tuberculosis in the adult who has already had a primary infection has been the subject of controversy. No one has been able to prove conclusively whether the tuberculosis is the result of spread from the original primary disease, or whether it represents a new infection with tubercle bacilli from outside the body. Because of this, a nonspecific term, such as *reinfection* or *postprimary* tuberculosis is used, simply indicating that further infection

has taken place in a patient who has had primary tuberculosis. In the present state of our knowledge, the terms superinfection and exogenous tuberculosis had best be avoided.

The Early Lesion. It was once thought that reinfection tuberculosis began in the apex of the lung and then spread downward. However, since the description by Wessler in 1918 and again in 1923, and the later contributions of Assmann, it has been recognized that reinfection tuberculosis generally begins in the upper lobe beneath the level of the clavicle. In the great majority of cases, the lesion begins in the posterior segment of the upper lobe.

The early phase of reinfection tuberculosis can be studied pathologically only in animals, as human specimens showing the onset are rare. In the few cases in which human lungs have been available for study, the early lesion was found to consist of an area of tuberculous bronchopneumonia characterized by consolidation and interstitial infiltration. From these studies it appears that the extent of the inflammatory process varies in different individuals. Whereas the size of the lesion may depend, in part, upon the intensity of the infection, it is most likely that the allergic response of a patient previously sensitized by a primary infection is largely responsible for extension of the inflammatory process far beyond the focus of the infecting bacilli.

Where the tubercle bacilli first implant themselves and are most numerous, caseation necrosis occurs, giving rise to a persistent lesion. The surrounding pneumonia, where the organisms are few or absent, may resolve completely. Not uncommonly, however, there is some destruction of tissue in this area, and a variable degree of fibrosis and inflammatory infiltration remains after the acute inflammation has subsided. The interstitial fibrosis may even be predominant. Obliteration of many small bronchi causes shrinkage of the diseased portion of the lung, while destruction of muscle and elastic tissue in the walls of larger bronchi involved in the tuberculous bronchopneumonia can result in bronchiectasis. These changes may be present even though there is only a minimal degree of fibrosis. The caseous foci become encapsulated and frequently calcify. Even in the absence of calcification these lesions usually remain indefinitely. Cavitation can occur within a few weeks of the onset of the disease if the caseous focus empties its contents into a bronchus.

ROENTGEN TECHNIQUES IN EARLY LESIONS. Since the majority of cases of early tuberculosis begin in the posterior segment of the upper lobe,

and the lesion is projected behind or beneath the outer part of the clavicle, the roentgen examination must be designed to demonstrate this area particularly well if a small lesion is not to be overlooked. On the frontal film, this area is partly obscured by overlapping shadows of the scapula, clavicle and of the upper ribs which cross each other in this region. The scapulas can be shifted off the lung fields by proper positioning of the patient, but sufficient exposure must be used to penetrate the scapular muscles which otherwise cast a shadow over the outer part of the upper lobe. Sufficient exposure is also needed to penetrate the clavicles and ribs so that a pulmonary lesion can be visualized through these structures. The shadow of the lesion can usually be projected beneath the clavicle if the roentgen tube is elevated and angled downward (Fig. 9A), or if the patient stands in a hypererect position (see p. 19). A similar result is accomplished with the apical lordotic view as the shadow of the clavicle is then projected over the dome of the thorax, while the shadow of the lesion remains in the same position relative to the posterior ribs as in the frontal projection (Fig. 15). The lesion is frequently more clearly outlined if a slight oblique projection (approximately 15 degrees) is made.

It is important, in terms of diagnosis, to determine whether or not a lesion seen in the infraclavicular region on the frontal film, is situated posteriorly. Smaller lesions in this region are usually not visible in the lateral projection but they can almost always be demonstrated on the appropriate oblique view (45 degrees). Tomograms disclose the character of the process and its extent in much greater detail than ordinary films. It is advisable to make films in positions that demonstrate the lesion to best advantage, in addition to tomograms, when a patient with tuberculosis is first studied, since these will serve as a baseline for comparison with films later in the course of the disease.

ROENTGEN APPEARANCE. The early lesion generally begins as a small, ill-defined area of consolidation and infiltration projected beneath

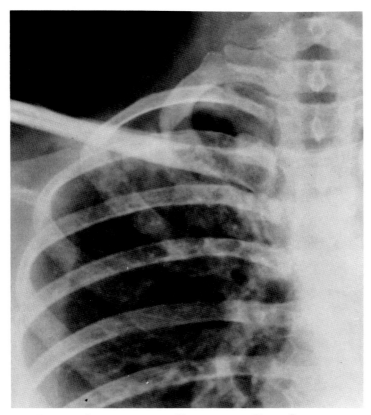

FIG. 281. INFRACLAVICULAR TUBERCULOSIS: EARLY INFILTRATE

The lobular consolidation in the infraclavicular region represents the early infiltrate of the reinfection type of tuberculosis. The area of increased illumination above and mesial to the shadow suggests a cavity. However, this appearance is caused by normally aerated lung outlined by thickened pleura over the apex. A film made several months previously was negative.

the outer part of the clavicle at the level of the third or fourth space posteriorly (Fig. 281). Most often the shadow is not completely homogeneous. Small nodules of varying size and density and streak-like shadows representing areas of interstitial infiltration or small foci of atelectasis are seen within it. Sometimes these shadows are distributed adjacent to a small, homogeneous density. In either case, the conglomeration of densities helps to differentiate the early tuberculous lesion from a peripheral bronchogenic neoplasm.

In some cases the early lesion consists entirely of consolidation. The shadow is then homogeneous and often quite large (Fig. 282), appearing the same as the shadow of a nonspecific pneumonia. The tuberculous nature of the disease may not become evident until subsequent examinations are made. Cavitation frequently occurs early, particularly in the case of larger lesions (Fig. 283). The cavities are usually thick-walled in the early stages when they are surrounded by a large area of tuberculous pneumonia but occasionally they are thin-walled, es-

pecially when they occur in association with small, more discrete lesions.

The location of the early lesion of reinfection tuberculosis in the axillary portion of the posterior segment of an upper lobe is so common that, except in certain specific instances, if the shadow is situated anywhere else, the diagnosis of tuberculosis is open to serious question (Fig. 271). When the lesion is seen more mesially, i.e., separated from the lateral chest wall by a distance of more than 3 or 4 centimeters, or when the shadow is situated in the paravertebral portion of the posterior segment, an additional lesion is usually present in the outer portion of the segment. Similarly, involvement of the apex of the lung without evident disease in the posterior segment beneath the level of the clavicle is quite rare.

Occasionally tuberculous lesions occur in atypical locations, in diabetics and in members of racial groups that are particularly susceptible to the disease. Of the atypical locations, the anterior segment of the upper lobe and the superior segment of the lower lobe, are the most common

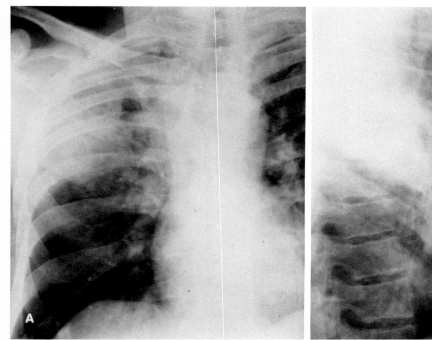
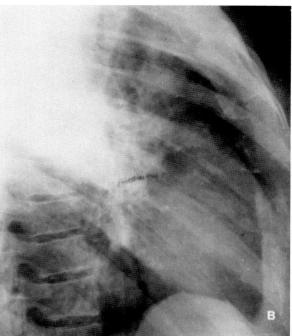

FIG. 282. TUBERCULOUS PNEUMONIA

A: There is a dense, homogeneous consolidation of the outer, upper part of the right upper lobe. The patient had high fever and signs of consolidation suggesting pneumococcal pneumonia. However, the sputum was positive for tubercle bacilli. *B:* The lateral view shows a large, wedge-shaped area of consolidation in the posterior portion of the right upper lobe. The sharply defined lower border corresponds to the upper portion of the long fissure. The lesion involved the posterior and apical segments.

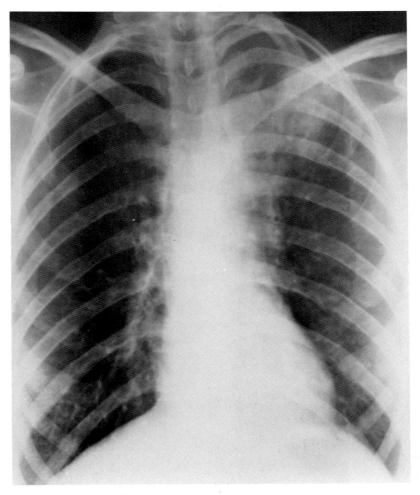

FIG. 283. EXUDATIVE TUBERCULOSIS

There is an area of consolidation in the left upper lobe extending from the apex to the level of the anterior portion of the second rib. The lucency at the level of the clavicle represents an early cavity. The left lung root is elevated. Pathologically, the lesion consisted of an atelectatic, caseous bronchopneumonia with obstruction of many small bronchi. The trachea is not displaced because there were no adhesions over the outer part of the upper lobe so that the lower lobe could undergo compensatory hyperinflation.

(Figs. 13 and 97). In our experience, reinfection tuberculosis in the middle lobe seems to occur particularly in older individuals. The fact that a lesion is tuberculous should be suspected if many tiny nodules are present in the neighborhood of a rather homogeneous density or a cavity, regardless of its location (Fig. 284).

Resolution. Contrary to the general impression, the early lesion shows a marked tendency to spontaneous resolution. Even large lesions may resorb without leaving a trace, within a period of a few weeks. This occurs when the patient's resistance is good and the lesion consists mainly of a gelatinous pneumonia, representing an allergic response to the infection with little necrosis of lung tissue. Rapid resolution occurs more frequently if treatment with antituberculosis drugs is begun early and it is further hastened by the administration of corticosteroids. Usually, however, absorption of the exudate proceeds slowly and the lesion does not diminish perceptibly in size for a period of 6 to 8 weeks after the institution of drug treatment. In some cases no change is noted for as long as 3 or 4 months. If corticosteroids are given together with the antimicrobial drugs, evidence of resolution may appear within 3 or 4 weeks. In some instances this form of treatment is indicated as a therapeutic test in differentiating tuberculosis from carcinoma.

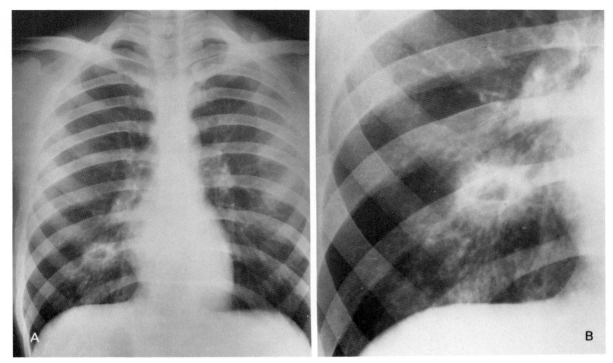

FIG. 284. BASAL TUBERCULOSIS

A: The cavity in the lower part of the right lung at the level of the posterior portion of the tenth rib was demonstrated on oblique and lateral views to be situated in the subapical segment of the right lower lobe. Because of its location and the presence of a fluid level, the appearance suggests a putrid abscess. *B*: A close-up shows numerous miliary infiltrations below the cavity. These are most unusual in pulmonary abscess and suggest tuberculosis. The sputum contained tubercle bacilli.

In most cases there is a significant amount of caseation necrosis and it is then impossible for resolution to be complete. Furthermore, persistence of tubercle bacilli in portions of the lesion produces chronic, indurative changes associated with the deposition of tuberculous granulation tissue and eventually scar tissue. The caseous foci themselves become surrounded by fibrous tissue, and remain in the form of nodular lesions which persist indefinitely. Complete stabilization of the process, leaving inactive areas of induration and encapsulated caseous foci showing neither further absorption nor extension, usually occurs within about 8 months after the institution of chemotherapy. In some instances stabilization is slower. In the absence of cavitation, it may generally be assumed that the maximum degree of resolution will occur within one year of chemotherapy. The treatment, however, does not insure against further reactivation, since viable tubercle bacilli may be demonstrated within the lesion in a majority of cases. Chemotherapy is therefore continued for a considerably longer period, during which time any remaining viable tubercle bacilli become well encapsulated by fi-brous tissue and thus are prevented from spreading the disease.

Bronchial Dissemination. Spread of the infection from the early tuberculous lesion occurs through the bronchi rather than by direct extension through the alveoli or through the lymphatics. Local spread of the infection usually occurs soon after the onset while more extensive spread occurs later, usually following formation of a cavity. Often spread of the disease is caused by aspiration of blood during a hemoptysis. The dissemination may then be widespread and result in a tuberculous bronchopneumonia affecting one or more lobes.

The individual lesions produce ill-defined, fairly large, mottled shadows (Fig. 285). When several patches of bronchopneumonia coalesce, a large, dense, homogeneous shadow results. The radiologic appearance of this caseous pneumonia may be indistinguishable from that of lobar pneumonia produced by other organisms (Fig. 286).

Large bronchi may also become involved as the disease spreads and, if they are severely inflamed, they can become obstructed by tena-

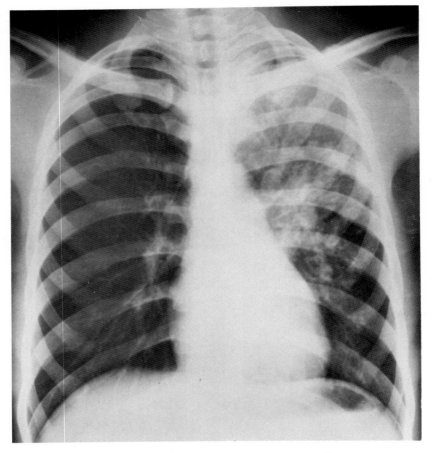

FIG. 285. TUBERCULOSIS SIMULATING RESOLVING LOBAR PNEUMONIA

The lobular consolidation throughout the left upper lobe and the superior segment of the lower lobe cannot be differentiated radiologically from lobar pneumonia during the stage of resolution. An extensive tuberculous process such as this results from bronchogenic spread and is usually associated with a visible cavity. In this case, the cavity is not seen. It apparently is filled with exudate which accumulated because of obstruction of the entering bronchus. The cavity was visualized on a later film made after bronchial drainage was established.

cious mucoid or mucopurulent exudate, resulting in atelectasis of one or more lobes. This is evidenced by diffuse clouding of the affected side, a shift of the mediastinum toward that side, and approximation of the overlying ribs (Fig. 287).

A less serious dissemination of the infection occurs in patients with greater resistance to the disease. The infiltrations are smaller and more discrete, and take the form of numerous small, rather well-demarcated, irregular nodules (Figs. 2 and 288). These represent localized areas of exudation and conglomerate tubercles involving individual acini (the portions of the pulmonary lobule supplied by the terminal bronchioles). Because of the acinar distribution of the nodules, Aschoff termed the condition "acinar-nodose tuberculosis." In some cases the nodules are uniform in size because they all represent inflam-

mation of individual acini. In others, the size of the lesions vary, although in general they are small. The larger ones represent disease involving two or more contiguous acini.

In contradistinction to the acinar nodules, the more diffuse, bronchopneumonic lesions are often complicated by cavitation and dense fibrosis. Acinar-nodose lesions disappear within a relatively short time after the institution of chemotherapy and even in the absence of drug treatment they may resolve within a period of 3 to 6 months. In either case, they have little tendency to spread or become confluent.

The nodules that are not absorbed diminish in size and are replaced by connective tissue. Some are transformed into small fibrocaseous foci within which tubercle bacilli are imprisoned and rendered harmless. Eventually some of these le-

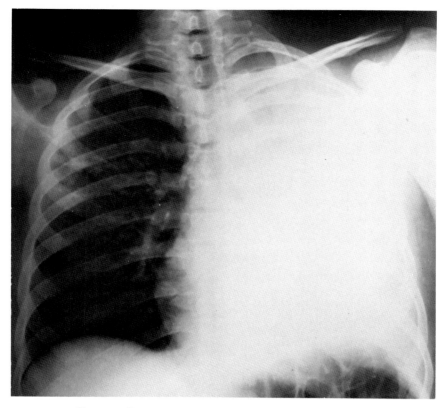

FIG. 286. TUBERCULOUS PNEUMONIA SIMULATING EFFUSION

The entire left hemithorax is opacified, suggesting a large pleural effusion. However, with an effusion of this size, one would expect the left leaf of the diaphragm to be depressed and the mediastinum displaced to the right. Since this is not the case, the differential diagnosis lies between atelectasis of the lung with an effusion, and consolidation of the lung. The acinar-nodose lesions and small lobular areas of consolidation in the outer part of the right upper lobe are typical of cross-infection tuberculosis.

sions calcify. Even repeated bronchogenous dissemination of this character cause little harm to the patient. Similar focal lesions may be the result of hematogenous dissemination. Since this usually occurs in patients with low resistance to the disease, they are of more serious import if not treated by specific drugs.

Caseation. The exudative tuberculous lesion representing the early infiltrate or the result of bronchial dissemination, may undergo more or less extensive caseation. The necrotizing, caseating process usually occurs in spotty fashion within the area of tuberculous pneumonia. While the purely exudative lesions can resolve completely so that the lung can return to a normal state with little or no fibrosis, the areas of caseation within it are not completely absorbed and leave permanent residua. Localized caseous foci usually become surrounded by a capsule of connective tissue and appear as dense, more or less sharply demarcated shadows on the film (Fig.

289). For a period, these may diminish in size as partial absorption takes place, but finally they become stabilized and the size of the foci remains constant (Fig. 290). Calcium is frequently deposited within the encapsulated caseous lesions, causing their shadows to become more and more dense over a period of years (Fig. 137).

Multiple nodules, representing fibrocaseous foci of tuberculosis, may be confused with metastatic neoplasms. However, they are easily recognized when they exist in conjunction with other tuberculous lesions, as is usually the case. On the other hand, when only the nodular foci are present, the differential diagnosis becomes more difficult. Their characteristic location in the upper lobes, the nonhomogeneous density of the individual shadows, their tendency to an irregular outline, and the recognition of deposits of calcium within the lesions, attests to the tuberculous nature of the process. Even in the absence of roentgen evidence of fibrosis adjacent

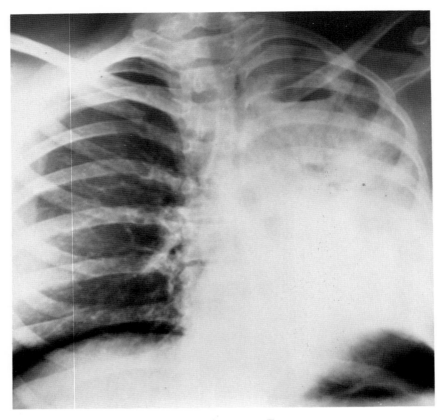

FIG. 287. BRONCHIAL SPREAD OF TUBERCULOSIS

A large cavity with a fluid level, in the left upper lobe, was the source of spread of the tuberculous infection throughout the left lung. The remainder of the upper lobe is involved in a caseous pneumonia. The lobe is consolidated and shows an air bronchogram. The lower lobe is completely collapsed. This was due to tuberculous bronchitis and bronchial obstruction by tenacious exudate. The heart and mediastinal structures are displaced to the left.

to the lesion, there frequently occurs a characteristic elevation of the lung root on the side of the larger lesions. This is caused by partial atelectasis of the affected upper lobe which occurred early in the disease. When the lesions are situated in the lower lobes or when they are scattered indiscriminately throughout the lungs, the diagnosis depends primarily on the demonstration of calcification within them. Although complete healing cannot be said to have taken place, such localized, sharply demarcated, irregular, round or oval areas of caseation and calcification are relatively benign. Bronchogenic dissemination rarely occurs from these foci.

This sequence of changes is the rule when the areas of caseation are small. It is not unusual therefore, to observe the dense shadows of a number of small calcified lesions in a lung which has been the seat of a previous tuberculous infection. Occasionally the same process occurs in lesions of considerable size and then there are large calcific deposits in the lung.

Cavitation. When the caseous foci are large, the necrotic material within them is often extruded through the bronchi, leaving one or more cavities. The cavities vary in size, depending mainly on the extent of the caseation. In the early stages, the cavity is represented by an area of rarefaction within the dense shadow of the consolidated lung tissue (Fig. 291). The cavity is usually irregular and often shows an air-fluid level (Fig. 292). As the exudate about the cavity is absorbed and the pulmonary tissue becomes aerated, the irregular cavity becomes round and more clearly demarcated. The fluid in the cavity diminishes in quantity and may disappear completely or remain only as an extremely thin, horizontal layer at the base of the cavity. Occasionally, the cavity wall is not clearly delineated because of surrounding infiltration or fibrosis and its identification may depend upon the presence of an air-fluid level, no matter how small.

The cavity in the early tuberculous lesion is usually situated in the posterior portion of the

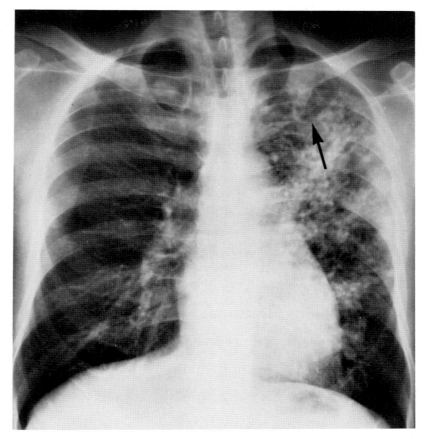

FIG. 288. BRONCHIAL DISSEMINATION OF TUBERCULOSIS: ACINAR-NODOSE LESIONS

The middle two-thirds of the left lung is studded with numerous small nodular shadows. A thin-walled cavity (arrow) is present beneath the left clavicle. The nodular lesions represent consolidated acini resulting from spread of the infection from the tuberculous cavity. The density projected through the mesial portion of the right clavicle represents spread to the right upper lobe.

upper lobe, below the level of the clavicle. Not infrequently, in the later stages of the disease, the cavity is situated above the level of the clavicle. It should not be concluded that this was the original site of the lesion. Tuberculous infections are often associated with atelectasis. Shrinkage of the tissues at the apex of the lung above the cavity causes its upward displacement. In these cases, the mediastinum will be displaced and the trachea sharply angulated toward the side of the lesion.

Occasionally, the cavity has a clover-leaf shape. Although this irregularity in contour is noted most frequently in the early stages of its formation, it is also found in chronic cases. Here it is most commonly due to coalescence of large, irregular areas of caseation.

The roentgen appearance of a cavity depends on many factors. The thickness of its wall varies with the extent of the inflammatory process about it. The presence or absence of fluid exudate within it and the amount of its content depend on the patency of the bronchus that enters the cavity, the position in which this bronchus lies in relation to the lower border of the cavity, and the extent of the caseous process within its walls. The shape and size of the cavity depend on the ability of air to make its exit from the entering bronchus as well as the extent of the original caseous penumonia.

THE ENTERING BRONCHUS. As a rule, there is a fairly wide opening of the bronchus into the tuberculous cavity (Fig. 126). This is sometimes visualized on ordinary roentgen films but is seen more frequently by tomography. In chronic cavities it is usually possible to demonstrate the free bronchial communication by bronchography performed in the Trendelenburg position. In this

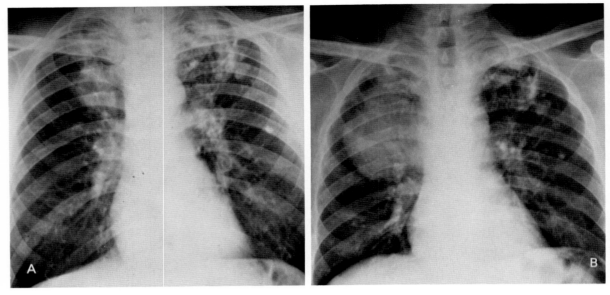

FIG. 289. PULMONARY CARCINOMA AND TUBERCULOSIS

A: The left upper lobe is studded with circumscribed caseous and partly calcified nodules. Infiltrations are present at the apex of the right lung, and beneath this there is a circumscribed oval density with an irregular border. It was obvious that the lesions in the left upper lobe represented tuberculous foci, but it was impossible from this examination alone to be certain whether the lesion in the right lung was a caseous focus or a primary carcinoma. *B*: Three months later. The increase in the size of the lesion in the right upper lobe indicates that it is a carcinoma. However, during the interval between the examinations, the patient developed metastases. It is unwise to await growth of a neoplasm to prove the diagnosis of a carcinoma. Where the roentgen findings are indecisive, the diagnosis should be made in some other way, if necessary by thoracotomy.

respect, a tuberculous cavity differs from an early lung abscess in which the contrast medium cannot be made to enter the cavity.

Because the tuberculous cavity is most often situated in the outer portion of the posterior segment of the upper lobe, it is drained by a branch of the posterior segmental bronchus which runs downward and inward from the base of the cavity. The basal position of the entering bronchus, its downward course and its free communication with the cavity tend to keep the tuberculous cavity empty. Usually, therefore, only a comparatively short time elapses between the formation of the cavity and the disappearance of the fluid level.

HIDDEN CAVITIES. Because the tuberculous cavity tends to be empty and therefore does not show a fluid level, it may be difficult to recognize roentgenologically, particularly when there is considerable surrounding inflammation or fibrosis. This difficulty is often accentuated by the presence of extraneous shadows resulting from pneumothorax treatment or a previous thoracoplasty, or because the lung is obscured by an overlying empyema. Since it is important in all cases of tuberculosis to recognize a cavity which may serve as an indication for surgical treatment,

special methods must be used to confirm or exclude its presence (Figs. 13, 15 and 21).

A cavity is more easily detected if there is an air-fluid level within it. The formation of a fluid level can be encouraged by permitting exudate to accumulate within the cavity. This is done by having the patient lie on the affected side overnight and by inhibiting the cough reflex with adequate sedation. The patient is transported to the X-ray Department, lying on that side, and films are made in the frontal, oblique and inclined or lateral decubitus positions in order to demonstrate a fluid level, if present. The fluid level may be extremely small and is easily mistaken for a slight flattening of the lower border of the cavity. However, a similar, horizontal shadow seen in the inclined or lateral decubitus views, will prove that it is really a fluid level.

BALLOON CAVITIES. The size and shape of a cavity depend on the condition of the entering bronchus. A small, irregular cavity may suddenly become large and round if the bronchus is narrowed or kinked. Kinking is not infrequent following induction of a pneumothorax, or a thoracoplasty (Fig. 293). The sudden ballooning of the cavity is the result of a check-valve mechanism, permitting air to enter the cavity, but blocking

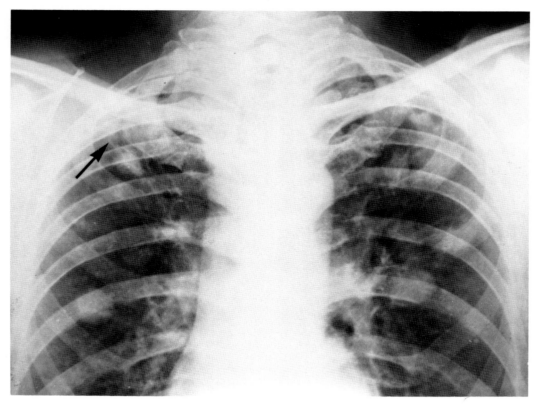

FIG. 290. NODULAR TUBERCULOSIS

A number of nodular shadows suggesting metastatic neoplasm are present in the upper two-thirds of each lung. Although they are well circumscribed, the ones beneath the left clavicle have an irregular contour. This is unusual in pulmonary metastases. Moreover, the fibrous streaks beneath the mesial half of the right first rib are indicative of inflammatory disease. The nodules proved to be encapsulated caseous foci. Such tuberculous lesions are relatively common in diabetics. The oblique, streak-like shadow (arrow), extending from the outer border of the oval lesion in the right upper lobe is a Fleischner line, which indicates that the lesion has occluded a small bronchus. This is one of the rare exceptions to the rule that a Fleischner line distal to a nodule is indicative of a primary carcinoma of the lung.

its exit. In this way the amount of air and, therefore, the pressure within the cavity increases after each inspiration. When the obstruction is relieved, the positive pressure within the cavity is released and the cavity diminishes in size. It then assumes an irregular or clover-leaf shape. Any fluid which accumulated during the stage of partial obstruction is usually eliminated and all that remains is an irregular area of rarefaction of smaller size, more or less sharply demarcated by the cavity wall. During the stage of blockage, there may be activation of the infection in the wall, causing marked thickening of the wall by caseating tissue. This can lead to extensive spread of the disease when the bronchial communication becomes free.

DISAPPEARANCE OF CAVITIES. If the entering bronchus becomes completely obstructed, either by a stricture or kinking, air can no longer enter

the cavity and as it is absorbed, the cavity tends to disappear. If the walls of the cavity are thin, they fall together and become agglutinated. In such cases a fibrous streak is often all that remains of the lesion. If, on the other hand, the wall of the cavity is thick and cannot collapse, it fills with exudate which may dissect into the adjacent lung if the local disease has not been well encapsulated by fibrous tissue. In other cases, the cavity simply remains filled and presents the roentgen picture of a localized nodule, simulating a neoplasm (Fig. 294). Gradually the exudate may be absorbed. In some cases it becomes inspissated, shrinks, and finally is calcified. Complete obstruction of the entering bronchus is undoubtedly the most important mechanism by which the cavity in tuberculosis is eliminated.

OPEN HEALING OF CAVITIES. Before the ad-

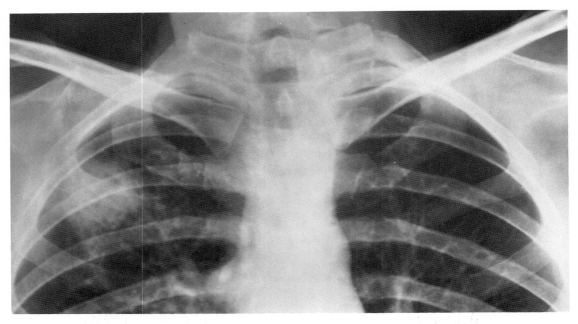

FIG. 291. TUBERCULOSIS: EARLY CAVITATION

The round density in the right infraclavicular region represents a tuberculous pneumonia. The irregular area of lucency within it indicates early cavitation. Air entered the lesion after caseous material was extruded through the communicating bronchus.

vent of specific drug treatment for tuberculosis, a persistent tuberculous cavity was almost always associated with active infection in its walls. The open cavity was therefore conducive to bronchogenic spread of the infection. Antimicrobial drugs in the early stage of the disease usually result in disappearance of the smaller cavities, and even large cavities frequently close completely.

If, instead of complete stricturing of the entering bronchus, epithelialization takes place at the bronchocavitary junction, the bronchial communication persists and the cavity remains despite adequate therapy. Nevertheless, the infection in the cavity wall and surrounding lung may be completely eliminated by the chemotherapeutic agents. This type of healing with persistence of the cavity is referred to as *open healing.*

Pathologically, the healed tuberculous cavity has a smooth, glistening lining and resembles a cyst. The wall may be extremely thin or thick, depending upon the degree of fibrosis of the lung about the cavity. If the infection is eliminated in the early stage, before extensive pericavitary fibrosis has taken place, the cavity is represented by an exteremely thin-walled, smooth, annular shadow. When healing occurs in the more chronic stage of tuberculosis, the wall of the cavity is thicker. The cavity is frequently irregular in shape, and its wall tends to merge in places with the surrounding dense, fibrotic lung. As in the case of a thin-walled cavity, there is no fluid level. Despite the thick wall, it may be difficult to visualize the cavity on ordinary films because of the density of the adjacent lung. The possibility of open healing must be considered in all cavities without an air-fluid level in patients who have been under adequate chemotherapy.

It might be expected that the cavity, after open healing, would persist unchanged indefinitely. However, changes do occur occasionally, as they may in persistent cavities from any cause. Secondary infection may result in the formation of an air-fluid level, and it may cause necrosis of the epithelial lining resulting in stricture at the bronchocavitary junction. It is then possible for the cavity to close permanently. The cavity may become filled or partly filled with blood clot if there is hemorrhage from its wall. Finally, the cavity may serve as a nidus for the proliferation of fungi which form a mycelial ball (Fig. 251).

SPREAD OF INFECTION FROM CAVITIES. In the patient who has not been treated with specific drugs, myriads of tubercle bacilli are present in the cavity. That an overwhelming spread of the disease from this source does not occur soon after the formation of a cavity is undoubtedly due to the fact that the patient has already acquired

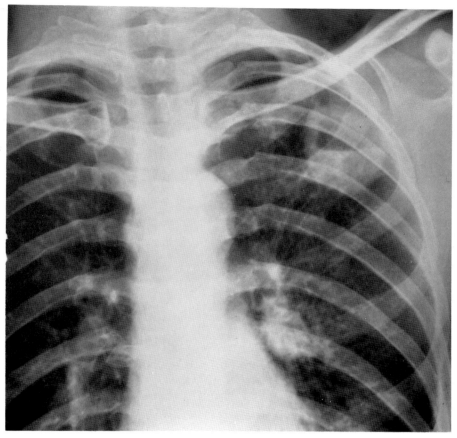

FIG. 292. CAVITARY TUBERCULOSIS

The single cavity beneath the left clavicle is partly filled with fluid. The fluid level and the absence of any infiltration about the cavity are more characteristic of a putrid abscess than of tuberculosis. The differential diagnosis cannot be made radiologically and depends upon the clinical history and the examination of the sputum. The thick wall is due to active caseation which is also responsible for poor drainage and the accumulation of fluid.

considerable resistance. If drugs are not administered, sooner or later there is a breakdown in this resistance and dissemination of the disease. This usually occurs first in the region of the cavity, but, at any time, the infection can spread through the bronchi to other portions of the lung.

In some cases, despite adequate treatment, the tuberculous cavity does not close or undergo open healing. Nevertheless, dissemination of the disease from the persistent, infected cavity is prevented by the chemotherapy in most instances. On the other hand, there always remains the danger of development of resistant tubercle bacilli and consequent spread of the infection.

Spread of the infection is usually manifested by the appearance of small areas of infiltration and consolidation in the region of the cavity. The infiltrations are frequently miliary or submiliary in size. The presence of such infiltrations adjacent to a cavity strongly suggests tuberculosis. This finding is particularly useful in differentiating a tuberculous cavity in a lower lobe from a lung abscess (Fig. 284).

Most cavities in reinfection tuberculosis are situated in the outer part of the posterior segment of the upper lobe. Usually the portion of the lung next affected is the mesial or paravertebral part of the posterior segment, soon followed by the apical segment of the affected upper lobe. The anterior segment of the lobe is less frequently involved. Focal spread of the disease to the lower lobe on the same side occurs most frequently to the superior segment. A localized spread to the opposite lung usually affects the outer part of the posterior segment of the upper lobe.

It is extremely important to recognize the fact that the apex of the lower lobe on the same side

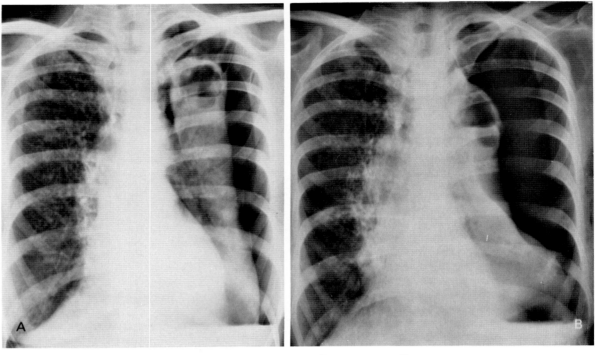

FIG. 293. PERSISTENCE OF TUBERCULOUS CAVITY DESPITE PNEUMOTHORAX

A: A pneumothorax was induced in an attempt to collapse the cavity in the left upper lobe. Although the pneumothorax was adequate, the cavity was held open by adhesions which prevented retraction of the involved portion of the lung. The linear shadows crossing the pneumothorax space represent attenuated portions of lung which are attached to the chest wall. Numerous fine tubercles throughout the right lung are due to bronchogenic spread of the disease. *B*: Following lysis of adhesions, the lobe is retracted from the chest wall, but the cavity remains and still shows an air-fluid level. This indicates that its bronchial communication is partially blocked, suggesting tuberculous bronchitis.

is involved, particularly if resection is contemplated. In such cases there is often a marked shrinkage of the upper lobe with a corresponding elevation of the upper part of the long fissure and of the apex of the adjoining lower lobe. This portion of the lower lobe may be situated so high that an area of consolidation within it appears to be within the upper lobe. Under such circumstances, only the lesion in the upper lobe may be resected, leaving the diseased portion of the lower lobe intact.

Quite frequently, examination in the lateral view will disclose the fact that the lower lobe is involved. However, in some instances, the long fissure is not visualized and the exact position of the apex of the lower lobe cannot be determined. Moreover, even if the long fissure is well outlined and the superior segment of the lower lobe appears clean, lesions within this segment may be obscured on the lateral projection by the shadows of the spine and chest wall. While the oblique views are helpful, tomography in the lateral view discloses the lobar distribution of the disease much more precisely. Lateral tomog-

raphy, therefore, should always be performed preliminary to resective surgery for upper lobe tuberculosis.

In all cases of pulmonary tuberculosis with cavitation, the outer part of the opposite upper lobe should be inspected carefully as this is the region where cross infections occur most frequently (Fig. 286). Cross infection on the left side usually occurs at the level of the axillary part of the second and third anterior costal spaces. On the right side, the lesions are generally situated somewhat higher, at the level of the first and second anterior intercostal spaces. The difference in the location of the contralateral spread is probably due to the difference in the bronchial distribution on the two sides.

Cross infections practically always originate from a cavity. If there is a dense shadow beneath one clavicle and a small, faint shadow on the other side in a characteristic location, the dense lesion should be studied carefully for the presence of a cavity (Fig. 295). If none is seen on ordinary films, tomography should be performed.

In the later stages of the disease, there are

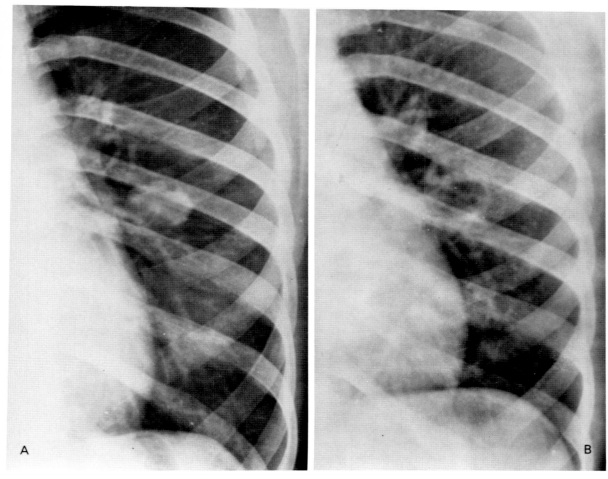

FIG. 294. BLOCKED TUBERCULOUS CAVITY

A: The nodule in the superior segment of the left lower lobe has a fairly well-defined, slightly irregular border. The appearance is most suggestive of a peripheral carcinoma. However, the possibility of an inflammatory lesion such as a tuberculoma or the residuum of a fungous infection is not excluded. *B*: Review of a film made 13 years previously when the patient had active tuberculosis shows a round cavity in the exact location of the present nodule. In the intervening years the entering bronchus became strictured and the cavity filled with inspissated exudate and caseous material.

usually areas of irregular fibrosis extending in fan-like manner to the upper, outer, axillary portion of the chest, and, not infrequently, areas of calcification are present about the lesion, indicating its tuberculous nature. Bilateral cavities in the upper lobes, or scars from a previous tuberculous infection are additional criteria for the diagnosis of tuberculosis.

Atelectasis in Tuberculosis. It has been emphasized that the early tuberculous lesion, even though small, is in the nature of a bronchopneumonia. Pathologic examinations in this stage have shown evidences of severe infection of the bronchi in the affected area. There is not only a destructive process in the walls of these bronchi but also plugging of the lumina by exudate. The

bronchial obstruction results in foci of atelectasis within the inflamed lung tissue. However, the entire lesion is usually so small in the early stage that evidence of shrinkage of the involved portion of the lung is usually not visible on the roentgen film.

When a larger area of lung is involved, whether it be in the early or late stage of the disease, the atelectasis that results from obstruction of the bronchi is more apparent. The roentgen manifestations of the atelectasis depend on the location of the lesion, the size and number of bronchi obstructed, and the presence or absence of pleural adhesions. In all instances of atelectasis, the vessels in the infiltrated area are more closely approximated than in the normal lung. The pres-

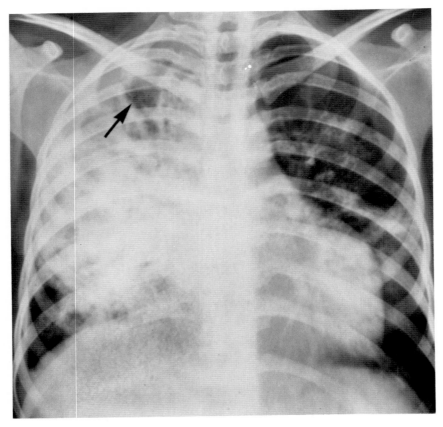

FIG. 295. TUBERCULOUS PNEUMONIA WITH CROSS INFECTION

There is confluent, lobular consolidation of the lower half of the right upper lobe, the middle lobe and the superior and subapical segments of the lower lobe. This represents spread of tuberculosis from the cavity (arrow) beneath the right clavicle. The infiltrations in the axillary portion of the left lung are also due to bronchogenous spread. Cross infections on the left side are usually situated at a lower level than those on the right (see Fig. 286).

ence of atelectasis is easily determined if the crowding of the blood vessels can be recognized on the film. In the more extensive lesions in the right upper lobe, the short fissure is often considerably elevated (Fig. 94). Elevation and forward displacement of the upper part of the long fissure may be disclosed on the lateral view. If the disease is rather extensive and the lung is adherent to the chest wall so that the upper lobe cannot retract toward the mediastinum, the trachea becomes displaced sharply to the side of the lesion (Fig. 73). It should be emphasized that these changes occur during the acute pneumonic stage of the disease as a result of bronchial obstruction and are not caused by retraction of scar tissue. The fibrous tissue that is laid down in the course of the disease simply serves to keep the partially atelectic lung from reexpanding.

Streak-like shadows are common in tuberculosis and appear to represent areas of fibrosis. They frequently appear in the early phases and,

in rare instances, may be the earliest roentgen manifestation of the disease. Actually, these streaks represent small areas of atelectasis. Frequently they disappear as the process resolves. However, if fibrous tissue is deposited in the area, the streak-like shadows become permanent.

The evidence of atelectasis is often more conspicuous after resolution of the disease, for at this time the pulmonary vessels can be more clearly seen. The extent of the tuberculous infection can be inferred from the degree of condensation of the vessels in the upper lobe. Often, after resolution of tuberculosis involving the apical as well as the posterior segments, all that is seen is a marked elevation of the lung root with only faint, strand-like shadows in the upper part of the lobe. The elevation of the root appears out of proportion to the paucity of roentgen signs (Fig. 95). This is explained by the fact that granulation tissue forms within the inflamed, atelectatic lung during the acute stage of the disease and the fine strands of scar tissue persist in the collapsed lung after resolution of the inflammatory process. These serve to keep the lung root elevated, particularly because the peribronchial and perivascular connective tissues, which are scarred, run largely in a vertical direction. The elevation of the lung root is due to loss of volume in the upper lobe and not to retraction of scar tissue. The distance between the root and the apex is shortened early because of the atelectasis and the shortening is maintained by the newly formed scar. Even though the fibrous scars are fine and cast little shadow on the film, they are sufficient to keep the lung root elevated.

Bronchiectasis in Chronic Tuberculosis. Extensive early infiltrates usually undergo considerable caseation. The caseous bronchopneumonia is regularly accompanied by more or less extensive disease of the bronchial branches whose walls are partly destroyed together with the parts of the pulmonary parenchyma which they supply. Many small caseous foci in the lung may be eliminated through these bronchi, leaving numerous small cavities.

The resulting roentgen picture mirrors the pathologic process. Numerous small, irregular areas of rarefaction which represent multiple bronchopulmonary cavities are seen within the shadow of the pneumonic area. The affected portion of the lung presents a moth-eaten appearance. Following further elimination of the caseous material, there is irregular absorption of exudate. However, resolution is incomplete and fibrosis takes place. Thus, a large amount of dense connective tissue is deposited throughout the involved region, giving rise to irregular opacities on the film. The atelectasis resulting from obstruction of many of the bronchi by exudate, together with some contraction of the scar tissue, causes marked shrinkage of the affected area. In spite of displacement of the surrounding structures to compensate for the diminution in the size of the partially destroyed and atelectatic lung, traction is exerted on the weakened bronchial walls, causing the bronchi to become dilated.

The resulting disease is a chronic one, complicated by the presence of numerous small tuberculous cavities and bronchial dilatations. The ulcerative tuberculosis is complicated by secondary infection of the widened bronchi whose walls are diseased and which are unable to eliminate their secretions properly.

Such an area of chronic tuberculosis, consisting of dilated bronchi entering into small caseous ulcerated areas of lung may serve as a source for infection of the remainder of the lung in the same way as does a persistent single large cavity. In some cases, however, the infection is held in check and the tubercle bacilli are either expectorated or destroyed. The ulcerative foci in the lung then become lined by a smooth epithelial layer which is continuous with the lining of the dilated communicating bronchi. The further course of this lesion then is that of nonspecific bronchiectasis (Fig. 296).

Bronchiectasis, with or without active tuberculous infection, is frequently associated with true, large tuberculous cavities in chronic tuberculosis. Nonspecific infection and induration of the lung by scar tissue and exudate complicate the roentgen picture by producing persistent shadows in addition to the areas of rarefaction. The bronchiectasis which persists even when the tuberculous infection has been controlled, leaves these shadows which cannot be differentiated radiologically from those caused by active tuberculosis. Only the inability to demonstrate tubercle bacilli in the sputum on many examinations enables one to exclude an active tuberculous infection.

Even small tuberculous lesions may leave bronchiectases in their wake. Regardless of the extent of the bronchiectasis, secondary infection is usually minimal or absent because the posterior and apical segments of the upper lobes, which are the ones most commonly involved in tuberculosis, drain well. Cough may be absent, but bleeding from the distal bronchi is not infrequent. Hemoptysis in these cases, therefore, is not necessarily indicative of active tuberculosis. In the absence of tubercle bacilli in the sputum or gastric contents, simple post-tuberculous bronchiectasis should be suspected as the cause of the hemoptysis. The bronchiectases may be demonstrated by tomography.

Occasionally, the bronchiectases in the upper lobe do become secondarily infected with pyogenic organisms. Extensive suppurative bronchiectasis, confined to an upper lobe, is usually the result of a tuberculous infection that has healed. In these cases the patient frequently expectorates a considerable amount of sputum without tubercle bacilli. The sputum is due to persistent, nonspecific infection in the deep sacculations. The diagnosis of post-tuberculous bronchiectasis is warranted only if bronchograms show no evidence of underlying bronchial obstruction.

Bronchostenosis in Tuberculosis. Obstruction of bronchi by tuberculous lymph nodes has been described in the section on Primary Tuberculosis. Obstruction of the larger bronchi occurs in reinfection tuberculosis as the result of a se-

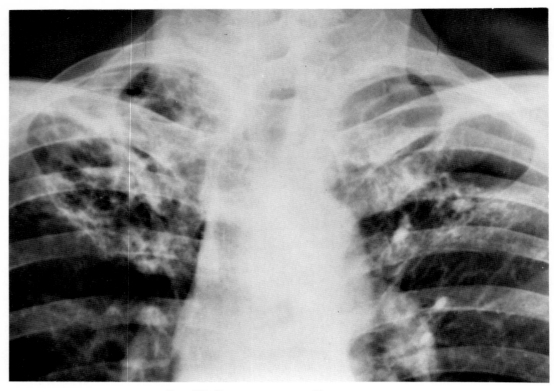

FIG. 296. BRONCHIECTASIS IN TUBERCULOSIS

The upper part of the right upper lobe presents a honeycombed appearance. The septa between the cavities are thin and there is little infiltration of the lung. The appearance represents the end state of an extensive tuberculosis in which the specific infection has been eliminated and all that remains is residual bronchiectasis. The trachea is sharply angulated to the right because of shrinkage of the right upper lobe. There are large bullae at the left apex and, beneath them, fine scars and calcific deposits of healed tuberculosis.

vere tuberculous bronchitis without disease of the adjacent lymph nodes. In some cases a granuloma forms in the wall of the bronchus and protrudes into the lumen to cause bronchial obstruction. More often the obstruction results from scar tissue formed within the wall of the affected bronchus, causing a stricture. In either case, obstructive emphysema or atelectasis may occur distally, depending upon the degree of obstruction.

It is important to recognize the bronchostenosis because it may influence the type of treatment to be employed. Collapse therapy is usually ineffective in tuberculous bronchitis with bronchial obstruction. Moreover, the obstruction of the bronchus is not infrequently complicated by pyogenic secondary infection which may be difficult to eradicate. Obstructive emphysema may cause troublesome symptoms. For these reasons, resective surgery may be indicated in patients with bronchial obstruction resulting from tuberculous bronchitis.

The presence of the stenosis is recognized roentgenologically by characteristic changes. The sudden appearance of a diffuse, homogeneous shadow of lobar distribution or of lobar emphysema in a patient with tuberculosis who develops dyspnea without any of the constitutional effects of a tuberculous pneumonia, suggests an occlusive type of tuberculous bronchitis. Examination during expiration and inspiration will yield further evidence of obstruction and should lead to bronchoscopic study for confirmation of the diagnosis.

In some cases, particularly when the left upper lobe is involved, bronchoscopy may be difficult and unrewarding because the distortion of the bronchus makes visualization of the lesion impossible. In such cases, bronchography can provide valuable diagnostic information and establish the location of the obstruction. Characteristically, the stricture resulting from tuberculous bronchitis appears as a rather long area of bronchial narrowing while strictures due to other causes, particularly those following the perforation of a lymph node show only a short zone of stenosis. Generally, the tuberculous stricture does not obstruct the bronchus completely and contrast material extends beyond it into dilated bronchi. A long, stenotic area, causing only partial obstruction, also occurs occasionally in malignant bronchial neoplasms, but the presence of a positive sputum confirms the diagnosis of bronchial tuberculosis.

Emphysema in Tuberculosis. The occurrence of obstructive emphysema as a result of partial occlusion of one of the larger bronchi has been mentioned. Obstructive emphysema may also result from repeated infections of the smaller bronchi throughout the lungs. These infections occur sporadically in cases of neglected cavities. They follow the aspiration into other parts of the lung of exudate from the cavities or of blood contaminated with tubercle bacilli during the course of a hemoptysis.

In many cases of chronic tuberculosis, there is also a secondary, nonspecfic bronchitis, particularly in individuals with an allergic background. This results in a generalized obstructive emphysema from nonspecific infection and spasm of the smaller bronchi. The emphysema, together with the atelectasis and destruction of lung tissue by the tuberculosis itself, causes considerable impairment of pulmonary function. One should recognize this type of emphysema in tuberculosis and differentiate it from the compensatory emphysema secondary to contraction of a portion of the lung. It is particularly important to make this differentiation when surgical treatment is considered. The obstructive type of emphysema accompanying tuberculosis is perhaps more easily diagnosed clinically. However, its roentgen appearance is also quite characteristic. The generalized distribution of the emphysema, the depression and flattening of the leaves of the diaphragm, and the irregularity and attenuation of the pulmonary vessels together with the presence of interstitial infiltrations and fibrosis, differentiate this form of emphysema from the compensatory type. In the latter, there is only straightening and spreading of the pulmonary vessels without any interstitial changes. The blood vessels are not narrowed and the diaphragm is not depressed.

Chronic Fibroid Tuberculosis. In certain cases of long standing tuberculosis, the roentgen appearance is dominated by dense, irregular shadows of fibrosis. The lesions are usually bilateral although they tend to be more marked on one side. The dense, more or less massive infil-

trations involve the upper portion of the lungs and in most cases include the apices. They extend downward for a variable distance, usually below the level of the second rib anteriorly. When the fibroid lesions are not obscured by other pathologic processes, they cast irregular, coarse, streak-like shadows extending from the periphery toward the root of the lung.

Fibroid tuberculosis is practically always associated with considerable atelectasis, evidenced by a sharp elevation of the lung root and, in most cases, displacement of the trachea to the more affected side (Fig. 297). Not infrequently, the displacement is marked and the trachea becomes sharply angulated. The upper ribs are often drawn together and pulled downward, causing a flattening of the dome of the thorax. As a result of the loss of volume in the upper lobe, there is compensatory emphysema of the lower lobe. This is manifested by some increase in the lucency of the lower lung fields, but the main roentgen sign is straightening of the lower lobe vessels as they traverse the increased distance from the elevated lung root to the diaphragm.

The pleura is usually thickened and produces a rather dense shadow over the lateral portion of the upper lobe. The pleura at the apex is often retracted by the fibrotic, atelectatic lung, causing an appearance simulating thickening of the apical pleura. The short fissure is clearly visualized because of the pleural reaction and fibrosis in the region. The fissure is generally elevated and bowed upward.

Between the dense fibrous streaks, there are irregular areas of increased illumination resulting from both compensatory and obstructive emphysema. One or more chronic tuberculous cavities may be clearly visualized on ordinary films or demonstrated by special methods. These chronic cavities often have large bronchial communications which can be demonstrated radiologically. In addition, bullae are frequently present. Single bullae at the apex of the lung or near the outer portion of the lung at the level of the clavicle may be difficult to differentiate from true tuberculous cavities. Multiple bullae are more easily recognized. Frequently the lesions have a honeycombed appearance resulting from small bronchiectatic sacculations.

Dense round or irregular shadows of varying size are interspersed among the bronchiectases and represent localized granulomas and encapsulated caseous foci. Calcific deposits, usually of small size, are scattered throughout the diseased area in many of the cases. The remaining lung, outside the region of dense fibrosis, commonly

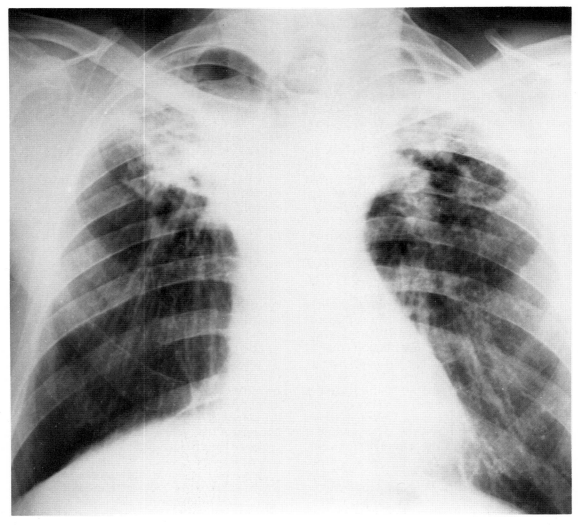

Fig. 297. Fibroid Tuberculosis

There are dense, irregular shadows in the upper part of each lung. These portions of the lung are shrunken as evidenced by marked elevation of the lung roots and the straightening of the blood vessels to the lower lobes. The trachea is sharply angulated to the right, the result of more marked shrinkage of the right upper lobe. The appearance is characteristic of tuberculosis of long standing. The irregular areas of increased illumination within the dense shadows are due to secondary bronchiectasis. The large lucent area at the right apex represents a bulla.

contains small nodular lesions of varying density, some of which are partly calcified. These may be associated with irregular, fine interstitial fibrosis and areas of obstructive emphysema in addition to the compensatory emphysema resulting from contraction of the upper lobe. Because of the generalized thickening of the pleura in chronic fibroid tuberculosis, the border of the mediastinum may appear sharply etched and its contour straightened. The cardiophrenic angle is frequently blunted, the diaphragm appears straightened and the costophrenic sinus becomes shallow.

The character of chronic fibroid tuberculosis is determined by several factors. Most important among these is the underlying bronchial disease. Evidences of bronchial obstruction and destruction are to be found in practically all of the cases. This accounts for the extensive atelectasis. While it is true that contraction of fibrous tissue over a long period plays some part in the shrinkage of the lung, close observation of the course of the disease by repeated roentgen films has shown that the atelectasis occurs suddenly, often during exacerbations of the infection. It must therefore be concluded that the contraction of the lung characteristic of fibroid tuberculosis is due to bronchial obstruction during active phases of the disease rather than to the gradual shrinkage of scar tissue.

The final picture of the fibroid lung in tuberculosis is usually the result of a smoldering infection which has not been completely controlled. This occurs in the form of persistent infected cavities or chronic bronchial tuberculosis. In the latter, ulcerated foci of active infection are usually present in one or more of the bronchiectatic sacculations. Repeated spread of the disease, involving only small areas in the neighborhood of the infected foci, are responsible for what appears to be a gradual increase in the size of the lesion. Without treatment, in most cases, there is eventually a breakdown in resistance, resulting in widespread tuberculous pneumonia. In others, the ulcerative process within one of the cavities results in rupture of a large blood vessel with consequent hemoptysis and aspiration spread of the infection to other parts of the lung. Usually, however, the resistance of the patient is sufficient to prevent widespread infection for a considerable period. During this time healing of repeated small local extensions of the disease occurs, resulting in increased fibrosis. Eventually, even without chemotherapy, the infection often is controlled, and the roentgen picture of chronic fibroid tuberculosis persists unchanged throughout the life of the patient.

Determination of Activity of the Infection. In every case of tuberculosis the question arises as to whether the disease is active. An active tuberculous lesion is one in which the tubercle bacilli are able to produce spread of the disease. The finding of tubercle bacilli in the sputum may be the only evidence of activity. However, patients may be quite ill from actively spreading tuberculosis while the sputum is negative for tubercle bacilli. Moreover, the disease may be actively spreading while the patient himself feels quite well, and the only way to determine that the disease is active is to visualize the lesion roentgenologically.

In addition to absence of tubercle bacilli in the secretions, proof of inactivity of the tuberculosis is obtained only by showing that the lesion remains stable. Where successive films show spread of the disease it is obvious that the disease is active. On the other hand, demonstration of recession of the lesions indicates that the inflammatory process, while undergoing resolution, is not at a standstill. Experience has shown that tubercle bacilli may still be present in the sputum during this stage of resolution and therefore the potential for spread of the disease remains. Un-

der the circumstances, one must consider resolution, as well as spread of the disease, as evidence of activity. The determination that the disease is inactive, therefore, must depend upon the demonstration that the lesions are stable, remaining unchanged over a period of time. Experience has shown that lesions which show no change on repeated x-ray examinations during a period of a year and in which a cavity cannot be demonstrated, prove, as a rule, to be inactive. However, the possibility remains in certain cases that the disease may become reactivated at a later date.

In many instances it is possible to judge from a single examination whether or not the disease is active. The presence of a few fine, streak-like shadows at the apex of the lung or immediately beneath the clavicle without any associated hazy densities, practically always denotes healed tuberculosis. Small or moderate sized, sharply defined calcific deposits invariably represent healed lesions. Even larger nodules up to 5 mm in diameter without demonstrable calcium are practically always inactive if they are sharply demarcated. However, if there is any haziness of the border, the lesion may be active.

Nodules up to 2 cm in diameter may be safely considered inactive if they are sharply defined and contain a considerable amount of calcium distributed throughout the lesion. Nodules of this size which do not contain calcium, or in which the calcium is deposited in one portion of the periphery, frequently represent active lesions. Some of them are really blocked cavities filled with inspissated, necrotic material and contain many tubercle bacilli. Lesions larger than 2 cm in diameter cannot be considered as inactive without prolonged observation.

Bullae are frequently encountered in healed tuberculosis, and may be disregarded in the consideration of activity of the disease if they can be differentiated from true tuberculous cavities. This is not always possible from the roentgen examination alone. However, if the areas of lucency are thin-walled and situated at the extreme apex, or if they are multiple and characterized by the presence of sharply outlined angular borders or septa, it is justifiable to conclude that they represent bullae rather than true cavities.

The presence of a true tuberculous cavity in a patient who has not undergone prolonged chemotherapy must be considered as evidence of active disease. A thin-walled cavity with little or no infiltration in the surrounding lung in a patient who has had treatment with antituberculosis drugs for a long period may represent a healed lesion (open healing). However, the conclusion that the disease is really inactive cannot be drawn from the roentgen appearance alone. In addition, it is necessary to show that tubercle bacilli have been absent from the sputum for a long time.

Hazy shadows with poorly demarcated borders (soft lesions) practically always indicate active disease. The same is true of denser lesions which do not contain sharply defined fibrous streaks or nodules. Large lesions which are made up mostly of fibrous streaks and nodules often prove to be inactive, but it is impossible to exclude activity of the tuberculous process unless repeated observations are made.

Except in those patients with obviously healed lesions, the x-ray examination of the chest should be repeated every 6 months in order to detect reactivation at a comparatively early stage. When there is any question concerning activity of the disease, the examination should be repeated more frequently. In such cases it is wise to make several views. Where the lesion is partly hidden by the clavicle or upper ribs, the lordotic view is essential. It is necessary to compare the appearance of every portion of each lesion with that seen on previous films. To do this effectively, films of comparable quality and projection are required. It is advisable to make tomograms at the initial examination for the detection of cavitation and to serve as a basis for comparison with future films. If the lesion is not well visualized on ordinary films, it is necessary to follow its course with tomograms. In any case, tomography should be repeated before deciding that a lesion has become stabilized.

The roentgen examination is not reliable in determining the activity of tuberculous lesions of the bronchi. Bronchial stenosis and its complicating atelectasis may be associated with either active or healed bronchial tuberculosis, and the differentiation may be possible only by bacteriologic or bronchoscopic examination. Similarly, it is impossible from the roentgen examination to determine whether the bronchiectasis which complicates bronchial tuberculosis is the seat of active disease or whether it represents a completely burned-out, healed lesion.

Classification of Reinfection Tuberculosis. Cases of reinfection tuberculosis have been categorized in different ways in order to indicate the extent of the disease, the activity of the process and the capability of the patient to spread infection.

The grouping of cases in accordance with the extent of the disease is exclusively a roentgenologic classification. The one in general use groups the cases as either minimal, moderately ad-vanced or far advanced. These have been rather thoroughly defined in a report from the American Thoracic Society. Minimal tuberculosis indicates unilateral or bilateral disease of limited extent without evidence of cavitation. The lesions must be of only slight or moderate density and involve an area no greater than that contained by the space between the apex of one lung to the second costal cartilage or the body of the fifth thoracic vertebra. Moderately advanced tuberculosis consists of lesions occupying an area equivalent to that of one lung, provided the lesions are disseminated and of slight to moderate density. If they are confluent and dense, the area involved should not exceed a third of one lung. The lesions may be unilateral or bilateral. Cavitation may be present, but the total of the diameters of all of the cavities should not exceed 4 cm. Far advanced tuberculosis signifies involvement in excess of the above.

The classification of tuberculosis according to its extent has been useful from a statistical and a public health standpoint. It was also valuable as an indication of the prognosis and as a guide to treatment before the advent of effective chemotherapy. Today this classification is of limited value in relation to the individual patient. Other factors frequently far outweigh the radiologic extent of the disease. Of particular importance is the observation of the response of the disease to chemotherapy.

Special criteria have been laid down by the American Thoracic Society for the classification of reinfection tuberculosis into active, quiescent and inactive cases. Cases are classified as *active* if the lesions are obviously recent, as determined by a single roentgenologic examination, if they show progression or if they diminish in size to any considerable degree during a period of 6 months' observation. The demonstration of tubercle bacilli in the sputum or gastric contents, or the presence of a tuberculous empyema, a bronchopleural fistula or evidences of active bronchial tuberculosis are also indications of active disease. Cases are classified as *quiescent* if the lesions show no increase in extent during a period of 6 months' observation and there is little or no diminution in their size. Cavitation may be present but monthly examinations of the sputum and gastric contents by culture or animal inoculation must not reveal the presence of tubercle bacilli. *Inactive* tuberculosis indicates that the lesion has been stable radiologically for a period of 6 months, although it may exhibit a slight degree of resolution during this period. The lesion must be free of cavitation and the sputum and gastric contents free of tubercle bacilli.

The terms *open* and *closed* tuberculosis are frequently used clinically. This classification is based solely on the presence or absence of tubercle bacilli in the secretions regardless of the appearance of the chest roentgenogram. If the sputum or gastric contents are positive for tubercle bacilli, the disease is considered open or active, even though the roentgen findings satisfy all the criteria of an inactive lesion.

Before the advent of chemotherapy, the great majority of patients whose films showed a tuberculous cavity were cases of open tuberculosis, and sooner or later tubercle bacilli could be demonstrated in the secretions. This does not hold true for cases under adequate chemotherapy, as cavities may undergo open healing. In such cases the cavities do not harbor tubercle bacilli and reactivation of the disease does not occur even after chemotherapy has been discontinued.

Hematogenous Tuberculosis

Miliary Tuberculosis. A mild, transient bacteremia probably occurs in practically all cases of primary pulmonary tuberculosis. The tubercle bacilli extend from the caseous foci in the mediastinal nodes by way of the lymphatics to the thoracic duct and then into the blood stream. As a rule, the patient's resistance is sufficient to prevent the development of significant disease from the relatively small number of bacilli that enter the blood stream. In some instances, however, there is massive bloodstream invasion. This can occur in several ways. Probably the most frequent is direct extension of the infection from a tuberculous mediastinal node into an adjacent pulmonary vein, resulting in a caseous, tuberculous endophlebitis. The thoracic duct may become directly involved in a similar manner. Another source of extensive blood stream contamination is a subintimal caseous focus in a vessel not directly related to an infected node. The pathogenesis of this lesion is uncertain.

Most often massive blood stream invasion in the child or adult is associated with a primary focus in the lung. Not infrequently, however, the source of the infection is an extrapulmonary focus, i.e., the genitourinary tract, the intestine, or one of the bones. Only occasionally does such extensive hematogenous dissemination occur in the reinfection type of tuberculosis.

The miliary tubercles consist of tiny granulomas situated in the interstitial tissues of the lung. The lesions are innumerable and are distributed more or less uniformly throughout the lungs, but they appear to be more numerous in the upper two-thirds of each lung where they are somewhat larger and therefore more prominent. At first the lesions are so tiny that they are barely visible. The cut section of the lung appears as if it had been sprinkled with tiny grains of pepper. After a period of a few weeks the tubercles increase in size to form easily visualized, round nodules varying up to 1 to 2 mm in diameter in the upper portions of the lungs, while those in the lowermost portion of the lungs appear to be distinctly smaller.

In extremely rare instances, miliary tubercles that have undergone caseation become calcified. The lungs are then uniformly studded with the tiny deposits. These tend to be more numerous than similar lesions in histoplasmosis.

From repeated roentgen examinations of the lungs in cases of miliary tuberculosis, it has been found that the lesions first become visible radiographically 2½ to 3 weeks after the hematogenous spread of the tubercle bacilli. It takes this long for the tubercles to become large enough to be visualized on the film. They then appear as faint shadows, the size of millet seeds, sprinkled diffusely throughout the pulmonary field (Fig. 298). The lesions are almost uniform in size, although those in the upper lobes may be somewhat larger. Rarely are they larger than the size of a pin head.

The individual lesions remain discrete and show little tendency to coalesce. In the terminal stages of the disease, collateral inflammation between the tubercles may cause them to be obscured in portions of the lung. Since the miliary spread usually occurs when the primary complex is still active, it occurs most commonly in children. Often a large hilar or paratracheal lymph node can be seen on the film together with the miliary tubercles. Large lymph nodes are much less frequently visible in the adult with miliary spread from the primary pulmonary complex. Miliary tuberculosis in the adult may also originate from an extrapulmonary focus, particularly in the genitourinary tract. In these cases the calcified primary complex or calcification of a mediastinal lymph node may be seen on the chest film. Since miliary tuberculosis is rare in association with reinfection tuberculosis, the finding of such calcification together with evidences of miliary tuberculosis should lead one to suspect an extrapulmonary source.

It is important to keep in mind the uniformity of the size of the lesions and their minuteness if other tuberculous lesions are not to be confused with miliary tuberculosis. A similar appearance may be caused by fine infiltrations in the lungs in chronic bronchitis and emphysema, pneumoconiosis, sarcoidosis, miliary carcinosis, and mi-

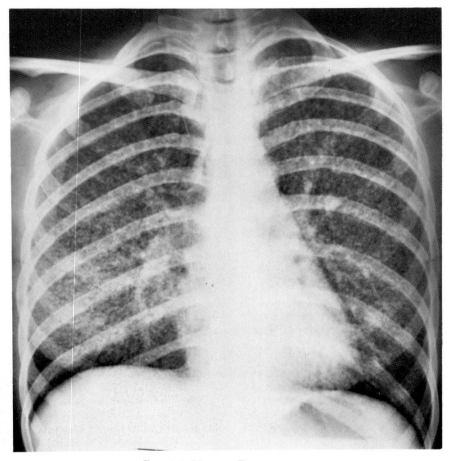

FIG. 298. MILIARY TUBERCULOSIS
The patient was admitted with evidences of meningitis. Both lungs are studded with innumerable miliary nodules. These are distributed uniformly throughout the lungs with the exception of the extreme bases. As in most cases of miliary tuberculosis, the primary lesion is not visible.

tral disease. Errors will usually be avoided if strict criteria for diagnosis are observed in accordance with the description given above. In the adult, the differentiation may be extremely difficult from the roentgen findings alone. However, the clinical history in conjunction with the roentgen findings generally leads to an accurate diagnosis.

Other Forms of Hematogenous Tuberculosis. Spread of tuberculous infection through the bloodstream may produce lesions of the lungs other than of the acute diffuse miliary variety. Where the patient's resistance is diminished, dissemination of only a few tubercle bacilli can produce significant disease. In some cases, typical miliary tubercles are formed but are limited to one or more local areas in the lung. In others, the lesions are larger (submiliary) and undergo caseation. The course of the lesions varies. Some

resolve completely, others become fibrotic and some of them progress and may undergo cavitation.

APICAL TUBERCULOSIS. For a long time the small lesions noted by the roentgenologist at the apex of the lung, and the retraction of the pleura associated with them, was thought to indicate clinically significant pulmonary tuberculosis. It is now known that these lesions, in themselves, are benign. When first seen on the film they are rarely recent, and represent a disease of minor importance which has been held in check by the natural defenses of the patient. The apical lesions usually make their appearance during adolescence and are probably the result of a sporadic hematogenous spread from caseous lymph nodes in the mediastinum. Just why the tubercle bacilli should implant themselves in the apices of the lungs is not clear. It is assumed by some, however, that the localization in the apex is the result of lymphatic spread from tuberculous lesions in the tonsil or pharynx.

In the early stages, the lesions often appear as miliary or submiliary nodules, usually bilateral, at the apex of the lung, associated with slight thickening of the overlying pleura (Fig. 299). Later the pleural thickening increases and the apical pleura is retracted as the lesions in the lung undergo fibrosis. These now appear as more or less irregular, small shadows above the clavicle. At times the lesions are large and cause irregular clouding of most of the apical region on one or both sides. They interfere with aeration of the apices. This is best detected on fluoroscopy, when the apices fail to light up during cough or deep inspiration as they do normally.

INFRACLAVICULAR LESIONS. The hematogenous lesions which appear beneath the clavicle are generally more important than the apical ones for they have a greater tendency to develop into larger foci. Not infrequently there is more or less extensive, although local, perifocal reaction, and, occasionally, cavity formation. The classical case of hematogenous infraclavicular tuberculosis is manifested radiologically by bilateral, more or less symmetrical infiltrations, situated mainly below the clavicle, often extending down to the level of the second space anteriorly. Frequently they are associated with fine tubercles in the apices.

Typical lesions consist largely of small nodules which may become more or less confluent. When they resolve the lesions may become completely absorbed although it is more common for fibrous streaks and a distortion of the vascular pattern to remain. In the case of larger tubercles, 3 to 5 mm in diameter, fibrocaseous nodules frequently persist as sharply demarcated, round shadows, some of which calcify. The final roentgen picture then consists of a number of small calcific foci in the infraclavicular regions, together with fine, irregular, fibrous streaks.

The hematogenous nature of these lesions is attested to by their not infrequent association with known extrapulmonary foci. The demonstration of calcific deposits in the spleen together with bilateral infraclavicular calcifications, in some cases, is additional evidence of the hematogenous origin of the pulmonary lesions.

The sudden appearance of the tubercles in both lungs is best explained on the basis of hematogenous spread. However, there are cases of unilateral infraclavicular tuberculosis which are undoubtedly also of hematogenous origin. These lesions can begin with the appearance of small tubercles beneath one clavicle. Soon thereafter a perifocal reaction may develop, producing a more diffuse shadow in which a cavity sometimes appears. Under such circumstances, the lesion cannot be differentiated from reinfection tuberculosis of bronchial origin. Because such cases have been observed, the opinion is held by many that the ordinary form of adult reinfection tuberculosis is endogenous in origin.

During the course of the hematogenous spread, one or more caseous tubercles on the surface of the lung may discharge bacilli into the pleura, resulting in tuberculous pleurisy. The tubercles in the lung are usually too small or too few to be visualized radiologically at the time of the pleural complication. They may be evident only when there is a perifocal reaction about a group of tubercles. This reaction is generally unilateral. If

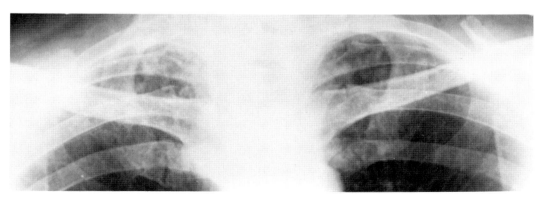

FIG. 299. BILATERAL APICAL TUBERCULOSIS

This is a remarkable case illustrating the hematogenous origin of apical tuberculosis. The patient developed diffuse miliary tuberculosis following resection of a kidney for renal tuberculosis. The miliary lesions throughout the lungs resolved spontaneously, leaving only conglomerate tubercles at each apex, casting small, irregular shadows within the circle made by the first rib and the clavicle on each side. These shadows gradually became smaller and finally disappeared after 4 years.

untreated, the patient with tuberculous pleurisy not infrequently later develops a classical picture of infraclavicular tuberculosis, simulating exogenous bronchial reinfection. This occurs in about 30% of the cases, usually within 5 years after the tuberculous pleurisy has resolved (Fig. 300).

EXTENSIVE PULMONARY DISSEMINATION. More extensive lesions in the lungs from hematogenous dissemination usually occur in cases of advanced extrapulmonary tuberculosis. In many instances the hematogenous spread involves the liver and spleen as well as the lungs.

The roentgen film is characterized by the presence of innumerable tiny nodules, somewhat larger than miliary tubercles, throughout the upper half or two-thirds of each lung (Figs. 40 &

301). The apices are involved as well as the infraclavicular regions. The lower portion of each lung may show few or no infiltrations. Characteristic of the lesions is the remarkable symmetry of their distribution. As the disease progresses, the nodules often increase considerably in size and exudation frequently takes place between them. However, this is usually not sufficient to obscure the nodules. The sputum is often negative at this stage and the disease is then easily confused with sarcoidosis.

In treated cases, rapid resolution of the process usually takes place. A distinct change for the better may be noted within a month after the onset of chemotherapy and almost complete resolution can occur within a period of 3 months.

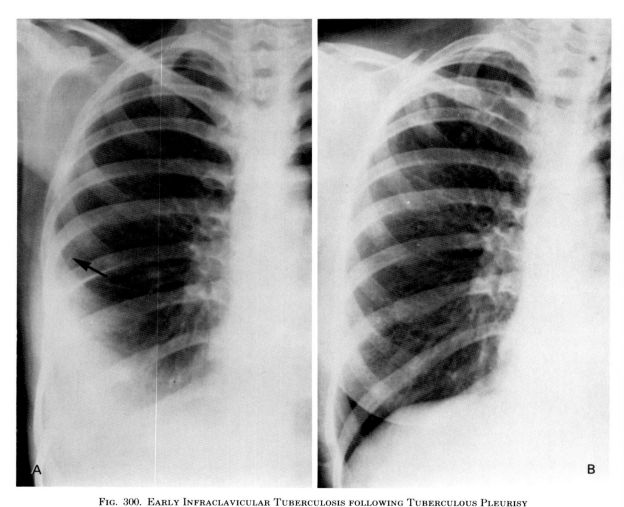

FIG. 300. EARLY INFRACLAVICULAR TUBERCULOSIS FOLLOWING TUBERCULOUS PLEURISY

A: There is a moderate-sized collection of fluid at the base of the right pleural cavity. Part of the long fissure is outlined by exudate (arrow). No lesion is visible in the lungs. The fluid resorbed without specific treatment. B: Sixteen months later. The right costophrenic sinus is clear. However, a small tuberculous lesion has appeared beneath the outer part of the clavicle. The sputum was now positive for tubercle bacilli.

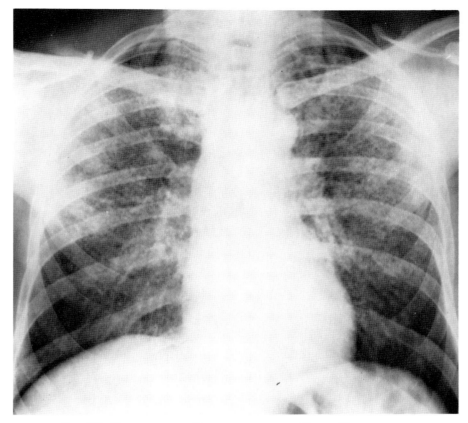

Fig. 301. Hematogenous Dissemination from Renal Tuberculosis

The upper two-thirds of both lungs are studded with miliary and submiliary tubercles. The character and distribution of the lesions and the absence of distortion of the blood vessels indicate a hematogenous spread of the disease. This sporadic dissemination is to be differentiated from acute hematogenous miliary tuberculosis in which the lungs are involved more uniformly and which runs a more acute and unfavorable course.

Most often, however, fibrous streaks and fibrocaseous nodules, some containing calcium, remain. In untreated cases, cavitation frequently occurs. The cavities often form in areas where the lesions have become confluent and the exudate has produced dense consolidation. In some cases the cavities are thick-walled and irregular. In many instances, however, perfectly round, thin-walled cavities appear in a lung which seems to be involved only by tubercles with little exudation.

Other Mycobacterial Infections

The term, pulmonary tuberculosis, is generally restricted to pulmonary disease caused by the *Mycobacterium tuberculosis* or *Mycobacterium bovis*. Other mycobacteria can cause pulmonary disease similar to tuberculosis. These infections are usually characterized by a high incidence of resistance to antituberculosis drugs and a lack of pathogenicity for guinea pigs. In addition, the organisms present cultural or morphological characteristics which differentiate them from those that are responsible for tuberculosis. These mycobacteria have been termed atypical or unclassified. However, they are divided into four groups depending on their cultural and antigenic characteristics.

Group I consists of the *Mycobacterium kansasii* (photochromogens). Group II are the scotochromogens. Group III is the Battey bacillus and Group IV consists of *Mycobacterium fortuitum* and other rapidly growing organisms. M. kansasii and the Battey bacillus are most frequently responsible for pulmonary disease. The scotochromogens and the rapid growers are less apt to cause disease. However, the former have been found in cases of lymphadenitis and the latter, on rare occasions, has been responsible for pulmonary as well as generalized disease (Fig. 302).

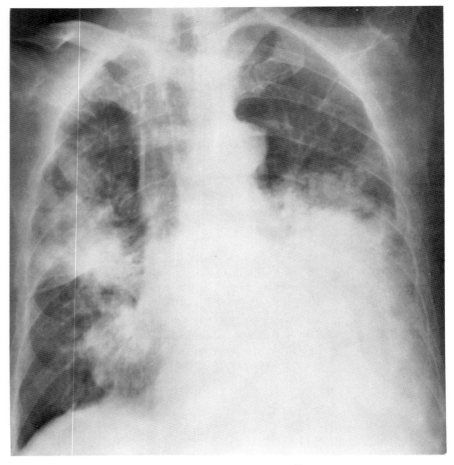

FIG. 302. *MYCOBACTERIUM FORTUITUM* PNEUMONIA

There is extensive consolidation of the lower half of the left lung, and patchy consolidation of the right lung. Culture of the sputum shows rapidly growing colonies of *M. fortuitum*. The disease progressed despite treatment with antituberculosis drugs.

Experience with the unclassified mycobacterial diseases has been insufficient to permit the formulation of any clear cut roentgen characteristics. In general, the roentgen picture cannot be differentiated from that of pulmonary tuberculosis (Fig. 303). Since the disease is not well controlled by chemotherapy, more cases of advanced chronic lesions are seen. As in tuberculosis, the lesions are predominantly in the upper lobes. Cavitation and evidence of fibrosis and contraction are common. Although chemotherapy is effective in less than a third of the cases, extensive bronchogenic spread is uncommon, and hematogenous dissemination is rare.

Thromboembolic Disease

Occlusion of a pulmonary artery, regardless of whether it is a small, peripheral branch or one of the major vessels, usually does not result in infarction because the collateral circulation of the lung is able to maintain adequate blood flow to the affected region. The blood supply of the lung is derived from two sources: the pulmonary artery which carries blood from the right side of the heart, and the bronchial arteries which arise from the descending aorta. There are numerous anastomoses between the two systems although most of them are not functional under normal circumstances. In addition, there is an extensive cross circulation between the smaller pulmonary arterial branches. The latter provide most of the collateral blood flow when peripheral pulmonary vessels are occluded by emboli while the bronchial arteries are of prime importance in occlusion of the central pulmonary arteries.

The fate of individual vessels occluded by blood clot varies. In some, the embolus is fragmented and eventually absorbed, while in others, the clot is canalized so that some degree of direct

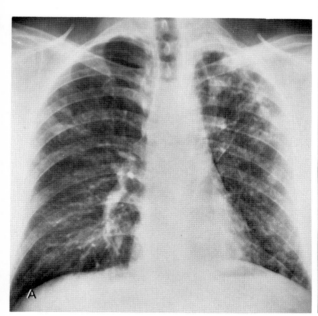
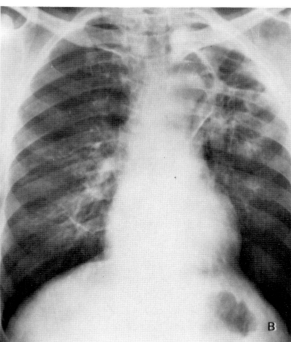

FIG. 303. ATYPICAL MYCOBACTERIAL INFECTIONS

A: Mycobacterium kansasii. There is extensive fibrosis throughout the left lung with cavitation and bulla formation in the upper lobe. Fine and coarse infiltrations and fibrosis are present throughout the lower lobe. A relatively small area of infiltration is present in the outer portion of the right upper lobe representing a spillover infection. Culture disclosed *M. kansasii.* *B: Mycobacterium avium-intracellulare* (Battey bacillus). The upper lobe is the seat of extensive fibrosis, cavitation and bulla formation. Shrinkage of the lobe has caused flattening of the dome of the hemithorax and elevation of the left lower lobe. Infiltrations are also present in the superior segment of the left lower lobe. There is recent infiltration in the upper part of the right lower lobe. Both leaves of the diaphragm are depressed as a result of emphysema. Culture of the sputum disclosed the Battey bacillus. (Courtesy of Dr. M. Ziskind, New Orleans, La.)

blood flow is reestablished. The thrombus in the remaining vessels becomes organized and the arteries may be permanently obliterated by the proliferating fibrous tissue. Thus, although a single shower of peripheral emboli rarely produces persistent impairment of lung function, the effects of multiple episodes are cumulative.

When the collateral circulation of the lung is inadequate because of preexisting pulmonary disease or congestive failure, the temporary ischemia of the portion of lung supplied by the occluded vessel may be severe enough to result in damage to the capillary bed. As collateral blood flow of the area increases, the weakened capillary walls may rupture and the alveoli become inundated with blood and edema fluid. Since there is no destruction of lung tissue associated with this pulmonary hemorrhage, the changes are completely reversible.

Infarction, which implies the death of lung tissue, is uncommon. Although it is not possible to accurately determine its incidence, the commonly accepted estimate is that infarction occurs in 10 to 15% of cases of thromboembolism. Infarcts occur more often in patients with congestive failure or pulmonary disease and are rare in young persons with normal lungs unless there are complicating factors such as immobilization in a cast or prolonged bed rest.

Pulmonary Embolization without Infarction

Because clotted blood has the same radiodensity as normal blood, a pulmonary embolus cannot be visualized with standard x-ray techniques. However, when the density of the blood is increased by the injection of contrast material, the embolus can often be recognized as a lucent filling defect within the opacified vessel. When the artery is completely occluded by the embolus, only the proximal margin of the clot can be identified, at the point where it causes an abrupt amputation of the contrast column in the vessel.

Except when the clot can be identified by angiography, the diagnosis of pulmonary embolization depends on demonstration of irregularities in local blood supply or changes in the lungs and pleura that develop secondary to the vascular occlusion. The isotope perfusion scan is the simplest and most accurate technique for detecting abnormalities in regional pulmonary blood flow. However, in an appreciable number of cases, standard films of the chest provide the first indication of thromboembolic disease. In addition, they are extremely useful in conjunction with the lung scan to detect false positive results.

Major Pulmonary Artery Emboli. The most striking feature of embolization of one or both pulmonary arteries is the disparity between the often catastrophic clinical picture and the benign roentgen appearance of the chest. Interruption of blood flow through a pulmonary artery results in oligemia of the affected lung. The vessels beyond the occlusion decrease in size, causing an increase in the radiolucency of the involved pulmonary field (Fig. 304). The significance of this appearance as an indication of a major pulmonary embolus was first described by Westermark. Not uncommonly, however, even where there is a significant decrease in pulmonary vascularity, the difference in density between the normal and abnormal lung is slight and is easily overlooked on films of less than optimal quality. In other cases, this sign is com-

pletely absent although the embolus occludes a major pulmonary artery. On the other hand, when one lung or part of a lung appears oligemic and a major pulmonary embolus is suspected clinically, the presence of increased lucency does not confirm the diagnosis with certainty unless previous films are available to show that the local hypovascularity is not the result of pulmonary or vascular disease.

Although a major pulmonary embolus can cause a precipitous rise in central pulmonary artery pressure, the hilar vessels usually do not dilate during the acute phase. Enlargement of these vessels when it does occur, is a late manifestation and is generally caused by increase in the size of the obstructing thrombus (Fig. 305).

Perfusion scans of the lung are always positive when an embolus lodges in a main pulmonary artery. However, the study is not specific for pulmonary embolism because a similar picture can be produced by any unilateral pulmonary disease that increases vascular resistance and causes a redistribution of pulmonary blood flow. Angiography is the most accurate method for establishing the diagnosis of an embolus in a main pulmonary artery. Although injection of contrast material into a peripheral vein or the right atrium may suffice to demonstrate the embolus in some cases, selective pulmonary arteri-

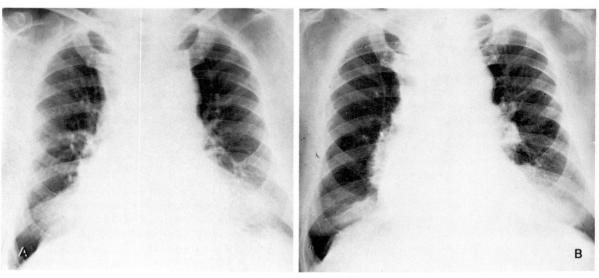

FIG. 304. MAJOR PULMONARY ARTERY EMBOLUS

A: This film was made shortly after the onset of severe tachypnea and chest pain. The heart is somewhat enlarged but the pulmonary vasculature appears normal. There is no difference in the vascularity of the two lungs. The hazy shadow at the base of each lung is caused by a pendulous male breast. Angiography at this time revealed a large pulmonary embolus which extended from the right to the left main pulmonary artery. Despite the marked decrease of blood flow to each lung, the patient responded to medical management. *B*: Five months later the patient is asymptomatic. At this time, however, there is marked decrease in the vascularity of the right lung. Presumably the right pulmonary artery is permanently occluded and the blood supply to the lung is derived mainly from the bronchial arteries.

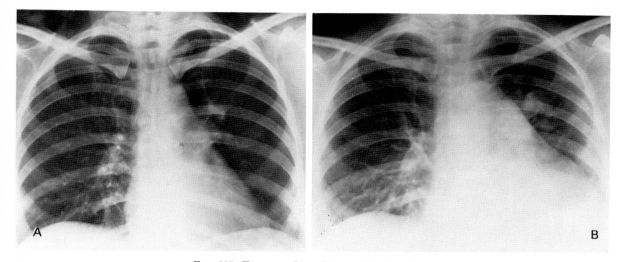

FIG. 305. EMBOLUS, LEFT PULMONARY ARTERY

A: Two weeks after occlusion of the left pulmonary artery by an embolus, the left lung appears lucent. This is due to a marked decrease in blood flow to that site. *B*: Six months later, the left diaphragm is elevated and the heart is displaced to the left as a result of shrinkage of the left lung. Presumably this occurred because adequate blood flow was not reestablished. The main arteries to both lobes are markedly dilated as a result of increase in size of the obstructing thrombus by accretion.

ography provides much better visualization of the vessels and is the method of choice. The right pulmonary artery is best studied in the frontal projection. The left pulmonary artery, which courses almost directly backward, is foreshortened in this view and often is not seen in its entirety. The vessel can be seen with the least distortion in the right posterior oblique projection.

Peripheral Pulmonary Emboli. Small pulmonary emboli occur in showers and produce obstruction of multiple peripheral pulmonary arterial branches. They frequently are scattered throughout the lungs but the majority occur in the lower lobes. Like major pulmonary emboli, blood clots in the peripheral arteries cause oligemia of the affected portions of the lung. However, these areas are small and the increase in their radiolucency is too slight to produce a recognizable change in the appearance of the lungs on standard films. Rarely, after multiple thromboembolic episodes, the outer portions of both lungs show a distinct decrease in vascularity. These cases are usually associated with a significant increase in central pulmonary pressure, dilatation of the main pulmonary arteries at the hilum and evidences of chronic cor pulmonale (Fig. 306). It has been estimated that more than 70% of the pulmonary arterioles must be obliterated before the resistance in the vascular bed is sufficiently elevated to produce pulmonary hypertension.

The most common roentgen manifestation of

a peripheral embolus is one or more Fleischner lines resulting from atelectasis of a pulmonary subsegment. The local ischemia beyond an obstructive arterial branch causes an impairment in the transfer of gases across the alveolar membrane and results in a change in the composition of the expired air in the regional bronchi. This can initiate a reflex spasm in the bronchus. The bronchospasm is accentuated because of histamine and serotonin released from platelets damaged in the process of clot formation. The sudden interruption of blood supply also results in congestion and edema of the bronchial mucosa. Lastly, there is a tendency for secretion to stagnate in the bronchi, particularly in the lower lobes, because of splinting of the chest and decrease in respiratory motion. These are related to the pleuritic pain usually associated with embolization. All of these factors contribute to produce obstruction of small bronchi which, together with local impairment of collateral air drift and a decreased production of surfactant, results in subsegmental atelectasis.

The Fleischner line is not a specific sign of a pulmonary embolus. The lines can be seen in many pulmonary diseases and indicate nothing more than atelectasis of peripheral areas of the lung. However, if simultaneous occurrence of Fleischner lines in both lungs is considered, the list of differential diagnoses becomes much smaller. The conditions that can produce bilateral Fleischner lines without any other roentgen sign of pulmonary disease are still fewer. This

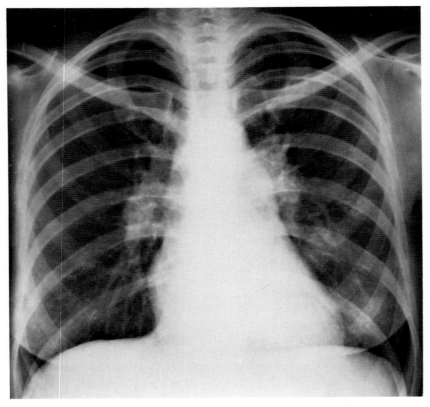

FIG. 306. PULMONARY HYPERTENSION RESULTING FROM REPEATED EMBOLIZATION

The hilar vessels are markedly dilated and the peripheral vessels constricted. The change in caliber of the pulmonary arteries occurs abruptly near the root of the lung. The picture is that of pulmonary hypertension. The electrocardiogram showed marked right ventricular hypertrophy.

can occur in association with asthma or fibrinous bronchitis and is fairly common in patients who do not move their diaphragms well, e.g., patients who are bedridden or those with peritoneal irritation from any cause. The reason for the atelectatic streaks in these cases is clearly indicated by the clinical history. Once these conditions are excluded, the presence of bilateral Fleischner lines can be considered as presumptive evidence of pulmonary embolization.

When a pulmonary subsegment collapses, it retracts from the surface and pulls in a double layer of visceral pleura, in essence, forming a new fissure in the lung. The Fleischner line is produced when this fissure is projected on end. If it is viewed obliquely or *en face,* the line will not be visible. A single film of the chest, therefore, is not adequate for the detection of many of these lines. In addition, because many of the atelectatic streaks involve the basal portions of the lungs, they are obscured on the frontal film by the diaphragm. For these reasons, when peripheral pulmonary emboli are suspected, oblique and

lateral films should also be obtained. In some instances, Fleischner lines at the bases are best seen through the shadows of the liver or spleen on abdominal films.

Peripheral emboli are often associated with a pleural effusion of small or moderate size. This probably reflects pleural irritation caused by subpleural infarcts that are not large enough to cast an identifiable shadow. Such infarcts are almost certainly the cause of many of the left-sided pleural effusions in congestive heart failure.

In some cases the roentgen picture produced by the effusion is fairly specific. Irritation of the pleura within a fissure can cause a local accumulation of fluid between two lobes of the lung. Interlobar effusions are usually associated with congestive failure. The increase in pulmonary venous pressure in this condition, results in a generalized weeping of all pleural surfaces. Loculation of fluid within a fissure results when there are adhesions around the periphery of the fissure, sealing it off from the general pleural cavity. Collection of fluid in only one of the fissures in the right lung indicates that the other fissure is obliterated by adhesions. The fissure is, therefore, thickened and can be visualized when viewed in the appropriate projection. An interlobar effusion on the right side without visible thickening of the other fissure signifies a local cause for the effusion, in most instances, a pulmonary embolus. A pleural effusion, even though small, on one side, in association with Fleischner lines in the opposite lung, has the same significance as bilateral Fleischner lines (Fig. 307).

The perfusion lung scan is the most sensitive method for the detection of peripheral pulmonary emboli. Occlusion of an artery causes a perfusion defect whose location and shape are consistent with the subsegmental anatomy of the lungs. However, defects in perfusion can also be produced by any disease of the heart or lungs that affects regional pulmonary ventilation in an irregular fashion, e.g., bronchopneumonia, pulmonary fibrosis, and congestive failure. These can be excluded if a chest film is obtained at the time of the scan or if a ventilation scan is also performed.

Angiography is of more limited usefulness and practicality in the diagnosis of peripheral emboli than of major embolus. The peripheral pulmonary arteries are so numerous that even with a selective injection of contrast material into the main pulmonary artery, it is difficult to separate the overlapping shadows enough to disclose occlusion of one or more small branches. The accuracy of the angiogram can be considerably increased if the branch arteries that supply the underperfused areas identified by scanning are superselectively catheterized, especially if the study is filmed with magnification techniques.

Pulmonary Infarction

Acute Phase. The characteristic roentgen picture of a pulmonary infarct is that of an area of consolidation whose shadow represents the densities of the alveoli filled with blood and edema fluid and the necrotic lung. If most of the alveoli are airless, the shadow is homogeneous whereas if there is patchy involvement of groups of alveoli, the shadow appears mottled. In either case, an air bronchogram is often apparent because the bronchi in the region are patent. When the bronchi become obstructed by clotted blood or retained secretion an air bronchogram is not seen. However, atelectasis is usually not a prominent feature in the early stages because the fluid filling the alveoli keeps them distended.

An infarct always involves an anatomic divi-

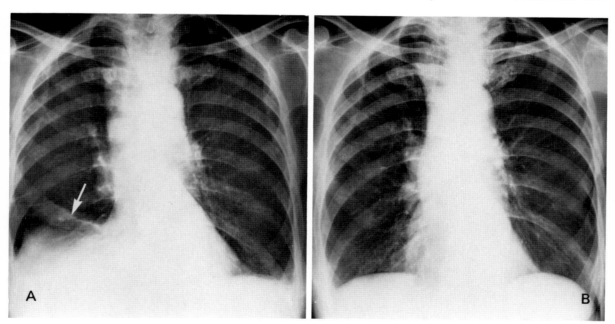

FIG. 307. ACUTE PULMONARY EMBOLIZATION

A: A film made soon after the onset of chest pain and dyspnea shows a small pleural effusion blunting the left costophrenic sinus and a broad Fleischner line (arrow) at the right base. The right leaf of the diaphragm is elevated because of splinting of the chest and basal atelectasis. The tented appearance of the outer portion of the diaphragm is caused by pleural retraction secondary to atelectasis of the adjacent pulmonary segment. *B*: Four months later the chest is clear and the evidences of subsegmental atelectasis have disappeared. The diaphragm now has a normal contour.

sion of the lung, one or more pulmonary lobules or as much as an entire segment. However, even when the lung is viewed in multiple projections, it is extremely rare to see a triangular shadow that corresponds to the shape of a pulmonary subdivision because the apical portion of the involved lung, which is nearest the hilum, is usually protected by collateral blood flow and does not become infarcted.

Infarcts can occur in any portion of the lung but are much more common in the lower lobes. Infarction of the outer portion of the anterior or lateral basal segment often produces a rather characteristic roentgen picture. The shadow of

the consolidated lung fills the lateral costophrenic sinus and presents a convex border directed toward the lung root, "Hampton's hump" (Fig. 308).

Almost without exception, infarcts extend to the visceral pleura. If viewed in the appropriate projection, the shadow of an infarct can be shown to abut on the parietes, the mediastinum, the diaphragm or an interlobar fissure. The pleura over the infarct is always inflamed and covered with fibrin. The layer of exudate causes considerable thickening of the pleura but this may be difficult to appreciate on the chest film unless it causes blunting or obliteration of a costophrenic

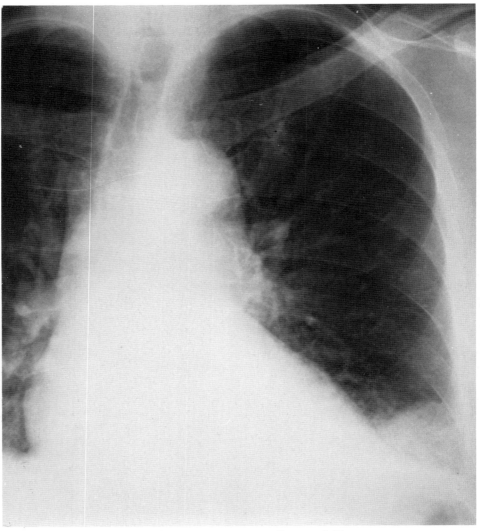

FIG. 308. PULMONARY INFARCT: HAMPTON'S HUMP

The homogeneous shadow in the left costophrenic sinus has a well-defined convex border that is directed toward the lung root. This was an 81 year old man with chronic heart disease who suffered a pulmonary infarction 2 weeks previously. Partial resolution of the infarct accounts for its sharp margination.

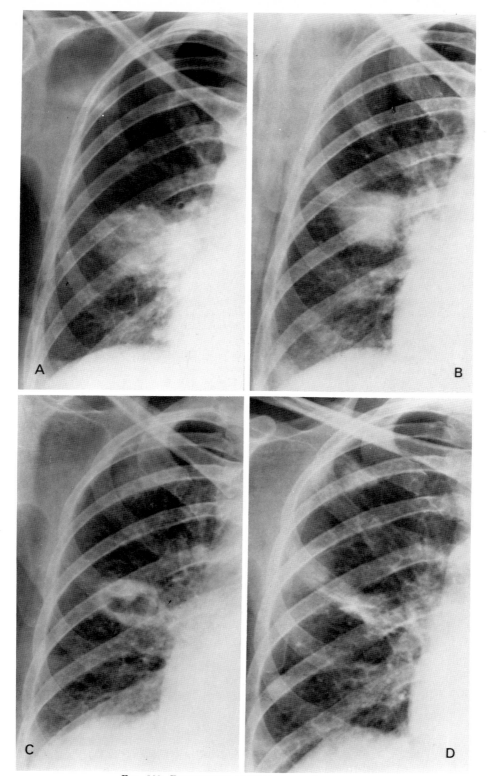

FIG. 309. RESOLUTION OF PULMONARY INFARCT

A: Sept. 15. The film made shortly after the onset of chest pain and hemoptysis shows a poorly defined area of consolidation in the midportion of the right lung. *B*: Sept. 22. The infarct has diminished in size and is more sharply demarcated. The short fissure crosses the shadow, indicating that the lesion is situated in the superior segment of the lower lobe. *C*: Oct. 7. The infarct has continued to shrink and has undergone cavitation. There was no fever or purulent expectoration indicating the absence of secondary infection of the infarct. The cavity is thick-walled, and on the single film cannot be differentiated from a broken-down neoplasm. A new area of consolidation has appeared beneath the outer part of the right clavicle. This was due to a second infarct. *D*: Oct. 30. The cavity has disappeared, leaving little more than a fibrous scar. The new infarct has shrunken and has partially resolved.

sinus, or thickening of an interlobar fissure. A pleural effusion is commonly associated with a pulmonary infarct. The fluid may be loculated by adhesions or lie free in the pleural space. In either case, there is nothing specific in the appearance of the effusion to indicate the underlying cause. However, the association of an effusion with an area of pulmonary consolidation should suggest the possibility of an infarct. An infarct in the lower lobe is often obscured by the pleural effusion.

Resolution. A pulmonary infarct resolves rather slowly and usually requires 3 to 5 weeks for complete clearing. The greatest change in the appearance of the infarct occurs in the first week or two during which time a goodly portion of the blood and edema fluid in the alveoli is absorbed. Healing of the necrotic lung occurs by fibrosis, which begins in the periphery. As the infarct matures, it becomes smaller and more sharply defined (Fig. 309). Many infarcts, even when large, heal without leaving any abnormality that can be detected on films of the chest (Fig. 310). In others, one or more fibrous scars remain after resolution.

Cavitation of an infarct usually indicates the presence of infection, either because the original embolus was septic in nature, or because of secondary invaders. However, a bland infarct can cavitate (Fig. 309). The two cannot be distinguished from their radiologic appearances. Once a communication with a bronchus is established, an air-fluid level may appear. Irregularities in this level or excrescences on the inner wall of the cavity can be caused by sloughing of the necrotic tissue of the infarct. Distinction from a neoplasm may be difficult but the infarct changes in appearance within a relatively short time, while the shadow of a carcinomatous abscess is more stable. The walls of the excavated infarct may become very thin as the necrotic lung is shelled out and expectorated. In some instances, the cavity ruptures through the pleura and can produce a bronchopleural fistula possibly with a tension pneumothorax. Bland, cavitary infarcts that are not secondarily infected undergo resolution in the same way as any other infarcts.

In rare instances, the necrotic tissue of an infarct is not liquefied or expectorated but undergoes calcification (Fig. 139).

Roentgen Diagnosis. The shadow of a pulmonary infarct is often identical to that of an area of consolidated pneumonia. However, a pleural effusion is a more common accompaniment of an infarct. The pleural reaction to an infarct is exceptionally severe and is accompanied by the exudation of a large amount of fibrin. Reflex elevation of the diaphragm occurs early

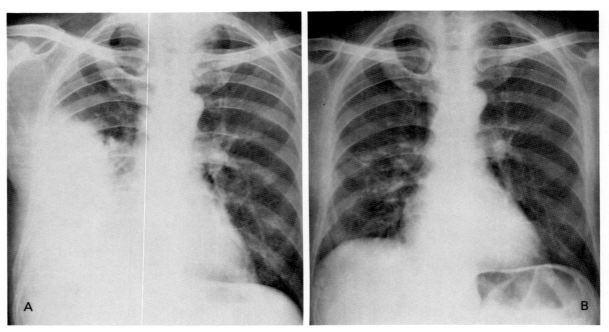

FIG. 310. PULMONARY INFARCT

A: The film was made soon after the onset of severe chest pain and hemoptysis. The area of opacification in the right lung represents a huge infarct together with fluid in the pleural cavity. *B*: A film made 6 months later shows complete resolution of the infarct. The only indication of previous disease is the presence of a few fine fibrous scars.

and its peripheral portion soon becomes adherent to the chest wall. A "hung up" diaphragm occurring soon after the appearance of a shadow in the lung strongly favors the diagnosis of infarction. Fleischner lines or a pleural effusion on the opposite side are presumptive evidence of pulmonary embolization.

Multiple infarcts can produce an appearance similar to that of pulmonary edema. This is especially confusing because both conditions are particularly common in cardiac patients. However, edema tends to involve the central portions of the lung and does not invariably extend to a pleural surface. In addition, the pattern of lung involvement by pulmonary edema tends to change from day to day.

The roentgen picture of pulmonary hemorrhage secondary to occlusion of an artery, is the same as that of an infarct except that the hemorrhagic area never undergoes cavitation. Distinction between the two depends on the rate of healing. A pulmonary hemorrhage clears completely within a week to 10 days and leaves no residual shadow while resolution of an infarct is considerably slower and may leave a scar. From a practical standpoint, the differentiation is not of much importance since both lesions are the result of pulmonary thromboembolic disease and this is the condition that requires treatment.

Emphysema

Emphysema has been defined by the Committee on Diagnostic Standards of the American Thoracic Society as an anatomic alteration of the lung characterized by abnormal enlargement of the air spaces distal to the terminal nonrespiratory bronchiole, accompanied by destructive changes of the alveolar walls. This definition is generally accepted. It serves to differentiate emphysema from simple hyperinflation of the lungs in which most of the alveolar walls are intact. Emphysema, as a pathologic entity, occurs in a diffuse and a local form. The clinical disease entity, emphysema, refers to the diffuse form.

Diffuse Emphysema

The diffuse form of emphysema involves all segments of the lungs. The cause is not entirely clear. Most cases are associated with chronic bronchitis, but since emphysema can occur without evidence of bronchitis, and since the majority of chronic bronchitics do not develop emphysema, other factors must be involved. An intrinsic weakness in the walls of the alveoli is probably important in the pathogenesis. In some instances this appears to be related to a deficiency of alpha$_1$ antitrypsin.

In most cases of emphysema, there is clinical evidence of obstruction to the expulsion of air from the lungs. Microscopic studies have shown occlusion of bronchioles by mucous plugs and by inflammation of their walls. Many of the bronchioles are permanently strictured. It has been postulated that air enters the alveoli distal to the obstructed bronchiole by means of collateral respiration. Interference with emptying of the alveoli during expiration causes them to distend. Weakening and inflammation of the alveolar walls from viral or bacterial infections, or intrinsic factors as yet unknown, then leads to destruction of portions of the alveolar septa which results in the formation of large confluent air spaces.

Disruption of the elastic tissue in the lung, which normally supports the smaller bronchiolar radicles, permits these air channels to be compressed by the adjacent distended alveoli during expiration. The narrowing of the bronchioles acts as a check valve and leads to further dilatation of the alveoli and disruption of their walls. Narrowing of small- and medium-sized bronchi from external pressure during coughing, when the intraalveolar pressure is markedly increased, contributes to progression of the disease.

Because of the diffuse nature of the process and the importance of the obstructive element, the disease has been termed, diffuse obstructive emphysema. Since it is irreversible, it is also called chronic obstructive pulmonary disease (COPD). It occurs in two forms, panlobular and centrilobular, which present different pathologic, clinical and roentgen pictures. In some cases, a mixture of the two is present.

Panlobular (Panacinar) Emphysema. This is the common variety of diffuse obstructive emphysema. It involves acini indiscriminately throughout the secondary pulmonary lobule, which is the smallest unit of lung bounded by connective tissue. The secondary lobules appear on the surface of the inflated, excised lung in the form of polyhedral areas measuring from 1 to 2 cm in diameter, sharply demarcated by fibrous connective tissue. They are particularly well outlined when the lymphatics of the interlobular septa are distended either by fluid in heart failure or by neoplastic cells in lymphangitic carcinosis. Each secondary lobule is supplied by a lobular bronchiole which divides into several intralobular branches that lead to the acini. In view of the distribution of the emphysema, it seems likely that obstruction of the terminal bronchiole supplying the acinus plays a part in the production of the disease.

The roentgen picture in the early stage varies. The lungs may appear entirely normal, even when the disease is moderately advanced. On the other hand, rather extensive roentgen changes may be present when the patient is relatively asymptomatic and shows few, if any, abnormal physical findings. The earliest changes often are simply a slight diminution in the excursion of the diaphragm and a tendency to flattening of this organ, related, in part, to an increase in the diameter of the chest. This may be evident only on the lateral view because the increase in size of the chest is proportionately greater in the anteroposterior direction than from side to side. In some cases, the enlargement of the anteroposterior diameter of the chest is not evident on physical examination but the lateral chest film will disclose an increase in the depth and lucency of retrosternal and retrocardiac spaces.

The changes become more marked as the disease progresses. The diaphragm, which at first appears flattened only in the lateral view, loses its normal curve in the frontal projection as well. The diaphragm is also depressed and its respi-ratory excursion increasingly diminished. The limitation of motion of the diaphragm usually mirrors the degree of disability. Eventually, the curve of the diaphragm disappears entirely and is replaced by a straight line which pursues an oblique course downward and outward from the mediastinum (Fig. 311). At its periphery, inter-digitations of the diaphragmatic musculature may be evident where it meets the chest wall.

As the lungs enlarge, the anterior lappets of the upper lobes insinuate themselves behind the sternum, displacing the mediastinal structures posteriorly. This is the cause for the widening and hyperlucency of the retrosternal space on the lateral view. It may be associated with an-gulation of the manubrium with the body of the sternum. In advanced cases, as the anterior lap-pets of the lungs become more distended, they extend further down and may completely sepa-rate the heart from the anterior chest wall.

Enlargement of the thoracic cavity is accomplished, in part, by elevation of the anterior portions of the ribs, causing widening of the intercostal spaces. In extreme cases, the aerated lung bulges into the intercostal spaces. This is seen especially in children and is best detected

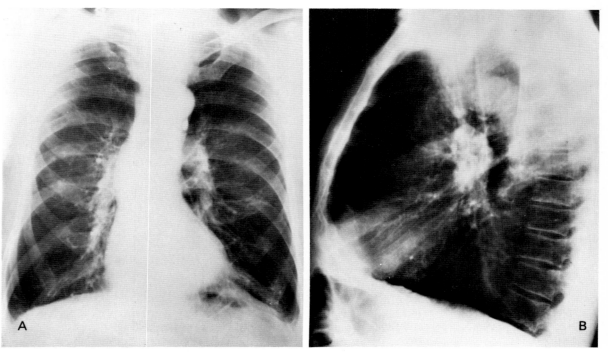

FIG. 311. PANACINAR EMPHYSEMA

A: Frontal view. The lungs are hyperlucent and the diaphragms are low and flattened. The peripheral pulmonary vessels are thinned and spread apart. The process is diffuse and no individual bullae can be identified. *B*: Lateral view. The anteroposterior diameter of the chest is considerably increased with marked widening of the retrosternal and retrocardiac spaces. The flattening of the diaphragm is more obvious than on the frontal view.

in the oblique projections. In many cases, dorsal kyphosis develops, further increasing the antero-posterior diameter of the chest.

As the diaphragm descends, the cardiac axis becomes more vertical and the heart more centrally placed. This, together with some increase in the transverse diameter of the chest, makes the heart appear smaller than normal on the frontal projection. Actually, the heart may diminish in size because of the decrease in systemic venous return caused by pressure of the overdistended lungs on the veins leading to the right side of the heart. In some cases, the outer part of the inferior surface of the heart is exposed because of the low position of the diaphragm. In the normal chest, the transverse diameter of the heart increases as the diaphragm rises during expiration. This no longer occurs in advanced emphysema because the movement of the diaphragm is so limited.

With proper exposure of the film, the pulmonary vessels are sharply outlined by contrast with the adjacent hyperaerated, hyperlucent lung. However, when there are peribronchial and interstitial infiltrations, resulting from repeated infections, the outlines of the vessels are not so clearly delineated. Normally, the pulmonary vessels fan out during inspiration and move together in expiration. When the lung is emphysematous and the diaphragmatic excursion limited, the vessels tend to remain splayed throughout both phases of respiration. In addition, the caliber of the vessels in the peripheral parts of the lungs is diminished because they are compressed by the distended alveoli surrounding them. This is a prominent feature in the later stages of emphysema but may also be noted in early cases. When the disease is advanced and the obstruction to blood flow through the lungs is significant, the central pulmonary arteries become dilated. Characteristically, there is then an abrupt change in the caliber of the arteries at the junction of the central and lateral two-thirds of the lungs (Fig. 119) and no vascular markings at all may be visible in the outer third of the chest. This is a common finding when the pressure in the pulmonary arteries is elevated and is associated with chronic cor pulmonale. The peripheral vessels become more prominent and nearer their normal size if the patient coincidentally develops left heart failure. The picture then differs from that of right heart failure associated with cor pulmonale because of the absence of the marked disparity in size between the central vessels and the peripheral ones.

Increased lucency of the pulmonary field is characteristic of this form of emphysema. However, the degree of lucency of the lungs is difficult to judge because it can be considerably affected by variations in filming technique. In simple hyperinflation, the overdistension of alveoli almost always involves only one lung or part of a lung so that the lucency of the normal lung is available for comparison. This is not the case in generalized emphysema when, as a rule, both lungs are more or less uniformly and diffusely involved. The hyperlucency is more easily appreciated when the parasternal or lower portions of the lung are inordinately overdistended.

Most films of emphysematous patients are too dark because they are overexposed. This results from the tendency to judge exposure solely from the measurement of the chest, which assumes that the increased diameter is due only to increased thickness of the chest wall. However, the chest wall is often thin in these patients, particularly in the advanced stages of the disease, because of wasting of the thoracic musculature.

Overexposure of the film obscures the pattern of the peripheral vessels and wipes away the density contributed by the ground substance of the lung. This can be compensated for by viewing the film with a strong light. The vessels in the middle third of the pulmonary field then appear thin, straight and sharply demarcated against the abnormally clear, adjacent lung. Even with the bright light, the finely stippled appearance of the outer third of the lungs, normally contributed by the multiplicity of fine peripheral vessels, is diminished or absent in advanced emphysema.

Films made in each phase of respiration provide a record of the diminished motion of the diaphragm, the lessened clouding of the lung during expiration and the persistent splaying of the blood vessels. These changes can be more accurately evaluated by fluoroscopy, partly because many patients fail to use their diaphragm to the best of their ability unless their breathing is watched and deficiencies in the use of the diaphragm are corrected by instruction.

Difficulty in roentgen diagnosis of emphysema is experienced in patients with naturally long, thin chests and low diaphragms. Such patients, particularly those with a sunken sternum, often show an angulation between the body and manubrium of the sternum which causes an increase in the depth of the retrosternal space. The heart, which is oriented vertically and tends to be centrally placed, appears small. All of these findings combined with a tendency to overexposure of the films because of the poor development of the musculature of the chest wall, leads to a suspicion of emphysema. However, the diaphragm is not flattened and its motion is not limited and the pulmonary vascular markings which may appear splayed on inspiration, approach each other normally on expiration as the diaphragm rises. When such a patient develops emphysema, the diagnosis may be quite difficult. It depends largely on observation of flattening of the diaphragm and limitation of its motion, and thinning of the peripheral vessels. This is best appreciated by comparison with previous films.

Centrilobular Emphysema. In centrilobular emphysema, the lesions are located primarily in the central part of the secondary lobule although here and there, the periphery of the lobule may also be involved. The disease affects respiratory bronchioles of the second and third order. The walls of these bronchioles are partially destroyed so that contiguous bronchioles may communicate with each other.

The underlying cause is a generalized bronchitis which involves both the bronchi and bronchioles. Cigarette smoking is probably the most common cause of the bronchitis. It can also result from viral or bacterial infections or exposure to irritating gases. In any case, aeration of the central portion of the lobule is interfered with because of narrowing or obstruction of the terminal bronchiole by plugs of mucous and exudate, inflammatory infiltration and stricture formation. Air enters the central portion of the lobule by collateral respiration and its exit is impeded by the obstructed terminal bronchiole. The accumulation of air, which is under increased pressure during coughing, causes overdistension of the bronchioles whose walls are weakened and partly destroyed. The alveolar ducts and alveoli are spared and surround the large air spaces which represent the ectatic and confluent bronchioles. The disease is usually widespread throughout the lungs but its distribution, in contrast to panlobular emphysema, is more patchy and spares many of the lobules.

In the early stage, no abnormality is visible on films. Since most of the alveoli of the secondary lobule are not affected, there is little enlargement of the lungs. The diaphragms are not flattened and their excursion is not limited. The peripheral blood vessels are normal in caliber and the vascular pattern is generally prominent. The vessels may appear somewhat irregular and poorly outlined as a result of inflammation and thickening of the peribronchial and interstitial tissues surrounding them.

Evidences of pulmonary arterial hypertension appear more commonly than in the panlobular form. The main pulmonary arteries of the lung roots are dilated and the outflow tract of the right ventricle becomes prominent. Although the right ventricle is hypertrophied, enlargement of the cardiac shadow is usually absent or minimal until right heart failure supervenes and causes dilatation of the right atrium.

Mixed Form. Centrilobular emphysema may be associated with a variable degree of panlobular involvement. It is uncertain whether the two conditions are concomitant or whether the disease in the periphery of the lobules follows and represents an advanced stage of centrilobular emphysema. As the disease progresses, the roentgen findings typical of panlobular emphysema become predominant. However, the tendency to pulmonary hypertension and cor pulmonale remains as in the uncomplicated centrilobular form.

Bullous Emphysema

It is unlikely that bullous emphysema represents a specific disease entity. Rather, it seems to be simply a relatively severe form of generalized emphysema. Bullous changes are common in advanced cases of panlobular emphysema although they are unusual in uncomplicated cases of the centrilobular form.

Bullae associated with emphysema tend to be multiple and scattered throughout the lungs. Smaller ones, 1 to 2 cm in diameter, are almost impossible to identify on conventional films. Even larger ones, particularly those situated in the periphery of the pulmonary field, may be difficult to detect because of the hyperlucency of the surrounding emphysematous lung. Thin, streak-like or angular hairline shadows representing the walls of the bullae can be seen when the bullae are adjacent to one another. Tenting of the diaphragm in a patient with generalized emphysema indicates the presence of bullae at the lung bases (see Fig. 322). The tenting is due to invagination of the pleura between the air cysts and may be the only roentgen sign of their presence.

Bullae, whether associated with emphysema or occurring in an otherwise normal lung, can grow large enough to interfere with respiration. Identification of those cases associated with generalized emphysema is extremely important in determining proper therapy. Resection of bullae that represent isolated abnormalities often results in marked improvement in pulmonary function as the remaining lung is no longer compressed. On the other hand, if the lung is emphysematous, the further distention of the already overexpanded lung to fill the space created by the removal of the bullae may cause the dyspnea to become worse.

Recognition of the presence of generalized emphysema may be difficult in the presence of multiple large bullae. When there are no bullae in the lower lobes, flattening of the diaphragm is indicative of generalized emphysema (Fig. 312). However, the converse is not true, and significant emphysema may be present even though the diaphragm has a normally rounded contour. Tomography may be helpful in disclosing the topography of the bullae and in demonstrating the vascular pattern in the remainder of the lung. When the lung is emphysematous, the vessels at a distance from the bullae will appear narrowed and stretched and splayed. In some cases, the findings on tomography are equivocal and pulmonary angiography provides more definitive information.

Local Emphysema

Chronic obstructive disease, although generalized, may not involve all parts of the lungs with equal severity. Thus, obvious roentgen evidence of emphysema may be seen in scattered parts of the lungs while the remainder appear normal. Similarly, bullae which represent local accentuation of the emphysematous process, may develop in only one region while moderately advanced emphysema in the rest of the lungs is not evident on films. In some instances, however, the emphysema is confined to only one part of the lung and there truly is no disease in the remainder.

Unilateral Emphysema of Swyer, James and Macleod. This is a form of obstructive emphysema usually confined to one lung. It is most probably the end result of a severe pneumonia and bronchiolitis in childhood with scattered areas of lung destruction, and obliteration and distortion of many of the small bronchial branches. Often, the growth and development of the affected lung fails to keep pace with the healthy one so that years later the abnormal lung appears small and hypoplastic (Fig. 273). The ultimate size of the lung is probably determined

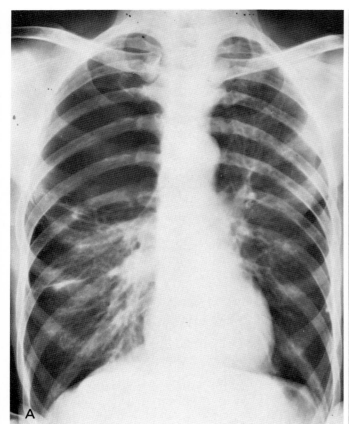
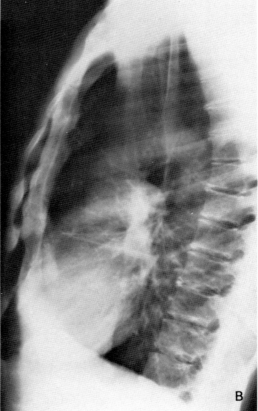

FIG. 312. BULLOUS EMPHYSEMA

A: Frontal view. Only a single large bulla is seen in the right upper lobe compressing the lower part of the lung. However, both leaves of the diaphragm are depressed and the lateral portions of the lower lobes show diminished vascularity indicating diffuse emphysema. *B*: Lateral view. The diaphragms are flattened as well as depressed. In the absence of basal bullae, these changes signify the presence of generalized emphysema.

not only by the severity and extent of the original infection but also by the age of the patient at the time of the pneumonia. The emphysema is a direct result of the bronchial obstructions and air which enters the alveoli by collateral air drift through the pores of Kohn cannot be completely expelled.

The involved lung appears hyperlucent because of marked diminution in its blood flow. The increased intrapulmonary pressure due to the obstructive emphysema results in compression of the smaller blood vessels within the interstitium of the lung, thus increasing the vascular resistance. Since resistance is a major determinant of blood flow, an inordinate proportion of the right ventricular output will be distributed to the normal lung. The affected lung is oligemic and, although its vessels can usually be seen, they are small in calibre. The imbalance in blood flow between the two lungs may result in opacification of the pulmonary artery only on the normal side on a venous angiogram. This appearance is easily misinterpreted as indicating absence of one pulmonary artery (Fig. 313). However, selective pulmonary arteriography will demonstrate a small main pulmonary artery and its branches on the involved side.

The cardinal roentgen feature of the Swyer-James syndrome is the demonstration of air trapping in one lung. During expiration, the lung cannot expel its air and remains expanded. The heart and other mediastinal structures shift towards the normal, collapsed lung. If the diseased lung is normal in size, the mediastinum will shift into the opposite hemithorax during expiration. If the lung is small, the mediastinum may be deviated so far towards the abnormal side in inspiration that it will not shift even as far as midline during expiration. In either case, however, the mediastinum shows a pendular movement as the patient breathes, toward the affected lung on inspiration and away from it on expiration (Fig. 313).

Bronchography reveals amputation of many of the smaller bronchial branches. In some, the cut-off is sharp, while in others, the peripheral branches end in club-shaped terminal dilatations. The bronchial branches are separated by clear intervening lung because of the absence of filling of many of the smaller bronchial radicles (Fig. 314).

Unilateral hyperlucency of one lung is, in itself, a nonspecific sign and can be produced by large bullae, agenesis of a pulmonary artery, a major pulmonary arterial embolus, or a ball-valve obstruction of a main or lobar bronchus from any cause. The presence of air trapping excludes all conditions but bronchial obstruction from consideration. If the hyperinflated lung is small, the diagnosis of Swyer-James syndrome is confirmed. If the lung is normal in size, bronchoscopy or bronchography may be needed to exclude obstruction of a large bronchus.

Lobar Emphysema. Most of the reported cases have been in newborn infants. In the great majority, an upper lobe was involved or, less often, the middle lobe. Involvement of a lower lobe is rare. In about half of the cases, evidence of an obstructive lesion was found in a major bronchus. Most often this was due to faulty development of the bronchial cartilages so that the bronchus collapses during expiration (Fig. 315). Less commonly the bronchial obstruction was due to pressure from an aberrant blood vessel. Considerably rarer causes are a bronchial stricture or a fold of redundant bronchial mucosa. The remainder, in which there was no evidence of large bronchus obstruction, probably represent true emphysema. In these, the presence of air trapping indicates that the obstruction lies at the bronchiolar level. Whether this is due to a congenital defect or is the result of a pulmonary infection as in the Swyer-James syndrome is not certain.

The roentgen picture is characteristic. The affected lobe is markedly enlarged and hyperlucent while the remaining lung on that side is compressed. The lobe may herniate across the mediastinum and can produce significant displacement of the heart to the opposite side. The normal lung often appears clouded as a result of compression atelectasis. Widening of the rib spaces and flattening of the diaphragm on the side of the emphysematous lobe prove that the hyperexpansion is obstructive rather than compensatory. Although a pneumothorax or large bullae can produce the same effect, the presence of vascular markings in the hyperinflated portion of lung excludes those possibilities.

Focal Emphysema. Emphysematous foci are not uncommon in mucoviscidosis, severe bronchitis or in association with bronchial pneumonia, particularly of the suppurative type. Partial obstruction of small bronchi leads to air trapping in lobules or portions of pulmonary lobules and the infection weakens the alveolar walls resulting in localized overdistention (Fig. 245).

Extensive destruction of alveolar walls can produce a large air space which rapidly increases in size as the result of a check-valve obstruction of the bronchus. The resultant cavity is rather

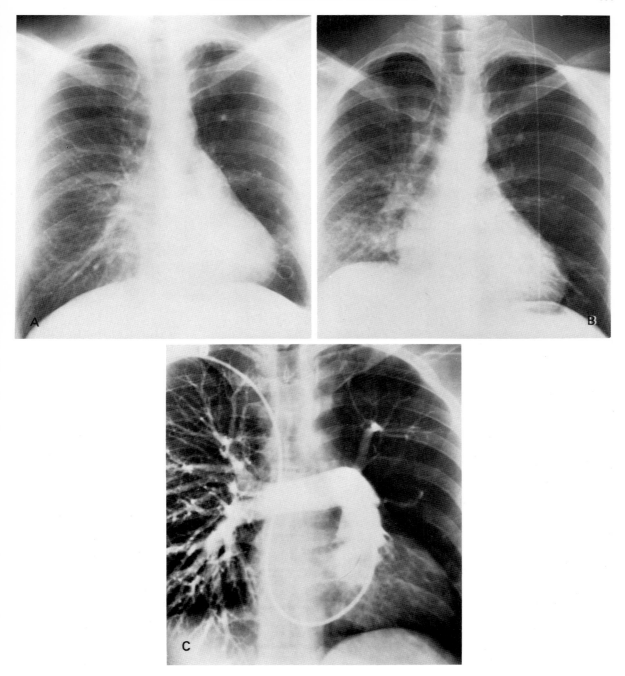

FIG. 313. UNILATERAL HYPERLUCENT LUNG: SWYER-JAMES SYNDROME

A: Inspiration. The heart and mediastinum are shifted to the left. The vasculature of the left lung is markedly decreased and only a few, small pulmonary vessels can be seen. The vasculature on the right side is increased. Except for the occasional ring shadow in the left lung, this picture is compatible with absence of the left pulmonary artery. *B*: Expiration. The right lung has become clouded as its air is expelled. The left lung remains fully inflated. The mediastinum has shifted toward the right. These findings indicate obstructive emphysema on the left side. The combination of emphysema and hypoplasia of a lung is indicative of the Swyer-James syndrome. *C*: Pulmonary arteriogram. Almost all of the right ventricular output goes to the right lung. The paucity of opacified vessels in the left lung does not necessarily indicate absence of the pulmonary arterial branches. The vascular resistance in an emphysematous lung is increased and therefore most of the blood is shunted to the opposite lung.

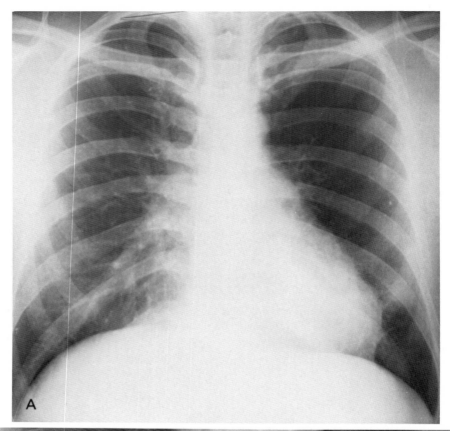

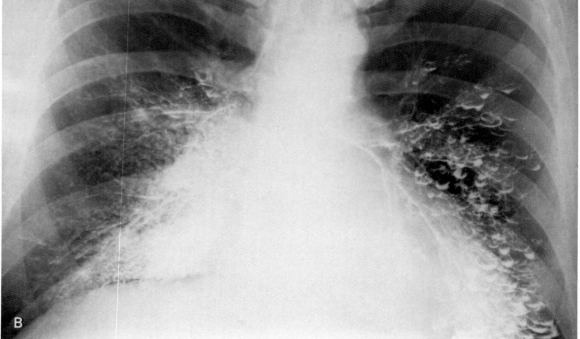

Fig. 314. Unilateral Hyperlucent Lung: Swyer-James Syndrome

A: The film made in complete inspiration shows the heart to be displaced to the left while the left lung is hyperlucent. Almost no blood vessels are seen in the left lung and those which are visible are markedly attenuated. During expiration the left lung did not empty and the heart was displaced toward the right. Obstructive emphysema in a hypoplastic lung is diagnostic of the Swyer-James syndrome. *B*: The bronchogram reveals thin-walled, sacculated dilatations of the terminal bronchi. These resulted from a severe bronchopulmonary infection in childhood. (Courtesy of Dr. B. Robinson, New York, N. Y.)

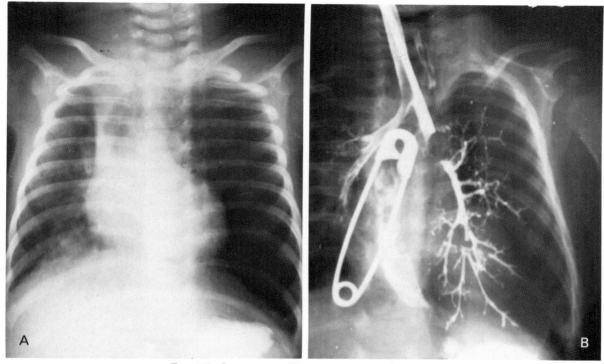

FIG. 315. OBSTRUCTIVE HYPERINFLATION IN INFANCY

A: The film of an infant in severe respiratory distress shows marked hyperinflation of the entire left lung. The diaphragm is depressed, the heart is markedly displaced to the right, and the anterior lappet of the lung has herniated across the mediastinum. *B*: At bronchoscopy, there appeared to be a complete occlusion of the left bronchus. However, it was possible to advance the bronchoscope past this point. The bronchogram made at this time shows marked narrowing of the main bronchus with abnormal distribution of its branches. The examination of the lung after pneumonectomy showed incomplete development of the bronchial cartilages just beyond the carina. Because of the lack of support of the bronchial wall, the pressure in the lung caused the bronchus to collapse during expiration. The safety pin is on the patient's gown.

large and similar to a bulla (Fig. 243) except that it usually shrinks and disappears as its bronchial communication becomes strictured during the course of the infection. This type of cavity, beginning as a focal area of emphysema and disappearing with subsidence of the infection is termed a pneumatocele. Once the cavity disappears, only a fine fibrotic streak may remain and often this is not detectable radiologically. On occasion, the pneumatocele persists after the infection clears and remains as a permanent air cyst within the lung (Fig. 240).

In tuberculous or fungous infections as well as in other granulomatous diseases, foci of emphysema are often present between the fibrotic and infiltrative lesions. These too, are probably due to obstruction of bronchioles as in the case of generalized emphysema, but are present only in the vicinity of the granulomatous lesions.

Bullae. A bulla represents a sharply demarcated, localized area of emphysema. Although bullae are often associated with generalized pulmonary emphysema, they also occur in an other-

wise normal lung. In either instance, they probably form as a result of partial obstruction of small bronchial branches. If the obstruction is in the nature of a check valve, air enters the alveoli during inspiration but cannot be completely expelled in expiration. The affected portion of lung becomes overdistended and the alveolar walls rupture and many of the small air spaces coalesce into one. It is often possible to enter such a bulla through the bronchus with a fine probe.

Bullae may be single or multiple. They are frequently found in areas of healed fibroid tuberculosis, fungous infections or other fibrotic or granulomatous diseases.

They commonly occur in association with some of the pneumoconioses, most notably silicosis, and in Boeck's sarcoid and histiocytosis X. Other bullae develop in the absence of roentgen evidence of any pulmonary disease. However, scarring of the lung is usually noted in the area on pathologic examination and the bullae probably form as the result of distortion of the bronchi and emphysema of the alveoli along the interlobular septa. Such bullae are most often situated in the upper lobes, particularly at the apices (Fig. 135) but also occur near the base of the middle lobe and lingula. They are situated immediately beneath the pleura and have a tendency to rupture and produce a pneumothorax.

Bullae are the most common cause of spontaneous pneumothorax. Most of them are too small to be detected on conventional films. They are better seen during expiration and sometimes can be visualized when the adjacent lung is collapsed by a pneumothorax. Larger bullae appear as localized avascular spaces demarcated by curved shadows of hairline thickness. When multiple bullae are situated adjacent to one another these fine linear shadows representing their boundaries may be straight or angulated. Sharply defined, thicker, linear shadows crossing the lucent area of the bulla are caused by septa which often contain blood vessels.

As a bulla enlarges, it compresses the adjacent lung, thus adding to the apparent thickness of its wall. A single large bulla can appear similar to a large air cyst, a bronchogenic cyst, or the residual cavity of a healed lung abscess or cystic bronchiectasis. The bronchial communication is usually so narrow that the bulla does not collapse during expiration as some air cysts do. Bullae may grow so large that the adjacent lung is compressed against the mediastinum or behind the heart, producing the picture of a "vanishing lung" (Fig. 316).

A fluid level can develop within a bulla if it becomes infected or when there is an inflammatory process in the adjacent lung. The infection need not be pyogenic and can subside spontaneously. The fluid may remain in the bulla for many weeks especially if the communication with the bronchial tree is sealed off. The bulla then shrinks as the air within it is absorbed and can disappear completely when the fluid is also absorbed.

Bullae are more clearly delineated by tomography. This is of particular importance in the differentiation of true tuberculous cavities from bullae associated with healed tuberculosis. A single bulla is thin-walled and round but multiple bullae tend to be facetted. In either case, the bullae are located in the most peripheral portion of the lung. The wall of the tuberculous cavity is usually thicker and irregular. However, it is possible for its wall to be thin either because of partial resolution of the inflammatory process or ballooning of the cavity. In such instances, the correct diagnosis may be impossible from the roentgen study.

Tomography is usually not required for the clinical management of bullous disease. If resective surgery is considered, pulmonary angiography can be of considerable value in distinguishing isolated bullae from those associated with generalized emphysema. Bronchography may help in the differentiation of an air cyst from a bulla since the radiopaque material rarely enters a bulla (Fig. 240). Bronchography may also be helpful in evaluating whether the remainder of the lung is emphysematous or if it is normal.

Interstitial Emphysema. Interstitial emphysema denotes the presence of air within the interlobular septa and the connective tissue about the bronchi within the lungs. It is caused by rupture of alveoli adjacent to the septa, usually resulting from a sudden marked elevation of alveolar pressure. This happens during the forced expiration required to expel air from the lungs through an obstructed airway. It is not uncommon in association with laryngeal obstruction in children as in laryngeal edema or croup, but also may be the result of narrowing of small bronchi. In rare instances, interstitial emphysema is caused by trauma to the chest with laceration of the lung.

The air in the interstitial tissues courses along the septa to the subpleural connective tissue where it forms blebs on the surface of the lungs. A bleb differs from a bulla in that it is situated within the intestitial connective tissue, between the superficial alveoli and the overlying pleura or within the layers of the visceral pleura, while a bulla is situated completely within the lung and consists of a number of communicating alveoli. Mesially, the air can proceed toward the mediastinum to produce mediastinal emphysema (see Fig. 356). The large air vesicles in the mediastinum or the blebs beneath the pleura can rupture to produce a pneumothorax. This is often bilateral.

At postmortem examination, the lung is crepitant and remains inflated after it is removed from the chest even if there is no bronchial obstruction. Air may escape from the alveoli, but the air trapped in the interstitial tissues keeps the lung distended.

Roentgenologically it is impossible to recognize interstitial emphysema of the lung unless there is a complicating mediastinal emphysema or pneumothorax. When interstitial emphysema occurs with laryngeal edema or croup, the hyperinflated condition of the lungs is presumed to be due to laryngeal obstruction. However, if the obstruction has been relieved by a tracheotomy and the lungs remain hyperexpanded during expiration and the diaphragm is limited in upward motion, interstitial emphysema is likely.

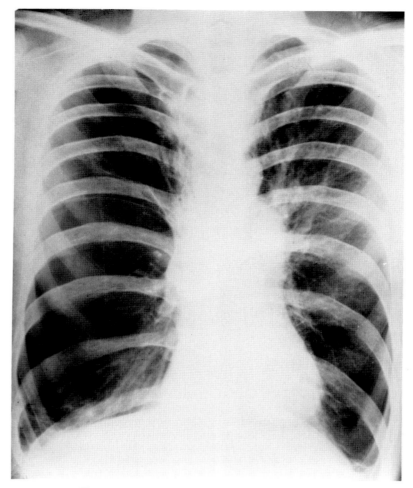

FIG. 316. BULLOUS EMPHYSEMA: VANISHING LUNG

The striking diminution of the pulmonary markings in the lower part of the right lung is due to a large bulla. The upper border of the bulla is seen as a sharp, curved line, paralleling the lower border of the posterior part of the seventh rib. The vessels of the right lower lobe are crowded together and displaced towards the cardiophrenic angle. Both leaves of the diaphragm are depressed, the posterior rib spaces are widened and the vessels in the left lower lobe are attenuated and spread apart. These findings indicate generalized emphysema in addition to the bulla.

The finding of mediastinal emphysema before the fascial planes have been opened during tracheotomy is presumptive evidence that there has been rupture of alveoli into the interstitial tissues. Once the laryngeal obstruction is relieved, persistence of the symptoms suggests interstitial emphysema even in the presence of a small or medium-sized pneumothorax. A pneumothorax of this size, even if bilateral, should not interfere that much with the mechanics of respiration.

Inhalation Diseases

Most inflammatory diseases of the lungs are caused by organisms which, although inhaled, produce infection by multiplying within the respiratory tract. Many of the bronchopulmonary diseases, however, result from the inhalation of inanimate chemical and physical agents. These are considered under the heading of inhalation diseases. They are broadly classified into three groups: those which result from the inhalation of dust (pneumoconioses), those resulting from the inhalation of irritating gases and fumes, and those resulting from the aspiration of liquids.

Rarely does the roentgen film present a pathognomonic picture from which an unqualified diagnosis of an inhalation disease can be made. It is necessary to obtain a history of inhalation of the offending agent in order to confirm the diagnosis. This history may not be volunteered by the patient because he does not connect it with his symptoms or does not realize that he has been exposed to a noxious agent. When the film suggests the possibility of an inhalation disease, it is essential that the patient be questioned meticulously concerning every possible inhalation exposure. On the other hand, it should be borne in mind that even an overt history of such an exposure is insufficient to warrant a conclusion that the roentgen findings are due to the inhalation. The possibility that the roentgen abnormalities may be due to some other cause must always be excluded.

The Pneumoconioses

The pneumoconioses, or dust diseases of the lungs, result from the inhalation of particulate material which accumulates in the lungs. The disease of the lungs and its roentgen features depend upon many factors. Among these are the nature of the dust, the size of the particles and their concentration in the atmosphere, the duration of the exposure, the susceptibility of the individual, and complicating infection.

Some dusts are relatively inert and cause little or no reaction in the lungs. Nevertheless, they may produce widespread shadows on the chest film because they are radiopaque. This is true of dusts containing the heavy elements, such as iron, barium and tin. In most cases of pneumoconiosis, there is an inflammatory reaction. In some instances, as in berylliosis, this may come acutely. In others, as in silicosis and asbestosis, a prolonged exposure is usually required.

It is necessary for the dust to be inhaled at least as far down as the respiratory bronchioles in order to produce disease. The finer the dust, the more apt it is to be retained in the lungs and cause an inflammatory reaction. Particles more than 15 micra in diameter are usually innocuous. In general, pneumoconiosis is caused by particles that are less than 5 micra in diameter.

There is an individual variation in susceptibility to pneumoconiosis. Many persons who are heavily exposed for many years do not develop any significant disease. The reason for this is not clear. However, it has been noted that previous disease of the lungs increases the tendency to pneumoconiosis. This is undoubtedly due to greater accumulation of the dust in the diseased areas, as well as the tendency to increased reaction.

In many of the pneumoconioses the dust remains in the lungs indefinitely and continues to produce disease. Progressive changes therefore occur in the lungs long after the patient is re-moved from the dusty environment. This occurs particularly in the case of silicosis and asbestosis.

The x-ray appearance of the pneumoconioses does not always reflect the clinical picture. Patients whose films show extensive shadows throughout the lungs may present few if any symptoms. In other cases the changes on the film may appear rather slight and are almost within normal limits while the patient suffers from severe respiratory disability. The disturbance in respiration appears to be related to the extent of the diffuse interstitial infiltrations of the lung and complicating emphysema. Where the interstitial fibrosis is fine it is not immediately noticeable on the films and yet may be responsible for severe disability. If the lesions are mainly nodular and unaccompanied by diffuse interstitial fibrosis or emphysema, the patient may not have any symptoms even though the pulmonary lesions are large and numerous.

Silicosis. Silicosis is caused by the inhalation of silicon dioxide often called *free silica*. Since ordinary sand is made up entirely of silicon dioxide and most rocks contain a large percentage of this material, workers in a great many occupations are exposed to dust containing silica. However, the concentration of tiny particles of free silica in the atmosphere is usually not great enough to produce disease. Generally, an atmosphere containing more than five million particles of less than 10 micra in size per cubic foot of air, is considered necessary for the development of silicosis. However, the constancy of the exposure is also a factor which influences the production of the disease so that the results of sporadic dust counts may be misleading. In some instances, two and a half million particles per cubic foot may cause silicosis, while in others a count of 50 million particles may not be significant.

Usually 2 or 3 years of exposure to the dust are necessary to produce a sufficient concentration of silica in the lungs to cause disease. However, the roentgen manifestations generally do not occur until several years later. Once established, the disease usually progresses from the silica that has already been deposited, but its progress is more rapid when inhalation of the dust continues. In certain occupations, where the atmosphere contains a high concentration of extremely fine particles, a shorter exposure is sufficient. In workers involved in the production of scouring powder, the clinical and roentgen manifestations of silicosis tend to appear earlier, the disease is more rapidly progressive and massive involvement of the lungs occurs more frequently (Fig. 317). Whether this is due solely to the silica

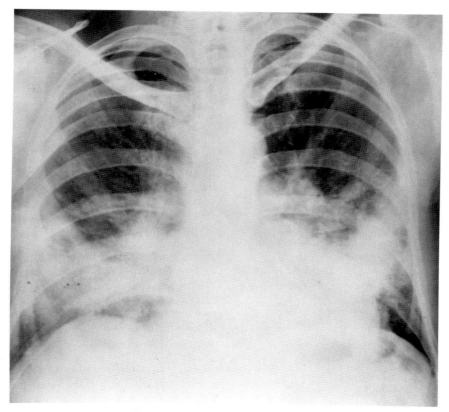

FIG. 317. SILICOSIS: PNEUMONIC FORM

The patient, who had been exposed to pumice dust, complained of severe dyspnea. There are large, homogeneous areas of opacification in the lower part of each lung. No nodular lesions are visible and there is no evidence of emphysema. This form of silicosis, which simulates an infectious pneumonia, is unusual and occurs particularly as a result of exposure to high concentrations of extremely fine particles of free silica.

in the fine dust, or to inhalation of additional irritants in the powder, is not certain.

Pathologically, the lesions of silicosis consist of nodules in the lungs, interstitial infiltrations and fibrosis, and inflammation and fibrosis of the lymph nodes in the hilum and mediastinum. The silica particles inhaled into the alveoli, are picked up by macrophages and transported to the regional and hilar lymph nodes where an inflammatory and fibroblastic reaction occurs. Some of the particles are arrested in lymphoid follicles in the interstitial tissues of the lungs, where they cause a similar inflammatory reaction. Here the characteristic lamellated fibrous silicotic nodules containing whorls of hyaline material are to be found. In addition, a more diffuse inflammatory reaction of the interstitial tissues of the lungs often takes place. This is associated with interstitial, perivascular and peribronchial fibrosis, and blockage of lymphatic drainage. Particles of silica are then transported peripherally toward the pleura and produce nodules in the subpleural

lymphoid tissue. The nodules vary in size from a fraction of a millimeter upwards. In some cases the nodules remain more or less discrete; in others they coalesce. The lesions of silicosis are characteristically bilateral and distributed symmetrically from the very onset of the disease.

In many cases, the earliest roentgen manifestation of silicosis is simply a slight increase in the density of the pulmonary markings, particularly in the region of the lung roots. While, pathologically, this is associated with the presence of innumerable small nodules in the interstitial tissues, they are too small to be recognized on the film. The hilar shadows may be slightly enlarged as a result of enlargement of the lymph nodes. The borders of the hilar structures are often poorly demarcated because of the convergence of the thickened interstitial tissues in this region. In other cases, the pulmonary markings and the hilar regions appear normal and the only abnormality is the presence of small nodules in the lungs. These are usually few in number, of varying size, and are situated mostly in the outer part of the upper portion of the lungs. In some cases a fine reticulation of the lungs is the earliest manifestation of the disease. This may be associated with a few tiny nodules in the upper parts of the lungs.

The later stage of the disease is often predominated by a more sharply defined reticular pattern caused by thickening of the pulmonary septa and the peribronchial and perivascular tissues. Thickening of the interlobular septa at the periphery of the lower part of the lungs produces short, parallel, horizontal streaks above the costophrenic sinuses, Kerley B lines (Fig. 318). These are often more clearly seen on the oblique view. They are usually 0.5 to 1.5 cm apart. In addition, longer, more angular lines may be seen radiating upward from the hilum, Kerley A lines.

The reticular and streak-like shadows are usually associated with the presence of numerous

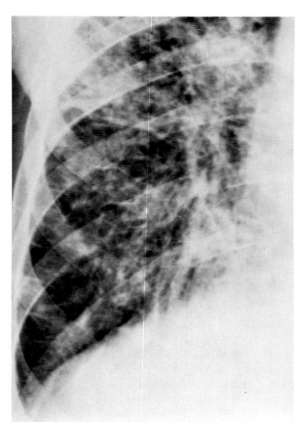

FIG. 318. SILICOSIDEROSIS

A close-up of the lower part of the right lung shows coarse, linear and nodular infiltrations. The lung has a reticular appearance. Fine, horizontal streak-like shadows are present above the costophrenic sinus, representing thickened interlobular septa. These are Kerley B lines. The patient had worked for many years in an iron mine.

nodular lesions measuring from 2 to 5 mm in diameter. The nodules tend to be larger and more numerous in the upper portion of the lungs below the clavicle. These changes, symmetrically distributed in both lungs, immediately suggest the presence of silicosis. When they are found, careful inquiry should be made into the patient's occupation with particular attention to exposure to free silica.

As the disease progresses, the reticular appearance of the lungs becomes more evident. The nodules increase in size and number, and now can be recognized throughout the lungs although they tend to be more numerous in the upper portions. In the late stages they become denser and more sharply demarcated although their borders remain irregular (Fig. 319). In some cases the density of the nodules approaches that of calcium. In fact, pathologic examination of extremely dense nodules usually discloses necrotic changes with deposition of calcium. The calcified nodules are no larger than the uncalcified ones. The calcification occurs in the absence of either tuberculosis or histoplasmosis.

The lymph nodes at the roots of the lungs become enlarged and often produce considerable prominence of the hilar shadows. Occasionally calcium is deposited in these nodes. The pattern of the calcification may be nonspecific, differing in no way from that which is seen in tuberculosis. Occasionally in silicosis, the calcium is deposited predominantly in the periphery of the nodes which then cast ring-like shadows (Fig. 320). This *eggshell* calcification of the nodes is quite characteristic of the advanced form of silicosis, although it may occur in milder cases of long duration. Only rarely is it encountered in the absence of this disease (Fig. 142).

Circumferential deposition of calcium can also occur within the pulmonary nodules of silicosis (Fig. 321). When the rim of calcium is rather thick, the nodule shows a sharply defined, lucent center. We have not observed this type of lesion in any disease other than silicosis. More commonly, larger eggshell calcifications, measuring up to 1.5 cm in diameter, are seen in the lung in advanced cases of silicosis. However, these are situated near the root of the lung and represent silicotic nodules within intercalated lymph nodes.

In the later stages of silicosis, there is usually considerable thickening of the pleura, often associated with dense adhesions to the parietes, diaphragm and pericardium. Marked thickening of the pleura is often most evident over the axillary portion of the lungs on the frontal projection. Calcification of the pleura is rare in pure

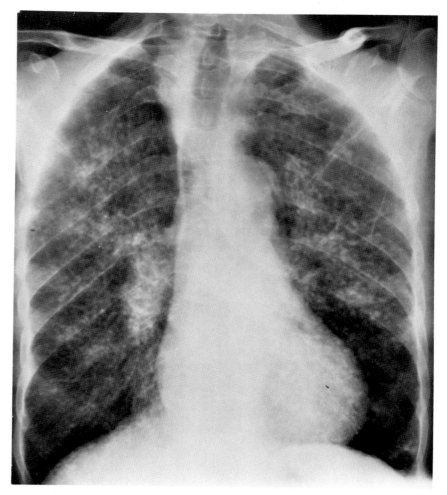

FIG. 319. SILICOSIS: DIFFUSE NODULAR FORM

Both lungs are studded with small nodular infiltrations, most numerous in the upper two-thirds. The hilar shadows are prominent because of enlargement of the lymph nodes as well as of the main pulmonary arteries. The patient was exposed to rock dust for a great many years.

silicosis, except over the upper portion of the lungs (Fig. 321).

Most cases of silicosis eventually become complicated by emphysema. This is due to partial obstruction of bronchioles and small bronchi by infection, spasm or the inflammatory reaction resulting from the irritating effect of the silica. Clinically, it is associated with cough, wheezing and shortness of breath. Radiologically, the evidences of emphysema are similar to those which occur in the emphysematous patient without silicosis. The leaves of the diaphragm become depressed and flattened, and their excursion is limited. On the lateral view, the anteroposterior diameter of the chest is seen to be considerably increased. There is an increase in the size and lucency of the retrosternal and retrocardiac spaces and an increase in the kyphotic curvature

of the dorsal spine. In this view the diaphragm appears more flattened than in the frontal. In addition to the generalized emphysema, bullous emphysema is frequently present. The bullae occur particularly at the apices and bases of the lungs (Fig. 322). Few nodules may be present in these areas even though the middle two-thirds of the lungs are thickly studded with them. The reason for this is obvious. Where there is little or no lung tissue present one can hardly expect to find interstitial infiltrations.

In some cases of silicosis, the roentgen picture simply shows innumerable, fairly well defined, somewhat irregular nodules throughout the lungs with a minimum of reticulation and no discernible evidence of emphysema. These patients may have little or no dyspnea despite most extensive involvement of the lung with the nodules. On the

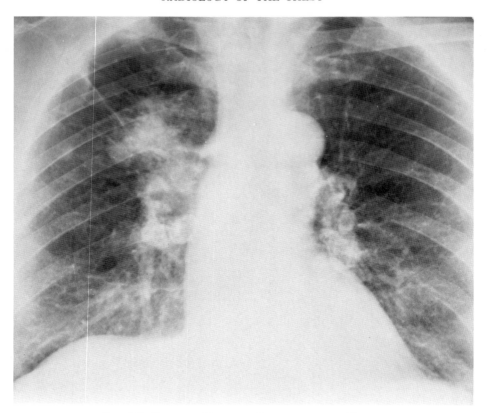

FIG. 320. SILICOSIS: EGGSHELL CALCIFICATION OF NODES

The lymph nodes at each hilum show the typical circumferential calcification associated with silicosis. Despite long exposure to silica dust, there is little evidence of involvement of the lung. The large, lobulated shadow near the root of the right upper lobe represents a coincidental bronchogenic carcinoma. The diagnosis of carcinoma can be made from the film because of the linear streak (Fleischner line) extending from the nodule to the periphery of the lung. The small, triangular shadow at its outer end represents an indrawing of the pleura. The massive lesions of silicosis are almost always bilateral and associated with emphysema.

other hand, there are cases in which the nodules are extremely small and barely evident on the film, even though the condition is of long duration and associated with dyspnea and marked emphysematous changes. In such cases, minute inspection of the films with the aid of optimal illumination will disclose fine reticulation throughout the lungs. This form of silicosis is seen particularly in molders. The clinical picture is usually characterized by disturbance in respiratory function far out of proportion to the roentgen findings.

The advanced stage of silicosis is often characterized by the presence of massive shadows in the lungs, *progressive massive fibrosis* (PMF). These lesions result from conglomeration and coalescence of smaller silicotic nodules (Fig. 323). The pathogenesis is not entirely clear, but it appears probable that blockage of lymphatic drainage contributes to their formation. This predisposes to infection and inflammation of the

lung. The inflammatory process in the bronchi leads to obstruction of many of the small branches and results in foci of atelectasis. Absorption of air from the lung between the nodules undoubtedly is the important factor in their coalescence. Once coalescence of the lesions has occurred, there is further interference with aeration and lymphatic drainage, resulting in progressive increase in the size of the lesions.

The roentgen appearance of the massive form of silicosis is fairly characteristic. It is almost always bilateral and rather symmetrical. The shadows are dense and usually irregular with ill-defined margins as a result of local infiltration of the lung. These densities are almost always situated in the upper third of the lungs, usually in the outer portions. In some cases the shadows are situated more mesially and appear to extend out from the upper part of each lung root in a butterfly pattern. In either instance, the massive shadows are not necessarily limited by the

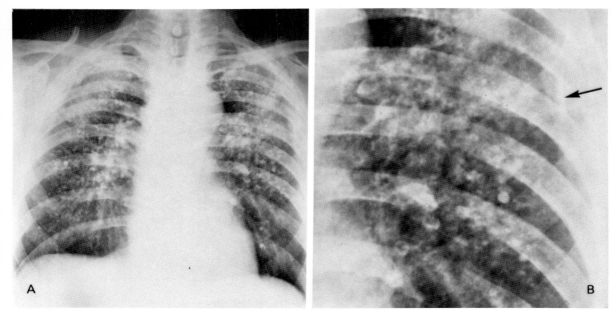

FIG. 321. CALCIFICATION IN SILICOSIS

A: Both lungs are studded with small nodules which are most numerous in the middle lung fields. Many of the nodules are calcified. There is coalescence of the lesions beneath each clavicle. The mesial portions of the upper lobes are emphysematous. *B*: Close-up of left midlung. The calcium is distributed diffusely within some of the nodules, while in others it is deposited only in the periphery in the form of a shell. The linear shadow (arrow) in the axillary portion of the upper left chest is due to calcification of the pleura.

boundaries of the lobes. In addition to the large densities, the surrounding lung exhibits the nodular infiltrations and reticulation typical of silicosis (Fig. 322).

Extensive emphysema is a most frequent accompaniment of the massive form of silicosis. In part, the emphysema is compensatory in response to the atelectasis that has occurred in the formation of the massive lesions. In addition, bronchial infection, which is almost constantly present in this form of the disease, also predisposes to obstructive emphysema. Bullae are frequently present at the apices and bases of the lungs. They also occur lateral to the massive lesions in the axillary portions of the lungs. Enlargement of the bullae displaces the lesions mesially (Fig. 324). The outer border of the lesion is usually sharply outlined, and is often smooth where it is in contact with the bullae.

A massive lesion may appear quite suddenly in a silicotic patient who contracts pneumonia. Consolidation then occurs between the nodules. Resolution is generally slow because of the underlying silicosis and is frequently incomplete, leaving a persistent, large, fibrotic, inflammatory lesion. The resultant density is often round and well demarcated. When the lesion is unilateral, it may be impossible to differentiate it from a

neoplasm unless repeated films show evidence of shrinkage.

Narrowing and closure of capillaries and small branches of the pulmonary artery occur regularly in the area of the silicotic nodules. However, in most cases there are a sufficient number of uninvolved blood vessels for the maintenance of a normal flow through the lesser circulation. Pulmonary hypertension and cor pulmonale are, therefore, rare in uncomplicated cases of nodular silicosis. When the disease is characterized by fine, diffuse interstitial infiltrations throughout both lungs, there is an appreciable degree of interference with the pulmonary circulation.

Pulmonary hypertension and cor pulmonale are not uncommon when the silicosis is associated with extensive emphysema. This is especially the case in the massive form of silicosis with extensive bulla formation. Obstruction to the circulation in this instance is due not only to the bullae but also to the narrowing of the blood vessels within the remaining atelectatic and fibrotic lung.

SILICOTUBERCULOSIS. There is a great predisposition for the development of pulmonary tuberculosis in patients with silicosis. Older studies suggested that between 60 and 75% of patients with silicosis eventually develop tuberculosis.

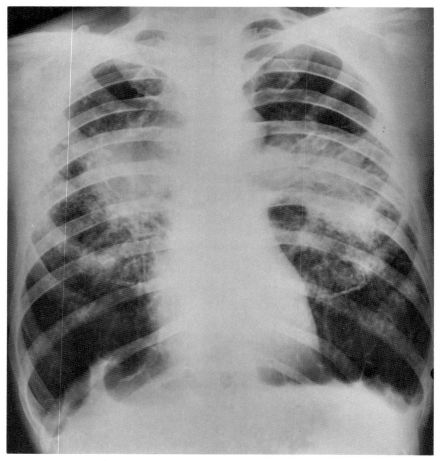

FIG. 322. SILICOSIS: MASSIVE FIBROSIS

The patient, a ceramics worker, was exposed to extremely fine particles of siliceous dust for many years. There is dense induration of the central portion of each lung. Fine nodulation and interstitial fibrosis are present beneath these areas. The apices and lower thirds of the lungs are free of infiltration because the pulmonary tissue is almost completely replaced by bullae. The irregularity of the diaphragm and its tent-like elevations are due to extensive pleural adhesions and focal areas of atelectasis between the bullae.

Today it appears that the incidence is considerably lower. Nevertheless, complicating tuberculosis is so common that it must be considered in all patients with silicosis. Because of this association and the fact that the clinical and roentgenologic characteristics of tuberculosis are modified by silicosis, the term *silicotuberculosis* is in common use.

The onset of complicating tuberculosis is usually obscure. Cough and bronchial infection with fever are common in patients with silicosis, as is the development of patchy lesions in the upper lobes without tuberculous infection. A definitive diagnosis of silicotuberculosis usually rests upon the demonstration of tubercle bacilli in the sputum or gastric contents. Repeated cultures are necessary in many cases to demonstrate the tubercle bacilli. Not uncommonly they are found only sporadically, but eventually, as the disease progresses, they are demonstrable in the sputum with ease at all examinations. In some instances, proof of the existence of complicating tuberculosis is not obtained until autopsy.

The radiologic diagnosis of tuberculosis is more evident in patients with diffuse infiltrative or nodular disease than in those with massive lesions. The appearance of a patch of consolidation or apparent coalescence of the silicotic nodules in an asymmetric manner, mainly in one upper lobe, is presumptive evidence of complicating tuberculosis and is an indication for additional studies. The gastric contents and the sputum should be cultured for tubercle bacilli and tomograms should be made in search of a cavity (Fig. 325). For practical purposes, the demonstration of a cavity in such a lesion may be considered to confirm the diagnosis of tuberculosis in patients with pure silicosis. While small cavities can be demonstrated at autopsy in patients with pure silicosis without tuberculosis, these are invariably filled with fluid and are not visualized radiologically. Exceptions to this are extremely rare. However, nontuberculous cavities are quite common in the anthracosilicosis of coal miners.

The question often arises in patients who have been exposed to free silica and who have an infraclavicular tuberculous lesion with nodules in the lungs, as to whether the patient really has underlying silicosis. Several facts should be taken into consideration in the diagnosis of silicotuberculosis in these cases. First, the history of the type and length of exposure to free silica must be considered. Second, an attempt should be made to locate previous films to determine whether the nodules visualized in other portions of the lung preceded the area of infiltration or cavitation in the upper lobe. Finally, the films should be observed from the standpoint of the distribution of the nodules. The acinar nodose form of tuberculosis, which complicates spread of infection from a tuberculous lesion, usually has a characteristic distribution. Most often the lesions are unilateral or more extensive on the side of the lesion from which the bronchogenic

dissemination occurred. When bronchogenic dissemination occurs to the opposite lung, nodules will be found mostly in its lower portion. If the nodules are seen to be more or less uniformly distributed throughout the lungs, or if they are more numerous and larger in the upper portion of each lung, the diagnosis of an underlying silicosis is justified in the patient who has been exposed to siliceous dust. Obviously, if the nodules respond to treatment with antituberculosis drugs, their infectious nature is established despite a history of intense and prolonged exposure to free silica.

The diagnosis of tuberculosis in the massive form of silicosis is more difficult. In previous years it was considered that most, if not all cases of silicosis with symmetrical massive shadows were tuberculous. Our experience has been that a tuberculous infection cannot be demonstrated in the majority of such cases. However, the incidence of proved tuberculosis increases in the cases in which the lesions are not symmetrical, i.e., in those in which there is an increase in the size of the dense lesion on one side. The demonstration of a cavity within the lung in silicosis either in, or adjacent to, the massive lesion, is quite diagnostic of active tuberculosis. In this connection it is necessary to differentiate between a bulla and a true tuberculous cavity since

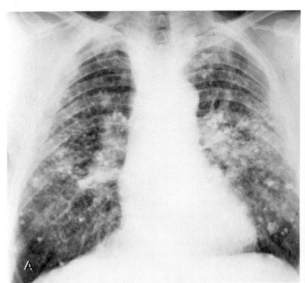 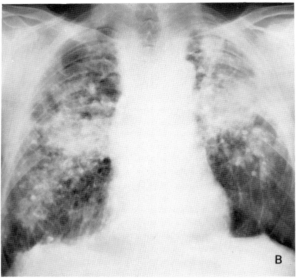

FIG. 323. SILICOSIS: PROGRESSIVE MASSIVE FIBROSIS

A: The film of this patient who had long exposure to dust containing free silica, shows the typical appearance of silicosis. Both lungs are studded with small nodules, some of which are calcified. The pulmonary markings are irregular as the result of interstitial infiltrations and fibrosis. The root shadows are accentuated, suggesting enlargement of the hilar nodes. *B:* Eleven years later, many of the nodules have coalesced and formed massive shadows in the perihilar regions. The lower half of each lung is emphysematous, accounting for the decrease in the number of nodules in these areas. In addition, there are bullous changes in both upper lobes.

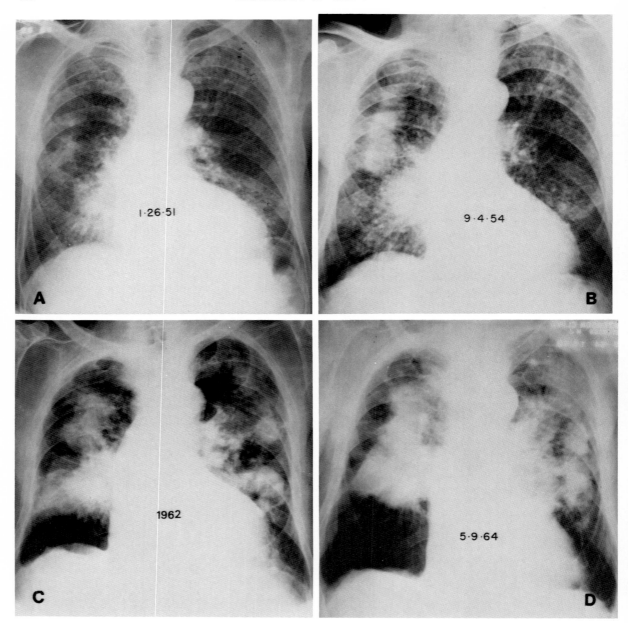

FIG. 324. PROGRESSIVE MASSIVE FIBROSIS

A: 1951. The film of a carbon black worker shows fine nodular infiltrations in the upper lobes with denser shadows in the lower lobes, particularly on the right. There is some confluence of the lesions in the lateral portion of the right upper lobe. *B*: 1954. Although there has been some progression of the disease in both lungs, the confluent lesion in the right upper lobe has become markedly larger. The fact that this lesion is seen in only one lung suggests the possibility of complicating tuberculosis. However, in tuberculosis, the infiltrate practically always is situated at a higher level. There is beginning emphysema at both bases. *C*: 1962. Massive lesions have developed in the left lung and the distribution in the chest is now symmetrical. There is extensive bullous emphysema and the massive lesion in the right upper lobe has been displaced mesially by the bullae. *D*: 1964. The large nodular lesions have become confluent to form a mass of shrunken, fibrotic lung with a corresponding increase in the severity of the emphysema.

bulla formation is so common in the massive form of silicosis. In any case, the possibility of concomitant tuberculosis must always be suspected in massive silicosis and the patient should

be observed from this standpoint by means of frequent x-ray examinations of the chest and intensive search for tubercle bacilli.

The response to drug treatment of tuberculosis

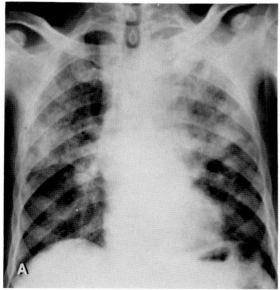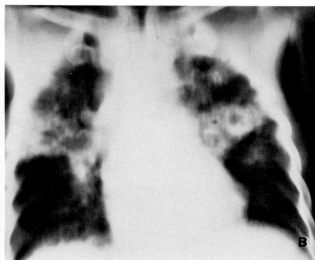

FIG. 325. SILICOTUBERCULOSIS

A: The film of this patient with known silicosis shows small nodular densities throughout the lungs and patchy shadows in both upper lobes. In addition, there is a dense area of consolidation in the uppermost portion of the left upper lobe without a corresponding lesion on the right side. The asymmetric distribution of the lesions, together with the absence of emphysema, strongly suggests complicating tuberculosis rather than progressive massive fibrosis. *B*: The tomogram reveals cavitary lesions in each upper lobe. The sputum was positive for tubercle bacilli.

in the silicotic is much less satisfactory than in ordinary tuberculosis. Cavities have a greater tendency to remain open, possibly because of the fibrosis caused by the silicosis. Although there may be initial improvement under therapy, relapses are extremely common. Because of the persistence of infection, often in smoldering form, drug-resistant organisms frequently emerge and cause rapid extension of the disease. Furthermore, there is good reason to believe that atypical mycobacteria are the infectious agents rather than tubercle bacilli in some of these refractory cases.

Coal Workers' Pneumoconiosis (Anthracosis and Anthracosilicosis). Most coal workers who suffer from pneumoconiosis have been exposed to free silica as well as coal dust. The manifestations and course of the disease are somewhat different from pure silicosis and the condition is best termed anthracosilicosis. Such exposure occurs particularly in anthracite mines where there is considerable exposure to dust from drilling through rock in addition to the coal dust. Considerably less exposure to silica occurs in the mining of bituminous coal, but here also, a certain amount of silica may be inhaled during the mining process. Workers at the coal face, where the silica content may be less than 1 or 2%, can be exposed to a much greater concentration of silica because of drilling of rock in the

vicinity. A minimal exposure to free silica occurs in coal handlers and coal trimmers. Yet, even these workers can develop a type of pneumoconiosis which is essentially pure anthracosis. Exposure to a significant quantity of silica together with carbon occurs in the handling of graphite.

In general, the pneumoconiosis resulting from inhalation of coal dust is characterized by the formation of extremely tiny, poorly demarcated nodules, distributed diffusely throughout both lungs. In the early stages of silicosis, on the other hand, a few larger, more sharply demarcated nodules are frequently visible in the outer portions of the upper lobes. The anthracotic pigment is deposited largely about the respiratory bronchioles which frequently become considerably dilated. Since the respiratory bronchioles are situated in the central portion of the pulmonary lobule, the picture is one of centrilobular emphysema. Although this may cause considerable disturbance in pulmonary function, the emphysematous areas are not well delineated on ordinary films. There is little fibrosis of the interstitial tissues in pure anthracosis, so that the reticular pattern of the pulmonary fields which occurs in silicosis, is unusual.

Most often the anthracosis of coal miners is combined with silicosis. Massive lesions occur more frequently in coal workers than in those exposed simply to silica. These lesions are usually bilateral and are situated mainly in the upper lobes and in the superior segments of the lower lobes. They consist of granulation tissue, alveoli filled with phagocytes containing coal dust, dense scar tissue and collections of coal pigment. The shadows cast by these lesions have been described as angel-wing densities when they are situated at the apices, as reniform shadows when adjacent to each lung root, or as cannonball shadows.

Cavitation takes place rather frequently within the massive lesions of coal miners' lung, even in the absence of tuberculosis. In many instances, particularly in the case of the cannon ball

shadows, liquefaction has already taken place, but the lesions appear solid where the bronchial communication has not yet been established. The cavities frequently become visible following expectoration of a considerable amount of inky black sputum. This condition has been called *phthisis nigra*, even in the absence of tuberculous infection (Fig. 326).

The cavity walls vary in appearance. Most often they are thick and irregular, but not infrequently they are thin and smooth. The cavities may be single or multiple, and may be empty or show an air-fluid level. Usually the bronchial opening is so small that radiopaque material

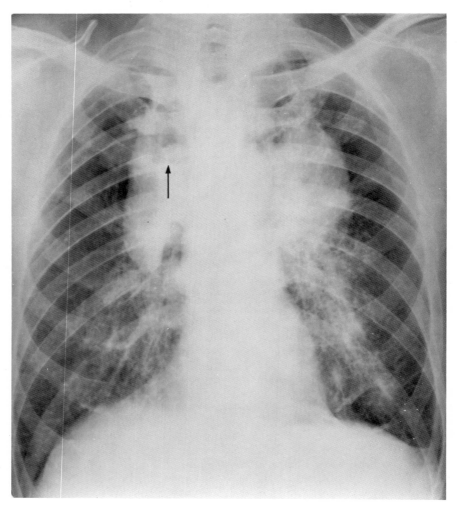

FIG. 326. ANTHRACOSILICOSIS: PHTHISIS NIGRA

The patient had been a coal miner for many years and recently expectorated black sputum. The film shows a dense shadow in the mesial portion of each upper lobe suggesting massive fibrosis. However, the outer border of each shadow is smooth and sharply demarcated and there is no evidence of emphysema in association with the lesions. There is an air-fluid level (arrow) within the lesion on the right side. The sputum was persistently negative for tubercle bacilli. The presence of a nontuberculous cavity together with expectoration of inky fluid is indicative of liquefaction of anthracotic lung (phthisis nigra). The lesion on the left side is similar, but has not extruded its contents through a bronchus. (Courtesy of Dr. I. J. Selikoff, New York, N. Y.)

cannot enter the cavity at bronchography. If the bronchial communication becomes blocked, the cavity refills, and again presents as a solid shadow.

Many of the blood vessels in the massive lesions of coal workers' lung are obliterated. The interference with blood supply probably contributes to necrosis within the lesion and formation of the cavities. Occasionally, a portion of infarcted lung tissue becomes separated and forms a sequestrum within a cavity. The appearance is then indistinguishable radiographically from a mycetoma. Closure of blood vessels also occurs in association with the progressive massive fibrosis of pure silicosis. Here also lung tissue may undergo liquefaction. However, unlike the coal worker's lung, the silicotic lung shows only small cavities or clefts filled with fluid. Rarely is there a free bronchial communication and, therefore, the cavities are rarely demonstrable radiologically except in those cases where they are the result of complicating tuberculosis.

As in silicosis, the massive form of pneumoconiosis that occurs in coal workers is often associated with bronchopulmonary infection which commonly leads to emphysema. The emphysema resulting from the bronchial disease is of the panacinar or diffuse type in contradistinction to the centrilobular emphysema that is associated with the simple pneumoconiosis caused by the deposition of coal dust in the lungs. The distribution of the panacinar emphysema in the massive lesions of the lungs in coal workers is similar to that which occurs in pure silicosis.

Rheumatoid Pneumoconiosis (Caplan's Syndrome). Caplan called attention to the occurrence of rather characteristic nodules in the lungs of coal miners who had rheumatoid arthritis in addition to pneumoconiosis. The nodules had a histological structure similar to subcutaneous rheumatoid nodules, entirely different from those caused by pneumoconiosis. These nodules were common among coal workers with rheumatoid arthritis, but rare in patients with rheumatoid arthritis without pneumoconiosis.

The extent of nodular involvement of the lungs bears no relationship to the degree of pneumoconiosis or to the severity of the rheumatoid arthritis. The nodules may appear concurrently with the onset of the rheumatoid arthritis, they may appear late in the disease, or months or even years before the rheumatoid symptoms. There is no increased incidence of rheumatoid arthritis among patients with pneumoconiosis. However, there is no doubt that the pneumoconiosis does result in a marked increase in the incidence of rheumatoid pulmonary nodules in

patients with generalized rheumatoid disease. While the great majority of the cases of Caplan's syndrome have occurred in patients with coal dust pneumoconiosis, a number of cases have been reported in conjunction with pure silicosis and with asbestosis.

The classical roentgen picture of Caplan's syndrome shows several rather well demarcated, round nodules distributed throughout the lungs with a tendency to greater accumulation in the upper portions. The more characteristic nodules are fairly large, measuring from 0.5 to 5.0 cm in diameter. Small infiltrations, reflecting the presence of the underlying pneumoconiosis are usually visible between the nodules. While this picture is quite characteristic of rheumatoid pneumoconiosis, it can occur in the absence of rheumatoid disease. It occurs occasionally in the massive form of pneumoconiosis and in pneumoconiosis complicated by tuberculosis or nonspecific infection.

The rheumatoid nodules usually have necrotic centers which frequently result in cavitation (Fig. 327) and calcification. The cavities are generally multiple, of moderate size and thin walled. As in tuberculosis, an air-fluid level is usually absent. The cavities in Caplan's syndrome rarely contain tubercle bacilli. This is in sharp contrast to the cavities in pure silicosis which are practically always tuberculous, and to those of coal workers' pneumoconiosis which frequently contain tubercle bacilli. The cavities often close spontaneously, leaving a small, faint, ill-defined density. In other instances no trace of the lesion remains.

In some cases the lesions involute without demonstrable intervening cavitation. Calcium is often deposited within the nodules. This occurs more frequently in rheumatoid nodules than in the lesions of silicosis.

A more nonspecific roentgen picture occurs in some cases. The nodules are smaller, more numerous and more diffusely scattered throughout the lungs. Although these nodules have the histological pattern of rheumatoid disease, the roentgen picture is indistinguishable from that of silicosis. Distinct nodules may be absent, and the roentgen picture is characterized simply by fine interstitial infiltrations similar to those that occur in the rheumatoid lung without pneumoconiosis.

In the later stages the larger nodules may coalesce. While the individual rheumatoid nodules can still be identified pathologically, the roentgen appearance is identical with that of progressive massive fibrosis of pneumoconiosis without rheumatoid disease. However, in many instances other characteristic round nodules are also evident to suggest Caplan's syndrome (Fig. 327).

It is important to keep in mind the possibility of Caplan's syndrome in patients with pneumoconiosis with multiple nodules in the lungs, even in the absence of outspoken symptoms of arthritis. The lesions may be confused with metastatic neoplasms. The predominance of the lesions in the upper lobes and the lack of progressive growth and the common occurrence of cavitation aid in the interpretation of the shadows. In some cases, observation of the patient over a period of time may disclose the occurrence of classical rheumatoid arthritis.

Asbestosis. Asbestos is a fibrous mineral consisting of a variety of silicates. The disease, asbestosis, which results from the inhalation of the fine fibers, is in essence a silicatosis, in contradistinction to silicosis which is caused by the inhalation of free silica. Asbestos is widely used in many industries, not only in roofing and insulation, but also in the manufacture of textiles, paper, and certain cements, putties and plastics. Injurious exposure to asbestos dusts can occur not only in those who work directly with asbestos products, but also in those in the immediate neighborhood. Thus, asbestosis is common among electricians and sheet metal workers who do not handle asbestos, but who work in the vicinity where pipes and furnaces are being covered with this material. The exposure to asbestos may therefore not be evident from a routine occupational history.

Inhalation of asbestos results in an inflammatory reaction in the interstitial tissues of the lungs and a relatively fine fibrosis. This involves mainly the lower half of the lungs. It is usually associated with a reaction in the pleura resulting in thickening and the formation of fibrous plaques, especially over the parietal pleura. Occasionally there is a small effusion which absorbs spontaneously.

As the disease progresses, the upper portions of the lungs also become involved, although to a lesser extent. The interstitial infiltrations and fibrosis become coarser and the lungs become stiffened and diminish in volume. While emphysema may complicate the picture in the later stages, this is largely compensatory and rarely causes an increase in lung volume. Occasionally there is bulla formation. Secondary infection may result in areas of persistent pneumonia and dense fibrosis, but such lesions are unusual.

Roentgen signs of asbestosis do not appear until a number of years after the onset of exposure to asbestos. However, during this period symptoms referable to pulmonary involvement may occur. A negative roentgen film, therefore,

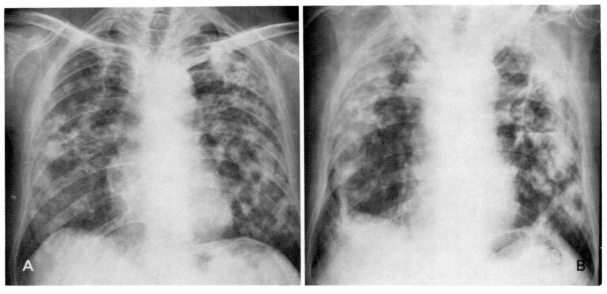

FIG. 327. CAPLAN'S SYNDROME

A: June 8, 1957. The patient was a coal miner with rheumatoid arthritis. The lungs show numerous nodules some of which are round and well circumscribed. In addition, there are generalized interstitial infiltrations. Bullae are present in both upper lobes. *B*: June 3, 1971. There has been marked progression of the disease. Many of the nodules have coalesced and a number of them have undergone cavitation. An air-fluid level has appeared in a large cavity on the left side. Focal areas of atelectasis are present at each base associated with tenting of the diaphragm. (Courtesy of Dr. I. J. Selikoff, New York, N. Y.)

does not exclude the possibility that asbestosis has been contracted. Not infrequently, roentgen manifestations of the disease first become evident several years after exposure to asbestos has ceased.

The earliest roentgen manifestation of asbestosis consists of a slight graying of the basal portions of the lungs caused by fine, diffuse infiltration and fibrosis of the interstitial tissues. The thickening of the interstitial tissues partly obscures the borders of the vascular shadows in the lungs, making them indistinct. This produces what has been called a ground glass appearance of the affected portions of the lungs (Fig. 328). When faint, it is frequently difficult to differentiate this from the normal lung. Films made during expiration accentuate the clouding of the lungs in striking fashion and are often useful where there is some doubt concerning the presence of interstitial infiltrations.

Various factors, such as differences in the roentgen exposure, the contrast of the film and the thickness of the patient may serve to obscure the infiltrations or to intensify the markings of the normal lung and mimic the presence of interstitial disease. In patients who work with, or in proximity to, asbestos, preemployment films made with a standard technique are desirable for comparison with future examinations.

Another manifestation of asbestosis which frequently occurs in the early stage of the disease is poor definition of the borders of the cardiac and diaphragmatic shadows. This is caused, in part, by thickening of the pleura but is also due to the interstitial infiltration in the subpleural portion of the adjacent lung. The rather characteristic blurring of the outline of the heart and diaphragm has given rise to the descriptive term, shaggy heart or shaggy diaphragm. Thickening of the pleura and an indistinct border of the heart or diaphragm may be present before the cloudiness of the lung or other manifestations of the interstitial infiltrations become evident radiologically.

The thickening of the pleura is also manifested as a band of increased density along the rib margins over the lower part of the chest. This is seen best in the oblique views. Despite the fre-

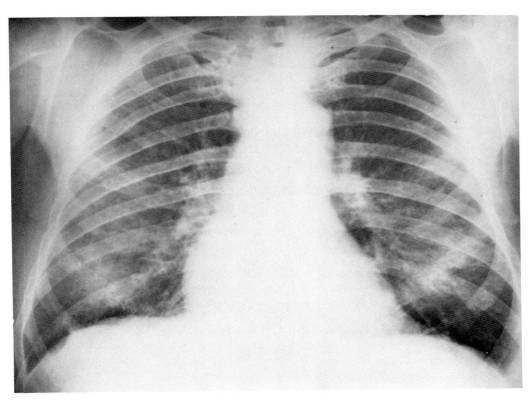

FIG. 328. PULMONARY ASBESTOSIS

There are extremely fine interstitial infiltrations throughout the lower two-thirds of each lung. These obscure the outlines of the blood vessels and impart a hazy appearance to the pulmonary fields. This is rather characteristic of asbestosis. The clear areas above the diaphragm are due to emphysema.

quency of pleural thickening, obliteration of the costophrenic sinuses is not common.

As the disease progresses, there is a tendency to coarser infiltration of the perivascular and peribronchial tissues and the interlobular septa. This results, at first, in the formation of fine striations and reticulation in the pulmonary fields. As the interstitial fibrosis becomes more pronounced, these shadows become thicker and denser. The shaggy appearance of the heart and diaphragm becomes accentuated. The cardiac border may appear spiculated as a result of the coarse interstitial fibrosis of the adjacent lung, producing an appearance described as the porcupine heart (Fig. 103).

Rarely, distinct nodules are formed as in silicosis. When they do occur, they are probably the result of the inhalation of free silica together with the asbestos. Enlargement of the hilar lymph nodes is also very unusual and calcification of the nodes does not occur. In rare instances, one or more dense, patchy shadows appear, comparable to the progressive massive fibrosis of silicosis. However, they are rarely associated with extensive emphysema. Most often they have the appearance of areas of consolidation, and are undoubtedly due to complicating, nonspecific inflammation. In contrast to silicosis, tuberculosis is not a complication of asbestosis.

After many years of exposure to asbestos dust, areas of emphysema are frequently interposed between the fibrotic strands. This is in part due to dilatation of the respiratory bronchioles (so-called bronchiolar emphysema) and results in the picture of honeycomb lung (Fig. 329). Occasionally fairly large bullae occur either at the apex or the base. However, despite the emphysematous changes, the lungs show little or no increase in volume and the diaphragms are therefore rarely depressed.

Calcified pleural plaques occur frequently, many years after the onset of exposure to asbestos. They rarely occur before 10 years but are found with increasing frequency as time goes on. Roentgenologically, the plaques have an appearance quite unlike that associated with other diseases. They are characteristically situated in the parietal pleura, most frequently over the diaphragm and the lateral chest wall. Usually the plaques are visible only when they are viewed on end (Fig. 330). They then appear as dense, linear shadows along the borders of the diaphragm, the chest wall or the mediastinum. Generally they measure about 1.5 to 2.0 cm in length. Even in the absence of pulmonary infiltration, such calcifications in the pleura should strongly suggest the possibility of asbestosis. When associated with interstitial infiltrations of the lower portions of the lungs, they may be considered as pathognomonic of this disease. So important is the recognition of these plaques that they should be sought for most carefully in all cases of diffuse infiltration of the lungs the cause of which is unknown. It is often necessary to make Bucky films in order to visualize the diaphragmatic plaques and oblique views for the demonstration of the calcific deposits over the lateral portion of the chest (Fig. 331).

In severe cases of asbestosis of long duration, the calcified plaques are more extensive. They may be distributed over large areas of the pleura and therefore are easily visible with the patient in any position. They are practically always bilateral and are generally characterized by irregular linear or interlacing annular shadows. Despite the extent of the calcification, the plaques may still be confined to the parietal pleura without adhesion to the visceral pleura. This is demonstrated fluoroscopically when the peripheral lung markings are seen to move independently of the calcified plaques during respiration. Frequently the costophrenic sinuses are not obliterated and the intercostal spaces are not narrowed. All of these characteristics aid in the differentiation of pleural calcification in asbestosis from calcification of the pleura in tuberculosis, hemothorax and old empyemas.

Carcinoma of the lung occurs anywhere from 8 to 15 times as frequently in patients with asbestosis as in the general population. The carcinomas arise from either the small bronchi or the lining cells of the alveoli and not from the larger bronchi. The roentgen shadows, therefore, are caused by the neoplasms themselves rather than by atelectatic lung or pneumonia secondary to bronchial obstruction. The lesions may be round and fairly well delineated or they may be poorly demarcated and suggest inflammatory consolidation. Since massive pulmonary fibrosis is rare in asbestosis, the appearance of a nodular or ill-defined, more or less homogeneous, density on the film of a patient who has been exposed to asbestos should immediately suggest the presence of primary carcinoma of the lung (Fig. 331).

It is now realized that most if not practically all cases of mesothelioma of the pleura are associated with asbestosis. The mesothelioma may present a more or less characteristic scalloped shadow on the pleura or it may be manifested simply by the presence of a pleural effusion. Although a pleural effusion may occur in the course of asbestosis without mesothelioma, it is usually small and is always transient. The presence of a large pleural effusion, or one which is

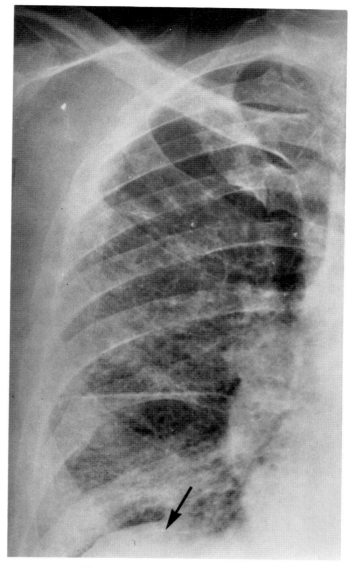

FIG. 329. ASBESTOSIS: HONEYCOMB LUNG

The lower two-thirds of the lung show a reticular pattern which is due to the presence of innumerable microcysts together with fine interstitial fibrosis, creating the appearance of a honeycomb. The short fissure is accentuated as a result of fibrous pleuritis. The paucity of markings in the right upper lobe is due to emphysema. A calcific plaque is seen on end (arrow) just below the dome of the diaphragm. This is characteristic of asbestosis.

persistent, in a person exposed to asbestos should suggest a complicating mesothelioma. Mesotheliomas of the peritoneum, as well as malignant neoplasms of other intraabdominal structures occur with increased frequency in association with asbestosis.

Talcosis. Talc is a nonfibrous, crystalline or granular form of hydrous magnesium silicate. It rarely occurs in a pure form. Mixed with the talc crystals are variable quantities of an asbestos-like, fibrous material, notably tremolite. In some instances, commercial talc contains an appreciable amount of free silica in the form of quartz. Although the contaminating materials undoubtedly influence the pathologic and roentgen picture of talcosis, talc alone can produce fibrosing disease of the lungs.

Talcosis is common in workers exposed to high concentrations of the dust over a long period of time. The disease is rare in those exposed for a period of less than 10 years or to a dust concentration of less than 20 million particles per cubic

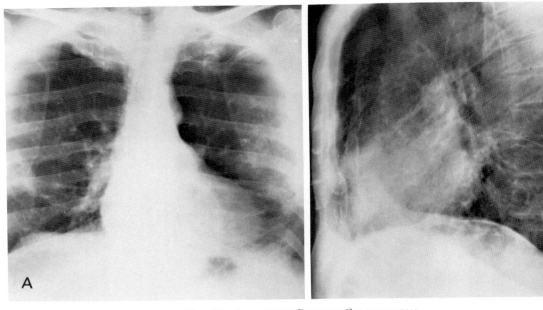

FIG. 330. ASBESTOSIS: PLEURAL CALCIFICATION

A: Frontal projection. The curvilinear shadows in the lower part of each lung represent focal areas of atelectasis. They sweep upward and outward and converge towards areas of pleural thickening. Similar shadows may be observed following severe fibrinous pleurisy from other causes but they are characteristically unilateral. Interstitial fibrosis is not visible. No calcification is seen over the diaphragm. *B*: Lateral view. The large calcific plaque over the left leaf of the diaphragm is diagnostic for asbestosis. Note that the costophrenic sinus is not obliterated. In addition, calcific plaques are seen on end over the anterior and posterior portions of the lung.

foot. Most of the cases have occurred in miners and millers of talc, and in the rubber industry where talc is used as a dusting powder.

The pathologic picture of talcosis consists essentially of interstitial inflammation and fibrosis of the lungs. The roentgen picture is similar to that of asbestosis. It affects chiefly the middle and lower portions of the lung. The early changes consist of a ground glass appearance of the involved portion of the lungs. As the disease progresses, coarser fibrosis of the peribronchial and perivascular tissues and the interlobular septa occurs, producing striation and reticulation of the pulmonary fields. In the more advanced cases, the upper portions of the lungs are also involved and poorly defined nodular densities may appear between the reticular and linear shadows. Massive fibrotic lesions also occur in advanced cases, but they are uncommon. In the late stages, bullae and honeycombing may develop (Fig. 332) and the heart may be enlarged as a result of cor pulmonale. As in asbestosis, thickening of the pleura and calcified pleural plaques are common (Fig. 333). There remains a question as to whether these are due to the talc itself or to the contaminating tremolite or other asbestos-like materials.

There is no apparent predisposition to tuber-

culosis as in silicosis. Thus far there has been no definite evidence of an increase in the incidence of carcinoma of the lungs or of mesothelioma of the pleura as in asbestosis.

Generally, talcosis cannot be differentiated roentgenologically from asbestosis. However, there is less tendency for the disease to be confined to the lowermost portions of the lung in talcosis and there is a greater tendency to coarse fibrosis and nodulation.

Other Silicatoses. Chief among the silicates, other than asbestos or talc, that can produce pulmonary lesions, is kaolin, a hydrated aluminum silicate used in pottery in the form of china clay. The roentgen appearance in most cases is characterized by the presence of micronodular lesions throughout the lungs. These usually measure 1 to 2 mm in diameter. Progression of the disease appears to be extremely slow. Confluence of the lesions in the upper lobes may occur after a number of years. Massive fibrosis is rare. Pleural calcification has been described but there remains some question as to whether this is caused by the kaolin itself. There is no known etiologic relationship to neoplastic disease and tuberculosis does not appear to be more frequent than in the ordinary population.

Pneumoconiosis rarely results from exposure

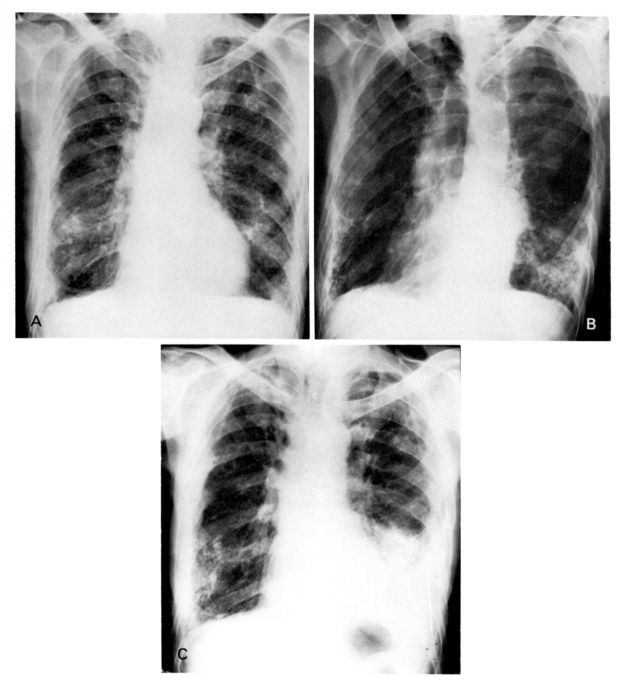

FIG. 331. CARCINOMA IN ASBESTOSIS

A: Frontal projection. Interstitial infiltrations are present throughout the lower half of each lung in a patient who had been exposed to asbestos dust for many years. There is marked thickening of the pleura over each lower lobe but the costophrenic sinuses are not obliterated. The densities at the anterior end of the fifth rib on each side present a geographic conformation suggesting calcific plaques on the pleura viewed *en face*. *B*: Left oblique view. The calcific pleural plaques are clearly demonstrated because they are viewed on end in this projection. *C*: Four years later, the film shows a poorly defined round shadow in the lower part of the left lung. The pleura on this side is now markedly thickened. There has also been an increase in the pleural calcification on the right side. A nodular shadow in the lung of a patient with asbestosis is practically always due to a complicating carcinoma.

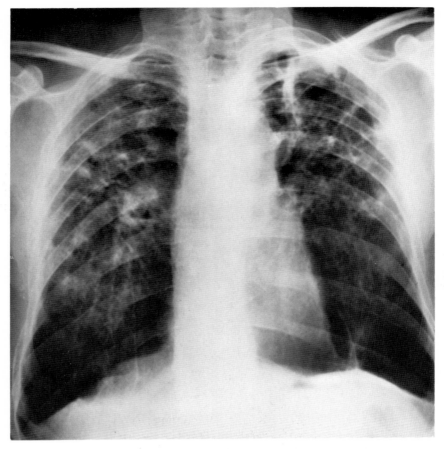

FIG. 332. TALCOSIS

Coarse fibrotic lesions are present throughout the upper half of each lung interspersed with small cystic areas. There are bullae at the bases. The patient had worked for 7 years as a talc miner. Although his exposure to injurious dust stopped 20 years ago, he has suffered increasing dyspnea since that time.

to other silicates, such as mica, sillimanite, etc. Calcification of the pleura is not uncommon in pneumoconiosis due to mica.

Diatomite Pneumoconiosis. Diatomite, also known as diatomaceous earth, consists of the fossilized remains of diatoms (bivalved unicellular plants). Natural diatomite consists of amorphous silicon dioxide. However, when this material is processed by heating and fluxing, some of the amorphous silica is changed to cristabolite, a form of crystalline silica which appears to be the injurious agent.

The early roentgen changes consist of an increase in the pulmonary markings in the upper portions of the lungs, beneath the clavicles. Tiny nodules, up to 1 to 2 mm in diameter, may be visualized in these areas, but the infiltrations are generally linear or reticular. The nodules do not seem to increase in size or density as in silicosis,

nor is there any tendency to calcification within them. As the disease progresses, the infiltrations become more coarse. Late in the course, coalescence takes place with the formation of large masses of induration and fibrosis. Emphysema is a common complication and occurs at the bases of the lungs as well as at the apices. It is often associated with the formation of large bullae which may rupture and produce spontaneous pneumothorax. In general, the roentgen appearance is not unlike that which occurs in molders, who are also exposed to cristobalite, formed as the result of exposure of sand to extreme heat.

Shaver's Disease. A pneumoconiosis described by Shaver occurs in workers exposed to fumes formed when bauxite is heated to high temperatures during the production of aluminum. In addition to the aluminum, the fumes contain a significant concentration of silicon dioxide in extremely fine particles. It appears most probable that the silica plays a major role in the production of the pneumoconiosis. Pneumoconiosis caused by inhalation of aluminum dust alone is quite unusual.

The course of Shaver's disease differs from the ordinary cases of silicosis in several ways. Well-developed disease has been reported after relatively short exposure, months rather than years. Massive shadows throughout the lungs are common, occurring in ill-defined patches as well as large areas of progressive fibrosis. Widening of the mediastinum as a result of involvement of the lymph nodes is common and may occur early. Bullous emphysema is a particularly frequent occurrence, and is often complicated by spontaneous pneumothorax.

Berylliosis. This disease results from the inhalation of compounds of beryllium. It is seen particularly in persons involved in the extraction of beryllium oxide from the ore, bery, and in the processing of substances containing beryllium, such as certain nickel and copper alloys. Beryllium used to be used in the manufacture of fluorescent tubes and the disease was encountered in persons exposed to dust from breakage

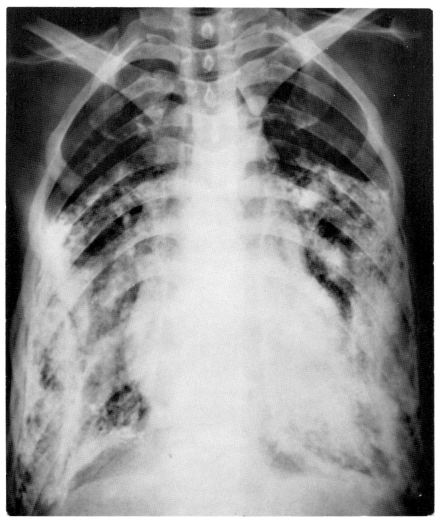

FIG. 333. PLEURAL CALCIFICATION IN TALCOSIS

Despite the extensive calcification of the pleura on both sides, the contour of the diaphragm remains regular and the costophrenic sinuses were not obliterated. This serves to exclude old tuberculosis or hemothorax from consideration. The patient had been exposed to talc for many years. Pleural calcification of this degree is more common in talcosis than in asbestosis.

of these tubes. Poisoning can result from the inhalation of minute amounts of beryllium and cases of berylliosis have been encountered in people who have no occupational contact with the material, but who merely lived in the general vicinity of a beryllium processing plant. Berylliosis occurs in an acute as well as a chronic form. The two are not necessarily related to each other.

ACUTE BERYLLIUM PNEUMONIA. An acute pneumonic reaction can occur as a result of intensive exposure to beryllium fumes. The pneumonia can be very severe and result in death, largely from asphyxia. The pathologic picture is that of an acute bronchitis and alveolitis with an outpouring of exudate in many of the alveoli throughout the lungs. In this respect the disease is similar to other chemical pneumonias. It differs from chronic berylliosis which is characterized by a granulomatous reaction.

The x-ray manifestations generally begin a number of days after the exposure and after the onset of cough and difficulty in breathing. The latent period may be as long as 3 weeks. The lesions are symmetrical and present as soft, poorly defined, patchy areas of consolidation in each lung. They may have the butterfly distribution often seen in pulmonary edema. There may simply be a slight haze in the hilar region on each side or both lung fields can become completely clouded. In some cases the film shows only a large patch of consolidation in the outer portion of the middle third of each lung. In others, each lower lobe presents a picture of irregular consolidation extending from the root to the diaphragm, similar to the picture of nonspecific bronchopneumonia. If the disease is confined to the apices, the appearance is like that of tuberculosis (Fig. 334).

Rarely, when both lungs become extensively involved, death occurs in the acute stage. In most instances, clearing occurs gradually, in patchy fashion, leaving irregular, poorly defined nodular shadows of varying size. These, in turn, usually resolve after a period of time, varying from several weeks to several months. In a relatively small percentage of cases, there is residual fibrosis and the disease may assume a chronic form.

CHRONIC BERYLLIOSIS. The onset of the chronic form of beryllium disease may be insidious and become manifest radiologically before the appearance of symptoms. Not all workers exposed to the dust develop the disease no matter how long the exposure, and there is a great variation in the extent and type of reaction in

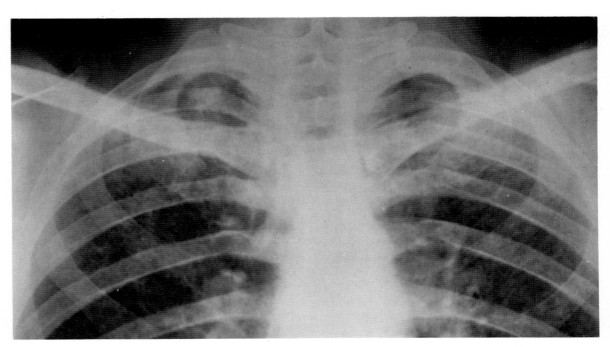

FIG. 334. BERYLLIOSIS: ACUTE FORM

Although berylliosis characteristically causes small nodular shadows which are distributed diffusely throughout the lungs, patchy lobular consolidations and diffuse interstitial infiltrations also occur, particularly during the acute phase of the disease. In this case, the distribution of the shadows at the apices and immediately beneath the clavicles causes an appearance identical with that of tuberculosis.

individuals who have been exposed to the same degree. Clinical and radiologic manifestations may not appear for a number of years after exposure to beryllium has ceased. Unlike other dust diseases, the lesions in chronic berylliosis may resolve to a considerable degree but complete clearing has not been reported.

Pathologically, chronic berylliosis is a granulomatous disease similar to other pneumoconioses. The granulomas are relatively small, usually less than 5 mm in diameter. In addition, there is inflammatory infiltration of the interstitial tissues of the lung, including the alveolar walls.

The roentgen picture in the early stages may disclose a granular, nodular, or reticular pattern. These changes generally involve the lung most intensively from the region below the clavicle downward almost to the level of the diaphragm. The granular pattern is caused by the faint shadows of multiple, minute granulomas, and is often associated with some degree of interstitial infiltration. The lungs may simply present a rather cloudy appearance, but close inspection of the film will usually reveal myriads of fine, stippled shadows. Larger nodules measuring anywhere from 2 to 5 mm in diameter may be present. They are poorly demarcated but are of rather uniform size in each individual case. In patients who have predominantly interstitial infiltrations throughout the lungs, nodules or granulations may not be evident, and the only change noted on the roentgen film is the presence of fine linear or reticular shadows.

In either case, there may be some areas of coalescence in the later stages, producing the appearance of consolidation. After a period of years, irregularly distributed areas of coarse, linear fibrosis, of variable density may appear. These are interspersed with areas of increased lucency, representing foci of emphysema. Occasionally the emphysema becomes quite marked, particularly at the bases. As a result of this and the contraction and coalescence of lesions in the upper portions of the lungs, the infiltration and fibrosis frequently are accentuated in the upper half of the pulmonary fields. Bullae may form at the bases and, in rare instances, a spontaneous pneumothorax occurs.

The hilar and mediastinal lymph nodes are involved in all stages of the disease, and often cause enlargement of the shadows at the lung roots. The appearance can be quite similar to sarcoidosis (Fig. 335). Calcification of the nodes has been described in a few instances. Superimposed respiratory infections are common, and can result in pulmonary insufficiency, particu-

larly in advanced cases. Cor pulmonale is not infrequent in patients with extensive fibrosis and emphysema and right heart failure may be the terminal event. The incidence of tuberculosis and neoplastic disease does not appear to be increased in berylliosis.

Thesaurosis. Thesaurosis is a name which has been applied to a disease thought to be caused by the inhalation of a synthetic resin used in hairsprays. The resin most commonly used is polyvinylpyrrolidone. The x-ray changes consist of either miliary or small nodular densities throughout the lungs which may be associated with streak-like shadows, representing more diffuse interstitial infiltrations and fibrosis. The hilar lymph nodes are enlarged in some cases. There is a tendency to resolution. Because of the similarity of the granulomatous lesions to those of sarcoidosis, the tendency to resolution and the low incidence among hairdressers, the question has been raised as to whether these are really cases of pneumoconiosis.

Benign Pneumoconioses. Benign pneumoconiosis refers to a condition in which inhaled particles are retained in the lungs without producing any reaction other than phagocytosis of the foreign material. There is no other evidence of inflammation and no fibrosis or granuloma formation. A certain amount of pneumoconiosis of this type is almost universal but rarely can be recognized except on pathologic examination. However, certain dusts, when present in the lungs in sufficient concentration, produce roentgen shadows which may present diagnostic difficulties. The dusts which cause the roentgen changes consist of heavy metals or their salts, and the shadows are due entirely to the accumulation of the radiopaque particles.

In view of the absence of reaction in the lung, it is generally considered that the benign pneumoconioses are not responsible for respiratory symptoms. Pulmonary function does not appear altered even in cases with extensive radiologic changes. Emphysema and chronic bronchitis, when present, are assumed to be purely coincidental. There is no increased incidence of tuberculosis in the benign pneumoconioses and, when it does occur, its course is not affected.

SIDEROSIS. Accumulation of iron, usually in the form of iron oxide, occurs in significant concentration in the lungs in a considerable percentage of workers who have had prolonged exposure to the dust. The iron oxide dust lies mainly in collections of phagocytes in the interstitial tissues of the lungs. Siderosis occurs in pure form in workers engaged in the manufacture of iron oxide, in metal grinders, and in metal polishers

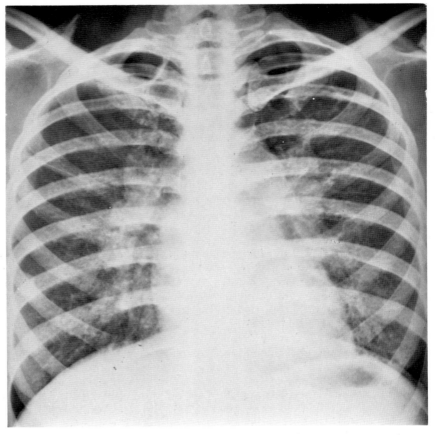

FIG. 335. CHRONIC BERYLLIOSIS

The hilar nodes are symmetrically enlarged. The lungs are studded with innumerable, extremely fine nodules. The vascular markings are obscured by the diffuse interstitial infiltrations. The short fissure is elevated and there is a large bulla at the right apex. The appearance cannot be differentiated from that of sarcoidosis.

who inhale rouge (ferrous oxide) used in the polishing operation. Iron ore miners may develop pure siderosis, but most often it is complicated by silicosis. The miners are exposed to free silica both from the quartz in the ore and from the dust produced by drilling operations through rock. Foundry workers who chip and grind castings and scale furnaces and flues, are generally exposed to silica as well as iron and therefore usually develop a mixed form of pneumoconiosis.

The x-ray appearance of the lungs in siderosis is characterized by the presence of tiny nodules, uniform in size and distribution, throughout the lungs. They rarely measure more than 2 mm in diameter and their outline appears to be quite regular. In addition, a fine reticular pattern may be observed in some cases (Fig. 336). There is no enlargement of the lymph nodes. The nodules do not tend to coalesce and there is no coarse reticulation or massive shadows from fibrosis. Since the iron oxide is largely situated within phago-

cytic cells, it is possible for the shadows to clear to some extent after exposure has ceased.

When there has been exposure to free silica in addition to iron dust and the roentgen changes consist only of small uniform nodules throughout the lungs, it is impossible to determine whether silicosis plays a part in the production of the roentgen shadows without prolonged observation. A marked increase in the size of the nodules, particularly in an irregular manner, or the development of coalescence or massive fibrotic lesions, or significant enlargement of the lymph nodes will indicate the presence of silicosis. Even in the absence of these changes, any enlargement of the nodules that occurs after the cessation of exposure to the dust likewise indicates silicosis.

STANNOSIS. Stannosis results from the inhalation of tin oxide, either from the handling of the raw ore (cassiterite) or from exposure to fumes during the smelting operation. The characteristic lesions of stannosis consist of extremely dense, discrete, small nodules, 1 mm in diameter, uniformly distributed throughout the lungs. There is no fibrous or inflammatory reaction and no evidence of emphysema. In addition to the nodules in the pulmonary parenchyma, there are also evidences of deposition of the tin oxide in the lymphatics. These are seen in the form of horizontal lines above the costophrenic sinuses, occasional short straight or oblique lines in other portions of the lung and a fine reticular pattern, representing networks of lymphatics containing accumulations of the dust. In some cases, the interlobar fissures and the borders of the mediastinum and diaphragm are partly outlined by a thin dense line caused by deposition of the radiopaque material in the subpleural lymphatics.

Since tin has a high atomic weight, even small nodules are extremely dense if they contain a high concentration of the dust. In the earlier stages, when the dust concentration is less, the nodules are not so dense. Larger nodules, up to 5 mm in diameter have been described in workers exposed to the fumes from molten ore. These are not very dense, but they can diminish in size and increase in density as they become older.

BARITOSIS. Baritosis occurs from the inhalation of dust containing barium sulfate crystals, either in the mining of the mineral (barite) or in the handling of barium sulfate in various indus-

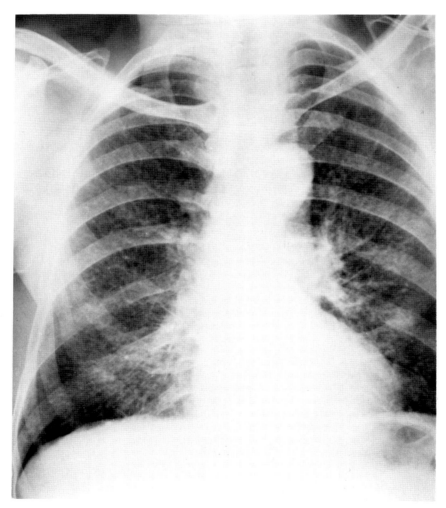

FIG. 336. SIDEROSIS

The patient was a welder for 45 years. Tiny nodules are distributed uniformly throughout both lungs. In addition, there are fine interstitial infiltrations producing a reticular pattern in places. The diaphragms show a normal curve and there is no evidence of emphysema. The hilar lymph nodes are not enlarged and the vessels at the lung roots are not dilated. Pulmonary function was not abnormal.

tries. The x-ray appearance is the same as that of stannosis. Of all the pneumoconioses, these two conditions produce the densest shadows. In each of them, as in some cases of siderosis, the nodules may diminish in size after cessation of exposure.

Diseases due to Organic Dusts

In general, two types of reaction to the inhalation of vegetable dusts can be distinguished. First, there is the typical asthmatic reaction associated with bronchial spasm and increased bronchial secretion, such as occurs in *byssinosis*. Second, there is the granulomatous bronchiolitis and diffuse interstitial reaction in the lungs characterized by *farmer's lung*.

Farmer's Lung. The clinical entity of farmer's lung consists of a disease of acute onset with dyspnea, cough, fever, chills, weight loss and severe sweats following exposure to moldy vegetation. The substances which usually cause the disease are moldy hay, fodder, silage and grain. The molds which are responsible for the disease are also found in tobacco, the dusts resulting from threshing (*thresher's lung*) and the compost used in growing mushrooms (*mushroom picker's disease*). Recently a similar condition has been found among pigeon breeders.

Pathologically, the disease is characterized by the presence of tiny granulomas distributed diffusely throughout the lungs, similar to the granulomatous lesions in sarcoidosis. In addition, there is a diffuse, fine infiltration of the alveolar walls and interstitial tissues of the lungs. In some cases, distinct granulomas are absent and the only pathologic manifestation is the diffuse infiltration of the interstitial tissues. The lymph nodes are not enlarged. The interstitial disease is responsible for the dyspnea.

The x-ray film of the chest can be negative even though pulmonary lesions are visible microscopically. As a rule, however, a fine stippling or granularity of the lungs is noted on careful inspection of the films. These changes are usually less marked at the extreme apices and the outer basal portions of the lungs. The remainder of the lungs appears to be more or less uniformly involved in most cases. In some cases the shadows present a more coarsely granular or even a nodular appearance similar to sarcoidosis (Fig. 337). However, the hilar lymph nodes are not enlarged. As a rule, the x-ray findings parallel the severity of the clinical symptoms.

The lesions progress as exposure to the vegetation continues. Coalescence of the infiltrations may occur with the production of large dense, homogeneous shadows. The symptoms subside after contact with the offending substances is discontinued, and this is accompanied by gradual resolution of the roentgen shadows. If exposure to the molds is continued over a long period, diffuse, irregular fibrosis occurs throughout the lungs together with emphysema, enlargement of the root shadows and cor pulmonale secondary to the pulmonary hypertension.

Bagassosis. Bagasse is the remains of the sugar cane after the sugar-containing juices have been extracted. Exposure to rotted bagasse produces a clinical, pathologic and roentgen picture identical with that of farmer's lung. As in farmer's lung, the disease is the result of a sensitivity reaction to molds and their products associated with decomposition of bagasse.

Maple Bark Disease. A number of cases of a condition apparently identical with farmer's lung has been described among workers engaged in stripping the bark off moldy maple logs. The mold has been identified as *Coniosporium corticale*.

Suberosis. This is an allergic alveolitis due to antigens in moldy cork dust. As with the other diseases in this group, the typical roentgen picture shows fine miliary densities throughout the lungs. These usually clear within a few weeks if the patient is removed from the offending dust. If the exposure continues, pulmonary fibrosis may result.

In some cases, where the clinical picture is that of acute asthma, the film may show evanescent patchy densities.

Byssinosis. Byssinosis differs from the diseases mentioned above in that it is characterized by typical asthma associated with bronchial spasm and increased bronchial secretion, usually without pulmonary infiltration. It is encountered principally in workers handling raw cotton, flax and hemp. It usually occurs after many years of exposure to the dust and is apparently the result of a sensitivity reaction. However, there remains some question as to the nature of the substance to which the body becomes sensitive. Whether the fibers themselves or molds or some other foreign material mixed with the fibers are the offending agents is the subject of controversy.

The symptoms usually develop in a characteristic pattern. They begin on return to work after a weekend. As the week goes on the asthma lessens and may disappear completely, although the exposure continues, only to recur at the beginning of the following work week. During this period there are no radiologic abnormalities except those that might be associated with acute asthma. After many years of continued exposure,

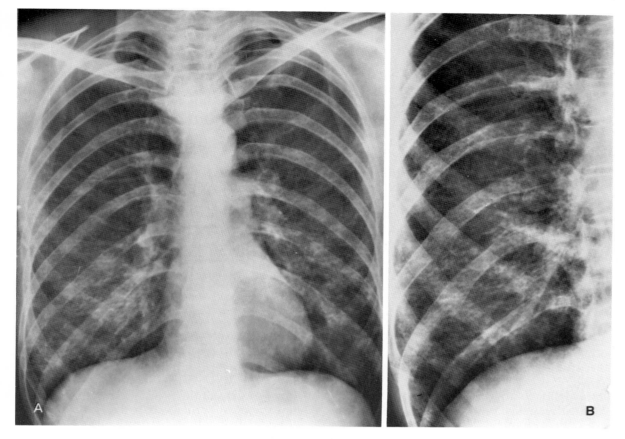

FIG. 337. FARMER'S LUNG

A 39 year old dairy farmer complained of shortness of breath during the winter months when he spent most of the day working in the barn. *A*: There are interstitial infiltrations throughout both lungs except for the extreme bases and apices. The hilar lymph nodes are not enlarged. *B*: Close-up of right lung, right oblique view. The infiltrations are more clearly defined. They consist of small nodules as well as fine, streak-like shadows. The lesions are distributed uniformly throughout the involved portions of the lungs.

the disease becomes chronic and is characterized by the changes associated with chronic bronchitis and emphysema and interstitial fibrosis of the lungs.

Irritative Gases, Fumes and Vapors

The reaction of the bronchi and lungs to these irritating substances depends upon the type of material inhaled as well as its concentration. In some instances there is an immediate reaction, characterized mainly by bronchial spasm and if the injury is severe, pulmonary edema. In others, the bronchial spasm is not so prominent a feature and the illness is characterized by an inflammatory reaction in the lungs. This may occur some time after the exposure.

Chlorine, Ammonia and Similar Irritants. Injurious exposure to these gases usually occurs

as a result of industrial accidents. Immediately after the inhalation of the gas, severe spasm of the bronchi frequently takes place, producing obstructive emphysema similar to that of an acute asthmatic attack. A varying degree of pulmonary edema then develops, depending upon the nature of the gas, its concentration and the duration of the exposure. The pathologic process usually consists of focal areas of hemorrhagic edema, and the roentgen film discloses small, ill-defined, patchy shadows distributed throughout the pulmonary fields. Foci of atelectasis are often present together with these shadows. Frequently there are areas of increased illumination of the lung between the edematous or atelectatic foci, representing local areas of obstructive emphysema. In the more severe cases the pulmonary fields appear gray as a result of more generalized edema of the lungs. Because of the replacement of the air by edema fluid in the alveoli adjacent to the blood vessels, the vascular markings are poorly delineated.

If the patient recovers from the acute stage, the edema fluid becomes absorbed and areas of consolidation, representing foci of chemical pneumonia, may become manifest. These areas assume the form of patches of lobular pneumonia of varying size. In some instances small nodular shadows similar to the acinar-nodose lesions of tuberculosis appear. The latter are the result of bronchiolitis which is associated with consolidation of pulmonary acini or single pulmonary lobules. When the medium-sized bronchi are severely inflamed, they are often plugged by exudate. Foci of atelectasis, represented by streak-like or broad, faint elongated shadows, may be present between the areas of consolidation. Secondary infection of the lung can result in a prolonged bronchopneumonia involving mainly the lower lobes. In some cases the pneumonia is suppurative in nature, and leads to bronchiectasis.

Severe destruction of the walls of the smallest bronchi and of the bronchioles is frequently followed by the formation of plugs of granulation tissue. These are the characteristic lesions of bronchiolitis obliterans. Partial obstruction of the finer bronchial branches may result in extensive bulla formation. One of the characteristics of the late effects of gas poisoning which we have encountered has been the presence of marked cylindrical bronchiectasis with a cutting off of the smaller bronchial branches. Distal to these, the lung appeared to be replaced by bullae and fine or coarse strands of fibrous tissue.

Phosgene. Phosgene was one of the poison gases commonly used during the first World War, and cases exhibiting the late results of this form of gas poisoning are still encountered. New cases of phosgene poisoning seen today usually occur from industrial accidents. Phosgene may be formed from contact of various chemicals with high heat. Thus, phosgene poisoning has occurred in the home from exposure of carbon tetrachloride and of paint thinners to high temperatures.

Exposure to phosgene frequently results in a delayed reaction in the lungs. No abnormality may be manifested for several hours following the exposure, after which outspoken pulmonary edema may develop. The roentgen changes are then the same as those which occur after the inhalation of chlorine and ammonia.

Silo-filler's Disease. Silo-filler's disease is a chemical pneumonia caused by the inhalation of nitrogen dioxide. The nitrogen dioxide is formed by the fermentation of chopped corn stalks or alfalfa in freshly loaded silos. The nitrogen dioxide forms for a period of only a week or 10 days, after which time it is usually dissipated.

Severe exposure to the gas may cause a fulminating illness resulting in death from pulmonary edema within a few days. Illness resulting from lesser exposure is characterized by cough and a feeling of tightness in the chest which improves within a few hours after removal from the gaseous atmosphere. The symptoms may then persist in a mild form for 2 to 4 weeks, only to be followed by the onset of more severe cough, chills, fever and dyspnea. Death from pulmonary insufficiency may then ensue, or the disease may gradually resolve. In some cases there is a latent period of several hours between the exposure and the onset of symptoms.

In the acute stage, the films usually show patchy shadows representing areas of pulmonary edema (Fig. 338). These are sometimes more marked in the upper lobes. The patches generally resolve gradually, but frequently leave small submiliary nodules resulting from a persistent bronchiolitis. The pathologic picture at this stage may be typical of bronchiolitis obliterans. Many of the densities may disappear over a period of 4 to 16 weeks and resolution proceeds until the lungs appear normal. In some cases, however, interstitial fibrosis persists and causes permanent roentgen changes. Sometimes the disease is progressive, there is confluence of the shadows with increasing opacification of the lungs, followed by death from pulmonary insufficiency.

Because silo-filler's disease and farmer's lung both occur in agricultural workers, and since the roentgen film in each may show small nodular densities throughout the lungs, these two diseases are often confused. It is even possible for a worker to develop farmer's lung from working in a silo. This happens when the silo is being emptied a considerable length of time after the nitrogen dioxide has been dissipated and the worker is exposed to the dust from moldy silage.

Nitrogen dioxide poisoning is occasionally encountered in occupations other than farming. Exposure to injurious amounts of the gas can occur in industries in which nitric acid is used, and in certain welding operations, especially those performed in confined spaces. The clinical, pathologic and roentgen features are identical with those of silo-filler's disease.

Mercury Vapor. Injurious exposure to mercury vapor has resulted from overheating metallic mercury. As in the case of phosgene, only mild respiratory symptoms may be present at first, and the patient becomes seriously ill with pul-

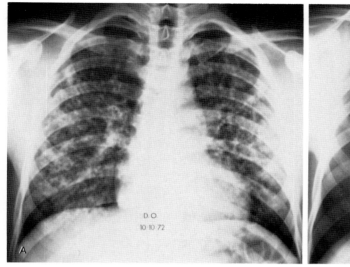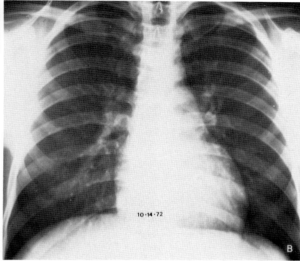

FIG. 338. SILO-FILLER'S DISEASE

A: The patient became extremely dyspneic shortly after being exposed to freshly fermented silage. Numerous small patches of consolidation are distributed throughout both lungs. Although the film is made in full inspiration, the diaphragm is depressed only to the level of the ninth rib posteriorly. *B*: Four days later, following treatment with steroids, both lungs are completely clear. The pulmonary compliance has returned to normal and the patient was able to lower his diaphragm to the level of the tenth rib. (Courtesy of Dr. A. Crummy, Madison, Wisconsin.)

monary edema a few hours later. Pathologically, the lungs show edema, infiltration of the interstitial tissues and a necrotizing bronchiolitis. The latter is responsible for obstructive emphysema which may be complicated by interstitial emphysema, mediastinal emphysema and pneumothorax.

In the few cases that have been described there were poorly defined densities intermingled with areas of increased lucency. In severe cases the pulmonary fields displayed a structureless haze resulting from pulmonary edema. In some cases death occurred within a short time, while in others there was complete resolution. We have observed a patient who developed persistent bronchitis with emphysema, but without pulmonary infiltration, after the initial inflammatory edema had disappeared.

Smoke and Flame. Most of our knowledge concerning the roentgen findings in injury to the bronchi and lungs by smoke and flame is derived from the experience in the Coconut Grove disaster (Schatzki). It is difficult to assess the relative roles of the smoke and the flame in the production of the lesions. In most of the patients there was definite evidence that flame was actually inhaled. However, smoke itself can cause pulmonary lesions. Hemorrhagic pulmonary edema has been produced experimentally by inhalation of smoke of relatively low temperature.

The pathologic picture is dominated by a se-

vere inflammatory reaction in the trachea, bronchi and bronchioles. The lungs themselves show areas of inflammatory edema of varying size together with foci of atelectasis and emphysema resulting from bronchial obstruction.

The roentgen changes that occur immediately are largely due to the pulmonary edema. These are characterized by ill-defined areas of patchy density or more diffuse clouding. This is soon followed by changes due to bronchial obstruction. Evidences of atelectasis may be seen within a few hours, but often do not appear until several days have elapsed. Apparently the obstruction of the bronchi is caused by secretions as well as by swelling of the bronchial mucous membrane. In some cases, complete collapse of one or more lobes occurs but generally the atelectasis is more focal in nature, resulting from the obstruction of smaller bronchi in both lungs. This produces fine streaks, either horizontal, oblique or vertical, representing plate-like areas of atelectasis viewed on end, or thicker, band-like shadows. Collapse of groups of lobules or portions of pulmonary segments may be manifested by more or less well-defined triangular shadows.

Foci of emphysema appear as small areas of increased lucency between the areas of atelectasis. Emphysema of an entire lobe may be caused by incomplete obstruction of a lobar bronchus by secretion. Two cases of mottling of the lungs with tiny shadows, similar to those of silo-filler's disease, have been described. These probably represent the lesions of bronchiolitis.

Complete clearing of the process usually occurs within 2 or 3 weeks but may be delayed for several months in exceptional cases.

Metal-Fume Fever. Chills and fever of short duration occur occasionally in workers exposed to the fumes of zinc, brass or magnesium. In contrast to poisoning from mercury vapor, no pulmonary lesions are demonstrable radiologically in these cases.

Inhalation of Liquids

Considerable quantities of bland isotonic liquids may be inhaled without obvious harm to the lung. Relatively large amounts of saline solution have been instilled into the bronchi without deleterious effects. However, the inhalation of large amounts of fluid in submersion produces asphyxia and reactive pulmonary edema. Inhalation of irritating liquids calls forth an inflammatory reaction and produces the roentgen appearance of a lobular pneumonia. The inhaled fluid may carry with it bacteria from the mouth or throat to produce infection in the lung. The susceptibility to infection is increased if the fluid is irritating and injures the lungs and bronchi.

Submersion. The roentgen picture of the lungs in near-drowning is caused by the rapid development of lobular areas of pulmonary edema. These produce puffy, ill-defined nodular shadows. In some instances, the densities are small and apparently involve only portions of lobules. In any case, the lesions are usually bilateral and symmetrical. Frequently the shadows are distributed uniformly throughout the lungs with some clouding of the lung between the nodules. In other cases, the middle third of the lungs is most involved with sparing of the apices and extreme bases. Although the lesions are bilateral, they may be preponderant on one side. There does not appear to be any difference between the roentgen findings of near-drowning in fresh water and sea water.

In the cases uncomplicated by infection, resolution generally occurs within a week but the shadows may clear within a day or two, leaving only a few atelectatic streaks. When severe infection is superimposed, the picture may be that of a suppurative bronchopneumonia. In patients with poor dental hygiene, inhalation of organisms from the mouth can result in a diffuse, gangrenous bronchopneumonia, or, if the infection is more localized, a putrid lung abscess.

Aspiration of Blood. When there is bleeding from a pulmonary cavity or from a bronchus, the blood is usually coughed up promptly. In some instances, blood is aspirated and may produce roentgen changes that complicate the picture. The blood produces roentgen shadows both because of its presence in the alveoli and because of blockage of bronchi. The alveolar inundation results in small fluffy shadows which have a tendency to confluence (Fig. 339). In massive bleeding these shadows may be bilateral, but they are usually unilateral, occurring on the side in which the bleeding originates. The shadows may be confused with extension of the disease which caused the bleeding, such as tuberculosis or neoplasm. However, absorption of the blood, which usually takes place rapidly, clarifies the diagnosis within a few days.

Aspirated blood may clot within a bronchus and produce either obstructive emphysema or atelectasis. While these changes are usually short lived, the blood clot may remain for one or more weeks. The persistent atelectasis resulting from this can easily lead to an error in diagnosis, particularly in cases of benign bronchial bleeding (Fig. 209).

Persistent or progressive nodular lesions have been reported in a few instances of aspiration of blood. These were found to be caused by tissue reaction to broken-down blood resulting in hemosiderosis. Such instances are exceedingly rare.

Aspiration of Gastric Contents. Inhalation of vomitus takes place most frequently during the course of surgical anesthesia or during alcoholic stupor. It can also occur in the conscious infant. The pathologic effect results from the action of the hydrochloric acid in the vomitus upon the lung and upon the bronchi. The irritating effect of the acid on the alveoli causes an inflammatory pulmonary edema, producing scattered, ill-defined densities in the lungs. The lesions are most often bilateral but not uncommonly are limited to only one lung or part of a lung. If the aspiration occurred when the patient was lying on his back, the superior segment of the lower lobe may be most intensively involved, while if the patient was lying on his side, the lesions may be confined to the outer portion of an upper lobe.

Severe injury to the bronchial mucosa by the acid produces a necrotizing bronchitis which results in bronchial obstruction of varying degree. The changes due to obstruction of bronchi are superimposed upon those resulting from the inflammatory edema. Areas of lucency representing obstructive emphysema become interspersed with the shadows caused by the chemical pneu-

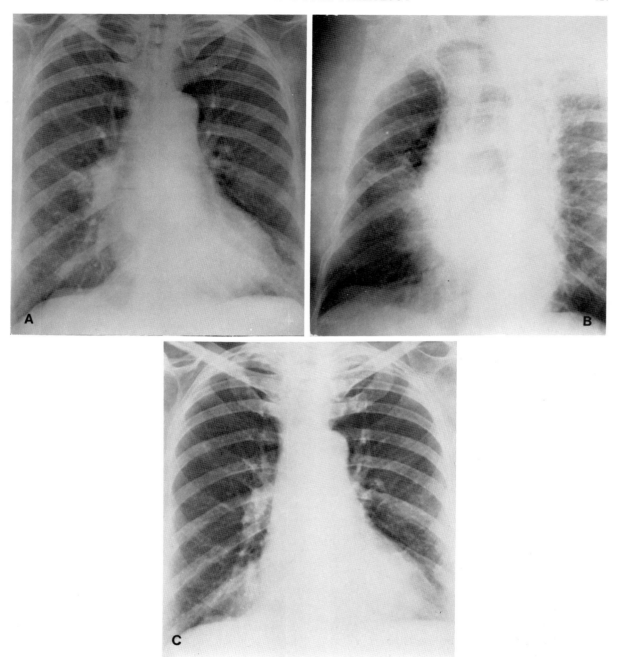

FIG. 339. BLOOD INUNDATION

A: A 45 year old woman with hypertension was admitted to the hospital following expectoration of a large amount of bright red blood. The frontal film shows a density at the root of the right lung suggesting a neoplasm. *B*: The left oblique view shows consolidation of the mesial segment of the middle lobe. In the frontal view, this shadow was projected over the hilum and simulated an abnormality of the lung root. Bronchoscopy disclosed blood clot adherent to the wall of the right bronchus but no endobronchial lesion. *C*: The film made several days later, during which time the patient coughed up a moderate amount of brownish sputum, shows the shadow over the right root to have disappeared. The absence of fever or other evidence of infection indicates that the shadow was due to filling of alveoli with blood resulting from the benign bronchial bleed, rather than pneumonia.

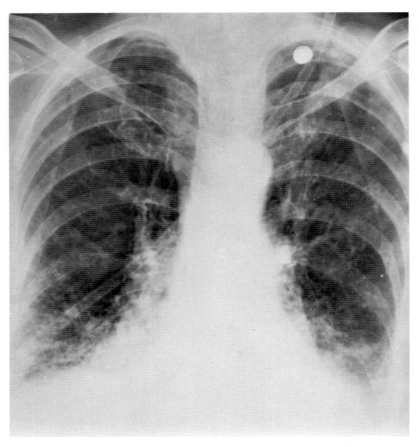

FIG. 340. MENDELSON'S SYNDROME

An 81 year old female with an organic mental syndrome vomited and became cyanotic immediately after aspiration of the vomitus. Coarse infiltrations are present at both bases with confluence of the shadows in the mesial part of the right lower lobe. Both lung roots are depressed indicating atelectasis in association with the bilateral pneumonia.

monia. Many small bronchi become completely occluded and this soon causes shrinkage of the involved portion of lung. The roentgen appearance then is that of an atelectatic pneumonia (Fig. 340). The bronchial obstruction may be accentuated by inhalation of solid particles in the vomitus.

The injury to the lung and small bronchi by the irritating gastric juice makes them more susceptible to infection by bacteria carried with the aspirate. This results in prolongation of the pneumonia which is often suppurative in nature.

The clinical and pathologic picture resulting from aspiration of acid gastric contents (Mendelson's syndrome) differs from the picture caused by aspiration from an esophageal diverticulum. In the latter instance only a relatively small amount of material, free of acid is aspirated. The roentgen film usually shows only a small area of pneumonia which is of bacterial rather than chemical origin. It is usually of a suppurative nature and tends to run a prolonged course.

Aspiration of Corrosive Liquids. This occurs most frequently in attempted suicides. The injury to the throat by the corrosive liquid interferes with the swallowing reflex and leads to aspiration of some of the material. We have seen localized areas of consolidation which have undergone necrosis and cavity formation following the ingestion of Lysol.

Hydrocarbon Pneumonia. Pneumonia following the ingestion of kerosene or other hydrocarbons, such as gasoline, turpentine, lighter fluid and insecticides occurs with considerable frequency in young children. The pneumonia is probably caused by aspiration of some of the material as it is being swallowed.

The radiographic changes have been observed within a half hour after the accident. They usually consist of soft, poorly delineated, mottled densities which have a tendency to confluence.

Most often these involve the basal portions of both lungs but not infrequently the lesions are confined to the right lower lobe. When the lesions are limited to the superior segment of the lower lobe, the roentgen appearance suggests perihilar infiltration. Resolution is slow and the shadows may persist for several weeks after the clinical symptoms have disappeared. Pneumatoceles occur in occasional cases, even in the absence of infection. They may be complicated by pneumothorax or pneumomediastinum.

Lipid Pneumonia (Mineral Oil Pneumonia). The term lipid pneumonia has been used to refer to two different conditions, one endogenous and the other exogenous. The endogenous disease is characterized by the deposition of fatty substances, mainly cholesterol, in the necrotic foci of suppurative pneumonia. The exogenous disease is due to the inhalation of oily substances. The most common of these is mineral oil. To obviate confusion it seems better to use the term "mineral oil pneumonia" when referring to the lesion produced by the inhalation of this material.

Persons who habitually take mineral oil, particularly in large doses, or those who use mineral oil in the form of sprays or nose drops over a long period of time frequently inhale some of the oil. Much of the aspiration takes place during sleep following regurgitation of oil ingested before retiring. It occurs mostly in the aged, particularly those with cerebral arteriosclerosis, whose laryngeal defensive mechanisms are not well coordinated. We have also observed several cases of mineral oil pneumonia in patients with cardiospasm and with esophageal diverticula.

Since the oil is bland, its passage into the lungs is unnoticed. However, it does incite a reaction within the lung, resulting in a chronic fibrosing pneumonia. The droplets of oil and the reactive elements are distributed in a focal manner in the portion of lung that is affected. The foci may be of acinar distribution or involve groups of alveoli between which normal air-containing alveoli are interspaced. A granulomatous reaction occurs not only in the alveoli, but in the small bronchi as well and there is a tendency to secondary infection. Eventually fibrosis takes place and is often progressive, even after the intake of mineral oil has ceased.

The portions of the lung that are affected are those which are dependent at the time of the aspiration. The basal segments of the lower lobes are the most frequent site of the disease. The middle lobe, the lingula, and the outer portions of the upper lobes, are not infrequently involved, presumably from aspiration of the oil while the patient was lying on the side. However, it is most unusual to have lesions in these locations without additional lesions in the lower lobes. Usually the lesions are bilateral although they may be more prominent on one side. Those in the left lower lobe may be overlooked because they are hidden behind the heart.

The roentgen picture is varied. The disease may be manifested by a fairly large, rather homogeneous shadow of moderate density at the base of one lung, with a few smaller, ill-defined, patchy densities at the opposite base. The homogeneous shadow usually has an unusual quality which distinguishes it from the consolidation of lobar pneumonia. Not only is it somewhat less dense but on careful inspection it appears to have a ground glass or spun glass appearance. This is due to the presence of numerous air-containing alveoli scattered throughout the diseased area. The patchy consolidation of the lower lobes may be associated with an additional small density in the outer portion of an upper lobe. Persistent shadows of this type and distribution, particularly in patients with few or no clinical symptoms should arouse the suspicion of mineral oil pneumonia (Fig. 341). The history of the use of mineral oil must be sought specifically. Rarely will it be volunteered by the patient because he does not associate his use of mineral oil with disease of the lungs.

As the disease progresses, there is increasing fibrosis which causes distortion of the pulmonary markings. Streak-like shadows may appear not only within the lesion but also in the outer portion of the lower lobes, representing fibrosis and infiltration in the interlobular septa (Kerley B lines). The lesions, in general, may become more sharply demarcated although irregular.

Occasionally the lesion appears to be single, dense and quite well demarcated. It is then indistinguishable from a primary bronchogenic neoplasm (Fig. 342). Careful inspection of the film may disclose additional small infiltrations in the lower portion of the outer part of the upper lobe or a lesion behind the heart. The latter may be visible only on the left oblique projection or by the use of tomography. The presence of such an additioal lesion will serve to exclude a primary carcinoma from consideration and suggest the possibility of mineral oil pneumonia. Several fairly well demarcated small, rather dense shadows, representing mineral oil granulomas, may resemble metastatic neoplasms. Not uncommonly one or more of the lesions has a bizarre shape, and usually most of them have an irregular border as a result of the interstitial fibrosis which characterizes granulomatous disease.

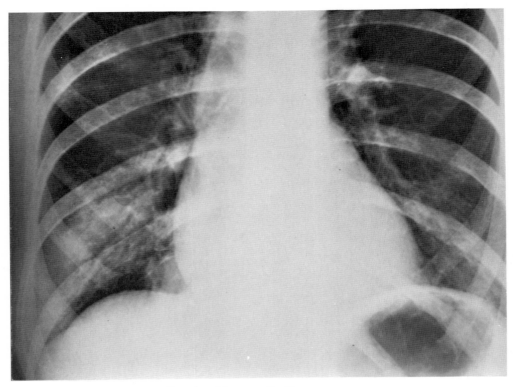

FIG. 341. MINERAL OIL PNEUMONIA

There is a triangular area of consolidation in the outer part of the right lower lobe together with nodular lesions in the mesial portion of the lobe and in the axillary part of the upper lobe. The left lung was free of disease. The shadows were present at a routine x-ray examination 2 years previously. The patient was asymptomatic and there was little change in the lesions during this period. He had been taking mineral oil for many years. The unilateral distribution was due to the fact that he always slept on his right side.

The lesions may increase in size and number over a period of years. A sudden increase in the size of the shadow is usually caused by superimposed infection. Shrinkage of the lesion may occur from granulomatous change involving the walls of the small bronchi, resulting in atelectasis. This, as well as progressive fibrosis, causes an increase in the density of the shadows. The lesions do not show a tendency to resolution. We have observed calcification to develop within the lesion in two cases.

Bronchographic Contrast Material. IO-DIZED OIL. Although the instillation of iodized oil into the bronchi is generally an innocuous procedure, cases are occasionally encountered in which there is a reaction to the oil. (Fig. 343). The reactions vary in severity. Most often they result in the formation of small foci of consolidation about collections of oil that have entered the alveoli. These are depicted as small nodular shadows not unlike the acinar-nodose lesions of tuberculosis. Careful examination of the shadows will show them to have a granular quality, caused by extremely dense, tiny areas within the nodules, representing oil in the alveoli. If the nodules are extremely small, they may be mistaken for miliary tubercles unless a careful search is made for the dense, granular deposits within them. In other cases there is a more severe reaction associated with more or less massive consolidation of the lung. If a large amount of oil is used, particularly in mapping the bronchi of both lungs, there may be a severe lobular bronchopneumonia, represented by ill-defined, patchy densities distributed throughout the lungs. This is largely due to a sensitivity reaction to the oil. In some cases the oil causes spread of a preexisting bronchopulmonary infection.

Oil that enters the bronchioles and alveoli may remain there for weeks or months without exciting an inflammatory reaction. Numerous small, sharply defined, extremely dense, irregular shadows, representing radioopaque material in clusters of bronchioles and alveoli, are seen in the periphery of the lung. Retention of the oil is most apt to occur in portions of the lung affected by chronic inflammatory disease and in the region of pleural adhesions, where motion and aeration of the lung are limited.

Errors can be made by confusing the shadows of iodized oil pneumonia with other diseases. Thus, erroneous diagnoses of metastatic neoplasm and of inflammatory diseases have been made when the roentgenologist was unaware that iodized oil had been injected. These errors may be avoided by inquiring concerning the previous injection of iodized oil whenever unusual shadows are found, by obtaining previous films for comparison, and by close examination of the film for the characteristic, sharply defined, extremely tiny, very dense granules of iodized oil within the shadows of alveolar consolidation.

Aqueous solutions of iodinated compounds have been used because they are rapidly absorbed. However, in general, they are quite irritating to the bronchi.

BARIUM SULFATE SUSPENSION. Barium sulfate is more inert than iodized oil and therefore causes less reaction. However, foreign body granulomas do occur and may persist for a long time. There is a greater tendency for retention of the barium within the alveoli and it may be visible on the film for many months in patients in whom the lung is otherwise normal.

Fibrosing Diseases of the Lungs

More or less extensive fibrosis occurs in the lungs in the chronic, suppurative diseases, such as bronchiectasis, lung abscess, and in fungous infections, as well as tuberculosis, chronic nonspecific bronchial infections, and pneumoconiosis. These diseases are considered separately because they have other important connotations. However, there remains a group of diseases in which fibrosis of the lung is the outstanding

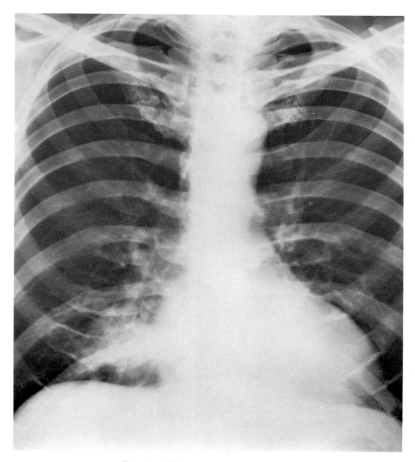

FIG. 342. MINERAL OIL PNEUMONIA

The shadow at the base of the right lung was thought to be a carcinoma. However, when specifically questioned, the patient admitted that he had been taking a large gulp of mineral oil directly from the bottle every night. A chest film made several years previously was located and showed the same shadow.

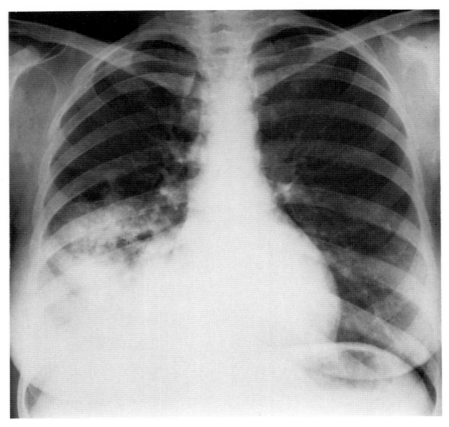

FIG. 343. LIPIODOL PNEUMONIA

The film made several days following bronchography shows confluent lobular areas of consolidation throughout the right middle and lower lobes. The fine, stippled densities within the upper part of the shadow represent oil retained in the alveoli. There was a severe febrile reaction following injection of the oil. Several weeks were required for resolution of the process.

feature. In practically all instances, the fibrosis is associated with some degree of cellular infiltration, so that the shadows on the film represent inflammatory infiltrate as well as fibrosis.

The fibrous tissue in the lungs in these diseases is situated mainly about the bronchi and blood vessels and in the interlobular and alveolar septa. The fibrosis, therefore, tends to result in linear densities that converge toward the lung root along with the shadows of the blood vessels. It is sometimes difficult to differentiate fibrosis from dilated vessels. The film may seem to show only accentuation of the pulmonary markings. However, in the case of fibrosis, the markings appear irregular and do not show the typical branching one would expect if they represented blood vessels. In addition, the lungs present a reticulated appearance, caused by the fibrosis of the finer septa. This is best seen in the outer portions of the pulmonary fields. Frequently the lung appears stippled with fine nodular shadows, representing either small granulomatous lesions or local accentuations of the fibrotic process. If, in addition, there has been organization of exudate within the alveoli or atelectasis from obstruction of small bronchi or bronchioles, coarse, thick, dense, fibrous strands or solid patches of fibrosis appear.

The focal contraction of innumerable small portions of the lung results in compensatory emphysema of the remaining pulmonary tissue. Partial obstruction of tiny bronchi and bronchioles produces small areas of obstructive emphysema throughout the lungs. Occasionally, sizeable bullae are formed.

Extensive fibrosis causes shrinkage of the lungs and results in elevation of the diaphragm if the associated emphysematous changes are not marked. Because of the rigidity and diminished compliance of the lungs, the diaphragm cannot descend to its usual level during inspiration. During expiration, however, the increased negative-pressure in the pleural space resulting from the diminution in lung volume causes a markedly increased elevation of the diaphragm. Therefore, the diaphragm is abnormally high in both phases of respiration, although its excursion may be normal even when fibrosis is extensive. If the fibrosis is associated with a considerable degree of obstructive emphysema, expiration is interfered with, the diaphragms do not rise properly and their excursion becomes smaller.

Kinking of smaller bronchi can result in the formation of bullae. Rupture of one of these produces a pneumothorax. Since all of the fibrosing diseases, with the exception of radiation fibrosis and some solitary granulomas, involve both lungs, bilateral pneumothorax is not rare.

Narrowing of the small pulmonary vessels is constantly present in these diseases. When extensive, obstruction to the flow of blood through the lungs results in pulmonary arterial hypertension with dilatation of the major pulmonary arteries and enlargement of the hilar shadows.

Sarcoidosis

Boeck's sarcoid, or sarcoidosis, is a generalized disease characterized by the formation of granulomas consisting of accumulations of noncaseating epithelioid tubercles. The cause is unknown. It is most common in the third and fourth decade but the disease has been found in early infancy and in elderly persons. It is particularly common in the negro race.

In the early stages of the disease, the most striking changes are usually found in the mediastinal and hilar lymph nodes, which frequently become markedly enlarged. At this time the lungs may also show more or less extensive infiltrations of the interstitial tissues with epithelioid tubercles. These may be conglomerated into granulomatous masses, or they may be scattered in the form of miliary tubercles. The bronchi are often involved, but the changes in the mucosa and within the bronchial wall may be detectable only by microscopic examination. Occasionally, bronchial obstruction results from a heaping up of the epithelioid granulomatous tissue which occludes the lumen, or by fibrotic stricture of the bronchial wall.

The disease often resolves spontaneously. In some cases, however, fibrosis occurs. The process may come to a standstill at this stage, leaving an interstitial, partly hyaline fibrosis without any evidence of activity. On the other hand, the epithelioid tubercles may increase in number as the fibrosis takes place, resulting in progressive sarcoidosis.

In many instances, the stage of fibrosis is associated with cystic changes in the lungs. Usually these take the form of bullae, but in some instances microcystic changes develop, producing the appearance of honeycomb lung. When the fibrosis is extensive, the pulmonary vascular bed is diminished, resulting in pulmonary hypertension, which can lead to right heart failure. Cardiac failure may also result from direct involvement of the heart muscle by the granulomatous disease.

Significant abnormalities are present on the roentgen film of the chest in the great majority of cases of sarcoidosis. Although the disease is a generalized one, and involves multiple organs, the lesions in the chest may be the only ones that are manifest. Not infrequently they are first found on a routine chest film in patients who have no clinical symptoms of any kind.

Sarcoidosis manifests itself radiologically in the chest in three main forms: first, that which is characterized by enlargement of the lymph nodes; second, cases showing pulmonary infiltrations with or without enlargement of the lymph nodes; and third, those in which pulmonary fibrosis is predominant.

Perhaps the most striking roentgen feature of sarcoidosis is the bilaterality and symmetry of the pulmonary and mediastinal lesions. In the occasional case when the lesions are unilateral, they usually represent a transient stage of the disease. Previous films may show the lesions to have been bilateral originally, or later films may show the lesions to become bilateral as the disease progresses.

Lymph Node Enlargement. The most frequent roentgen manifestation of sarcoidosis is enlargement of the lymph nodes. This is the sole finding in about half of the cases at the first roentgen examination. In over half of the remainder, enlarged nodes are recognizable in addition to pulmonary infiltrations and fibrosis. In only about 20% of the cases are changes in the lungs seen without detectable lymph node enlargement at the time of the first examination.

Characteristically, the films show enlargement of multiple groups of nodes rather than a single large mass jutting out from the mediastinum. Coalescence of these groups of nodes frequently results in the formation of large, bilateral, lobulated masses to which the term, Kartoffelknoten (potato nodes), has been applied (Fig. 344).

The hilar nodes are practically always involved on both sides in symmetrical fashion. The symmetry of the lesions is clearly demonstrable in the case of the bronchopulmonary lymph nodes which jut out from the lung roots and often simulate large pulmonary vessels. Above them, the shadows of large tracheobronchial nodes are

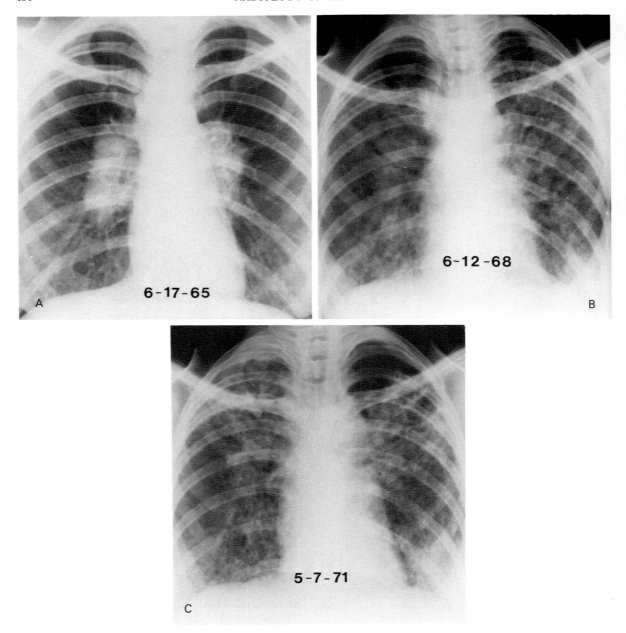

FIG. 344. SARCOIDOSIS: PROGRESSIVE CHANGES

A: The nodes at both hila are symmetrically enlarged. They are extremely large and lobulated. In addition, there is a bulge of the right border of the superior mediastinum and the aortic knob is obscured, indicating enlargement of the paratracheal lymph nodes. The lungs appear normal. This pattern of nodal enlargement is extremely rare in anything but sarcoidosis. *B*: Three years later, coarse infiltrations are present throughout both lungs. The hilar nodes have receded but the paratracheal nodes are still enlarged. *C*: After another 3 years without treatment, the shadows in the lungs appear more streak-like and are better defined, indicating that fibrosis has taken place. Bullae have developed in the upper part of the left upper lobe.

practically always visible, although they are more easily recognizable on the right side. Enlargement of the paratracheal nodes is less common. They are much more frequently seen only on the right side, possibly because the left paratracheal chain is often obscured by the aorta. Demonstrable enlargement of the paratracheal nodes alone is rare. There is almost always concomitant enlargement of the hilar lymph nodes. The subcarinal nodes are regularly involved in the disease but are usually not recognizable on the films.

Enlarged hilar nodes have a knobby appearance. Often their contour is composed of a series of convex arcs, differing from the shadows of the vessels at the hilum. The latter may have a partly convex border when they run at an angle to the plane of the film, but have straight sides where they lie in a parallel plane. When the hilar vessels are dilated, they may simulate enlarged lymph nodes in the frontal projection. However, examination in a slight oblique view or in kyphotic or lordotic projections will almost always disclose tapering and branching of the shadows when they represent the pulmonary vessels. Enlarged lymph nodes maintain their knobby appearance in all views. Tomograms are helpful in making the differentiation. Enlargement of the hilar nodes is sometimes best appreciated on the lateral view, but care must be taken to differentiate them from hilar vessels, in this projection. In general, the shadows of the lymph nodes are larger than those of the blood vessels and extend posterior as well as anterior to the bronchus.

Enlarged right paratracheal nodes often produce only a small localized protuberance along the straight border of the upper mediastinum. This should not be confused with the shadow of a prominent azygos vein, which is situated lower down, at the tracheobronchial angle.

Large nodes in the left tracheobronchial region are more difficult to recognize. They may be identified by careful examination of the aortic knob. If the nodes are very large, they can be confused with the aortic knob. However, the shadow of the knob, which lies posterior to the nodes, is usually visible within the shadow produced by the nodes if the film is not underexposed. When the nodes are not large, they do not extend beyond the knob and do not form the border of the mediastinum. In this instance, the density of the aortic knob, which should be homogeneous, is often uneven because the dense, irregular shadow of the mass of enlarged nodes is projected within it.

There are a few lymph nodes in the mediastinum adjacent to the superior surface of the left side of the aortic arch. When these nodes are enlarged, they fill in the normally sharp angle between the superior aspect of the aortic knob and the left border of the upper mediastinum. Since they lie in the same plane as the aorta, the mesial portion of the superior border of the knob is obscured. In some instances the shadow of the knob appears to run upward and mesially to merge with the superior mediastinum.

When there is extensive pulmonary fibrosis, the outlines of enlarged nodes are frequently obscured. Demonstration of these nodes may be crucial in the differential diagnosis of the fibrosing disease. Enlargement of the nodes can frequently be recognized because of an increased density of the mediastinal shadow in the frontal projection, or an increase in the width of the normal paratracheal shadow in the oblique view. When the subcarinal nodes are very large, they often produce an increase in the density of the upper part of the cardiac shadow immediately below the tracheal bifurcation. The film may show splaying of the interbronchial angle with elevation of the left main bronchus.

The development of enlarged nodes seems to occur over a short period of time. Usually, by the time the roentgen film of the chest is made in a patient with sarcoidosis, the lymph nodes have reached their maximum size and distribution. Patients have been observed with the full-blown roentgen manifestations of sarcoidosis only several months after a normal routine chest film.

Most commonly, the nodes undergo spontaneous regression. The period of nodal regression is comparatively prolonged. Nevertheless, in the majority of cases the nodes return to normal size within 1 or 2 years. In some instances, regression takes place over a period of 5 or more years and, occasionally, the nodes remain enlarged indefinitely. Frequently they regress when pulmonary infiltrations appear (Fig. 344). After spontaneous regression is complete, recurrence of lymph node enlargement is not to be expected.

The picture of symmetrical enlargement of the hilar lymph nodes, with or without enlargement of the paratracheal nodes on one or both sides, is almost pathognomonic of sarcoidosis. Exceptions are rare, but do occur, particularly in berylliosis (Fig. 335), lymphatic leukemia, reticulum cell sarcoma and infectious mononucleosis. Enlargement of the mediastinal shadow in the right paratracheal region without concomitant enlargement of the hilar lymph nodes on both sides is unusual in sarcoidosis. Unilateral involvement of the hilar nodes (Fig. 345) is even more uncommon. Unilateral enlargement of the lymph nodes, regardless of their level, is more characteristic of pulmonary tuberculosis, Hodgkin's disease or bronchogenic carcinoma. Lymphosarcoma usually produces a single large mass in the mediastinum rather than enlargement of individual groups of nodes. Bilateral lymph node involvement occurs occasionally in tuberculosis, but it is rarely symmetrical. The anterior mediastinum is characteristically spared in sarcoidosis even when the disease is most extensive. This is in contradistinction to Hodgkin's disease

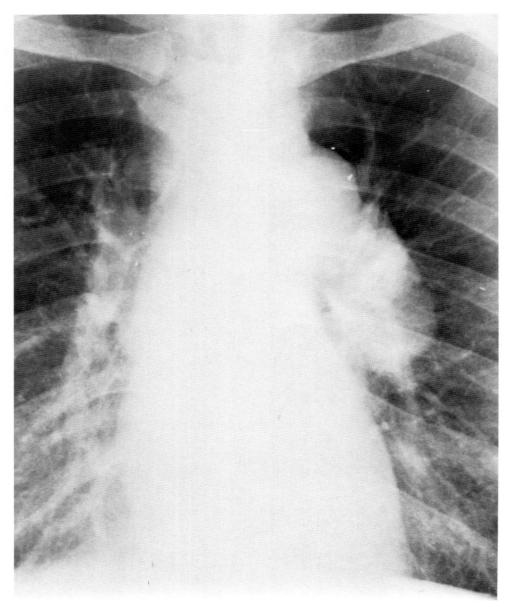

FIG. 345. UNILATERAL NODE ENLARGEMENT IN SARCOIDOSIS

The mass at the left hilum represents a group of large lymph nodes. The lower portion of the mass is separated from the heart by a strip of radiolucent lung. This is a rather common finding in sarcoidosis and is indicative of involvement of intercalated lymph nodes. The patient was thought to have Hodgkin's disease. Mediastinoscopy was uninformative. The diagnosis of sarcoidosis was made at thoracotomy.

and bronchogenic carcinoma. The lateral view, for inspection of the anterior mediastinum, is therefore most valuable in the differential diagnosis.

Pulmonary Infiltration. The interstitial tissues of the lung are the seat of infiltration with noncaseating tubercles in almost all cases of sarcoidosis. However, the pulmonary infiltrations cannot be visualized on the roentgen film in half of the cases when first seen, even though large lymph nodes are clearly evident. Pulmonary function studies performed on patients whose films show only large hilar or mediastinal nodes disclose interference with diffusion of oxygen through the alveolar walls, indicating significant involvement of the lungs in most of them.

In some cases, extremely fine infiltrations can be seen early in the disease, particularly in the neighborhood of the lung roots. In others, the pulmonary infiltrations become manifest later. The infiltrations are practically always bilateral and symmetrical in distribution. They are usually either in the form of miliary shadows, or larger nodules associated with coarse irregular infiltrations. Discrete, large, nodular lesions, patchy densities or massive lesions also occur.

Miliary infiltrations are tiny, measuring 1 mm or less in diameter. It is difficult to visualize the individual lesions, but because they are so numerous, they impart a granular appearance to the pulmonary fields. The miliary deposits occur either with or without demonstrable enlargement of hilar and mediastinal nodes. They may be distributed uniformly throughout the lungs (Fig. 346), but most frequently appear confined to the midlung fields.

The miliary lesions usually resolve completely within a year, but sometimes an extremely fine interstitial fibrosis remains. Rarely, the miliary shadows persist as tiny, well-demarcated nodules.

Coarse nodulation and infiltration of the lungs also occur with or without concomitant enlargement of the lymph nodes. The nodules usually measure up to about 5 mm in diameter. They may begin as extremely soft, patchy shadows, as in bronchopneumonia, and later become more defined. However, more commonly, they remain poorly demarcated and irregular, and are associated with diffuse, coarse or fine interstitial infiltrations throughout the lungs. The lesions tend to be most predominant in the midlung fields but they may be more numerous at the bases. Involvement of the basal portion of the lungs alone is extremely rare. In some cases, coarse infiltrations are limited to the infraclavi-

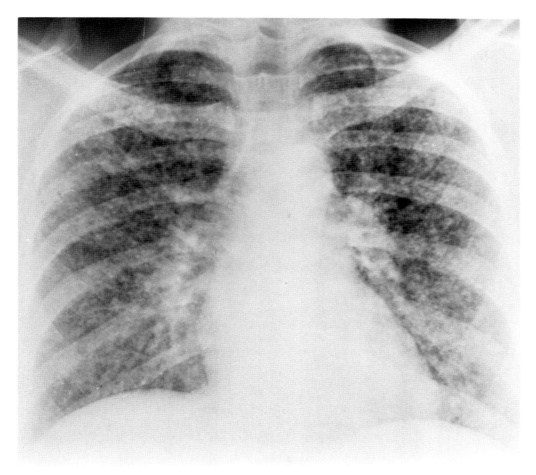

FIG. 346. DIFFUSE MILIARY SARCOIDOSIS

Both lungs are uniformly studded with miliary and submiliary nodules. There is no enlargement of the hilar or mediastinal nodes.

cular region of each lung. Although such an appearance occurs in hematogenous tuberculosis, this pattern of infiltration is much more common in sarcoidosis. In hematogenous tuberculosis, the apices are almost always involved (Fig. 299). In sarcoidosis the infraclavicular lesions are often associated with diffuse miliary nodules distributed throughout the remainder of the lungs (Fig. 347), although the apices are usually spared. In bronchogenous spread of tuberculosis, a cavity is almost always demonstrable and the lesions are not apt to be symmetrical.

Larger nodular lesions, measuring up to a few centimeters in diameter, are unusual. They are generally few in number and are irregularly distributed (Fig. 348). The margins are almost always indistinct and are usually associated with diffuse interstitial infiltrations. The indistinctness of the margins of the nodules and the concomitant diffuse pulmonary infiltration should lead to a suspicion of sarcoidosis rather than metastatic neoplasm. On extremely rare occasions, however, the nodules have a sharply demarcated border, making the differentiation from metastatic neoplasm impossible from the roentgenograms.

Massive lesions having the appearance of large areas of consolidation also occur. The shadows are rather homogeneous and poorly demarcated. While the massive lesions are sometimes unilateral, they are always associated with lesser densities in both lungs. As in silicosis, the massive lesions may form from the coalescence of smaller nodules but can also result from a complicating nonspecific pneumonia.

Calcification of the lesions in sarcoidosis is extremely rare. We have observed deposition of calcium within miliary lesions in one instance. Kerley has described eggshell calcifications of the mediastinal lymph nodes and central calcification within the pulmonary nodules.

Cavitation within a sarcoid nodule is also extremely rare and probably results from ischemic necrosis. When lucencies are seen on the film, they almost always represent bullae rather than true pulmonary cavities. In some instances, cavitation occurs within an area of suppurative bronchopneumonia complicating the sarcoidosis.

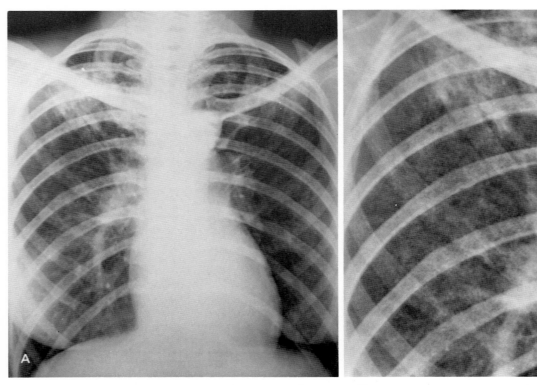

FIG. 347. SARCOIDOSIS SIMULATING TUBERCULOSIS

A: There is a patchy area of confluent infiltration beneath each clavicle. Extremely fine infiltrations are present throughout the remainder of the lungs. The apical regions are clear. There is some accentuation of the hilar shadow on the right side but this is insufficient for the diagnosis of large lymph nodes. *B:* Close-up of the right upper lobe shows the fine infiltrations to be made up of miliary nodules.

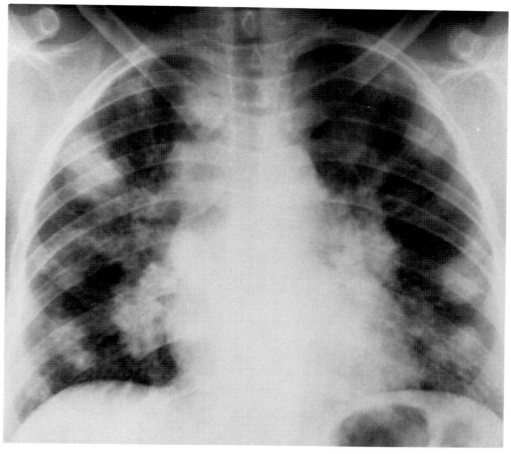

FIG. 348. LARGE NODULES IN SARCOIDOSIS

Several rather poorly demarcated nodules of varying size are present in both lungs. There is marked enlargement of the right paratracheal nodes. The hilar nodes are also enlarged. Despite the extent of the pulmonary lesions, there is relatively little diffuse interstitial infiltration.

Fibrosis. If the pulmonary infiltrations do not resolve completely, fibrosis eventually takes place. Fibrosis may be manifested by extremely fine shadows that are easily overlooked, or by coarse, dense, strandlike shadows. The fibrotic stage of the disease is frequently associated with emphysema and occasionally with multicystic disease of the lungs (Fig. 349).

Fine fibrosis may represent the residuum of the disease in which the inflammatory infiltration and tubercles have disappeared. This occurs most frequently following healing of the miliary form of sarcoidosis but can occur after absorption of the coarser nodular and interstitial infiltrations. Attention may be called to the fine fibrosis by poor definition of the mediastinal borders. This is caused by superimposition of the fibrotic strands in the overlapping lung. The fibrosis may impart a fine reticular appearance to the pulmonary fields or produce thin straight or irregular, wavy linear shadows. In many instances, the shadows of the fibrous tissue itself are not clearly visualized, but the presence of fibrosis is evidenced by the distortion and obscuration of the pattern of the small and medium-sized vessels throughout the lungs.

The shadows caused by coarse fibrosis are quite evident (Fig. 344C). They are preceded by coarse infiltrations. The shadows become more dense, irregular and sharply demarcated as fibrosis takes place, and the individual lesions frequently assume a stellate appearance. Concomitantly, there is usually marked distortion of the vascular pattern together with evidences of emphysema and shrinkage of the lung. The lung roots and the short fissure are frequently elevated and descent of the diaphragm is impeded.

A characteristic pattern is formed by condensation of the fibrotic strands or coalescence of the fibrosing masses about the elevated lung

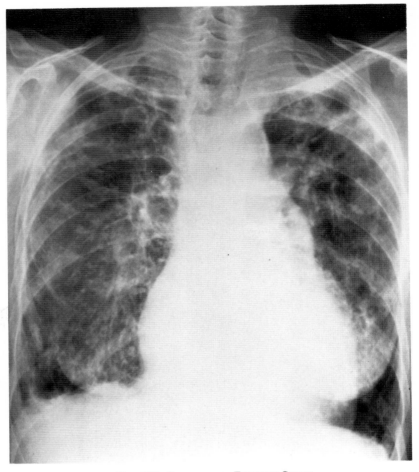

FIG. 349. SARCOIDOSIS: FIBROTIC STAGE

There is severe interstitial fibrosis throughout both lungs with bullous changes in their upper portions. The leaves of the diaphragm are moderately depressed because of emphysema. The hilar and mediastinal nodes are not enlarged. This picture is often referred to as the "burnt-out" stage of sarcoidosis.

roots. These lesions often extend horizontally outward from the mediastinum and are frequently associated with overinflation of the apices and lower lobes. As the massive lesions undergo fibrosis, their borders tend to become sharply irregular and assume a stellate appearance. A similar stellate configuration is also seen on the lateral view of the chest, projected over the hilum. This is especially prominent if the hilar nodes are enlarged.

The dense shadows seen in the fibrotic stage of sarcoidosis are rarely due to fibrosis alone. Persistent infiltration of the lung by active disease contributes to the roentgen appearance. Moreover, it may be difficult to determine whether there is fibrosis in addition to coarse pulmonary infiltrations. In general, it may be assumed that at least some fibrosis is present when the infiltrations have persisted for at least

2 years. However, it is possible for shadows to disappear even after a period of 4 or 5 years. On the other hand, one may be certain of the presence of fibrosis if the lesions persist for a longer period.

Emphysema is a common accompaniment of fibrosis in sarcoidosis. Focal areas of emphysema are interspersed between the fibrotic and infiltrative lesions. These are manifested by areas of increased lucency which contribute to the distortion of the vascular pattern. In the late stages of the disease where marked shrinkage of the lung has occurred, extensive emphysema may be present. This may be localized to the apical and basal regions, above and below the densely scarred lung which has become contracted into the middle third of the chest. The appearance, then, is similar to certain cases of silicosis (Fig. 322).

Despite the presence of marked emphysema,

the total volume of the lung is rarely increased because of contraction of the infiltrated and fibrotic portions of the pulmonary tissue. The diaphragms, therefore, are usually not depressed or flattened (Fig. 350). Occasionally, a more uniform, diffuse type of emphysema occurs, especially in patients with extremely fine fibrosis. The diaphragms may then be depressed. The differential diagnosis between this type of sarcoidosis and chronic bronchitis and emphysema may be impossible from the roentgen examination in this stage.

Multicystic disease of the lung is a common finding at necropsy in patients dying from chronic sarcoidosis, but is not so frequently recognized roentgenologically. Most evident on the films are bullae, usually situated at the apices and associated with coarse fibrotic lesions (Fig. 344). However, it is possible for the bullae to form in the acute stage before fibrosis becomes evident. They behave in the same manner as bullae complicating other fibrosing diseases. They may develop a fluid level as a result of secondary infection, they may disappear, or they may rupture and produce a pneumothorax.

Microcystic disease producing the picture of

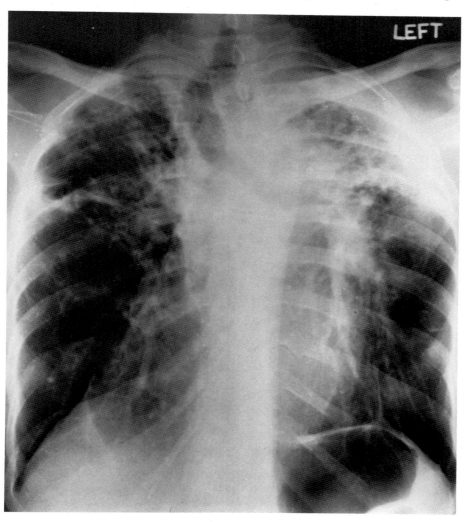

FIG. 350. ASPERGILLOSIS COMPLICATING SARCOIDOSIS

The patient has a late stage of sarcoidosis with marked shrinkage of the upper lobes and emphysema of the lower lobes. The trachea is sharply angulated to the right because of extreme shrinkage of the right upper lobe. The pleura over the apex and axillary portions of the left upper lobe is extremely thick. In addition, there are coarse infiltrations in the left upper lobe. The asymmetry of the lesions and the marked local thickening of the pleura are strongly suggestive of invasive aspergillosis, a not uncommon complication of advanced sarcoidosis. The marked hyperaeration of the lungs without depression or flattening of the diaphragm are indicative of compensatory emphysema.

honeycomb lung is much less common and is
usually not recognized on the films because the
small cystic areas are overshadowed by the dense
fibrotic lesions. Uniform involvement of the
lungs by tiny, thin-walled cavities in the absence
of dense fibrosis can occur in sarcoidosis (Fig.
351), but is rare. Such a picture is most commonly due to histiocytosis X. Honeycombing in
the presence of coarse fibrosis is more characteristic of idiopathic fibrosis of the lungs (Hamman-
Rich syndrome). However, if the changes are
confined to the middle third of the lungs, sarcoidosis should be strongly considered.

Bronchial Involvement. The bronchi are affected frequently in sarcoidosis and become obstructed either by active granulomatous disease
or by fibrotic strictures. The small bronchi in the
foci of coarse infiltration are particularly involved. This results in the formation of numerous
small areas of atelectasis within the lesions.
These are reflected in a gross shrinkage of the
involved portions of the lungs. Because the upper

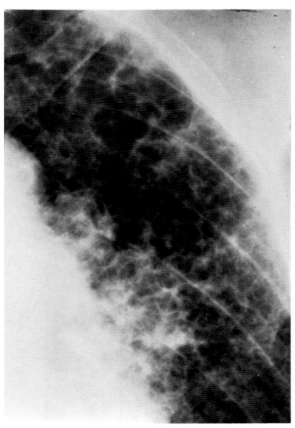

FIG. 351. HONEYCOMB LUNG IN SARCOIDOSIS
Close-up of the left lung shows numerous small thin-walled
cavities. The hilar shadows are indistinct because of denser
fibrosis in this region.

portions of the lungs are usually more involved,
there is frequently an upward retraction of the
lung root. This may occur in the early stage of
the disease and persist indefinitely once fibrosis
takes place. Since the process involves both lungs
in symmetrical fashion, both hila are elevated
and the trachea remains in the midline, as a rule.

The emphysema in relation to the atelectatic
foci is only partly compensatory. Numerous
areas of emphysema interspersed among the foci
of infiltration and atelectasis are caused by partial obstruction of small bronchi. These together
with the atelectatic lesions are responsible for
distortion of the vascular pattern regardless of
the presence of fibrosis. The latter simply causes
accentuation and sharpening of the abnormal
pulmonary markings.

The atelectatic foci may be manifestated by
fine streak-like shadows running in various directions. Tenting of the diaphragm is caused by
atelectatic foci at the base of the lung.

Disease of the larger bronchi is also common,
but rarely causes bronchial obstruction and,
therefore, is usually not detectable on roentgen
examination. When it does occur, the obstruction
is produced either by active granulomas or fibrous stricture. It is not caused by pressure, or
by erosion of adjacent diseased lymph nodes as
in tuberculosis or histoplasmosis, but is due to
the bronchial disease itself.

Obstruction of the main bronchi, with the exception of the middle lobe bronchus, is extremely
rare. Segmental bronchi are occasionally occluded, producing a triangular shadow of atelectasis and infiltration, similar to that which occurs
in bronchogenic carcinoma. Obstruction of these
bronchi occurs in a haphazard fashion. Since
there is no symmetry to the obstructing lesions,
the atelectasis may occur on only one side and
result in displacement of the mediastinum.

Occasionally, bronchiectasis occurs distal to
partial obstruction of one of the larger bronchi.
However, it can also occur without evidence of
gross bronchial obstruction. It is then usually
situated in the lower lobes and is probably the
result of a complicating nonspecific suppurative
bronchopneumonia rather than the sarcoid disease. Bronchiolectasis, giving rise to a microcystic or honeycomb appearance of the lung is probably due to partial obstruction of the smallest
bronchi.

Pleural Involvement. Pleural complications
are unusual in sarcoidosis. Although pleural effusions occur, they are generally small. Not infrequently the effusion is not due to the sarcoid
disease itself but rather to complicating tuberculosis, cardiac failure or a secondary, nonspe-

cific infection of the lung. Thickening of the pleura occurs more frequently. It is usually localized to the base and associated with obliteration of the costophrenic sinus. Marked thickening of the pleura in the apical and subapical regions is usually due to complicating aspergillosis (Fig. 350). Spontaneous pneumothorax may result from rupture of a large bulla or a small air cyst.

Course of the Disease. The most common early roentgen manifestation of sarcoidosis is enlargement of the hilar and mediastinal lymph nodes. This is the sole manifestation in about half of the cases when first seen. Roughly one-fourth of the cases show infiltrations of the lungs in addition to the lymph nodes at this time. There is a great tendency for resolution of the disease in the nodes even in the face of the emergence of infiltrations in the lungs. Fine miliary infiltrations of the lungs have a similar tendency to resolution, but the coarser lesions are more apt to undergo fibrosis.

Once the lesions resolve, either in the lymph nodes or in the lung, there is little tendency for them to recur. Exceptions to this rule occur when the resolution takes place during the course of treatment, particularly with steroids, or during pregnancy. Recurrence of the lesions is common when the steroids are discontinued before the disease has run its course.

Cor pulmonale develops in a considerable percentage of the cases of extensive fibrosis and is manifested by an enlargement of the right side of the heart and prominence of the pulmonary vessels. The latter may be most difficult to differentiate from large lymph nodes. Generalized enlargement of the heart may be caused by diffuse involvement of the heart muscle by the granulomatous disease. This results in left heart failure. Congestion and edema of the lungs can then contribute to an increase in the extent and density of the shadows in the lungs.

The diagnosis of sarcoidosis often depends upon observing the course of the disease on serial roentgen examinations. It is, therefore, most important to obtain previous films of the chest for comparison when the patient is first observed. Spontaneous disappearance of the lymph nodes serves to differentiate the disease from lymphoma. Diffuse pulmonary infiltrations are most probably due to sarcoidosis if previous films reveal only enlargement of the hilar lymph nodes, even in patients exposed to harmful dusts.

Difficulty is experienced in the recognition of pulmonary diseases superimposed upon sarcoidosis. This problem arises especially in patients treated with steroids, for they are prone to complicating tuberculosis and fungous infections. In this connection it is helpful to bear in mind the fact that exacerbation of the pulmonary lesions once they have begun to undergo resolution is unusual in sarcoidosis and is an indication of an additional pulmonary disease.

Other Fibrosing Pulmonary Diseases

Cystic Fibrosis of the Pancreas (Mucoviscidosis). Cystic fibrosis of the pancreas is a familial disease which is associated with abnormally viscid bronchial secretions. The pulmonary manifestations are caused by obstruction of bronchi by thick secretions and secondary infection. The pulmonary lesions may become evident during the first few months of life although they usually appear in early childhood. In recent years more and more cases have been detected in adults.

Obstruction of bronchi by the tenacious secretion is responsible for atelectasis and emphysema. Secondary infection causes thickening of the bronchial walls and foci of pneumonia of varying size. The latter are frequently suppurative and lead to cavitation and bronchiectasis. The infections have a tendency to great chronicity and are characterized by recurrences and exacerbations, eventually resulting in fibrosis. They may be complicated by spontaneous pneumothorax, mediastinal and subcutaneous emphysema and cor pulmonale.

No abnormality is seen on the roentgen film until evidence of bronchial obstruction or infection occur. A common early manifestation is the sudden appearance of emphysema as in acute tracheobronchitis of infants. In older children or in adults, atelectasis is due to obstruction of segmental or subsegmental bronchi but in infants, because of the small size of the bronchi, lobar atelectasis may occur. Thickening of the bronchial walls and peribronchial tissues is a regular feature of the disease after infection has set in. The thickened tissues create fine linear shadows between the blood vessels, radiating outward from the hilum. Parallel linear shadows (tram lines) represent the walls of the thickened bronchi.

The disease is characterized by persistent, diffuse, interstitial infiltrations. As it progresses, the vascular pattern becomes distorted with areas of emphysema and atelectasis (Fig 352). Frequently the process is more marked in the upper lobes, and is sometimes associated with elevation of the lung roots.

The course of the disease is punctuated by the occurrence of patchy areas of consolidation, often

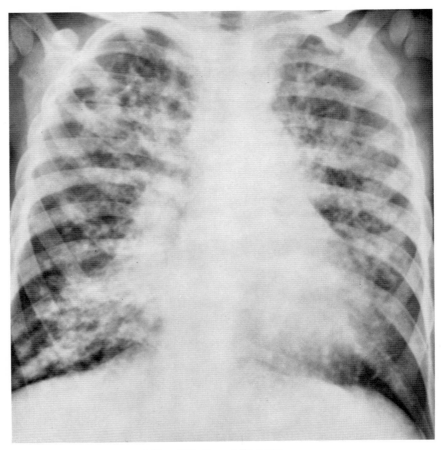

FIG. 352. CYSTIC FIBROSIS

A 9 year old boy with a history of repeated respiratory infections developed gradually increasing dyspnea. The film shows diffuse, coarse, interstitial infiltrations interspersed with areas of hyperaeration. Both leaves of the diaphragm are depressed. Cystic areas are present in the right upper lobe. The finger-like densities at the base of the right lung represent dilated bronchi filled with secretion.

representing foci of suppurative bronchopneumonia due to *Staphylococcus aureus.* They tend to be small and confined to the distribution of small bronchi.

The lesions resolve slowly and frequently result in fibrosis. A few may persist indefinitely as chronic, suppurative foci which drain through the bronchi. The resulting cavities may become lined by bronchial epithelium producing the picture of small sacculated bronchiectases. They differ from most cases of bronchiectasis in that the sacculations tend to be irregularly scattered with relatively good lung between them. Thin-walled cavities may be visualized as ring shadows on ordinary films, but are better delineated on tomograms. When filled with thick secretions, which are not easily eliminated, they result in persistent densities.

Larger areas of pneumonia also occur. In contrast to the small patchy lesions, which are usu-

ally widespread, the larger lesions may be unilateral. The pneumonia is also suppurative in nature, and may result in the formation of one or more cavities. When the lower lobes are involved, the large pneumonic lesions can result in bronchiectases which do not differ from those of ordinary suppurative bronchiectasis.

Persistent peribronchial infection and recurrent suppuration result in interstitial fibrosis. The fibrosis caused by the peribronchial inflammation is usually fine, but that which follows in the wake of diffuse suppurative foci is coarse, and produces rather dense, irregular shadows throughout the lungs.

The diagnosis of cystic fibrosis should be suspected in all children with recurrent pneumonias. When the film shows diffuse, persistent infiltrations interspersed with areas of emphysema and foci of atelectasis, cystic fibrosis is the most probable diagnosis. The diagnosis should also be considered in adults whose films present a similar picture, particularly when bronchography discloses the presence of scattered sacculated bronchiectases.

Diffuse Idiopathic Interstitial Pulmonary Fibrosis (Hamman-Rich Syndrome).

In 1944, Hamman and Rich described four cases of an interstitial pneumonia of unknown etiology, characterized by fibrosis and running a rather acute, fatal course. Since then a chronic form of the disease has been recognized. It consists of a fibrosing interstitial pneumonia which may begin acutely, but more often has an insidious onset and a slowly progressive course with constantly increasing fibrosis.

The essential pathologic lesion is an inflammatory process with infiltration and fibroblastic changes in the alveolar walls and the peribronchiolar and other interstitial tissues of the lungs, all of which become markedly thickened. In the early stage of the disease, there is an outpouring of fluid and mononuclear cells into the alveoli. This exudate is mostly absorbed. However, the thickening and fibrosis of the alveolar septa and interstitial tissues gradually increases and encroaches upon the alveoli, many of which become disorganized and unrecognizable as air spaces. In the late stages, other groups of alveoli and their communicating bronchioles become distended and form tiny air cysts. The resultant picture is that of a carnified lung in which fibrosis, bronchiolectasis and an increase in smooth muscle, together with infiltration with round cells and plasma cells, are the component features. Depending upon whether the emphasis is on the dilated bronchioles or on the increase in the smooth muscle, the terms *bronchiolectasis, bronchiolar emphysema* and *muscular cirrhosis* of the lungs have been applied to this late stage of the Hamman-Rich syndrome.

Most frequently, the disease first becomes manifest in the fourth or fifth decade, but its onset has been noted in young infants as well as in very old people. Early, when the inflammatory process is presumably more active, the pathologic changes are represented on the film by a ground glass appearance with extremely fine stippling of the affected portions of the pulmonary field. With rare exceptions, the disease affects both lungs from the beginning. Characteristically, the changes first appear at the bases, extending upward as the disease progresses, the basal lesions remaining more prominent (Fig. 353). In some, the disease is evenly distributed throughout both lungs, except for the extreme apices. In rare instances, the condition appears to involve the upper portions of the lungs pri-

marily, but in most of these, close inspection of the film reveals changes in the lower portions as well. Usually, even in the early stages of the disease, there is a reduction in the volume of the affected portions of the lungs, manifested by crowding of the blood vessels and incomplete descent of the diaphragm during inspiration.

When the acute inflammatory reaction subsides and the exudate in many of the alveoli resorbs, the interstitial fibrosis produces a network of fine, linear densities, imparting a reticular appearance to the pulmonary fields (Fig. 105). As the disease progresses, coarser infiltrations appear, and the fine stippling and diffuse haziness of the intervening lung may not be so evident. Usually the infiltrations in the lower part of the lung are more coarse and dense than those in the upper portion. Increasing fibrosis is reflected by an increase in the extent and density of the shadows together with greater restriction of pulmonary expansion and increasing elevation of the diaphragm. One or more homogeneous shadows may appear, gradually increasing in size as time goes on. These represent large areas of fibrous replacement of alveoli or a persistent pneumonia resulting from a complicating infection.

At first the pulmonary vascular pattern is composed of the usual regular, branching shadows, but the outlines of the individual vessels become fuzzy because of the fine interstitial fibrosis. As the disease progresses and the alveoli become disorganized and fibrotic, the vascular pattern becomes grossly distorted. Eventually, the increasing fibrosis narrows the vascular bed, resulting in pulmonary arterial hypertension. The main pulmonary arteries dilate as the peripheral vessels are constricted, and in many instances right heart dilatation and failure follow.

Although pleural adhesions are frequently found at necropsy and at thoracotomy late in the disease, evidence of pleural thickening is usually absent on the films.

The course tends to be progressive in the great majority of cases. Death usually occurs within 2 to 6 years, although some patients have survived for a considerably longer interval. In fact, occasionally the disease appears to come to a standstill, and in some instances a certain degree of resolution may take place in the early stages. This has been observed particularly in patients treated with steroids. This form of treatment, however, has been effective in only a relatively small percentage of cases, and even in these, recrudescence of the disease usually occurs after discontinuing the drug.

In patients who survive a few years, evidence

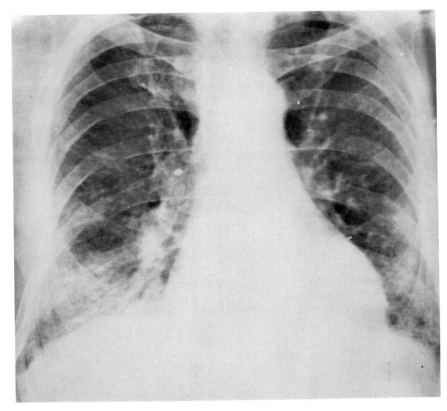

FIG. 353. HAMMAN-RICH SYNDROME

Coarse infiltrations are present throughout the lower portion of each lung. The vessels at the right base are drawn together indicating shrinkage of the lung in this region. The patient had a mild chronic cough productive of a minimal amount of clear sputum. The roentgen changes were detected 1 year ago and have progressed since that time. The diagnosis of idiopathic interstitial fibrosis was made by open lung biopsy.

of bronchiolectasis appears on the films. The bronchiolectases are generally 2 to 5 mm in diameter but some measure as much as a centimeter. They appear on the film as lucencies, often sharply defined, within the infiltrated lung, and impart a honeycomb appearance to the diseased areas. Usually the changes are seen in the lower or midlung fields. Frequently they are more clearly visible along the border of the chest on the oblique view, and in the anterior part of the chest on the lateral projection. The honeycombing is often more evident on well-exposed Bucky films, and is particularly well seen through the shadow of the liver on films of the abdomen. Large air cysts or bullae are rare.

Bronchography discloses a crowding together of the bronchi as a result of shrinkage of the lung. The bronchi may be slightly widened and sometimes there is bulging of the walls between the cartilages, such as occurs in chronic bronchitis. Bronchiectasis, in the usual sense, is rarely encountered. The dilated bronchioles, which are

responsible for the honeycombing, can usually be demonstrated in the form of small, globular saccules at the ends of the bronchi. The clear area, normally interposed between the ends of the opacified bronchi and the border of the chest, no longer exists. The alveoli, which should occupy this area, are largely gone, so that the bronchi, some of which are amputated, and others which end in racemose collections of contrast material, now extend to the border of the lung.

Despite the great number and superficial location of the microcysts, spontaneous pneumothorax rarely occurs. This is probably due to the thickness of the walls of the bronchiolectases, which consist of fibrotic, collapsed and disorganized alveoli.

Idiopathic Pulmonary Hemosiderosis. Pulmonary hemosiderosis is a consequence of recurrent or prolonged bleeding from the pulmonary capillaries into the lungs. The most common cause is mitral stenosis (Fig. 354). It also occurs with renal disease (Goodpasture's syndrome) and in association with pulmonary vasculitis. Pulmonary hemosiderosis is also encountered in patients with no other known disease and is then termed idiopathic.

The condition occurs most commonly in children below the age of 7, but a number of cases have been observed with an onset in the third and fourth decades. The disease is characterized by recurrent hemoptysis, low grade fever and anemia.

The bleeding apparently takes place from numerous capillaries throughout the lungs. A considerable portion of the blood is not coughed up and remains in the alveoli where the red cells degenerate and are engulfed by macrophages. These deposit blood pigment in the form of hemosiderin in the alveolar walls and interstitial tissues. The hemosiderin eventually incites the formation of fibrous tissue. Death is most often due to recurrent pulmonary hemorrhage rather than to right heart failure secondary to the fibrosis.

The initial roentgen changes result from inundation of the alveoli by blood. The films show patchy areas of consolidation in both lungs. These are distributed mainly in the midportion of the pulmonary fields. The lesions may extend to the diaphragm but the apices are practically always spared and the costophrenic sulci are usually clear. The areas of consolidation are depicted as poorly defined, mottled densities of varying size, representing acini, lobules or groups of lobules filled with blood, macrophages and proteinaceous fluid. Usually, clearing takes place in 1 to 2 weeks, although it may be delayed for several months.

As the hemorrhages continue and hemosiderin collects in the interstitial tissues and alveolar walls, evidences of fibrosis appear. The fibrosis is characteristically fine and imparts a ground

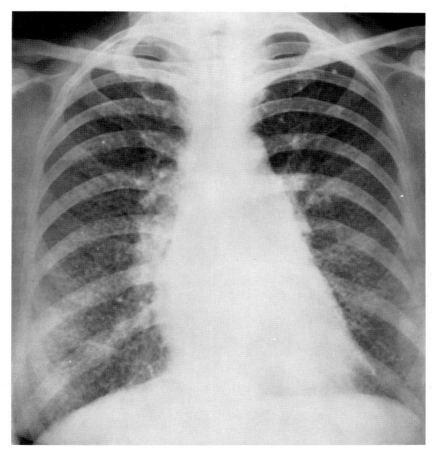

FIG. 354. HEMOSIDEROSIS IN MITRAL STENOSIS

The lower two-thirds of the lungs are studded with tiny shadows. The appearance of the lesions suggests miliary tuberculosis. However, in tuberculosis the lesions are most numerous in the upper portions of the lungs. The distribution of the fine nodular lesions in this case is typical of the hemosiderosis associated with stenosis of the mitral valve.

glass appearance to the pulmonary fields. On close inspection this can be seen to be caused by extremely fine stippled shadows. Coarser stippling, simulating miliary tuberculosis and a fine reticular appearance about the hila, may also be present (Fig. 355). These changes persist indefinitely. Patchy densities are superimposed on this background during subsequent episodes of bleeding. Rarely, the disease is manifested at first on only one side, but, eventually, changes become visible in both lungs.

The hemosiderosis is progressive and may result in pulmonary hypertension with enlargement of the major pulmonary arteries and the right side of the heart. The x-ray picture may then suggest mitral disease, but the left atrium is not enlarged.

It is not always possible to differentiate idiopathic pulmonary hemosiderosis from Goodpasture's syndrome before evidence of renal disease appears. This may be delayed for several months. It should be noted that Goodpasture's syndrome does not seem to occur before the age of 16. In general, it may be concluded that, in the absence of evidences of mitral stenosis or diffuse vascular disease, the occurrence of diffuse mottled densities in a young person with hemoptysis is indicative of idiopathic pulmonary capillary hemorrhage. The later occurrence of miliary lesions or fine reticulation with chronic anemia confirms

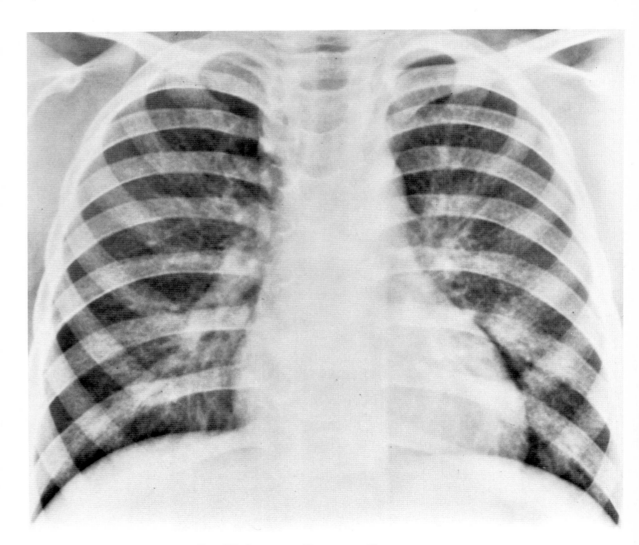

FIG. 355. IDIOPATHIC PULMONARY HEMOSIDEROSIS
The frontal film of a 6 year old child with a previous history of hemoptysis shows fine nodular densities scattered throughout both lungs. Lung biopsy revealed hemosiderin deposits in the interstitial tissues. Incidentally, an azygos lobe is present.

this diagnosis. Older children and adults should be observed for a period of time for evidence of renal disease before excluding the possibility of Goodpasture's syndrome.

Histiocytosis X. The term histiocytosis X was promulgated by Lichtenstein in 1953 to encompass the conditions previously described as eosinophilic granuloma of bone, Hand-Schüller-Christian disease and Letterer-Siwe disease. His conclusion that these diseases are manifestations of a single entity representing a histiocytic reaction to an unknown agent, has been generally accepted. Eosinophilic granuloma of the lung is now also included in the same category.

The differences between these diseases appear to lie in their clinical manifestations rather than in the basic pathologic process. Letterer-Siwe disease represents an acute, disseminated, rapidly progressive condition occurring in children, usually under 3 years of age, and generally is fatal. Hand-Schüller-Christian disease occurs in young adults as well as in children, runs a chronic or subchronic course, and is usually characterized by lytic lesions in the skull, exophthalmos and diabetes insipidus. Eosinophilic granuloma is the more localized form of histiocytosis X. It occurs primarily in adults, and affects chiefly the bones and the lungs.

In histiocytosis X, the lungs may be involved alone, or in combination with lesions elsewhere in the body. The earliest pathologic change in the lungs is a diffuse infiltration of the interstitial tissues by aggregates of histiocytes, lymphocytes, plasma cells and a variable number of eosinophiles. As the infiltration increases, small granulomas may form. These can resolve completely although more often they persist and become fibrotic. Small cystic cavities are usually present in association with the fibrosis and may dominate the pathologic picture. They seem to be most prominent in the periphery of the lungs.

In the earlier stages, the infiltrations cause a haziness of the pulmonary fields or produce an ill-defined reticular pattern. Nodular lesions then appear. These are generally small and produce soft, poorly circumscribed shadows which may measure up to 5 mm in diameter. The reticular pattern persists as a background to the nodular densities.

Characteristically, the lesions are rather uniform in size and evenly distributed throughout the lungs from apex to base. In the early stages, they may appear to be confined to the upper lobes or perihilar regions, only to become more disseminated as the disease progresses. Occasionally complete resolution takes place and the chest film reverts to normal. When resolution is

incomplete, the nodules may disappear, but fine linear and reticular shadows, representing interstitial fibrosis, persist. In contradistinction to the early lesions, these shadows are rather sharply defined.

In other cases the lesions progress, and the fibrosis is associated with the formation of numerous small, cystic spaces producing honeycombing of the lungs. The cysts are small, practically always less than 1 cm in diameter, and usually appear thin-walled (see Fig. 439). As in the case of the infiltrations that precede them, the cystic changes are evenly distributed throughout the lungs. The cysts may be easily overlooked because their thin walls cast only faint shadows. However, they can be clearly demonstrated by tomography, or through the liver shadow on abdominal films. Lateral or oblique projections often show the outlines of the cysts more definitely than the frontal view.

The microcysts are not filled during bronchography. In this respect they differ from the bronchiolectases encountered in the Hamman-Rich syndrome. Apparently in histiocytosis X they are largely alveolar in origin, as in scleroderma. Pneumothorax from rupture of a cyst occurs in about one-fourth of the cases. If the cyst ruptures into a pulmonary septum, interstitial emphysema ensues, frequently complicated by pneumomediastinum (Fig. 356) and pneumothorax.

Occasionally the films show larger, patchy shadows in the early stages of the disease, simulating the ill-defined shadows of lobular pneumonia. This is more frequent in Letterer-Siwe disease. Fibrosis is uncommon in this type of histiocytosis X because the disease usually runs a rapidly fatal course. We have observed large, irregular, well-defined nodular lesions, up to several centimeters in diameter in a case of Hand-Schüller-Christian disease (Fig. 357). Although the hilar and mediastinal lymph nodes may be involved, they are rarely large enough to be recognized radiologically. Pleural effusions do not occur in the absence of pneumothorax, and thickening of the pleura is not notable.

The diagnosis of histiocytosis X is suggested by the uniformity in size and distribution of the lesions. The lungs tend to be evenly involved from apex to base, regardless of whether the shadows are characterized by reticulation, nodulation or honeycombing. Sharp definition of the nodules or the presence or irregular, coarse fibrosis suggests some disease other than histiocytosis X. Faint infiltrations or microcysts in conjunction with a pneumothorax point to eosinophilic granuloma (Fig. 358) or scleroderma.

Whenever the findings on the chest film sug-

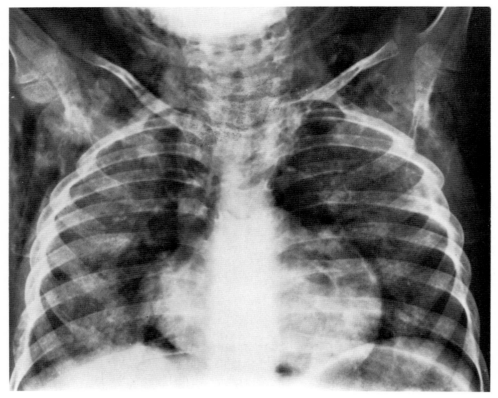

FIG. 356. MEDIASTINAL AND SUBCUTANEOUS EMPHYSEMA: HAND-SCHÜLLER-CHRISTIAN DISEASE
The diffusely infiltrated lungs are separated from the heart and other mediastinal structures by air in the mediastinum. This is depicted as a sharply outlined band of radiolucency on either side of the mediastinum. The air has dissected upward into the neck causing a mottling of the soft tissue shadows. From here the emphysema has spread over the upper part of both sides of the thorax.

gest the possibility of histiocytosis X, a bone survey should be made in a search for characteristic lytic lesions. The presence of diabetes insipidus together with a nodular pattern in the lungs is strongly suggestive of histiocytosis X. This combination is rarely encountered in sarcoidosis. Microcystic changes in the lung are also unusual in the latter condition.

Nonspecific Granulomas. Occasionally, a rather irregular, moderately well demarcated nodule, as large as 4 or 5 cm in diameter, is found on a routine chest film in a patient with no pulmonary symptoms. Pathologic examination of the nodule may show only evidence of chronic inflammation in the form of a granuloma with no clue to its etiology. Radiologically, the appearance of the lesion is similar to that of a primary carcinoma. If it is situated in the posterior part of the upper lobe, the possibility of a tuberculoma or of a blocked tuberculous cavity is suggested. particularly if the patient is below cancer age. A histoplasmoma or a coccidioidoma can present the same appearance.

The only characteristics pointing to a granuloma are a grossly irregular shape, unlike that of most circumscribed nodular neoplasms, and the absence of growth of the lesion over a period of time. However, on occasion, a granuloma can increase considerably in size in a relatively short time. When multiple lesions are present, they suggest metastatic neoplasms. This possibility can be excluded if comparison with previous films shows no increase in the shadows over a long period.

Radiation Pneumonia. What is generally called radiation fibrosis begins as a pneumonia following injury to the lung by x-rays. This pneumonia is almost universally associated with granulation tissue formation. It usually results in permanent pulmonary fibrosis of varying extent.

The pneumonia affects primarily the interstitial tissues and results in thickening and hyalinization of the walls of the alveoli and bronchi. In the early stage there is an outpouring of fluid and cellular exudate into many of the alveoli and bronchioles, together with evidence of diffuse vasculitis. These changes are soon accompanied by proliferation of fibroblasts. Resolution of the acute inflammatory process eventually takes place, although it may be long delayed. However, the fibrosis does not disappear and, in general, tends to become more extensive. The intensity of the reaction varies with the individual patient and the condition of the lung before radiation, but the prime factors are the quality of radiation employed, the total dose, the dose rate and the size of the field.

Radiation changes usually become evident from 1 to 3 months after completion of treatment, but may be delayed for as long as 6 months. The reactions which occur early, within 6 weeks after treatment, tend to be more severe and, if the treatment field was large, may even prove fatal. The reactions which appear late are often insidious and show more evidence of fibrosis than pneumonia.

In the hyperacute cases, the radiologic appearance is essentially one of consolidation of the lung. The shadow is dense and homogeneous.

The boundary of the consolidated area is related to the field of irradiation without regard to the borders of the lobes or segments of the lung. The edge of the consolidated area is sometimes sharply defined. In the less acute cases, the lesion is not as dense and appears as a haze through which the shadows of the pulmonary vessels are visible. Mottled shadows of consolidation and linear streaks are apparent within the involved area.

There is usually some evidence of resolution of the pneumonic process within 2 or 3 months, at which time fibrosis and shrinkage of the lung occurs. The sharp border of the densely consolidated lesion becomes indistinct because of the irregularity of the process of resolution and distortion of the lung by fibrosis. Maximum clearing usually occurs within a year, but may be delayed for several additional months. Subsequently, the condition usually remains stationary. Complete resolution of the pneumonia without evidence of residual fibrosis is unusual.

As the lung shrinks, the vessels are drawn

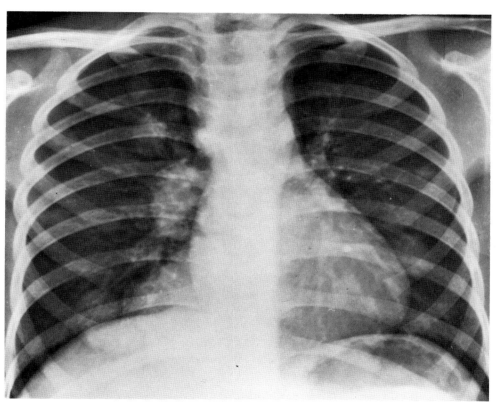

FIG. 357. GRANULOMATOUS LESIONS IN HAND-SCHÜLLER-CHRISTIAN DISEASE

There are large, irregular nodules at the base of the right lower lobe near the root of the lung and in the mesial portion of the right upper lobe. Smaller nodules are visible in the left lung. The paratracheal nodes on each side are enlarged. The patient also had osteolytic lesions in the bones. The diagnosis was proven by biopsy.

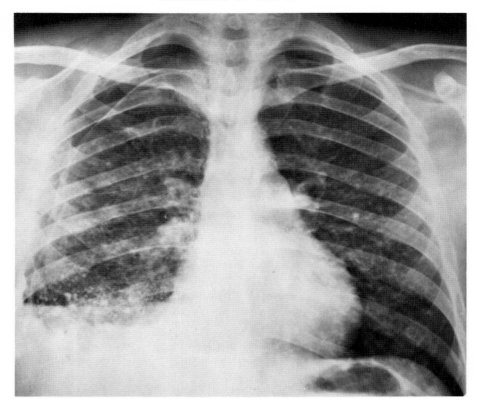

FIG. 358. EOSINOPHILIC GRANULOMATOSIS: INTERSTITIAL INFILTRATIONS AND SPONTANEOUS PNEUMOTHORAX
Both lungs show fine, streak-like and nodular shadows. There is a small pneumothorax on the right side. The border of the lung is sharply defined by a coating of Lipiodol which was injected into the pleural cavity to produce symphysis of the pleura. A small air-fluid level is seen at the right base. Roentgen survey of the bones disclosed areas of rarefaction and the diagnosis of eosinophilic granulomatosis was confirmed by biopsy of a tooth socket.

together, the ribs become approximated, the mediastinum is displaced toward the side of the lesion, and the diaphragm is elevated (Fig. 359). The fissures become retracted towards the shrunken portion of the lung. If the upper part of the lung is affected, the hilum is elevated. The amount of shrinkage is not always related to the intensity or extent of the disease as seen on the film. The shadows in the lungs may be minimal, while the shrinkage of the lung is marked. Contraction of the thorax, in some instances, is due largely to an associated fibrous pleuritis and peripleuritis rather than the disease in the pulmonary parenchyma.

The lung is usually shrunken despite the presence of secondary emphysema which occurs in focal areas within the fibrotic lung. Occasionally, bullae of varying size are present. One of these may rupture to produce a spontaneous pneumothorax.

Evidences of marked thickening of the pleura are frequently visible, particularly in patients treated with rays of relatively low kilovoltage or through fields tangential to the chest wall. In contradistinction to the lesion in the lung, thickening of the pleura usually extends beyond the field of irradiation. Frequently it is associated with a small pleural effusion. The fluid absorbs spontaneously within a few months, while the thickening of the pleura generally persists. Often the border of the mediastinum becomes indistinct and irregular because of exudate on the pleura together with interstitial infiltrations and fibrosis of the lung adjacent to the mediastinum. Fibrosis of the pleura results in ironing out of the mediastinal contours.

The outer portion of the diaphragm is frequently elevated and the costophrenic sinus obliterated. The contour of the diaphragm may form a continuous curve with the vertical shadow of the thickened pleura along the outer border of the chest. When there is a severe radiation reaction, this band-like shadow can measure as much as a centimeter in thickness.

The midportion of the diaphragm is frequently drawn upward in triangular fashion for a distance of several centimeters. This tenting of the diaphragm is quite characteristic of radiation pneumonia. Although it is seen in association with changes in the pleura, it occurs early and is due primarily to atelectasis of a subsegment of the basal portion of the lung. The diaphragmatic changes may occur even when the treated area and pulmonary reaction are limited to the upper part of the chest (Fig. 360). The basal atelectasis is related to restriction of diaphragmatic motion caused by the pleuritis. This results in diminished aeration of the basal portion of the lung and consequent obstruction of a small bronchus by mucus.

Severe reactions of the pleura are usually associated with extensive fibrosis of the peripleural tissues in the chest wall. This results in retrac-tion, increased obliquity and approximation of the ribs. When the fibrosis occurs over the upper lobes, the outer part of the dome of the thorax becomes flattened. This is associated with marked thickening of the pleura at the apex. The ribs may show irregular areas of increased denisty, representing a necrotizing osteitis from the radiation injury. The affected ribs are weakened and tend to fracture (Fig. 165) particularly from traction by the shrunken, fibrotic, peripleural tissues. The fractures occur most commonly at the bends of the ribs where the strain is greatest.

The shadows of radiation pneumonia and fibrosis are easily confused with extension of the neoplastic disease for which the treatment was given. It is essential to recognize the radiation changes to avoid additional treatment which

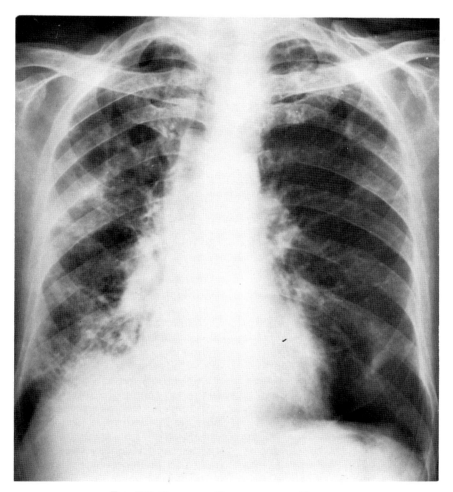

FIG. 359. RADIATION PNEUMONIA AND FIBROSIS

Coarse and fine infiltrations are distributed throughout the lower two-thirds of the right lung. The volume of the lung is considerably decreased, which accounts for the contracture of the right chest, the elevation of the right diaphragm, and the displacement of the trachea and other mediastinal structures to the right. This film was made several weeks after completion of a course of grid radiotherapy for a squamous cell carcinoma in the mesial portion of the right middle lobe.

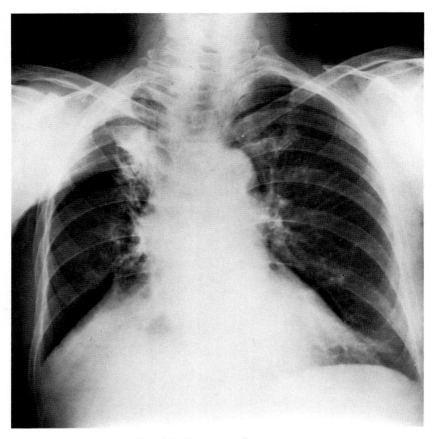

FIG. 360. RADIATION REACTION

The patient had a course of radiotherapy following a radical mastectomy, and was very dyspneic. The shadow in the mesial portion of the right upper lobe represents an area of dense pulmonary fibrosis, and the clouding of the lateral part of the chest is caused by thickened pleura. The right border of the mediastinum is irregular because of superimposition of adjacent fibrotic lung. The right leaf of the diaphragm is elevated and tented and the right hemithorax is considerably shrunken. All of these changes indicate a severe radiation reaction. The oblique line crossing the right upper lobe is cast by the soft tissues of the chest wall that remain after radical mastectomy.

may result in severe pulmonary insufficiency. For this purpose, it is advisable to make an x-ray examination of the chest on completion of the course of irradiation and at monthly intervals for a period of 6 months.

Radiation reaction within the lung is confined to the treated area, and in the early stage often conforms to the shape of the field of radiation. It is therefore necessary to know the exact location of the irradiated area in addition to the other factors employed in the treatment. The sudden appearance of a shadow within the zone of treatment after a free interval of up to a few months following radiotherapy, is indicative of radiation pneumonia rather than spread of the neoplasm. Partial resolution during the ensuing months will confirm the diagnosis.

Differentiation between a cancerous pleural effusion and one due to irradiation is especially difficult. An association with marked tenting of

the diaphragm is strong evidence for radiation reaction. Usually, when the pleural effusion is secondary to radiotherapy, evidences of radiation pneumonia are also present. However, the pneumonia may resolve before the effusion. Serial films following completion of radiotherapy will disclose the sequence of events. Later films showing resorption of the fluid confirm the diagnosis.

Whenever the question arises as to whether a shadow in the lung is due to radiation reaction, special attention should be paid to the ribs over the lesion. Evidences of osteosclerosis will indicate the presence of radiation reaction in the underlying tissues.

The Autoimmune Diseases

Included in this chapter is a group of diseases of unknown etiology in which there is evidence of some form of immune reaction to the patient's own tissues. Although rheumatic fever is the result of an immune reaction to an extrinsic agent, namely the streptococcus, it is also included in this chapter because of its similarity to the autoimmune diseases. The exact role played by the autoimmune process in the production of these diseases remains obscure. Most of them involve multiple organs, and the abnormality in the lungs represents only one phase of the systemic disease. In some, as in eosinophilic pneumonia or in certain cases of scleroderma, the pulmonary manifestations are predominant, while in others, they are incidental. In either case, the occurrence and type of pulmonary lesions in these systemic diseases should be appreciated, both as an aid in the diagnosis of the underlying disease and for the avoidance of errors in the interpretation of the shadows seen on the films.

Progressive Systemic Sclerosis (Scleroderma). Scleroderma is a disease characterized by progressively increasing fibrosis and sclerosis of many organs in addition to the skin. Involvement of the lungs is quite common. In many cases, the x-ray examination of the chest discloses evidences of pulmonary fibrosis before the typical manifestations of scleroderma appear in the skin. In some, the only extrapulmonary manifestation is Raynaud's syndrome or a disturbance of esophageal motility. Either condition may precede the pulmonary lesions.

The earliest change in the lungs usually consists of an extremely fine fibrosis at the bases. At first, this appears simply as an increase in the pulmonary markings, but close observation reveals fine, linear infiltrations between the vessels, extending to the periphery. Fibrosis is also present in the upper portion of the lung at this stage, but is not visible radiologically until later when the disease appears to extend upward. However, the apices are practically always spared. Later, the infiltrations become coarser (Fig. 361), and may show some tendency to nodulation.

In rare instances the infiltrations are visible only in the upper lobes beneath the clavicles, and suggest the possibility of tuberculosis. However, the symmetry of the lesions and absence of coarse, irregular nodules of acinar or lobular consolidation, make the possibility of tuberculosis unlikely.

With advancing fibrosis, the lungs become less compliant and the descent of the diaphragm is

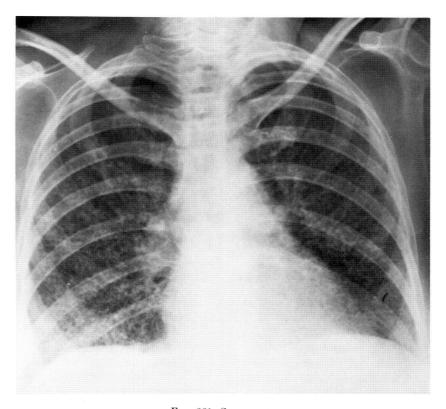

FIG. 361. SCLERODERMA

There are fine interstitial infiltrations throughout both lungs, most dense at the bases. The infiltrations are more extensive than in most cases of scleroderma.

restricted. As there is no obstruction to expiration, the upward movement of the diaphragm is not affected and the total excursion of the organ can remain within normal limits. The diaphragm simply reaches a higher position than usual during full expiration.

Cystic changes resulting from distention or rupture of the alveolar walls often occur in the late stages of the disease. The cysts are quite small, but may attain a diameter of 1 to 1.5 cm. Because of their alveolar origin the microcysts in scleroderma are thin-walled in contradistinction to those of the Hamman-Rich syndrome, which represent distended bronchioles surrounded by thick walls of collapsed alveoli. The cysts in scleroderma are more diffusely distributed throughout the lungs.

The honeycomb shadows of the microcysts in systemic sclerosis are often difficult to recognize on conventional chest films. They are more clearly delineated within the shadow of the liver on films of the abdomen and on tomograms. They may be visible on oblique and lateral views even though they cannot be recognized on the frontal projection.

Occasionally, overdistention of one or more cysts results in the formation of a pneumatocele. Rupture of one of the microcysts or of a pneumatocele produces a pneumothorax.

The diagnosis of scleroderma of the lung cannot be made from chest films alone. However, the roentgen pattern is often sufficiently suggestive to warrant study of other organs for more characteristic alterations.

The disease usually involves the small arteries and arterioles. Myxomatous and fibrous tissue is deposited in the intima of these vessels, narrowing the lumen. Eventually, pulmonary arterial hypertension may develop, manifested by prominence of the arteries at the root of the lungs and enlargement of the right side of the heart. Generalized enlargement of the heart can result from involvement of the myocardium by the sclerosing process. Pleural effusions are rare unless caused by heart failure.

Because scleroderma often interferes with esophageal motility, aspiration pneumonia is not uncommon. This causes patches of consolidation superimposed on the background of interstitial fibrosis. Suppuration may supervene.

There appears to be an increased incidence of bronchiolar carcinoma of the lung in association with scleroderma. Therefore, if a single round shadow or multiple discrete densities develop in a patient with scleroderma, the presence of a carcinoma should be seriously considered.

Dermatomyositis. Dermatomyositis is also a generalized disease and affects many organs in addition to skin and muscle. However, involvement of the lungs is rare. There may be an increase in the markings at the bases similar to that which occurs in scleroderma, but we have also noted scattered, irregular, nondescript mottled shadows in various portions of the pulmonary fields. Honeycomb changes have been described. The heart may be dilated, and the respiratory movement of the chest wall and diaphragm restricted as a result of muscular involvement.

Systemic Lupus Erythematosus. Abnormalities on the chest film are encountered frequently in lupus erythematosus. Changes referable to disease of the heart, pleura and pericardium occur in about half of the cases at some time during the course of the disease. However, the pulmonary lesions that are visible on the film are almost always due to a complicating pneumonia rather than the disease itself.

A pleural or pericardial effusion is often the first abnormality to be seen. The pleural effusions are usually small to moderate in size and are frequently bilateral, especially when associated with fluid in the pericardium. The effusion may be accompanied by marked thickening of the pleura at the bases of the lungs. A fairly characteristic finding is a homogeneous shadow at one or both bases with considerable elevation of the diaphragm. The latter is frequently immobile. The appearance, which suggests a pleural effusion, is caused simply by dense, fibrinous exudate. When the border of the diaphragm is not completely obscured, its hazy outline, in association with the shadow over the adjacent lung, suggests pneumonia, especially when the pleural process is combined with foci of atelectasis. This occurs frequently in lupus because of splinting of the diaphragm and chest wall.

The pleural effusions have a tendency to absorb spontaneously, leaving only fine adhesions which obliterate the costophrenic sinus and accentuate the fissures. The shadows caused by dense, fibrinous pleurisy at the bases usually clear more slowly, but even these resolve, leaving comparatively little evidence of pleural thickening. As in any severe pleurisy, generalized adhesions do form, but are usually manifest only in the costophrenic sinuses and interlobar fissures. The effusions disappear very rapidly under steroid therapy but may reappear when treatment is stopped or during exacerbations of the disease.

A pericardial effusion may occur alone or together with fluid in the pleural cavity. When the associated pleural effusion is unilateral, it is practically always situated on the left side. This is in contrast to the unilateral effusion of heart failure, which characteristically occurs on the right side. The pericardial effusion is usually moderate in amount but is sometimes quite large. It tends to resorb together with the pleural effusion. Frequently it results in the formation of pericardial adhesions. These tend to iron out the normal curves of the cardiac silhouette. Slight or moderate enlargement of the heart in systemic lupus may be due to causes other than pericarditis, such as anemia, renal disease, or involvement of the myocardium.

Perhaps the most common roentgen finding in the lungs is the presence of one or more atelectatic streaks at the bases. These are usually associated with pleurisy, even if there is no effusion. Less common are patchy areas of consolidation of varying size, situated anywhere in the lungs. They usually resolve, often as a result of treatment, but tend to recur in different places. Whether these lesions are an integral part of the disease or whether they are due to secondary infection by pyogenic organisms, is not certain. Some of them may represent infarcts secondary to thrombosis of small pulmonary arteries.

Larger areas of consolidation, often associated with partial atelectasis, undoubtedly are the result of complicating infection to which patients with lupus are especially susceptible. These pneumonias are often hemorrhagic and accompanied by a severe necrotizing bronchitis which is responsible for the atelectasis. Suppuration in the pneumonic area is not uncommon. Rarely, this results in empyema and bronchiectasis.

Nonspecific pulmonary edema occurs frequently as a terminal event, but occasionally it is a transient phenomenon. In some cases, necropsy has shown basophilic fluid in the alveolar walls and interstitial tissues, similar to that seen in the early stage of scleroderma. Collections of this fluid may cause the pulmonary markings to become indistinct and impart a hazy appearance to the pulmonary field. Small areas of interstitial infiltration and fibrosis have frequently been noted at necropsy, but are generally insufficient to alter the roentgen picture. Diffuse fibrosis, causing persistent infiltrations, are rare in lupus erythematosus.

In patients with lupus complicated by thrombocytopenia and cutaneous purpura, blotchy shadows, simulating lobular pneumonia, may be present. These represent hemorrhagic foci in the lungs. Such lesions have also been described in the absence of thrombocytopenia, and are apparently related to infarction or bleeding from disease of the smaller blood vessels. A rare complication of lupus erythematosus is pulmonary hypertension secondary to thrombi in many of the peripheral arteries.

Since most patients with lupus erythematosus are treated with steroids for a long period of time, they are susceptible to reactivation of latent tuberculosis. It is important, therefore, to study the film carefully before steroids are administered. The slightest evidence of an old tuberculous lesion, even if presumably healed, is an indication for prophylactic treatment with antituberculosis drugs. Steroids also increase the susceptibility to fungous infections. The occurrence of any persistent infiltration in the lungs or enlargement of the hilar or mediastinal lymph nodes should suggest the possibility of complicating mycotic or tuberculous infection.

Polyarteritis Nodosa (Periarteritis Nodosa). Polyarteritis nodosa is a particular form of widespread necrotizing angiitis, characterized by distinct foci of inflammatory infiltration around the small and medium-sized arteries, imparting a nodular appearance to the vessels. There is destruction of the media with a tendency to aneurysm formation. About 25 % of the cases develop demonstrable pulmonary lesions secondary to the polyarteritis at some stage of the disease.

Involvement of the lungs in polyarteritis can become manifest roentgenologically in several forms. In some cases, a single area of consolidation and infiltration, like that of a nonspecific pneumonia, is seen. This clears spontaneously but is followed by the appearance of one or more similar lesions elsewhere in the lungs. Several such areas may be noted at the first examination, some clearing while others progress.

In other cases, the roentgen film shows simply an accentuation and thickening of the shadows of the blood vessels as a result of the extensive perivascular infiltration. These occur particularly in the lower lobes and may be present in association with areas of consolidation.

A third form consists of dense, lobular areas of consolidation which are persistent and may be confluent (Fig. 362). These represent areas of both infarction and pneumonia in relation to the vascular lesions. They may appear as multiple, fairly well circumscribed, round shadows, growing up to 5 cm in diameter and suggesting metastatic neoplasms. Necrosis and liquefaction may take place and result in the formation of either thin- or thick-walled cavities.

In the majority of instances, the lesions are

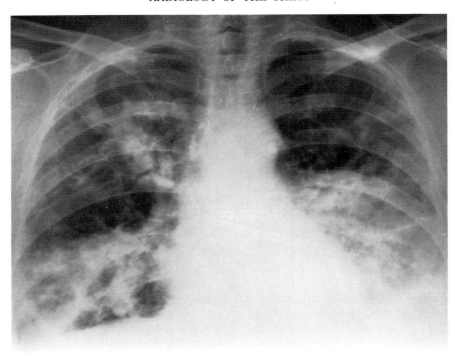

FIG. 362. PERIARTERITIS NODOSA

The film of a 62 year old female with persistent cough and fever shows gross confluent areas of consolidation in both lungs. A small effusion is present at the left base. The diagnosis was established by lung biopsy. The patient responded to steroid therapy.

bilateral but occasionally they affect only one portion of a lung. They may be associated with a small or moderate-sized pleural effusion which is sometimes bilateral. Small effusions can be present without roentgen evidence of underlying pulmonary disease and without enlargement of the heart.

When the lungs are extensively involved by the arteritis, pulmonary hypertension develops, and can produce the picture of cor pulmonale. A number of cases have been described in which the arterial lesions were confined to the lungs, with death from right heart failure.

In addition to the lesions which are the direct consequence of the pulmonary arteritis, changes occur secondary to involvement of the heart or kidneys. The cardiac shadow may be enlarged either because of cardiac dilatation or a pericardial effusion. The vascular pattern of the lungs may be accentuated simply as a result of pulmonary congestion from cardiac failure. Pulmonary edema from heart failure or renal disease can produce a typical butterfly shadow. A pleural effusion may result from cardiac failure rather than from the periarteritis. Bronchopneumonia can occur terminally from secondary infection by a variety of organisms.

It is frequently impossible to differentiate the pulmonary lesions of polyarteritis nodosa from other diseases associated with generalized vasculitis without a biopsy or postmortem examination. Certain cases of polyarteritis nodosa are associated with considerable eosinophilia in the peripheral blood. If, in addition, there are fleeting infiltrations in the lungs, the roentgen picture is indistinguishable from eosinophilic pneumonia (Löffler's syndrome). Conversely, cases of eosinophilic pneumonia which clinically show evidence of vascular disease in other organs are easily misdiagnosed as polyarteritis nodosa unless a biopsy is made. When the pulmonary lesions in Wegener's granulomatosis are multiple, differentiation from polyarteritis nodosa may be impossible roentgenologically.

Eosinophilic Pneumonia. In a variety of diseases the pulmonary lesions occur together with an increased number of eosinophils in the blood. They have been grouped under the heading of PIE syndrome (Pulmonary Infiltration with Eosinophilia). However, this combination may be coincidental, as in an allergic individual with an eosinophilia who develops pneumonia. The eosinophilia in these instances is moderate, usually under 10%. A higher degree of eosinophilia may be due to an allergic reaction to drugs used to combat pulmonary disease already present, especially penicillin and paraaminosalicylic acid.

Sulfonilamide, nitrofurantoin (see Fig. 382) and several other drugs can cause pulmonary infiltration together with an eosinophilia (PIE syndrome). In the parasitic infestations that produce the syndrome, notably ascariasis and tropical eosinophilia, the pulmonary lesions are due to the organisms themselves, rather than to vasculitis. Mycotic infections, particularly aspergillosis, when complicated by asthma, may be associated with a considerable degree of eosinophilia. About 10 % of patients with polyarteritis nodosa have been reported to have pulmonary lesions and eosinophilia.

Of particular interest are the cases of pulmonary infiltrations with eosinophilia described by Löffler. These patients were largely asymptomatic and their infiltrations cleared spontaneously in 1 to 3 weeks. Twenty-five per cent of them were eventually proved to have ascariasis. In the remaining cases a specific etiology could not be demonstrated. This benign transient condition may be properly termed *Löffler's pneumonia.*

There is another group of cases with similar pulmonary lesions and an eosinophilia of over 15%, in which the infiltrations are either persistent or recur over a long period of time. In these there is usually evidence of an underlying allergic state and often a history of bronchial asthma. This group of cases will be referred to as *eosinophilic pneumonia.* In addition to the prolonged course, the cases differ from those described by Löffler in that the disease is frequently associated with disseminated inflammatory vascular lesions, and before the advent of steroid therapy, 25% proved fatal. The vascular lesions differ from those of polyarteritis nodosa in that they are not associated with a well-defined periarterial mantle of inflammatory cells or aneurysm formation. Included in the category of eosinophilic pneumonia are the cases described by Harkavy under the heading of *vascular allergy,* and those of asthma, fever and high eosinophilia described by Churg and Strauss under the name of *allergic angiitis and granulomatosis.* Pathologically, these cases show disseminated, necrotizing, vascular lesions and small granulomas.

The roentgen changes in eosinophilic pneumonia consist of areas of consolidation and infiltration. When first seen, there may be only a single, ill-defined, small patch of consolidation in one lobe. However, soon, one or more additional densities usually appear in other parts of the lung. More commonly, the lesions are bilateral

when the patient is first observed. Streak-like shadows are often present within the consolidated area, suggesting foci of atelectasis secondary to obstruction of small bronchi. In addition, tiny, poorly demarcated nodular shadows and faint interstitial infiltrations are present about the larger lesions and may be scattered throughout the lungs. Individual lesions tend to clear, usually showing some degree of resolution within 10 days, while new lesions appear in other places. Some of the foci progress and may become quite large, at times involving the greater part of a lobe. When the upper lobe is involved, the appearance simulates tuberculosis (Fig. 363), particularly when there are streak-like densities, partial atelectasis, tiny nodules and interstitial infiltrations. In rare instances, cavitation occurs. Pleural effusions are not uncommon and may be bilateral (see Fig. 555).

There is often a characteristic shadow that we have rarely seen in any disease other than eosinophilic pneumonia. This consists of an oblique, linear streak in the outer part of the upper lobe. The shadow may be thin or rather broad (Fig. 364). It courses downward and outward, more or less parallel to the lateral border of the upper chest and separated from it by a variable distance. The shadow may clear on one side and then appear on the other, or it may be bilateral. It suggests a focus of atelectasis or a streak of exudate on the pleura. However, its direction is unlike that of focal atelectasis in this location, and it can be shown to lie within the lung rather than on the pleura. The appearance of the shadow is so characteristic that its presence justifies a presumptive diagnosis of eosinophilic pneumonia. A similar shadow can occur in silicosis, but tends to be broader and more dense and is separated from the upper part of the chest wall by a system of emphysematous bullae. Here the shadow represents silicotic lung which is displaced mesially and condensed by the bullae (Fig. 324). In eosinophilic pneumonia there are no bullae lateral to the oblique streaks.

The course of the disease varies. Resolution may take place in a month or two, although without treatment, the disease usually persists for a longer time and frequently recurs. Recurrences may take place over a period of years. There is usually a dramatic response to steroid treatment, and lesions that have been present for weeks or months can disappear within a few days. However, there is a tendency to relapse within a few weeks unless steroid treatment is continued for a considerable period.

Roentgenologically, it is not possible to differentiate the migrating infiltrations of eosinophilic

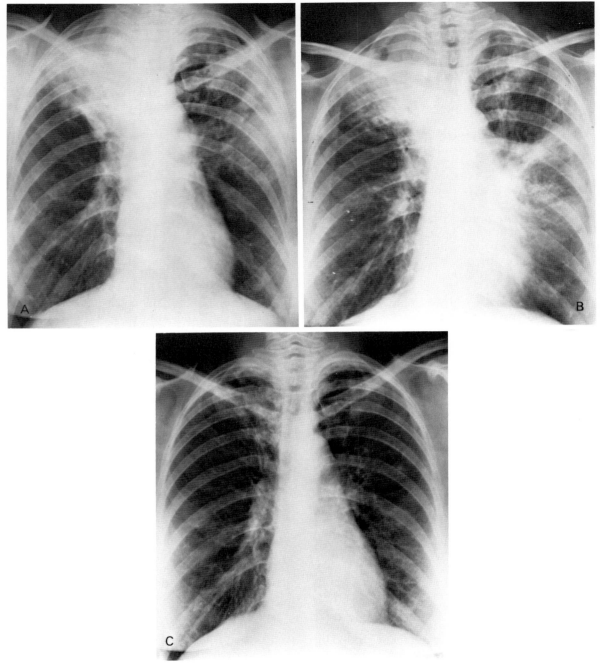

FIG. 363. EOSINOPHILIC PNEUMONIA

A: There is a dense shadow of consolidation in the upper part of the right upper lobe. Within this are a few irregular areas of radiolucency. In addition, there is consolidation of the outer part of the left upper lobe and fine and coarse infiltrations extending to the apex. The roentgen appearance at this single examination cannot be distinguished from that of tuberculosis. There was a high blood eosinophilia and the sputum, which was negative for tubercle bacilli, contained many eosinophils. *B:* A few weeks later, the shadow in the axillary portion of the left upper lobe is condensed and forms a streak-like shadow characteristic of segmental atelectasis. The lucency of the lung above this area is increased as the result of compensatory hyperinflation. The infiltrations at the left apex remain. In addition, there is now extensive infiltration in both lingular segments, partially obscuring the left border of the heart. *C:* Four months later. The lungs are now clear except for faint infiltrations at the apices. The course in the interim was characterized by clearing of the infiltrations in one area and the appearance of new infiltrations in other places.

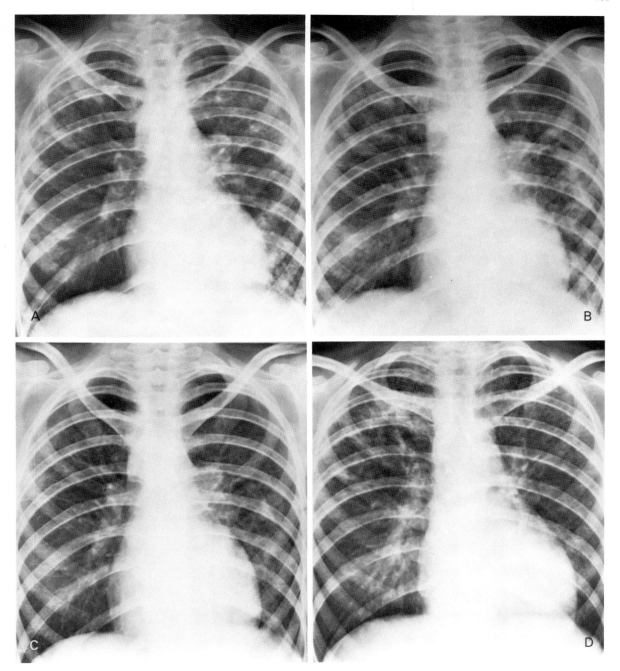

FIG. 364. EOSINOPHILIC PNEUMONIA: INTERSTITIAL INFILTRATIONS AND OBLIQUE STREAKS

A: October 14. The patient had fleeting infiltrations in the lungs and recurrent fever for two years. At this time there are interstitial infiltrations in the upper lobes with condensation of the shadows in the left axillary region. There are also patchy shadows at the bases. *B:* October 20. Little change has occurred on the right side. The infiltrations in the left upper lobe have largely cleared. Two oblique streaks, roughly parallel to the outer border of the chest, have appeared in the midportion of the left lung. These shadows are characteristic of eosinophilic pneumonia. We have rarely seen them in any other condition. Both costophrenic sinuses are obliterated by pleural exudate. A blood smear showed 40% eosinophils. *C:* October 25. Shortly after the institution of steroid therapy, there was marked clearing of all of the infiltrations and the pleural reaction in the costophrenic sinuses. Only a small, single streak remains in the left lung. *D:* November 30. Following cessation of steroid therapy, the patient's symptoms returned. Interstitial infiltrations have appeared in each upper lobe, more marked on the right. This patient was observed before the need for prolonged steroid therapy was appreciated.

pneumonia from those of polyarteritis nodosa. However, thus far, we have not encountered the oblique, streak-like shadows in the latter disease.

Necrotizing Granulomatosis (Wegener's Syndrome). Wegener described a group of cases characterized by a necrotizing granulomatous process involving the upper air passages and the lungs, associated with diffuse vascular lesions and focal glomerulitis. More recently several cases have been reported with identical granulomatous and vascular lesions limited to the lungs. In the disease termed *lethal midline granulomatosis*, similar lesions are found predominating in the upper respiratory tract. All of these conditions may be considered under the single heading of *necrotizing granulomatosis*.

The pulmonary lesions consist essentially of necrotizing granulomas associated with a granulomatous, ulcerative type of bronchitis. The granulomas are fairly well circumscribed, but the borders are irregular. Frequently they undergo central necrosis and form irregular cavities (Fig. 365) which communicate with one or more ulcerated bronchi. There is usually granulomatous thickening of the major bronchi, the trachea, larynx and the lining of the paranasal sinuses.

Ulceration is common and may involve the bone about the sinuses. The kidney lesions consist of focal glomerulitis, frequently in conjunction with granulomas outside the glomeruli. The necrotizing angiitis involves not only the arteries and veins in relation to the granulomas, but distant blood vessels as well.

The nodular form of the disease is manifested by one or more densities in the lungs. When only a single lesion is present, it usually measures no more than 2 to 3 cm in diameter when first observed. It may be situated in any part of the lung and casts a dense shadow with an irregular, rather indistinct outline. Rarely, the nodule is round and sharply demarcated (Fig. 366). The lesion tends to persist and undergo cavitation. The cavity is frequently quite large and irregular, and is usually surrounded by a zone of dense granulomatous lung. Occasionally, the entire granuloma is infarcted and liquefied, resulting in a round, thin-walled cavity (Fig. 367). A fluid level is not as common as in a pyogenic abscess. At any stage the appearance may be identical to that of a carcinoma.

When multiple, the lesions are generally smaller and usually appear as dense, patchy

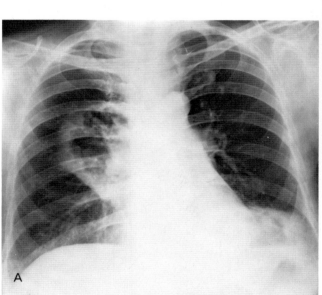
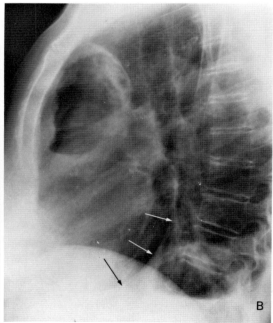

FIG. 365. WEGENER'S GRANULOMATOSIS

A: Frontal film. There is a large, thick-walled cavity with an irregular lining in the mesial part of the right lung. A similar cavity is seen at the base of the left lung behind the heart. This shows a fluid level. *B:* Lateral view. The cavity in the right lung is situated in the anterior segment of the upper lobe and extends across the short fissure to involve the adjacent portion of the middle lobe. The cavity at the left base is associated with diminution in the volume of the left lower lobe, as evidenced by posterior bowing of the long fissure (arrows). The walls of the trachea appear normal.

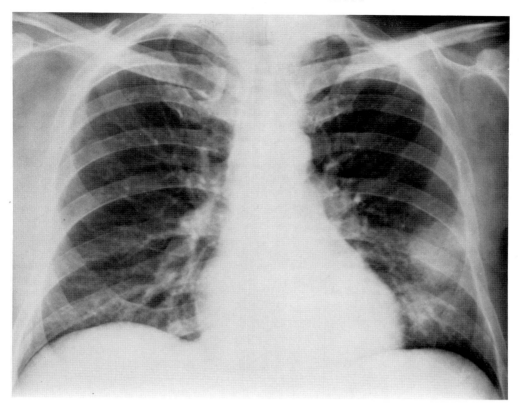

FIG. 366. WECENER'S GRANULOMATOSIS

The nodule in the left lower lobe is lobulated and has an indistinct border, resembling a primary bronchogenic carcinoma. However, the lesion was observed to grow rapidly and had doubled in size in the previous 2 months. In addition, the patient was febrile and the hazy density below the nodule appeared during this time. These facts suggested an inflammatory disease such as Wegener's granulomatosis rather than neoplasm. Lobectomy was performed. The patient was treated with steroids and remains well 4 years later.

shadows with irregular margins. Some of the shadows may represent infarcts secondary to the arteritis rather than granulomas. Cavities may form in one or more of the lesions. Frequently the densities diminish in size under steroid therapy and some disappear completely. Eventually, however, many of them recrudesce and new lesions appear, especially if the steroid dosage is diminished. Although the disease is progressive and often fatal, spontaneous regression and cure do occur.

In some instances, the disease affects mainly the bronchi, the pulmonary component consisting only of fine interstitial infiltrations involving one or more lobes and simulating viral pneumonia. The granulomatous disease causes an irregular thickening of the walls of the trachea and bronchi and may result in bronchial obstruction (Fig. 368) with segmental or, occasionally, lobar atelectasis, especially of the middle lobe. Tomograms often demonstrate the thickening of the bronchial and tracheal walls, which appear

denser than normal, and can show scalloped intrusions on the air column. These changes can also be shown by bronchography. In addition, the bronchogram often demonstrates a relative paucity of medium-sized and smaller bronchi, many of which are obstructed or totally destroyed. The ulcerative bronchitis can lead to bronchiectasis. This differs from ordinary bronchiectasis in that the dilated bronchi tend to be club-shaped rather than saccular, and the lumina of the proximal bronchi are narrowed and wavy in outline because of the marked thickening of their walls.

Fleeting shadows may appear in the lungs as the result of small areas of infarction. Pulmonary edema, seen in the later stages of the disease, is a complication of renal insufficiency. Pleural effusions occur occasionally. Although granulomatous disease of the lymph nodes is not uncommon, the nodes are rarely large enough to be detected on the film. The interstitial infiltrations may be so fine that they cannot be visualized on

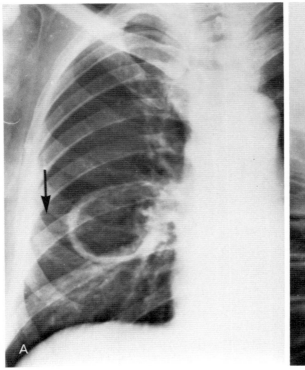
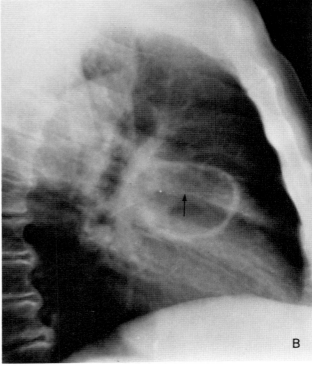

FIG. 367. WEGENER'S GRANULOMATOSIS

A: Frontal view. The relatively thin-walled cavity has a smooth contour. It overlies the short fissure (arrow). Bronchoscopy revealed thickening of the mucous membrane of the lower part of the trachea with marked narrowing of the intermediate bronchus. Biopsy disclosed Wegener's granulomatosis. *B:* Lateral view. The fact that the cavity lies at the root of the lung rather than at the periphery excludes a pyogenic abscess from consideration. The cavity also straddles the short fissure in this view. The lesion cleared on steroid therapy.

the films even though they are sufficiently extensive to interfere with pulmonary function and can be demonstrated on lung biopsy.

A definite diagnosis of necrotizing granulomatosis is usually not possible from a single roentgen examination. However, it should be suspected whenever the films show a number of persistent, irregular densities, especially when one or more undergo cavitation. Evidences of granulomatous disease in the upper respiratory tract may confirm the diagnosis.

Rheumatoid Disease of the Lungs. Rheumatoid arthritis is a generalized disease despite the fact that the clinical manifestations are usually limited to the joints. The lungs and pleura are often involved and frequently exhibit classical rheumatoid nodules on microscopic examination.

The pulmonary lesions are manifest either as interstitial inflammation and fibrosis or in the form of discrete nodules. The interstitial lesions are more common. They vary from extremely fine infiltrations to dense fibrotic deposits. They

are bilateral and more pronounced in the basal portions of the lungs (Fig. 369). Frequently the changes are so slight that they are difficult to recognize on the roentgen film, appearing simply as an increased haze over the lower third of the pulmonary fields. This is accentuated on films made during expiration.

The fact that the lungs are abnormal may not be realized unless previous films are compared with the present ones. In most cases, close inspection will then reveal fine, streak-like densities or innumerable pinpoint nodules between the blood vessels. The tiny nodular shadows may be as small as miliary tubercles. Frequently the interstitial infiltrations or fibrosis impart a reticular appearance to the involved portions of the lungs.

As the disease progresses, the infiltrations become coarser. They are largely confined to the lower portions of the lungs and represent dense fibrosis as well as infiltration with inflammatory elements. They are somewhat more irregularly distributed than the finer shadows, and are as-

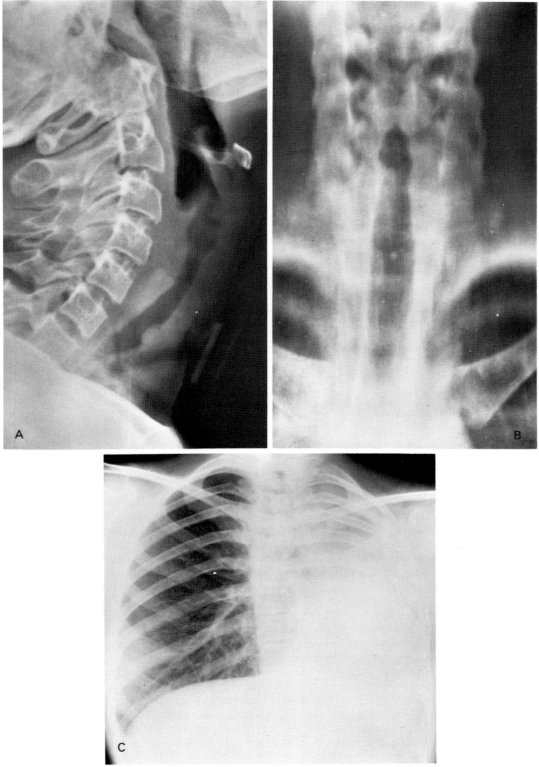

FIG. 368. WEGENER'S GRANULOMATOSIS

A: The disease was confined mainly to the trachea and bronchi. The lateral view of the neck shows narrowing and marked irregularity of the trachea beginning immediately below the larynx. The diagonal lucency in the lower anterior portion of the neck represents a plastic tracheotomy tube. *B:* The frontal tomogram of the trachea shows an irregular narrowing of the lumen and thickening of the tracheal wall. At this time there was no abnormality in the lungs. *C:* A year later extension of the disease into the major bronchi has produced complete atelectasis of the left lung.

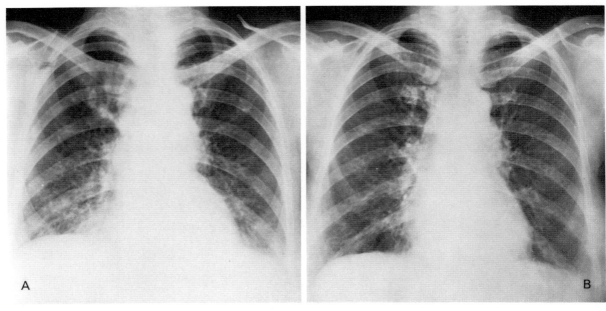

FIG. 369. RHEUMATOID DISEASE

A: The patient, who had rheumatoid arthritis for several years, presented with cough and dyspnea. There are fine interstitial infiltrations throughout the lower half of each lung. The high position of the diaphragm on this film, made in maximum inspiration, is due to limitation of distensibility of the lungs. *B:* Three years later. The symptoms have been relieved by treatment with prednisone. The pulmonary lesions have resolved and the patient is able to take a full inspiration, indicating return of normal lung compliance.

sociated with distortion of the vascular pattern and, not infrequently, with evidences of thickening of the pleura. Microscopic examination of the lung in the late stages of the disease often discloses numerous tiny, cystic cavities which are usually not demonstrable on the films. The roentgen picture of honeycomb lung is not common.

The interstitial infiltrations produce a nonspecific picture, pathologically as well as radiologically. They tend to progress and lead to fibrosis with little tendency to spontaneous resolution. Steroids or chloroquine may result in considerable clearing if the drugs are administered during the acute inflammatory stage before extensive fibrosis has taken place.

Irregular densities, varying up to 3 or 4 cm in diameter, suggesting patches of lobular pneumonia, may appear quite suddenly and represent an acute form of pulmonary involvement. They tend to persist and form irregular areas of fibrosis. A single, larger, irregular density may appear in association with fever, and at first be mistaken for a nonspecific infection. Failure of resolution of the shadow may then suggest a neoplasm. However, the association with rheumatoid arthritis should bring to mind the possibility of rheumatoid pneumonia. These lesions should respond to steroid treatment.

Nodular lesions in the lungs with the same histological structure as the subcutaneous rheumatoid nodules are less common than diffuse interstitial infiltrations. The nodules are few in number and vary from 0.5 to 5 cm in diameter. They are often round and sharply demarcated (Fig. 370) but are sometimes oval in shape with rather indistinct borders. They can occur anywhere in the lung, but are situated mostly beneath the pleura. They may regress spontaneously or with steroid therapy. Cavitation is rather common. The wall of the cavity is often thick (Fig. 371) but when more extensive shelling-out of the nodule occurs, only a thin wall remains. The cavities usually close spontaneously. Rarely, one ruptures to produce a pneumothorax.

Occasionally, the lungs are diffusely studded with numerous, smaller nodules, 0.3 to 1.0 cm in diameter. When the nodules have been present for a long time, they may show calcification on histologic examination, but the calcium deposits are not so evident on roentgen films.

Involvement of the pleura is common in rheumatoid arthritis even in the absence of pulmonary lesions. Pathologically the pleura is often thickened and may show typical rheumatoid nodules on microscopic examination. However, the pleural thickening is usually not evident ra-

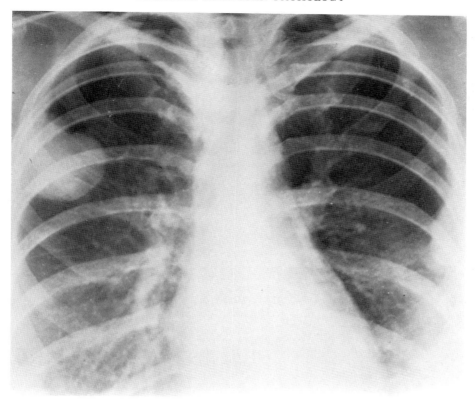

FIG. 370. RHEUMATOID NODULES

There is a sharply demarcated, round, homogeneous density in the outer part of the right upper lobe, based against the pleura. A similar but flatter nodule is seen in the axillary portion of the left chest. The patient had rheumatoid arthritis, and biopsy of one of the pulmonary lesions showed the typical picture of a rheumatoid nodule. The differentiation from metastatic neoplasm cannot be made from the single film without the clinical findings. (Courtesy of Dr. William Martel, Ann Arbor, Mich.).

diologically. Effusions are not uncommon at some stage of the disease and may be bilateral. They are usually small or moderate in size and not encapsulated even when present for a long time. The fluid frequently lies between the lung and the diaphragm and is easily overlooked. Rarely, a small or moderate-sized pericardial effusion occurs. Frequently it is associated with fluid in the pleura and may be present without any roentgen evidence of involvement of the lungs.

Cor pulmonale can result from extensive pulmonary fibrosis which interferes with the circulation through the lungs. Narrowing of the pulmonary arterial bed also occurs from diffuse inflammation of the smaller pulmonary vessels, which is part of the rheumatoid process. Although vasculitis is rarely a prominent feature of the disease, it may constitute the major pathologic process in the lungs. In fact, death from cor pulmonale secondary to the vasculitis has been reported even in the absence of roentgen evidence of pulmonary infiltrations.

The pulmonary infiltrations may precede the joint symptoms or occur considerably later. The diagnosis of rheumatoid disease of the lung cannot be made from the roentgen films alone. The interstitial infiltrations cannot be differentiated from many other inflammatory diseases, the multiple nodules suggest metastatic neoplasm, and the persistent single lesion is easily mistaken for a primary bronchogenic carcinoma. The diagnosis depends largely on the association of the pulmonary lesions with rheumatoid arthritis. However, it should be borne in mind that patients with rheumatoid arthritis are not immune to other diseases of the lungs. Characteristics which suggest specific pulmonary involvement are bilaterality and predominantly basal distribution of the interstitial infiltrations, their chronicity and their frequent association with small pleural effusions. Regression of the nodular lesions, either spontaneously or in response to steroids, will exclude neoplastic disease. The occurrence of cavitation in one or more of the multiple nodules makes the possibility of metas-

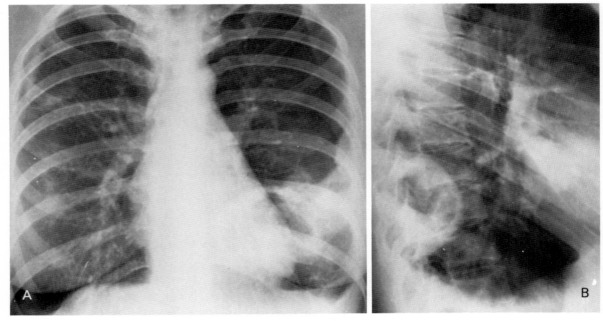

FIG. 371. CAVITATION OF RHEUMATOID NODULES

A: There is a large, irregular, thick-walled cavity in the posterior basal segment of the left lower lobe. A second small cavity is present above and lateral to this. The left costophrenic sinus is obliterated as a result of rheumatoid pleuritis. In addition, there is a scalloped shadow in the left axillary region, representing a pulmonary nodule based against the pleura. An elongated, nodular density obscures the right cardiac border. In the periphery of the right lung are two indistinct nodules which represent areas of fibrosis. *B:* Lateral view shows the large thick-walled cavity in the left lower lobe to be situated peripherally. Below this there is a small collection of fluid in the posterior costophrenic sinus. The elongated nodule seen against the right border of the heart on the frontal film lies within the middle lobe abutting on the long fissure. (Courtesy of Dr. William Martel, Ann Arbor, Mich.)

tic neoplasm unlikely. Differentiation from other inflammatory nodules may not be possible roentgenologically.

CAPLAN'S SYNDROME. Caplan reported the association of unusual nodules in the lungs of coal miners with anthracosilicosis and rheumatoid arthritis. The lesions had the classical picture of rheumatoid nodules on microscopic examination. Subsequently the same type of nodules have been noted, on rare occasions, in patients with silicosis and asbestosis. Studies have indicated that the incidence of rheumatoid disease is no different in patients with pneumoconiosis than in the general population. However, the incidence of rheumatoid nodules in the lungs is much greater when the two conditions coexist. In some cases the pulmonary nodules precede the arthritic symptoms by as much as several years.

The roentgen appearance of the nodules is the same as the ones occurring in rheumatoid disease without pneumoconiosis. Rheumatoid disease should be suspected when a few round, fairly well demarcated nodules, varing up to 5 cm in diameter, are found against a background of smaller, diffuse infiltrations of pneumoconiosis.

The sudden appearance of such nodules, which tend to come out in crops, makes the diagnosis of Caplan's syndrome most likely. The lack of symmetry in their distribution and the presence of cavitation without tubercle bacilli in the sputum also suggests rheumatoid disease. While the nodules in phthisis nigra may also be spherical and sharply demarcated, they are usually considerably larger and few in number.

The rheumatoid nodules may coalesce to form large, irregular densities which have the same appearance as those of progressive massive fibrosis if they are bilateral, or of complicating tuberculosis if unilateral. In such cases the diagnosis of Caplan's syndrome can be made only if previous films are available showing the discrete nodules before they have coalesced (Fig. 327).

Rheumatic Pneumonia. X-ray films of the chest in the acute stage of severe cases of rheumatic fever often show abnormal shadows in the lungs. At postmortem examination, the picture is frequently dominated by the presence of edema and hemorrhage. However, there are areas in which the alveoli are filled with round cells, contributing to patchy consolidation of the lungs. While these alveolar collections also occur in congestion and edema from other causes, there are additional changes in the lungs which indicate that they are really inflammatory in origin. The alveolar septa are often moderately thickened by infiltration with round cells, and areas of fibrinoid necrosis and fibroblastic proliferation can be seen in the walls of the alveoli and alveolar ducts. Therefore, it is reasonable to conclude that, in addition to the edema, there is a distinct pneumonic reaction in many cases of rheumatic fever.

The roentgen picture varies considerably, from changes that cannot be differentiated from pulmonary edema to patchy densities having the appearance of lobular pneumonia or infarction. The patchy shadows represent consolidated groups of lobules. Generally the densities are rather homogeneous with fading borders. The patches are often confluent and may involve most of a lobe. They are usually multiple and bilateral, and are frequently confined to the middle and upper thirds of the pulmonary fields (Fig. 372). They may clear in one place and appear in another, but usually resolve after a few weeks as the patient recovers. The lesions cannot be distinguished radiologically from those of infarction. Bacterial pneumonia can produce a similar appearance, but need not be considered because nonspecific infection of the lung is rare during the acute stage of rheumatic fever.

Pulmonary edema secondary to left heart failure occurs commonly in acute rheumatic fever, and may be present without enlargement of the

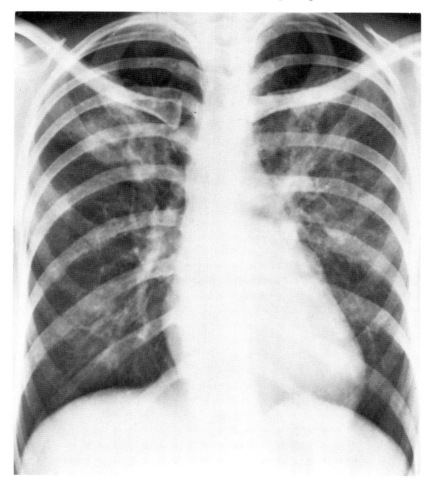

FIG. 372. RHEUMATIC PNEUMONIA

The lobular consolidation beneath the right clavicle and the interstitial infiltrations in the left upper lobe extending out from the lung root were associated with a recurrence of acute rheumatic fever. The prominence of the left atrial appendage is indicative of enlargement of the left atrium. In addition, the heart is elongated downward and to the left because of left ventricular enlargement. Clinically, the patient had disease of both the mitral and aortic valves. The pulmonary lesions resolved completely when the patient recovered from the acute phase of rheumatic fever.

heart. When the edema is largely confined to the central portions of the lung, typical butterfly shadows are produced. In more generalized edema, there are scattered fluffy densities, more pronounced at the bases (Fig. 373). When the lungs are congested there is accentuation of the shadows of the pulmonary vessels which can give rise to a stippled appearance resembling miliary tuberculosis. In such instances it is difficult, if not impossible, to determine radiologically whether there is edema, or consolidation and infiltration from rheumatic pneumonia as well.

A small or moderate-sized pleural effusion, either unilateral or bilateral, sometimes accompanies the rheumatic pneumonia. However, the effusion can occur in the absence of any demonstrable infiltration of the lungs. When it occurs without cardiac failure or pulmonary infarction it is due to rheumatic pleuritis.

Goodpasture's Syndrome. Goodpasture's syndrome consists of a combination of pulmo-nary hemorrhage and glomerulitis. The condition occurs predominantly in young adult males. Hemoptysis is usually the first symptom, while evidence of renal disease may not appear until several months later. The hemoptyses are intermittent but the renal insufficiency tends to be steadily progressive. A severe anemia, out of proportion to the amount of hemoptysis or the severity of the renal disease, is frequently present. The disease is usually fatal within a year but occasional recoveries have been reported.

The changes in the lungs in Goodpasture's syndrome are referable to three distinct pathologic processes. The first is inundation of the alveoli with blood. The second is an inflammatory reaction secondary to deposition of hemosiderin into the interstitial tissues resulting from breakdown of blood in the alveoli. Finally, there are changes secondary to the renal failure. Any or all of these processes may be responsible for abnormalities on the roentgen film.

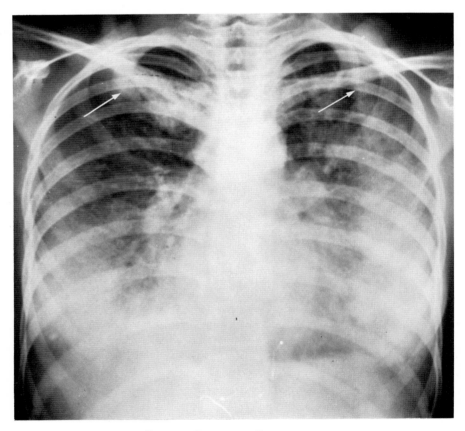

FIG. 373. RHEUMATIC PNEUMONIA

An 11 year old girl with acute rheumatic fever. There are confluent areas of consolidation throughout the upper portions of the lungs. The heart is not enlarged. There is no pleural effusion. It is not possible from the single film to determine how much of the density is due to rheumatic pneumonia and how much to pulmonary edema. The irregular densities over the upper lobes (arrow) are artifacts due to braids.

The stage of acute hemorrhage in the lung is almost always associated with hemoptysis. The hemoptyses may be large or small and bear no direct relationship to the extent of the roentgen shadows. The inundated portions of the lung cast rather large, homogeneous shadows which are usually bilateral and simulate areas of pneumonic consolidation. The shadows are usually not quite as dense as those of lobar pneumonia because many of the alveoli are not filled with blood and remain aerated. Typically, the shadow appears as a rather hazy cloud which, on close inspection, shows a granular texture. In other cases, the shadows are quite dense and homogeneous (Fig. 374). However, in most instances, the outlines of the blood vessels can be distinguished within the lesion because of the presence of air in many of the adjacent alveoli. Occasionally,

denser shadows are seen within the diffuse hazy areas.

Small, multiple shadows, up to 2 or 3 cm in diameter, are the result of many small hemorrhages in the lungs. They are irregularly distributed throughout both lungs but practically always spare the apices. The bases, also, are often clear. The shadows are poorly defined and, in places, confluent, but occasionally they are fairly well demarcated. When the densities are small, measuring no more than 1 cm in diameter, they are more uniformly distributed throughout the lungs. These may coexist with large diffuse shadows.

The episodes of bleeding are short-lived and the shadows usually clear completely within a week or 10 days, and sometimes even more rapidly. New densities appear with subsequent hem-

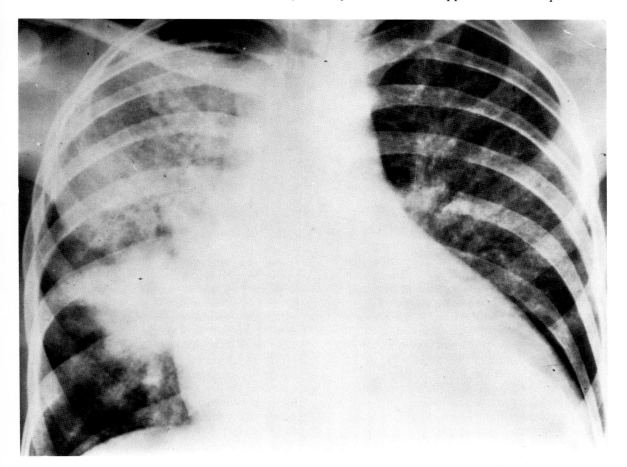

FIG. 374. GOODPASTURE'S SYNDROME

A young man presented with massive hemoptysis and evidence of glomerulonephritis. The films show patchy areas of consolidation in the upper part of the right lung. The homogeneous density in the lower part of the lung is the result of more uniform filling of the alveoli. The left lung is congested and the left ventricle is markedly enlarged. The appearance could be due to unilateral pulmonary edema in heart failure. However, the presence of the renal disease together with massive hemoptysis is indicative of Goodpasture's syndrome. The consolidation was due to intrapulmonary hemorrhage.

orrhages. Hemosiderin is deposited within the lung in the same manner as in idiopathic pulmonary hemosiderosis. It calls forth a foreign body reaction resulting in interstitial fibrosis. The roentgen appearance is then characterized by a fine, sharply etched reticular pattern with punctate densities that impart a granular appearance to the film.

When renal failure supervenes, the picture may become complicated by the occurrence of pulmonary edema. This can produce the typical butterfly pattern of central edema of the lungs or ill-defined, scattered patchy densities, sometimes more numerous on one side. The pulmonary vessels are generally widened and hazy in outline. A pleural effusion is frequently present and may be bilateral. Although the heart may be enlarged, it is often normal in size.

The roentgen picture of the lung in Goodpasture's syndrome, before the pulmonary congestion and edema associated with renal failure occur, is identical with that of idiopathic pulmonary hemosiderosis. However, four-fifths of the cases of idiopathic pulmonary hemosiderosis occur in patients before they reach the age of 16, while Goodpasture's syndrome must be extremely rare, if it occurs at all, before that age.

Miscellaneous Diseases

Pulmonary Alveolar Proteinosis. Pulmonary alveolar proteinosis is a disease of unknown etiology, characterized by filling of alveoli with a proteinaceous, eosinophilic, P-aminosalicylic acid-positive substance, rich in lipid, with little or no involvement of the alveolar walls. The involved portion of the lung is not homogeneously affected, many of the alveoli adjacent to those filled with the proteinaceous material remaining free. The disease is most common between the ages of 20 and 50, but it has been noted in children as young as 2½ years of age. There may be few or no symptoms even when the lungs are extensively involved.

The roentgen picture is most commonly characterized by the presence of flocculent, soft densities simulating pulmonary edema. The shadows are not as dense and homogeneous as those of lobar pneumonia because numerous alveoli remain aerated. The blood vessels, therefore, are visible within the affected area although their outlines are indistinct. The lesions are almost always bilateral and the shadows appear to be concentrated in the region of the lung roots. Often they extend from here to the bases, but may remain localized to the perihilar region, producing the butterfly shadow usually associated with central pulmonary edema.

Less commonly, the disease is manifested by densities of a more patchy character, scattered throughout the lungs. These vary in size, up to 2 cm in diameter. They are irregular and their borders are indistinct. As in the case of the more diffuse central lesions, the shadows are not very dense because many of the alveoli remain aerated. Rarely, almost all the alveoli in the involved portion are filled, and then the patches are denser, more sharply circumscribed and present a nodular appearance.

When only small groups of alveoli are involved, the roentgen picture is characterized by numerous miliary or submiliary densities, or simply by a finely granular pattern. The appearance is determined by the size of the alveolar groups involved and the amount of aerated lung tissue between them. The tiny densities may be distributed throughout the lungs but are more frequently situated in the perihilar regions or at the bases (Fig. 375). There is no reticular pattern because the interstitial tissues are not involved.

Rarely the lesions are unilateral. Fine densities localized to the base of one lung present the picture of viral pneumonia. A case has been reported in which there was dense, homogeneous consolidation of the lingula, simulating lobar pneumonia radiologically. We have observed a case in which nodular lesions were confined to the apical portion of one lung, simulating tuberculosis.

The appearance may remain unchanged for years, but there is generally a tendency to gradual progression, with coalescence and increasing density of the shadows and extension of the lesion throughout the lungs. Granular or stippled shadows may become transformed into irregular patches of consolidation.

Partial resolution is not uncommon with or without treatment. The peripherally situated lesions tend to clear first, although in some instances resolution begins in the region of the lung roots. Clearing may occur on one side while the disease spreads on the other. Occasionally the shadows disappear completely, but this does not necessarily mean that the disease is entirely cured. A necropsy performed on a patient with complete radiological clearing disclosed persistent disease.

In the progressive cases death frequently results from pulmonary insufficiency caused by widespread filling of the alveoli with the proteinaceous material. Interstitial fibrosis has been found at autopsy in addition to the alveolar-

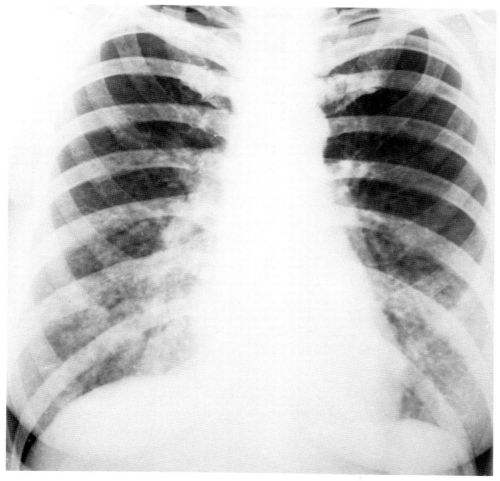

Fig. 375. Alveolar Proteinosis

The lower part of each lung field appears clouded as the result of numerous, poorly defined nodular densities. These represent groups of alveoli filled with proteinaceous material. The diagnosis was proved by lung biopsy.

filling process, sometimes with cor pulmonale.

Patients with alveolar proteinosis are susceptible to secondary infection, particularly by fungi. Nocardiosis is inordinately frequent. The complicating infection may be completely masked by the underlying proteinosis. However, it may be manifested radiologically by the presence of a pleural effusion or enlargement of lymph nodes, neither of which occurs in uncomplicated proteinosis. In several instances the complicating fungal infection in the lungs was not apparent until subcutaneous lesions or symptoms referable to a brain abscess appeared.

The diagnosis of alveolar proteinosis cannot be made from the x-ray films alone. Most often the roentgen picture suggests pulmonary edema. However, the absence of cardiac enlargement, azotemia, marked dyspnea or other clinical manifestations of pulmonary edema exclude this condition from consideration and should suggest the possibility of alveolar proteinosis.

Desquamative Interstitial Pneumonia. This is a chronic disease of the lungs, described by Liebow, Steer and Billingsley, who reported the details of 18 cases and mentioned 14 additional ones. Twelve additional examples of this entity were described by Gaensler and his coworkers. The disease is characterized by proliferation and desquamation of masses of large alveolar cells into the distal air spaces. The alveolar walls become infiltrated with proliferating cells and, in the later stages, with fibroblasts and focal collections of lymphocytes. There is no destruction of lung tissue or necrosis of the desquamated cells. The main symptom of the disease is dyspnea, which is slowly progressive and eventually results in pulmonary insufficiency. None of the patients was under 16 years of age.

The x-ray films in most of the cases of desquamative interstitial pneumonia show a bilateral, symmetrical, hazy opacification of the mesial portion of the lower lobes. The shadows seem to extend downward from the hilar region to the diaphragm, usually not reaching the lateral chest wall. The blood vessels are poorly outlined and are drawn together, indicating shrinkage of the involved portion of the lung. This occurs particularly in the later stages when there is an increase in the interstitial infiltration together with fibrosis. The shrinkage of the lung is due to obstruction of the bronchioles by infiltration of their walls or plugging by masses of desquamated cells, and is manifested by elevation of the leaves of the diaphragm. In some instances, the lesions are more punctate and involve the lungs diffusely. Coarse, strand-like shadows, extending downward and outward from the lung roots are late manifestations. Although the roentgen changes are mainly in the lower portion of the lungs, biopsies have shown the upper lobes to be involved even when they appear perfectly clear on the roentgen films.

The disease tends to persist and progress over a long period of time but complete resolution can take place, particularly under steroid therapy. Spontaneous pneumothorax occurs occasionally in the later stages of the disease as a result of rupture of dilated air spaces. Evidences of pleurisy have been found in several cases. In one, there was extreme thickening of the pleura. Bilateral pleural effusions have also been observed, and one case of pericardial effusion has been reported.

Pulmonary Alveolar Microlithiasis. Pulmonary microlithiasis is characterized by the presence of concretions of calcium salts (calcospherites) in the alveoli throughout the lungs. Half of the reported cases have been familial. The concretions are lamellated and are similar in appearance to corpora amylacea. There is usually little or no reaction in the alveolar walls, although some fibrosis occurs in the later stages.

The most striking feature of this disease is the lack of any correlation between the symptoms and the degree of involvement of the lungs. In most cases the pulmonary abnormality is first noted at a routine x-ray examination in a patient who has few or no symptoms referable to the disease. The lungs may be extensively involved at this time and the pulmonary fields diffusely clouded by fine, granular opacities of calcific density (Fig. 376). The individual opacities are usually less than 1 mm in diameter but may be as large as a pinhead. The fine, punctate character of the shadows may be recognizable on ordinary films, but usually the overlapping of the individual densities results in a generalized, more or less homogeneous clouding of the lungs. The borders of the heart and diaphragm are obscured and the pulmonary vascular pattern is indistinct. The appearance resembles that of an underexposed film. Actually, the ordinary exposure is insufficient to disclose detail because the lungs are so dense. Bucky films reveal the characteristic discrete, punctate nature of the lesions.

Even when first observed, the lesions are distributed throughout the lungs from the apex to the base, although the upper portions are somewhat less involved. In the earlier cases the lung above the costophrenic sinus appears to be less dense, possibly because the anteroposterior diameter of the lateral part of the chest is less than that of the central portion.

As the disease progresses, the opacity of the lungs increases so that all structural detail is lost. The density of the lung is frequently so great that the contour of the diaphragm once more becomes visible, but this time because the density of the abdominal structures is *less* than that of the lungs. Similarly, we have observed the reappearance of the cardiac silhouette as a relative lucency in contrast to the adjacent lung. As more and more alveoli become filled with calcospherites, the density of the lung above the costophrenic sinuses increases. The apices may become completely opacified, leaving a rim of lucency within the curve of the upper ribs, formed by the extrapleural fat and connective tissue. The upper portions of the lungs may remain clear because of the presence of bullae in the apices.

In some cases there is increased accumulation of the microliths in the subpleural alveoli. This results in the formation of a dense, linear shadow outlining the pleural surface of the lung. The pulmonary fissures then become visible and a dense line may be seen running along the inner border of the chest wall. A similar line can appear along the surface of the diaphragm and along portions of the mediastinal border. The lateral view may provide a striking picture of the line of subpleural calcification behind the sternum.

It is a peculiar fact that when first observed, the disease has always been quite extensive. This suggests the possibility that its development may be quite rapid in the early stage. However, once established, the course of the disease is slowly-progressive over a period of many years. There is no tendency to clearing of the lesions at any time. More and more alveoli become involved, culminating in death from pulmonary insufficiency or cor pulmonale. While acute respiratory

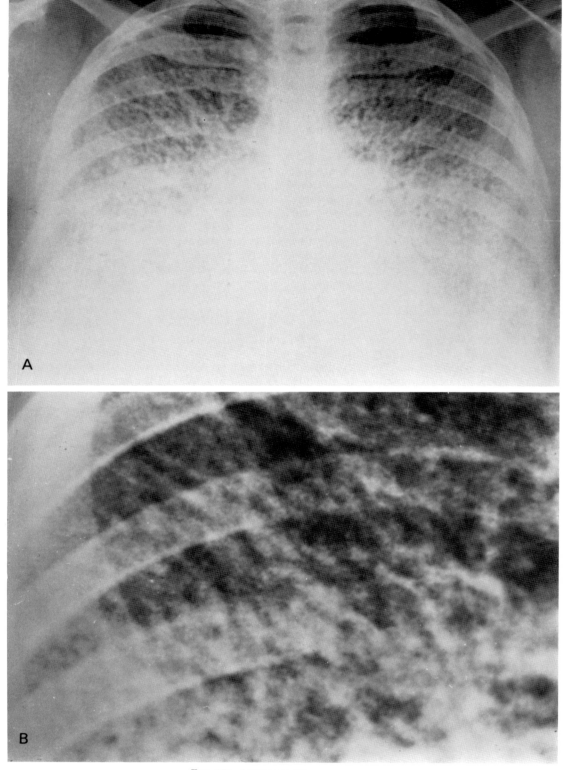

FIG. 376. ALEVOLAR MICROLITHIASIS

A: Both lungs are diffusely studded with dense, tiny nodular lesions. These are more numerous at the lung bases. The opacification of the lung is so great that the cardiac borders are obscured. *B:* A close-up of a Bucky film shows the densities to be formed by multiple, fine calcific nodules. This picture is pathognomonic for alveolar microlithiasis.

infection may contribute to the final outcome, there does not appear to be any increased incidence of secondary respiratory infections in this disease.

The diagnosis of pulmonary alveolar microlithiasis is immediately suggested by the density of the diffuse symmetrical shadows in the lungs. Bucky films provide a pathognomonic picture, disclosing the punctate calcific components of the shadow. These are smaller and more numerous than the calcific deposits occurring in histoplasmosis, tuberculosis, silicosis or mitral stenosis. The density of the calcium differentiates microlithiasis from other miliary diseases. The lymph nodes and pleura are not involved. The costophrenic sulci are free even in the presence of dense subpleural lines. The lesions of stannosis and baritosis are denser than those of microlithiasis since they are metallic rather than calcific. In addition, the individual lesions in these diseases tend to be larger, and more numerous in the upper lobes.

Amyloid Disease. Secondary amyloidosis, which occurs in the course of a chronic infection, does not cause gross changes in the lungs. Pulmonary amyloidosis is a manifestation of the *primary* form of the disease, and occurs independent of any known underlying cause. It may be confined to the lung or involve the trachea and major bronchi, in addition to other organs.

Primary amyloidosis can affect any part of the lower respiratory tract. Most commonly, there is diffuse involvement of the tracheobronchial tree, sometimes together with deposition of amyloid in the walls of the pulmonary vessels and the interstitial tissues of the lungs. Less frequently, the disease assumes a more circumscribed form, manifested by localized amyloid tumors in the trachea, bronchi or pulmonary parenchyma. Amyloidosis of the lungs, in all its forms, is a disease of older people, affecting mostly those over the age of 50.

The lungs may be involved diffusely, or by one or more amyloid nodules. In either instance, the disease may be confined to the lungs, although the diffuse form is often associated with amyloid deposits elsewhere in the body.

Localized pulmonary amyloidosis usually appears radiologically in the form of several slow-growing nodules in both lungs. They vary in size and have been reported as large as 8 cm in diameter. The nodules may be round and sharply demarcated, but often have an irregular, less distinct border. Occasionally their margins are spiculated, like the shadows of inflammatory granulomas. Most of them extend to the surface of the lung. Some are broad-based against the pleura like metastatic neoplasms, but unlike these, their borders tend to be irregular rather than in the form of smooth scallops. Like malignant neoplasms, amyloid tumors may grow through the pleura into the chest wall or through a fissure to involve an adjacent lobe. While most amyloid tumors contain microscopic deposits of bone, only occasionally is there sufficient calcification to be detected on the roentgen film. The bone is deposited irregularly throughout the nodules, and when it is abundant the appearance is similar to that of metastases from an osteogenic sarcoma. When the nodule is single, the calcific deposits produce an appearance similar to that of a hamartoma.

Solitary nodular amyloid tumors are less frequent. As in the case of metastatic neoplasms, only one nodule may be visible on the film while additional ones are found either at operation or at autopsy. Tomograms of both lungs may show additional small nodules not seen on the films. If the tomograms do not disclose calcification within a solitary amyloid nodule, the lesion cannot be differentiated radiologically from a primary bronchogenic neoplasm.

The diffuse form of amyloid disease of the lungs is more often associated with amyloidosis of the remainder of the respiratory tract than of other organs. The infiltrations involve the interstitial tissues of the lungs, particularly about the blood vessels, as well as the alveolar walls. The roentgen appearance is characterized by diffuse nodulation and reticulation of the lungs (Fig. 377). The nodules form a miliary or submiliary pattern. In the latter, the nodules are larger, poorly defined and irregular in shape. The combination of reticulation with tiny nodules suggests pneumoconiosis.

Condensation of the shadows at the lung roots from extensive amyloid deposits about the major blood vessels in addition to the pattern of infiltration in the lungs often suggests lymphangitic carcinomatosis. Involvement of the hilar nodes may contribute to the dense shadows at the lung roots but usually the lymph nodes are not involved to any great extent. The heart may be enlarged as a result of cor pulmonale but more frequently the cardiac enlargement is secondary to deposition of amyloid in the myocardium.

Neonatal Respiratory Distress. In about half the cases of respiratory distress in the newborn, the cause lies outside the chest and no pulmonary abnormality is found on the films. However, difficulty may be experienced in determining whether or not the lungs are normal. Allowance must be made for the pulmonary markings which are normally prominent in the

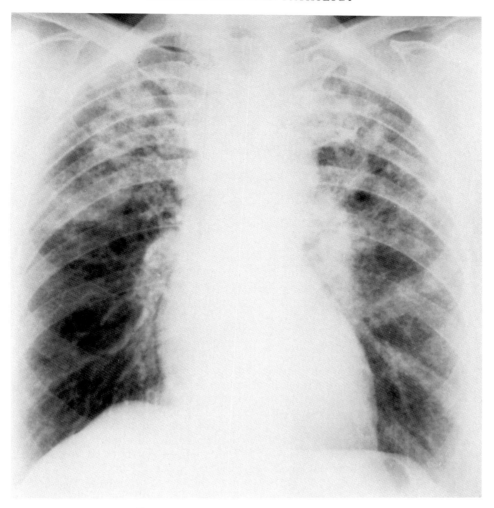

FIG. 377. PRIMARY PULMONARY AMYLOIDOSIS

There are a number of indistinct nodules in each upper lobe together with interstitial infiltrations. Similar infiltrations are present throughout the lower half of the left lung. The diagnosis was proved by lung biopsy. There was no evidence of amyloidosis elsewhere in the body.

newborn. This is due to the relatively large anteroposterior diameter of the chest at the time and the fact that the x-ray beam is frequently centered low so that the rays are angled, and traverse a greater depth of lung tissue. Special care must be taken to make the films in full inspiration since those made in expiration show diffuse clouding of the pulmonary fields, easily confused with pulmonary disease. To accomplish this, the exposure should be triggered during the deep inspiration that follows a burst of crying.

Chief among the diseases of the chest that are responsible for respiratory distress in the newborn are cardiovascular anomalies, the effects of aspiration, and hyaline membrane disease. Less common, but especially interesting, is the Wilson-Mikity syndrome. Other causes of respiratory distress, i.e., anomalies of the trachea, bronchi, lungs and diaphragm, are described in other sections.

ASPIRATION SYNDROME. The primary effect of aspiration of amniotic fluid or meconium is bronchial obstruction, producing emphysema and atelectasis. These changes may be lobar, segmental or subsegmental in distribution, and are apparent immediately after birth. Increased secretion and mucus plugs cause further obstruction, and secondary infection results in complicating pneumonia. A similar picture can occur later in the neonatal period from aspiration of milk or vomitus.

In some cases, the roentgen abnormality consists solely of lobar emphysema or atelectasis. Usually, however, the changes are more diffuse, although the lesions are not uniformly distributed throughout the lungs. Patchy shadows, varying considerably in size, are present in both lungs, characteristically interspersed with lucent areas. These represent multiple foci of atelectasis and emphysema. The pneumonia may follow immediately upon aspiration if the amniotic fluid is infected.

Pneumonia may also occur independent of aspiration, as the result of hematogenous spread of infection from the mother. The inflammatory foci are then more uniform in size and distribution. The roentgen films show small patchy shadows which may be confluent, but are not associated with evidences of atelectasis or emphysema.

HYALINE MEMBRANE DISEASE. Hyaline membrane disease in the newborn is a distinct pathologic entity characterized by the presence of an eosinophilic, hyaline substance lining many of the alveoli, alveolar ducts and terminal bronchioles, often with necrosis of the underlying epithelium. Many of the alveoli are collapsed, while other alveoli and alveolar ducts are overdistended and may be filled with proteinaceous material. In addition, some degree of pulmonary edema is present in most cases. The lung remains approximately normal in size even though its air content is diminished.

The disease occurs most frequently in premature infants, in children of diabetic mothers and in those delivered by cesarean section. Dyspnea and cyanosis may be absent at birth, but invariably appear within the first 8 hours of life. If the disease pursues a fatal course, death almost always occurs within 72 hours. If the infant survives this period, the lungs gradually clear and resolution is usually complete within a week.

The most common roentgen manifestation is simply a rather uniform clouding of the pulmonary fields as a result of poor aeration of the lungs. Frequently the lungs present a diffuse granular appearance, produced by the intermingling of groups of emphysematous alveoli with those that are atelectatic or filled with fluid or proteinaceous material. The radiolucent air-filled bronchi are usually clearly visualized because of contrast with the dense adjacent lung, producing an air bronchogram (Fig. 378). In more severe cases, the irregular opacification of the lung may result in blurring of the borders of the heart and diaphragm. Rarely the lungs are opaque as in complete atelectasis of the newborn.

The appearance of the roentgen changes may not coincide with the onset of clinical symptoms. Occasionally the film is normal when the respiratory distress first becomes manifest and the roentgen changes become evident shortly thereafter. On the other hand, these changes have been observed prior to the respiratory difficulty. If the infant survives, the shadows begin to clear within a few days and the film rapidly reverts to normal. Occasionally, rupture of alveoli results in interstitial emphysema complicated by pneumothorax or pneumomediastinum (see Fig. 481). These conditions also tend to resolve quickly.

A roentgen appearance similar to that of hyaline membrane disease occurs in patients with congenital pulmonary lymphangiectasia and total anomalous pulmonary venous drainage. In the former, the lymphatic channels in the interlobular septa and about the bronchi and blood vessels are markedly dilated and appear increased in number, giving rise to a microscopic picture of diffuse lymphangiomatosis. The abnormal lymphatics, filled with fluid, cause diffuse clouding, reticulation or granularity of the pulmonary fields.

When the pulmonary veins do not enter the left atrium, they usually form a common trunk which communicates with the systemic venous circulation. The common trunk may be compressed, particularly if it passes through the diaphragm to drain into the portal system. This causes congestion and edema of the lungs, while the heart is not enlarged. The condition can be differentiated from hyaline membrane disease if the widened pulmonary veins are recognized. This requires films of extremely fine quality.

WILSON-MIKITY SYNDROME. This is a pulmonary disease of premature infants, characterized by multiple small foci of emphysema and small areas of atelectasis or incompletely formed alveoli with thickened septa, mingled with areas of normal lung. There is also evidence of incomplete formation of the pulmonary capillary network. The entire pathologic picture suggests incomplete maturation of the lung.

While dyspnea and cyanosis are often present at birth, the onset of these symptoms may be delayed for a considerable period, occasionally for several weeks. The symptoms gradually increase and about half of the children die, usually in 2 to 4 months, often from right heart failure. In most of the survivors, the chest returns to normal in 6 to 12 months.

The x-ray appearance of the chest may vary at different stages, but the full-blown picture is characteristic of the disease. It consists of innumerable cyst-like areas of lucency, measuring up to 1 cm in diameter, distributed rather uniformly throughout both lungs. Between these emphysematous foci are poorly defined, coarse septa, representing atelectatic lung or incompletely

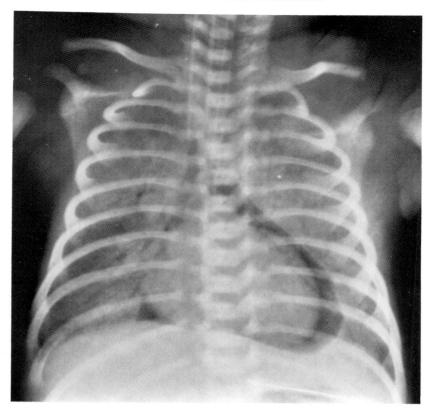

FIG. 378. HYALINE MEMBRANE DISEASE

A one day old premature infant in severe respiratory distress. Both lungs are clouded and, in places, have a granular appearance. The lucent streaks radiating outward from the root of the right lung represent air in the bronchi indicating consolidation of the lung rather than atelectasis. This picture is characteristic of hyaline membrane disease. There is a complicating pneumopericardium. (Courtesy of Dr. J. Rose, New York, N. Y.)

formed alveoli with thickened walls. At first the cystic areas may not be well defined. The evidences of emphysema may be present only at the bases, while the remainder of the lungs have a coarse, reticular appearance, sometimes studded with very small, indistinct nodules (Fig. 379).

X-ray examination has disclosed the presence of the disease before the onset of symptoms. This is to be expected if the condition is truly one of pulmonary dysmaturity, as is generally believed. If the patient survives, the cystic changes gradually regress, leaving some thickening of the interstitial tissues which eventually become normal. Enlargement of the heart occurs in the children who develop pulmonary hypertension and right heart failure.

The Wilson-Mikity syndrome differs from hyaline membrane disease in several respects. Its onset is often late, its course more prolonged, and the emphysematous foci are larger, imparting a characteristic bubbly appearance to the pulmonary field.

Traumatic Injuries of the Lung. The pulmonary changes caused by penetrating wounds of the lungs are similar to those caused by blunt trauma. However, in the case of penetrating injuries, the changes in the lung are usually obscured by an accompanying hemothorax or by collapse of the lung by a pneumothorax. Blunt trauma may cause only a contusion of the lung, but if the injury is severe, the lung can be lacerated as well.

The distribution of the lesions caused by blunt force is influenced by the type and severity of the trauma. In blast injuries the lesions tend to be multiple, involving both lungs. In the more localized types of injury, the lesion is usually single and situated directly under the point of trauma. However, in some instances the opposite portion of the lung is the only area affected. This *contrecoup* injury is most frequently situated adjacent to the posterior part of the chest because this is the most rigid portion of the thoracic cage.

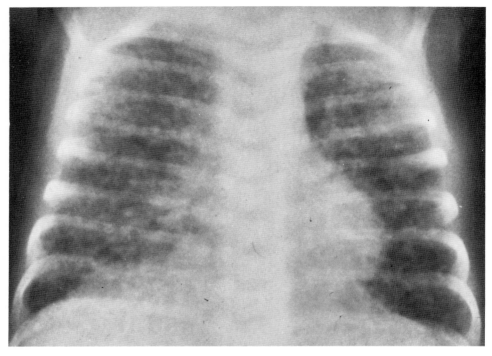

FIG. 379. WILSON-MIKITY SYNDROME

The film of a 2 week old premature infant in respiratory distress shows numerous poorly defined nodular densities throughout the lungs. These represent small areas of atelectasis and incompletely developed acini. The lung bases are hyperlucent because of emphysema and cystic changes.

Most often the injury to the lung is associated with fractures of the ribs, but extensive damage to the lung can occur even though the ribs are intact. Hemothorax, pneumothorax, pneumomediastinum, tracheal or bronchial rupture, or a diaphragmatic hernia can also result from blunt trauma and complicate the picture.

CONTUSION OF THE LUNG. A pulmonary contusion results from rupture of small vessels with extravasation of blood in the perivascular, peribronchial and interstitial tissues, as well as into the alveoli. It is associated with a variable amount of local pulmonary edema.

The contusion appears radiologically as an ill-defined area of consolidation (Fig. 380). It may be large or small, depending on the extent of the injury. The shadow may be of uniform density as in lobar pneumonia, but if only some of the alveoli in this area are filled with blood, the shadow is mottled. In severe crushing injuries, multiple, irregular, patchy shadows of varying density may involve a considerable portion of the lung (see Fig. 441).

The contusion is evident on films made soon after the accident. During the next few days the shadows may increase in size and density before they begin to recede. Resolution is gradual and

is usually complete in 1 to 3 weeks, without residual shadow. In exceptional instances, large densities have been noted to disappear completely in a day or two. In such cases, it is assumed that the abnormality was almost entirely due to edema rather than to hemorrhage. A shadow lasting more than 3 weeks indicates a laceration and hematoma of the lung rather than a simple contusion.

PULMONARY HEMATOMA. This represents a collection of blood within a space in the lung resulting from laceration of the pulmonary tissue. It differs from a simple contusion, which is caused by seepage of blood into the pulmonary tissue with comparatively little tearing of the lung. Thus, a pulmonary contusion is comparable to an ecchymosis rather than to a hematoma. Although pulmonary hematomas are generally due to traumatic injuries, they may also follow segmental or wedge resection due to accumulation of blood in the space left in the lung.

A cavity forms immediately after a laceration because of retraction of the torn elastic tissue. Thus, a comparatively large, round cavity may form even though the tear in the lung is small and irregular. Larger or multiple lacerations can result in the formation of irregular cavities.

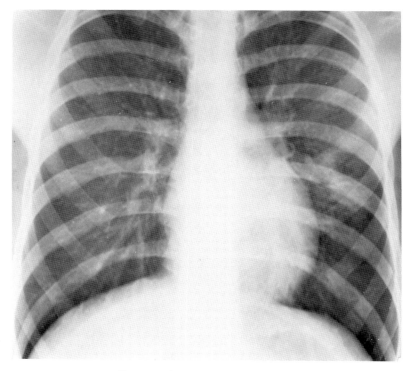

FIG. 380. CONTUSIONS OF THE LUNG

The patient received a sharp blow to the left side of the chest during a wrestling match. Films show no evidence of rib fracture. However, there is an irregular area of consolidation in the left mid-lung. Although this cannot be distinguished from a pneumonia, it did occur immediately after blunt chest trauma and the patient had no fever or other signs of sepsis. The shadow cleared completely within a week leaving no residuum.

Blunt trauma sufficient to cause a laceration of the lung also causes contusion of the surrounding pulmonary tissue. The shadow seen on the film immediately after the injury is mainly the result of pulmonary contusion, but part of the density may represent a cavity filled with blood. A lucent area within the more diffuse shadow represents air within a partially filled cavity. If no air is present, the cavity cannot be recognized roentgenologically.

The cavities are usually 2 or 3 cm in diameter. Occasionally they are considerably larger. Most often the cavity lies well within the shadow of the surrounding contusion. When it is peripherally placed, the picture simulates a suppurative bronchopneumonia complicated by a pneumatocele.

Usually there is a considerable amount of consolidated lung about the cavity, so that its wall appears very thick. However, if the surrounding lung is clear, the cavity is thin-walled and is represented simply by a fine annular shadow. Irregularly loculated cavities are the result of more extensive laceration and may be multiple in severe crushing injuries. Communications between the cavities can produce a multicystic appearance.

Because of bleeding in association with the tear in the lung, an air-fluid level is commonly present soon after the injury (Fig. 381). If there is a wide bronchial communication, the level disappears rapidly as the contents of the cavity are expectorated. Similarly, a secondarily infected hematoma frequently shows a fluid level but this usually appears for the first time a week or more after the accident.

When the blood within the cavity clots, the roentgen appearance of the hematoma remains unchanged unless air is also present. The clot is then visualized as a round, well demarcated density in the most dependent portion. The air is represented by a crescent-shaped lucency above the clot. Since the clot lies free within the cavity, it can shift with a change in the position of the patient. Radiologically, the appearance is identical to that of an intracavitary fungus ball. The differential diagnosis depends primarily on a history of recent injury.

Frequently the shadow of the hematoma increases in size within the first few days, probably

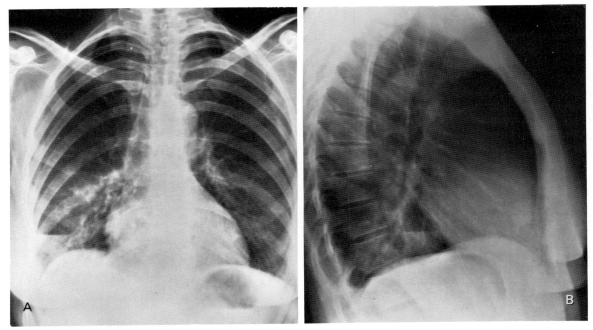

FIG. 381. LACERATION OF THE LUNG

A: The film made several hours after an automobile accident in which the patient sustained blunt trauma to the chest shows a cavity with an air-fluid level in the right lower lobe. Small patches of consolidation are present above and mesial to the cavity, representing areas of contusion. The patient was afebrile and coughed up blood immediately after the accident. *B:* Lateral view. The cavity is situated in the anterior portion of the lateral basal segment. The patient was discharged without specific treatment. A film made several weeks later showed no abnormality in the lungs.

as a result of continued blood seepage and reactive edema in the lung about the laceration. While the surrounding contusion may soon begin to undergo resolution, the laceration itself heals slowly. The air within the cavity is absorbed rapidly, but the accumulation of blood disappears gradually. The entire shadow becomes smaller and more sharply defined as the hematoma is encapsulated and the surrounding contusion resolves, leaving a round or oval, nodular shadow. Clearing of the hematoma usually requires many weeks, and complete resolution may not occur for a full year. Usually no trace of the hematoma remains, although fibrous streaks or thickening of the pleura may persist.

Since the roentgen appearance is not specific, the diagnosis of pulmonary hematoma depends, in large degree, upon the history of an injury. The patient who is found to have a lesion of the lung shortly after an alcoholic bout, may not recall any injury, and the hematoma may be mistaken for a pneumonia or a lung abscess. Occasionally, a nodular shadow is found some time after an accident, a history of which is not volunteered by the patient because it appeared trivial. The lesion may then be confused with a primary neoplasm if it is single, or metastases if more than one shadow is present. If there is evidence of one or more rib fractures, even if healed or at a distance from the lesion, the possibility of a hematoma should be considered. The history should be gone into thoroughly, especially with regard to hemoptysis associated with an accident.

ATELECTASIS AND EMPHYSEMA. Atelectasis of a lobe, or even of an entire lung, occurs occasionally after trauma to the chest. In the absence of any demonstrable injury to the lung itself, it had been thought that the collapse of the lung was neurogenic. However, it appears more probable that the atelectasis is due to bronchial plugging by blood or secretions. The injury to the chest wall inhibits deep breathing and coughing, thereby interfering with clearing of the bronchial tree. Obstructive emphysema occurs under the same conditions if the obstruction is incomplete. Both atelectasis and obstructive emphysema are less common in contusion than in laceration of the lung where there is a greater tendency for accumulation of blood in the bronchi.

TORSION OF THE LUNG. This is a rare complication of a crushing injury to the chest, and has been reported only in children. The lung is twisted 180° about its root so that the lower lobe extends to the apex of the hemithorax and the upper lobe is displaced to the base. Apparently it is necessary for the inferior pulmonary ligament to be torn before torsion can occur.

The shadows of the vessels are very prominent and appear unusual. Films made soon after the accident have shown the shadows of the large vessels of the lower lobe to extend upward and outward from the lung root in the position usually occupied by the smaller vessels of the upper lobe. Later, granular or mottled shadows appear in the lungs, representing edema due to the circulatory disturbance resulting from torsion of the vessels. Finally, the lung may become diffusely opaque as atelectasis supervenes because of twisting of the main bronchus.

Drug-Induced Lung Disease. An ever-increasing number of drugs are being recognized as a potential cause of pulmonary disease. In some cases, the damage results from a hypersensitivity reaction, but in the majority of instances, the mechanism by which the lung is injured is not known. As a rule, discontinuation of the offending medication causes arrest or regression of the pulmonary changes.

Unfortunately, the causal relationship between the drug and the pulmonary disease is often not obvious. Not uncommonly, the pulmonary manifestations do not appear until after the drug has been taken for months or even years and then the clinical picture is nonspecific. The roentgen appearance of the drug-damaged lung resembles that of pulmonary edema with patchy areas of consolidation, or the picture of interstitial pulmonary fibrosis from any cause. In either case, the shadows in the lung are easily mistaken for lesions of the underlying disease for which the drug was administered. This may lead to an increase in the drug dosage which will cause the patient's condition to worsen and possibly can initiate chronic or irreversible changes in the lungs.

NITROFURANTOIN (FURADANTIN). This antibiotic is commonly used in the treatment of urinary tract infections. It can cause an acute pulmonary reaction or a chronic pneumonitis. The two seem to be totally separate disease entities.

The acute disease most probably represents a hypersensitivity reaction and usually occurs in patients who are receiving the drug intermittently. Typically, the patient develops a high fever, often with an associated peripheral eosinophilia, within hours or days of resumption of the drug. Indistinct, patchy areas of increased density may be present throughout both lungs, occasionally together with a small collection of fluid in the pleural space. The roentgen picture is much like that of pulmonary edema. The appearance of the chest reverts to normal within 24 to 48 hours after discontinuation of the drug.

The chronic reaction to nitrofurantoin occurs in patients on continuous, prolonged therapy. The onset of the disease is insidious, occurring months to years after the drug is begun. Unlike the acute reaction, it is not associated with peripheral eosinophilia or pleural effusion. The roentgen picture is that of a diffuse interstitial pneumonitis (Fig. 382), or pulmonary fibrosis. The lung changes tend to clear slowly once the drug is withdrawn but steroids may be needed for complete recovery.

HEROIN AND METHADONE. Acute intoxication due to an overdose of these drugs can produce the characteristic clinical and roentgen picture of pulmonary edema (Fig. 383). However, the heart is not enlarged. Fluffy areas of consolidation are distributed in the perihilar regions or may be scattered diffusely throughout the lungs. This does not appear to be a hypersensitivity reaction because it occurs only with an overdose of the drug. In almost all cases, the patient is comatose or has just recovered consciousness. It is unlikely that the central nervous system depression is the cause because such findings do not occur, for example, with barbiturate overdosage.

The edema usually responds promptly to continuous positive pressure breathing, oxygen therapy and steroids. If the roentgen changes persist for more than 24 to 48 hours, the possibility of secondary infection should be strongly considered. Similar noncardiogenic pulmonary edema has also been encountered with overdosages of propoxyphene hydrochloride (Darvon) and aspirin, to name a few.

METHOTREXATE. Some patients receiving this drug develop a pneumonitis with fever, cough, dyspnea and interstitial pulmonary infiltrations. Other patients simply show a decrease in pulmonary function without any roentgen changes in the lungs. The time of onset of the pulmonary disease is quite variable and has been reported as early as 2 weeks after the beginning of therapy or as late as 4 or 5 years. It does not appear to be dose related. The pulmonary manifestations usually clear once the drug is stopped, especially if steroids are given. However, in some cases, the pulmonary infiltrates and symptoms resolve completely even though the methotrexate therapy is continued without any decrease in dosage.

BUSULFAN AND CYCLOPHOSPHAMIDE. The pulmonary disease produced by these alkylating agents is different from most drug-induced diseases because it is associated with cytologic

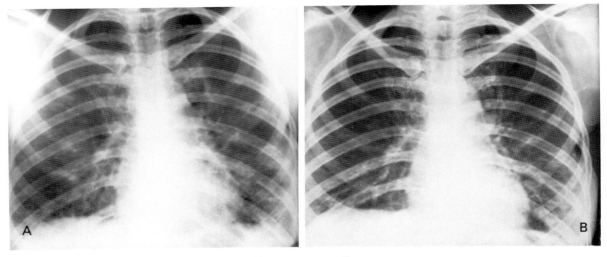

FIG. 382. NITROFURANTOIN PNEUMONIA

A: The patient had severe shortness of breath, a dry cough and fever of 3 weeks' duration. She had been taking Furadantin for several months because of a urinary tract infection. Patchy infiltrations are present throughout both lungs. *B:* The symptoms subsided promptly after discontinuing the Furadantin. The film made 3 weeks later shows resolution of the infiltrates except those in the left lower lobe. These subsequently cleared on steroid therapy.

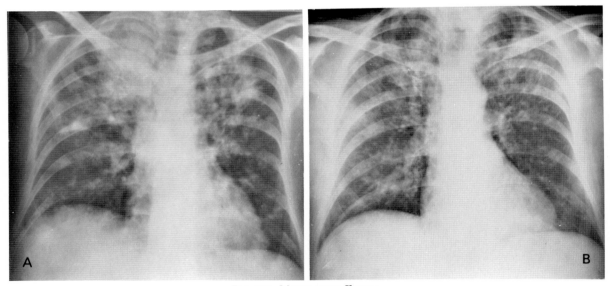

FIG. 383. METHADONE EDEMA

A: Portable film of a comatose patient following overdose of methadone. The hazy, ill-defined shadows in the mid-lung fields are characteristic of pulmonary edema. The heart is not enlarged. The cardiac silhouette is magnified because this is an anteroposterior projection and because the x-ray tube was relatively close to the patient. *B:* Erect, 6 foot posteroanterior film. Four days later. The patient responded rapidly to treatment and the heart and lungs appear normal.

changes. Atypical cells, having an almost neoplastic appearance, are found in the alveolar walls and, on occasion, may be detected in bronchial washings or in the sputum. Pulmonary symptoms and roentgen changes have been reported in 2 to 10 % of patients receiving long term therapy with these drugs. Histologic

changes without clinical evidence of disease are considerably more common. The average time of onset of symptoms is about 4 years after the beginning of therapy. The disease is a progressive one and often results in death from respiratory insufficiency. In some cases it is arrested or may even regress if the drug is discontinued but in other instances, the disease progresses even after the drug is stopped. Steroids may be of help.

The chest film shows a combination of interstitial pulmonary fibrotic lesions and indistinct, nodular areas of consolidation (Fig. 384). The pulmonary changes tend to be most prominent in the perihilar regions. The appearance may be indistinguishable from that of an opportunistic infection such as *Pneumocystis carinii* or from leukemic infiltrations in the lungs. A definitive diagnosis can be established by finding the atypical pneumocytes in the sputum or on lung biopsy.

BLEOMYCIN. This antitumor antibiotic can produce a fatal pneumonitis very similar to that caused by busulfan. Most of the reported cases have been in patients receiving large doses of bleomycin. Prior radiotherapy to the lungs and, possibly, even therapy limited to the mediastinum, predispose to bleomycin pulmonary toxicity.

Pulmonary Neoplasms

The x-ray examination of the chest is the most sensitive method for the detection of pulmonary neoplasms. Circumscribed carcinomas are readily discernible radiologically in the early stages, before they produce symptoms and when there is a fair chance for surgical cure. In patients who do have pulmonary symptoms, x-ray studies are essential to determine whether or not the pulmonary lesion is neoplastic. In addition, the roentgen examination is often helpful in deciding the mode of therapy to be employed.

Benign Pulmonary Neoplasms

The hamartoma is by far the most common benign tumor of the lung. They arise from embryonic rests and are characterized by an overgrowth of one or more of the tissues normally present in the lung. Strictly speaking, they are malformations rather than neoplasms and are therefore discussed under the heading Anomalies of the Lung (p. 270).

Benign neoplasms of the lung are extremely rare and consist of lipomas, hemangiomas, fibromas and neurinomas. Actually, some of these may really be hamartomas. They are characterized by their sharp circumscription and the homogeneity of the round or oval shadow they cast on the film (Fig. 385). While these characteristics serve to differentiate them from most cases of bronchogenic carcinoma, they cannot be distinguished radiologically from the peripheral form of bronchial adenoma or a solitary metastasis.

Benign Lymphoma of the Lung. Certain lymphomatous tumors of the lung appear to be benign. They have been observed to persist unchanged for a long time without evidence of lymphoma elsewhere in the body. In addition,

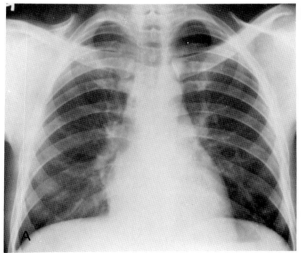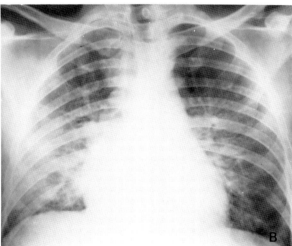

FIG. 384. BUSULFAN LUNG

A: The patient had been receiving busulfan for several years for chronic myelogenous leukemia. The film, made shortly after the onset of low grade fever and dyspnea, shows diffuse streak-like and fine nodular infiltrations suggesting interstitial pneumonia with alveolar filling. There is some confluence of the shadows behind the clavicles. *B:* One month later, while the patient was still taking the drug, the film shows a large area of consolidation in the right middle lobe and patchy areas of alveolar filling throughout the remainder of the lungs. The diagnosis was established at autopsy, histologic examination of the lungs revealing a characteristic pattern of fibrosis and cellular atypism.

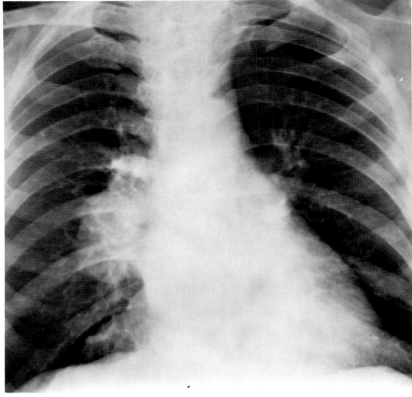

Fig. 385. Lipoma of the Lung

The sharply demarcated density seen at the root of the right lung on this projection was also demonstrated at the lung root on the lateral view. Because of its shape and location, it was thought to represent a tumor of the hilar lymph nodes, and a course of radiotherapy was given. It did not respond to this treatment and the patient subsequently died of pulmonary embolism. At necropsy the lesion proved to be a lipoma of the lung. The shadow in the right cardiophrenic angle was caused by herniated properitoneal fat.

the cells are uniform, mitoses are absent, and they have been resected without recurrence.

Radiologically, the benign lymphoma of the lung casts a round or oval shadow of variable size. In the three cases that we have observed, the tumors were not encapsulated. Nevertheless, the border was very sharply demarcated in one. The other two were not so well defined and appeared more like nodular peripheral carcinomas. Although these cases seem to be examples of benign lymphoma, comparable to the benign lymphoma of nodes described by Castleman, the possibility that they really represent variants of primary lymphosarcoma of the lung cannot be denied.

Bronchogenic Carcinoma

It is presumed that primary carcinomas of the lung, with the possible exception of the neoplasm referred to as pulmonary adenomatosis, alveolar cell carcinoma, or bronchiolar carcinoma, arise from the bronchial epithelium. The point of origin can be demonstrated by careful dissection of the bronchi in the majority of cases. In most of the remainder, the microscopic findings suggest a bronchial origin. Some of the others probably arise from the lining cells of the pulmonary alveoli.

Pathologically, pulmonary neoplasms may be grouped according to the gross site of origin or the microscopic cell type. In any case, the topography of the growth, its manner of spread through the lungs, and the complications resulting from bronchial obstruction are of prime importance in determing the x-ray picture.

Topography in Relation to Site of Origin. The tumors that arise from the main or root bronchi are usually of an infiltrative nature. Early in the course of their growth they extend beyond the bronchial wall and tend to involve the mediastinal lymph nodes. Dissemination into the lung and, in some cases, to the pleura, occurs by way of the peripheral lymphatics. At any stage the tumor may obstruct the bronchus partially or completely, causing complications such as obstructive emphysema, atelectasis, bronchiectasis or pneumonia (Fig. 101).

Neoplasms arising from the medium-sized bronchi are either diffusely infiltrating or of a more localized type. The diffuse infiltration may be confined to one portion of the lung, but the bronchial lymph nodes and the pleura are often involved early in the disease. Sometimes lymphatic spread of the neoplasm occurs rapidly throughout both lungs. The more localized type of neoplasm arising from a branch bronchus is quite similar to one which originates from a bronchus so small that the point of origin of the tumor may not be visible. The growth takes a nodular form which is fairly well demarcated from the surrounding pulmonary parenchyma. There is comparatively little tendency for the tumor to spread mesially. Spread to the lymph nodes usually occurs late and may not occur at all.

The small bronchus in which the tumor originates is soon obstructed and the area of lung which it supplies becomes atelectatic. As this portion of the lung collapses, it retracts from the surface and draws in the overlying visceral pleura. In most cases, therefore, the surface of the inflated lung will show one or more deep clefts or puckers, at the base of which the carcinoma is situated (see Fig. 398).

When the neoplasm originates more peripherally, it can extend to the pleura without causing atelectasis. While the mesial part of the growth may remain well demarcated from the adjacent normal lung, its peripheral portion not infrequently grows through the pleura to invade adjacent structures. If it abuts on an interlobar fissure it may grow into the neighboring lobe. If it is situated on the costal surface of the lung, it can grow through the parietal pleura into the chest wall and erode or completely destroy one or more of the overlying ribs. Similarly, when it is situated on the mesial surface of the lung, it may directly invade the mediastinum, and when it is situated at the base it can infiltrate the diaphragm.

Relation of Topography to Cell Type. Most of the bronchogenic carcinomas can be classified into four groups: (1) squamous cell or epidermoid carcinoma, (2) adenocarcinoma, (3) small or oat-cell carcinoma, (4) anaplastic carcinoma.

Neoplasms arising from the larger bronchi are mostly of the squamous cell type. The more mature ones are apt to be localized and produce obstruction largely by endobronchial growth. They do not tend to spread diffusely by way of the lymphatics. Marked enlargement of the lymph nodes at the lung roots is common in small cell carcinomas and often there are large masses in the mediastinum and diffuse infiltration of the lung and pleura. Anaplastic and adenocarcinomas of the large bronchi behave in a similar manner. The potential for diffuse infiltration exhibited by the less mature squamous cell carcinoma lies between that of the mature squamous cell carcinoma and other growths.

The majority of localized peripheral growths are adenocarcinomas, although some are epidermoid. It is very unusual for the small cell or anaplastic variety to take this form.

The manner of growth and spread of a carcinoma of the lung depends largely on whether it originates in the hilar or peripheral portion of the lung. Those which arise in the periphery tend to produce localized nodular growths regardless of cell type. On the other hand, in the case of carcinomas of the larger bronchi, the tendency to rapid spread is influenced by the cell type. The small cell, anaplastic and adenocarcinomas tend to spread extensively and rapidly, while the growth and extension of squamous cell carcinomas in this location is related to the maturity of the neoplasm.

Root Bronchus Carcinoma. The roentgen appearance of carcinomas arising in the main or lobar bronchi depends largely on the presence or absence of bronchial obstruction. When the bronchus is occluded, the appearance is dominated by the effects of the obstruction. If the bronchus is patent, the growth itself is usually seen.

STENOSING TYPE. The stenosing tumors of the main or lobar bronchi frequently cause atelectasis of the obstructed lobe or lung before the patient is first examined (Figs. 71 and 83). The presence of a dense shadow at the root of the atelectatic lung (Figs. 77, 79 and 420) or enlargement of hilar nodes is indicative of an underlying bronchial carcinoma. Paralysis of the diaphragm on the side of the lesion has the same significance (see Fig. 516).

Frequently, the lung distal to the obstruction is infected and shows changes associated with suppuration in addition to those of atelectasis (Fig. 70). A lobe which is completely collapsed generally casts a homogeneous shadow of only moderate density. The density increases when infection supervenes (Fig. 170). When the lobe is partially collapsed, the evidences of infection are visible in the form of streak-like and irregular patchy shadows. However, such shadows can also be caused by retained secretion in the bronchi distal to the obstruction (Fig. 386). Infection

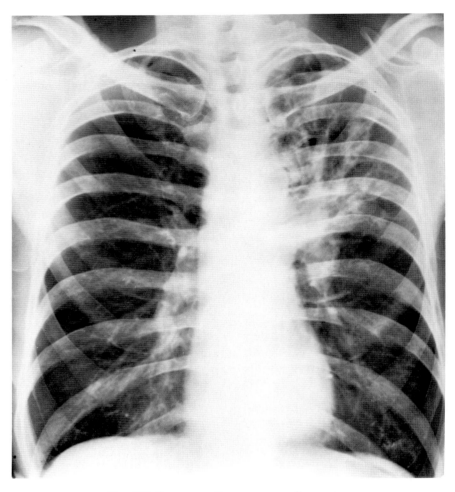

FIG. 386. STENOSING BRONCHOGENIC CARCINOMA

The left hilar shadow is enlarged, dense and elevated as the result of an obstructing carcinoma of the left upper lobe bronchus. The branching shadows radiating from the root were found to be caused by dilating bronchi filled with mucopurulent secretion distal to the obstruction.

distal to a completely occluding bronchial carcinoma may be manifested by fever without any respiratory symptoms. The cause of the fever may then be disclosed only by roentgen examination. However, films of good technical quality must be obtained if an inflamed, atelectatic left lower lobe, projected within the shadow of the heart is not to be overlooked (Fig. 69). Properly exposed films will disclose either obliteration, clouding or irregularity of the vessels seen through the cardiac shadow. The shadow of the infected atelectatic lobe is projected clear of the cardiac silhouette in the lateral and left oblique views (Fig. 69B). Depression of the hilum and relatively increased aeration of the corresponding upper lobe are indications of atelectasis of a lower lobe.

The infected lung distal to the stenosing neoplasm may contain one or more cavities. If only a single large cavity is seen, it can simulate a chronic lung abscess, and may or may not show a fluid level. When there are several small cavities, the appearance suggests simply a suppurative bronchopneumonia, and if the lower lobe alone is involved, the differentiation from suppurative bronchiectasis is often impossible.

The neoplasm itself may become necrotic and form a cavity. The cavities resulting from pulmonary infections are situated in the periphery of a lobe. If the cavity is visualized in the vicinity of the lung root on all views, an excavated carcinoma should be suspected. The presence of an irregular shadow projecting into the cavity from its mesial wall (Fig. 387) is additional evidence of a neoplasm. The protuberance represents the neoplasm arising from the entering bronchus.

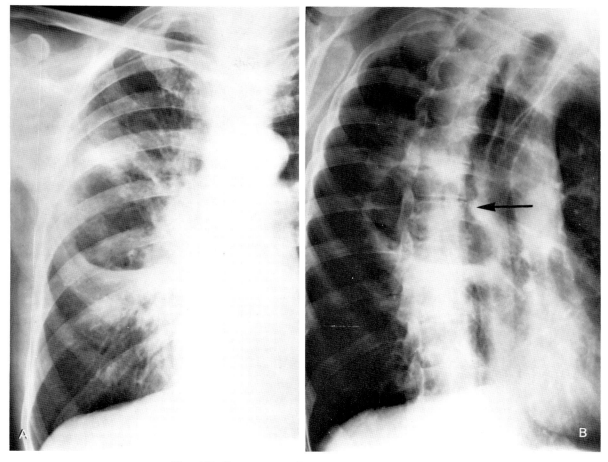

FIG. 387. CAVITATION IN BRONCHOGENIC CARCINOMA

A: There is a large, thick-walled cavity in the midportion of the right lung. It extended to the root of the lung in all views. The appearance in this view is nonspecific and could be caused by either an excavated carcinoma or a lung abscess. *B:* Right oblique view. The cavity is seen to be situated anteriorly. It extends both above and below the level of the fourth rib which is the normal position of the short fissure, indicating that the lesion involves both the upper and middle lobes. The nodular protuberance on the mesial border of the cavity (arrow) points to a bronchogenic carcinoma as the underlying cause.

A pleural effusion associated with obstructive atelectasis of one or more lobes is most frequently due to a bronchogenic carcinoma (Fig. 88). The effusion usually obscures the shadow of the atelectatic lung, but the presence of underlying bronchial obstruction is indicated by displacement of the heart and mediastinal structures to the side of the fluid. Bronchial obstruction should also be suspected when the heart remains in its normal position despite the presence of a large effusion. Approximation of the ribs on the side of the effusion is additional evidence of obstructive atelectasis (Fig. 388).

The stenosing neoplasm may act as a check valve and produce obstructive emphysema rather than atelectasis. The air trapping may not be recognizable on routine chest films since these are made in complete inspiration and both lungs may, therefore, be equally expanded. However, the presence of obstruction becomes quite evident during expiration. The affected lobe or lung remains expanded while the normal lung becomes clouded as its air is expelled. Swing of the mediastinum away from the more lucent side during expiration is also a characteristic of obstructive emphysema (Fig. 389). If the growth is mainly endobronchial no other changes may be noted.

Eventually, as the bronchus becomes completely occluded, atelectasis takes place. Although the narrowing of the bronchus occurs gradually, atelectasis can appear suddenly if the bronchus becomes plugged by mucus or exudate.

NONSTENOSING TYPE. A nonobstructing car-

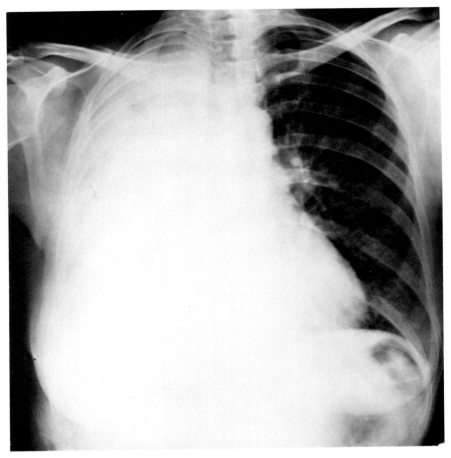

FIG. 388. BRONCHOGENIC CARCINOMA

The right hemithorax is almost completely opacified. If this were due simply to a large pleural effusion, the heart would be shifted to the left. Not only is the heart in its normal position but the ribs on the right side are drawn together, the intercostal spaces are narrowed and the dome of the hemithorax flattened. These signs reflect a decreased volume of the right hemithorax indicating atelectasis of the underlying lung. Bronchoscopy revealed an obstructing carcinoma in the right main bronchus.

cinoma at the root of the lung may be completely hidden by the mediastinal structures and the film show no abnormality. Sooner or later, however, evidences of lymphatic extension of the tumor in the lung or mediastinum appear.

Lymphangitic spread in the lung is manifested by nodular or strand-like shadows fanning out from the root. The infiltrations are coalescent and more dense at the hilum and fade out peripherally. The entire lung or only one lobe may be involved in this manner. At a single examination the appearance may be identical with that of viral pneumonia, but if the shadow is persistent, the picture is characteristic of a nonstenosing large bronchus neoplasm, and is hardly to be confused with any other disease (Fig. 106). When the infiltrations are associated with large lymph nodes at the lung root, the diagnosis of lymphangitic spread of the carcinoma becomes evident (Fig. 390). Not infrequently, however, there is

massive involvement of the regional lymph nodes with little or no visible infiltration in the lung. The primary tumor and its pulmonary extension may not be visible even when the mediastinal lymph nodes are only moderately enlarged.

One of the characteristic forms assumed by the nonstenosing root bronchus neoplasm is a triangular shadow with its base at the hilum and the apex extending into the middle of the pulmonary field (Fig. 391). The shadow is cast by the locally infiltrating neoplasm and large hilar nodes. It is more frequently noted on the right side and is then almost always associated with marked thickening of the short fissure by the spreading carcinoma. Often there is elevation of the corresponding leaf of the diaphragm which is paralyzed because of local invasion of the phrenic nerve.

The carcinoma often extends by way of lymphatics to involve the pleura, producing one or

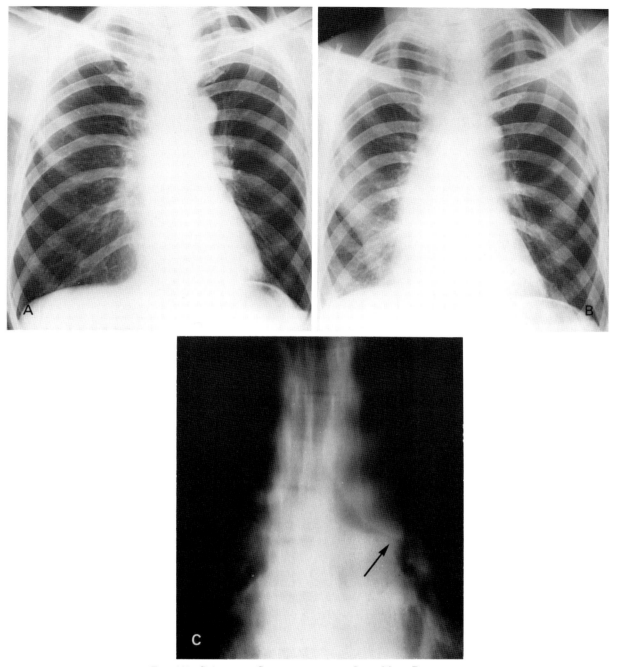

FIG. 389. STENOSING CARCINOMA OF THE LEFT MAIN BRONCHUS

A: The frontal film made in inspiration had been reported as negative. However, in retrospect, the vascular markings in the left lung appear significantly less prominent than on the right. *B:* Because of the presence of a loud rhonchus, the examination was repeated in expiration. The right lung is normally clouded, but the left remains fully aerated. The heart and mediastinal structures are shifted to the right, indicating obstructive emphysema of the left lung. *C:* Frontal tomograms show a mass within the left main bronchus (arrow). The bronchial air column is visualized distal as well as proximal to the lesion, indicating that the narrowing is real and not created by the plane of the section.

more scalloped shadows (see Fig. 563) or an effusion. When the pleural involvement is secondary to a carcinoma arising from a large bronchus it is almost always associated with recognizable infiltrations in the lung. When the effusion is large, it may be necessary to aspirate some of the fluid in order to disclose the underlying disease.

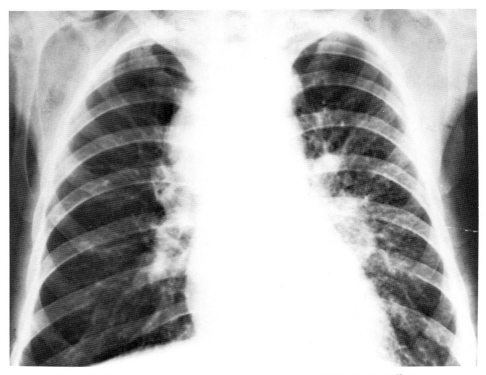

FIG. 390. BRONCHIAL CARCINOMA: MEDIASTINAL AND LYMPHANGITIC FORM

There is a mass of large lymph nodes projecting from both sides of the mediastinum. The left lung is poorly aerated because of permeation of the lymphatics by the carcinoma. The primary neoplasm in the bronchus is not visible. The clinical impression in this case was Hodgkin's disease, but the roentgen appearance, with innumerable tiny nodules following the course of the septa and blood vessels is that of a carcinomatous lymphangitis. The fact that this involves only one lung indicates the bronchial origin of the neoplasm.

Peripheral Carcinoma. A carcinoma originating in a segmental or subsegmental bronchus tends to form a localized tumor and may present radiologically as a circumscribed, round density. In some cases the neoplasm spreads by way of the lymphatics to produce more or less extensive, irregular infiltration of the lung.

NONCIRCUMSCRIBED FORM. The roentgen appearance of the noncircumscribed tumors originating in the segmental or subsegmental bronchi varies according to the manner of their growth. Those which cause bronchial obstruction are often complicated by infection of the segment of the lung that is involved. The picture then is that of an atelectatic segmental pneumonia, usually of the suppurative type (Fig. 69). Despite the presence of suppurative foci within the diseased segment, roentgen evidence of cavitation is usually lacking because the obstructing tumor prevents the egress of exudate and entrance of air in the inflamed area. While the roentgen picture is often simply that of a persistent pneumonia, the tumor itself is frequently visible at the root of the involved segment. The presence of a mass at

the mesial extremity of a segmental area of pneumonia is diagnostic of a bronchogenic neoplasm.

When there is local spread of the tumor through the regional lymphatic channels, the peribronchial and perivascular tissues and the interlobular septa become infiltrated. Even though the lesion consists entirely of tumor tissue, the roentgen appearance is often indistinguishable from that of a segmental bronchopneumonia. The primary tumor is not delimited and there may be no distinct mass at the root of the involved segment (Fig. 106). The regional lymph nodes or the nodes in the mediastinum are practically always involved, but often are not large enough to be visualized on the film. The combination of a shadow suggesting a bronchopneumonia and enlargement of the hilar or mediastinal nodes in a patient of cancer age points to bronchogenic carcinoma (Fig. 392).

The primary tumor and its local extension may be quite small and yet produce marked enlargement of the mediastinal nodes. In addition, the neoplasm may spread beyond the nodes and invade the mediastinum diffusely. The roentgen

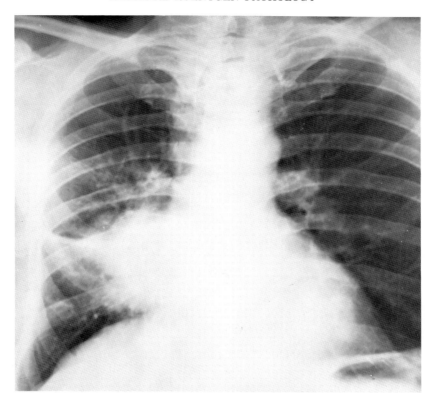

FIG. 391. ROOT BRONCHUS CARCINOMA

The triangular shadow at the root of the right lung was due to atelectasis and infiltration of the lung together with invasion of the regional lymph nodes by carcinoma. At necropsy, the broad streak which extends laterally was shown to represent carcinomatous invasion of the pleura forming the short fissure. The bronchus to the lower lobe was not obstructed.

picture then is one of a mediastinal neoplasm (Fig. 174). The small, poorly demarcated primary bronchogenic carcinoma can easily be overlooked, and if it is situated in the mesial portion of the chest, it may be invisible.

A carcinoma arising from one of the smaller bronchi can spread through lymphatic channels to involve both lungs in a diffuse manner. The spread usually occurs while the primary tumor is still small, and often not recognizable. The film shows streak-like shadows throughout the lungs, frequently together with small, irregular nodules. Usually the lesions are more numerous and the shadows more dense at the root of the involved lobe (see Fig. 411). This contrasts with the symmetric distribution of the shadows in lymphangitic carcinosis resulting from spread of a carcinoma from some other organ (see Fig. 436). Despite the widespread involvement of the lymph channels in the lungs, the mediastinal nodes may be small and not visible on the film.

Because of the great tendency of the noncircumscribed carcinomas to spread through the lymphatics, the neoplasm often extends beyond the confines of the lung. The mediastinum is most commonly involved but its shadow is not always widened. Invasion of the mediastinum may be manifested simply by paralysis of the diaphragm, indicating involvement of the phrenic nerve. In other cases, splaying of the angle of the carina or distortion of the tracheo-bronchial angle may be the only sign of enlarged mediastinal lymph nodes (see Fig. 421). Enlarged subcarinal nodes often cause local posterior displacement of the esophagus or indentation of its anterior wall. Similarly, narrowing of the esophagus may be the only manifestation of diffuse involvement of the mediastinum (see Fig. 422). Involvement of the pleura may occur early, either in the form of scalloped shadows or a pleural effusion. If the collection of fluid is large, it usually obscures the neoplasm. If the effusion is small, or if some of the fluid is aspirated, the underlying neoplasm may be visualized as a poorly demarcated, irregular shadow.

Pleural scallops, indicating the cancerous nature of the effusion, are frequently visible only in the oblique views or in the decubitus position

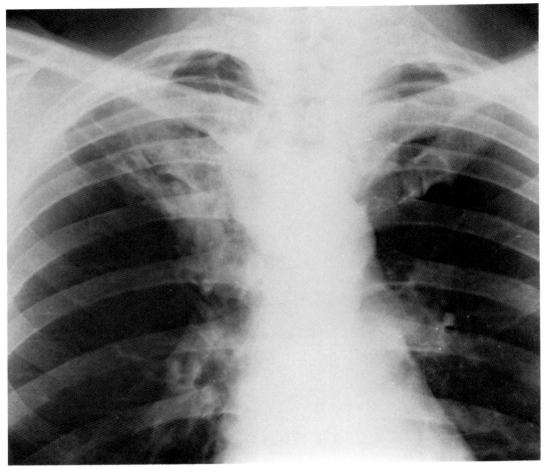

FIG. 392. CARCINOMA SIMULATING PNEUMONIA

The infiltrations beneath the right clavicle appear to represent nonspecific inflammatory disease. However, the right side of the manubrium is abnormally dense. This is due to enlarged paratracheal lymph nodes. The combination of a pulmonary infiltrate and large regional nodes in a patient of cancer age is almost always due to bronchogenic carcinoma.

with the involved side uppermost. In questionable cases, air injected into the pleural cavity at the time of thoracentesis will help to disclose nodules on the parietal pleura (see Fig. 562), particularly on films made in the oblique and lateral decubitus positions.

The pleural involvement may be so extensive that it dominates the roentgen picture even in the absence of an effusion. The tumor may spread diffusely throughout the pleura to envelop the lung in a dense, cancerous encasement. Marked thickening of the pleura produces a homogeneous shadow, most dense at the base, often obscuring the underlying lung. In the upper part of the chest, lucent lung may be visible, bounded laterally by the thickened pleura. The hemithorax is usually contracted, its contour flattened, and the rib spaces drawn together (Fig. 393).

The infiltrating tumor occasionally spreads to the pericardium. While this is usually the result of direct extension from a mediastinal mass, the mediastinal component may be too small to be visualized on the film. Involvement of the pericardium may be manifested only by an unusual straightening of a portion of the cardiac border (Fig. 394). More often, however, it results in a pericardial effusion of considerable size. This can obscure the shadow of the underlying pulmonary neoplasm. The possibility of metastasis from a bronchogenic carcinoma should be considered in any pericardial effusion of unknown etiology in a patient of cancer age.

The invading carcinoma usually produces nodular thickening of the pericardium together with the effusion. The nodules can be demonstrated on films made after replacing the pericardial fluid with air.

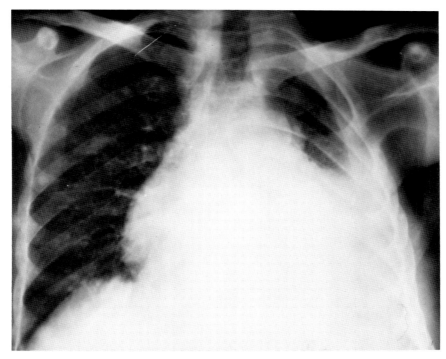

FIG. 393. BRONCHOGENIC CARCINOMA: PLEURAL FORM

The left chest is flattened and the ribs are drawn together and shingled over each other as the result of carcinomatous involvement of the pleura. The marked thickening of the pleura is best noted in the upper part of the chest. The carcinoma also involved the pericardium and invaded the mediastinum, but both the clinical and radiologic pictures were dominated by the invasion of the pleura. Radiologically, this picture cannot be distinguished from that of a mesothelioma. At postmortem examination, there was a carcinoma *en cuirasse* over the lung. The origin was demonstrated in the left lower lobe bronchus.

CIRCUMSCRIBED OR NODULAR TUMORS. Most of these tumors arise from small bronchi although the point of origin may not be demonstrable on gross examination of the specimen. In the early stage the growth presents as a nondescript, faint, poorly outlined, smudge-like density. The shadow is frequently so faint that it is easily overlooked on routine examination, particularly since there usually are no symptoms at this time. When an abnormal shadow is noted, its significance is often not appreciated and is considered to be inflammatory because of its poor demarcation. Occasionally, the density is more apparent and more sharply delineated on the oblique or lateral projections.

The character of the shadow changes as the tumor grows. When it attains a diameter of 1.5 to 2 cm, it becomes denser, its borders become more circumscribed and the appearance is more characteristic of a neoplasm. Just why the tumor should first be manifested as a smudge-like shadow and later as a circumscribed nodule is not entirely clear. However, bearing in mind that the tumors practically always originate in a bronchus, it appears quite probable that the roentgen

appearance in the early stage is caused not only by the growth but also by atelectasis of the portion of lung distal to it. As the tumor grows, it involves the collapsed portion of the lung. The border of the advancing growth then makes up the circumference of the roentgen shadow.

Usually the tumor is 2 or 3 cm in diameter when first recognized. At this time the shadow is fairly dense and homogeneous in appearance. Its border is round or somewhat lobulated and fairly well defined (Fig. 395). A portion of the circumference may show an extremely sharp demarcation from the surrounding lung, but the remainder of the shadow of a primary bronchogenic carcinoma is not so well defined. An exquisitely regular, sharp border about the entire circumference is more characteristic of a benign neoplasm, a cyst, a sarcoma, or a metastasis.

Lobulation occurs because the tumor does not grow evenly. Usually the lobulation is confined to only one part of the circumference so that the shadow has an irregular shape even though most of its contour is round. When the lobulation occurs on the anterior or posterior surface, the shadow of the tumor does not appear homoge-

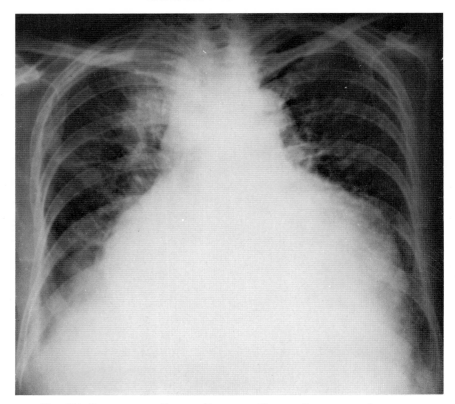

FIG. 394. INFILTRATING BRANCH BRONCHUS TUMOR: PERICARDIAL INVASION

The patient presented with symptoms of constrictive pericarditis. Roentgenologically, the diagnosis of bronchogenic carcinoma with metastases to the pericardium was suggested by the irregular infiltration in the apex of the right lung, the enlargement of the cardiac shadow and the angular contour of the left heart border. At postmortem examination, the neoplasm was found to arise in the apical division of the right upper lobe bronchus. It was diffusely infiltrating and involved the mediastinum as well as the pericardium and heart.

neous on the frontal view because of the local increased density caused by the protuberance. When the lobulation is prominent, it may produce a round, circumscribed density within the larger shadow of the tumor, suggesting the presence of two masses, one projected over the other. However, the true shape of the mass becomes evident on the oblique or lateral view.

Rigler has described a notch on the mesial border of the shadow of a nodule which he considered indicative of a bronchogenic carcinoma. The notch represents a cleft between lobulations (Fig. 396). Since a lobulated density in the lung usually represents a primary carcinoma, the sign is a valid one. However, it should not be considered pathognomonic since the notch, as well as other evidences of lobulation can occur in other lesions, some of which are benign.

Manner of Growth. The rate of growth of the neoplasm is extremely variable. Some attain a diameter of 8 to 10 cm within a few months (Fig. 289), while others show little increase in size over a period of years. Furthermore, the rate of growth of individual tumors frequently varies during their development. They may show little or no discernible growth for a period of a year or more and then suddenly begin to increase rapidly in size. This often occurs in association with the sudden development of extensive metastases. Because of this, it is not advisable to wait for growth of the shadow before deciding that the lesion is malignant. However, a short delay is justifiable to determine whether the lesion diminishes in size under treatment, indicating that it is inflammatory.

Every effort should be made to obtain previous films to determine whether there has been a change in the size of the lesion. It is important to make actual measurements because even a slight difference in the density of the films can affect the apparent size of the shadow. Generally, the lesion appears larger on a light film. It should be borne in mind that benign lesions, such as hamartomas, histoplasmomas and tuberculomas

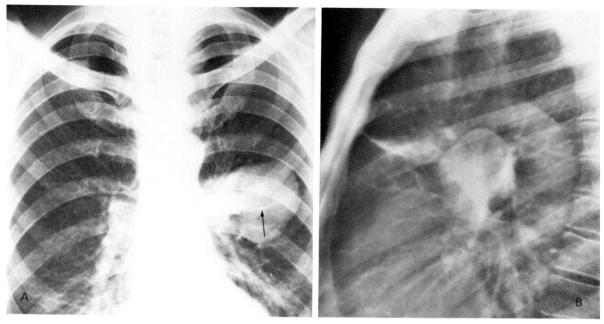

FIG. 395. CIRCUMSCRIBED CARCINOMA OF BRANCH BRONCHUS

A: Frontal projection. The lobulated, circumscribed growth in the left lung is situated at the root of the anterior segment of the left upper lobe. Although the tumor is well demarcated, it is not sharply outlined throughout its entire circumference as would be expected with a benign growth. The horizontal line (arrow) crossing the tumor is caused by a focal area of atelectasis. *B:* Lateral projection. The area of focal atelectasis extends from the tumor to the anterior pleural surface.

can increase in size, although slowly, over a period of years.

The peripheral carcinoma grows largely by expansion as well as by local infiltration of the lung and tends to maintain its shape as it increases in size (Fig. 289). It is characteristic of the circumscribed tumor that it remains circumscribed as it grows. It appears to have no tendency to infiltrate the lung beyond the immediate vicinity, or to grow into the lymphatic channels to produce the picture of lymphangitic carcinosis. As it enlarges, it does not tend to infiltrate adjacent bronchi, but pushes them aside, as is well demonstrated by bronchography. Thus, these tumors rarely cause lobar atelectasis from secondary obstruction of a large bronchus. On the other hand, tumor cells may spread from alveolus to alveolus to involve an entire lobe, resulting in lobar consolidation. The picture differs from that of lobar pneumonia in that it is associated with a bulging of the interlobar fissure (Fig. 397). The appearance then is similar to some cases of Friedländer's pneumonia.

Involvement of the hilar and mediastinal lymph nodes is usually a late complication of the circumscribed peripheral carcinoma of the lung. Occasionally, especially in small cell carcinomas, the lymph nodes are involved early and the roentgen film may show evidence of extensive involvement of the mediastinum. In most cases, however, there is no evidence of enlargement of the nodes even though the neoplasm is quite large and has been present for a considerable length of time. In fact, the nodes may be free of tumor even when the neoplasm involves an entire lobe.

The Fleischner Line. In most cases the circumscribed tumor originates in a small bronchus at some distance from the pleural surface of the lobe. This bronchus is soon obstructed, and the lung distal to it collapses, drawing the visceral pleura inward. When the expanded lung is examined, a cleft is seen on its surface at the point where the pleura is infolded (Fig. 398). At the base of the cleft lies the tumor, covered by a thin layer of atelectatic lung. The cleft is absent when the specimen is not inflated. The neoplasm, which is actually situated at an appreciable depth, then appears to be superficial because the lung distal to it is collapsed.

The films show the tumor to be separated from the chest wall by an appreciable distance in all views. In at least half of the cases, the tangential projection of the double layer of infolded visceral pleura casts a linear shadow (Fleischner line, or atelectatic streak), extending from the tumor to

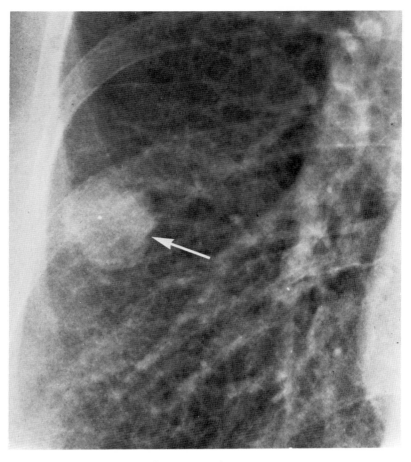

Fig. 396. Peripheral Adenocarcinoma

The mass in the outer portion of the right lower lobe shows a notch (arrow) on its mesial aspect. This has been described by Rigler as a sign of bronchogenic carcinoma. In addition, there are indentations on the upper and outer border of the tumor. The indentations are due to the lobulated nature of the tumor.

the chest wall (Fig. 399). The Fleischner line peripheral to a circumscribed density is a definitive diagnostic sign of primary bronchogenic carcinoma. One or more atelectatic streaks in association with a noncircumscribed density, however, have little diagnostic significance, as they are frequently seen with inflammatory disease in which small bronchi are obstructed.

A solitary granuloma of the lung, such as a tuberculoma or histoplasmoma, is the residual of an area of peripheral consolidation. Although one or more small bronchi are obstructed, the lung does not collapse because the alveoli distal to the obstruction are filled with exudate. Hamartomas of the lung and metastatic tumors originate outside the bronchi. We have never seen a Fleischner line distal to a hamartoma and very rarely in association with a granuloma (Fig. 290) or metastatic neoplasm, whereas we have seen the line in literally hundreds of primary carcinomas arising in small bronchi.

The Fleischner line is so important from a diagnostic standpoint that it should be carefully looked for in association with all solitary pulmonary nodules. The line is visible only in that projection in which the pleural cleft lies parallel to the x-ray beam. It is thin and sharply defined and usually measures 1 to 4 cm in length.

The relationship of the line to the shadow of the neoplasm depends upon the view in which the cleft is visualized. The classical picture is seen when the line is projected lateral to the tumor (Fig. 400). When the pleural cleft extends anteriorly or posteriorly, the line crosses the shadow of the tumor in the frontal projection and its extension to the chest wall cannot be seen in this view (Figs. 95 & 401). However, it can be demonstrated in other projections (Fig. 395).

Oblique or lateral views should be made when a Fleischner line cannot be visualized in relation to a nodule in the lung on the frontal projection. If the line still cannot be demonstrated, tomo-

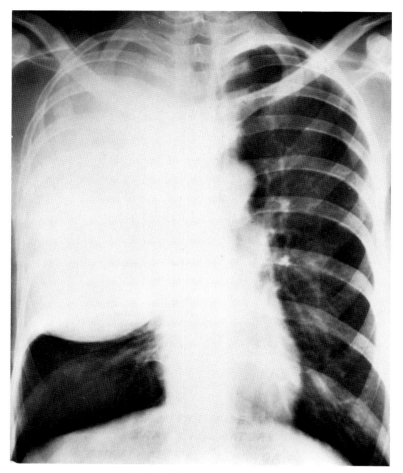

FIG. 397. LOBAR CARCINOMA

The mass in the right upper lobe had been observed to grow over a period of 2 years. Although the autopsy specimen disclosed an anaplastic carcinoma, the mediastinal lymph nodes were not involved. The upper lobe was actually consolidated by the carcinoma and the major bronchi were not infiltrated. The roentgen appearance differs from lobar pneumonia in that there is a downward bulge of the short fissure.

grams should be made. It should be borne in mind that if the cleft extends anterior or posterior to the nodule, the line will not be seen on the same section in which the tumor is most sharply defined, but will appear on adjacent sections in which the mass may not be visualized at all (Fig. 402). Sometimes more than one line is present, and these often cross each other.

Cavitation. Cavitation in relation to a peripheral neoplasm results from necrosis of the tumor itself. On the other hand, cavitation associated with a tumor of a large bronchus occurs in the lung distal to the obstructing carcinoma and is secondary to infection.

The peripheral carcinoma which has undergone cavitation may appear identical to an abscess of the lung. However, certain characteristics are often present which point to the diagnosis of neoplasm. Cavitation rarely occurs before the tumor has attained a diameter of 3 cm. The wall is usually thick and well defined, whereas the wall of a noncarcinomatous abscess is generally thin. If there is extensive inflammation of the lung around an inflammatory abscess, the wall may appear thick but it is poorly demarcated. The irregular inner border of the carcinomatous cavity remains unchanged over a period of weeks (Fig. 403), whereas the inner contour of an inflammatory abscess usually changes within a matter of days. In rare instance, an inflammatory cavity has a thick, irregular wall and cannot be differentiated from a broken-down neoplasm. This occurs particularly in Wegener's granulomatosis. However, inflammatory lesions are usually multiple.

A nodular protuberance frequently projects into a carcinomatous cavity from its mesial aspect, at the site of the entering bronchus. This

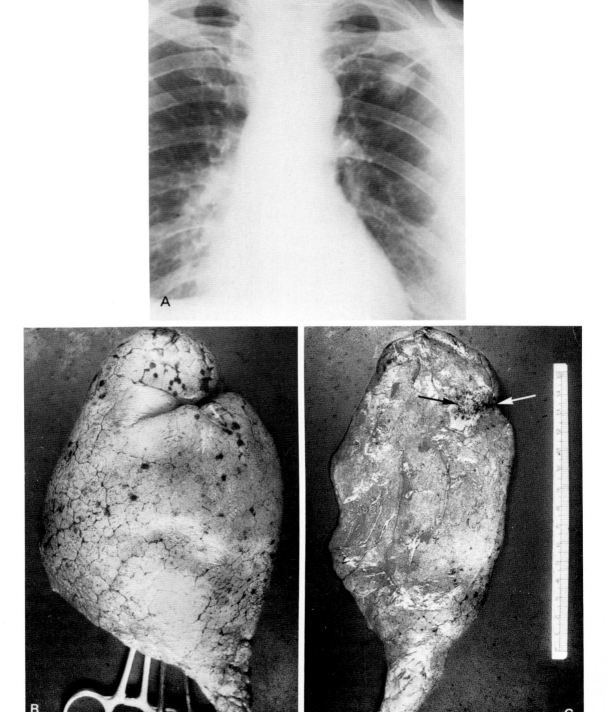

FIG. 398. FLEISCHNER LINE IN BRONCHOGENIC CARCINOMA

A: A carcinoma of the thyroid had been resected several years earlier. The nodule in the left upper lobe was first seen on this examination. It was considered to be a primary bronchogenic carcinoma and not a metastatic tumor because of the distal Fleischner line. The left upper lobe was therefore removed. *B:* The inflated specimen shows a deep cleft in the surface of the lung with indrawing of the visceral pleura. The mass was palpated at the base of the cleft. *C:* Cut section of the upper lobe reveals the tumor (black arrow) at the base of the newly formed pleural fissure (white arrow). There was extensive anthracosis within the tumor indicating its origin in lung.

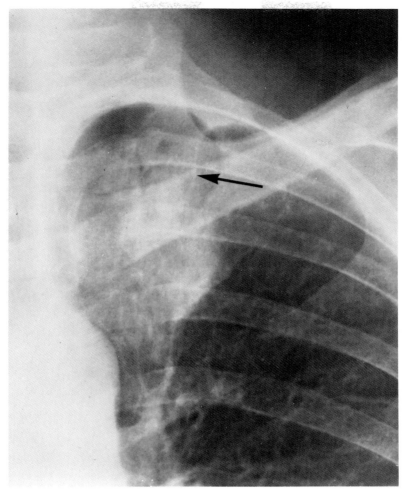

FIG. 399. FLEISCHNER LINE IN BRONCHOGENIC CARCINOMA

A fine, linear streak (arrow) extends outward from the ill-defined mass in the left upper lobe. The streak represents a double layer of infolded pleura, resulting from atelectasis of the lung peripheral to the mass. A Fleischner line distal to the mass in the lung is characteristic of a primary bronchogenic carcinoma. The triangular shadow at the extremity of the Fleischner line is caused by retraction of the extrapleural tissue as a result of the atelectasis.

may be obscured by even a small amount of fluid in the cavity. Tomograms may be required to demonstrate this protuberance which is diagnostic of a carcinoma. In rare instances, a persistent scallop is present within the lateral border of the cavity (Fig. 404), while the remainder of the lining of the cavity is smooth. The scallop represents local involvement of the pleura. It is unusual because most circumscribed tumors do not extend to the chest wall. Inflammatory cavities regularly abut on a pleural surface, but they do not show a protuberance in this location.

In some cases, these characteristic findings are not present, and a distinction cannot be made between a carcinomatous and a noncarcinomatous cavity. For example, if most of the carci-

noma is destroyed, its wall can become quite thin. The cavity can then balloon out and reach the periphery of the lung. Despite the absence of distinguishing features, persistence of a cavity with little change, in a patient whose sputum is negative for tubercle bacilli, should suggest the likelihood of an underlying carcinoma.

Peripheral Invasion. Some nodular carcinomas infiltrate peripherally while their mesial surface remains sharply demarcated from the adjacent lung. These growths tend to spread through the pleura to involve the chest wall. Although the pleura is traversed by the neoplasm, effusions are uncommon. As the tumor advances into the visceral pleura, it incites a local fibrinous reaction with the formation of adhesions. The tumor ex-

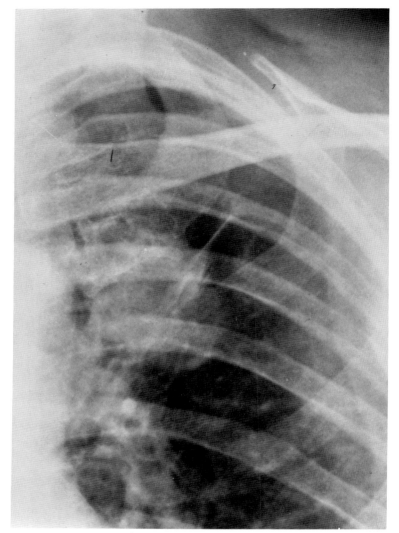

Fig. 400. Bronchogenic Carcinoma: Fleischner Line

Because the pleural cleft in this case is directed laterally rather than forward or backward from the carcinoma in the left upper lobe, the Fleischner line extends from the lateral border of the mass toward the chest wall.

tends through this area of pleurodesis to reach the chest wall without contaminating the free pleural space (Fig. 405).

Once the tumor has advanced beyond the parietal pleura, it extends in all directions. It may grow in sheet-like fashion in the tissue plane outside the parietal pleura or it may infiltrate the chest wall and involve one or more adjacent ribs. If the invasive tumor is situated on the mediastinal surface of the lung, it may involve the phrenic nerve and produce diaphragmatic paralysis.

A neoplasm that has invaded the extrapleural tissues may lose its sharp demarcation except when viewed tangentially. Tumors situated in the anterior or posterior portion of the chest are seen *en face* in the frontal view and are poorly delineated. In the proper oblique or the lateral projection, the inner border, where the mass abuts on the lung, is sharply outlined. The tumors that lie against the lateral chest wall are sharply defined in the frontal projection. They appear semicircular in shape with the base against the chest wall. The angle where the mass meets the parietes is frequently blunted because of the extrapleural extension of the tumor.

Involvement of a rib is often first manifested by a small erosion of one border. Further destruc-

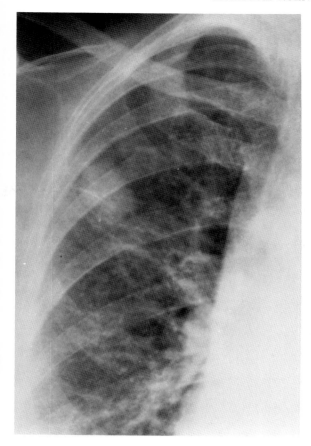

FIG. 401. BRONCHOGENIC CARCINOMA: FLEISCHNER LINE

The sharply etched linear shadow crossing the nodule in the right upper lobe is a Fleischner line resulting from a focal area of atelectasis which extends backward from the tumor to the posterior chest wall. Therefore, the line is projected over the tumor in the frontal view and its peripheral extension is not seen.

tion may occur rapidly and the tumor can extend through the entire width of the rib in a few weeks. One or more ribs over the tumor can be destroyed in this fashion (Fig. 160). However, the area of rib destruction does not extend beyond the confines of the shadow of the tumor. In this respect a peripherally invasive lung carcinoma differs from many cases of primary or metastatic tumor of a rib. Absence of periosteal reaction or new bone formation helps to differentiate neoplastic invasion of the rib from inflammatory disease.

Apical Carcinoma and Pancoast Syndrome. Peripheral neoplasms at the apex of the lung frequently present special characteristics. These tumors have a great tendency to invade the extrapleural tissues, and generally do not pro-

duce a large mass within the lung. In fact, the pulmonary component may be quite small despite extensive peripheral invasion. As the growth infiltrates the extrapleural tissues adjacent to the spine, it often invades the upper thoracic nerve roots, the paravertebral sympathetic chain, the overlying ribs and the spine. The resulting Horner's syndrome, together with pain radiating down the arm, was first described by Pancoast as a distinct clinical entity.

In the early stage, the tumor frequently shows a sharply defined, concave lower border, in the frontal projection, more or less parallel to the curve of the posterior portion of the second rib. The shadow then resembles a local thickening of the pleura, the so-called pleural cap attributed to healed tuberculosis. However, the pleural cap resulting from tuberculosis is due to hematogenous spread of the disease and therefore is practically always bilateral (see Fig. 495).

As the tumor extends downward extrapleurally, its lower border is no longer projected tangentially in the frontal view, and becomes indistinct (Fig. 406). A sharply defined, convex lower border, characteristic of a tumor, can be demonstrated on films made in the apical lordotic projection. This is also true when the tumor appears in the frontal view simply as a well defined apical cap (Fig. 407). A definite diagnosis of Pancoast tumor may be made when there are destructive changes in the adjacent ribs or spine. The upper ribs are poorly visualized on conventional films because they overlap each other and are partly obscured by the shadow of the tumor. Even extensive rib destruction can be overlooked unless Bucky films are made.

In the absence of evidence of extrapleural involvement, differentiation from tuberculosis may be difficult. The presence of an apical cap on only one side without fibrosis or calcification in the adjacent lung is presumptive evidence of a Pancoast tumor. We have never observed cavitation in this type of neoplasm. An apical carcinoma does not displace the trachea unless it is quite large, and then the displacement is toward the opposite side. A shift of the trachea towards the side of the lesion excludes the possibility of this type of tumor (Fig. 408).

Tumors in the chest wall, whether primary or metastatic, may be differentiated from carcinomas of the apex of the lung by reexamination after a pneumothorax has been induced. If the lung is separated from the shadow at the apex, the tumor is obviously extrapulmonary. On the other hand, if the apex of the lung remains adherent to the dome of the chest, no conclusion is

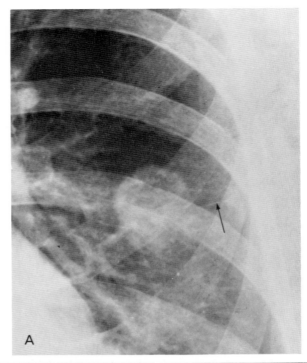

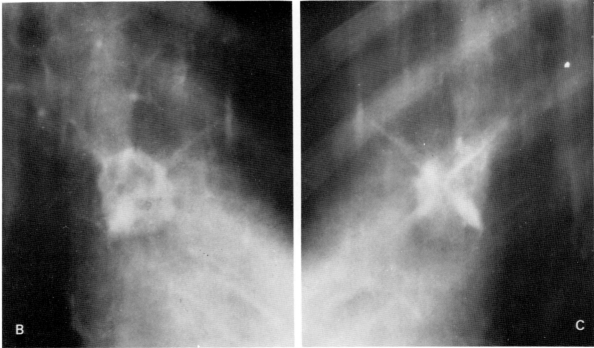

FIG. 402. FLEISCHNER LINES IN BRONCHOGENIC CARCINOMA

A: In the frontal view the ill-defined nodule in the left midlung shows an eccentric lucency, indicative of cavitation. An extremely fine streak (arrow) extends laterally from the nodule. *B:* Because the streak was not clearly shown on frontal sections, lateral tomograms were made. This section, through the center of the nodule, demonstrates its irregular border and the cavity within it. A Fleischner line cannot be seen. *C:* A section made lateral to the nodule clearly shows two Fleischner lines which cross each other. If tomography is performed at right angles to the course of the Fleischner line, the line and the tumor from which it extends do not appear on the same section.

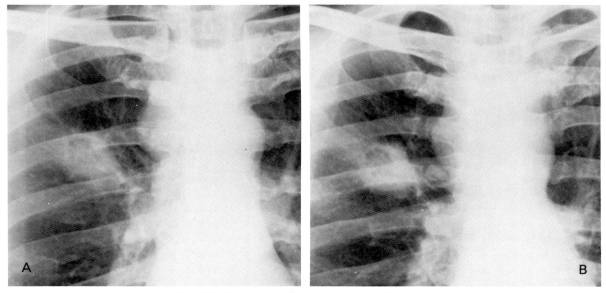

FIG. 403. CAVITATING CARCINOMA OF THE BRONCHUS

A: The cavity in the anterior segment of the right upper lobe has an irregular wall, thickest in its mesial portion toward the lung root. The bulging shadow in the right paratracheal region represents a group of large lymph nodes. *B:* Two weeks later the cavity has an identical appearance. This is indicative of a neoplasm rather than an abscess or an infarct, since it is extremely unlikely that either of the latter conditions would remain stable for this period of time.

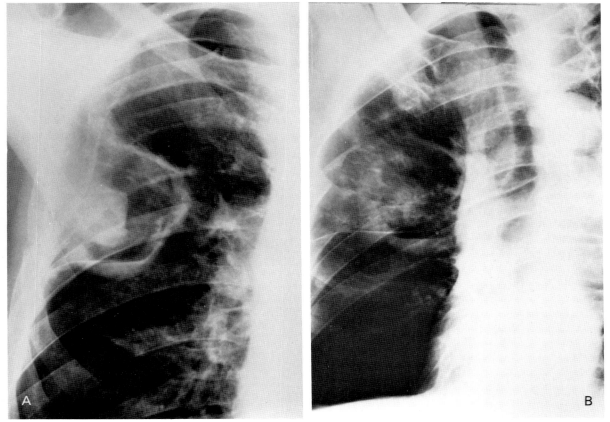

FIG. 404. CARCINOMATOUS LUNG ABSCESS

A: The frontal projection shows a relatively thin-walled cavity with a small air-fluid level at its base. A sharply demarcated mass projects into the cavity from its lateral aspect. This establishes the diagnosis of a carcinomatous abscess. *B:* The left oblique view discloses destruction of the posterolateral portions of the fourth, fifth and sixth ribs over the lesion. Destruction of multiple contiguous ribs over the lesion without periosteal proliferation is indicative of a primary carcinoma of the lung invading the chest wall.

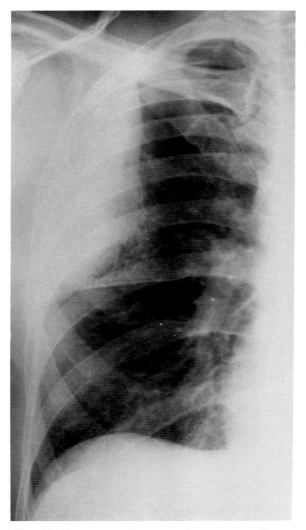

FIG. 405. PERIPHERAL CARCINOMA INVADING THE CHEST
WALL

The large mass in the lateral portion of the right upper
lobe represents a peripheral bronchogenic carcinoma. Although the tumor extended through the pleura to involve the
chest wall, there is no pleural effusion. This is common in
peripherally infiltrating carcinomas because they incite a
local inflammatory reaction which obliterates the pleural
space over the tumor. A large portion of the mesial border of
the neoplasm is sharply demarcated from the pulmonary
parenchyma.

warranted as to the origin of the growth since
adhesions may be present, whether the tumor
originates in the lung or the chest wall.

A tumor at the apex of the lung is not necessarily pulmonary in origin. It is possible for a
mass of large cervical lymph nodes to depress
the parietal pleura at the dome of the thorax and
indent the apex of the lung without invading it.
We have seen this in Hodgkin's disease and

metastatic carcinoma of the cervical nodes. The
roentgen picture is indistinguishable from that of
an apical carcinoma of the lung (Fig. 409).

Calcification in Peripheral Carcinoma. Calcification within a nodular shadow in the lung
makes the possibility of bronchogenic carcinoma
unlikely. However, it is necessary to demonstrate
that the calcium is situated within the tumor and
not simply projected over it. On occasion, one or
more calcific deposits are present within a carcinoma. These almost always represent preexisting calcifications within the lung, engulfed by the
growing neoplasm, rather than calcification of
the tumor itself. The calcium is not situated in
the exact center of the shadow as in a tuberculoma or histoplasmoma and it is not distributed
throughout the lesion as in a hamartoma (Fig.
410). It is conceivable that calcification could
occur within a necrotic carcinoma but this must
be exceedingly rare.

Pulmonary Spread of Carcinoma. LOCAL
GROWTH. The nodular tumors arising from the
smaller bronchi increase in size largely by expansion as well as by local infiltration. Even though
they may spread peripherally to invade the chest
wall, they remain fairly well demarcated from
the surrounding lung and retain a nodular character throughout their entire course. The neoplasms arising in the large bronchi have a greater
tendency to spread widely by way of the lymphatics but they also grow locally, often extending through the bronchial wall to form a mass.
In the case of tumors arising from the segmental
bronchi, the mass appears in the lung at the root
of the affected segment. The extrabronchial mass
originating in a lobar or a main bronchus is
situated at the root of the lung.

Bronchial obstruction occurs from either endobronchial or intramural growth of the tumor.
A tumor of a segmental or lobar bronchus may
first cause atelectasis of only a segment of the
lung. As the tumor extends proximally it can
obstruct a lobar bronchus and cause atelectasis
of an entire lobe. Further extension of the growth
in the bronchial wall may result in incomplete
obstruction of the adjoining lobar bronchus producing obstructive emphysema of the adjacent
lobe. Finally this lobe may also become atelectatic.

LYMPHATIC EXTENSION. Involvement of the
lymphatic channels around the tumor is very
common with carcinomas of the larger bronchi
and is responsible for the irregularity of their
shadows. Some tumors arising from the small
bronchi also have a marked tendency for lymphatic extension from the very beginning and
never form a circumscribed growth. Both types
of carcinoma can extend widely by lymphatic

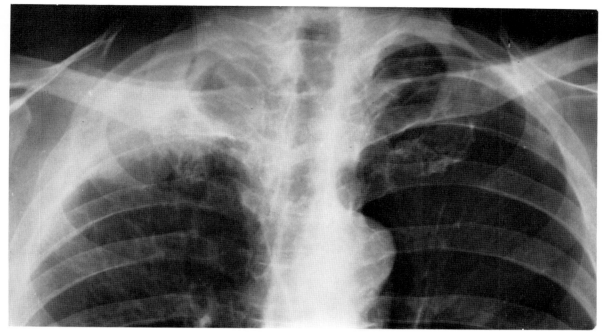

FIG. 406. APICAL CARCINOMA: PANCOAST SYNDROME

The right apex is opacified, suggesting an old fibrotic tuberculous lesion. However, the absence of any deviation of the trachea to that side makes this diagnosis somewhat unlikely. If the individual ribs in this region are traced, it can be noted that the third rib on the right side has been destroyed. This indicates the presence of a peripheral carcinoma of the lung that has invaded the chest wall. The classical syndrome of pain behind the shoulder radiating down the arm, and miosis and enophthalmos, described by Pancoast, was present in this case.

permeation and may involve a lobe (Fig. 106), an entire lung or even both lungs (Fig. 411). In places, the tumor cells grow through the walls of the lymphatics and form multiple, irregular, small nodules. These produce a snowflake appearance on the film, superimposed on the linear pattern of lymphangitic spread. Not infrequently, a pleural effusion or pleural nodules develop as a result of involvement of the pleural lymphatics (see Fig. 563).

Lymph node involvement is very common in association with the noncircumscribed tumors, whether they arise from a small or a large bronchus. Enlargement of the hilar and mediastinal nodes can dominate the picture and completely obscure the primary tumor on the film. In contrast to this, a circumscribed tumor can be present for a long time and attain considerable size without involving the hilar or mediastinal nodes (Fig. 397).

HEMATOGENOUS SPREAD. Hematogenous dissemination of a bronchogenic carcinoma to the lungs is not common. Occasionally one or more rather small, well-demarcated, round nodules are found in the lung peripheral to a carcinoma at the root (Fig. 412). These probably represent metastases resulting from invasion of a branch of the pulmonary artery adjacent to the primary

growth. Involvement of both lungs by hematogenous metastases probably occurs from seeding of the blood in the superior vena cava via the thoracic duct. The lungs are then studded with small, fairly well demarcated nodules varying from a few millimeters to a centimeter in diameter. Large cannonball metastases do not seem to occur.

Occasionally a second nodule of considerable size is encountered with a bronchogenic carcinoma, or in a patient who has had one removed. If the appearance suggests a neoplasm, the question arises as to whether the nodule represents a solitary hematogenous metastasis or a second primary carcinoma. Definite pathologic proof is available to support the concept of a second primary growth. Peripheral adenocarcinomas have been found in patients whose original tumor was of the squamous cell type arising from a large bronchus. We have even observed three nodular tumors in the same lung, each with a different histologic picture. One was a squamous cell carcinoma, the second an adenocarcinoma, and the third a small-cell carcinoma of the oat-cell type.

Special Diagnostic Methods. Other views, in addition to the conventional frontal projection, are often helpful in the diagnosis of carci-

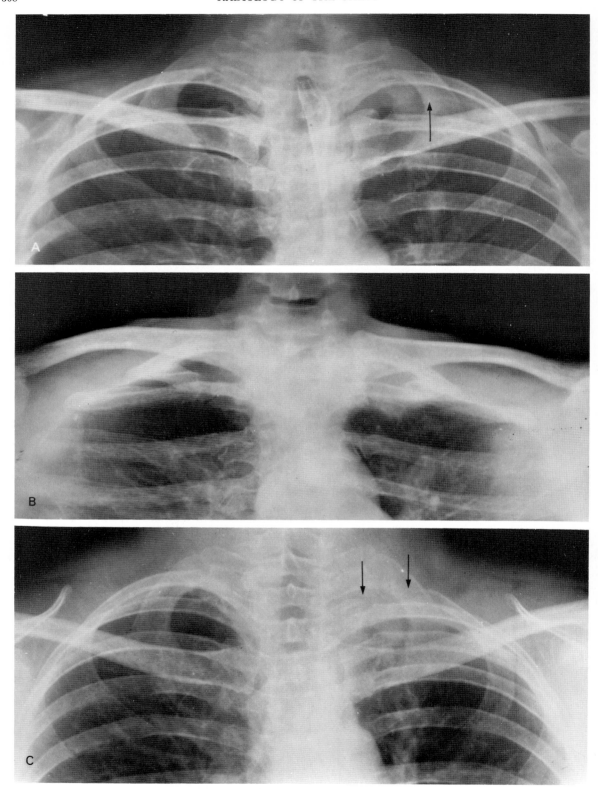

FIG. 407. APICAL CARCINOMA

A: The frontal view shows a density at the left apex with a concave lower margin (arrow), simulating thickening of the apical pleura. The right apex is perfectly clear. A unilateral apical cap is very unusual in tuberculosis. *B:* The apical lordotic view shows the lesion at the left apex to represent a mass rather than thickening of the pleura. The true shape of the lesion is apparent on this view because the posterior part of the dome of the thorax is not foreshortened as it is on the frontal projection. *C:* Eight months later the entire supraclavicular region is clouded. The posterior portion of the second rib is destroyed (arrows). At this time the patient had all of the symptoms of the Pancoast syndrome.

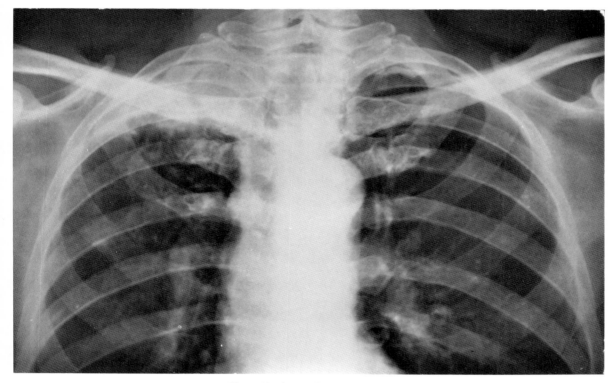

Fig. 408. Apical Tuberculosis

The dense shadow at the right apex could be due to an apical carcinoma. However, the trachea is drawn toward the lesion which excludes a Pancoast tumor and is indicative of tuberculosis. In addition, the right lung root is elevated and there is a pleural cap on the left side. The sputum was positive for tubercle bacilli.

noma of the lung. Lateral and oblique projections are frequently needed for localization of the lesion. Thus, a density which appears to be situated at the hilum and resembles an enlarged node on the frontal view, may be shown to represent a nodule in the periphery of the lung. Localization of the lesion in the anterior rather than the posterior segment of an upper lobe favors the diagnosis of carcinoma over that of tuberculosis. In addition, minor degrees of displacement of the long fissure, indicative of atelectasis and suggesting an obstructing lesion, may be clearly visualized only in these views (Fig. 180). The lordotic projection is most useful in the recognition of apical neoplasms (Fig. 407). Fluoroscopy or films made in expiration and inspiration are often needed to disclose the presence of obstructive emphysema. Bucky films in either the oblique or lateral view may reveal a tumor projecting into the lumen of one of the main bronchi (Fig. 175). In some cases more specialized roentgen techniques are required.

TOMOGRAPHY. The demonstration of calcification within a nodular lesion, usually indicating that it is benign, is frequently impossible without tomography. Even when a central density is seen within a mass on conventional or Bucky films, tomograms may be needed to confirm the finding and to determine whether it represents a calcific deposit or a blood vessel viewed on end. Tomograms in an additional projection may be required to make this distinction. Tomography is also useful in demonstrating a Fleischner line distal to a nodule, identifying it as a bronchogenic carcinoma (Fig. 413).

Often the interlobar fissures are clearly demonstrated only by lateral tomography. This may disclose local retraction of the fissure adjacent to a density in the periphery of a lobe, signifying segmental or subsegmental atelectasis (Fig. 414). This is most often due to a peripheral carcinoma. Lateral tomograms may also be required to determine whether a lesion is situated in the central portion of the lung or whether it extends to the periphery. This cannot always be recognized from the frontal projection and the shadow may not be sufficiently well visualized on the conventional lateral view. A lesion confined to the root of a lobe or a pulmonary segment is practically always neoplastic while inflammatory lesions extend to the periphery.

The diagnosis of carcinoma of a large bronchus

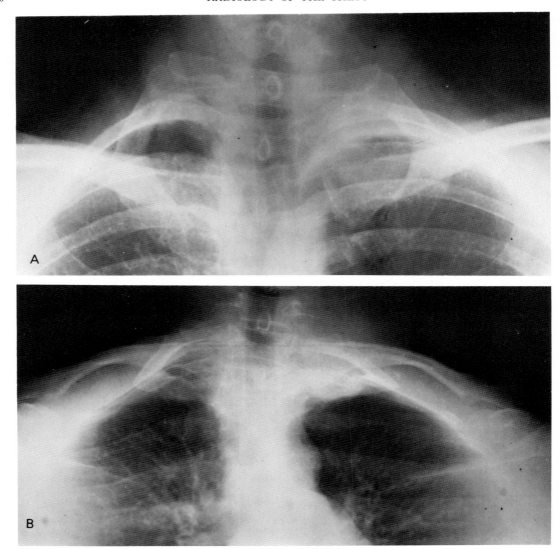

FIG. 409. HODGKIN'S DISEASE MIMICKING APICAL CARCINOMA

A: There is a curvilinear density at the dome of the left thorax simulating an apical pleural cap. The apical pleura on the right side is not thickened as would be expected in tuberculosis. The most common cause of a unilateral apical cap is a carcinoma at the apex of the lung. *B:* The lordotic view shows a mass with a well demarcated, convex lower border indistinguishable from a carcinoma. There is some fullness of the soft tissues of the left side of the neck. The biopsy disclosed Hodgkin's disease.

may depend largely upon the findings on tomography, particularly in patients who cannot withstand bronchoscopy. Often the shadow of a neoplasm within or about the bronchial wall can be clearly demonstrated (Fig. 22). In other cases an irregular narrowing of the bronchial lumen can be seen. In interpreting the tomograms, it should be borne in mind that when a normal bronchus courses at an angle to the plane of the section, it is cut obliquely and may appear funnel-shaped, simulating narrowing by tumor. To be certain

that the lumen is really compromised, the bronchus above and below the point of narrowing should be visualized on these sections (Fig. 389).

BRONCHOGRAPHY. Bronchography is occasionally useful in the diagnosis of bronchogenic carcinoma. Characteristically, a carcinoma produces a long, irregular, funnel-shaped narrowing of the involved bronchus, giving a rattail appearance to the column of contrast material within its lumen (Fig. 182). This results from submucosal extension of the tumor which occludes the orifices of

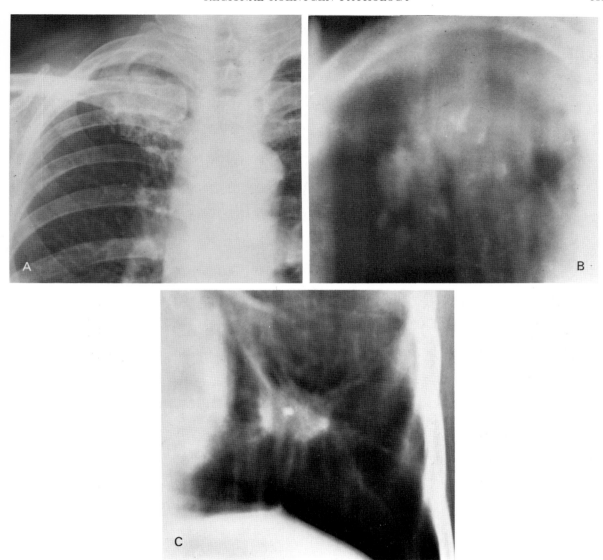

FIG. 410. CALCIFICATION IN BRONCHOGENIC CARCINOMA

A: A poorly defined mass is seen in the right upper lobe. The appearance is most suggestive of a primary carcinoma of the lung. However, because of irregularity in the density of the mass, tomograms were made. *B:* On the frontal tomogram, three calcific deposits are seen in the mesial portion of the mass. Since a carcinoma can grow around a preexisting calcific deposit in the lung, the presence of calcification within a mass, if eccentrically distributed, does not exclude the possibility of malignancy. *C:* Tomogram of a histoplasmoma shown for comparison. In this case the calcific deposit lies directly in the center of the mass.

the smaller branches. In some cases the endobronchial component of the growth produces a localized, irregular protrusion into the lumen. In others, there may simply be a local area of irregular narrowing of the lumen.

Obstruction of a segmental bronchus is easily detected when the narrowing is gradual or when the occlusion occurs distal to the origin of the bronchus so that its stump is visible. When the bronchus is completely occluded at its orifice, its

absence on the bronchogram may be easily overlooked. It is important, therefore, to identify each segmental bronchus to make certain that all of them are accounted for.

In the case of peripheral tumors, the small bronchi are frequently splayed around the mass which grows largely by expansion. This sign is not pathognomonic for carcinoma since it does occur occasionally in inflammatory lesions. The subsegmental bronchus leading to a carcinoma is

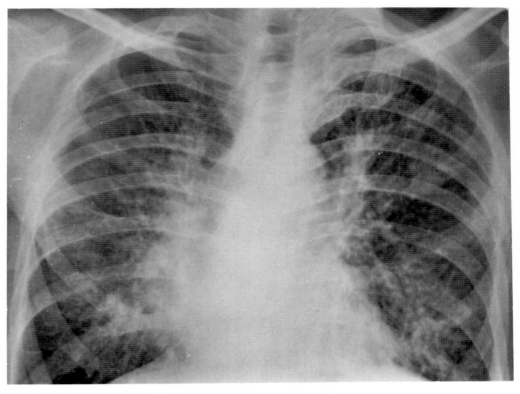

FIG. 411. BRONCHOGENIC CARCINOMA: LYMPHANGITIC FORM

Both lungs are poorly aerated and are permeated by streaks which extend out from each hilum. These represent carcinoma growing within the lymphatic channels. A dense shadow is noted near the root of the right lower lobe where the carcinoma originated. Here, there is a coarse, dense, more localized infiltration by the growth. The patient's respirations were rapid and shallow, undoubtedly because inspiration was restricted by the strands of carcinoma coursing throughout the lungs.

usually cut off, but if the bronchus is not completely occluded its branches within the tumor appear narrowed and bare of subdivisions. Dilatation of these branches, found frequently in chronic inflammatory diseases, is rare in peripheral carcinomas. Obstruction of a bronchus leading to a cavity does not signify that the lesion is neoplastic. It occurs commonly in lung abscess, especially in the acute phase. However, an irregular narrowing of the bronchus proximal to the cavity is indicative of an underlying bronchogenic carcinoma.

ANGIOGRAPHY. A bronchogenic carcinoma frequently compromises blood flow to the involved portion of lung, resulting in diminished opacification of the vessels on an angiogram. Although venous angiography can provide fair delineation of most of the pulmonary vessels, far better detail is obtained by selective pulmonary arteriography. Failure to visualize a main pulmonary artery or one of its branches on a venous study does not necessarily indicate that the vessel is occluded, since a local disturbance in pulmonary ventilation can divert the flow of blood away from the

affected area. However, irregularity or abrupt obstruction of the lumen of a major pulmonary artery is indicative of invasion or occlusion of the vessel (Fig. 415). Involvement of a main pulmonary artery usually signifies that the tumor cannot be entirely resected.

Carcinomas of the lung derive the major part of their blood supply from the bronchial arteries. These vessels can be catheterized and selectively opacified. A vascular pattern, characteristic of neoplasm, can occasionally be demonstrated, particularly in the case of central lesions. However, the patterns show considerable variation, and the technique has not been particularly useful in distinguishing inflammatory from malignant lesions. Furthermore, serious neurological complications can occur from injection of the spinal arteries, whose orifices are in close relation to the bronchial arteries.

DENSIMETRY. Densimetry is a technique whereby minute changes in the radiolucency of a portion of the lung are continuously measured and recorded. It is possible by this means to demonstrate a pulsatile increase in the density

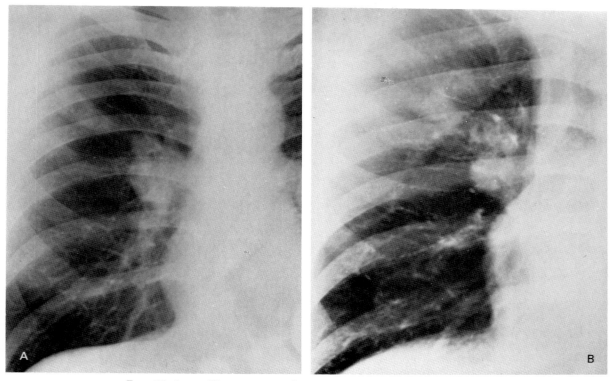

FIG. 412. LOCAL HEMATOGENOUS SPREAD OF BRONCHOGENIC CARCINOMA

A: Frontal view. A lobulated shadow is present at the upper part of the right hilum. In addition, there is a poorly defined density projected over the anterior part of the third rib. *B:* In the right oblique projection the density at the right hilum is separated into two masses, the lower of which proved to be an oat cell carcinoma of the bronchus with invasion of contiguous lymph nodes. The upper mass and the lesion seen over the anterior part of the third rib on the frontal projection were found to lie in the distribution of the pulmonary artery which was involved by the tumor and was the origin of these metastases.

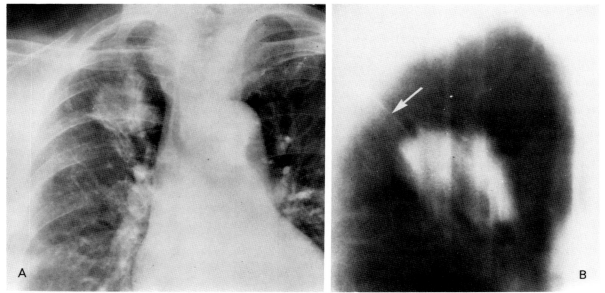

FIG. 413. BRONCHOGENIC CARCINOMA: FLEISCHNER LINE

A: A 77 year old female with rheumatoid arthritis. The irregular mass in the right upper lobe is most suggestive of a carcinoma. The bulge in the right paratracheal region is caused by a tortuous innominate artery and does not represent enlarged nodes. *B:* The frontal tomogram shows a fine Fleischner line (arrow) extending outward from the mass. This confirms the roentgen diagnosis of bronchogenic carcinoma.

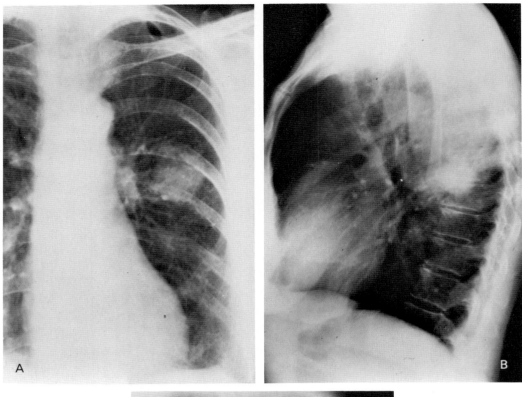

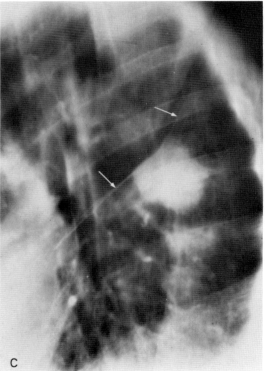

Fig. 414. Peripheral Carcinoma: Use of Tomography

A: The poorly circumscribed, round density in the left lung is most suggestive of a primary carcinoma. *B:* In the lateral view the lesion is located within the superior segment of the lower lobe. *C:* The lateral tomogram reveals retraction of the long fissure (arrows) over the lesion. This indicates that the mass has produced a local area of atelectasis and therefore is obstructing a bronchus. The diagnosis of a bronchogenic carcinoma can now be made with a considerably greater degree of certainty.

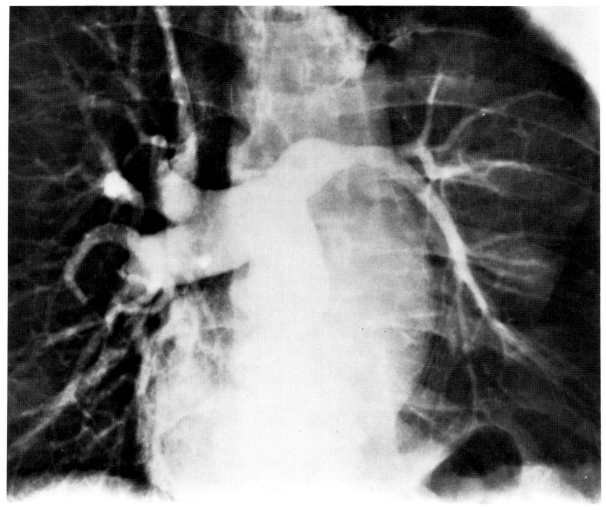

FIG. 415. ANGIOGRAPHY IN BRONCHOGENIC CARCINOMA

The carcinoma completely obstructed the left upper lobe bronchus. A venous angiogram shows an irregular narrowing of the left main pulmonary artery indicating invasion of the vessel wall by the neoplasm. However, because the most proximal portion of the artery and the main pulmonary artery appear uninvolved, the lesion may still be completely resectable. The artery to the left upper lobe is not visualized. Whether this is due to obstruction of the vessel or to diminished flow as a result of the atelectasis of the upper lobe could be determined only by selective pulmonary angiography.

of the lung during each systolic thrust of blood into the pulmonary arteries. The pulsations are diminished over a primary bronchogenic neoplasm whereas a normal pattern has been observed over benign and metastatic tumors. However, diminished pulsations also occur over inflammatory lesions.

Diagnostic Clues. Frequently the diagnosis of bronchogenic carcinoma is quite evident on casual examination of the roentgen film. However, often the diagnosis is not as clear. In these instances we have found the following observations to be useful.

Not infrequently a carcinoma of the lung presents as a pneumonic shadow (Fig. 392). Since at least part of the shadow is cast by the tumor, it never resolves completely. It is therefore essential to follow the patient with pneumonia with serial chest films until the lungs are entirely clear. This must be done even though the patient is free of symptoms, if an underlying carcinoma is not to be missed.

Recurrences of pneumonia in the same portion of the lung, even though complete clearing has occurred between episodes, should suggest the possibility of partial obstruction of a bronchus, which may be due to a carcinoma. It is, therefore, important to document every case of pneumonia by roentgen examination in order to determine whether the same area is involved if the patient again develops pneumonia (Fig. 416).

Visualization of air-filled bronchi within an area of *segmental* consolidation of the lung eliminates bronchogenic carcinoma from consideration. However, the open bronchus sign does not have the same significance when an entire lobe is consolidated or atelectatic. It is possible for a carcinoma to partially obstruct a lobar bronchus and still permit air to enter its branches even though there is a complicating distal suppurative atelectatic pneumonia. On the other hand, the caliber of a segmental bronchus is such that it is completely obstructed by even a very small carcinoma. The open bronchus sign has been most useful in differentiating a persistent pneumonia in the anterior segment of the upper lobe from a neoplasm. The anterior segmental bronchus is seen on end on the frontal view and, when patent, casts a small, perfectly round, annular shadow (Figs. 33 and 417).

The earliest roentgen manifestation of a peripheral carcinoma is a small, nondescript, smudge-like shadow. This usually measures less than 2 cm in diameter. As the tumor becomes larger, it tends to become more circumscribed. A smudge-like shadow, situated in the outer part of the posterior segment of the upper lobe is more characteristic of tuberculosis. However, anywhere else in the lung, this shadow, in a person of cancer age, is usually due to a carcinoma originating in a small bronchus. Occasionally, such a shadow represents a pneumonia or an infarct, but a short period of observation will usually suffice to exclude these conditions.

The presence of a large lymph node at the root of the lung, or one jutting out from the mediastinum, in combination with a smudge-like density or a larger pneumonic shadow in a person of cancer age favors the diagnosis of primary bronchogenic carcinoma (Fig. 392). The paratracheal region should be inspected carefully whenever a lesion is seen in the lung. A slight protuberance in the right paratracheal region, or a faint density within the aortic knob or obscuring its upper border, should immediately give rise to a suspicion of involvement of the mediastinal nodes by carcinoma. Hodgkin's disease or the primary complex of tuberculosis or histoplasmosis can also give rise to a similar combination of shadows but they are quite uncommon in patients over 45 years of age.

Extremely sharp demarcation of the margin of a nodular shadow in the lung indicates either a benign or a metastatic lesion. At least part of the border of a nodular carcinoma is less well defined.

A distinct nodule less than 1.5 cm in diameter, even if not exquisitely demarcated, rarely represents a primary bronchogenic carcinoma.

A nodular shadow identical to that of a bronchogenic carcinoma can be caused by an inflammatory lesion (Fig. 232) or an infarct (Fig. 418) even in a patient with relatively few symptoms. Therefore, it is a good rule to postpone thoracotomy for a week or 10 days after discovery of a nodular shadow and to repeat the roentgen examination immediately before surgery (Fig. 67). Any decrease in the size of the shadow excludes neoplasm from consideration. Because a diminution in the size of the shadow may be more apparent than real, it is necessary to check the size of the lesion by calipers or actual measurement.

Detection of an area of erosion or destruction in a rib overlying a nodular lesion in the lung is extremely important in the recognition of a peripheral carcinoma. Often the lesion in the rib is overlooked because the attention is focused on the shadow in the lung. The course of each rib should be traced within the shadow. Obviously, films must be made with sufficient penetration to visualize the ribs in this location. Bucky films may be required (Fig. 160).

Some inflammatory lesions may extend through an interlobar fissure to affect the adjoining lobe. This happens particularly in tuberculosis, lung abscess and fungous infections, notably actinomycosis. However, they appear as pneumonic rather than circumscribed shadows, while the peripheral carcinoma retains its nodular character even when it extends through an interlobar fissure. The relationship of the lesion to the fissures is best seen in the lateral view.

The presence of a Fleischner line peripheral to a nodular shadow is practically diagnostic of primary bronchogenic carcinoma. Exceptions to this rule are rare. All nodular lesions, therefore, should be examined carefully for this line. Films made in different projections and even tomograms may be required for its detection.

Bilateral thickening of the pleura at the apices is generally the result of an old tuberculous infection. On the other hand, apparent pleural thickening over the apex of one lung, in the absence of tuberculous scarring beneath it, is strongly suggestive of a carcinoma and always requires further investigation.

Except for traumatic hemothorax and empyema in children, nonmalignant pleural effusions rarely fill an entire pleural cavity. Films made in the erect position almost always disclose a portion of aerated lung above the fluid. Opacification of an entire hemithorax by a nontrau-

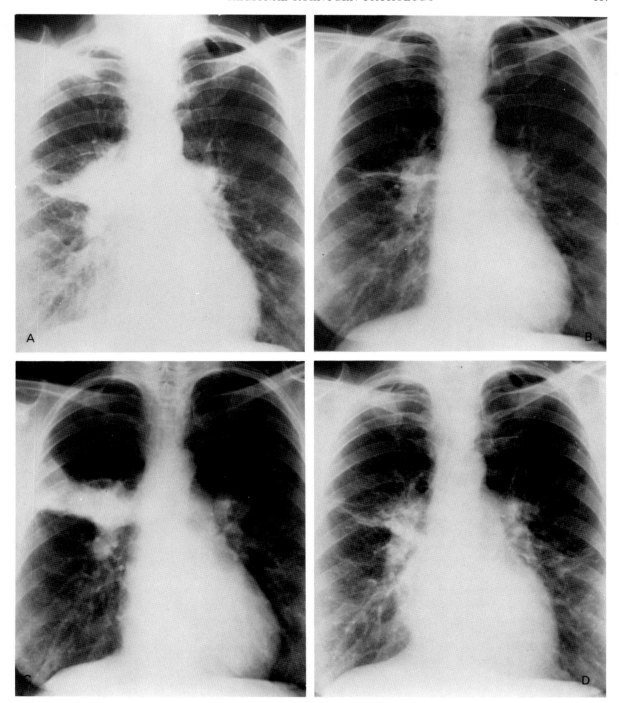

FIG. 416. RECURRENT PNEUMONIA

A: April 9, 1969. The patient had clinical evidence of a pneumonia with sudden onset. The film shows consolidation and atelectasis of the anterior segment of the right upper lobe. *B:* June 19, 1969. Following antibiotic treatment the patient was asymptomatic. The pneumonia had resolved leaving a thickened short fissure and an area of discoid atelectasis. The prominence of the hilar shadows was due to increased pulmonary blood flow, the result of an atrial septal defect. *C:* December 2, 1969. There has been recurrence of the pneumonia in the anterior segment of the right upper lobe. *D:* January 10, 1970. Resolution again occurred rapidly under antibiotic therapy. Because the pneumonia recurred in the same segment, the patient was bronchoscoped. A carcinoma was found in the right upper lobe bronchus, occluding the anterior segmental branch.

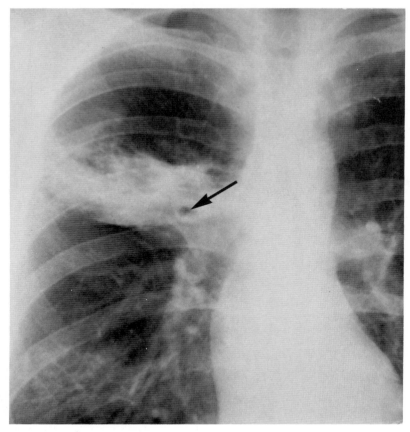

FIG. 417. OPEN BRONCHUS SIGN

The lower border of the shadow in the right lung is sharply demarcated and straight, indicating that it is bounded by the short fissure and therefore must involve the anterior segment of the right upper lobe. However, the bronchus to the anterior segment is patent (arrow). The lesion proved to be a primary tuberculous infection.

matic pleural effusion in an adult indicates the presence of neoplastic disease (Fig. 388). Although such an effusion is sometimes caused by metastasis from a neoplasm elsewhere in the body, if unilateral it is usually due to a primary tumor of the lung or pleura.

Evidence of periosteal new bone formation in the extremities in conjunction with a lesion in the lung is an indication of primary bronchogenic carcinoma. Although clubbing of the fingers is common in lung abscess and bronchiectasis, bone changes (so-called pulmonary osteoarthropathy) are very rare in these conditions. Likewise, periostopathy is most unusual in metastatic neoplasm of the lungs.

When the mediastinum is not displaced, it may be difficult to differentiate between lobar atelectasis and consolidation on the frontal film. Emphysema of the adjoining lobe indicates that the density is due, at least in part, to atelectasis (Fig. 101). The presence of atelectasis of a lobe can be confirmed by examination in the lateral view, in which the fissures are best seen. Lobar atelectasis in older patients is strongly suggestive of an obstructing bronchial carcinoma.

A mediastinal mass in a person of cancer age is usually secondary to bronchogenic carcinoma even though no lesion can be visualized in the lungs. If the cases with obvious aortic aneurysm and those in which the mass is situated in the anterior mediastinum and abuts on the sternum are excluded, over 90% will prove to be primary bronchogenic neoplasms.

Carcinoma of the lung is a frequent complication of asbestosis. Calcific pleural plaques on the diaphragm, over the mediastinum, or over the lower portion of the lung without obliteration of the costophrenic sinus are indicative of asbestosis even in the absence of visible pulmonary infiltrations. A nodular lesion within the lung in association with such calcifications or other evidence of asbestosis practically always represents a primary bronchogenic carcinoma (Fig. 331).

Patients with hemoptysis, persistent cough or

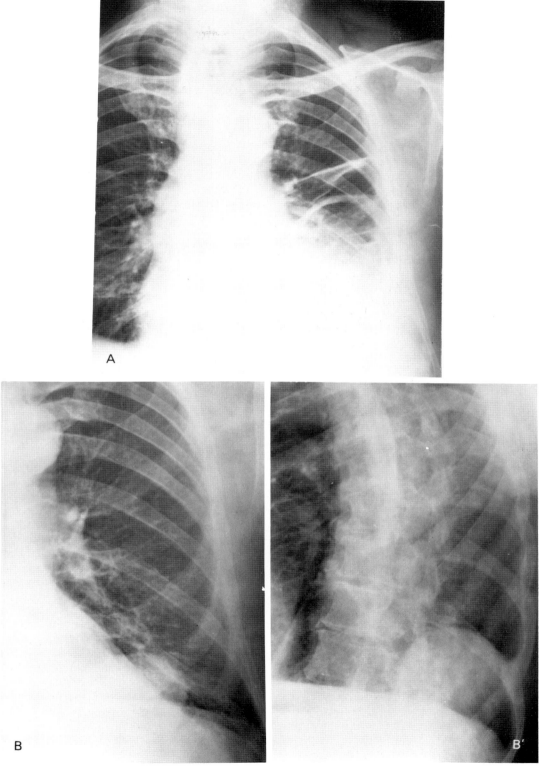

FIG. 418. PULMONARY EMBOLIZATION AND INFARCTION

A: The frontal film shows an effusion at the left base with several Fleischner lines above it. The latter represent foci of atelectasis and are the most common manifestations of pulmonary embolization. An effusion of this size in pulmonary embolization rarely occurs without infarction. *B:* Two months later the frontal and left anterior oblique views show complete clearing of the effusion and the Fleischner lines. There remains a sharply circumscribed, round density in the posterior basal segment of the lower lobe. Because of the possibility of a neoplasm, the lesion was resected. It proved to be an infarct with a partly liquefied center.

a constant rhonchus with an apparently negative chest film require further roentgen study from the standpoint of bronchogenic neoplasm. The film, which is customarily made in inspiration, may show no obvious abnormality. However, careful examination with special attention to the vascular pattern may disclose thinning of the blood vessels, suggesting obstructive emphysema of a lobe or of an entire lung. The presence of an obstructing lesion is more clearly demonstrated on films made in expiration (Fig. 389).

It is important to bear in mind that the posterior costophrenic sulcus can extend more than 4 inches below the dome of the diaphragm. Any tumor in the posterior lappet of the lower lobe is therefore often projected over the liver, stomach or colon and is often first detected on films of the abdomen (Fig. 419). It may be difficult to demonstrate the lesion on chest films without special views such as the kyphotic or oblique or by tomography.

Roentgen Evaluation of Resectability. A resectable carcinoma is one that can be completely removed at operation. The roentgen examination often reveals changes that indicate spread of the tumor beyond the limits of resectability. However, it is necessary to be extremely conservative in classifying a lesion as nonresectable if the error of withholding operation in cases in which the tumor can be removed is to be avoided. On the other hand, it is obvious that the absence of such changes does not guarantee that the tumor can be completely resected.

Resectability should not be confused with operability. Operation may be indicated for palliation, and may prolong life even though neoplasm is left behind.

MEDIASTINAL INVOLVEMENT. Diffuse invasion of the mediastinum or metastases to the mediastinal lymph nodes indicates nonresectability. Mediastinal involvement may result in diffuse widening of the mediastinal shadow or simply a small protuberance in the paratracheal region (Fig. 420). Local displacement of the lower end of the trachea toward the uninvolved side with a resultant hook-shaped tracheobronchial angle, is indicative of involvement of the tracheobronchial lymph nodes (Fig. 421). Widening of the tracheal bifurcation by enlarged subcarinal lymph nodes or the shadow of the mass of nodes, can sometimes be demonstrated on Bucky films. These should be made in the upright position because the normal carinal angle appears widened when the patient is supine. Enlargement of the hilar lymph nodes does not have the same significance as involvement of the mediastinum

because the hilar nodes can be removed together with the lung.

Invasion of the phrenic nerve is usually indicative of nonresectability since it is most often associated with extensive involvement of the mediastinum. However, in the case of a circumscribed carcinoma abutting on the mediastinum, the mediastinal invasion may be only local and even though the phrenic nerve is involved, the entire tumor may be resectable.

Tomography is sometimes useful in the detection of mediastinal masses and in revealing the extent of involvement of the bronchi and, possibly, the trachea. However, caution must be observed in interpreting the tomograms, particularly in relation to densities at the lung roots. The shadows of the hilar vessels often appear inordinately large on tomograms and are easily confused with large lymph nodes. Similarly, it should be borne in mind that the normal mediastinum appears wide on tomograms because the films are made with the patient recumbent.

A barium study of the esophagus is advisable before deciding that a bronchogenic carcinoma is amenable to resection because this may yield the only evidence of involvement of the mediastinum. Indentation or local displacement of the esophagus just below the level of the tracheal bifurcation indicates that the subcarinal lymph nodes are enlarged. An irregularity of the esophageal wall, a stricture, or a fistula into the trachea or main bronchus signifies direct invasion of the esophagus by the tumor (Fig. 422).

Mediastinography can be employed to determine whether the mediastinum is invaded. Permeation of the gas throughout the fascial planes indicates that the mediastinum is free of gross invasion by the tumor. However, either complete or partial obliteration of these planes is not necessarily diagnostic of tumor invasion since the planes may be obliterated by a previous or concomitant inflammatory process. This procedure is, therefore, rarely used.

Invasion of the mediastinum may be associated with involvement of the mediastinal blood vessels. Superior vena caval obstruction indicates that the tumor is not resectable. This is best demonstrated by venous angiography. Narrowing or irregularity of either main pulmonary artery indicates that the mediastinum is invaded. However, poor visualization of one pulmonary artery by venous angiography is not conclusive evidence that the artery is obstructed. In the absence of definite deformity of the vessel, the lack of filling may be related to disturbed function in the lung, so that the presence of obstruc-

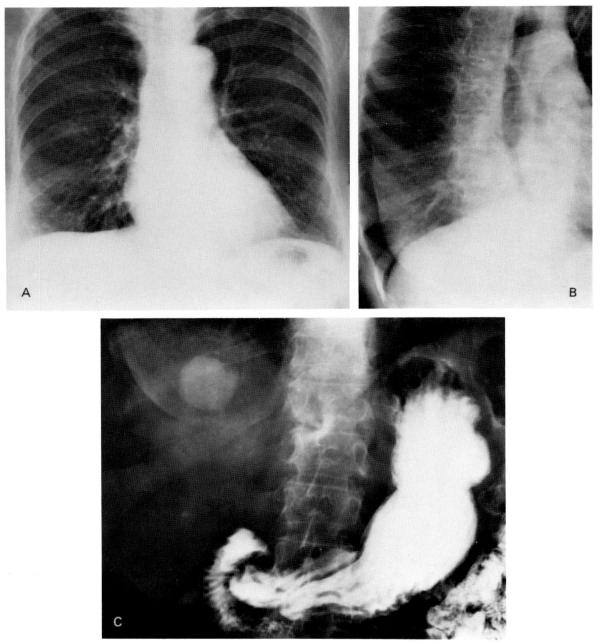

FIG. 419. PERIPHERAL CARCINOMA, RIGHT LOWER LOBE

A: Frontal view. No abnormality is seen in the lungs. *B:* Right oblique view. The posterior costophrenic sinus appears clear. However, there still remains a portion of the lower lobe which is obscured by the liver. The hazy shadow over the lower part of the right chest is cast by the breast. *C:* The lesion was detected accidentally on an abdominal film made as part of an x-ray examination of the stomach. The nodule in the right upper quadrant is clearly demarcated and therefore must be denser than the material surrounding it. Since it is composed of soft tissue, it cannot be within the liver which has a similar density. Therefore the nodule must be situated within the lung where it contrasts with the air around it. The lesion could not be visualized on the lateral view of the chest even in retrospect.

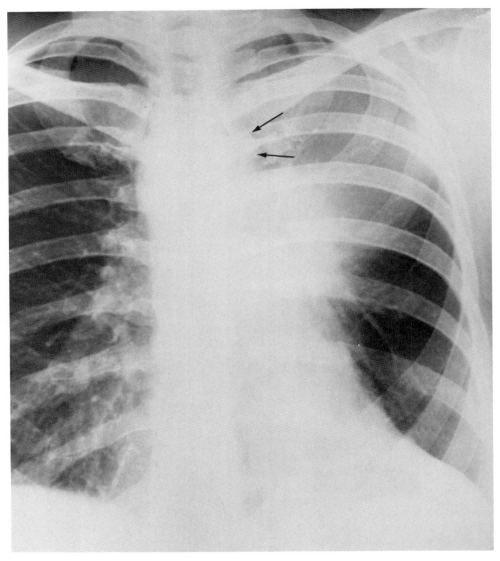

FIG. 420. STENOSING CARCINOMA OF THE LEFT UPPER LOBE

The veil-like shadow over the upper part of the left lung with shift of the heart and mediastinum to the left and elevation of the left leaf of the diaphragm indicates atelectasis of the left upper lobe. There is compensatory emphysema of the left lower lobe. The irregular density in the mesial portion of the atelectatic lobe represents an obstructing carcinoma. Because of adhesions over its anterior surface, the upper lobe collapsed in a forward direction so that the aortic knob (arrows) is not obscured. The localized bulge in the right paratracheal region indicates involvement of the mediastinum by neoplasm.

tion should be confirmed by selective pulmonary arteriography. Involvement of lobar or segmental vessels does not affect resectability since they are intrapulmonary and are removed together with the lung.

Obstruction of the azygos vein indicates infiltration of the mediastinum. The azygos vein can be clearly delineated by percutaneous injection of contrast material into the marrow of one of the lower ribs (Fig. 29). This examination is particularly useful when the findings referable to

involvement of the mediastinum are not conclusive and require confirmation before deciding that the tumor is not resectable.

PLEURAL INVOLVEMENT. The presence of a pleural effusion is almost always an indication that the carcinoma is not resectable since most of the effusions are caused by diffuse neoplastic involvement of the pleura. In some cases the effusion is caused by lymphatic obstruction secondary to involvement of the mediastinum (Fig. 423). On occasion, however, a pleural effusion

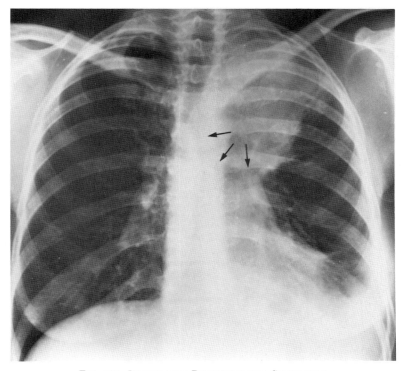

FIG. 421. INOPERABLE BRONCHOGENIC CARCINOMA

The shadow in the upper part of the left chest represents an atelectatic left upper lobe. The heart is displaced to the left and the left main bronchus is elevated. Despite this, the lower end of the trachea is displaced to the right, producing a hook-shaped tracheobronchial angle (arrows). The displacement of the trachea away from the atelectatic lobe indicates involvement of the mediastinal lymph nodes. The small effusion at the left base could be due either to infection of the lung secondary to bronchial obstruction or to spread of the carcinoma. The pleural effusion by itself, therefore, does not indicate nonresectability.

associated with an obstructing carcinoma is due simply to infection of the lung distal to the growth. In this instance, the tumor may be completely removable (Fig. 424).

In the absence of bronchial obstruction, a pleural effusion indicates that the carcinoma is not resectable even though malignant cells cannot be demonstrated in the fluid or on needle biopsy. The same is true of an obstructing carcinoma if there is no clinical evidence of infection. One or more scallops on the pleura also indicate pleural involvement by the neoplasm. They may be present in the absence of an effusion.

BONE INVOLVEMENT. Direct invasion of one or more ribs overlying the tumor does not necessarily prevent complete resection of the growth as it is often possible to remove the involved portion of the chest wall together with the carcinoma. However, in some cases, the growth spreads along the parietal pleura for a considerable distance beyond the area of rib destruction. This extension is best evaluated on films made with the rays tangential to the involved portion

of the rib. The extrapleural spread is manifested by blunting of the angles between the shadow of the tumor and the chest wall. Its extent above and below the tumor is judged from the length of the thickened soft tissue separating the ribs from the lung.

Carcinomas involving the ribs in the paravertebral region are rarely resectable. They usually cannot be freed completely from the spine even if the x-ray examination fails to reveal any involvement of the vertebrae.

Other Primary Malignant Neoplasms

Bronchiolar Carcinoma (Alveolar Cell Carcinoma, Pulmonary Adenomatosis). These names have been used to denote a special type of pulmonary neoplasm which has a characteristic microscopic appearance. It is composed of columnar cells, many of which are of the goblet type, resting on a basement membrane which appears to represent the alveolar wall. The cells are more or less uniform and the nuclei rather regular. The lung architecture remains relatively

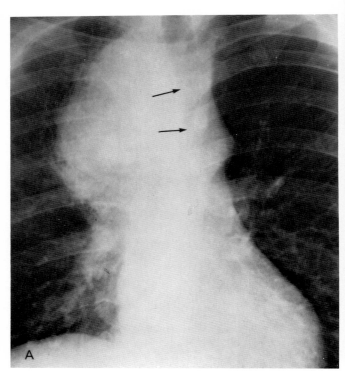
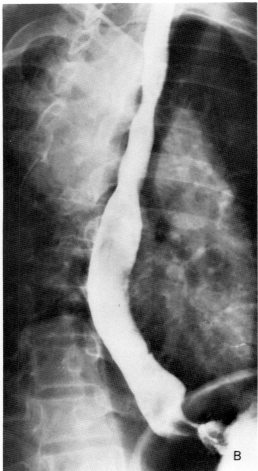

FIG. 422. MEDIASTINAL INVASION BY BRONCHOGENIC CARCINOMA

A: There is a large mass in the right upper lobe abutting on the mediastinum. The displacement of the trachea (arrows) suggests that the mediastinum is involved. *B:* Barium swallow shows an irregular, elongated narrowing of the upper esophagus caused by invasion of the neoplasm around the organ.

undisturbed. There is little fibrous tissue within the tumor and the bronchi are not involved. The term alveolar cell carcinoma has been used because of the fact that the tumor cells line alveolar walls, and the term adenomatosis has been applied because the gland-like structures present a benign appearance. On the other hand, the tendency of the tumor to spread widely throughout the lungs is indicative of a more malignant process. The term bronchiolar carcinoma is the one most commonly used because it reflects the malignant nature of the lesion and because the cells resemble bronchiolar epithelium rather than the lining cells of the alveoli.

Bronchiolar carcinoma manifests itself in three different forms. It may exist in the form of a single nodule, one or more diffuse areas of consolidation, or multiple small nodules throughout both lungs.

The border of the solitary nodule is usually rather indistinct (Fig. 425). It is never exquisitely demarcated as in the case of benign growths, and tends to be less well defined than most peripheral carcinomas. In some cases, because of extension of the tumor into neighboring alveoli, the contour of the nodule is spiculated and has been described as having a sunburst appearance. Often it is impossible to differentiate the solitary nodular form of bronchiolar carcinoma from a circumscribed peripheral bronchogenic carcinoma. However, since the growth does not originate in a bronchus, the atelectatic streak (Fleischner line) that is characteristic of many cases of bronchogenic carcinoma, does not occur in association with the bronchiolar neoplasm.

When the disease is more diffuse, the involved lung, which is consolidated with tumor cells and secretion, presents the appearance of a pneu-

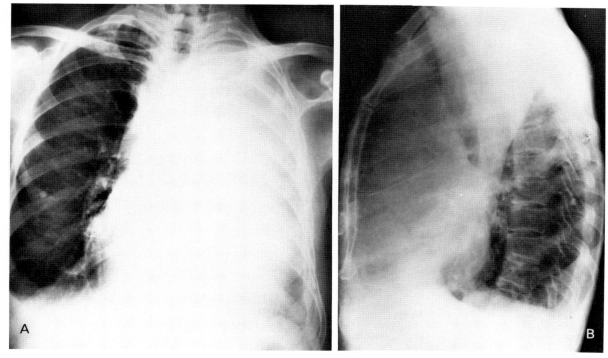

FIG. 423. STENOSING BRONCHIAL CARCINOMA: MEDIASTINAL INVASION

A: The patient had a carcinoma of the left main bronchus which completely occluded the bronchus to the upper lobe. The flattening of the dome of the left side of the thorax, the increase in obliquity of the ribs, and narrowing of the intercostal spaces indicate loss of volume of the left lung. The mediastinum was fixed by neoplastic invasion and could not shift toward the affected side. Most of the shadow on the left side was caused by the densely infiltrated upper lobe and thick pleura. There was only a small effusion. At postmortem examination, the pleura on the right side was free of metastases. The effusion on the right side was due to obstruction of lymphatic drainage. *B:* The lateral view shows the long fissure displaced upward as the result of atelectasis of the left upper lobe. The retrosternal space is clouded and the trachea is pushed backward by the neoplasm which has invaded the anterior mediastinum. The remarkable clarity in the region of the lower lobe in this view is striking in comparison with the appearance on the frontal projection.

monia both on x-ray examination and gross inspection of the specimen (Fig. 115). The roentgen film usually shows a large, poorly defined area of homogeneous opacification which may be confined to a single pulmonary segment. More commonly, by the time the disease is detected, it involves portions of adjacent segments and may extend throughout one or more lobes (Fig. 426). Since the bronchi are not involved, they remain patent and an air bronchogram is often seen within the area of consolidation (see Fig. 428).

The growth spreads from alveolus to alveolus, involving some and sparing others in an irregular fashion. As a result, the lung at the periphery of the homogeneous density often appears stippled. The entire shadow may have a granular appearance in the early stages of the pneumonic form as well as in the more localized form that eventually develops into a single homogeneous nodule.

The homogeneity of the lesion is due, in part, to the accumulation of secretion within the

spaces lined by tumor cells. The secretion is characteristically thin and watery and large amounts are frequently expectorated. When this occurs, the dense, pneumonic shadow of the bronchiolar carcinoma may become less homogeneous as though it were beginning to undergo resolution. However, the spaces are soon filled again and the shadow once more becomes homogeneous.

When an entire lobe is consolidated, the roentgen picture can be identical to that of lobar pneumonia. However, not uncommonly, as the tumor expands, the lobe becomes larger than normal and causes bulging of the adjacent fissure. In this respect, the appearance is similar to that of Friedländer's pneumonia. Sooner or later the disease spreads, probably through the bronchi, to form one or more similar lesions in an adjacent lobe or in the opposite lung (Fig. 427). At first the newly formed lesions cast faint, poorly demarcated shadows but soon they become large and dense. Eventually the areas of

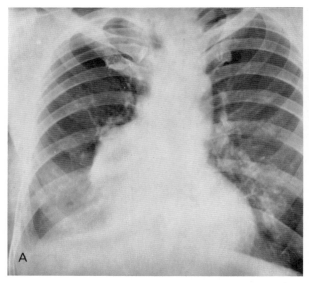
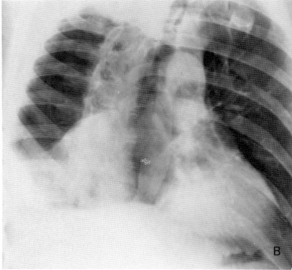

FIG. 424. BRONCHOGENIC CARCINOMA WITH SYMPATHETIC EFFUSION

A: The mass at the hilum of the right lung is associated with a veil-like shadow over the lower lobe and compensatory hyperaeration of the upper lobe. These signs indicate atelectasis of the lower lobe due to obstruction of its bronchus by the mass. A small effusion blunts the right costophrenic sinus. Bronchoscopy revealed a primary carcinoma in the lower lobe bronchus. *B:* In the oblique view, the effusion is seen to be of considerable size. Because the patient had fever, it was assumed that the lung beyond the obstructed bronchus was infected. A pleural tap showed the fluid to be clear. At operation, there was no gross or microscopic evidence of pleural involvement by the neoplasm.

consolidation coalesce and can involve most of both lungs.

The least common presentation of bronchiolar carcinoma is characterized by numerous nodules diffusely studding both lungs. The nodules are rather uniform in size varying up to 1.5 cm in diameter. Sometimes one of the nodules is larger than the others, suggesting that this may be the primary growth. In general, the multinodular forms of bronchiolar carcinoma cannot be differentiated from metastatic neoplasms from other organs. However, the nodules are not delineated by an extremely sharp border as are some metastatic tumors.

Cavitation occasionally occurs in both the nodular and pneumonic forms of the disease. It is seen more commonly in the pathologic specimen than on the film because the cavities are usually filled with secretion. After expectoration of secretion, the cavities may be visualized as areas of increased lucency within the shadow of the tumor (Fig. 428). We have not observed fluid levels within them. It is difficult to differentiate between a cavity and a lucent area representing a group of uninvolved alveoli.

Bronchography has been reported to disclose a characteristic picture in this disease. The bronchus leading to the tumor is not obstructed, and the larger bronchial branches within the tumor are patent. However, the latter are often irregularly thinned because of extrinsic pressure and present a dead tree appearance. There is a paucity of ramifications because the small bronchi and alveoli are plugged with tumor cells and secretions, and do not fill with contrast material. This appearance is not entirely specific for bronchiolar carcinoma since it has been observed in other diseases, particularly lymphosarcoma of the lung.

Enlargement of the hilar and mediastinal nodes is rarely noted on the roentgen film despite widespread involvement of the lungs. In fact, in a large percentage of the cases the lymph nodes have been found to be free of tumor on pathologic examination. Similarly, involvement of the pleura is unusual and pleural effusions are rarely seen. Involvement of the chest wall has been reported but is also extremely rare.

The diagnosis of bronchiolar carcinoma cannot be made from a single roentgen examination. It should be suspected when there is a persistent pneumonic shadow which gradually enlarges locally and finally becomes complicated by the appearance of additional irregular areas of consolidation. Bronchiolar carcinoma should also be suspected when a single, poorly demarcated nodular shadow persists unchanged or grows slowly over a period of years, or when the film of the

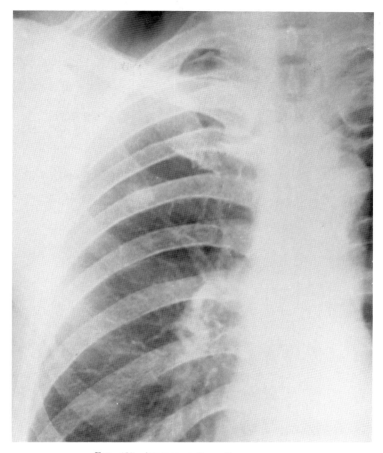

FIG. 425. ALVEOLAR CELL CARCINOMA

There is a poorly defined, small nodule in the right upper lobe, projected over the anterior portion of the second rib. Neither calcium nor a Fleischner line could be demonstrated by tomography. The lesion cannot be differentiated from a peripheral bronchogenic carcinoma or granulomatous disase. It proved to be an alveolar cell carcinoma.

chest shows numerous, rather poorly demarcated nodular shadows without evidence of a primary growth elsewhere. Bronchiolar carcinoma is unlikely if the lesion becomes increasingly demarcated, if it shows a persistent decrease in size or density, or if it is associated with lymph node enlargement or pleural effusion.

Sarcoma. Almost all the microscopic types of sarcoma found elsewhere in the body also occur as primary tumors in the lung. Some arise from the bronchial wall but most of them originate in the pulmonary connective tissue.

The bronchial sarcomas appear to originate mainly from the large bronchi. Most of them are polypoid, but they infiltrate the bronchial wall and usually involve the surrounding pulmonary tissue. The roentgen picture is dominated by atelectasis and infection of the lung beyond the obstructing tumor. The endobronchial growth may be visualized on the films in the same man-

ner as in the case of bronchial carcinoids. An obscuring pleural effusion may be due either to infection or spread of the tumor to the pleura. The mediastinum is frequently uninvolved.

The parenchymal sarcoma usually presents as a rather large, well demarcated, round mass. Even when small, the tumor tends to be well circumscribed and in this way differs from the smudge-like shadow of an early, bronchogenic carcinoma. The tumor grows largely by expansion and therefore remains circumscribed as it increases in size (Fig. 429). Some grow very slowly while others become large in a relatively few months. Because of its extremely sharp, circumscribed border, the shadow of a pulmonary sarcoma is quite similar to that of a benign lesion or a solitary metastasis. In rare instances, a circumscribed sarcoma erodes into a neighboring major bronchus to form an intraluminal polypoid mass. If this causes complete obstruction of the

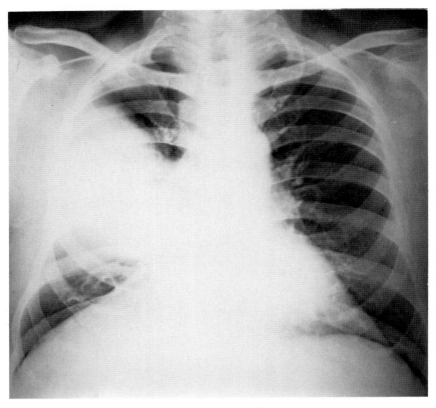

FIG. 426. ALVEOLAR CELL CARCINOMA

There is a large area of homogeneous consolidation involving the anterior segment of the right upper lobe and most of the middle lobe. The distribution of the lesion is unusual because diseases characterized by consolidation of the lung are almost always limited by the interlobar fissures. In this case, the consolidation was due to alveolar cell carcinoma which had spread by contiguity from the upper to the middle lobe because the short fissure was absent.

bronchus, the resulting atelectasis obscures the underlying tumor and the appearance is then no different from that of a bronchial carcinoma.

Occasionally a sarcoma of the lung is more invasive and its border is indistinct. Like a carcinoma, it can extend across the pleural fissure to involve an adjacent lobe. The distinction between the invasive type of sarcoma and a carcinoma of the lung cannot be made radiologically.

Sarcomas of the lung differ from some peripheral carcinomas in that they do not invade the chest wall, even when extremely large. Large mediastinal lymph nodes are very rare and the neoplasm does not seem to metastasize to bone. Pleural effusions may occur in the later stages.

Angiosarcomas behave somewhat differently from the other sarcomas. When the angiosarcoma arises from the pulmonary parenchyma it tends to infiltrate the lung irregularly rather than to grow in the form of a circumscribed nodule. If it involves only a single lobe, the lesion resembles a pneumonia. In some cases multiple lesions are present throughout the lungs and appear either as diffuse infiltrations or as scattered, irregular, poorly defined nodules. In these respects, the roentgen appearance of the neoplasm resembles that of bronchiolar carcinoma.

Lymphomatous Diseases. Only a small percentage of malignant lymphomas are primary in the lung. The most common is lymphosarcoma; reticulum cell sarcoma is less frequent, and primary Hodgkin's disease of the lung is extremely rare.

Radiologically, the lesion most often appears as a round or oval density whose border is not sharply demarcated. The edge of the shadow tends to be hazy and fade into the surrounding lung. Because of its poor definition, distinct lobulation of the mass is usually absent. The shadow appears homogeneous but, in rare instances, a cavity is present. Usually the lesion is quite large, measuring over 4 or 5 cm when first seen.

Lymphosarcoma and reticulum cell sarcoma do not tend to produce obstruction of any but

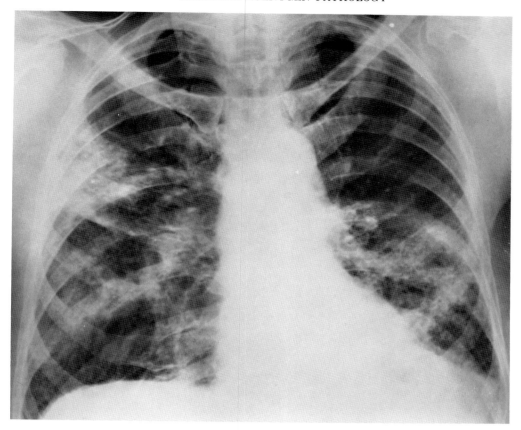

FIG. 427. BRONCHIOLAR CARCINOMA

This is a late stage of the disease when the patient was bringing up large quantities of clear, watery secretion. The carcinoma involves both lungs. The patchy shadows represent consolidation by neoplastic cells. In places the shadows appear stippled because the alveoli are not uniformly involved.

the smallest bronchi so that tomograms usually disclose air-filled bronchi coursing through the mass. Bronchograms show the pattern of the bronchi unaltered except for a dead tree appearance similar to that seen in bronchiolar carcinoma. On the other hand, Hodgkin's disease, which is a more desmoplastic tumor, tends to occlude the larger bronchi within the lesion.

In some cases, particularly when the lesion is extensive, the appearance suggests pneumonic consolidation. This may involve an entire lobe and may extend into an adjoining lobe.

It is impossible to make a diagnosis of primary lymphoma of the lung from the roentgen examination alone. A lymphoma should be considered when the film shows a persistent area of homogeneous consolidation in the absence of symptoms suggesting inflammatory disease.

Primary lymphoma of the lung does not differ in appearance from the pulmonary lesions in generalized lymphomatous disease. The diagnosis of primary lymphoma, therefore, is not justi-fied unless other possible sites of involvement have been excluded.

Plasmacytoma. Only a few cases of plasma cell tumors of the lung have been reported. Most of them appear to be granulomas rather than neoplasms. As in the case of plasmacytomas involving the upper air passages, some of the true plasma cell neoplasms of the lung appear to be benign, while others show characteristics of malignancy. A pulmonary plasmacytoma may exist as a solitary lesion or be a part of multiple myelomatosis. It is, therefore, advisable to make an x-ray survey of the bones in all cases of plasmacytoma of the lung.

When encapsulated and apparently benign, the plasmacytoma appears as a sharply demarcated round mass. However, when the tumor is invasive, its borders are poorly demarcated. One case has been reported in which large and irregular dense areas representing deposits of bone were present throughout the shadow of the tumor.

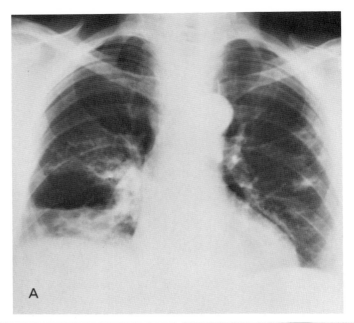

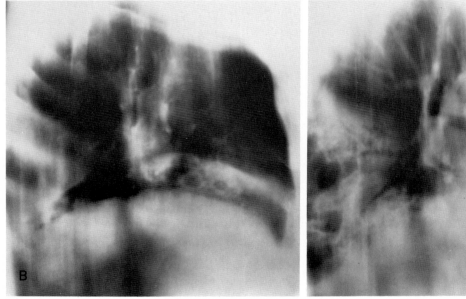

FIG. 428. BRONCHIOLAR CARCINOMA

A: There is a large cavity within an area of consolidation in the right lower lobe. Several smaller cavities are present in the lung just above the diaphragm. There is also an irregular patch of consolidation in the midportion of the left lung. The patient was afebrile and was expectorating large amounts of clear, thin, salty sputum. Biopsy revealed bronchiolar carcinoma. *B:* A lateral tomogram shows the multiple smaller cavities to lie within the middle lobe of the right lung. *C:* A more mesial section reveals a large area of consolidation in the posterior portion of the right lower lobe. The bronchi within this area are patent and are seen as branching lucencies within the opacified lung (air bronchogram).

Metastatic Neoplasms

Metastatic neoplasms of the lung rarely give rise to abnormal physical signs. However, they are readily disclosed by roentgen examination even when quite small. Therefore a film of the chest should be made before instituting treatment for a malignant tumor anywhere in the body. In some cases, the demonstration of metastases in the lungs provides the first indication of a primary tumor elsewhere.

Metastatic neoplasms may be roughly divided

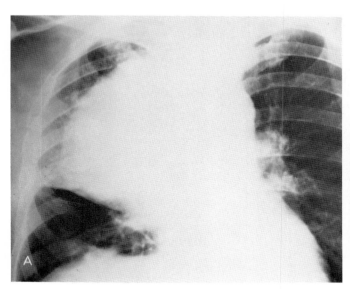
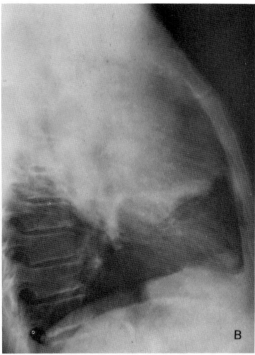

FIG. 429. SARCOMA OF THE LUNG

A: A 56 year old man presented with a history of hemoptysis for 3 months and pain in the extremities secondary to periostopathy. The frontal film shows a huge, homogeneous mass in the right upper lobe which displaces the short fissure downward. *B:* In the lateral view, the upper part of the long fissure is displaced backward by the mass. Although a bronchogenic carcinoma can present a similar appearance, the possibility of a sarcoma must be considered because of the size of the lesion and its circumscription.

into three types, according to their roentgen appearance: nodular, lymphangitic and pneumonic.

Nodular Metastases. Nodular metastases to the lungs are almost always multiple and usually appear as numerous round densities of varying size throughout the pulmonary fields. They are either evenly distributed, or more numerous in the lower part of the chest (Fig. 430). In this way they differ from nodular tuberculous lesions, which are practically always more numerous in the upper portion of the pulmonary field, and from many cases of nodular silicosis and sarcoidosis which tend to have a similar distribution.

When the metastases are numerous, the lesions are usually more or less uniform and of moderate size (Figs. 430 and 431). When few in number, they often differ greatly in size (Fig. 3). In the rare cases where the tumor is single, it may assume large proportions (Figs. 432 and 433).

Frequently the metastatic nodules are perfectly round and sharply circumscribed. In other cases their shape is rather irregular and their borders are not so well demarcated. Metastatic

carcinomas tend to fall in the latter group and although they are of fairly uniform density, they usually are not absolutely homogeneous. In these respects they differ from the sarcomas, whose shadows are more uniform and whose borders are sharply circumscribed and regular. Similar sharply circumscribed densities also occur in the case of pulmonary metastases from carcinoma of the thyroid, melanoma, endometrial carcinoma and trophoblastic and testicular tumors (Fig. 3).

The nodular metastases grow mostly by expansion and retain their nodular character without diffuse infiltration. An exception to this is the metastatic chorioepithelioma which may show a tendency to irregular infiltration of the lung in the later stages. The presence of irregular infiltrations in association with large, round, circumscribed nodules is more characteristic of anthracosilicosis (miner's lung) or Caplan's syndrome.

SOLITARY METASTASES. Metastases to the lung are almost always multiple. A small, single density in the lung in a patient with a neoplasm elsewhere in the body often represents an inflam-

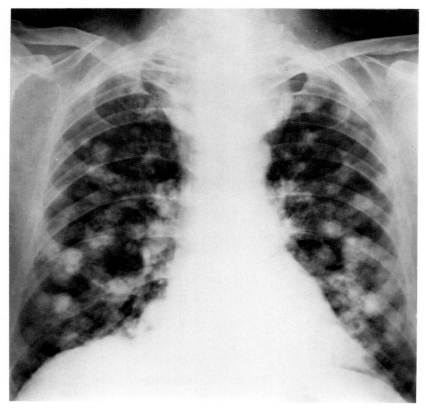

FIG. 430. METASTATIC CARCINOMA: NODULAR TYPE

Both lungs are studded with numerous, fairly well demarcated nodules. The shadow in the superior mediastinum represents a carcinoma of the thyroid which was the primary growth.

matory lesion or a benign hamartoma. The finding of such a nodule, therefore, does not justify withholding operation for the primary neoplasm. However, experience has shown that it is very easy to overlook additional nodules which establish the diagnosis of metastatic disease.

Systematic scrutiny of all parts of the pulmonary fields may disclose other nodules whose shadows are very faint even though they are sharply defined. Oblique views are helpful. However, the possibility of multiple nodules cannot be excluded without tomograms of both lungs.

The nodular type of metastasis rarely causes bronchial obstruction, and the round shadow which it casts on the film is rarely associated with an atelectatic streak (Fleischner line). The presence of this line distal to a nodule is practically always indicative of a primary bronchogenic carcinoma. In the absence of such a streak, however, it is impossible to differentiate between a solitary metastasis and a primary tumor. In the case of an extremely sharply demarcated, round, homogeneous density, such as occurs in metastatic sarcoma, the appearance is similar to that of a fluid-filled pulmonary cyst (Fig. 433).

When a single round density appears in the lung of a patient who has had a malignant tumor resected, the question arises as to whether the mass in the lung should be removed. Many surgeons advocate waiting for a period of up to 2 or 3 months before performing resection for fear that the patient may have additional metastases which are not yet visible. We feel that this plan is justifiable in the case of a small nodule but not in the case of a large one, for the latter has undoubtedly been present for some time in order to attain its size. It remains necessary only to exclude the presence of other metastases. For this purpose it is advisable to make tomograms of both lungs. Since we are looking for very small nodules which cast faint shadows, the films should not be heavily exposed.

CAVITATION. Occasionally cavitation occurs in one or more metastatic nodules, but it is extremely rare in a solitary metastasis. Cavitation in a solitary nodule practically always indicates either inflammatory disease, a broken-down primary bronchogenic carcinoma or an infarct.

In the reported cases, cavitation occurred most frequently in metastases from adenocarcinomas

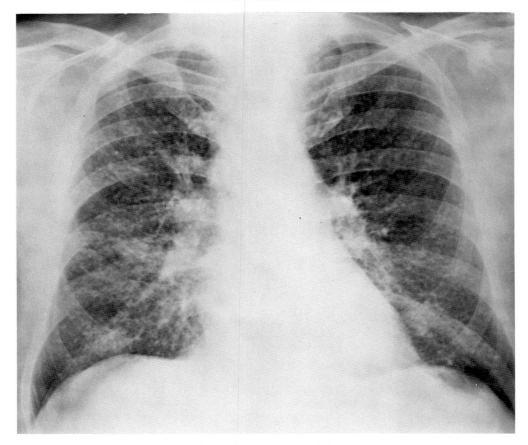

FIG. 431. METASTATIC CARCINOMA, MILIARY FORM

Both lungs are diffusely studded with innumerable tiny nodules and there is a mass of enlarged lymph nodes in the right paratracheal region. Both the parenchymal and nodal lesions represent metastatic spread from a primary carcinoma of the pancreas.

of the intestine or in squamous cell carcinomas, particularly those from the head and neck. Cavitation has been observed in untreated cases as well as after radiotherapy or chemotherapy.

In most instances, the cavities are thick-walled and have an irregular inner border. Usually a fluid level is absent. In rare cases the cavity is almost completely filled with necrotic tumor tissue. The upper border of the necrotic mass may be delineated by a crescent-shaped lucency as in the case of a mycetoma. In rare instances the cavity is extremely thin-walled and smooth, suggesting the cavity of inflammatory disease, such as tuberculosis, coccidioidomycosis, a healed lung abscess or a pneumatocele.

CALCIFICATION. Most frequently, calcific deposits within nodular pulmonary metastases are indicative of metastatic osteogenic sarcoma which contains bone (Fig. 434). The calcium tends to be irregularly distributed within the nodules. Some of the smaller nodules may appear to be entirely replaced by calcium, while in the

larger ones the calcium is usually distributed in a flocculant fashion. Less often calcification occurs in metastatic chondrosarcoma. In rare instances, calcification occurs in metastases from carcinoma of the thyroid. Since nodular metastases grow almost entirely by expansion, they do not engulf previously existing calcific deposits in the surrounding lung as does a primary bronchogenic carcinoma.

MILIARY NODULES. Studding of the lungs with innumerable, very small, or miliary nodules occurs occasionally. We have seen this type of metastasis in association with carcinomas of the lung, thyroid, prostate, kidney, pancreas and in malignant melanoma (Fig. 435).

SPONTANEOUS PNEUMOTHORAX. Spontaneous pneumothorax in association with nodular pulmonary metastases has been observed with significant frequency in osteosarcoma and in Ewing's and Wilm's tumors. Of the other neoplasms in which spontaneous pneumothorax has been reported, sarcomas have been predominant.

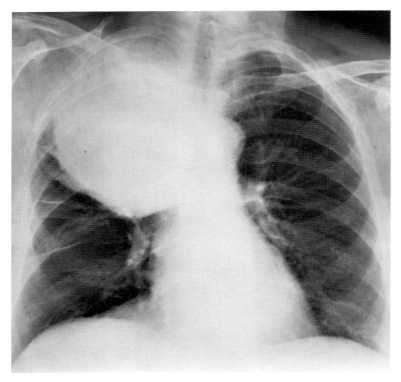

FIG. 432. SOLITARY METASTASIS TO THE LUNG

The clearly defined mass in the right upper lobe represented a metastasis from a fibrosarcoma of the rectus sheath. This is a tumor of low grade malignancy. An extremely sharp demarcation, such as this, is unusual for a primary carcinoma of the lung.

The mechanism of production of the pneumothorax is not entirely clear. In most cases there was no evidence of cavitation within the metastases. Blebs and bullae have been noted in association with these tumors and it seems most probable that rupture of one of them is responsible for the pneumothorax. The air in the pleural cavity can resorb in the same manner as a pneumothorax without neoplastic disease. Rupture of a broken-down pulmonary metastasis into the pleura has been a more unusual cause of pneumothorax.

Lymphangitic Metastasis. Nodular metastases to the lungs can occur as a result of *transport* of malignant cells through either the blood stream or the lymphatic channels. Spread of the tumor by *permeation* of the lymphatic channels produces interlacing cords of neoplastic tissue giving rise to the picture of carcinomatous lymphangitis.

The lymphangitic form of pulmonary metastasis occurs most frequently from carcinomas of the stomach and lung. Less frequently, the primary origin is in the breast or pancreas. Other primary sources are rare. In most cases the pulmonary involvement is bilateral. When unilateral, the primary tumor is almost always in the lung or in the breast on that side.

The radiologic picture is produced primarily by lymphatics distended with strands of tumor and by extensions of the tumor through the walls of these channels. The proliferating carcinoma is associated with a varying degree of fibrous tissue reaction. Since the lymphatics of the lungs are situated mainly about the bronchi, blood vessels and interlobular septa, the shadows of these structures become thickened.

At first, there is only a slight accentuation of the pulmonary markings, particularly at the roots of the lungs. Growth of the tumor is usually rapid and results in diffuse streaking and fine mottling between the shadows of the blood vessels within a few weeks. Tiny nodules are formed where the neoplastic cells break through the lymphatic channels and grow within the surrounding tissues. These streak-like and nodular shadows converge with the lymphatics toward the hilum of the lungs and the shadows are therefore more dense in this region (Fig. 436). The lymph nodes at the hilum are usually not visibly enlarged and may prove to be free of tumor on pathologic examination.

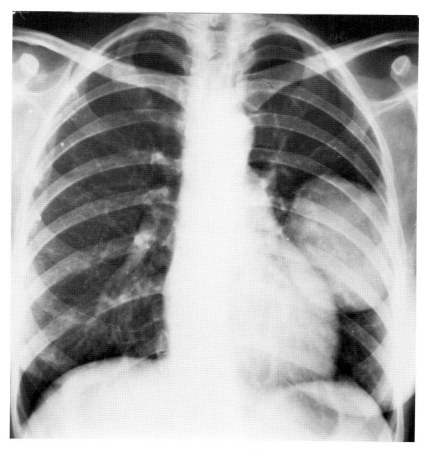

FIG. 433. CHORIONEPITHELIOMA OF THE LUNG

The sharply circumscribed oval mass, whose shadow overlaps the heart, does not obscure the cardiac border. It is therefore situated behind the heart in the left lower lobe. Not all chorionepitheliomas of the lung are sharply demarcated. Often part of the border is obscured because of hemorrhage into the surrounding pulmonary tissue. The primary lesion could not be identified at necropsy, but the tumor probably originated in the uterus.

The distinction between lymphangitic permeation and congestive failure may be difficult because both produce thickening of the interstitial tissues and can show Kerley's A and B lines. However, the linear shadows of lymphangitic metastasis are usually more sharply defined and often are coarser than those of congestion and interstitial pulmonary edema. The shadows of lymphangitic permeation tend to be much more dense at the lung roots. When they are more prominent in the periphery of the lungs, they are frequently patchy in distribution and are not associated with dilated vessels at the hilum. Enlargement of the heart is almost always present when interstitial changes or a pleural effusion are due to congestive failure.

The picture of lymphangitic carcinosis may be dominated by diffuse stippling of the lungs or by tiny nodules similar to hematogenous metastases. Careful examination will usually disclose evidence of irregular thickening of the vascular shadows to indicate involvement of lymphatics about these structures. Not infrequently, larger nodules appear together with the pattern of interstitial infiltration. Although these may be caused by concomitant blood stream invasion, more often they result from the growth of carcinoma through the walls of the lymphatic channels.

Frequently the lower portions of the lungs are the most extensively infiltrated, but both lungs are almost always involved symmetrically. However, in bronchogenic carcinoma the infiltration is most dense on the side of the primary tumor. This also occurs in some cases of breast carcinoma.

Because carcinomatous tissue in the lymphatics and the accompanying reactive connective

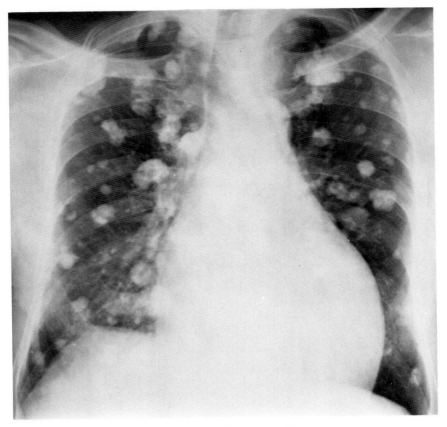

FIG. 434. METASTATIC OSTEOGENIC SARCOMA
Most of the nodules throughout the lung are extremely dense because they contain bone.

tissue form a network of guy ropes extending from the root of the lung to the periphery, they interfere with complete expansion of the lungs. This is manifested clinically by diminution in the vital capacity and tachypnea on exertion. The lessened expansibility of the lungs is manifested radiologically by diminished downward excursion of the diaphragms and decreased illumination of the lungs on full inspiration. During expiration the diaphragm ascends higher than normal and clouding of the lung during this phase is accentuated because the residual air is diminished. These changes become more marked as the lesions progress and the lung becomes more and more contracted.

Although the pleural lymphatics are always extensively involved, they cannot be visualized as individual shadows. The pleural fissures, however, may appear thickened because of superimposition of the shadows of many lymphatics filled with tumor. Pleural effusions are a common complication, particularly in the later stages of lymphangitic carcinosis. They are usually bilateral.

Pneumonic Form. Metastatic neoplasms of the lungs occasionally assume the roentgen appearance of localized areas of bronchopneumonia. Although the rather diffuse, ill-defined shadows of these metastases are usually multiple, they may be confined to one portion of the lung. Perhaps the most common site of origin of this type of metastatic carcinoma is the breast, but it is also encountered in metastases from the pancreas, stomach, intestine or prostate.

Pathologically, the lesion presents the picture suggested by the name, "pneumonia carcinomatosa," a form of carcinoma in which the alveoli are filled with neoplastic cells. The analogy of this condition to simple pneumonia, in which the alveoli are filled with inflammatory exudate, is obvious and the similarity in the appearance of the two conditions on the roentgen film is not surprising. Differentiation at a single roentgen observation is usually impossible. However, the persistence or gradual expansion of the process is sufficient to arouse the suspicion of a metastatic neoplasm.

Metastases from chorioepithelioma usually present themselves as well-defined, round nod-

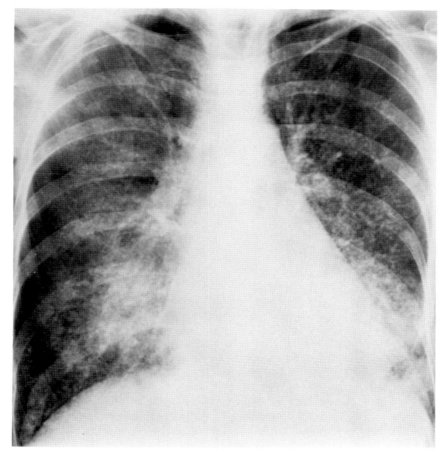

FIG. 435. MILIARY METASTASES

The fine nodular lesions throughout both lungs represent metastases from a malignant melanoma.

ules, but some cases are characterized by diffuse infiltration and consolidation of the lung producing poorly defined shadows simulating pneumonia. The poor definition of the lesions and the confluence of the shadows is due to extravasation of blood into the alveoli around the metastatic deposits.

Regression of Metastases. Occasionally, metastatic neoplasms in the lungs diminish in size or even disappear without any specific treatment. Regression of shadows in the lungs, therefore, should not be taken as conclusive proof that they do not represent metastatic tumors. A number of instances of disappearance of metastases from hypernephroma have been recorded after removal of the primary growth. Moreover, we have observed this to occur even when the primary tumor was not disturbed. Similarly, pulmonary metastases from trophoblastic tumors have been noted to disappear without hormone treatment or resection of the uterus or ovaries. We have also observed a patient with carcinoma

of the thyroid in whom some of the pulmonary metastases disappeared spontaneously while others diminished in size and some remained unchanged over a period of several years. In addition, we now have under observation a patient with pulmonary metastases from an endometrial carcinoma in whom some of the metastases have disappeared while others have continued to grow in the absence of any specific treatment.

Generalized Malignant Disease

In certain types of malignant neoplastic disease, the process appears to develop independently in several organs. The course suggests a multicentric origin of the tumors rather than metastases from any one site. In this sense, multiple tumors in the same organ may also represent independent growths rather than metastases from a single primary. The tumors that are usually associated with such multifocal neoplas-

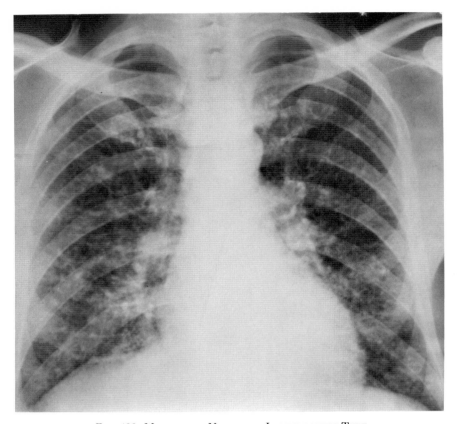

FIG. 436. METASTATIC NEOPLASM: LYMPHANGITIC TYPE

Fine, streak-like shadows and tiny nodules are present throughout both lungs. The distribution is characteristic of lymphangitic disease, but it is impossible to differentiate between an inflammatory and a neoplastic process from the roentgen films alone. The primary neoplasm was a carcinoma of the stomach. Clinically, a pneumonia was suspected because of fever and tachypnea.

tic changes are those which arise from the blood-forming and vascular tissues.

Hodgkin's Disease. The lungs are frequently involved in Hodgkin's disease, particularly in the later stages when the pulmonary lesions become manifest in one-half to three-quarters of the cases. However, the lungs may be affected earlier and, in rare instances, the pulmonary lesions may be the only abnormality on the film.

The pulmonary lesions of Hodgkin's disease can be divided into four types: hilar, pneumonic, nodular and pleural. Each of these may occur alone or in combination with one or more of the others. They may be unilateral or bilateral, single or multiple. When there are several lesions, they usually vary in size and each of the lesions tends to grow independently of the others. One may progress while others remain stationary.

The *hilar* type of Hodgkin's disease usually occurs in association with enlargement of the mediastinal and hilar lymph nodes. The disease tends to extend beyond the confines of the lymph nodes to involve the connective tissue of the mediastinum and the tissues about the bronchi and blood vessels at the root of the lung (see Fig. 472). The process in the lung is usually unilateral. The neoplasm spreads along the peribronchial and perivascular tissues and the interlobar septa to produce the picture of dense, interstitial infiltration similar to that of a locally spreading carcinoma of a root bronchus. As in bronchogenic carcinoma, the wall of the main or lobar bronchus is frequently infiltrated, narrowing the lumen. A funnel-shaped stenosis is often demonstrable by tomography or bronchography. A well-defined endobronchial mass is rarely encountered. Atelectasis supervenes when the bronchial obstruction becomes complete (Fig. 76). The shadow of the involved lung is then homogeneous and obscures the infiltrative nature of the underlying process.

The *pneumonic* type appears in the form of patchy densities which are poorly demarcated. Some are small, while others involve an entire lobe or most of the lung. The densities are usually multiple and bilateral (Fig. 108), but occasionally there is only a single area of involvement. The lesions begin as local areas of interstitial infiltration which tend to conglomerate as they enlarge, compressing alveoli to produce a picture simulating consolidation. The essentially interstitial nature of the disease is indicated by the presence of fine infiltrations of the lung along the borders of the dense shadows. The roentgen picture is quite similar to that of pneumonia. However, fibrosis is often evident in portions of the lesion, and may involve an entire lobe. Portions of the lung undergo contraction as a result of involvement of the small bronchi.

The *nodular* type of pulmonary Hodgkin's disease is characterized roentgenologically by the presence of one or more round or oval densities (Fig. 437). They are usually few in number and vary up to 6 to 8 cm in diameter. Even though the lesions frequently obstruct small bronchi, they are not associated with Fleischner lines

because they characteristically originate immediately beneath the pleura. In this way they differ from many peripheral carcinomas. In contradistinction to most metastatic neoplasms, the borders usually have a hazy outline. When the lesions are flat against the pleura, their shadows may be rather faint unless projected tangentially.

The *pleural* lesions of Hodgkin's disease occur either in the form of localized plaques or as a more diffuse thickening of the pleura. When the pleural plaques are viewed *en face,* their shadows are very faint and may not be visible on films of standard density. However, when the plaques are projected tangentially, they appear as sharply defined, scalloped shadows or as irregular, localized, flat densities lying against the contour of the chest wall.

More diffuse involvement of the pleura usually occurs at the base, in relation to the diaphragm and about the lower portion of the lung. These

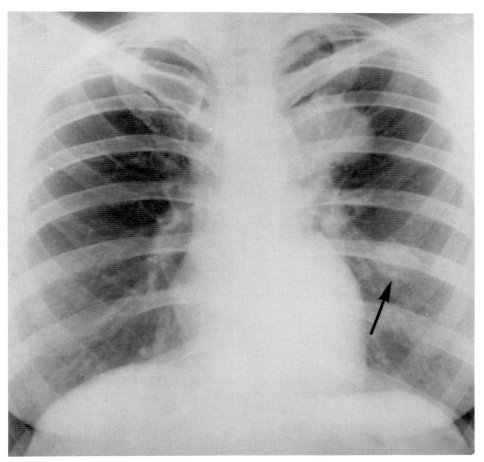

FIG. 437. HODGKIN'S DISEASE: PULMONARY NODULES

There is a large, well-circumscribed nodule in the anterior mesial portion of the left upper lobe. The arch of the aorta is visible within the shadow. A second mass is seen overlying the posterior portion of the eighth rib (arrow). The poor definition of this mass is more characteristic of the nodular form of Hodgkin's disease of the lung. There is no enlargement of the mediastinal lymph nodes. The diagnosis was made by biopsy of a supraclavicular lymph node.

structures are frequently involved together with the pleura and become fused into a solid mass. The homogeneous density then seen at the base of the pulmonary field fades out gradually in its upper portion, simulating a collection of fluid. Such lesions are often bilateral.

Pleural involvement by Hodgkin's disease is often associated with an effusion which may obscure the individual lesions on the pleura. The latter may be visualized if the examination is repeated after the fluid is withdrawn, particularly if replaced with air. On the other hand, it is possible for an effusion to form as a result of blockage of the lymphatics within the mediastinum without pleural involvement by the tumor. That this is not uncommon is indicated by the disappearance of the effusion in many cases after radiotherapy directed only to the mediastinum.

Cavitation occurs occasionally within the pulmonary lesions. Most often the cavities result from necrosis of the tumor caused by irradiation or chemotherapy, but cavitation can also take place spontaneously. The cavities may form within fairly well defined nodules or within the more diffuse, dense infiltrative lesions. The wall is usually thick (Fig. 76), but may be extremely thin in the case of a circumscribed nodule. The inner contour of the cavity may be irregular or smooth. Fluid levels are uncommon.

Lymphosarcoma. Pulmonary involvement is rarely an early manifestation of lymphosarcoma. The lungs are occasionally affected in the terminal stages, but not nearly as often as in Hodgkin's disease. The pulmonary lesions may appear as more or less round, fairly well circumscribed, medium-sized or large nodules. Numerous small nodules of uniform size, distributed throughout the lungs, are more frequently seen in follicular lymphoblastoma. We have observed miliary involvement of the lungs in the small-cell type of lymphosarcoma (Fig. 438). In rare instances, dense, patchy areas of infiltration, having the appearance of pneumonic consolidation, occur in lymphosarcoma but they are more commonly seen in reticulum cell sarcoma.

As in Hodgkin's disease, the pulmonary lesions are most frequently found in association with involvement of the mediastinum. Pleural effusions are common, but are frequently due to blockage of the lymphatics in the mediastinum

rather than to disease of the pleura itself. In general, as in leukemia, the shadows that appear in the pulmonary fields during the course of lymphosarcoma are usually due to complicating conditions, such as infection or infarction.

Leukemia. Leukemic infiltrations are often found in the lungs at necropsy, but are rarely large enough to be visible on the roentgen film. When the lesions can be seen, they usually appear as local infiltrations simulating pneumonia, or as numerous tiny miliary or submiliary nodules studding both lungs.

The shadows in the lungs of patients with leukemia are almost always due to complicating conditions and not to the leukemia itself. The leukemic patient is especially prone to pulmonary infections, particularly when treated with chemotherapeutic agents which tend to suppress the immune mechanisms. Hemorrhagic and necrotizing pneumonias are common in acute leukemia, while in chronic leukemia there is a tendency for recurrent episodes of pneumonia which produce patchy areas of consolidation in different parts of the lungs. These may persist over a period of several weeks despite antibiotic treatment. In such instances, it is easy to misinterpret the inflammatory lesions as true leukemic infiltrations. Fungous infections of the lung occur occasionally in leukemic patients who are treated with steroids, and bizarre necrotizing pneumonias occur in patients treated with antimetabolites. Pulmonary infarction is also common and may be mistaken for leukemic infiltration.

Kaposi's Sarcoma. Originally described as a hemorrhagic, pigmented sarcoma of the skin containing vascular elements, and noted particularly over the lower extremities, Kaposi's sarcoma is now considered to be a more generalized disease which may involve almost any organ in the body. Visceral lesions may precede those in the skin. Their distribution suggests a multicentric origin rather than metastasis from a single focus.

Some of the pulmonary lesions have been described as nodular on pathologic examination. However, in the four cases that we have observed, they appeared as irregular infiltrative lesions, characterized radiologically by poorly defined densities suggesting patches of pneumonia with interstitial fibrosis.

DISEASES OF THE MEDIASTINUM

Conventionally, the mediastinum has been defined as the space between the pleural cavities. However, the posterior border of this space corresponds to the anterior border of the bodies of

the thoracic vertebrae. The space between the pleural cavities posterior to this boundary is occupied by the spine and adjacent structures, and properly belongs to the chest wall. From the

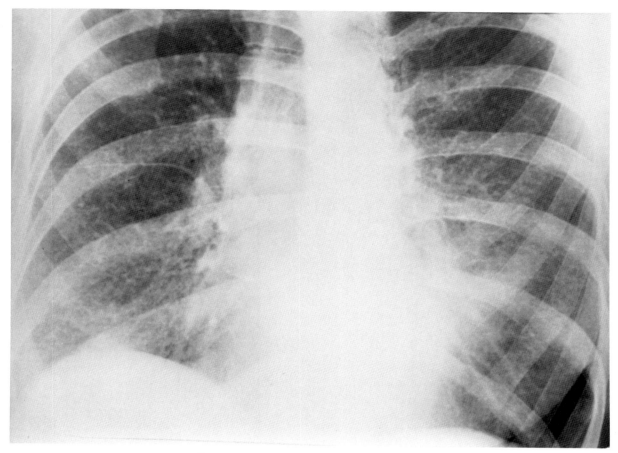

FIG. 438. LYMPHOSARCOMA: MILIARY FORM

A 62 year old female who had a small bowel resection for lymphosarcoma a few years previously, now presented with numerous miliary nodules throughout the lungs. The biopsy showed small-cell lymphosarcoma.

standpoint of the anatomist the lower two-thirds of the mediastinum is divided into an anterior, middle and posterior portion, while the upper third or superior mediastinum is not divided into compartments. From the standpoint of radiologic diagnosis, however, it is most helpful to divide the superior mediastinum into an anterior, middle and posterior portion as well. The anterior portion corresponds to the region in front of the trachea. The middle portion includes the trachea and paratracheal region, and the posterior portion extends from here to the anterior borders of the vertebrae.

The mediastinum is a region of considerable complexity because of the number of different structures which it contains. However, as a whole, this part of the chest presents itself favorably for roentgen examination since it is clearly outlined by the adjacent air-containing lungs and because many of its component structures can be well delineated on conventional films or by special roentgen techniques.

The trachea is outlined by the radiolucent air within it, demarcating it from the surrounding solid structures. The esophagus can be sharply delineated by the ingestion of radiopaque material. Both the ascending and descending aorta form parts of the mediastinal border and therefore can be brought into outline against the adjacent lung by examination in appropriate positions. Moreover, the pulsations of the aorta help to identify it. When the intrinsic pulsations of the vessels in the mediastinum cannot be recognized on fluoroscopy, angiography can be utilized to determine decisively whether an obscure mediastinal shadow is of vascular origin. The lymph nodes of the mediastinum are usually not recognizable under normal circumstances, but when enlarged they may appear as lobulated shadows projecting into the pulmonary fields. Tomography is helpful in the study of some mediastinal lesions, particularly for the disclosure of their position on the lateral view and for the delineation of their borders. Transverse tomography may be especially helpful in this regard. Finally, gas introduced into the mediastinum can outline the tissue planes to disclose the anatomic relationship between an abnormal shadow and the various mediastinal organs.

From the position of the lesion in the mediastinum and the characteristics of its roentgen shadow, it is often possible to make a precise diagnosis of the underlying disease. In the exposition of the diseases that affect the mediastinum, it is best to consider the mediastinal structures separately; first, the diseases which involve the connective tissues that hold the organs of the mediastinum together, and then the diseases of the individual organs.

Mediastinal Tissues

Mediastinal Emphysema. Air can enter the mediastinum from a perforation or rupture of the esophagus, trachea or a bronchus, or from the dissection of air into the mediastinum from interstitial emphysema of the lungs (Fig. 356). The latter is due to rupture of alveoli either as the result of obstructive emphysema or trauma to the chest. Interstitial emphysema is particularly common following assisted respiration at the time of birth and in conditions that cause respiratory distress of the newborn. In older infants and in young children it occurs most frequently as a complication of croup, acute tracheobronchitis or asthma.

Air rarely extends into the mediastinum from a lesion in the chest wall but can be easily sucked in from a wound at the root of the neck. This occurs particularly during the course of a tracheostomy for laryngeal obstruction associated with forced respiratory mevements (Fig. 547). These increase the negative pressure in the thorax so that air is drawn in through the incision. Mediastinal emphysema occurs frequently after diagnostic retroperitoneal air insufflation and following sympathectomy and other operations during which the mediastinal space is opened. Finally, it may be related to the induction of a pneumoperitoneum. During this procedure, air may be introduced inadvertently into the properitoneal tissues or it may enter this plane by seepage through the needle tract from the peritoneal cavity. The air in the properitoneal region courses upward deep to the abdominal muscles and between the diaphragm and the parietal peritoneum which covers its undersurface. From here, it may enter the mediastinum through one of the natural openings in the diaphragm.

Roentgenologically, the condition is manifested by vertical streaks of radiolucency just within the lateral borders of the mediastinal shadow. The parietal pleura is peeled off from the mediastinal structures and is seen as a fine linear shadow, parallel to and separated from the heart and mediastinum by the band of translucent air (Fig. 439). This is best seen on the left side. The line is often faint and easily overlooked. However, when identified, it is a certain sign of mediastinal emphysema. Unless the underlying lesion continues to leak air into the mediastinum, the lucent shadow disappears within a week to 10 days. During this time, there is sufficient absorption of the air to allow reapposition of the parietal pleura.

Air in the mediastinum dissects along the tissue planes and may outline the component structures. The thymus is displaced laterally and upward. This is most striking in the newborn and in young infants because the thymus is large and the collection of air in the mediastinum is relatively great. In the frontal projection, the lobes of the thymus are separated from the cardiac shadow by a zone of lucency. The collection of air in the mediastinum may be unilateral and displace only one lobe of the thymus. When the thymic lobe is widely displaced, it may have a crescentic shape which has been likened by Moseley to that of a windblown spinnaker sail (Fig. 440). In some cases, displacement of the thymus is so great that its lateral border reaches the chest wall. The appearance may then be confused with consolidation or collapse of the upper lobe (see Fig. 481).

Extension of the air through the mediastinum results in mottled areas of increased illumination at the root of the neck and, eventually, in the parietes of the chest, sometimes reaching as far as the abdominal wall. Often the air appears in the form of streaks outlining the muscular and fascial planes (see Fig. 496). The subcutaneous emphysema in the neck may be extensive and produce a striking roentgen picture, while the mediastinal emphysema which precedes it is slight and easily overlooked. Occasionally, the air dissects downward along the aorta and esophagus, through their respective openings in the diaphragm, to enter the retroperitoneal space.

Although the collection of air in the mediastinum appears to be relatively greater in infants, extension into the neck and subcutaneous tissues is considerably less marked than in older children and adults. Pneumothorax secondary to mediastinal emphysema is much more common in the infant. The rupture of the mediastinal air vesicles into the pleura is probably due, in part, to the inability of the mediastinum to decompress itself

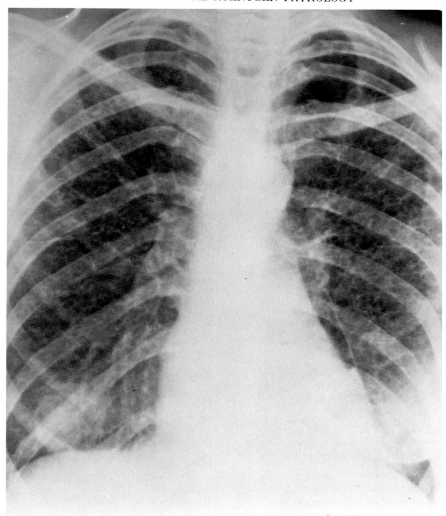

FIG. 439. HISTIOCYTOSIS X: PNEUMOMEDIASTINUM

Both lungs show evidence of diffuse, fine interstitial fibrosis with microcystic changes. The thin, linear density paralleling the left cardiac border represents the parietal pleura which has been dissected off the heart by air in the mediastinum. The poorly demarcated shadow above the right diaphragm is caused by the breast which was displaced mesially when the patient was positioned against the cassette.

because it is difficult for the air to dissect into the fascial planes of the neck.

The streak-like areas of radiolucency produced by air in the mediastinum are sometimes more clearly seen in the lateral and oblique views. In these, the borders of the heart, aorta, and thymus appear more sharply outlined than on the conventional frontal projection (Fig. 24). Air surrounding the thymus gland is a pathognomonic sign of mediastinal emphysema. This is best seen on an across-the-table lateral view with the patient supine. The air appears as a zone of lucency separating the thymus from the sternum and pericardium. This sign may be present even when there is no evidence of air in the mediastinum on the frontal projection. It is seen especially in infants. In adults, the thymus is usually atrophic and cannot be identified so that a pneumomediastinum produces only an increase in the depth and lucency of the retrosternal space.

Mediastinal Hematoma. Trauma is the most common cause of hematoma of the mediastinum. The hematoma can result from a blow or crushing injury as well as from a penetrating wound of the chest. It can follow a laceration of a large blood vessel at the root of the neck, the blood

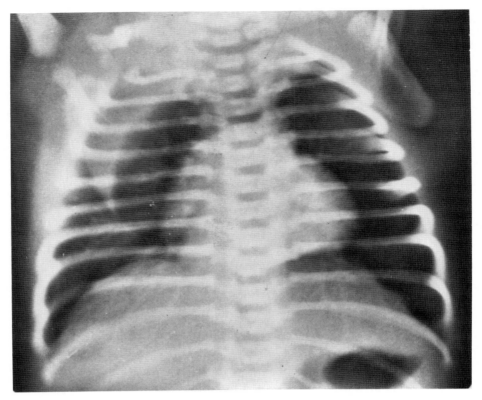

FIG. 440. THYMUS IN PNEUMOMEDIASTINUM

Newborn with respiratory distress. The crescentic density over the outer part of the right lung, which resembles a spinnaker sail, represents the right lobe of the thymus which has been displaced by a large collection of air in the mediastinum. This appearance is pathognomonic for pneumomediastinum. (Courtesy of Dr. J. E. Moseley.)

being drawn downward into the loose areolar tissue of the mediastinum by the negative pressure in the thorax. A hematoma of the mediastinum can also occur spontaneously, particularly from rupture of a dissecting aneurysm of the aorta.

In most cases, the blood collects in the anterior portion of the upper mediastinum. It causes widening of the superior mediastinal shadow, generally on both sides (Fig. 441). Even when the hematoma is quite large, the borders of the mediastinum usually appear straight. The shadow is sharply demarcated by the mediastinal pleura which is displaced laterally. When the hematoma is small, the mediastinal widening may be minimal and the only appreciable change is simply an obliteration of the normal mediastinal contours. Occasionally the hematoma produces a rounded bulging of the mediastinal borders. Rarely the bulge is unilateral, and if it is situated in the lower mediastinum, it may appear to be associated with the heart (Fig. 442). In any of these instances the hematoma may rupture into the pleura to produce a hemothorax.

Postoperative hematomas of the mediastinum frequently occur after removal of a substernal thyroid through the neck, as well as after mediastinotomy through a sternal-splitting incision. The shadow caused by the hematoma may be quite similar to that of a mediastinal tumor (see Fig. 493). This problem does not arise after an operation on the mediastinum through an ordinary thoracotomy incision because the blood drains into the pleural space and does not collect in the mediastinum.

Inflammation of the Mediastinum. Mediastinitis, whether acute or chronic, results from disease of an organ within the mediastinum or spread from an infection of one of the neighboring structures. The roentgen appearance is variable. In many cases there is nothing specific to differentiate this condition roentgenologically from other mediastinal lesions. On the other hand, characteristic changes may be observed from which a definite diagnosis can be established from the roentgen examination alone.

ACUTE MEDIASTINITIS. Acute mediastinitis occurs in three forms: (1) mediastinal lymphad-

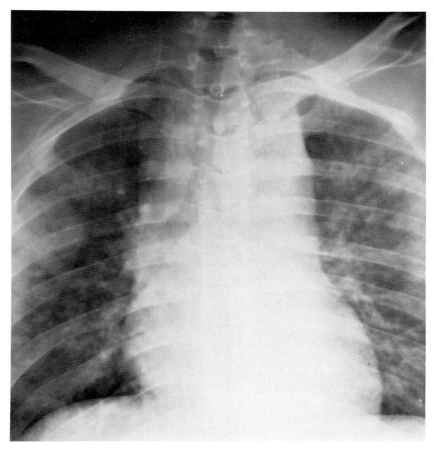

FIG. 441. MEDIASTINAL HEMATOMA

A supine film made shortly after an automobile accident shows the mediastinum to be markedly widened. Its borders are relatively straight and demarcated. This appearance following trauma to the chest strongly suggests a hematoma of the mediastinum. Angiography revealed a rupture of the proximal portion of the descending aorta. The mottled shadows in both pulmonary fields and the confluent areas in the axillary regions are due to contusions of the lung.

enitis, (2) phlegmonous mediastinitis and (3) mediastinal abscess.

Mediastinal lymphadenitis is generally secondary to disease in the lungs or bronchi, but is sometimes the result of severe pharyngeal infection which extends downward into the posterior mediastinum. The lymph nodes are usually not large enough to be discernible on the roentgen film. However, on occasion, they cause a widened mediastinal shadow with lobulated borders. Large paratracheal nodes may appear as discrete, bulging shadows on the right border of the mediastinum. At times, the shadows of enlarged tracheobronchial lymph nodes are seen near the roots of the lungs. When there is a large mass of agglutinated, suppurating lymph nodes, the roentgen picture may be undifferentiable from that of an abscess of the superior mediastinum. However, in most cases, the convex outlines of the individual nodes produce a scalloped or lob-

ulated border which does not occur in mediastinal abscess. Lymph nodes in the lower mediastinum are not visible on the frontal film, although it is possible to visualize them in the oblique view.

Phlegmonous mediastinitis results either from downward extension of a cervical phlegmon or from perforation of the esophagus. It also occurs from perforation of the trachea. In certain fulminating cases there may be no visible widening of the mediastinum, and the only roentgen change is referable to an accompanying lymphangitis of the lungs. This may spread to the pleura and cause a bilateral effusion.

In most cases, however, phlegmonous mediastinitis results in a diffuse widening of the superior mediastinal shadow. The outlines of the structures that make up the normal contour of the mediastinum are obscured, and the widened mediastinum is bounded by straight vertical bor-

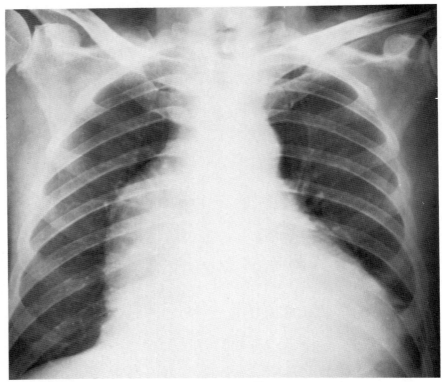

FIG. 442. MEDIASTINAL HEMATOMA

The bulge on the right side of the mediastinum appeared after operation for aortic stenosis. It involves the lower two-thirds of the mediastinum. Its border is sharply demarcated and, for the most part, is straight and vertical. The shadow extends too high to be caused by the heart and too low for the aorta. Angiography disclosed the aorta to be displaced to the left. The right atrium was compressed. Thoracotomy revealed a large hematoma of the mediastinum arising from a small leak at the suture line in the aorta.

ders. Superiorly, the shadow of the widened mediastinum appears to spread out over the apex of the lungs. Lateral views of the neck usually show widening of the retrotracheal space, often extending to the retropharyngeal region where the infection commonly originates (Fig. 46).

Abscesses of the mediastinum usually result from downward extension of an abscess in the neck or from perforation of the esophagus. Rarely the abscess is caused by perforation of the trachea or from direct extension of an abscess in the lung, osteomyelitis of the spine, or upward extension of a retroperitoneal abscess.

In the early stage of an abscess of the upper mediastinum, the roentgen picture is indistinguishable from that of phlegmonous mediastinitis, but rapid widening of the shadow and the formation of a bulging border indicate an abscess. In our experience, widening of the superior mediastinal shadow in association with an abscess in the neck has always proved to be due to an abscess of the mediastinum rather than to diffuse mediastinitis. The cervical abscess extends

downward through the superior aperture of the thorax along the fascial plane in front of the vertebral bodies, displacing the esophagus and trachea forward. As a rule, the posterior mediastinal space becomes sealed off at the level of the tracheal bifurcation, limiting further downward spread. However, in unusual instances, the abscess can reach the diaphragm. In fact, we have observed it to extend into the retroperitoneal region, and in one instance, to present as a bulging mass below the costovertebral angle.

An upper mediastinal abscess usually bulges toward the right. Protrusion of the abscess to the left is usually limited by the aortic arch, and the left border of the abscess is hidden within the shadow of the mediastinum (Fig. 443). On occasion, however, the abscess bulges from both sides of the mediastinum.

Since mediastinal abscesses are usually due to perforation of the esophagus or descent of an infection from the prevertebral space in the neck, the abscess is practically always situated in the posterior mediastinum. In the unusual case of

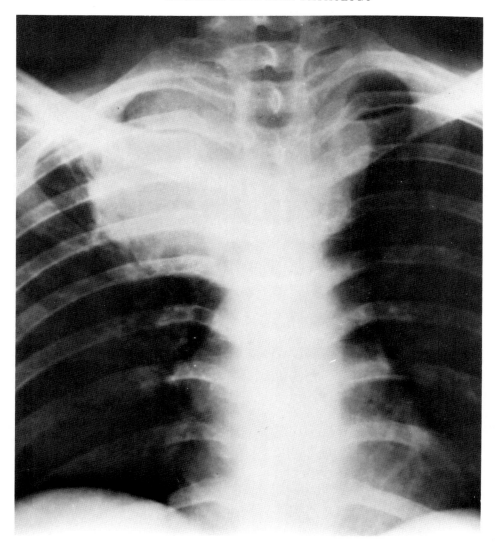

FIG. 443. MEDIASTINAL ABSCESS

There is a large shadow projecting from both sides of the superior mediastinum. The patient had an acute pharyngitis complicated by suppuration in the neck. The association of the mediastinal shadow with cervical suppuration is indicative of mediastinal abscess. As usual, this was situated posteriorly. It was cured by drainage through a posterior mediastinotomy.

perforation of a lung abscess into the mediastinum, the mediastinal infection can be situated more anteriorly. However, we have seen only a single case of such an abscess in the anterior mediastinum.

Most frequently the tissues of the neck are also involved, either because they were the site of the original infection, or because an abscess of the mediastinum extended upward. Anterior displacement of the trachea is clearly demonstrable on lateral views of the neck, which disclose a widening of the prevertebral space (Fig. 46). In questionable cases the diagnosis of mediastinitis may depend largely upon the demonstration of

widening of this space at the level of the lower cervical spine. In such instances lateral views of the neck should be made daily until the diagnosis is clarified.

An abscess of the lower mediastinum is almost always due to perforation or spontaneous rupture of the esophagus or, more rarely, to perforation of an adjacent lung abscess. In either case, the mediastinal abscess often shows a fluid level. When a fluid level is present in the lower part of the mediastinum, it is difficult to differentiate between an abscess and a hiatus hernia without a barium swallow. However, a mediastinal abscess in this location is usually associated with evidence of pleural reaction. In the absence of a fluid level, the abscess cannot be differentiated from a paramediastinal effusion unless it extends to both sides.

As a rule, when a mediastinal abscess follows perforation of the esophagus, there is evidence of air in the mediastinum or at the root of the neck. The mediastinal emphysema may be manifested on the frontal projection by separation of the parietal pleura from the underlying structures by air and, on the lateral view, by vertical lucent streaks in the posterior mediastinum. Occasionally a fluid level is present at the root of the neck, but most frequently the air appears in the form of one or more globules of lucency within the widened retrotracheal space.

An abscess confined to the mediastinum itself rarely shows a fluid level. A fluid level may be present once the abscess perforates into the lung. The abscess then is situated partly in the mediastinum and partly within the lung. The fluid level crosses the mediastinum and usually ex-

tends beyond the border of the translucent trachea (Fig. 444). An abscess of the lung whose fluid level crosses the trachea must be considered to involve the mediastinum and generally originates in the latter region. It is to be differentiated from a pyopneumothorax. The latter may displace the mediastinum toward the opposite side and may suggest widening of the mediastinal shadow, but the fluid level does not extend beyond the tracheal border (see Fig. 546). A Zenker's diverticulum can exhibit a fluid level in the upper mediastinum, and a barium swallow may be required to differentiate it from a mediastinal abscess. A perforated bronchogenic or paratracheal cyst can also produce a fluid level in the mediastinum. However, in a partially emptied paratracheal cyst the fluid level does not extend entirely across the trachea. The bronchogenic cyst that is confined to the mediastinum is situated immediately beneath the tracheal bifurcation. This is an exceedingly rare location for a mediastinal abscess.

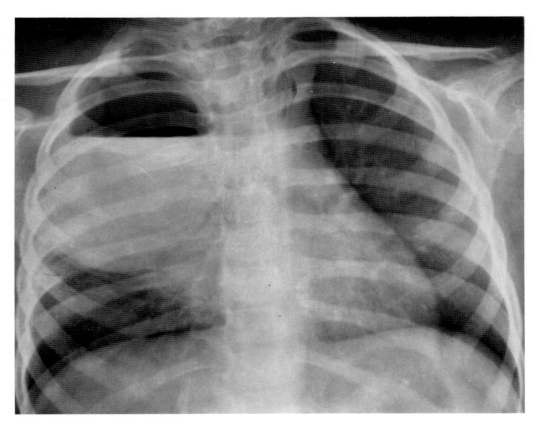

FIG. 444. MEDIASTINAL ABSCESS: PERFORATION INTO THE LUNG

There is a large abscess in the upper part of the right lung. However, the air-fluid level crosses the shadow of the trachea, which is not displaced. This indicates that the abscess involves the mediastinum. The fluid level of an abscess confined to the lung does not extend beyond the border of the mediastinum. A large pyopneumothorax can extend beyond the midline but it displaces the mediastinum so that the fluid level does not cross the trachea (see Fig. 546).

Perforation of a mediastinal abscess into the pleura results in a pyopneumothorax or an empyema which can become chronic. The cause of the pleural infection may not be suspected unless review of the clinical history, or films made early in the disease, disclose evidence of mediastinitis. A persistent sinus may follow drainage of the empyema because of the underlying infection in the mediastinum. In such instances, radiopaque material injected into the sinus tract will enter the mediastinum and usually ascend and descend within it (Fig. 27). In two of our cases, the injected lipiodol ascended in the prevertebral space to reach the base of the skull. The mediastinitis that caused the empyema in these instances undoubtedly originated from an infection in the nasopharynx.

MEDIASTINAL ADHESIONS. Adhesions between the mediastinal pleura and the visceral pleura over the mesial surface of the lung, and between the mediastinal pleura and the parietal pleura lining the anterior chest wall may result from acute or chronic inflammation of the mediastinum. However, far more commonly they are due to the pleuritis associated with infections of the lung or radiotherapy.

The borders of the mediastinum appear extremely sharp on the frontal projection because the adhesions obliterate the narrow pleural space in front of the upper mediastinum. The adhesions also cause an ironing out of the contours of the mediastinum, blunting of the cardiophrenic angle and thickening of the pleura over the mesial portion of the apices of the lungs (Fig. 75).

CHRONIC MEDIASTINITIS. Chronic mediastinitis may be divided into three types: first, a granulomatous form; second, a relatively localized fibrotic form; and third, diffuse fibrous mediastinitis.

The *granulomatous form* of chronic mediastinitis occurs principally in histoplasmosis and tuberculosis. It results from spread of infection into the mediastinal tissues from lymph nodes which have undergone caseous necrosis or abscess formation. The disease may be limited to the connective tissues about the involved nodes, but often extends to affect adjacent structures.

When the infection originates in the paratracheal or tracheobronchial lymph nodes on the right side, the superior vena cava may become obstructed. When the subcarinal nodes are involved, they may indent the anterior wall of the esophagus. Perforation of one of these nodes into the esophagus results in the formation of a so-called traction diverticulum. If the granulomatous disease extends about the entire circumference of the esophagus it can produce a stricture. Spread of the disease into the walls of the large bronchi in the mediastinum can result in bronchostenosis. Significant involvement of the trachea is rare. However, in children, a tuberculous lymph node can perforate into the trachea and cause obstruction. In adults, luetic tracheal stenosis may result from extension of the infection from a gumma of the adjacent lymph nodes.

Granulomatous mediastinitis occasionally occurs in certain mycotic diseases, such as actinomycosis, nocardiosis, blastomycosis and mucormycosis. In these diseases, the infection extends directly from the lung into the mediastinum without intermediate involvement of the lymph nodes.

The more limited form of granulomatous mediastinitis can produce a local widening of the mediastinal shadow. This is most frequently seen on the frontal view as a bulge in the right paratracheal region, usually associated with clouding of the retrosternal space. The lesion consists of a mass of granulomatous and fibrous tissue together with inflamed lymph nodes. A similar mass in the subcarinal region is more easily detected in the lateral or oblique projections. Here it is seen to encroach upon the posterior mediastinal space, and it may impinge on the anterior border of the esophagus. On the frontal view the subcarinal mass may be represented only by a local increase in the density of the upper portion of the cardiac shadow. When large, it can displace both main bronchi upward and outward, widening the angle of the tracheal bifurcation. However, the mass is not so clearly outlined as in the other views.

When necrosis and caseation take place within the mass, as in histoplasmosis or tuberculosis, calcification frequently occurs. The calcific foci often appear as poorly demarcated, irregular flecks which can best be recognized on Bucky films and tomograms. As the calcification becomes more extensive, large, well-defined densities are readily visualized.

The *localized fibrous form* of mediastinitis without distinct granulomas probably represents a late stage of the granulomatous form of the disease. Most cases are due to histoplasmosis or tuberculosis, but in some there is no indication of either disease and the etiology remains obscure. The latter are similar, in some respects, to idiopathic retroperitoneal fibrosis. As in granulomatous mediastinitis, this form may be complicated by superior vena caval obstruction and esophageal deformity and stricture. Instances of encasement and narrowing of the pulmonary arteries or veins by dense fibrous tissue have been described. There may be a concomitant constrictive pericarditis.

Normally, there is only loose areolar tissue

between the arch of the aorta and the trachea at the point where the aorta crosses over the left main bronchus. This permits independent movement of the two structures. In fibrous mediastinitis, however, they may be bound together. The aortic arch, then, will rise together with the trachea during the act of swallowing. This *aortic swallowing sign* also occurs in neoplastic disease or any other condition producing adhesions between the aortic arch and trachea (p. 56).

The least pronounced roentgen changes in chronic mediastinitis occur in the *diffuse fibrotic form*. The shadow of the mediastinum simply becomes dense, the borders become sharply outlined and the normal indentations are blunted. When the disease is more extensive, the superior mediastinum is widened and its borders are straightened. Frequently the cardiophrenic angles are obliterated.

Adhesive and constrictive pericarditis may be associated with this form of mediastinitis. It may be the result of tuberculosis or histoplasmosis of the subcarinal lymph nodes, but in most cases the etiology remains unknown. Calcification of the pericardium is common in association with constrictive pericarditis.

Frequently the roentgen picture is dominated by involvement of one of the mediastinal organs. Especially common is obstruction of the superior vena cava. This contributes to the widening of the superior mediastinal shadow, particularly on the right side. When the obstruction is below the entrance of the azygos vein, this vessel becomes the main collateral channel and may dilate sufficiently to produce a local bulge at the right tracheobronchial angle.

Bronchial stricture is a fairly common complication of mediastinitis caused by tuberculosis or histoplasmosis, and the roentgen picture may be due entirely to the effects of bronchial obstruction. An inflammatory stricture of the esophagus, confined to the level of the tracheal bifurcation, is usually the result of chronic mediastinitis secondary to infection of the subcarinal nodes.

In rare cases, chronic mediastinitis causes narrowing of the pulmonary arteries or veins. Obstruction of the pulmonary artery may be evidenced by diminished vascularity of the affected lung and by enlargement of the right side of the heart. Narrowing of the pulmonary veins results in congestion of the portions of the lung which they drain.

A *chronic abscess* of the mediastinum can result from an infection of the mediastinal lymph nodes or spine, a poorly drained acute mediastinal abscess, or a bronchial or esophageal fistula. Chronic abscesses originating in the spine or lymph nodes are almost always tuberculous. Bronchial fistulas generally occur as a complication of resective pulmonary surgery.

A chronic mediastinal abscess usually cannot be differentiated from the localized granulomatous or fibrous form of mediastinitis unless there is a bronchial or esophageal communication. A fluid level in the mediastinum, or demonstration of an esophageal communication proves the presence of an abscess. Obviously, the esophageal communication exists from the very beginning when the abscess results from rupture of the esophagus. However, a communication can form secondarily when a mediastinal abscess, due to some other cause, ruptures into the esophagus.

When the abscess is secondary to infection of a vertebra, the shadow usually bulges on both sides of the mediastinum. Evidence of the underlying bony disease is practically always visible on x-ray films of the spine (Fig. 155).

Mediastinal Cysts. A cyst of the mediastinum generally appears on the roentgen film as a sharply demarcated round or oval density. It can be situated anywhere in the mediastinum, depending upon its point of origin. With the exception of the Echinococcus cyst, pancreatic pseudocysts which extend into the thorax from the abdomen, cysts of the thyroid and some cystic lesions of the thymus, they are congenital in origin. The last two lesions will be considered in the sections on thyroid and thymus.

BRONCHOGENIC CYSTS. The bronchogenic cyst develops from an anomalous bronchial bud and usually does not communicate with the bronchial tree. The cysts that develop from the main bronchi and trachea are situated in the mediastinum. The ones that develop from the smaller bronchi are situated in the pulmonary field and are discussed under the heading, Anomalies of the Lung (see p. 267). The cyst is usually lined with ciliated epithelium and contains mucoid secretion. Smooth muscle, fragments of cartilage, and mucous glands may be found within its wall. In some cases, the cyst communicates with the bronchial tree, usually as a result of perforation following infection.

Most of the cysts bulge outward from the mediastinum into the pulmonary field. However, those which arise from the medial wall of the main bronchus are situated in the subcarinal region and may be completely buried within the mediastinum. The cyst which projects into the pulmonary field appears on the frontal projection as a homogeneous, semicircular density with a sharply outlined, smooth outer border (Fig. 220). The inner border of the mass merges with the shadow of the mediastinum. It may be situated anywhere between the thoracic inlet and lower portion of the lung root.

The *paratracheal cyst* is identical with the bronchogenic cyst except that it arises from the trachea. It is situated in the uppermost part of the mediastinum and cannot be differentiated radiologically from a noncalcified substernal or intrathoracic thyroid (Fig. 445). Like the thyroid, the paratracheal cyst rises on swallowing because of its attachment to the trachea. When it is located in the thoracic inlet, it displaces the trachea and esophagus to the opposite side. When it is completely within the thorax, these structures maintain their normal positions.

The bronchogenic cyst that is situated at the hilum, lies in the middle mediastinum and, therefore, overlies the trachea and main bronchus on the lateral projection (Fig. 220). In this view the cyst appears as a homogeneous, well-defined, oval or circular density with a smooth, regular border which differentiates it from a mass of large hilar nodes or a bronchogenic carcinoma.

A *subcarinal cyst* tends to splay the tracheal bifurcation, elevating both main bronchi (Fig. 446). When the cyst is moderate in size, it may be completely hidden by the heart in the frontal projection. However, it causes an increase in the density of the upper portion of the cardiac shadow. Obscuration of the intervertebral spaces beneath the tracheal bifurcation, on an adequately exposed film, indicates the presence of a subcarinal mass. When the subcarinal cyst is larger, it may project beyond the right cardiac border. In either case, the cyst bulges into the

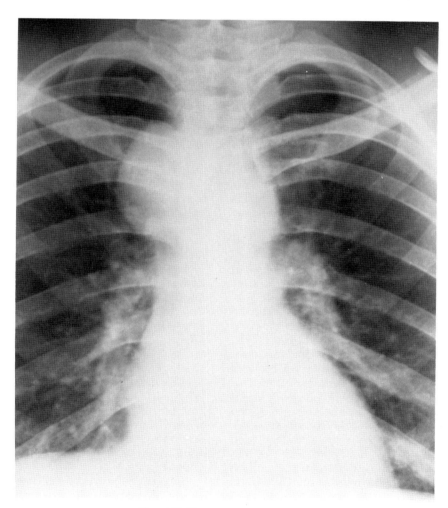

FIG. 445. PARATRACHEAL CYST

The mass in the right paratracheal region was found on a routine x-ray examination. At mediastinoscopy, the mass appeared flaccid and opalescent. Aspiration yielded 90 cc of clear, colorless fluid. The cyst was removed through the mediastinoscopy incision.

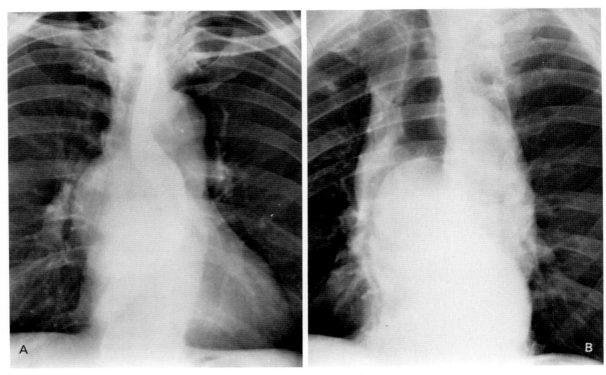

FIG. 446. BRONCHOGENIC CYST

A: Frontal projection. A sharply outlined, round mass projects from the right side of the mediastinum and displaces the esophagus to the left. *B:* The mass is situated in the subcarinal region and splays the main bronchi.

posterior mediastinum and indents the anterior wall of the esophagus, simulating an enlarged left atrium. A large cyst can displace the esophagus laterally, like a paraesophageal cyst.

Occasionally, a mediastinal bronchogenic cyst exhibits an air-fluid level, indicating communication with the airway (Fig. 447). Such a cyst is invariably infected, and its smooth outline may be obscured, making differentiation from a mediastinal abscess difficult. However, a fluid level localized to the subcarinal region usually signifies the presence of an infected bronchogenic cyst.

The cysts usually remain stationary in size for a long period, but may enlarge slowly. They can exert sufficient pressure on a bronchus to narrow its lumen, especially in the presence of bronchomalacia. This may result in atelectasis which obscures the cyst, or in obstructive emphysema. Gross calcification of the cyst wall has been described pathologically, but apparently the deposition of calcium is not sufficient for recognition on the roentgen films. However, calcium salts may be precipitated within the fluid content of the cyst and settle at its base. The resulting interface between the cyst fluid and the precipitated calcium salts remains horizontal when the patient is tilted, and thus simulates an air-fluid level.

ENTEROGENOUS CYSTS. Enterogenous cysts of the mediastinum, also known as paraesophageal, gastroenteric or duplication cysts, originate as evaginations of the primitive foregut. They are lined by mucous membrane which contains elements similar to that of the esophagus, stomach or intestine and are usually filled with mucoid material. When the cyst wall contains functioning gastric mucosa, acid may be secreted into the cyst and cause ulceration. This can lead to perforation into the esophagus, trachea, lung or pleura.

The majority of the cysts are discovered during the first year of life because of symptoms due to rapid enlargement or perforation. In infants the large cysts occupy so much space in the hemithorax that they often compress the esophagus, trachea or a bronchus to produce dysphagia or respiratory distress. In the adult the cysts are usually asymptomatic and are discovered incidentally.

Enterogenous cysts lie in the posterior mediastinum adjacent to the esophagus, mostly along its middle third. The great majority project into the right pulmonary field, probably because the descending aorta limits their extension to the left. The cysts are generally oval in shape with their long axis in a vertical direction. On the

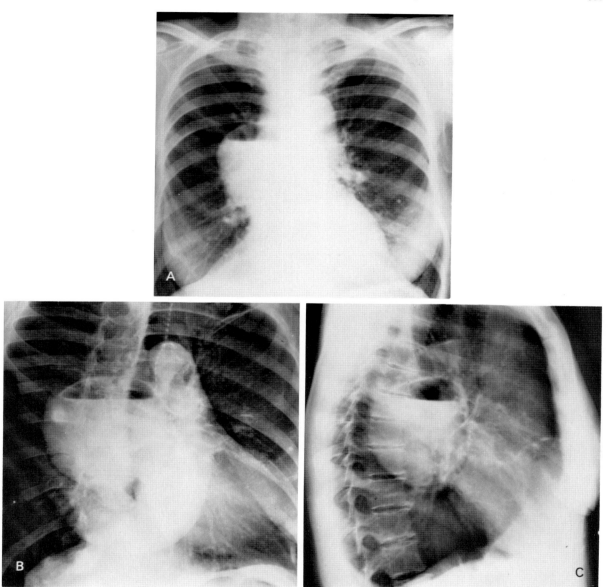

FIG. 447. BRONCHOGENIC CYST

A: The frontal view shows a large cystic structure at the root of the right lung. The fluid level extends over the right part of the mediastinum. *B:* Right oblique view. The cyst is circular in shape and extremely well circumscribed. Its wall, which is visible above the fluid level, is thin and smooth. The tracheal cartilages are calcified. *C:* The lateral view shows the mass to extend from the middle to the posterior mediastinum. At operation this was found to be a bronchogenic cyst which communicated with the right main bronchus. Although the cyst was infected, there was little inflammatory reaction about it. (Courtesy of Dr. I. A. Sarot, New York, N. Y.)

frontal projection the mesial border is hidden by the mediastinal structures, while laterally the cyst is bounded by a sharply outlined, smooth, semielliptical border (Fig. 448). On the lateral view the entire circumference of the cyst is usually visible. In this projection it overlies the esophagus. When large, it extends posteriorly to

overlap the vertebral bodies. Erosion of a vertebra is rare.

The cyst regularly causes an indentation on the lateral wall of the esophagus and sometimes displaces it to the opposite side. Occasionally the esophagus is displaced forward as well. Barium studies of the esophagus show the indentation

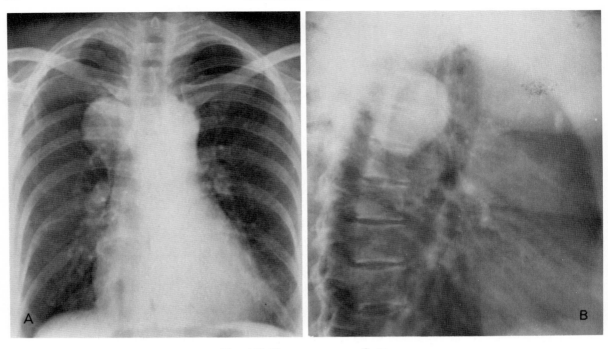

FIG. 448. PARAESOPHAGEAL CYST

A: The sharply outlined, round mass in the right side of the superior mediastinum proved to be a paraesophageal cyst. The congenital origin of the lesion is suggested by the anomalies of the posterior portions of the third and fourth ribs on that side. *B:* The lateral view shows the characteristic location over the posterior mediastinum. The mass is separated from the posterior chest wall, where neurofibromas occur, and does not extend to the middle mediastinum, where intrathoracic goiters and bronchogenic or tracheal cysts are found.

produced by the cyst to be smooth and elongated, tapering gradually at its upper and lower borders. In rare cases the cyst lies within the wall of the esophagus. The indentation is then more acute and identical with that produced by an intramural neoplasm of the esophagus (Fig. 449).

The intact cyst casts a homogeneous shadow. Although calcification of the wall can occasionally be demonstrated pathologically, it is not visible on roentgen films. Rupture of the cyst occurs particularly in infants, most commonly into the esophagus. An air-fluid level then becomes evident unless the cyst empties completely, in which case an annular shadow is seen. An esophageal communication can be demonstrated only after rupture of the cyst. Similarly, bronchography may disclose a communication with the airway when the cyst ruptures into the trachea or a bronchus. Rupture into the pleura results in a pleural effusion, and the emptied cyst cannot be seen.

The differentiation between an enterogenous cyst and a bronchogenic cyst of the mediastinum is generally made by observing the position of the cyst on the lateral view. The enterogenous cyst is situated more posteriorly. Splaying of the tracheal bifurcation, seen with a subcarinal bronchogenic cyst, is not associated with an enterogenous cyst. While indentation of the lateral wall of the esophagus is characteristic of the enterogenous cyst, it occasionally occurs in association with a large bronchogenic cyst of the mediastinum.

NEURENTERIC CYSTS. These are similar to the enterogenous cysts in that they are also lined by gastrointestinal mucosa. However, the neurenteric cyst develops at an earlier period in fetal life from the neurenteric canal which connects the primitive foregut with the notochord. Persistence of this canal causes a defect of the vertebral bodies and a deformity of the spine. The anomaly may take the form of a circumscribed tunnel through one vertebral body or it may involve several of the vertebrae, resulting in anterior spina bifida, hemivertebra or other malformations.

The neurenteric cyst lies between the esophagus and the spine, and is usually connected with the meninges by a fibrous cord extending through the defect in the vertebral body. The cyst itself may extend posteriorly as far as the spinal canal.

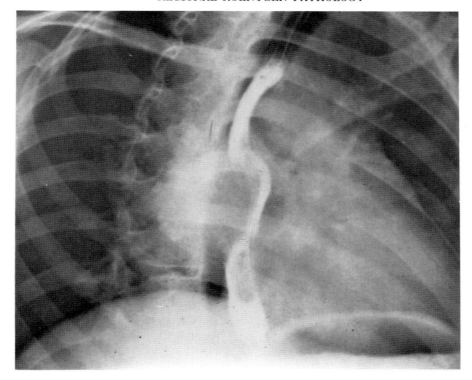

FIG. 449. DUPLICATION CYST OF THE ESOPHAGUS

The right oblique view shows a well-circumscribed mass in the posterior mediastinum, displacing the esophagus anteriorly and to the left. The sharp angulation of the esophagus indicates that the mass is intramural. The paraesophageal cyst was resected.

The roentgen picture is characterized by the association of a mediastinal mass with a deformity of the spine. Most of the cysts are located in the upper part of the mediastinum. They usually project to the right and have a smooth, curved, or lobulated contour. They are of homogeneous density unless there is a persistent communication with the gut, in which case air can be demonstrated within the mass. Since the cyst lies between the esophagus and the spine, it displaces the esophagus forward as well as to one side. Occasionally, the cyst arises in the abdomen and is connected with the small intestine rather than the esophagus, but it may extend upward through the diaphragm into the mediastinum.

Generally, the defects involve the bodies of the upper dorsal or lower cervical vertebrae. Attention is frequently called to the spinal abnormality by an associated scoliosis. However, a neurenteric cyst may be present without an obvious deformity. An x-ray examination of the spine should therefore be made in the case of all posterior mediastinal masses. An intrathoracic meningocele may be associated with similar vertebral anomalies. However, a meningocele can be filled with contrast material during myelography, while a neurenteric cyst does not communicate with the spinal canal.

PERICARDIAL CYSTS. Pericardial cysts are congenital in origin and develop from an abnormal septation of the thoracic portion of the celomic cavity during the formation of the pericardium. They are, therefore, often termed parapericardial celomic cysts. The term, spring-water cyst, has also been used because of the characteristic limpid quality of its fluid content.

Most pericardial cysts are situated in the cardiophrenic angle, more frequently on the right side. About 20% are somewhat higher, at the level of the auricular appendages, but practically never above this level. Although they are congenital, pericardial cysts are rarely seen in children. Frequently they are observed to increase in size over a period of years, and occasionally they may be found in patients whose previous films show no evidence of the lesion. When first recognized, they usually measure 4 to 8 cm in size. Significantly larger ones are rarely encountered.

The cysts at the cardiophrenic angle usually present a quadrantic outline in the frontal projection. In this view, the mesial border merges with the shadow of the heart while the lateral border is smooth, round and sharply demarcated. On the lateral view, the anterior border of the density merges with the shadow of the anterior chest wall. The upper and posterior borders may form a sharply outlined curve extending from the lower portion of the sternum to the diaphragm. More commonly, the cyst is poorly defined on the lateral view and its shadow merges imperceptibly with that of the heart (see Fig. 570).

Some of the cysts are pedunculated and extend outward along the diaphragm. The upper border then appears more flattened and the area of contact between the shadow of the cyst and that of the heart is small. It may be possible to visualize the pedicle by tomography or by examination after the induction of a pneumothorax. A pedunculated pericardial cyst may insinuate itself into the base of the long fissure and is then seen, on the lateral view, as a triangular or pear-shaped shadow with its broad, lower portion extending to the anterior costophrenic sulcus (Fig. 450).

Pericardial cysts situated at a higher level are also more commonly observed on the right side. On the frontal view, a cyst in this location appears as a rounded, sharply demarcated, localized bulge on the lateral border of the cardiac shadow (Fig. 451). If the cyst is large, it may extend to the diaphragm. However, because it is fixed to the heart it does not descend with the diaphragm so that the cardiac contour below the cyst is uncovered during inspiration. This is also well demonstrated in the appropriate oblique view. A high pericardial cyst is usually not well demarcated on the lateral view because its shadow merges gradually with that of the heart. In the rare instance when the cyst arises at the level of the pericardial reflection over the great vessels, its appearance is like that of a mediastinal bronchogenic cyst.

The wall of a pericardial cyst is thin and is easily stretched by the pulsation of the heart. The cyst, therefore, is usually flaccid and may vary in shape with the phase of respiration (Fig. 452) and changes in the position of the patient. The alteration in the contour of the cyst is most evident in the Trendelenburg position. A greater

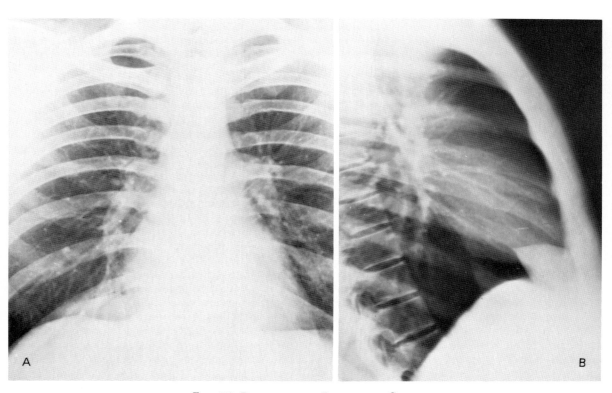

FIG. 450. PEDUNCULATED PERICARDIAL CYST

A: The shadow above the mesial portion of the right leaf of the diaphragm was discovered at a routine examination. Its upper border is flat, smooth and sharply demarcated. The mass obliterates the contiguous portion of the cardiac silhouette but does not obscure the dome of the diaphragm. *B:* In the lateral view, the mass is seen within the base of the long fissure. At operation, it was found to be a flaccid cyst connected to the pericardium by a short, broad pedicle. The cyst had insinuated itself between the middle and lower lobes.

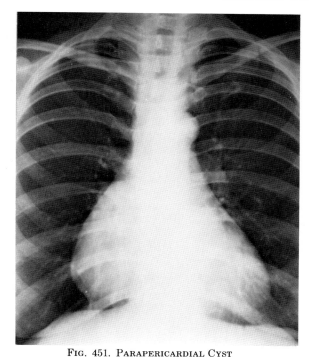

FIG. 451. PARAPERICARDIAL CYST

A large, sharply outlined, pear-shaped mass obliterates the right border of the cardiac silhouette, indicating that it is in contact with the heart. On the lateral view, the shadow of the mass merged imperceptibly with that of the heart. At operation, a flaccid parapericardial cyst was removed. The flattening of the border of the shadow indicates that the cyst is not tense.

change occurs when the cyst is pedunculated than when it is broad-based. Small cysts are more firm and do not vary in shape.

A cyst in the cardiophrenic angle may simulate an epicardial fat pad. However, the latter is more apt to be triangular in shape and is often bilateral. The fat pad is more lucent than a cyst and permits the cardiac border to be visualized through it. A mass of propericardial fat or a propericardial lipoma protruding into the cardiophrenic angle produces a more rounded shadow, but its border is generally not as smooth or as sharply demarcated as that of a cyst.

More difficulty is encountered in differentiating a cyst in this location from a hernia through the foramen of Morgagni. In most instances, the hernia contains only properitoneal fat or omentum. It bulges out from the cardiac silhouette in the right cardiophrenic angle. On the lateral view the hernia fills in the anterior costophrenic sinus and presents a quadrantic border which is frequently absent in a pericardial cyst. An irregularity of the border is indicative of fat herniation. Like a cyst, the hernia may insinuate itself into the long fissure, producing a triangular shadow at its base. In rare instances, a lucency is visible within the shadow, indicating the presence of a portion of the alimentary tract in the hernia, most often a loop of intestine. Barium studies may be required to demonstrate this. Occasionally, a portion of the transverse colon is angu-

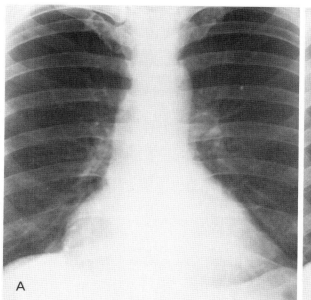
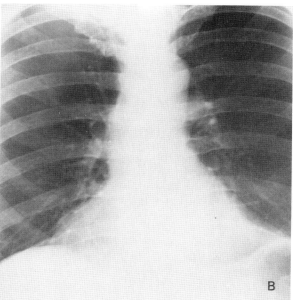

FIG. 452. PERICARDIAL CYST

A: A film in full inspiration shows a sharply defined quadrantic density in the right cardiophrenic angle. The right border of the heart is obliterated. B: With a lesser degree of inspiration, the cardiophrenic mass appears flatter. The change in shape with respiration indicates that the mass is flaccid and contains fluid.

lated upward because of impaction of omentum in the hernia. A communication between the hernia and the peritoneal cavity can usually be demonstrated by induction of a pneumoperitoneum.

The outer border of a cyst situated at a higher level can be mistaken for the border of the heart. However, if the cyst does not extend along the full length of the heart, angles are formed where its shadow meets the cardiac silhouette. The angles at the upper and lower borders of the cyst can frequently be visualized on the ordinary frontal projection but are usually better demonstrated on the oblique view. An aneurysm of the left ventricle can produce a similar sharply delineated bulge on the cardiac contour but it usually exhibits paradoxical pulsations.

A low lying thymic tumor can appear exactly like a pericardial cyst on the frontal film (Fig. 484). However, lobulation of the contour, or calcific deposits within the mass, exclude a pericardial cyst from consideration. Variation of the shape of the mass or change in its position during inspiration make a thymic tumor unlikely. A pericardial cyst can often be recognized by means of ultrasonography.

A loculated pericardial effusion can simulate a pericardial cyst. Its development during a febrile illness or its association with other evidences of pericarditis usually make the diagnosis quite clear. A chronic localized pericardial effusion may be associated with calcification of the pericardium, which is absent in a congenital cyst.

LYMPHANGIOMATOUS CYSTS (CYSTIC HYGROMA). These cysts are the result of a congenital overgrowth of the lymph vessels. Most of them are confined to the neck (hygroma colli). Mediastinal hygromas are rarely confined to the mediastinum and usually involve the neck as well. The cysts are usually single and may be uni- or multilocular. Occasionally they are multiple. Some are localized, extremely well defined, and round or oval in shape. Others, particularly those which are mutlilocular, have an irregular contour and intermingle with the mediastinal structures which they envelop. The cysts are usually quite large when first discovered and may assume massive proportions. Rapid enlargement may result from hemorrhage within the cyst.

Cysts that are confined to the mediastinum are usually not discovered until adult life and often are entirely asymptomatic. Most of them occur in the anterior mediastinum, projecting to one side, generally the right. The borders are well-defined and smooth, although they may be lobulated. A lymphangiomatous cyst which is confined to the mediastinum cannot be differ-

entiated radiologically from a dermoid cyst or a thymic tumor. The presence of calcification within the lesion makes the possibility of a lymphangiomatous cyst most unlikely.

The lymphagiomatous cysts that involve both the neck and mediastinum (cervicomediastinal type) are usually discovered in infancy because of the swelling of the neck. They frequently produce symptoms from pressure on the trachea and esophagus at the thoracic inlet. The shadow is more diffuse than that of the purely mediastinal form. It is most evident in the upper portion of the mediastinum although the lesion may extend down to the diaphragm (Fig. 453). It may present simply as a generalized widening of the mediastinum, but more often there is a localized bulge on one or both borders of the mediastinal shadow. Although the anterior mediastinum is practically always involved, the lesion frequently extends far backward and may reach the posterior border of the chest.

The cervical portion of the cyst frequently causes a bulging of the contours of the neck and obliterates the normal supraclavicular soft tissue planes. Even if a mass cannot be identified in the neck, displacement of the trachea and esophagus indicates the presence of a cervical component. The mediastinal portion of the cyst may become smaller on straining and coughing as some of the fluid is forced into the neck.

The combination of a large mass in the mediastinum and evidence of involvement of the neck in an infant or a young child, is usually indicative of a cervicomediastinal hygroma. In older persons a similar appearance is more frequently caused by Hodgkin's disease, other lymphomas, or a carcinoma of the thyroid or lung with mediastinal invasion.

THORACIC DUCT CYSTS. Cysts of the thoracic duct are extremely rare. They may occur anywhere along its course and may be multiple. The cyst presents itself as a round or oval density with a sharply defined border, adjacent to the esophagus. The roentgen picture is similar to that of a gastroenterogenous cyst. Since the lower two-thirds of the thoracic duct is located in the angle between the esophagus and the bodies of the vertebrae, the cyst is apt to produce an indentation on the posterolateral wall of the barium-filled esophagus. The cyst is generally rather small. Those reported have measured between 3 and 8 cm in their long diameter. On the lateral view, the cyst extends backward from the posterior mediastinum for a short distance over the bodies of the vertebrae. Since the cysts are not large, those situated immediately above the diaphragm may be completely hidden in the

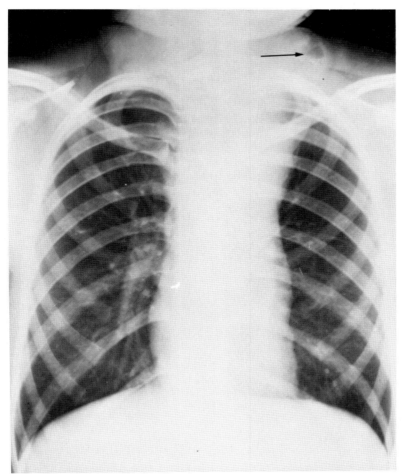

FIG. 453. CERVICOMEDIASTINAL LYMPHANGIOMA: HYGROMA COLLI

A 7 year old child presented with a swelling of the left side of the neck. The film shows a large, elongated mass with a sharply outlined border on the left side of the mediastinum. Although a cervicomediastinal mass in the adult usually represents a goiter or a lymphoma, these are uncommon in young children. The localized collection of air (arrow) in the neck is the result of a recent biopsy at this site. The mass was resected and proved to be a cystic hygroma.

cardiac shadow in the frontal projection if the heart is not adequately penetrated.

A communication between the afferent portion of the duct and the cyst can usually be demonstrated pathologically, but a connection with the thoracic duct above the cyst may be absent. In one of the cases observed by us this resulted in dilatation of collateral lymph channels including those in the lungs which caused an accentuation of the interstitial pulmonary markings. The cyst may be demonstrable by lymphangiography.

OTHER MEDIASTINAL CYSTS. Other mediastinal cysts are exceedingly rare. A few echinococcus cysts of the mediastinum have been described. Most were situated in the paravertebral region and were of the dumbbell type extending mesially into the spinal canal.

An acquired cyst of the pancreas (pseudocyst)

may extend upward in the retroperitoneal region through the esophageal hiatus to produce a cystic mass of considerable size in the posterior mediastinum. As in the case of a hiatal hernia, the supradiaphragmatic extension of the cyst may extend to both sides of the spine. It may be associated with a pleural effusion.

Developmental Neoplasms. Developmental neoplasms of the mediastinum arise from primordial germ cells, and usually include tissues from all three primitive layers. They are generally classified as teratomas. The dermoid tumors, so called because they characteristically contain hair, sebaceous glands and other ectodermal derivatives, are usually cystic and benign. The other teratomas are malignant and are similar to the germinal neoplasms of the testicle. Most of them have the appearance of mixed tumors, but in some, chorioepitheliomatous or seminomatous tissue predominates and, occasionally, is the sole constituent.

DERMOID CYSTS. Dermoid cysts comprise the great majority of teratomas of the mediastinum. They originate near the midline of the upper portion of the anterior mediastinum. Since they are intrinsically benign and do not invade the surrounding tissues, they tend to gravitate downward and become pedunculated. The tumor remains in the anterior mediastinum but is displaced to one side by the heart and great vessels.

Dermoid cysts have a tendency to increase in size. The most rapid growth appears to occur at about the time of puberty and this probably accounts for the fact that most of them are first discovered in young adults. The cyst presents as a rounded shadow, bulging out from the medias-

tinum, more frequently on the right side. Most are situated at about the level of the lung root or somewhat higher. The shape of the shadow is roughly hemispherical or semielliptical in the frontal projection, but often its contour is pear-shaped because the upper portion, where the tumor originates, is narrow and elongated. Occasionally the border is lobulated. In all instances the uncomplicated cyst is extremely well demarcated. On the lateral view it appears as a homogeneous, round or oval mass close to the sternum. Of the reported cases of thoracic dermoid cysts, only 1% have been situated entirely in the middle or posterior mediastinum.

Linear densities on the border of the shadow occur occasionally and represent calcified plaques in the capsule (Fig. 454). They are much less common in thymic neoplasms and do not

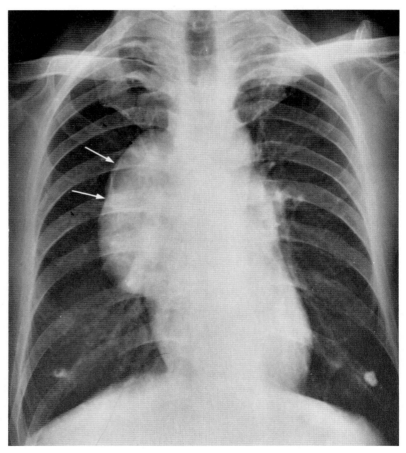

FIG. 454. DERMOID CYST

The sharply outlined, oval mass on the right side of the mediastinum obscures the right cardiac border and the ascending aorta, indicating that it lies anteriorly. The pulmonary arteries which lie behind the mass can be visualized through it. A portion of the circumference of the mass is outlined by a curvilinear calcific deposit (arrows). This differs from the calcification in thymomas which almost always is situated within the body of the lesion. The calcific deposits in the lower lobes represent old primary tuberculous foci.

occur in lymphomas. In rare instances the entire circumference of the cyst may be calcified. Teeth and bone, which are fairly common in dermoid cysts of the ovary, are rarely seen in mediastinal dermoids (Fig. 455).

The dermoid cyst usually contains a considerable amount of oily fluid in addition to cellular detritus. The latter has a tendency to settle to the bottom of the cyst if the patient remains stationary. The layering of the relatively lucent oily fluid over the denser sediment can produce a fairly well defined horizontal level. This is easily confused with an air-fluid level. However, the oily fluid is not as lucent as air, the interface is not so sharply defined, and it may disappear temporarily when the patient is tilted. This sign, described by Phemister *et al.,* is pathognomonic of a dermoid cyst.

Complications. Dermoid cysts occasionally become infected. Radiologically this may be evidenced by a sudden enlargement of the cyst as exudate accumulates within it. The borders of the cyst may lose their sharp definition as a result of inflammation of the overlying pleura. Occasionally there is a small pleural effusion.

The infected cyst can perforate into one of the neighboring structures, a bronchus, the trachea, pleura or pericardium. Rupture into one of the air passages may result in the production of a distinct air-fluid level within the cyst. As the cyst empties its contents, it becomes smaller and often less defined, and simulates an abscess of the lung. If the cyst discharges all of its contents it appears as an irregular, thick-walled, empty cavity. In some cases, air is not demonstrable within the cyst without tomography, and the lesion presents as a rather small, nondescript density on the conventional film. If the cyst perforates into the pleura, an effusion results. This may obscure the cyst, which, of course, contains no air. Similarly, perforation into the pericardium is heralded simply by the occurrence of a pericardial effusion. However, if the residual cyst is thick-walled, it may possibly be visualized as a mass abutting upon the enlarged cardiac silhouette.

Malignant change in a dermoid cyst of the mediastinum is rare. A benign dermoid can increase in size but it will maintain its original shape as it enlarges. The appearance of a nodular excrescence on its border should suggest the possibility that it has become malignant. This may be complicated by the occurrence of a pleural effusion resulting from implantation of malignant cells on the pleura.

Differential Diagnosis. The radiologic distinction between a dermoid cyst and a tumor of the

thymus gland is often impossible. A thymic tumor is more apt to be lobulated whereas a dermoid tends to be pendulous, hanging from a narrow pedicle. As a result, the angle formed between the upper border of a dermoid and the mediastinum is usually obtuse (Fig. 456). A thymoma, which usually is more fixed in position, tends to form a sharper angle with the mediastinum in this location. Calcific plaques within the capsule of a thymoma are exceedingly rare, whereas they are not infrequent in the capsule of a dermoid. On the other hand, irregular calcific densities within the substance of the lesion are fairly common in thymic tumors, benign or malignant, but are almost never seen in a dermoid. Ring-like calcifications within an anterior mediastinal mass are characteristic of tumors of the thymus or thyroid and are never seen in a dermoid cyst.

A dermoid cyst may be confused with an aneurysm of the aorta or a dilated main pulmonary artery when it lies adjacent to either of these vessels. It is often extremely difficult to differentiate between the expansile pulsations of an aortic aneurysm and pulsations transmitted through a dermoid. Furthermore, an aneurysm may pulsate poorly or not at all if its wall is markedly thickened by lamellated clot. Angiography may be required for the differential diagnosis.

A ruptured dermoid cyst is easily differentiated from a mediastinal abscess for the latter is practically always situated in the posterior mediastinum. However, differentiation from a lung abscess situated in the anterior medial portion of the upper lobe is difficult. The diagnosis becomes evident when previous films are available. The presence of a homogeneous, circumscribed density in the mediastinum on one of these films indicates a dermoid cyst, while a negative film excludes this from consideration. A thick, well-demarcated wall also favors the diagnosis of a dermoid.

MALIGNANT TERATOMAS. These are solid growths occurring almost solely in males, and are usually detected in the third and fourth decade. Since the tumors are malignant from their inception and invade the surrounding tissues, they remain fixed and do not shift to one side, as do the benign tumors. Rather, they expand into both pulmonary fields where they present as fairly well demarcated, lobulated masses, often with irregular borders (Fig. 457). Occasionally, on standard films, the lobulated tumor may appear to jut out on only one side of the mediastinum. However, the fact that the tumor is present on the other side of the mediastinum can

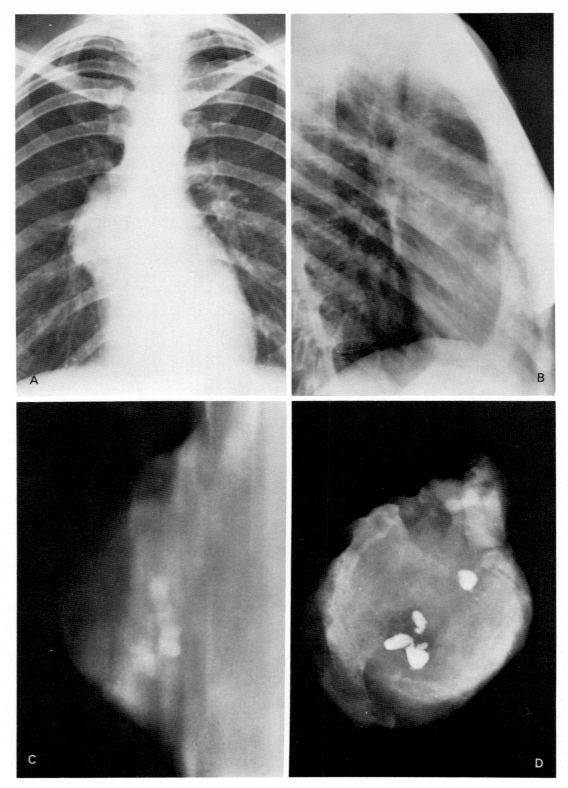

FIG. 455. MEDIASTINAL DERMOID

A: Frontal view. The mass projecting from the right side of the mediastinum has a sharply defined, wavy border. The contour of the ascending aorta is obliterated, indicating that the mass is situated anteriorly. *B:* Lateral view. Several calcific densities are seen within the anterior mediastinal mass. Tomography was performed for better definition. *C:* Frontal tomogram. Five calcific densities are seen within the mass. They are more or less round and uniform in size. A small, central lucency is seen within three of them, suggesting that they represent teeth. They differ from calcific deposits in a thymoma which appear either ring-like or grossly irregular. *D:* X-ray film of the excised specimen. The lesion proved to be a dermoid cyst which contained five teeth. These cast extremely dense, homogeneous shadows because they are composed mostly of enamel.

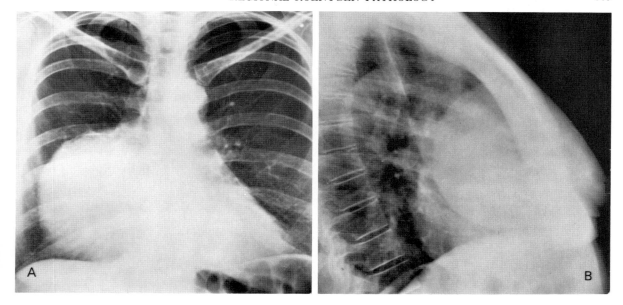

FIG. 456. DERMOID CYST OF THE MEDIASTINUM

A: The sharply circumscribed, homogeneous density projecting from the right side of the mediastinum obliterates the right cardiac border, indicating that it is situated anteriorly. The upper border of the mass joins the mediastinum at an obtuse angle. *B:* The lateral view shows the mass to be within the anterior mediastinum. The posterior border is smooth and exquisitely outlined. This excludes the possibility of a pericardial cyst and makes a thymoma unlikely. At operation, the lesion proved to be a dermoid cyst with a long pedicle arising in the superior mediastinum.

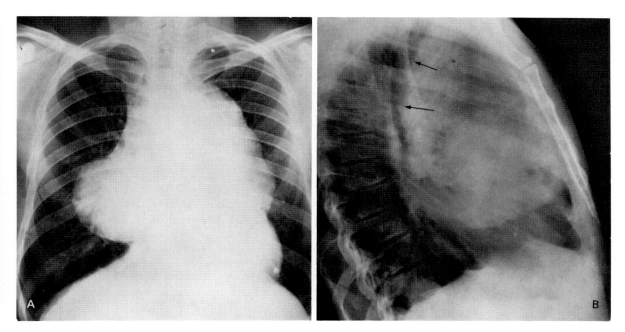

FIG. 457. MALIGNANT TERATOMA OF THE MEDIASTINUM

A: Frontal view. There is a large, sharply demarcated, lobulated mass extending out from both sides of the mediastinum. The irregularity of the mass and its extension to either side differentiate a malignant from a benign teratoma (dermoid cyst). *B:* Lateral view. The trachea (arrows) is displaced far backward by the tumor which is situated in the anterior mediastinum. The upper part of the retrosternal space is clouded, but is not as dense as the lower portion where the tumor is much wider.

be demonstrated on films made with increased exposure. Calcification does not take place on the circumference or within the body of the growth.

Because the malignant growth is fixed in the mediastinum, it exerts pressure on adjacent organs as it enlarges. The trachea is generally displaced backward and is sometimes greatly compressed (Fig. 457). Benign tumors are more mobile, and although when large they may displace the trachea, they rarely compress it, unless situated in the thoracic inlet.

The tumors usually increase rapidly in size and end fatally after a comparatively short course. In the late stages an effusion may occur in the pleura or pericardium as the result of local invasion.

It is difficult to differentiate a malignant teratoma of the mediastinum from a lymphoma, particularly Hodgkin's disease, which has a predilection for involving the anterior mediastinum. This is especially true when the teratoma is composed mainly of seminomatous tissue which is sensitive to radiotherapy in the same manner as the lymphomas (Fig. 458). The other malig-

nant teratomas are quite resistant to radiation. Those containing a considerable amount of chorioepitheliomatous tissue can be recognized because they secrete gonadotropins which can be detected in the urine.

Neurogenic Tumors. The neurogenic tumors arise from either the cells of the nerve sheaths (neurilemmoma, schwannoma), the nerve fibers themselves (neurofibroma), the sympathetic ganglion cells (neuroblastoma and ganglioneuroma) or the cells of the paraganglionic system (pheochromocytoma and chemodectoma). With the exception of the rare tumors arising from the vagus or phrenic nerves, and the chemodectomas, the growths are situated in the costovertebral gutter behind and lateral to the anterior borders of the vertebral bodies which represent the posterior boundary of the mediastinum. They are therefore not true mediastinal tumors, but are considered here because they usually appear to be situated in the mediastinum on frontal films. For the same reason, and because they bear a relationship to the nervous system, thoracic meningoceles and chordomas are also discussed in this section.

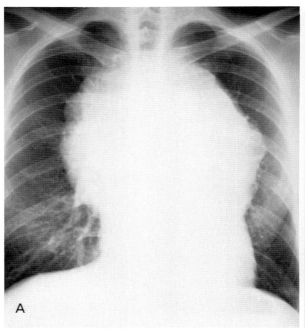 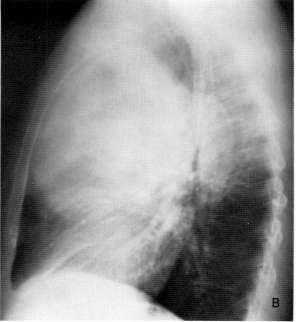

FIG. 458. MEDIASTINAL SEMINOMA

A: The frontal film of a 40 year old male who had been coughing for a few weeks shows an extremely large lobulated mass extending from both sides of the mediastinum. The trachea is not displaced. It is impossible to differentiate between a teratoma and lymphomatous disease. *B:* Lateral view. The mass occupies the anterior mediastinum, making lymphosarcoma unlikely. The trachea is pushed far backward. This is more characteristic of teratoma than Hodgkin's disease because the latter tends to infiltrate around the trachea rather than to displace it. Biopsy of the mediastinal mass revealed a seminoma. The testicles were not involved and lymphangiography showed no involvement of the pelvic or paraaortic nodes.

NEUROFIBROMA AND NEURILEMMOMA (SCHWANNOMA). These are the most common of the thoracic neurogenic tumors. In some instances they occur as part of the diffuse neurofibromatosis of von Recklinghausen. Most of them originate near the roots of the intercostal nerves as they emerge from the spine. Occasionally they involve the vagus or phrenic nerve. The neurofibromas and neurilemmomas will be considered together because their roentgen appearance is essentially the same, and because there may be some uncertainty concerning the pathologic classification of individual cases.

Paraspinal Neurofibromas. These tumors arise from the roots of the intercostal nerves at their exit from the intervertebral foramina. Some of them originate within the foramen and grow outward, adjacent to the spine. They can also extend into the spinal canal to produce a dumbbell tumor. They occur in all age groups but mostly about the third decade. The tumors are practically always benign, and, except when associated with diffuse neurofibromatosis, there is little tendency to malignant change.

On the frontal film, the neurofibroma appears as a homogeneous, semicircular density with its base against the spine. The mesial border of the shadow merges with that of the mediastinum, while the outer border is extremely sharp. It is most commonly situated in the upper portion of the chest above the sixth dorsal vertebra. On occasion the lesion is more elongated and its upper and lower borders merge with the spine in an obtuse angle so that the shadow appears more or less spindle-shaped.

On the lateral projection, the mass is located far posteriorly. Its anterior border is usually rounded and sharply demarcated against the lung, while its posterior border blends with the shadows of the chest wall. The tumor may not extend as far forward as the anterior border of the vertebral bodies but, when large, it can project over the posterior mediastinum. In extremely rare instances, particularly when in the upper part of the chest, it can reach the anterior chest wall. In the case of a more elongated, spindle-shaped tumor, the outline of the mass may not be visible on the lateral view. The only clue to the location of the tumor in this projection may simply be a slight increase in the density of the vertebrae at the level of the growth. If such a tumor is situated behind the heart, it can be overlooked on the frontal view as well.

Since the diagnosis of neurofibroma is based on the position of the mass in relation to the spine, it is sometimes necessary to resort to tomography for exact localization. When the tumor is situated in the uppermost part of the chest, the inclined lateral view may be helpful in this respect (Fig. 6). Because the neoplasm is fixed in the costovertebral angle, its position with relation to the spine remains unchanged on films made in the supine position in expiration and in the erect position in inspiration. This is in contrast to benign esophageal tumors and nonadherent pulmonary and pleural neoplasms situated in the same location.

Occasionally the border of a large neurofibroma is lobulated. Calcification can occur in tumors which have undergone necrosis or cystic degeneration, but this is unusual. In extremely rare instances, a pleural effusion is present even though the lesion is benign. This is due to necrosis of the tumor and irritation of the overlying pleura.

The growth frequently causes changes in the adjacent bones. The ribs over the mass are often spread apart and may be thinned as a result of pressure atrophy. This is associated with a condensation of the cortex rather than destruction of the bone. The head of the rib above the tumor may be displaced upward, dislocating the costovertebral articulation. Pressure from the tumor can cause scalloping of the lateral borders of the vertebral bodies. When the mass extends into the intervertebral foramen, the pedicle is thinned and the foramen becomes widened (Fig. 171). More than one of the foramina may be enlarged by ingrowth of the tumor. In the dumbbell variety with a large intraspinal component, scalloping of the posterior part of the vertebral body may be evident on the lateral view. Scoliosis is unusual. Because of the importance of the bony changes in the diagnosis of neurofibroma, films of the spine should be made whenever this condition is considered. Tomograms may be necessary for adequate visualization of the intervertebral foramina.

Neurofibroma of the Vagus. Neurofibromas of the vagus nerve are situated in the middle mediastinum. On the frontal projection they have the same appearance as the neurofibromas of the dorsal nerve roots. On the lateral view, they lie more anteriorly and the entire circumference of the lesion is well demarcated. The round or oval shadow can simulate a bronchogenic cyst. When situated in the upper mediastinum, the neurofibroma has the same appearance as a paratracheal cyst or an intrathoracic goiter. Unlike these lesions, the neurofibroma remains stationary on swallowing although it may displace the trachea and esophagus. Since, unlike tumors of the paraspinal nerves, it is not attached to the chest wall, it rises readily on coughing.

When the tumor is situated on the left side it can simulate a large aortic knob, and angiography may be required to exclude the possibility of an aneurysm. This possibility is suggested particularly when the tumor involves the left recurrent nerve and produces vocal cord paralysis. In the absence of paralysis of the vocal cord, the possibility of a bronchogenic cyst, a chemodectoma or a lymphoma must be considered (Fig. 459).

Von Recklinghausen's Neurofibromatosis. Intrathoracic neurofibromas are not uncommon in generalized neurofibromatosis. Most often they are single and appear identical to the isolated neurofibroma. They are apt to occur somewhat earlier in life and the majority are detected in the second decade.

In a considerable number of instances of Von Recklinghausen's disease, the intrathoracic neurofibroma takes the form of a cirsoid, tangled, plexiform mass of nerve tissue involving the posterior mediastinum and the paravertebral regions. Frequently the neurofibroma involves both sides of the mediastinum and forms an elongated shadow which mimics lymphomatous disease. In association with this, there may be bilateral, circumscribed, hemispherical masses representing neurofibromas in the dorsal nerve roots. In addition to these, there may be multiple neurofibromas situated more peripherally in the intercostal nerves. These have a tendency to produce notching on the inferior surfaces of the adjacent ribs (Fig. 168). The vagus or phrenic nerves may also be involved in Von Recklinghausen's disease, either singly or in combination with other intrathoracic neurofibromas. The combination of hemispherical shadows at the domes of the thoracic cavities together with an elongated widening of the mediastinal shadow, notching of the ribs and scalloped shadows in the periphery of the pulmonary fields, constitutes a rare but pathognomonic picture of diffuse neurofibromatosis, not to be confused with any other condition.

Neurofibromas on the skin over the thorax can cast shadows over the lungs, and when they are associated with a mediastinal neurofibroma, the frontal chest film may suggest a primary bronchogenic carcinoma with metastases in the lungs. However, when the patient is rotated to the oblique or lateral positions, many of the nodular

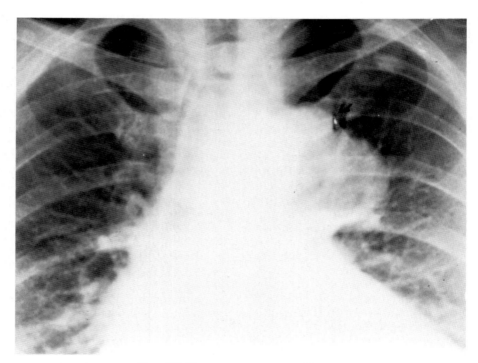

FIG. 459. NEUROFIBROMA OF THE VAGUS

The lobulated mass extending from the left side of the mediastinum was projected over the middle mediastinum in the lateral view. Differential diagnosis should include bronchogenic carcinoma, lymphoma, an aneurysm of the arch of the aorta, a chemodectoma or a neurofibroma of the vagus. The vocal cord was not paralyzed. A benign tumor of the vagus nerve was completely removed.

densities are projected outside the thoracic cage and seem to disappear unless attention is paid to the soft tissue shadows of the chest wall. The location of these lesions should strongly suggest the diagnosis of Von Recklinghausen's disease. A rounded paravertebral shadow in association with diffuse neurofibromatosis does not justify the diagnosis of neurofibroma. A meningocele, which casts a similar shadow, is a more frequent accompaniment of Von Recklinghausen's disease.

The intrathoracic neurofibromas associated with Von Recklinghausen's disease differ from the isolated neurofibromas of the dorsal nerve roots in that they have a much greater tendency to malignant change. Such change is usually impossible to recognize radiologically until the later stages when there is diffuse involvement of the pleura.

GANGLIONEUROMA. The ganglioneuromas that originate alongside the dorsal spine usually appear similar to the neurofibromas of the dorsal nerve roots. Both present sharply demarcated, homogeneous, semicircular shadows based on the spine, often associated with pressure changes in the adjacent ribs and vertebrae. However, certain differences have been noted. Ganglioneuromas generally occur in a younger age group. Most of the cases described have been in patients under the age of 10, and three-quarters under the age of 20. They are frequently more elongated and flatter against the spine. The junction of the shadow of the ganglioneuroma with the spine then forms an obtuse angle and the upper border of the shadow may be indistinct on the frontal projection, and its anterior border invisible on the lateral view. This view may disclose simply an increased density of the shadows of the vertebrae overlain by the tumor.

Ganglioneuromas tend to occur at a lower level than neurofibromas. When situated behind the heart they may be easily overlooked on the frontal as well as on the lateral projection. Occasionally calcification occurs, appearing either as punctate densities throughout the tumor or as linear densities on its periphery. Scoliosis is more commonly associated with ganglioneuromas than with neurofibromas but is less frequent with either of these lesions than it is with meningoceles.

Ganglioneuromas usually grow slowly and sometimes become very large (Fig. 460). Partic-

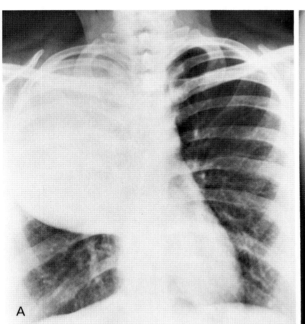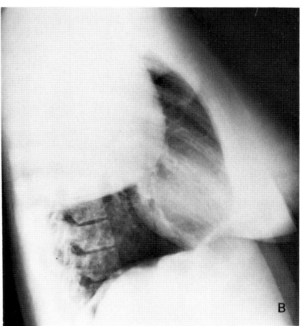

FIG. 460. GANGLIONEUROMA

A: Frontal view of a 27 year old woman shows a huge mass occupying the upper two-thirds of the right chest. Its lower border is sharply circumscribed, with a smooth regular border. The mass had been observed to grow slowly over a period of 12 years. *B:* The lateral view shows the mass to be based against the posterior chest wall. The location is suggestive of a neurogenic tumor although a fibroma of the visceral pleura can give an identical appearance. The mass was resected and proved to be a ganglioneuroma.

ularly in young children, the tumor may occupy a large portion of the chest, displacing the trachea and esophagus to the other side. Rapid enlargement occurs occasionally. Usually this is due to cystic degeneration of the tumor but may reflect malignant transformation. Perhaps 10% of ganglioneuromas undergo malignant change, in sharp contrast to the isolated neurofibroma which rarely becomes malignant.

NEUROBLASTOMA. Neuroblastomas are malignant tumors which arise from the sympathetic ganglia. They occur almost exclusively in infants and young children. When situated in the chest, they usually appear roentgenologically as lobulated masses against the spine. The border may be poorly demarcated. Calcification is common despite the malignant nature of the tumor. The calcium usually appears in the form of irregular densities scattered throughout the growth.

As in the case of a neurofibroma, the ribs over the growth may be spread apart, and the rib above the tumor may be narrowed and show condensation of the cortex of its lower border as the result of pressure by the tumor. Destruction of the overlying ribs indicates actual invasion of the chest wall by the growth. The tumor may metastasize widely at a relatively early stage so that nodular lesions in the lungs, enlargement of the hilar and mediastinal nodes, and destructive lesions in the bones may all be present while the primary tumor is still quite small. Metastasis to the pleura can cause an effusion large enough to obscure the primary neoplasm.

Although the tumor is malignant, it may grow very slowly and, in fact, may remain stationary in size for a long period. Occasionally the neoplasm matures and is transformed into a benign ganglioneuroma even though distant metastases have already appeared.

PHEOCHROMOCYTOMA. Pheochromocytes, the specific cells of the adrenal medulla, develop from embryonic cells that wander out from the neural crest. They may be situated anywhere along the paravertebral sympathetic chain. Tumors of these cells may therefore occur alongside the thoracic spine as well as in other locations. The tumors produce epinephrine and norepinephrine, and usually cause hypertension which may be paroxysmal. Even extremely small pheochromocytomas can be associated with hypertension. In occasional cases hypertension is not present, but may be evoked by handling the tumor at operation. Most pheochromocytomas are benign, but malignant ones have been observed in the abdomen. It is therefore presumed that a malignant pheochromocytoma can occur in the chest as well.

Radiologically, a thoracic pheochromocytoma appears as a well-defined, semicircular shadow alongside the spine in the costovertebral gutter identical to that of a paravertebral neurofibroma (Fig. 461). The diagnosis of pheochromocytoma should be suspected in paravertebral tumors associated with hypertension, especially if paroxysmal or in a young person. However, the absence of hypertension does not exclude the possibility of pheochromocytoma.

Since the tumor arises from the sympathetic chain alongside the spine rather than in relation to the nerve roots, there appears to be little tendency to pressure changes of the spine or ribs. We have not encountered calcification in an intrathoracic pheochromocytoma although conceivably this can occur, since large pheochromocytomas in the abdomen are often hemorrhagic and can undergo cystic degeneration with calcification.

AORTIC BODY TUMOR (CHEMODECTOMA). These tumors, which have been considered as nonchromaffin paragangliomas, arise from groups of cells connected with branches of the vagus nerve. They are found in relation to the inferior surface of the aortic arch near the ligamentum arteriosum, the upper anterior surface of the aortic arch near the origin of the left subclavian artery and the root of the aorta near the left coronary artery. Intrathoracic chemodectomas are rare. Most of them are encapsulated. Local invasion is common but distant spread is unusual.

The tumor casts a round or ovoid, sharply demarcated shadow, projecting either to the right or left side of the mediastinum. Most are situated anteriorly in the superior mediastinum and some extend into the neck. Those that arise near the root of the aorta or near the ligamentum arteriosum lie more posteriorly, in the middle mediastinum. A mass situated in this location may project on both sides of the mediastinum. Because of its proximity to the aorta, the tumor generally displays prominent pulsations. Angiography may be required to exclude the possibility of an aneurysm.

A malignant chemodectoma may be well circumscribed, but becomes poorly demarcated as invasion of the surrounding tissues increases. We have observed such extensive spread of the growth over the pleura that the original tumor was obscured.

INTRATHORACIC MENINGOCELE. An intrathoracic meningocele results from herniation of the meninges through an intervertebral foramen or through a defect in a vertebral body. The meningeal sac communicates with the spinal canal and

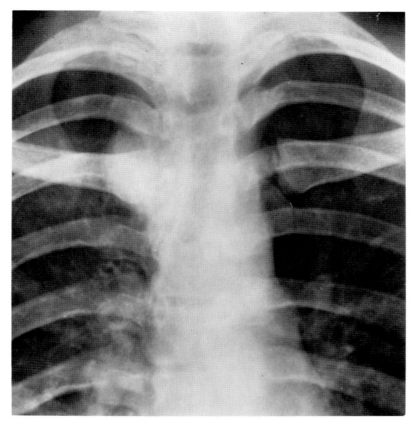

FIG. 461. THORACIC PHEOCHROMOCYTOMA

A 15 year old girl with hypertension had an abdominal pheochromocytoma removed previously. Following surgery, the blood pressure returned to normal but recently became elevated once more. The chest film which had been negative in the past, now shows a well-defined mass in the right paravertebral region. The appearance is identical to that of a neurofibroma. The hypertension was alleviated following removal of the thoracic pheochromocytoma.

is filled with spinal fluid. Although it may occur in infancy, it is almost always first detected later in life, most frequently about the age of 40. Two-thirds of the cases are associated with Von Recklinghausen's neurofibromatosis. Congenital defects of the spine, particularly spina bifida or hemivertebra, often occur in association with the meningocele.

Lateral Meningocele. Lateral meningoceles occur at any level of the thoracic spine, but are probably more frequent in the upper portion. They protrude through the intervertebral foramen to lie in the costovertebral gutter in a manner similar to neurofibromas. They vary in size, from those that are quite small to the ones that fill an entire hemithorax. A meningocele may remain stationary in size or enlarge slowly over a period of years. It presents radiologically as a homogeneous mass with an exquisitely sharp, round, outer border, while its mesial border merges with the shadows of the mediastinum

and spine. In rare instances, meningoceles are multiple.

The great majority of lateral meningoceles are associated with secondary changes in the adjacent bones, the most frequent of which is an increase in the size of the intervertebral foramen at the level of the mass. The foramina above and below this level may also be enlarged. The ribs are frequently spread apart by the meningocele and often undergo pressure atrophy as with a neurofibroma. In some cases, upward displacement of the posterior portion of the rib results in dislocation of the costovertebral junction. A lateral view of the spine may disclose concave scalloping of the posterior border of one or more of the vertebral bodies as the result of pressure of the meningocele (Fig. 462). Kyphosis or kyphoscoliosis occurs frequently, either from an associated congenital defect of the spine or from changes caused by the meningocele itself.

Anterior Meningocele. This is an uncommon

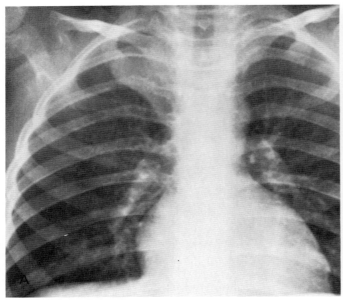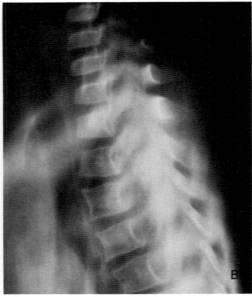

FIG. 462. LATERAL MENINGOCELE

A: A 4 year old child with generalized neurofibromatosis. The large homogeneous density extending outward from the right side of the mediastinum is sharply circumscribed. In the lateral projection, the mass was seen posteriorly, in the costovertebral gutter. *B:* A lateral tomogram shows erosion of the posterior margin of the vertebral bodies of D_1 through D_5. Ultrasonographic examination revealed the mass to be cystic. (Courtesy of Dr. J. F. Holt, Ann Arbor, Mich.)

form of intrathoracic meningocele. It results from anterior herniation of the meninges through a defect or cleft in one or more of the vertebral bodies. The meningocele then lies in the true posterior mediastinum and produces a shadow similar to that of a neurenteric cyst. The shadow usually projects to one side of the spine. On the lateral view the esophagus is seen to be displaced forward. When the lesion is situated in the superior mediastinum the trachea may be similarly displaced.

Diagnosis. The roentgen picture of an intrathoracic meningocele is quite similar to that of a paraspinal neurogenic tumor both in the position and appearance of the mass and the changes in the ribs and spine. It is important to differentiate between these two lesions because operation is often unnecessary in the case of a meningocele. A definitive diagnosis of meningocele depends upon the demonstration of a communication between the mass and the fluid in the spinal canal. This is done by myelography.

Certain roentgen characteristics aid in the differential diagnosis prior to myelography. A vertebral anomaly, such as spina bifida or hemivertebra, is indicative of a meningocele rather than a neurofibroma; kyphosis or scoliosis localized to the level of the mass, also favors the diagnosis of meningocele. In general, a meningocele is apt to be less dense than a neurogenic tumor of the

same size but the difference is difficult to evaluate in individual cases. The demonstration of calcium within the lesion excludes meningocele from consideration. Peculiarly enough, an association with generalized neurofibromatosis favors a meningocele rather than a paraspinal neurofibroma.

It is difficult to differentiate an anterior meningocele from a neurenteric cyst since both lie in the true posterior mediastinum and are associated with anomalies of the vertebral bodies. The presence of a characteristic round, tunnel-like defect in the vertebral body, air within the mass, or other evidence of communication of the mass with the gut is indicative of a neurenteric cyst. Myelography may reveal a communication between the spinal canal and the stalk of a neurenteric cyst, but filling of the cyst itself with contrast material is extremely rare, while it is the rule in a meningocele.

CHORDOMA. A chordoma is a locally invasive tumor which arises from a notochordal remnant in the fully developed spine. Although it is not a neurogenic tumor, it is considered here because it is sometimes confused with neurogenic tumors related to the spine and mediastinum.

The dorsal region is a rather uncommon location for a chordoma. However, when it does occur at this level, it grows forward and usually projects as a round tumor in the posterior mediastinum. On the frontal projection it may extend out from one or both sides of the mediastinal shadow. The tumor is generally homogeneous. Its border may be lobulated and not as sharply demarcated as a neurogenic tumor. Calcified plaques are not infrequently seen at the margin of the growth. On the lateral view, the esophagus and the trachea may be seen displaced forward by the advancing tumor. The anterior or lateral portions of the spine are often eroded, but in contrast to the meningocele or the neurofibroma, the posterior border of the vertebral bodies is not affected.

Tumors of Mesenchymal Origin. This group of tumors consists of a variety of neoplasms, both benign and malignant. It includes lipomas, fibromas, angiomas, and their malignant counterparts. Also included in this group are the extremely rare instances of mixed tumors designated as mesenchymomas. The tumors occur at any age. In general, the benign ones are apt to be very large when first discovered as they rarely produce symptoms. The malignant forms produce symptoms by invading and compressing adjacent structures.

There is a predilection for the growths to occur in the anterior mediastinum, but involvement of the middle and posterior mediastinum is not rare, particularly in the case of fibromas or fibrosarcomas. Tumors in the upper mediastinum may extend into the neck. Those that are situated posteriorly, even though benign, may extend into the spinal canal through an intervertebral foramen. Either the benign or the malignant variety can fill an entire hemithorax. Both can cause a pleural effusion which can be large enough to obscure the primary lesion. The diagnosis of the type of tumor is impossible roentgenologically except in certain specific instances.

Lipomas are usually less dense than other mediastinal tumors because fat is more radiolucent than other tissues. The tumor may be smooth or lobulated and its border is well defined. Although usually unilateral, the mass may project outward from both sides of the mediastinum (Fig. 463). Lipomas are most commonly situated in the anterior mediastinum alongside the heart and can simulate a parapericardial cyst. However, because they are more radiolucent, they may not obliterate the cardiac silhouette in spite of their anterior location. Those situated at the cardiophrenic angle have an appearance identical with that of properitoneal fat herniated through the foramen of Morgagni. A *liposarcoma* is more apt to be irregular in shape and occurs anywhere in the mediastinum.

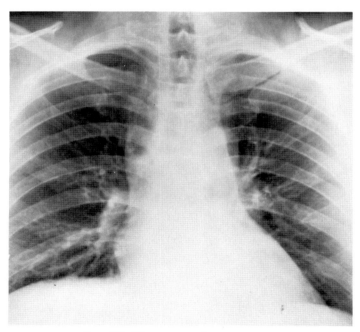

FIG. 463. MEDIASTINAL LIPOMATOSIS

The superior mediastinum is widened. However, its density is less than expected with an inflammatory or neoplastic process of this size. The contour of the aortic knob is seen clearly through the mediastinal shadow. The lucency of the shadow and its regular borders suggest fatty replacement of thymus or lipomatosis of the mediastinum. The latter diagnosis was proven by biopsy.

Fibromas and *fibrosarcomas* are extremely rare in the mediastinum. They cast a dense, sharply defined, round or oval shadow which may be lobulated. Like liposarcomas, they occur anywhere in the mediastinum. The fibroma grows slowly, while the fibrosarcoma tends to increase rapidly in size. However, the latter tumor has been observed to remain dormant for a long period before suddenly enlarging. Erosion of the spine from invasion by a posterior mediastinal fibrosarcoma has been reported.

Mixed tumors of mesenchymal origin, *mesenchymomas,* are extremely rare in the mediastinum. They may contain any of the tissues derived from the anlage of the mediastinum. Both benign and malignant forms occur and have a radiologic appearance identical with that of the fibroma and fibrosarcoma.

Both *hemangiomas* and *hemangiosarcomas* occur in the mediastinum either as isolated lesions or in conjunction with blood vessel tumors elsewhere in the body. Not infrequently they occur in young children. Most of them are situated in the anterior mediastinum. They present either as a sharply demarcated, round or oval mass projecting outward from one or both sides of the mediastinum or simply as a diffuse widening of the mediastinal shadow. The vascular tumor may produce a bruit or exhibit expansile pulsations. Angiography may then be required to exclude an aortic aneurysm. The angiomatous tumors are not likely to opacify.

The only pathognomonic roentgen sign of a tumor of mesenchymal origin is the demonstration of phleboliths within a hemangioma. Like phleboliths elsewhere, they appear as sharply defined, round or oval calcific densities, a few millimeters in diameter, often with a lucent center. This is the only form of calcification described in the mesenchymal tumors.

Xanthomatous tumors are rare. They are benign and encapsulated. Most of them have been noted in the paravertebral region and present an appearance identical to the neurofibromas which arise from the dorsal nerve roots. It is quite possible that many of them really represent neurofibromas which have undergone xanthomatous degeneration. Those observed in the anterior mediastinum have been reported as either xanthofibromas or xanthogranulomas. They jut out from either side of the anterior mediastinum, are sharply demarcated and appear as a round density behind the sternum on the lateral view.

Miscellaneous Tumors. A number of pathologic conditions, not necessarily neoplastic, are associated with the formation of masses in or adjacent to the mediastinum. Some are located in the paravertebral region, but are discussed here because they may have the appearance of mediastinal tumors on ordinary roentgen films.

EXTRAMEDULLARY HEMATOPOIESIS. In chronic anemias, blood cells are frequently formed outside of the bone marrow. Usually, this extramedullary hematopoiesis occurs in the liver, spleen and lymph nodes. However, in rare instances, masses of heterotopic marrow are formed in connective tissue outside of these organs. In the chest they occur adjacent to the spine and present as masses in the costovertebral gutters. This condition is encountered most frequently in patients with hereditary spherocytic anemia and thalassemia. It has also been described in conjunction with myelosclerosis, pernicious anemia and other diseases affecting the bone marrow.

The hematopoietic tumors appear radiologically as sharply defined, homogeneous, round or ovoid densities alongside the spine (Fig. 464, *A* and *B*). In most cases they are multiple. When single, the shadow appears identical with that produced by a paraspinal neurogenic tumor. The multiple tumors are often symmetrically distributed. There may be a single tumor on each side of one of the vertebrae or several tumors on one or both sides. They show no predilection for any particular level of the dorsal spine. In some cases the masses lie adjacent to each other along the course of the vertebrae, forming a continuous chain of nodules (Fig. 464C). The lesions are often quite large and, on the lateral view, may be seen to extend anterior to the vertebral bodies.

The diagnosis depends upon the association of the lesion with a disease affecting hematopoiesis. It should be strongly suspected whenever multiple masses are found in the costovertebral gutters. Appropriate hematologic studies should be made in all such cases, even in the absence of clinical evidence of bone marrow disease. When the mass is single, a blood-forming tumor should be suspected if the patient is known to have a chronic anemia or if the left leaf of the diaphragm is elevated by an enlarged spleen. The diagnosis is rendered more certain when the chest film reveals changes in the bones suggesting osteosclerosis or thalassemia.

Since thoracotomy is not required in the case of these hematopoietic tumors, it is important to differentiate them from other paraspinal growths. Even in the rare instances where the hematopoietic tissue extends into the spinal canal and compresses the spinal cord, surgical treatment may not be required since the tumors respond rapidly to radiation treatment. Unlike the neurogenic tumors, the masses of heterotopic

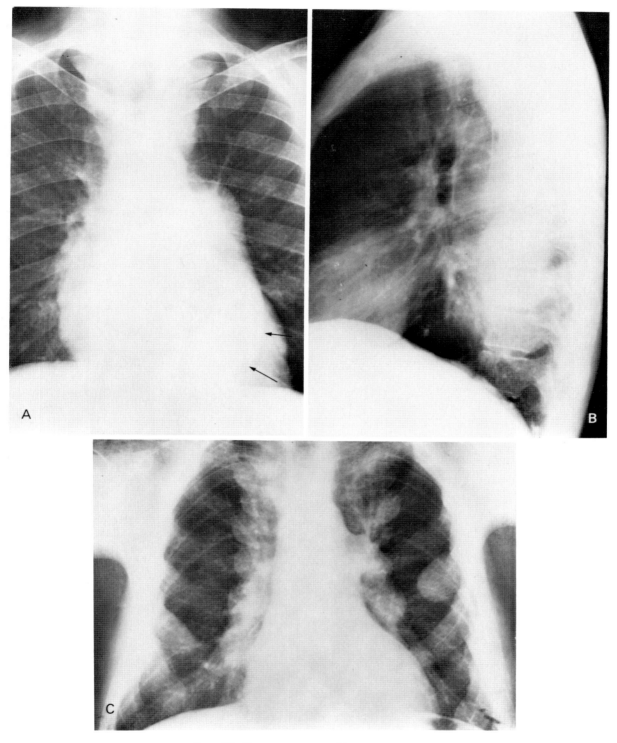

FIG. 464. EXTRAMEDULLARY HEMATOPOESIS

A: A 27 year old man with thalassemia. Bilateral masses are seen in relation to the cardiac silhouette. On the left side, the mass (arrows) is projected through the shadow of the heart and overlies the region of the main pulmonary artery, while on the right side, the lobulated mass extends beyond the right cardiac border. In addition, paravertebral masses are present above the level of the aortic knob. *B:* The lateral view shows the masses to be situated posterior to the mediastinum in the paravertebral gutter. The diagnosis was proven by biopsy. *C:* In another patient with severe chronic hereditary anemia, the hematopoetic tissue forms a symmetrical chain of nodules on either side of the spine. Additional masses are present in relation to the ribs and produce the appearance of diffuse scalloped thickening of the pleura. The ribs are widened as the result of marked increase in the marrow space and thinning of the cortex.

bone marrow do not produce pressure changes on the ribs or vertebrae and there is no tendency for calcification. The final diagnosis can be made by a scintiscan of the chest following tagging of the active bone marrow by a radioactive isotope, such as Au[198].

MEDIASTINAL CARCINOID. Carcinoids, similar in all respects to those of the bronchus and the intestine, have been found as primary growths in the mediastinum, completely separate from the bronchi or lung. Of the five cases that have been described, four were in the anterior mediastinum and one was situated in the lower part of the posterior mediastinum behind the heart. In one case a large tumor was present on each side of the anterior mediastinum and in another the carcinoid was found within the wall of a congenital cyst of the anterior mediastinum.

LIPOMATOSIS IN CUSHING'S SYNDROME. Atypical distribution of fatty tissue is characteristic of Cushing's syndrome, and is encountered most frequently as a result of steroid therapy. When it occurs in the chest, the fat tends to accumulate in the mediastinum and in the epicardial region.

The mass of fatty tissue in the upper mediastinum usually lies anteriorly and produces a roentgen picture similar to that of a hyperplastic thymus. The mediastinal shadow is symmetrically widened and has straight, smooth borders. The outer portions of the widened mediastinum are relatively radiolucent, suggesting the presence of adipose tissue. Large epicardial fat pads at the apex of the heart and in the region of the right cardiophrenic angle may also be present. The association of these shadows in the mediastinum with osteoporosis of the ribs or spine, or spontaneous fractures of these bones, should suggest the possibility of steroid lipomatosis. We have observed a case in which the mediastinal mass resembled a hyperplastic thymus on pneumomediastinography as well as on ordinary films.

PLASMACYTOMA. Most plasmacytomas are true neoplasms, consisting of plasma cells arranged in palisade formation with a connective tissue stroma, but some appear to be inflammatory in nature and are better described as plasma cell granulomas. The majority are situated in the upper air passages. Those involving the thorax are usually associated with multiple myeloma and, in the majority of instances, are situated in the ribs. However, a few cases have been noted within the mediastinum unassociated with evidence of multiple myeloma. They appeared as well-circumscribed, round or lobulated masses projecting from either side of the mediastinum, without any particular site of predilection, and it was impossible to differentiate them radiologically from other mediastinal tumors.

AMYLOID TUMOR. Involvement of the mediastinum in amyloid disease usually occurs in conjunction with bronchial and pulmonary amyloidosis, frequently with involvement of the lymph nodes. The disease in the mediastinum may take the form of a single mass or a generalized infiltrate in the connective tissues. In the latter instances, the roentgen films may disclose simply a widening of the mediastinal shadow. As in amyloidosis elsewhere, calcium deposits may occur in the lesion.

Mediastinal Lymph Nodes

Roentgen Anatomy

Distribution of the Mediastinal Nodes. From a roentgen standpoint it is useful to divide the mediastinal lymph nodes into seven groups:

1. *Paratracheal nodes,* arranged in a chain along either side of the trachea.

2. *Tracheobronchial nodes,* in the angle between the trachea and main bronchus on each side, immediately below the paratracheal chain.

3. *Hilar lymph nodes,* at the root of each lung, and more peripherally, in the region of the roots of the individual lobes. The most peripheral of the hilar nodes are imbedded in the lung substance and are called *intercalated nodes.*

4. *Subcarinal nodes,* immediately beneath the tracheal bifurcation, bounded behind by the esophagus and in front by the pericardium. They are often called the bifurcation or interbronchial nodes.

5. *Subaortic nodes,* a small group between the arch of the aorta and the pulmonary artery in the region of the ligamentum arteriosum.

6. *Posterior mediastinal nodes,* along the course of the esophagus.

7. *Anterior mediastinal nodes,* in front of the trachea and pericardium. These are few in number.

The *internal mammary nodes* are related to the anterior chest wall rather than to the mediastinum. They follow the course of the internal mammary artery on each side. The *paravertebral lymph nodes* are also situated beyond the limits of the mediastinum. They lie in the costovertebral gutters and are really related to the posterior chest wall.

Recognition of Enlarged Mediastinal Nodes. Although they contribute to the density of the shadows of the mediastinum and the lung roots, normal lymph nodes are not discernible radiologically. Even when moderately enlarged, the nodes are usually not recognizable. Thus, enlarged lymph nodes are regularly found at necropsy in association with severe pneumonias, but are rarely visible on the chest film except in young children. Therefore, lymph nodes large enough to be detected radiologically, are clinically significant.

Fairly large individual nodes or groups of nodes are easily recognized as prominent shadows projecting outward from the mediastinum. However, smaller nodes are easily overlooked. For their detection it is essential to have a thorough knowledge of the variations of the normal mediastinal contours and of the hilar shadows in the different projections. It is important to scan each component of the mediastinum for abnormal bulges or indistinctness of the borders, a local increase in density, and distortion or displacement of the mediastinal organs—any of which might indicate enlargement of the nodes. Comparison with previous films often proves helpful in questionable cases.

Further studies are indicated when the changes noted on routine films are equivocal. They are also advisable when the presence or absence of large nodes is decisive for diagnosis or treatment, even if the routine films appear normal. These studies include oblique views of the chest, Bucky films, barium studies of the esophagus, and the performance of Valsalva and Müller maneuvers during fluoroscopy. In some cases angiography, particularly azygography, is helpful. On the other hand, peripheral lymphangiography is rarely useful because the radiopaque material is carried into the thoracic duct by lymphatic channels which bypass the mediastinal nodes.

PARATRACHEAL NODES. Large paratracheal nodes are more frequently observed on the right side than on the left (Fig. 465). This is due to the fact that the right paratracheal chain contains more lymph nodes, and those on the left are apt to be obscured by the shadow of the aorta.

Enlargement of the *right paratracheal* lymph nodes may produce only an increase in the width of the right side of the mediastinum without distorting its border. This can simulate a dilated superior vena cava, but usually the shadow of the enlarged nodes is more irregular and less distinct.

Caution should be exercised in evaluating the width of the mediastinum by tomography. Tomograms are generally made with the patient recumbent and with a short tube-to-patient distance. This causes the mediastinal shadow to appear broadened. Venous angiography can be helpful in detecting enlarged paratracheal nodes by demonstrating lateral displacement or indentation of the superior vena cava.

In the frontal view, the paratracheal nodes are projected over the manubrium and the mesial end of the clavicle. Enlargement of the paratracheal nodes adds to the density of the shadows of these structures. This may be the only abnormal sign, even though the paratracheal nodes are of considerable size (Fig. 392). In some cases, widening of the right side of the mediastinum can be clearly demonstrated in a slight left oblique projection (10 to 15 degrees), when the findings on the frontal view are questionable. When there is discrete enlargement of the individual nodes along the paratracheal chain, the border of the mediastinum presents a scalloped outline. If the nodes are matted together, their shadows fuse to produce a single large bulge on the mediastinal contour. If the group of nodes is small, the bulge may be almost imperceptible. However, it can be clearly demonstrated on fluoroscopy, either by rotating the patient slightly or by observing elevation of the suspected area during swallowing or coughing.

A single large node or group of nodes may partially overlap the trachea in the frontal projection and suggest an intratracheal lesion. The differentiation can be made on Bucky films in which the entire tracheal lucency is more clearly visualized, or on oblique views in which the nodes are projected clear of the trachea.

The paratracheal nodes lie within the middle mediastinum and even when markedly enlarged, they rarely encroach on the anterior mediastinum to any considerable degree. In this respect, enlarged paratracheal nodes differ from thymic or teratoid tumors of the mediastinum. An intrathoracic goiter, however, may lie in the same position as the paratracheal lymph nodes, but its border is smoother, more rounded and more sharply demarcated.

Enlargement of the *left paratracheal* nodes is easily overlooked. Nodes above the aorta frequently do not appear as a well-defined mass, but simply fill in the angle between the aortic knob and the mediastinum, obscuring the mesial portion of the upper border of the knob (Fig. 466). Their presence may also be inferred if there is an increase in the density of the mesial portion of the clavicle, the manubrium, or the vertebral ends of the upper ribs on the left side. Often the border of the enlarged nodes can be visualized in a partial right oblique view even when it is not discernible on the frontal projection.

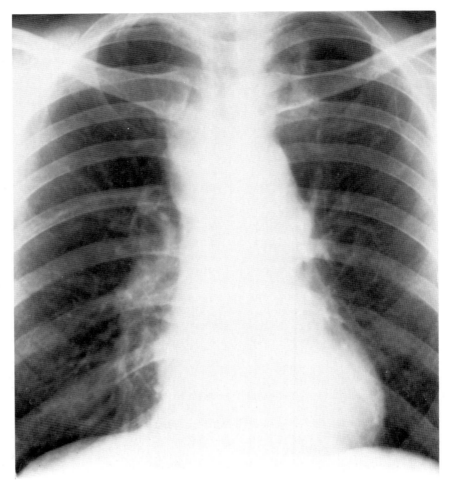

FIG. 465. HODGKIN'S DISEASE OF THE MEDIASTINUM

The shadow on the right side of the upper mediastinum is caused by large paratracheal lymph nodes. There is also a small bulge on the left border of the mediastinum immediately below the arch of the aorta, representing enlarged tracheobronchial nodes. A small scar of a healed tuberculous lesion is present at the left apex. The first rib on each side is incompletely developed. The one on the left is barely visible.

A small mass of nodes may be completely hidden by the arch of the aorta but frequently can be disclosed within the shadow of this structure on films made with sufficient penetration. A large group of nodes may extend beyond the aorta and resemble a large aortic knob, but the border is usually irregular or angulated. The aortic knob itself may be visualized within the shadow of the nodes, especially on Bucky films.

Large paratracheal nodes within the mediastinum usually do not displace the trachea. Displacement does occur when the nodes within the thoracic inlet are also enlarged. In this case, the cervical nodes, as well as those in the mediastinum, are involved.

TRACHEOBRONCHIAL NODES. Even moderately enlarged tracheobronchial lymph nodes on the right side are clearly visible on the frontal projection. These nodes appear as a small or slightly lobulated, rounded mass jutting out from the right border of the mediastinum at the tracheobronchial angle (Fig. 278). The possibility of a tumor of the anterior or posterior mediastinum is excluded by examination in the lateral view which shows the mass to be situated in the middle mediastinum overlying the trachea. It rises on swallowing and coughing.

The shadow of a node which is only moderately enlarged, is easily confused with that of a prominent azygos vein. This vein begins in the posterior mediastinum and arches forward over the right main bronchus to enter the superior vena cava. On frontal films its arch is often projected on end as an oval density in the same position as the tracheobronchial nodes. However, the long axis of the oval shadow of the vein is usually oriented downward and outward at an angle of about 45 degrees. Enlarged tracheobronchial nodes usually extend for a greater distance upward along the trachea so that their long axis tends more to the vertical. Differentiation between the shadow of the azygos vein and that of a large tracheobronchial node can frequently be made by observing the effect of the Valsalva maneuver. The shadow of an azygos vein will diminish in size during straining, while that of a node remains unchanged. Tomograms are often helpful in the differentiation. The sections may show the anterior or posterior limbs of the arch of the azygos vein whereas an enlarged lymph node appears simply as a nodule. If necessary, intraosseous venography can be utilized to opacify the azygos vein (see Fig. 514).

Lymph nodes at the left tracheobronchial angle are not visible roentgenologically unless they are quite large, because they are hidden by the

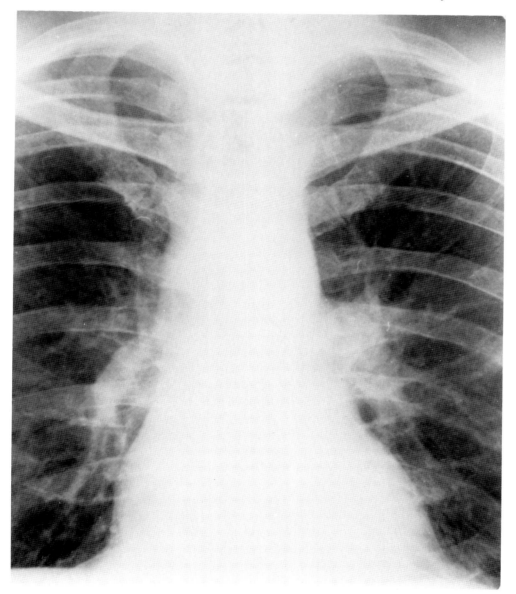

FIG. 466. ENLARGEMENT OF LEFT PARATRACHEAL NODES: HODGKIN'S DISEASE

The mediastinal shadow appears straightened. On the left side this is due to filling in of the angle above the aortic knob by a large lymph node. There is also some enlargement of the paratracheal nodes on the right side.

heart and great vessels. However, the outer border of the nodes may be seen within the shadows of these structures on adequately penetrated, or Bucky films. Only when the nodes form a large mass do they project beyond the overlying structures. Even then it is possible to confuse the shadow of the nodes with that of a prominent pulmonary artery. In such instances, the border of the main pulmonary artery may be visualized within the shadow of the nodes because the artery lies anterior to the tracheobronchial angle.

A mass of tracheobronchial lymph nodes on the left side frequently displaces the proximal portion of the left main bronchus mesially so that its course is more vertical, narrowing the angle between the main bronchi. The distal portion of the left main bronchus becomes more horizontal as it sweeps under the mass to reach the hilum of the lung (Fig. 421). This type of bronchial deformity is never produced by a large pulmonary artery, although it can be caused by an aneurysm of the arch of the aorta.

HILAR LYMPH NODES. It is difficult to identify the hilar lymph nodes radiologically unless they are considerably enlarged. Moderately enlarged nodes are easily confused with the shadows of the hilar blood vessels. Comparison of the density of the hilar shadows on the two sides is often helpful in determining the presence of unilateral hilar adenopathy. Normally the density of the hilar shadows is approximately the same on both sides. An increase in the density on one side suggests that the lymph nodes are enlarged even though the hilar shadow is of normal size. Often the enlarged nodes are better seen on the lateral view as a dense, well-demarcated shadow of considerable size (Fig. 24) even when not recognizable on the frontal projection.

The main problem in the identification of moderately enlarged hilar nodes is their differentiation from the normal blood vessels. Not infrequently the pulmonary artery on one or both sides appears as a round, nodular shadow on the frontal projection. Careful examination of adequately penetrated films will frequently show the shadow to be composed of branching blood vessels. Its vascular nature is usually best appreciated on films made in 5 to 10 degree oblique projections. In these views, the vascular shadows are uncoiled, disclosing their straight linear branchings. The same may be accomplished, in some cases, with a kyphotic or lordotic view. On the lateral view, enlarged hilar vessels do not cast as dense or sharply demarcated shadows as do large nodes.

Fluoroscopic examination is most useful in differentiating enlarged hilar nodes from vessels.

Expansile pulsations and diminution in the size of the hilar shadows during the Valsalva maneuver prove their vascular nature. Since the chest can be viewed in every conceivable angle during fluoroscopy, dissection of the vascular shadows to disclose their branches is easily accomplished.

Extreme caution should be exercised in making the diagnosis of large lymph nodes from frontal tomograms. The shadows of the blood vessels at the lung roots are magnified on these films because of the short tube to film distance. Furthermore, the branchings are often not visible because they lie in different planes. Each component of the hilar shadow should be carefully followed from section to section to discover branching that would indicate a blood vessel rather than a lymph node. In general, shadows with straight, sharp borders are more suggestive of blood vessels. On lateral tomograms, enlarged hilar vessels are projected anterior to the trachea and main bronchi while a mass of hilar nodes can extend behind as well as in front. The distinction between hilar vessels and enlarged nodes is best made from 55 degree posterior oblique tomograms (Fig. 23).

When the hilar nodes are considerably enlarged, they appear as smooth or lobulated masses at the lung roots (Fig. 344). If the nodes at the outer part of the hilum, the intercalated nodes, are enlarged, while the more central nodes are relatively unaffected, they seem to be separated from the hilum and suggest an intrapulmonary lesion. The mass of intercalated nodes may be situated directly lateral to the hilum or just above or below this region, at the root of the upper or lower lobe. The presence of such a mass indicates rather discrete involvement of the lymph nodes. This occurs particularly in sarcoidosis (Fig. 345), leukemia and infectious mononucleosis. Its occurrence in association with a bronchogenic carcinoma does not necessarily signify inoperability because the intercalated nodes can be completely removed together with the lung.

A neoplasm or localized inflammatory disease within the lung anterior or posterior to the hilum, can simulate large nodes on the frontal projection. That the lesion is located within the lung can be demonstrated in the oblique or lateral views.

SUBCARINAL NODES. Even grossly enlarged subcarinal nodes are usually not visualized on standard frontal films of the chest because the shadow of the mediastinum is not sufficiently penetrated. Like a large left atrium, a mass of subcarinal nodes can cause an increase in the density of the upper portion of the cardiac shadow and elevate the left main bronchus. The intervertebral spaces projected through the cardiac silhouette tend to be obscured in the region of the nodes, while those at a lower level remain visible. If the mass of nodes is very large, both main bronchi may be elevated, widening the angle of the tracheal bifurcation and blunting the carina. When extremely large, the nodes may project beyond the right border of the mediastinum and present as a bulge along the right side of the heart. Both main bronchi may be narrowed as a result of pressure on their lower mesial borders. These changes are particularly well delineated by tomography.

As the subcarinal nodes enlarge, they encroach on the posterior mediastinum. This is best seen in the right oblique or the lateral view. If the mass of nodes is moderate in size, the only abnormal roentgen sign may be a localized indentation on the anterior wall of the barium-filled esophagus (Fig. 467) similar to that caused by a subcarinal bronchogenic cyst. Larger nodes displace the entire esophagus posteriorly at the level of the tracheal bifurcation.

SUBAORTIC NODES. These nodes are visualized on the frontal projection only when they are quite large. They may then produce a protuberance on the left side of the mediastinum between the aortic knob and the pulmonary artery (Fig. 189). Smaller nodes can often be seen within the aortic window, especially in the left oblique projection. The entire aortic window is apt to be obscured if the nodes are large.

POSTERIOR MEDIASTINAL NODES. A large mass of matted esophageal nodes produces a shadow in the posterior mediastinum and tends to cause local displacement and distortion of the esophagus. Smaller and more discrete nodes are usually not demonstrable radiologically.

ANTERIOR MEDIASTINAL NODES. Like the posterior mediastinal nodes, these are not visualized radiologically unless they form a large mass. This is rare. Clouding of the anterior mediastinum in association with disease of the anterior mediastinal lymph nodes is practically always due to diffuse invasion of the mediastinal connective tissue rather than to the diseased nodes themselves.

INTERNAL MAMMARY NODES. Enlargement of these nodes produces a characteristic roentgen shadow on the lateral view. When the nodes are discrete, they appear as a vertical chain of scalloped shadows along the posterior border of the sternum (Fig. 468). When the nodes are matted together, they produce a thick, rind-like shadow in the same location. Large internal mammary nodes are poorly defined on the frontal view and

appear simply as a faint hazy shadow adjacent to the border of the sternum. This shadow may be localized to a small area or extend along the length of the sternum. Occasionally, all that is seen on the frontal view is an apparent increase in the density of the sternum.

PARAVERTEBRAL NODES. Moderate enlargement of these nodes may cause only lateral displacement of the paraspinal pleural reflection (Fig. 469). In the extremely rare instances when the nodes are considerably enlarged, they appear as well-demarcated paravertebral masses which simulate neurogenic tumors or extramedullary hematopoiesis.

Diseases of the Mediastinal Nodes

Tuberculosis and Histoplasmosis. While the lymph nodes are not affected in the reinfection type of tuberculosis, they are always involved secondary to the pulmonary lesion in the first infection type of this disease. This is true in adults as well as children. Since the *primary tuberculous infection* usually begins as a single focus in the lung, only the single group of lymph nodes that drains the pulmonary lesion is directly involved (Fig. 277). The infection may then spread through lymphatic channels to neighboring groups of nodes, but most often the extent of involvement of the nodes is limited. Bilateral disease of the lymph nodes, extensive enough to be visualized on the films, is unusual and when it occurs, the distribution is not apt to be symmetrical as in sarcoidosis.

If the primary lesion is in the upper lobe, the tracheobronchial lymph nodes on the same side are involved, although the infection frequently extends upward to the paratracheal nodes. Often the primary focus in the lung is not visible. The appearance then is similar to that of Hodgkin's disease (Fig. 279). However, Hodgkin's disease is rare before adolescence.

In primary tuberculosis of the middle lobe or a basal segment of the right lower lobe, the adenopathy may be confined to a small group of nodes in the angle between the middle and lower lobe bronchi. From here the infection can extend to the hilar and carinal nodes. Disease of the superior segment of a lower lobe is associated with involvement of the hilar lymph nodes. Although the carinal nodes are frequently diseased regardless of the location of the primary focus, they are rarely large enough to be visible on ordinary films.

In *histoplasmosis* also, the lymph nodes are affected together with the pulmonary parenchyma (Fig. 260). However, unlike primary tu-

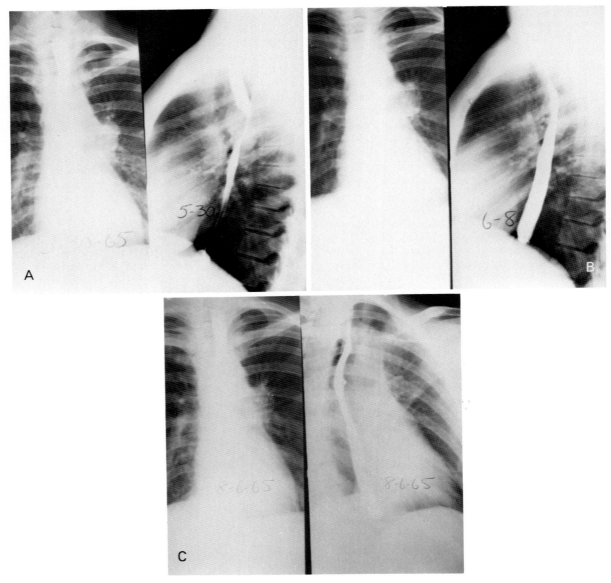

FIG. 467. DEVELOPMENT OF ESOPHAGEAL DIVERTICULUM

A: May 30, 1965. The conventional film shows a mass at the root of the left lung. Because the patient had dysphagia, an esophagram was performed. The esophagus is indented by a mass at the level of the carina. *B:* June 8, 1965. Shortly before scheduled bronchoscopy and esophagoscopy, the symptoms disappeared. The hilar mass remains unchanged. However, the indentation on the esophagus is no longer present. The sequence of events is indicative of extrusion of a diseased lymph node into the esophagus. The tuberculin test was negative and the histoplasmin skin test positive. *C:* August 6, 1965. The mass at the left root is smaller and a "traction" diverticulum has appeared at the point where the node perforated into the esophagus.

berculosis, this disease frequently begins with multiple pulmonary foci. The lymphadenopathy, therefore, is not so apt to be confined to a single group of nodes. Bilateral lymph node enlargement is not infrequent. Otherwise, the manifestations and complications of the nodal involvement in the two diseases are the same.

A common complication of lymphadenitis in

both tuberculosis and histoplasmosis is spread of the infection to the pleura overlying the mediastinum with consequent thickening of the pleura or an effusion. The latter is usually small and frequently is demonstrable only in the lateral decubitus position. If suppuration occurs, the lymph nodes enlarge rapidly and produce a well-demarcated bulbous protrusion from the mediastinum, simulating neoplastic disease. Suppuration in the subcarinal region causes an appearance similar to that of a subcarinal bronchogenic cyst.

Direct extension of the disease from the lymph nodes to the bronchial wall often results in bronchostenosis with atelectasis or obstructive emphysema. Atelectasis is most common in the upper or middle lobes. Nodes that occlude the upper lobe bronchus can also cause partial obstruction of the intermediate or lower lobe bronchus, thus producing atelectasis of the upper lobe together with obstructive emphysema of the remainder of the lung. As the disease resolves, the obstruction is usually relieved, but a permanent stricture can remain. Perforation of a caseous or suppurating subcarinal node into the esophagus results in a so-called traction diverticulum (Fig. 467). If the node perforates into a bronchus as well, a bronchoesophageal fistula is established.

The caseous nodes in tuberculosis or histoplasmosis have a tendency to calcify (Fig. 143). Calcification often occurs earlier and is more extensive in the lymph nodes than in the primary lesion in the lung. Large deposits of calcium usually consist of a number of concretions which impart a characteristic speckled appearance to the shadows of the nodes. Broncholithiasis results from involvement of a bronchus by a caseous node which undergoes calcification.

Other Infections. Although the hilar lymph nodes are usually enlarged and edematous in viral and bacterial pneumonias, they rarely attain sufficient size to be recognized radiologically.

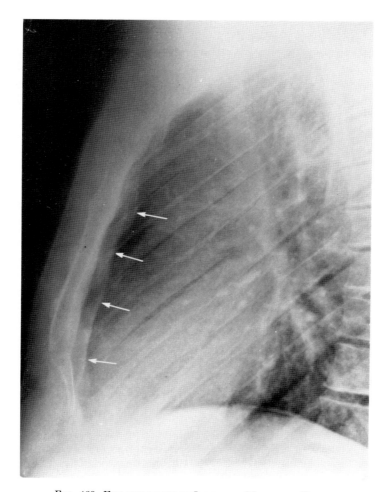

FIG. 468. ENLARGEMENT OF INTERNAL MAMMARY NODES

A lateral film of a patient with Hodgkin's disease shows a band-like scalloped shadow (arrows) immediately behind the sternum. This picture is caused by involvement of the internal mammary nodes and the internodal connective tissue. The anterior mediastinum is clouded because of infiltration of the connective tissue by the neoplasm, a common finding in this disease.

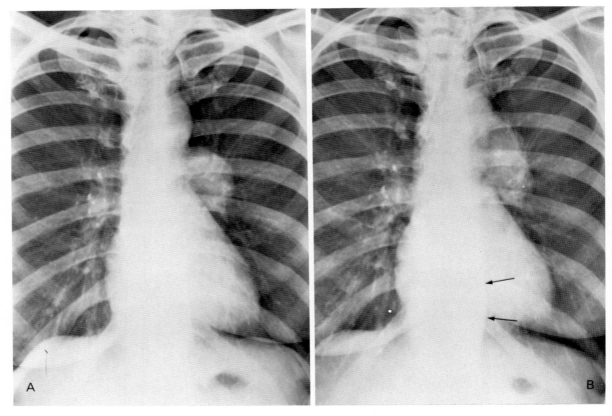

FIG. 469. LYMPHOSARCOMA

A: The mass at the left hilum was first noted on a film when the patient had an acute upper respiratory infection. A presumptive diagnosis of bronchogenic cyst was made and no treatment was instituted. *B:* Ten months later. The mass has increased in size and now involves the subaortic nodes as well as the hilar nodes. In addition, an outward bulge of the left paraspinal line (arrows) has appeared, indicating enlargement of the paravertebral lymph nodes. The diagnosis of lymphosarcoma was proved by biopsy of an axillary node.

Occasionally, slight enlargement of the lymph nodes is noted in children with nonspecific pneumonia but the nodes recede quickly as the pneumonia resolves. Considerable enlargement of the nodes occurs in the suppurative lymphadenitis associated with acute interstitial streptococcal pneumonia (Fig. 235). The nodes tend to become matted together as a result of periadenitis, and when an entire chain is involved, the mediastinal shadow may be diffusely widened.

Marked enlargement of the mediastinal nodes frequently accompanies the pneumonic form of tularemia. Large nodes may also be visible in several of the fungal infections of the lung but, except in histoplasmosis and coccidioidomycosis, they are not a prominent feature. Occasionally, large nodes are seen in infectious mononucleosis. These nodes have a tendency to be discrete and produce comparatively small, well-localized protuberances on the border of the mediastinum. Enlargement of intercalated nodes produces a circumscribed nodule at the root of a lobe. Rare causes of enlargement of the mediastinal nodes encountered in this country are leprosy, trypanosomiasis and syphilis.

Sarcoidosis. Enlargement of the mediastinal lymph nodes is a prominent feature of most cases of sarcoidosis at some stage of the disease. When the nodes are enlarged several groups are almost always involved in symmetrical fashion. The nodes tend to remain discrete so that each group presents as a separate, well-demarcated mass. The most characteristic picture is that of enlargement of the nodes at each hilum (Fig. 344). This symmetry rarely occurs in other diseases. In addition, the paratracheal nodes are often enlarged, but may be visible only on the right side.

When, as is frequently the case, the nodes become extremely large, the shadows of the various groups tend to merge to form a lobulated mass extending from the thoracic inlet to the lower part of the lung root on each side. Marked enlargement of the subcarinal nodes is more commonly due to sarcoidosis than any other inflammatory disease. Despite the extensive lymph node involvement, the lateral view shows the anterior mediastinum to be clear. This is due to the paucity of nodes in this region and the fact that sarcoidosis does not involve the thymus or the mediastinal connective tissue to any significant degree. In this respect it differs from many cases of Hodgkin's disease or bronchogenic carcinoma.

Most often the nodes in sarcoidosis regress spontaneously. Recurrent enlargement is then rare. However, if the regression is induced by drugs, the nodes may enlarge again when treatment is discontinued. Unlike tuberculosis and histoplasmosis, calcification of the nodes is not a feature of sarcoidosis.

Pneumoconiosis. Enlargement of the mediastinal lymph nodes is noted particularly in berylliosis and in silicosis. Although the lymph nodes are involved in other forms of pneumoconiosis, they are rarely large enough to be visualized on roentgen films.

Enlargement of the mediastinal and bronchopulmonary lymph nodes is a common feature of the acute stage of berylliosis. The nodes may remain enlarged in the chronic stage of the disease (Fig. 335) but more frequently they regress when the acute phase subsides.

In silicosis the lymph node enlargement occurs gradually and does not become manifest for many years. Once the nodes are enlarged, they never become smaller. The silicotic nodes are rarely sharply outlined on the films because their borders are obscured by the fibrosis in the overlying lung. They are evidenced, as a rule, by an increased density and enlargement of the shadows of the hilum and the mediastinum. Eventually calcification takes place in many of the nodes. In some cases the calcification occurs predominantly in the periphery of the nodes, producing a characteristic eggshell appearance, rarely encountered in any other disease (Figs. 142 and 320).

Benign Lymph Node Hyperplasia (Castleman's Disease). Castleman's disease is characterized by the development of a circumscribed mass of lymphoid tissue which is usually encapsulated and has the structure of a large lymph node with well-developed follicles. Apparently the disease is not inflammatory since the lesions always consist of a single nodule, unassociated with any abnormality of the adjacent lymph nodes or lung. The lesion is certainly not malignant, since its growth is limited, it may not increase in size for many years, it does not infil-

trate or produce metastases and, once removed, it does not recur. Whether or not it represents simple lymphoid hyperplasia, a benign neoplasm, or a hamartoma, has not been established. The fact that 60% of the reported cases have been found in patients between 15 and 30 years of age favors the possibility of hamartoma.

The disease is essentially symptomless and is usually detected on chest films as an incidental finding. Although, in the majority of cases, one of the paratracheal, tracheobronchial or hilar lymph nodes has been the seat of the disease, atypical locations are not uncommon. The lesions have been noted in the costovertebral gutter, the anterior mediastinum and in the internal mammary nodes.

Radiologically, the lesion appears as a single, round or oval, well-demarcated, homogeneous density (Fig. 470). Since the tumor represents diffuse enlargement of a single node, its margin is rarely lobulated. The masses are usually of moderate size but have been reported up to 16 cm in diameter. When situated anteriorly, the nodule can simulate a thymoma, and it is possible that the tumor develops within the thymus itself. A large hyperplastic node, situated in the costovertebral gutter, can have an appearance identical to that of a neurofibroma and may cause pressure atrophy of adjacent ribs and vertebrae.

A large, intercalated lymph node at the root of the lung or one of the lobes has been found in about one-fourth of the reported cases. On the frontal film the mass is then separated from the mediastinum and resembles a neoplasm of the lung. However, on the lateral view, the density is projected across the position of the fissures at the root of the lung. The lack of conformity to an anatomic division of the lung suggests that the lesion is extrapulmonary.

If the tumor is very large, it can indent the esophagus, displace the trachea or even cause compression of a main bronchus. Focal areas of calcification have been detected on pathologic examination, but no evidence of calcification has been noted on the films.

Lymphomas. It is usually impossible to differentiate the various types of lymphoma of the mediastinum, with any degree of certainty, from their radiologic appearance alone. However, the x-ray picture may suggest the proper diagnosis because the individual diseases tend to differ in their manner of growth, their distribution and their predilection for certain age groups.

Certain characteristics are common to all lymphomas and help to differentiate them from other diseases of the mediastinal nodes. In general, the lymphomas are radiosensitive, and the

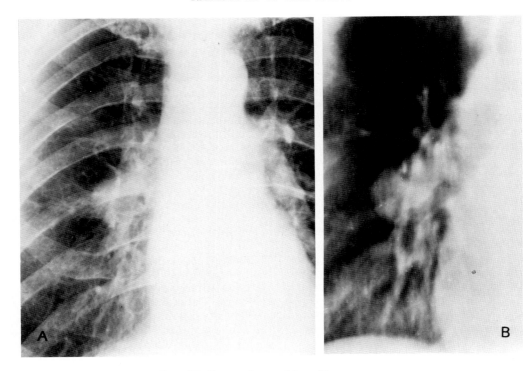

FIG. 470. BENIGN LYMPH NODE HYPERPLASIA

A: The round nodule at the root of the right lung produced no symptoms and was first detected at a routine x-ray examination. *B:* The tomogram shows the nodule to have a sharply demarcated, regular border, and to be separate from the intermediate bronchus and the pulmonary artery. It is impossible from these films to be certain whether the lesion is situated in the lung or represents a large hilar lymph node. Thoracotomy disclosed a single, large lymph node immediately behind the root of the lung. The microscopic examination revealed the characteristic pattern of Castleman's disease.

masses diminish rapidly in size following moderate doses of radiation. This distinguishes them from most metastatic carcinomas, which usually respond only to large doses. However, anaplastic and small-cell bronchogenic carcinomas behave more like lymphomas in this regard. The presence of a large spleen suggests lymphoma rather than carcinoma. Enlargement of the spleen should be suspected if the gastric air bubble is displaced mesially or if the left leaf of the diaphragm is elevated in the absence of a large air bubble in the stomach or a distended splenic flexure. Although the lymphomas are invasive and produce large masses in the mediastinum, involvement of the phrenic nerve is extremely rare. This is in contrast to other primary malignant mediastinal tumors and bronchogenic carcinomas, which not infrequently cause paralysis of the diaphragm.

HODGKIN'S DISEASE. The majority of cases of Hodgkin's disease become manifest between the ages of 20 and 40. Onset before the age of puberty or after the age of 60 is rare. The most common picture of the disease in the early stages shows mainly enlargement of the right paratracheal

lymph nodes (Fig. 465). Another characteristic form of Hodgkin's disease is caused by more diffuse involvement of the paratracheal nodes, producing symmetrical widening of the mediastinum which is delimited by rather straight, vertical borders (Fig. 466).

As the disease progresses, the tracheobronchial, hilar and subcarinal nodes may become involved in continuity. This produces a large, lobulated mass projecting from one or both sides of the mediastinum (Fig. 471). Enlargement of the tracheobronchial or hilar nodes without concomitant enlargement of the paratracheal nodes is unusual. Symmetrical enlargement of the lymph nodes at the lung roots, even in association with enlarged paratracheal nodes, such as occurs in sarcoidosis, is rare (Fig. 472).

The large, lobulated mass projecting outward from the upper mediastinum is frequently associated with diffuse clouding of the retrosternal space on the lateral view (Fig. 473). This is usually due to extension of the growth beyond the nodes, diffusely invading the connective tissue and matting together the anterior mediastinal structures. Such extension throughout the

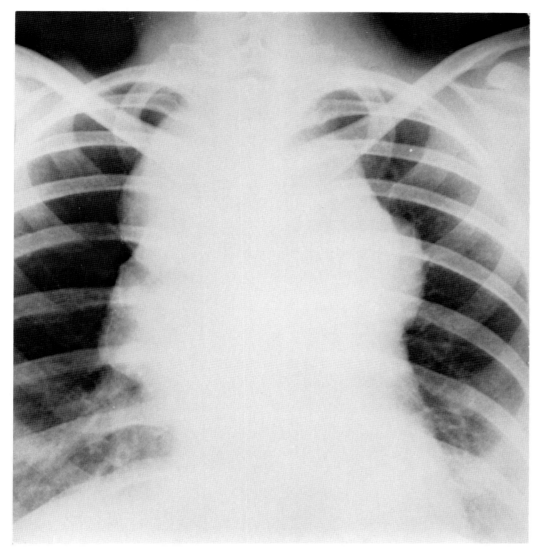

FIG. 471. HODGKIN'S DISEASE

The mediastinum in this young female is markedly widened by a huge lobulated mass projecting from both sides. The appearance is typical of matted groups of enlarged lymph nodes and is characteristic of a lymphoma. On the lateral view, the anterior mediastinum was uniformly clouded, indicating invasion by the tumor. This is very unusual in lymphosarcoma and is rather common in Hodgkin's disease.

connective tissue in the anterior mediastinum is characteristic of Hodgkin's disease in contradistinction to lymphosarcoma. The presence of large lymph nodes in association with diffuse clouding of the anterior mediastinum in patients below the age of 50 is indicative of Hodgkin's disease. Over this age, the combination is more suggestive of bronchogenic carcinoma.

A more unusual cause of obliteration of the anterior mediastinal space in Hodgkin's disease is involvement of the thymus (Fig. 24). This can occur in the absence of any lymph node involve-

ment or with only minor enlargement of the nodes, not visible roentgenologically. The appearance, then, is identical with that of a thymoma (Fig. 474). When Hodgkin's disease is completely confined within the capsule of the thymus gland, the entire lesion can be removed surgically. Involvement of the thymus gland does occur occasionally in lymphosarcoma, but almost exclusively in children.

Hodgkin's disease may extend from the anterior mediastinum directly into the sternum. At first, only the cortex on the posterior aspect of

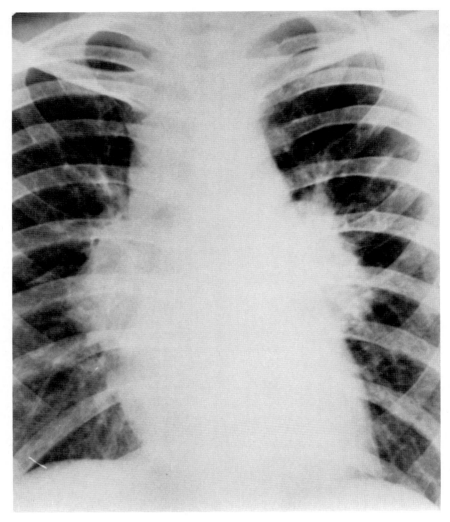

FIG. 472. HODGKIN'S DISEASE: SYMMETRICAL LYMPH NODE ENLARGEMENT

The nodes at both hila are markedly enlarged and are matted together to form irregular masses. Their borders are indistinct because of infiltration of the adjacent lung. The widening of the right side of the mediastinum and the obliteration of the aortic knob on the left indicate bilateral enlargement of the paratracheal nodes. The appearance is identical with that of sarcoidosis except for the agglutination of the nodes and perinodular pulmonary infiltration.

the bone is destroyed. As the disease extends, the anterior cortex is also eroded and a bulge may appear in the soft tissues of the anterior chest wall. It is also possible for the sternum to be involved primarily, rather than by extension through the mediastinum. Extension of the disease through the posterior surface of the sternum can produce a localized, spindle-shaped mass protruding into the anterior mediastinum, or a band-like density immediately behind the sternum leaving the remainder of the anterior mediastinum clear. A similar broad density or a series of scalloped shadows in the retrosternal region can also be produced by enlargement of the internal mammary chain of nodes (Fig. 468).

Involvement of the sternum and the retrosternal tissues can be easily overlooked if the x-ray beam is not directed tangential to the sternum. It is therefore essential that the patient be placed in a true lateral position with the tube centered on the anterior chest wall.

Neither necrosis nor hemorrhage occurs spontaneously within the mediastinal lesions in Hodgkin's disease. Therefore, there is no tendency for deposition of calcium if the lesions are undisturbed. On the other hand, we have observed calcification after biopsy of an anterior mediastinal mass in this disease, and calcification following radiotherapy is not unusual (Fig. 475). It is conceivable that similar calcification might occur after chemotherapy. In treated cases the calcium has occurred as an irregular deposit, ranging up to 3 cm in diameter, situated in the anterior mediastinum. The appearance is similar to calcification in a thymoma or a lymph node. When calcification has been observed in untreated cases, it has invariably occurred within nodes alongside the trachea or at the hilum and represented the residuum of unrelated inflammatory disease, most probably tuberculosis or histoplasmosis. If a calcific deposit is seen within a mass in the anterior mediastinum in an untreated patient, a thymoma or a teratoma should be suspected rather than Hodgkin's disease.

Pleural effusions are usually a late complication of Hodgkin's disease and are often bilateral. They may be due to direct involvement of the pleura or simply to blockage of the lymphatics within the mediastinum. In the latter instance the effusion can disappear when only the mediastinal lymph nodes are treated. Spread to the pericardium is common as a terminal event. While the pericardial effusion is usually small, it can attain considerable size. Resorption can follow irradiation or chemotherapy.

Involvement of the bones of the thoracic cage or of the spine occurs with or without disease of the mediastinal nodes. The lesions may be either osteolytic or osteoblastic or a combination of both. A characteristic manifestation of Hodgkin's disease is dense sclerosis of a single vertebra.

When the lesion is predominantly lytic, the vertebral body may collapse. The roentgen appearance differs from that of Pott's disease in that the adjacent intervertebral disc spaces are maintained.

LYMPHOSARCOMA. In contradistinction to Hodgkin's disease, lymphosarcoma is more likely to produce a single large mass in the mediastinum (Figs. 100 and 476) than enlargement of individual groups of nodes. Lymphosarcoma tends to involve the nodes alone without extensive invasion of the surrounding tissues (Fig. 469). Since most of the nodes lie in the middle mediastinum, the disease rarely causes clouding of the anterior mediastinum. When the anterior mediastinum is involved by lymphosarcoma, the disease appears to be situated within the thymus gland. The condition is really lymphosarcoma of the thymus. It occurs particularly in children and is rare in adults.

Follicular lymphoblastoma, which may be considered a form of lymphosarcoma, has a greater tendency to involve separate groups of lymph nodes. In this respect it behaves more like Hodgkin's disease. However, there is no predilection for involvement of the right paratracheal nodes.

RETICULUM CELL SARCOMA. In most cases of reticulum cell sarcoma the x-ray picture cannot be distinguished from Hodgkin's disease. Discrete enlargement of the nodes at each lung root, similar to Boeck's sarcoid, is more common in

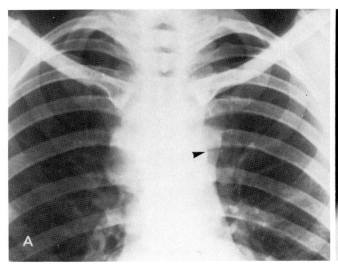
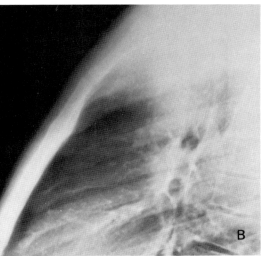

FIG. 473. HODGKIN'S DISEASE

A: The lobulated mass projecting from both sides of the mediastinum does not obliterate the contour of the aortic knob (arrow) and, therefore, is situated anteriorly. The differential diagnosis lies between a malignant thymoma or teratoma and Hodgkin's disease. A rhomboid notch is present on the undersurface of each clavicle. *B:* Lateral view. The upper portion of the anterior mediastinum is clouded from the manubrium to the trachea. The latter is displaced backwards. The indistinctness of the lower margin of the mediastinal shadow favors the diagnosis of Hodgkin's disease.

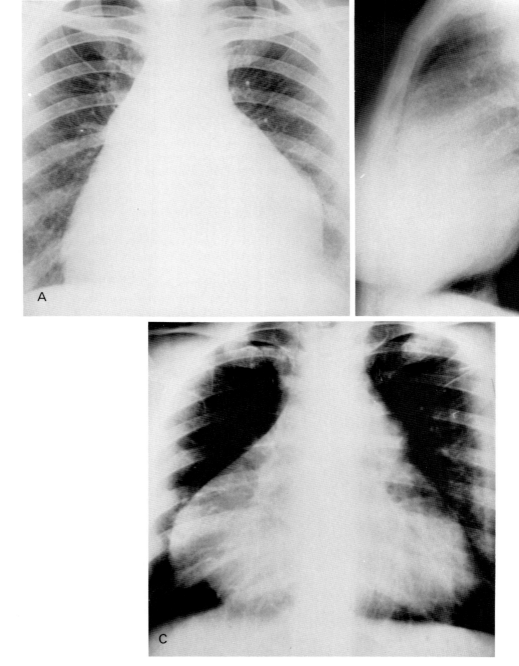

FIG. 474. HODGKIN'S DISEASE OF THE THYMUS

A 35 year old, asymptomatic female was referred because of a large mediastinal mass found on routine x-ray examination. It was considered to be a pericardial cyst. *A:* Frontal view. There is a large, sharply outlined mass involving both sides of the mediastinum. On the right it is seen as a localized protuberance at the level of the third rib anteriorly. On the left the mass extends beyond the border of the heart. The upper border of the mass is too high for a pericardial cyst and, furthermore, bilateral pericardial cysts are extremely rare. *B:* The lateral view shows the mass to fill almost the entire anterior mediastinum. The roentgen diagnosis lies between a tumor of the thymus, a mediastinal lymphangioma, and a teratoma. *C:* Lordotic view. A sharp notch is now visualized between the mass and the right cardiac border. This is characteristic of a large thymus gland. At operation the thymus was found to be enormous. Histological examination of the gland and a few adjacent lymph nodes showed Hodgkin's granuloma. The patient had a course of radiotherapy and is well 12 years later without any other treatment.

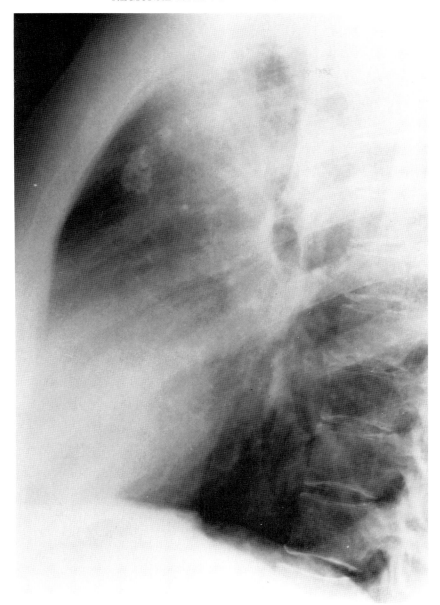

FIG. 475. CALCIFICATION IN HODGKIN'S DISEASE
Several irregular calcific deposits are present in the anterior mediastinum. The mediastinum was irradiated several years previously for Hodgkin's disease. There is no evidence of recurrence of the disease.

reticulum cell sarcoma than in Hodgkin's. A large mass of nodes, or a chain of enlarged paratracheal nodes may be present in Ewing's sarcoma. However, in this disease there is practically always detectable bone involvement by the time the lymph nodes become enlarged.

Leukemia. The lymph nodes of the mediastinum are often involved in leukemia, but only rarely are they large enough to be seen on the roentgen film. Detectable enlargement of the nodes is more common in lymphatic leukemia than in myeloid leukemia. In chronic lymphatic leukemia, which is more common in the older age group, the characteristic picture is that of discrete masses of nodes on both sides of the mediastinum. When these affect the hilar nodes in symmetrical fashion, the appearance is indistinguishable from sarcoidosis or reticulum cell sarcoma (Fig. 477).

In children, acute lymphatic leukemia may be

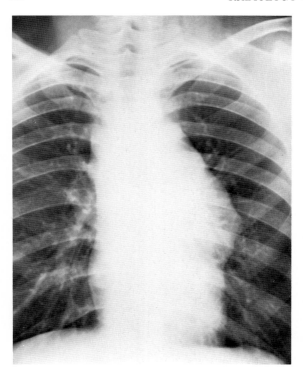

FIG. 476. LYMPHOSARCOMA OF THE MEDIASTINUM

There is a large, irregular mass protruding from the left side of the mediastinum, and a small bulge in the right paratracheal region. On the frontal view alone the appearance cannot be distinguished from a tumor of the thymus. However, the lateral view showed the retrosternal space to be clear.

atelectasis or infiltration of the lung is present to indicate the pulmonary origin of the disease.

Metastases to the mediastinal lymph nodes are frequently found at postmortem examination in patients with a distant neoplasm, but usually the nodes are of insufficient size to be seen roentgenologically. On occasion, the mediastinal nodes become considerably enlarged. This happens particularly with carcinoma of the breast, larynx, thyroid and scirrhous carcinoma of the gastrointestinal tract. A hypernephroma can be responsible for extensive enlargement of the mediastinal lymph nodes, and this may be the first outward manifestation of the disease.

There is no characteristic pattern of involvement of the lymph nodes by metastatic neoplasm. Most often only a single group of large nodes is demonstrable radiologically even though the nodes throughout the mediastinum are involved. In the case of carcinomatous lymphangitis of the lungs secondary to extrapulmonary disease, the lymph nodes at each hilum may be enlarged. More or less extensive involvement of the internal mammary nodes occurs characteristically from carcinoma of the breast.

THYMUS

The thymus gland is situated in the anterior part of the upper mediastinum, immediately behind the sternum. The normal thymus is not visualized on conventional films in the adult, and even when it is hyperplastic or the seat of a tumor it may not be demonstrable without special studies. In infants, however, the normal thymus occupies a relatively greater portion of the chest and often forms a recognizable component of the mediastinal shadow.

Thymus in Infancy. There is a great variation in the size of the normal thymus during the first 2 years of life. It may be quite small and invisible on the chest film or it may be so large that it suggests a tumor of considerable size. Usually the thymus in the infant causes a widening of the shadow of the upper mediastinum obscuring the outline of the other mediastinal structures. The shadow of the gland extends to both sides of the mediastinum in about half of the cases, usually projecting more to the right than to the left. In the remainder the thymic shadow is usually seen only on the right. Rarely does it present solely on the left.

Most often the shadow of the thymus has straight vertical borders. When large, the thymus tends to bulge outward into the pulmonary field in convex fashion. The shadow may then simulate a mediastinal tumor or cyst. The thymic

manifested by a large mass extending out from both sides of the mediastinum. The borders of the mass are usually lobulated, but when they are straight the appearance is that of a diffusely widened mediastinum. A similar large mass in the anterior mediastinum, perhaps involving the thymus gland, has been noted in acute myeloid leukemia, particularly in adolescents (Fig. 478). The mediastinal mass in acute leukemia is extremely radiosensitive, and even very large ones can disappear within a few days after the onset of treatment.

A large mass composed of leukemoid cells may be present in the anterior mediastinum with few or no abnormal white cells in the peripheral blood. Because the pathologic characteristics are suggestive of a malignant neoplasm, this condition has been classified as leukosarcoma.

Metastatic Neoplasms. Metastatic involvement of the mediastinal lymph nodes occurs most frequently with the infiltrating type of bronchogenic carcinoma. The involved nodes may be so large that they completely overshadow the primary tumor in the lung. Usually, however,

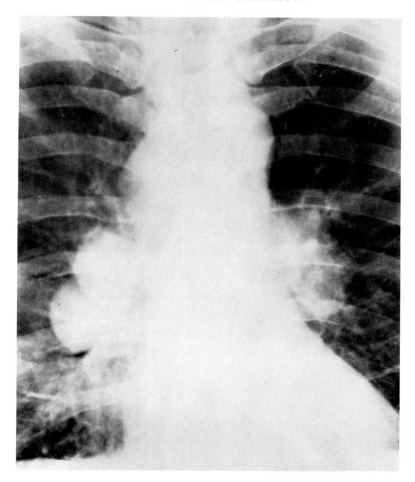

FIG. 477. LYMPHATIC LEUKEMIA

The right paratracheal lymph nodes and the hilar nodes on both sides are enlarged. The discreteness and sharp demarcation of the shadows in the right hilum and their extension into the pulmonary field indicate that they represent intercalated nodes. While this is most commonly seen with sarcoidosis, it also occurs in leukemia.

shadow is more prominent during expiration and appears particularly large after a deep expiration, as at the end of a prolonged cry. In exceptional cases the entire hemithorax can then be opacified. A large thymus displaces the trachea backward but does not compress the organ and rarely displaces it laterally.

The large thymus occasionally has an undulating or wavy border (*thymic wave sign*) (Fig. 479). It results from bulging of the thymic tissue into the spaces between the anterior ribs. This sign serves to differentiate the shadow of the thymus gland from that of a mediastinal cyst. However, it does not exclude an infiltrative disease of the thymus, such as lymphatic leukemia.

The lower part of the thymus spreads over the heart, and its inferior border tends to produce a sharp notch where it meets the cardiac shadow. The angular silhouette of the lower portion of

the gland has been likened to that of a sail (Fig. 480). This *sail sign* is pathognomonic of the thymus gland. It is best seen in the lordotic (Fig. 474) or oblique projections (Fig. 45). The thymic notch is usually evident only on films made during complete inspiration.

In the absence of a thymic notch or a wave sign, it may be difficult to differentiate between a prominent thymus gland and some other mass in the mediastinum, such as a cyst or neoplasm, or the vascular shadow produced by anomalous pulmonary venous drainage into the left innominate vein. Reexamination after a period of corticosteroid therapy may solve this difficulty. Steroids, in adequate dosage, usually cause notable shrinkage of the thymus within a week or 10 days. It is important to reexamine the patient soon after the steroid treatment is completed because the thymus can regenerate within a few

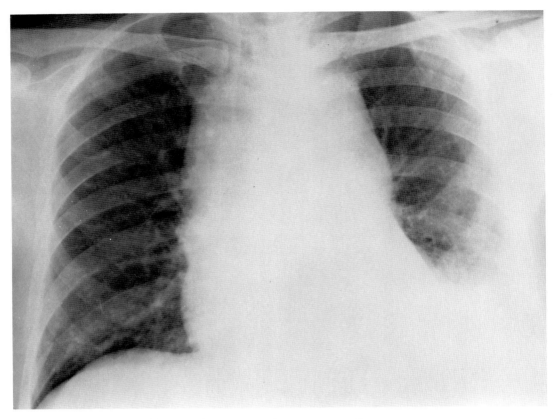

Fig. 478. Mediastinal Involvement in Leukemia

The large mass involving both sides of the mediastinum cannot be differentiated from Hodgkin's disease or lymphosarcoma. This patient had acute myelogenous leukemia. There is an effusion in the left pleural cavity, most likely due to obstruction of the mediastinal lymphatics or to complicating pulmonary infarction.

days. Of course, it is essential that the films be made in the same phase of respiration as the ones before the treatment.

The shadow of the thymus gland is often altered in the presence of a *pneumomediastinum*, which may cause a problem in roentgen interpretation. The air in the mediastinum forces the mediastinal pleura outward and separates one or both lobes of the thymus from the heart. The thymus is displaced upward and outward and produces a shadow which can simulate atelectasis of the upper lobe (Fig. 481). If the shadow of the thymus does not extend to the lateral chest wall, it resembles the shape of a spinnaker sail (Fig. 440). This may be the only indication of pneumomediastinum on the frontal projection. Differentiation from upper lobe atelectasis is more difficult when the gland reaches the lateral chest wall. The diagnosis of pneumomediastinum with displacement of the thymus as a cause of the shadow then depends upon examination in the lateral view. This must be done either in the erect position or with the infant supine, directing

the x-ray beam across the table in order to demonstrate the air in the anterior mediastinum.

Hyperplasia of the Thymus. Visualization of the thymus in the adult indicates that it is abnormal. Diffuse enlargement of the gland is most often due to hyperplasia. This may occur as an isolated abnormality, but is commonly seen in association with myasthenia gravis and, occasionally, with hyperthyroidism, Addison's disease or acromegaly.

The large thymus separates the anterior lappets of the upper lobes of the lungs, displacing them laterally. Since it is these lappets that produce the area of radiolucency behind the sternum on the lateral view, it is understandable that the retrosternal space in this projection should become clouded when the thymus is enlarged. When the thymus is hyperplastic the entire anterior mediastinal space is clouded uniformly and the anterior border of the ascending aorta is obscured (Fig. 482).

While a moderately enlarged thymus is usually apparent on the lateral view, even a considerably

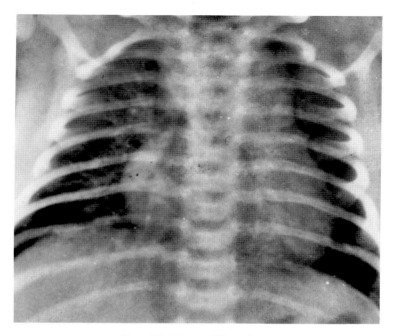

FIG. 479. THYMIC WAVE SIGN

The frontal film of a newborn infant shows a mass involving both sides of the superior mediastinum. The left side of the mass has an undulating border. The indentations correspond to the crossing of the anterior ribs. This picture is pathognomonic for a large thymus.

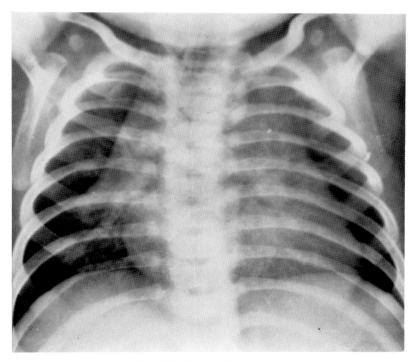

FIG. 480. THYMIC SAIL SIGN

The frontal film of an infant shows a large shadow extending from each side of the mediastinum. The lower part of the shadow on the right side ends abruptly, creating the appearance of a sail. This is pathognomonic for a large thymus gland and is normal in infancy.

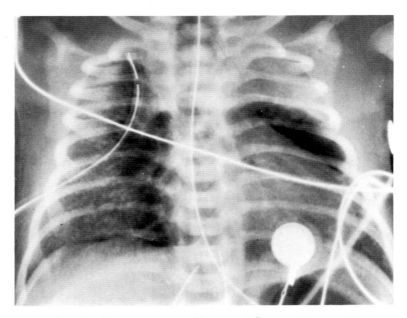

FIG. 481. DISPLACEMENT OF THYMUS BY PNEUMOMEDIASTINUM

Portable film of a newborn with hyaline membrane disease. The homogeneous shadow in the upper part of the left chest, at first thought to represent an atelectatic left upper lobe, really represents the left lobe of the thymus displaced laterally by the air in the mediastinum. The right lobe of the thymus is also displaced but it is considerably smaller than the left lobe. The lucent zones on either side of the heart are caused by the pneumomediastinum. The granular appearance of the right lung and the air bronchogram are typical of hyaline membrane disease.

enlarged gland may be overlooked on the frontal projection. The shadow of the thymus can be quite faint in this view, and may cause only a straightening of one or both borders of the superior mediastinum. Because the aortic knob is situated posteriorly, its shadow can be seen within the straight mediastinal border caused by the enlarged thymus gland. Even when the mediastinal shadow is not widened, an increase in its density should lead to the suspicion of a mediastinal mass. The entire superior mediastinum may be abnormally dense or there may be only an increased opacity of one or both sides of the manubrium.

When the thymus is large, it usually projects outward from both sides of the mediastinum, although the shadow is more evident on the right side. When the gland is very large and its lobes extend to the diaphragm on both sides, its borders run obliquely downward and outward. The gland then overlies the heart and its shadow obscures the cardiac silhouette. The contour of the shadow then simulates a pericardial effusion. However, the shadow extends beyond the upper limits of the pericardial sac. The pericardial reflection is situated below the level of the aortic knob so that widening of the mediastinal shadow above this excludes a simple pericardial effusion.

The thymic notch, or sail sign, occurs in adults as well as children. However, in the adult it signifies a hyperplastic rather than a normal thymus. The hyperplastic thymus often produces considerable posterior displacement of the trachea and may even cause posterior bowing of this organ. Nevertheless, it does not cause displacement to either side. In this respect the hyperplastic thymus differs from many other mediastinal tumors.

Thymic Cysts. In the adult, a cyst of the thymus is almost always due to hemorrhage or necrosis in a thymoma. In children, thymic cysts are practically always developmental in origin, although some have been considered inflammatory in nature because of an occasional association with congenital syphilis. The cysts may be extremely large and extend to the diaphragm. They may project to either side of the mediastinum. When situated on the right side, the thymic cyst obscures the right border of the heart. Because of its smooth, sharp outer border and its location in the anterior mediastinum, it cannot be differentiated radiologically from a dermoid cyst, a more common lesion in children.

In adults, regardless of whether the cyst is developmental or acquired, it cannot be differentiated radiologically from a thymoma (Fig. 483).

Thymoma. A considerable proportion of thymomas are malignant, but it is often difficult to differentiate them from the benign ones, even on microscopic examination. The benign thymoma is completely encapsulated. Extension of the tumor through the capsule indicates that it is malignant even though the histologic appearance is that of a perfectly benign growth. Because of the difficulty in determining whether a thymoma is malignant, the tumor should never be considered benign on clinical grounds. Either a benign or a malignant thymoma may undergo necrosis and hemorrhage, changes which lead to calcification and cyst formation (see Fig. 487).

The malignant tumors spread locally and only rarely metastasize to the mediastinal nodes or distant organs. Frequently they grow through the overlying parietal pleura and invade the adjacent lung, sometimes producing paralysis of the diaphragm by direct invasion of the phrenic nerve. Involvement of the pericardium is common, especially as a terminal event. Often tumor cells drop into the pleural cavity and form implants on the surface of the lung or on the parietal pleura.

About three-quarters of thymomas occur in patients with myasthenia gravis. Association with other diseases is unusual. However, thymomas have been found in about 50% of cases of aregenerative erythrocytic anemia and, to a lesser extent, in acquired hypogammaglobulinemia. Cases associated with Cushing's syndrome have been described.

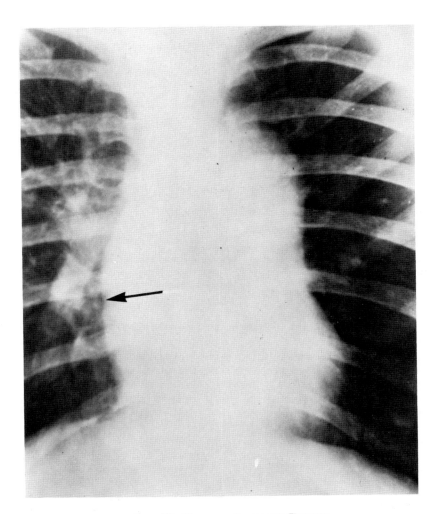

FIG. 482. HYPERPLASIA OF THE THYMUS

A: A routine film of a 17 year old male shows a dense, homogenous shadow over the upper two-thirds of the mediastinum. On the left side, this obscures the main pulmonary artery. On the right side of the mediastinum, there is a sharply outlined bulge which forms a notch (arrow) where it meets the cardiac border. The notch is characteristic of an enlarged thymus.

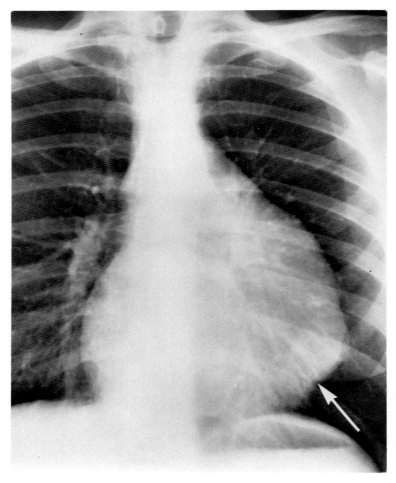

FIG. 483. THYMIC CYST

The pear-shaped shadow on the left side is situated in the anterior mediastinum and therefore obliterates the cardiac contour. A notch is seen on the undersurface of the shadow where the border of the mass joins that of the left ventricle (arrow). The mass extends to the level of the aortic knob. It is impossible to differentiate between a large thymus and a dermoid cyst. At operation this proved to be a single thymic cyst filled with limpid fluid.

Most thymomas are located in the upper two-thirds of the mediastinum, but they may be situated as low as the diaphragm, especially on the right side (Fig. 484). In general, benign thymomas are not fixed and are displaced to one side of the mediastinum. When a thymoma appears on both sides, it indicates that it is adherent within the mediastinum, suggesting that it is malignant (Fig. 485). However, since a malignant thymoma may not be infiltrative from its inception, it can appear on only one side of the mediastinum, like a benign thymoma. Paralysis of the diaphragm in association with a thymoma is due to invasion of the phrenic nerve and indicates that the tumor is malignant (Fig. 486).

On the frontal projection a thymoma appears as a sharply demarcated, round or lobulated density projecting from the mediastinum into the pulmonary field. Those that have an irregular border are usually malignant (Fig. 487). When a malignant thymoma infiltrates the lung, part of its border may become poorly demarcated.

Some thymomas produce only a small bulge on the mediastinum. This is easily overlooked when it is projected over the pulmonary artery or azygos vein, or when it is overshadowed by the aorta.

In some cases the border of the thymoma is not visualized on the frontal view and the tumor may cause only an increase in the density of the shadow of the sternum or transverse processes of the spine on one side.

The lateral view is essential whenever a thymoma is suspected. It may disclose clearly a small thymoma which cannot be visualized at all on the frontal projection (Fig. 488). The lateral view also serves to demonstrate the fact that the mass is situated in the anterior mediastinum, distinguishing it from a variety of mediastinal tumors that occur more posteriorly.

When a thymoma is small, its entire circumference is usually well outlined in the lateral view. The upper border of a large tumor in the upper part of the mediastinum may be poorly demarcated, while it is well delineated in tumors situated at a lower level. In some instances the entire substernal space is diffusely clouded as in the case of a hyperplastic thymus (Fig. 489). Since simple hyperplasia of the thymus is unusual in old people with myasthenia gravis, diffuse clouding of the anterior mediastinum in these patients is usually due to a thymoma.

Frequently the lateral view discloses posterior displacement or posterior bowing of the trachea. The observation of such displacement or distortion should always suggest the possibility of a lesion of the thymus. The thymoma is practically always seen to touch the sternum on films made in a true lateral position. Although, on occasion, a thymoma does not abut on the sternum, the possibility of some other lesion, such as an aneurysm of the ascending aorta or a peripheral carcinoma of the lung should be the first consideration when a space is seen between the sternum and an anterior mediastinal mass.

Calcification does not occur in a diffusely hyperplastic thymus and, when present, is indicative of a thymoma. The calcium is frequently demonstrable in malignant as well as benign thymomas. Most commonly it appears as one or more irregular, amorphous, dense, patchy shadows within the tumor. This type of calcific

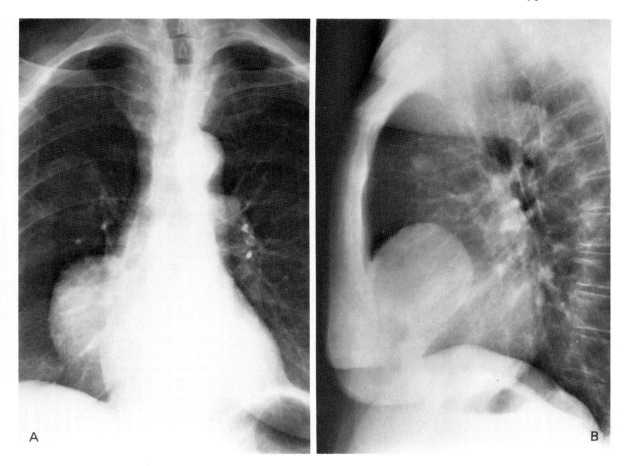

FIG. 484. LOW LYING THYMOMA

A: A sharply demarcated mass abuts on the heart and obliterates part of the right cardiac contour. *B:* The lateral view confirms the anterior position of the mass. The sharply demarcated posterior border excludes a pericardial cyst from consideration. Although tumors of the thymus gland are usually in the upper part of the mediastinum, such a low position is not rare.

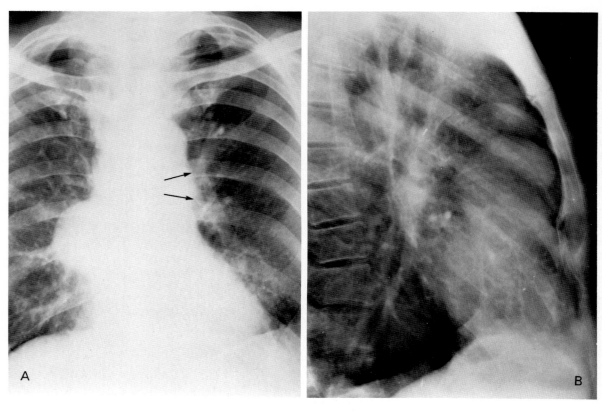

FIG. 485. MALIGNANT THYMOMA

A: The frontal film shows a well-circumscribed semicircular density with a smooth border projecting from the right side of the mediastinum. The right border of the heart is obliterated, indicating that the mass is situated anteriorly. The appearance is compatible with a benign thymoma. However, the left side of the mediastinum is also involved. The border of the mass (arrows) is superimposed upon the shadow of the left pulmonary artery. Presentation of a thymoma on both sides of the mediastinum is indicative of malignancy. *B:* The lateral view shows two distinct lobulations of the tumor. The upper one corresponds to the mass seen on the left side of the mediastinum. Marked irregularity of the mass is also indicative of a malignant tumor.

shadow is quite characteristic of thymoma (Fig. 489), although, in rare instances, it is encountered in mediastinal teratomas, in Hodgkin's disease following treatment, and in substernal thyroid adenomas. Curvilinear densities on the periphery of the growth are indicative of calcification of the capsule. They are usually confined to a limited area on the surface of the tumor, and only rarely completely encircle the growth as in some dermoid cysts. More commonly a ring-like density occurs within the substance of a thymoma. This is due to calcification in the wall of a cystic cavity formed as a result of local necrosis in the tumor (Fig. 487). A similar type of annular shadow can be seen in a thyroid adenoma in the periphery of which calcium has been deposited.

Pleural implants occur either spontaneously or following resection of a malignant thymoma. The implants may appear several years after the operation even though there is no local recurrence

of the tumor in the mediastinum (Fig. 490). Frequently the implants take the form of flat, plaque-like masses which may be difficult to visualize radiologically, and often are invisible unless they lie in a plane tangential to the x-ray beam. When observed on end, the pleural implants appear as one or more sharply demarcated, scalloped shadows along the inner border of the chest wall (Fig. 486). When seen *en face,* their shadows are faint and their borders indistinct. If the implant is situated on either the anterior or the posterior bend of the ribs, its mesial border is sharply demarcated on the frontal projection, while the lateral border fades off imperceptibly.

Implants on the diaphragm are often overlooked even when quite large, because the normal diaphragm frequently has a scalloped appearance (Fig. 490). They should be suspected when the scallops appear irregular. The shadows produced by the implants are usually best delineated on the lateral view. Despite the tendency of malignant thymoma to spread to the pleura, an effusion is uncommon except in the late stages. Similarly, pericardial effusions are quite rare, although the pericardium is frequently invaded.

ECTOPIC THYMOMA. In rare instances, thymomas develop in ectopic thymic tissue and are found in various locations in the thorax outside the anterior mediastinum. They have been described in the middle mediastinum, within the lung, or in the extrapleural tissues. Ectopic thymomas have been encountered in the form of a solitary nodule in the lung, a scalloped shadow bulging from the chest wall into the pleura, and as a tumor near the lung root. The possibility of an ectopic thymoma should be borne in mind whenever a mass is seen anywhere in the chest of a patient with myasthenia gravis when the anterior mediastinum is clear. However, the condition is so rare that it should not be considered in the absence of myasthenia.

THYMOMA AND MYASTHENIA GRAVIS. About 75% of patients with a thymoma, either benign or malignant, have evidence of myasthenia gravis. The symptoms of myasthenia may be minor and go unnoticed unless special attention is called to this possibility by the finding of a tumor in the anterior mediastinum. Conversely, a thymoma may be small and overlooked unless attention is focused on the anterior mediastium because the patient has myasthenia. About 15% of patients with myasthenia gravis have a thymic tumor.

The symptoms of myasthenia often regress after removal of a thymoma, only to reappear at a later date, even though there is no recurrence of the growth. Occasionally, return of the myasthenic symptoms is associated with the development of pleural implants which are demonstrable radiologically. In some cases, symptoms of myasthenia gravis first appear a considerable time after complete removal of a thymoma. Out of 30 patients reported by Osserman and Genkins, without evidence of myasthenia when a thymoma was removed, six subsequently developed distinct manifestations of the disease.

Other Abnormalities of the Thymus. Several other pathologic conditions can be associated with enlargement of the thymus. Lymphosarcoma of the thymus appears to occur almost exclusively in children, and may be limited to this organ. It causes generalized enlargement of the gland which may fill the entire anterior mediastinal space and displace the trachea back-

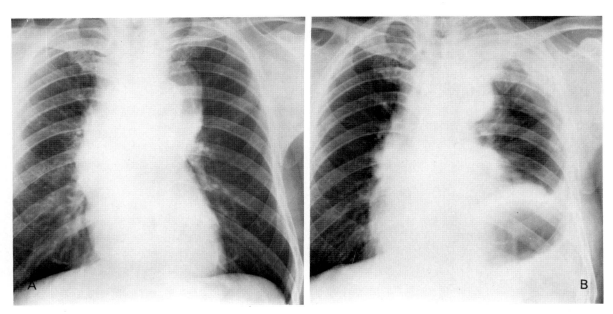

FIG. 486. MALIGNANT THYMOMA

A: There is a mass in the superior mediastinum extending more to the left than the right. It does not obliterate the silhouette of the aortic knob, indicating that the mass is situated anteriorly. Needle biopsy proved it to be a thymoma. Because of its extension to both sides ot the mediastinum it was considered most likely that the tumor was malignant. *B:* Ten months later. The mediastinal mass has become smaller following radiotherapy. However, scalloped shadows, representing pleural metastases, are present over the left upper lobe and the diaphragm. The left costophrenic sinus is obliterated by a small effusion. Marked elevation of the left leaf of the diaphragm is due to paralysis from invasion of the phrenic nerve by the growth.

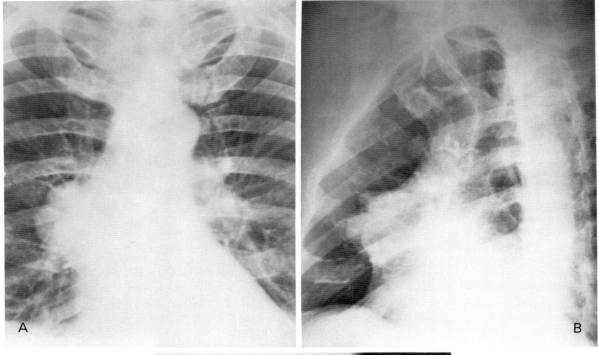

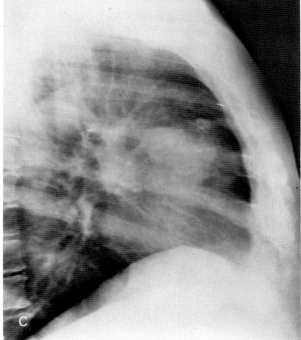

FIG. 487. CALCIFICATION IN MALIGNANT THYMOMA

A: The frontal film of a 51 year old male shows a lobulated mass at the right border of the mediastinum. The right border of the heart is obliterated, indicating that the lesion is situated anteriorly. Whether the mass originates in the mediastinum or the lung cannot be determined from this view. *B:* Left oblique projection. The shape of the lesion in this view is more suggestive of a mediastinal tumor, most probably a thymoma. The marked irregularity of the border indicates that it is, in all probablility, malignant. *C:* The lateral view shows a ring-like calcific density within the anterior portion of the mass. This type of calcification in the mediastinum is practically always due to hemorrhagic necrosis in a thymoma. It can occur in malignant as well as in benign thymomas. Operation disclosed a malignant thymoma which invaded the adjacent portions of the upper and middle lobes.

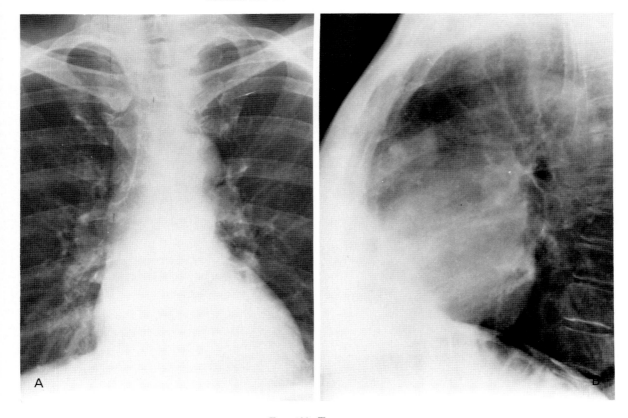

FIG. 488. THYMOMA

A: The frontal film of this patient with myasthenia gravis shows no abnormality. *B:* The lateral view reveals a well-circumscribed density immediately behind the sternum. The appearance is characteristic of a thymoma.

ward. Involvement of the thymus by Hodgkin's disease is much more common, but occurs during or after adolescence. Clouding of the anterior mediastinum in Hodgkin's disease is usually due to infiltration of the thymus in association with more generalized involvement of the lymphatic system. Only rarely is the disease limited to the thymus gland and then cannot be differentiated from a thymoma or a teratoma of the anterior mediastinum. In fact, some teratomatous tumors of the anterior mediastinum may actually arise from the thymus gland.

Acute leukemia in children and adolescents may be associated with dense infiltration of the thymus by immature white blood cells. The gland can be markedly enlarged but retains its shape and presents as a symmetrical shadow on both sides of the mediastinum. It may exhibit the thymic wave sign. The shadow can disappear within a few days after the institution of radiotherapy.

A local nodule of moderate size, representing benign lymphatic hyperplasia (Castleman's disease), may be present in the thymus. Radiologically, it cannot be distinguished from a thymoma.

Diffuse enlargement of the thymus may result from hemorrhage within the gland. This occurs occasionally in children following thoracotomy through a sternum splitting incision. The shadow disappears within a few weeks as the hematoma is absorbed.

Technical Considerations. Thymic tumors are not evident in the frontal projection in fully 25% of the cases. However, most of them can be seen on the lateral view, even when quite small. During this exposure the patient's arms should be in a vertical position so that no part of the anterior mediastinum is obscured. If the arms cannot be raised to this degree, they should be dropped and folded behind the back and the shoulders squared in order to clear the anterior mediastinum.

A true lateral projection is required to determine the exact relationship of a mediastinal shadow to the sternum. A hyperplastic thymus and most thymic tumors abut upon this bone. When the films are made at a distance of less than 6 feet, it is best to direct the central ray to the sternum. If the tube is centered over the middle of the chest, as is the usual practice, a

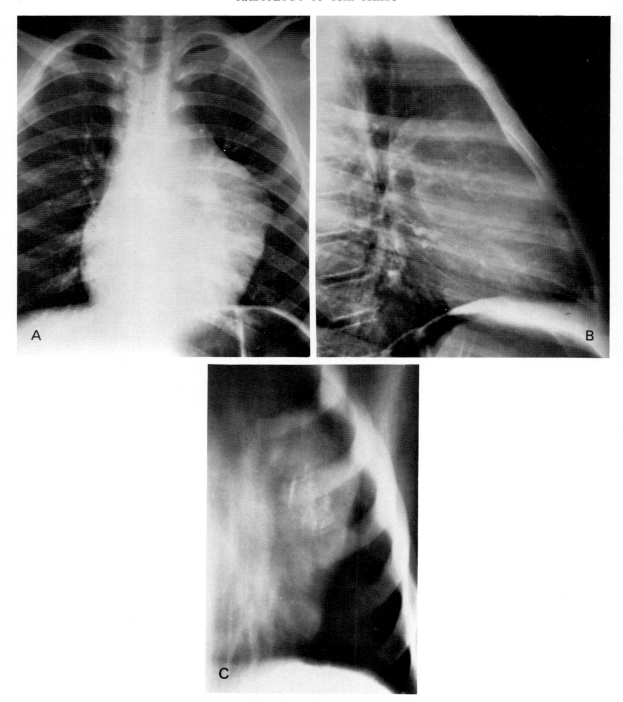

FIG. 489. CALCIFICATION IN BENIGN THYMOMA

A: The frontal film of a 14 year old asymptomatic boy shows a sharply demarcated, lobulated mass in the left side of the mediastinum. The mass obliterates the left cardiac border, indicating that it is situated anteriorly. The arch of the aorta and the pulmonary artery are visualized within the shadow of the mass. *B:* Lateral view. The anterior mediastinum is diffusely clouded by the tumor which contains two irregular areas of calcification. *C:* The frontal tomogram shows the calcium to be deposited in small patches. The anterior portions of the ribs are sharply outlined, indicating that this is an anterior section.

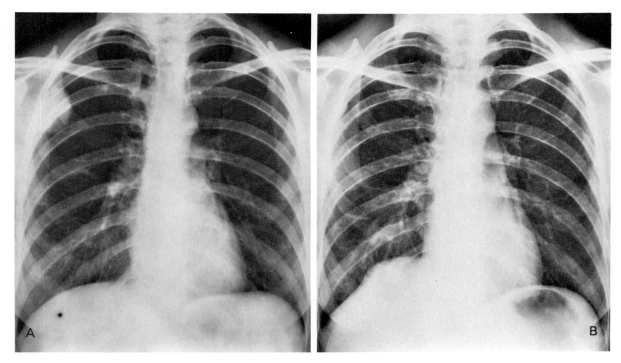

FIG. 490. MALIGNANT THYMOMA: PLEURAL IMPLANTS

A: Six years after removal of a thymoma, thought to be benign histologically, a solitary pleural mass is seen over the right upper lobe. At thoracotomy, in addition to this lesion, there were multiple flat nodules, all of which involved the parietal pleura. There was no evidence of recurrence of the tumor in the mediastinum. A right pleurectomy was performed. *B:* Three years later there is a localized bulge on the right diaphragmatic contour. At a single examination this would be considered to represent a local eventration. However, the diaphragm had a normal contour on previous films. This proved to be another pleural implant.

true picture of the retrosternal space is not obtained. Care should also be taken in the choice of exposure factors because the shadow of a hyperplastic thymus may be lost on an overexposed film, while on an underexposed film even the normal anterior mediastinum frequently appears clouded.

Oblique films are useful when there is a question regarding clouding of the anterior mediastinum on the lateral projection. In the oblique view, an anterior mediastinal mass is projected lateral to the middle mediastinal structures, so that it is well outlined against the air-containing lung. A partial oblique view, 15 to 30 degrees, is usually best, but the optimum degree of obliquity for the demonstration of the tumor can be determined by fluoroscopy. This view is often required, particularly in the adult, to disclose the thymic notch which is diagnostic of a hyperplastic thymus. The notch is also demonstrable on the lordotic view and on frontal films made in the supine position, but is revealed most strikingly in the lordotic oblique projection (Fig. 474).

Although calcific deposits in the thymus gland are usually best seen on the lateral view, particularly when a Bucky grid is used, the oblique views are helpful in determining whether the calcium is really within the thymus. Oblique views are also useful for the recognition of thymic implants on the pleura, not visible on the frontal and lateral views.

Fluoroscopic observation during swallowing can aid in the diagnosis of myasthenia gravis. Persistent puddling of barium in the vallecular spaces, with prompt emptying after administration of Tensilon or a drug with similar action, constitutes strong evidence of myasthenia gravis. Dysphagia is common in myasthenia, although there is no organic obstruction of the esophagus even when the thymoma is extremely large.

Lateral tomography is indicated whenever the other studies are inconclusive. It is important that midline sections be obtained, centering over the sternum. Sections made more laterally may give the erroneous impression of a clear space between the sternum and the mediastinal mass.

Pneumomediastinography discloses the thymus very clearly (Fig. 24). However, it is rarely required for the diagnosis of thymic disease, and can be dangerous in the presence of myasthenia.

THYROID

The normal thyroid is not visualized on films of the chest. However, hyperplastic or adenomatous goiters, even though situated entirely within the neck, are frequently seen on the frontal film. They often seem to be within the chest because the anterior part of the base of the neck is projected below the posterior portions of the upper ribs. Actually, the plane of the thoracic inlet is tilted forward so that the anterior boundary between the neck and the chest is at the level of the clavicles and jugular notch. Since the thyroid is an anterior structure, it is entirely cervical if it does not extend beneath the clavicle and the upper border of the sternum.

When the enlarged gland extends through the thoracic inlet, it is known as a cervicomediastinal thyroid. If the goiter lies completely within the chest and is connected with the neck only by a narrow stalk, it is called an intrathoracic or mediastinal goiter. An ectopic or aberrant thyroid is one that develops within the chest without any connection with the cervical region. It receives its blood supply from vessels in the mediastinum rather than from the thyroid axis.

Cervical Goiter. A hyperplastic thyroid or one which is enlarged by bilateral adenomas usually casts a faint haze over the mesial portion of the supraclavicular space on each side of the trachea. Large goiters cast a denser shadow which is more clearly delineated. In the case of unilateral adenomas or where the adenomas predominate on one side, the trachea is displaced and often shows a distinct curve with the convexity to the opposite side (Fig. 519). At first glance all that may be noted is displacement of the trachea. On closer inspection a hazy density can usually be seen in the mesial portion of the supraclavicular space even when the exact border of the goiter cannot be visualized. Sometimes there is only an apparent increase in the density of the mesial portion of the ribs above the clavicle.

Cervicomediastinal Goiter. This form of goiter results from extension of a large cervical thyroid down through the thoracic inlet. Most often it enters the anterior mediastinum (substernal thyroid). Occasionally it descends into the posterior portion of the mediastinum behind the esophagus. In rare instances, part of the gland lies between the esophagus and trachea. The mediastinal component is usually more

apparent than the cervical portion. On the frontal film it appears as a homogeneous density with a smooth, curved border, projecting outward from the superior mediastinum. Most often the mass appears confined to the right side. Even when the goiter presents on both sides of the mediastinum, it is apt to be more prominent on the right because the arch of the aorta and the great vessels interfere with its extension to the left. Similarly, an adenoma arising from the left lobe of the thyroid is often deflected to the right side as it descends into the mediastinum.

On the lateral view, the mediastinal portion of the goiter is usually situated immediately behind the sternum and displaces the trachea backward. In some instances, the goiter descends alongside the trachea and does not cause posterior displacement. When the adenoma descends in the posterior mediastinum, the esophagus and trachea are displaced forward (Fig. 491). In the rare instances in which the goiter insinuates itself between the trachea and esophagus, the structures become separated by the mass which bows the trachea forward and displaces the esophagus backward (Fig. 492).

As the goiter traverses the thoracic inlet, it exerts pressure on the structures within this confined space, displacing and occasionally narrowing the trachea and esophagus (Fig. 493). No matter whether the mediastinal portion is situated anteriorly or posteriorly, the trachea and esophagus are almost always displaced to one side because the anteroposterior diameter of the superior thoracic aperture is so narrow. The esophagus, being more mobile, is usually displaced to a greater degree. The deviation of the trachea by a cervicomediastinal goiter differs from that caused by a purely cervical thyroid. In the latter the trachea is displaced only in the neck and returns to the midline at the thoracic inlet. When the goiter extends into the chest the tracheal displacement continues into the mediastinum (Fig. 234).

Often the cervical portion of the goiter is not clearly visualized on the film but its presence may be inferred from the displacement of the trachea or the esophagus in the neck. Displacement of the trachea without evidence of disease in the adjacent lung is usually due to a large thyroid. Marked displacement of the trachea by a large cervicomediastinal goiter is often associated with tracheal compression, sometimes sufficient to cause respiratory difficulty. Paradoxically, the trachea may be displaced toward the mediastinal mass. This occurs only in the case of a large adenoma arising from the left lobe of the

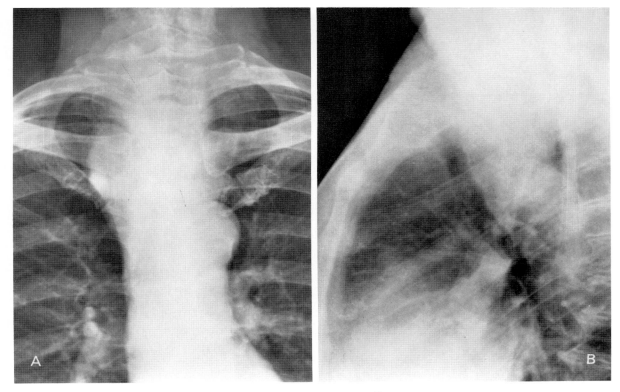

FIG. 491. CERVICOMEDIASTINAL GOITER

A: The upper border of the mass on the right side of the mediastinum fades out above the level of the clavicle, indicating that it is situated anteriorly. Because the tumor lies within the thoracic inlet, the trachea is displaced to the left. This picture is characteristic of a cervicomediastinal thyroid. *B:* Lateral view. The mass does not occupy the retrosternal space as in the usual form of cervicomediastinal goiter. In this case the thyroid adenoma has descended behind the trachea and displaces it forward.

thyroid. The goiter extends to the right side of the mediastinum because of the intervention of the aorta, and carries the trachea with it.

After the removal of a substernal thyroid, one may be greatly surprised to note that the shadow in the superior mediastinum persists. However, if attention is directed to the trachea, it is noted that this organ is no longer displaced laterally (Fig. 493). The reason for the persistence of the shadow is the presence of a dead space filled with blood and exudate in the bed from which the thyroid was removed. The dead space exists because the negative pressure in the pleura on either side of the mediastinum draws the walls of the thyroid bed outward. The mediastinal shadow disappears in a few weeks, when the blood and exudate within the space absorb.

Since the thyroid is attached to the trachea, it rises together with this structure and the larynx during the act of swallowing. Even a large cervicomediastinal thyroid rises on deglutition. Ex-

ception to this rule is rare and is encountered only when the mediastinal thyroid is situated posteriorly and becomes impacted in the thoracic inlet. This is usually associated with compression of the superior vena cava. It does not occur with a substernal thyroid because this type of goiter is situated anteriorly where there is room for it to rise. Therefore, an anterior mediastinal mass which remains stationary on swallowing should be considered to represent another type of tumor rather than a goiter.

Intrathoracic Goiter. This form of goiter also arises in the neck but descends completely into the mediastinum, being attached to its point of origin only by a narrow stalk which contains its vascular supply. There is, therefore, no displacement of the trachea at the root of the neck. Because the stalk permits relatively free movement of the mass, the latter tends to move away from the sternum and swing laterally alongside the trachea. As in the case of other movable

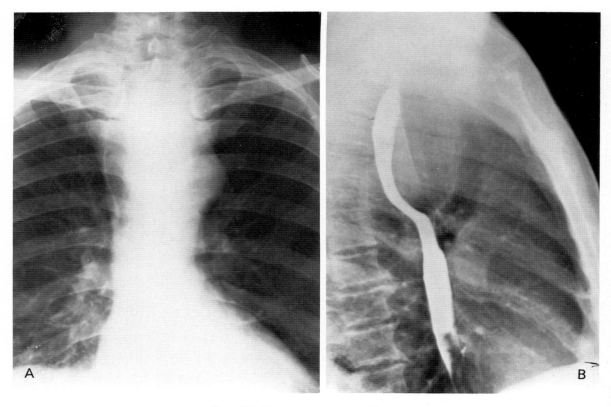

FIG. 492. CERVICOMEDIASTINAL GOITER

A: The lower part of the cervical trachea and the entire intrathoracic trachea are displaced to the right by a large mass. On the left side, the mass protrudes from the mediastinum and has a smooth, round contour. The appearance is characteristic of a cervicomediastinal goiter, although in rare instances it can be seen with a cystic hygroma. *B:* The esophagus has been displaced posteriorly while the trachea is bowed forward by the mass which proved to be an adenoma of the left lobe of the thyroid.

mediastinal tumors, it usually presents on the right side. Occasionally it descends behind the trachea or esophagus and then is more fixed.

On the frontal view, the intrathoracic goiter presents as a sharply circumscribed, semicircular mass similar to that of a cervicomediastinal goiter. The trachea may be displaced within the thorax but not in the neck or in the thoracic inlet (Fig. 494) unless an additional goiter is present within the portion of the gland remaining in the neck. On the lateral view, the mass is practically always projected over the trachea and is separated from the sternum. Because of its attachment in the neck, the intrathoracic goiter rises on swallowing except in the rare case when it is impacted behind the trachea.

Difficulty may be experienced in differentiating an intrathoracic goiter from an aneurysm of the aorta or a tortuous innominate artery. This difficulty can be resolved by angiography. However, care must be taken in interpreting the angiograms because goiters are often extremely

vascular and may be opacified by the contrast material.

Ectopic Thyroid. Thyroid tissue can develop ectopically in the chest whether or not there is a thyroid in the neck. The vascular supply of the aberrant thyroid is derived from neighboring vessels instead of the thyroid axis. Ectopic thyroids that are visualized radiologically are extremely rare, and are practically always the seat of goiterous change.

The ectopic thyroid may be situated almost anywhere in the mediastinum. The great majority lie in the superior mediastinum, but they have been described as low as the diaphragm. They may be situated in relation to the trachea, as in the case of ordinary goiters, but many are separated from this organ and therefore do not rise on swallowing. Some are located anteriorly in relation to the pericardium. These differ from substernal goiters in that there is no component in the thoracic inlet, and from intrathoracic goiters by their location near the sternum. Posteriorly an ectopic thyroid may lie between the trachea and the esophagus or further back, behind the esophagus.

Calcification. A considerable proportion of thyroid adenomas contain one or more calcific deposits. Characteristically, the calcium is laid down in the periphery of an area of necrosis and hemorrhage, and produces a ring-like or eggshell-shaped shadow (Fig. 495). More flocculant, irregular, dense shadows may also be produced by areas of calcification. When the characteristic shadow of thyroid calcification is found in the neck, it may be concluded that the patient has a thyroid tumor, most probably an adenoma, and that an associated shadow in the mediastinum represents either a cervicomediastinal or an intrathoracic goiter. Ring-like calcifications in the mediastinum also occur in thymomas, and in the mediastinal lymph nodes in silicosis.

A collection of numerous, small, round, faint calcific densities are sometimes encountered in carcinoma of the thyroid. These are similar in appearance to the psammoma bodies that occur within a carcinoma of the ovary. When seen in the neck, they are diagnostic of thyroid carcinoma. Because the shadows are faint, soft tissue technique is usually required to demonstrate them clearly. Tomography may possibly disclose this type of calcification when the tumor of the thyroid is situated in the mediastinum.

Carcinoma of the Thyroid. Only a small percentage of thyroid carcinomas can be differentiated from benign goiters radiologically. Thyroid carcinoma is more apt to produce obstruction of the trachea because of its tendency to invade the tracheal wall. A portion of the carcinoma may actually grow through the tracheal wall to present as a sharply demarcated intraluminal mass. This can usually be seen on oblique or lateral projections but may be clearly demonstrated on Bucky films or tomograms in the frontal projection as well.

Cervicomediastinal or intrathoracic thyroid carcinomas may differ from benign goiters by irregularity of their borders or by unusual lobulations. The presence of one or more ring-like calcifications within the thyroid mass does not exclude the possibility of a carcinoma. It is not

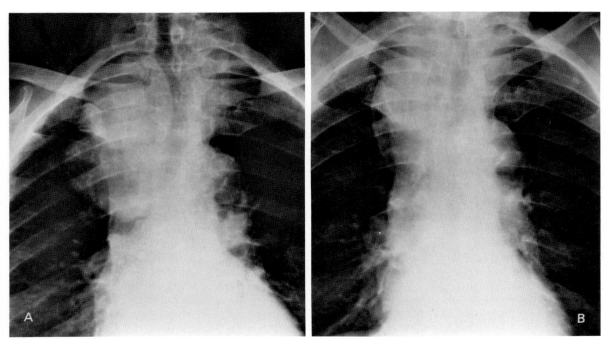

FIG. 493. SUBSTERNAL THYROID

A: There is a large mass on the right side of the mediastinum. The trachea is displaced to the left in the thoracic inlet, indicating that the mass is also present in the root of the neck. The displacement of the trachea makes the diagnosis of a substernal thyroid almost certain. *B:* Although the substernal thyroid had been removed 9 days previously and the wound closed without packing, the shadow on the right side of the superior mediastinum has diminished very little in size. However, the trachea has returned to the midline. The mediastinal shadow is caused by an accumulation of blood and exudate in the dead space within the bed of the enucleated gland. The trachea returned to its normal position because there was no longer a solid mass to displace it.

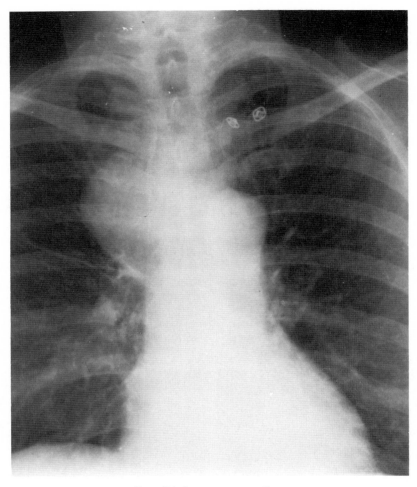

FIG. 494. INTRATHORACIC GOITER

The well-circumscribed mass in the right paratracheal region displaces the thoracic portion of the trachea to the left. However, the trachea in the neck and within the thoracic inlet is in its normal position. Fluoroscopic examination showed the mass to rise on swallowing. An I¹³¹ scan was positive. At operation, the thyroid adenoma was found to derive its blood supply from the neck through a long, thin pedicle.

unusual for the carcinoma to occur in a gland that has been the seat of one or more adenomas for many years during which there has been ample opportunity for calcification to occur.

PARATHYROID

Parathyroid masses which are large enough to be recognized radiologically represent neoplasms rather than simple hyperplasia. Most of them are adenomas. Only about 7% of adenomas of the parathyroid have been situated partly or wholly in the mediastinum. The remainder, which are confined to the neck, are not visualized directly on the roentgenogram, but may displace the esophagus and trachea.

A mediastinal parathyroid adenoma can orig-

inate in the neck and drop into the mediastinum because of its weight and the negative intrathoracic pressure. It may also originate in the mediastinum, in an aberrant gland.

The inferior parathyroids develop from the third branchial cleft, usually coming to rest in the posteroinferior portion of the lateral lobes of the thyroid. Occasionally, they descend into the anterior mediastinum together with the thymus gland.

Mediastinal parathyroid adenomas have been reported up to 12 cm in size, but most are much smaller, averaging 3 to 4 cm in diameter. The majority lie partly in the neck, and even those that are completely in the mediastinum are confined to the upper part of this region. About two-thirds are situated anteriorly.

Most of the adenomas cannot be visualized on conventional films. When the adenoma is large, it may present on the frontal film as a mass projecting outward from the mediastinum, usually to the right. Its outer border is curved and sharply demarcated, but its superior margin often merges with the shadows of the neck. On the lateral view, the mass is most frequently observed in the uppermost part of the anterior mediastinum like a substernal thyroid, but it may lie somewhat lower, like a thymoma. A sizable parathyroid can displace the trachea backward. An adenoma situated posteriorly usually lies in front of the vertebral column and pushes the trachea and esophagus forward. When the adenoma lies between these two or-

gans, the trachea is bowed forward and the esophagus is displaced backward. In any case, the tumor usually causes lateral displacement as well. Although cystic changes occur in parathyroid adenomas, calcification has not been described.

ESOPHAGUS

Most esophageal lesions do not produce any abnormality on films made without the aid of a contrast medium. Only the diseases of the esophagus associated with shadows in the mediastinum or the lungs will be discussed.

Perforation. Perforation of the esophagus into the mediastinum results in infection of the

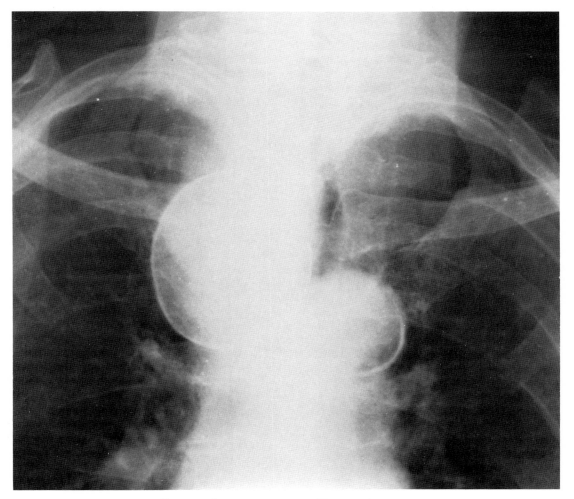

FIG. 495. CERVICOMEDIASTINAL THYROID ADENOMA

The sharply circumscribed mass with a fine calcific rim, on the right side of the superior mediastinum, extends above the level of the clavicle. The trachea is displaced to the left, indicating that the mass is situated anteriorly and lies within the thoracic inlet. The dense curvilinear shadow on the left side of the mediastinum represents calcification within the aortic knob. The irregular thickening of the apical pleura on both sides is the result of an old, healed tuberculosis.

mediastinal tissues and is usually associated with pneumomediastinum. The mediastinal shadow is widened more or less symmetrically. Within the shadow, irregular longitudinal streaks of air are often seen. In some cases the parietal pleura is displaced away from the mediastinum and is represented by a fine, sharp, more or less vertical line like that seen in mediastinal emphysema from other causes. In these instances, air may be seen in the soft tissues at the root of the neck (Fig. 496). In other cases the roentgen film shows the localized bulge of a mediastinal abscess, with or without a fluid level. When the perforation occurs in the lower part of the esophagus, a fusiform shadow is visible behind the heart on films made with adequate exposure, and this may simulate an aneurysm of the descending aorta or a Pott's abscess.

Perforations of the upper part of the esophagus produce anterior displacement of the trachea.

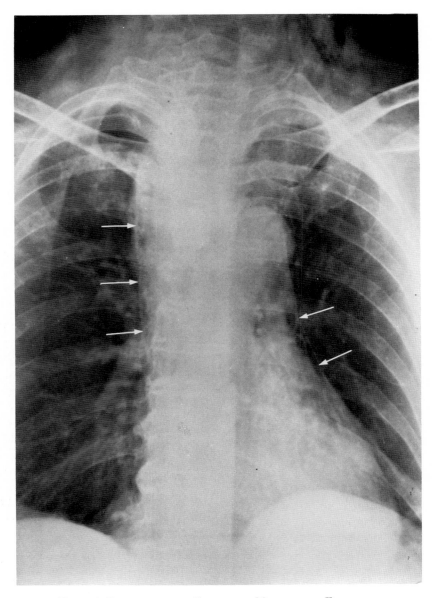

FIG. 496. PERFORATION OF ESOPHAGUS: MEDIASTINAL EMPHYSEMA

The patient developed severe pain during esophageal dilatation for achalasia. The film made shortly afterwards, shows broad, streak-like lucencies at the root of the neck representing air in the fascial planes. The mediastinal pleura (arrows) is separated from the underlying structures by the air that has dissected throughout the mediastinum.

This is best seen on the lateral view of the neck and is recognized by a widening of the retrotracheal space (Fig. 46). Small, round areas of radiolucency, representing bubbles of air within this space, serve to confirm the diagnosis of esophageal perforation. A large collection of air in this region appears as a longitudinal lucent streak, frequently extending upward as far as the base of the skull.

A large perforation of the lower part of the esophagus usually follows instrumentation, but it may occur spontaneously even though the esophageal wall is normal (Mallory-Weiss syndrome). In either instance, the parietal pleura over the esophagus may also be torn and air together with the esophageal contents enters the pleural cavity. This occurs most frequently on the left because of the proximity of the esophagus to the mediastinal pleura on that side. The cause of the collection of fluid and air in the pleural cavity is usually not evident on the film, but if there is evidence of mediastinal emphysema in addition to a large collection of fluid and air in the pleural cavity, the diagnosis of ruptured esophagus is most likely. If the pleural complications follow instrumentation of the esophagus, the diagnosis is evident. The possibility of spontaneous rupture of the esophagus should be considered if there is a sudden onset of severe pain, dyspnea and collapse after a heavy meal, especially if the patient has taken considerable quantities of alcohol and has been retching.

Achalasia (Cardiospasm). The widened mediastinal shadow caused by the dilated esophagus of cardiospasm often presents a confusing picture on a conventional chest film (Fig. 497). The right side of the mediastinum appears prominent. The shadow may extend from the root of the neck down to the diaphragm, but in some cases it appears as a localized bulge on either the upper or lower part of the right mediastinal border. In addition, there is often a fusiform shadow on the left side behind the heart. This is easily mistaken for an aortic aneurysm.

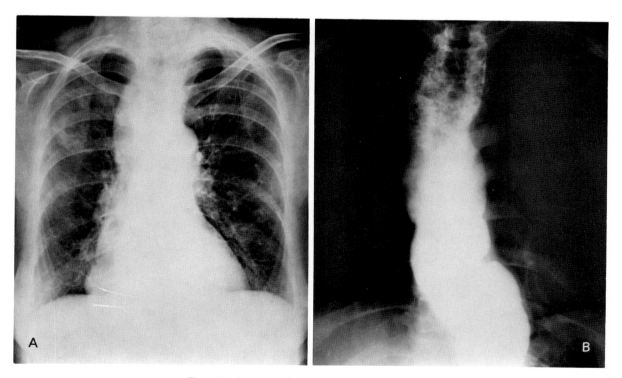

FIG. 497. DILATED ESOPHAGUS IN CARDIOSPASM

A: The density along the entire right side of the mediastinum does not obliterate the right border of the cardiac silhouette and therefore is situated posteriorly. It has an undulating contour. Although there is no air-fluid level, its upper portion appears rather lucent, suggesting that it represents a viscus containing air. No air is visible in the stomach. This combination of findings is characteristic of long standing esophageal obstruction. Dilatation of this extent is indicative of cardiospasm rather than carcinoma of the esophagus. The patchy shadow in the right upper lobe represents an area of aspiration pneumonia. *B:* The diagnosis is confirmed by barium swallow. The mottled appearance of the upper part of the esophagus is due to admixture of air with retained food and fluid.

If the film is made with sufficient exposure, the diagnosis is usually clear even before the ingestion of barium. The admixture of fine bubbles of air with the food and fluid in the esophagus usually produces a characteristic mottling of the shadow. Often a fluid level is seen in the upper portion of the dilated esophagus. Because of its diagnostic significance, the fluid level should be sought whenever there is widening of the right side of the mediastinum or when the shadow of the superior mediastinum appears unusually dense even though it is not widened. Since the fluid level is situated in the midline it may be mistaken, on casual inspection of the frontal film, for the border of a vertebral body or the upper margin of the manubrium. (Fig. 498).

The characteristic wavy outline of the tortuous, dilated esophagus is usually disclosed on highly penetrated films. It runs downward on the right side of the mediastinum and courses to the left along the diaphragm to the region of the esophageal hiatus. Because the esophagus is situated posteriorly, the right border of the ascending aorta can be visualized within the mediastinal shadow. This aids in the differentiation from aneurysm. Lateral and oblique projections often disclose the characteristic sausage-shaped conformation of the shadow of the dilated esophagus. The air-fluid level is more easily identified on these views than on the frontal projection.

Because the column of fluid retained in the esophagus serves as a barrier, air that is swallowed fails to enter the stomach. This explains the absence of a stomach bubble, a finding characteristic of cardiospasm.

Diverticula. Esophageal diverticula are of the traction or pulsion variety. Most traction diverticula are situated near the level of the tracheal bifurcation. They result from perforation of the esophagus by a necrotic subcarinal lymph node involved by tuberculosis, histoplasmosis or nonspecific infection (Fig. 467). The diverticulum represents the epithelialized remnant of the sinus tract together with distortion of the esophagus by local fibrosis. Since these nodes are situated in front of the esophagus, the diverticula are always situated anteriorly. Traction diverticula may also occur anywhere in the course of the esophagus as a result of perforation from other causes. Since they are small, traction diverticula are rarely seen on conventional films.

Pulsion diverticula occur characteristically in the superior mediastinum (Zenker's diverticulum), and immediately above the diaphragm (epiphrenic diverticulum). *Zenker's* diverticulum originates in the posterior wall of the pharynx and often descends through the thoracic inlet, behind the esophagus, into the posterior mediastinum. Here it produces a density projecting to either or both sides. It usually exhibits an air-fluid level and the appearance may be quite similar to that of a mediastinal abscess (Fig. 499). If the diverticulum is completely filled with fluid or food, the appearance suggests a neoplasm. The roentgen diagnosis depends upon demonstrating the sac-like diverticulum originating above the cricopharyngeus muscle, by means of a barium swallow. This procedure should be performed whenever a mass is seen in the posterior part of the superior mediastinum.

The *epiphrenic* diverticulum arises a short distance above the diaphragm and practically always projects to the right side. It appears as a sharply demarcated, round shadow in the posterior mediastinum and may or may not have a fluid level. Because of its location near the esophageal hiatus, it is easily mistaken for a hiatus hernia. However, it is quite unusual for a hiatus hernia to present only on the right side. As in the case of cardiospasm, mottling of the shadow, caused by its frothy contents, indicates that it is connected with the alimentary tract (Fig. 26). The diagnosis is established by barium swallow.

Neoplasms. It is unusual for a carcinoma of the esophagus to produce a mediastinal shadow that is visible on the frontal film of the chest (Fig. 500). However, occasionally, the shadow of the neoplasm is seen encroaching on the posterior mediastinal space in the lateral or oblique projections.

Benign tumors or myosarcomas of the esophageal wall usually do not encircle or constrict the esophagus and may attain considerable proportions before they produce dysphagia. In contrast to carcinomas, therefore, they are more likely to appear as a mass on the chest film at the first roentgen examination. The tumor presents as a sharply demarcated, circumscribed, round or oval density in the posterior mediastinum, and may involve any portion of the esophagus. When situated in the supradiaphragmatic region, it is obscured by the shadow of the heart on the frontal view, unless a sufficiently penetrated film is obtained. The location of the mass in the posterior mediastinum and its sharp, round, outer border may cause difficulty in differentiating such a tumor from a paravertebral neurofibroma. This can be resolved by making an additional film in expiration with the patient supine. An upward displacement of the tumor in relation to the vertebrae, in comparison with the erect film made during inspiration, will exclude the possibility of a paravertebral neurofibroma.

A carcinoma involving the lower portion of the

esophagus usually represents upward extension of a carcinoma of the stomach. In rare instances the tumor is large enough to be visualized through the shadow of the heart. That the neoplasm originates in the stomach may be inferred if a mass is seen indenting the mesial border of the stomach bubble. The mass represents the carcinoma of the cardia intruding into the gastric lumen.

As in the case of achalasia, obstruction of the esophagus from other causes can also result in a fluid level in the esophagus, sometimes with ab-

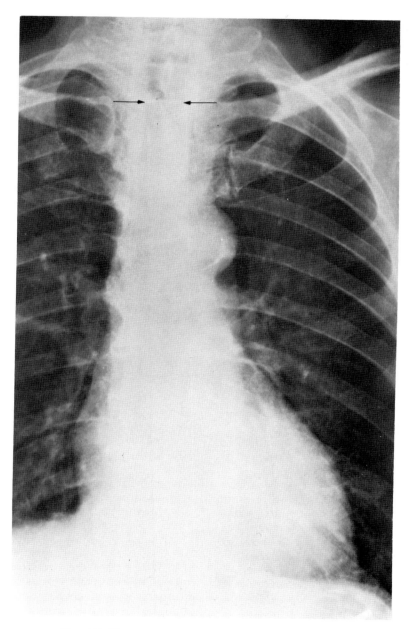

FIG. 498. FLUID LEVEL IN CARCINOMA OF THE ESOPHAGUS

The straight, horizontal line (arrows) is easily mistaken for the upper border of a vertebral body. However, there is a sudden change in the density of the mediastinum at this point, indicating that the line represents an air-fluid level. The presence of air in the stomach, the normal size of the esophagus above the fluid level, and the absence of the shadow of a widened esophagus below, make cardiospasm most unlikely. In this case the esophageal obstruction is due to a carcinoma at the esophagogastric junction.

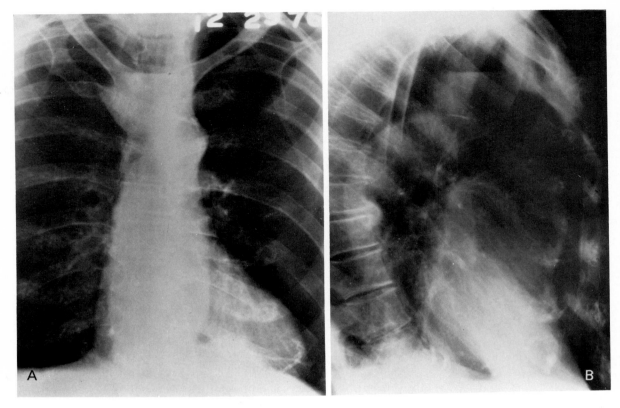

FIG. 499. ZENKER'S DIVERTICULUM

A: The frontal view shows an area of increased density behind the manubrium with an air-fluid level at its upper border. A localized collection of air and fluid in the upper mediastinum can be due to achalasia, a mediastinal abscess or a Zenker's diverticulum. *B:* In the lateral view, the trachea is seen to be bowed forward by the collection of air and fluid. Localized displacement of the trachea such as this is not seen with achalasia. The differential diagnosis between a mediastinal abscess and a diverticulum depends on the clinical picture and a barium swallow.

sence of a stomach bubble (Fig. 501). However, in obstructive lesions of relatively short duration, such as a carcinoma or foreign body, there is comparatively little dilatation of the esophagus above the point of obstruction (Fig. 498).

It is not uncommon for a carcinoma of the esophagus to perforate into the trachea or main bronchus and cause an aspiration pneumonia. This may involve either one or both lungs. The pneumonia is usually of lobular distribution. If the patient survives long enough, suppuration may take place with the formation of one or more cavities within the lung. This may occur without any roentgen or clinical evidence of mediastinitis.

In the absence of aspiration pneumonia, the presence of an infiltrating lesion in the lung in a patient with esophageal obstruction favors the diagnosis of bronchogenic neoplasm with invasion of the mediastinum and secondary esophageal obstruction. The roentgen appearance of the esophagus in these cases is rather typical. Because the esophageal obstruction is secondary to invasion of tissues about the esophagus by extension of the bronchial carcinoma into the mediastinum, the esophageal narrowing is funnel-shaped with smooth, regular walls. In contrast, an obstructing carcinoma of the esophagus usually protrudes irregularly into the lumen and there is often evidence of ulceration of the tumor.

Although acquired bronchoesophageal fistulas are usually due to carcinoma of the esophagus (Fig. 207), they are occasionally produced by ulcerating bronchial carcinomas. The diagnosis of a primary bronchial carcinoma is most likely if, in the presence of a bronchoesophageal fistula, there is evidence of obstruction of a large bronchus.

THE GREAT VESSELS

Abnormalities of the great vessels frequently cause shadows that simulate neoplasms in the mediastinum. In many instances their vascular nature can be determined from examination of conventional films and fluoroscopy, particularly after distention of the esophagus with barium. However, angiography is often required for a definitive diagnosis and to determine the exact type of vascular abnormality. Only the conditions that have the appearance of a mediastinal tumor will be discussed here.

Anomalies. RIGHT AORTIC ARCH. Normally, the aorta ascends on the right side of the mediastinum and then arches to the left in front of the trachea. The distal portion of the arch curves posteriorly over the left main bronchus and lies alongside the left border of the trachea. The upper portion of the descending aorta is in contact with the left side of the esophagus. As the aorta proceeds downward, it courses toward the midline, so that at the diaphragm it is situated

behind and slightly to the right of the esophagus. The esophagus and the descending aorta are attached to each other by loose connective tissue.

The aortic knob represents the shadow of the distal portion of the arch as it curves downward and posteriorly. Its lateral border is silhouetted against the air-containing lung and protrudes from the left side of the mediastinum above the bulge of the pulmonary artery. The mesial border of this portion of the arch usually indents the left side of the esophagus and in older persons often displaces the trachea to the right. In most instances the shadow of the descending aorta can be recognized along the left side of the spine.

At an early stage in embryonic development there are two aortic arches. Both arise from the single ascending aorta and curve posteriorly, one over the right main bronchus and the other over the left, to join behind the esophagus and form

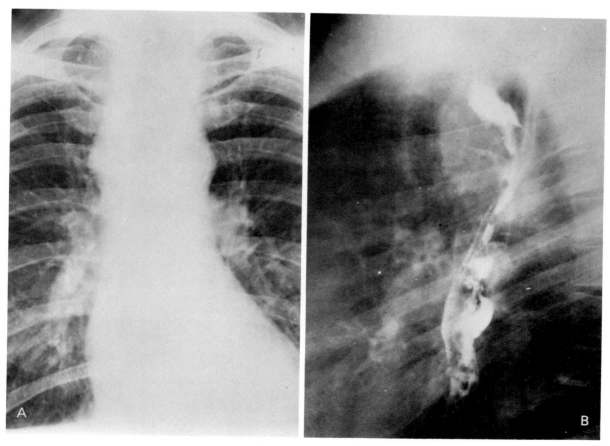

FIG. 500. CARCINOMA OF THE ESOPHAGUS

A: The sharply circumscribed mass in the right paratracheal region resembles enlarged lymph nodes. Because the patient complained of some difficulty in swallowing, a barium study was performed. *B:* In the lateral projection, the trachea is seen to be bowed forward and the esophagus displaced backward by a large soft tissue mass. The lumen of the esophagus is irregularly narrowed. Biopsy disclosed a squamous cell carcinoma. The presence of such a large extrinsic mass is unusual in carcinoma of the esophagus.

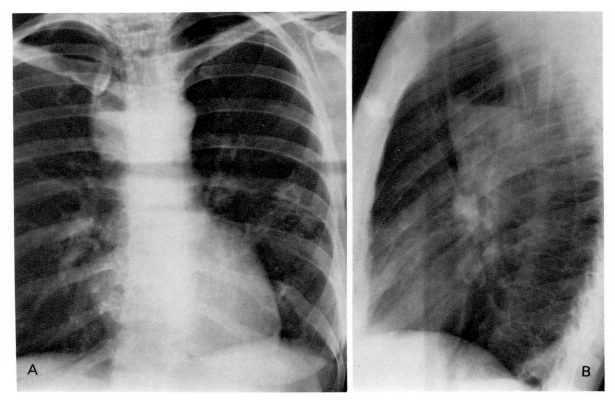

FIG. 501. MEDIASTINAL AIR-FLUID LEVEL

A: The shadow bulging from the right side of the superior mediastinum contains an air-fluid level. The level extends across the air column of the trachea. This is frequently seen with a mediastinal abscess (Fig. 444). In this case, the air and fluid are situated within the esophagus which is almost completely obstructed by a carcinoma in its midportion. The infiltration in the outer part of the left lung is the result of an aspiration pneumonia. *B:* In the lateral view the air-fluid level is seen behind the trachea which is displaced forward. Such dilatation of the esophagus is uncommon in carcinoma. Note the absence of a gastric air bubble.

the descending aorta. Normally, the right aortic arch regresses and only the left develops. If the left arch becomes obliterated, the right persists as the mature aortic arch. The aortic knob then protrudes from the right side of the mediastinum, indents the right side of the esophagus and may displace the trachea to the left. The descending aorta courses for a variable distance along the right side of the mediastinum and then crosses the midline to assume its normal position on the left at the level of the diaphragm. The presence of a bulging shadow on the right side of the upper mediastinum in the absence of an aortic knob on the left, should always suggest the possibility of a right aortic arch (Fig. 502). The diagnosis is confirmed if the shadow of the descending aorta is seen along the right side of the spine.

There are two types of right aortic arch. Both indent the right border of the esophagus. In the first type, examination in the lateral view fails to disclose any abnormality of the barium-filled esophagus (Fig. 503). The origin of the great vessels from the arch of the aorta is usually the mirror image of the normal. The first branch is the left innominate artery which gives rise to the left subclavian and carotid arteries, followed by the right carotid and lastly, the right subclavian artery. This type of right aortic arch is usually associated with congenital heart disease, most often tetralogy of Fallot. The second type, which is considerably more common, is associated with a rather large, smooth indentation on the posterior wall of the esophagus at the level of the aortic arch (Fig. 504). This is caused by a diverticulum of the aorta which represents the residuum of the left aortic arch. The diverticulum may be large enough to protrude from the left side of the mediastinum and simulate a normal aortic knob. There is no innominate artery and the left subclavian artery arises from the diverticulum as the fourth branch of the arch. This type of arch is not associated with congenital

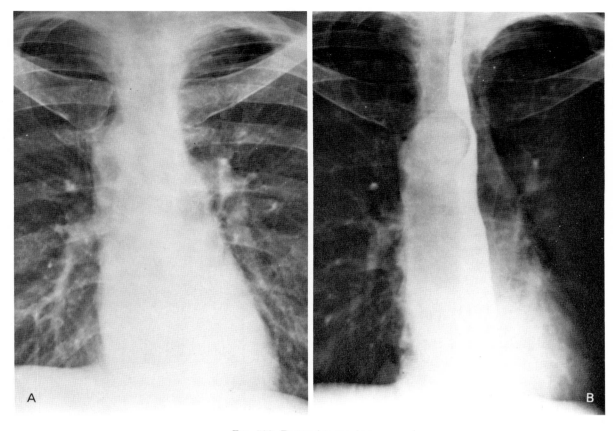

FIG. 502. RIGHT AORTIC ARCH

A: The patient had sarcoidosis. Following resolution of the hilar nodes, a shadow persisted on the right side of the superior mediastinum and was thought to represent residual involved lymph nodes. However, the shadow extends straight down beyond the hilum and no aortic knob is visible on the left side. *B:* The diagnosis of right aortic arch is confirmed by a barium swallow. The aortic arch indents the right side of the esophagus and displaces it to the left.

heart disease but may form a vascular ring around the esophagus and trachea.

DOUBLE AORTIC ARCH. In this condition both aortic arches persist. The left, which is situated anterior to the trachea, usually is the smaller of the two. Both arches join together behind the esophagus to form the descending aorta. This completes a vascular ring about the trachea and esophagus. On the frontal film a prominence is seen on both sides of the mediastinum, suggesting a superior mediastinal mass. Characteristically, there is an indentation on each side of the barium-filled esophagus. The indentation by the right arch is usually situated higher than the one on the left. The lateral view shows a large indentation on the posterior wall of the esophagus, produced by the posterior component of the ring. In some cases, the left arch causes sufficient compression of the anterior wall of the trachea to be recognizable on the lateral view. Occasionally the trachea is pushed backward by this arch

and produces a shallow depression on the anterior border of the esophagus.

COARCTATION OF THE AORTA. Congenital stenosis can occur in any portion of the aorta. The degree of coarctation varies widely, ranging from slight narrowing to almost complete interruption of the lumen. The most common location is at the level of the ligamentum arteriosum, distal to the origin of the left subclavian artery. The effects of the coarctation on the aorta and subclavian artery, and the secondary changes produced by the collaterals which bridge the coarcted segment, produce roentgen changes that are usually quite characteristic.

The left subclavian artery originates from the aorta more distally than normal, immediately above the narrowed segment. The artery then courses directly upward before turning toward the left arm. This artery is almost always dilated and forms the left border of the mediastinum, partially or completely obscuring the aortic knob.

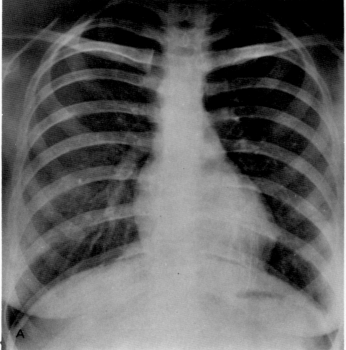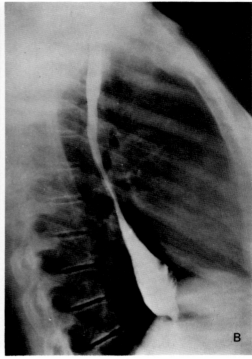

FIG. 503. MIRROR IMAGE, RIGHT AORTIC ARCH

A: A film of a 27 year old, mildly cyanotic female, shows a localized bulge in the right paratracheal region. The trachea at this level is deviated to the left and there is no evidence of a left aortic knob. These findings indicate the presence of a right aortic arch. *B:* In the lateral view, the barium-filled esophagus appears normal. Cardic catheterization and angiocardiography revealed a tetralogy of Fallot with a bidirectional ventricular shunt.

The straightening of the left border of the mediastinum and the obliteration of the shadow of the aortic knob form the most constant roentgen signs of coarctation (Fig. 166).

Not uncommonly, the lateral border of the descending arch presents a bilobed appearance, with two distinct curves separated by a sharply angulated niche. The niche represents the site of the coarctation, and is usually best seen in the left anterior oblique projection, although it is also visible on the frontal view. The upper curve is formed by the aortic knob and the dilated left subclavian artery, while the lower curve represents the widened aorta distal to the coarctation (poststenotic dilatation) (Fig. 505). In some cases, the bulge produced by the poststenotic segment is sufficiently prominent to mimic a normal aortic knob, but at a somewhat lower level. A barium swallow is often helpful in establishing the diagnosis. Characteristically, a double indentation is seen on the left border of the esophagus, the upper being produced by the aortic knob, while the lower is caused by the dilated aorta beyond the stenosis.

The collateral circulation which bypasses the narrowed segment of the aorta consists mainly of anastamoses between the branches of the subclavian artery above the coarctation and the intercostal arteries below. The intercostals become dilated and tortuous because of the increased blood flow through them. The pulsations of these tortuous vessels against the ribs produce notches on their inferior margins as a result of pressure atrophy. The notches have fine sclerotic margins. The posterior portions of the third to the eighth ribs are most commonly involved (Fig. 166). The notching is almost always bilateral. However, if the coarctation involves the midportion of the arch proximal to the left subclavian artery, only the right subclavian functions as a collateral and the notching is limited to the right side. If the coarctation is at the usual site and the right subclavian artery has an anomalous origin beyond the coarctation, rib notching is present only on the left side. Notching of the ribs is not commonly seen in infants and small children, and its absence, even in the adult, does not exclude coarctation.

The intercostal arteries near the aorta can undergo aneurysmal dilatation. If the aneurysms

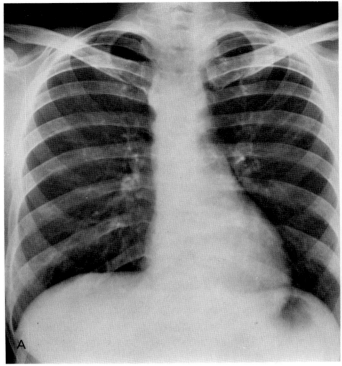
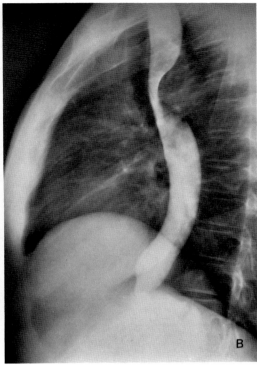

Fig. 504. Right Aortic Arch with Posterior Diverticulum

A: The frontal film of an asymptomatic man shows a right aortic arch. The picture is indistinguishable from that in the previous illustration. *B:* There is a large indentation on the posterior aspect of the barium-filled esophagus. The indentation is too large to be caused by an anomalous subclavian artery and indicates the presence of an aortic diverticulum extending behind the esophagus. The patient had no cardiac disease.

become calcified, they can appear as annular shadows on either side of the spine, measuring as much as 1 cm in diameter. Tortuous, dilated internal mammary arteries involved in the collateral circulation, may be visualized on the lateral view as elongated, wavy, retrosternal densities.

Persistent Left Superior Vena Cava. At an early stage in embryonic development, the venous system draining the upper portion of the body is symmetrical, with an anterior cardinal vein on each side. Normally, the left cardinal vein regresses, while the right develops into the superior vena cava. If the left cava persists, it courses vertically downward from its origin at the juncture of the left subclavian and jugular veins behind the pulmonary artery to empty into the coronary sinus. The persistent left cava casts a relatively faint density with a smooth, well-demarcated border along the left side of the mediastinum. This tends to obliterate a portion of the superior margin of the arch of the aorta and, on rare occasions, obscures the entire aortic knob. Although the shadow is not very dense, it can be mistaken for enlarged paratracheal and

tracheobronchial lymph nodes. However, there is no distortion of the tracheobronchial angle and no indentation or displacement of the esophagus. A persistent left superior vena cava may not be recognizable on conventional films, especially in infants and young children with a prominent thymus.

Total Anomalous Pulmonary Venous Drainage. In this anomaly, the pulmonary veins, instead of entering separately into the left atrium, form a common trunk which empties into a large systemic vein. The common pulmonary vein usually drains into the upper portion of the persistent left superior vena cava which empties into the left innominate vein. The left vena cava produces a bulge along the left border of the superior mediastinum. Dilatation of the right superior cava causes a similar bulge on the right side of the mediastinum. Widening of this vessel is due to increased blood flow comprising the venous return from the lungs as well as from the upper part of the body. The bilateral bulge of the superior mediastinum together with the silhouette of the heart produces a shadow resembling a figure-of-eight (snowman heart), characteristic

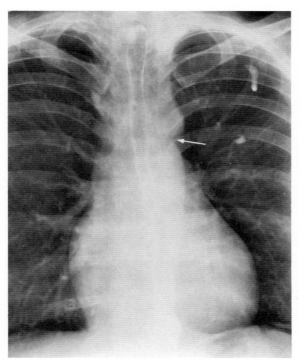

FIG. 505. COARCTATION OF THE AORTA

Young female with Turner's syndrome. There is a notch (arrow) just beneath the aortic knob, producing a figure-of-three conformation. This is pathognomonic of coarctation of the aorta. The upper border of the aortic knob is obscured by the dilated left subclavian artery. The bulge below the notch is due to poststenotic dilatation of the aorta. (From M. G. Baron: *Circulation, 43:* 311, 1971.)

of total anomalous pulmonary venous drainage (Fig. 219). The upper component of this shadow usually shows expansile pulsations. An increase in the pulmonary vasculature accompanies this anomaly, which, in essence, is a left-to-right shunt.

ANOMALOUS ORIGIN OF LEFT PULMONARY ARTERY (PULMONARY SLING). When the left pulmonary artery arises from the right pulmonary artery, it arches over the right bronchus and then runs transversely to the left, between the trachea and esophagus, to enter the hilum of the left lung. The anomalous left pulmonary artery is hidden within the mediastinum and cannot be identified on the frontal film. On the lateral view it is visible as a nodular, round or oval density behind the trachea. Because of the pressure of the artery on its soft posterior wall, the trachea is often narrowed. The artery also produces an indentation on the anterior border of the esophagus.

Tortuosity of the Arteries. The two vessels that most commonly produce confusing shadows in the mediastinum are the innominate artery and the aorta. When these arteries undergo degenerative changes, they often increase considerably in length with relatively little change in their diameter. As they elongate, the vessels become tortuous and bulge outward from the mediastinum. Their shadows may then simulate a neoplasm or an aneurysm.

AORTA. The aorta is anchored at several points; at the aortic valve, at the arch where the great vessels arise, at the ligamentum arteriosum, and at the diaphragmatic hiatus. Elongation of the aorta produces tortuosity between these points.

As the ascending aorta lengthens, it bulges forward and to the right. In the frontal view it confers a convexity to the right border of the mediastinum. This may be continuous with the curve of the right cardiac border, but it is usually demarcated by a slight indentation. Elongation of the ascending aorta is more apparent on the lateral view. Its anterior border is sharply outlined and produces a distinct bulge which encroaches on the retrosternal space. The nature of the shadow is evident if there are dense linear streaks along its borders, representing calcification of the wall of the aorta. This is characteristic of syphilitic aortitis (Fig. 506) but occurs occasionally in arteriosclerosis.

Tortuosity of the arch is characterized by an increased prominence of the aortic knob which enlarges upward and to the left. The large knob may mimic an aneurysm. Tortuosity of the arch can impart a double contour to the aortic knob on the frontal projection and suggest a mass of large mediastinal lymph nodes. Both possibilities can often be excluded by examination in the oblique and lateral projections which uncoil the shadow of the aorta and demonstrate its contour and caliber.

Elongation of the descending aorta results in a sharply demarcated bulging shadow to the left of the spine behind the heart. The lower portion of the tortuous aorta courses mesially to the aortic hiatus at an acute angle to the diaphragm. Its shadow can be confused with that of a hiatus hernia on the frontal projection but because the aorta lies behind the dome of the diaphragm its border can frequently be seen to extend below the level of the diaphragm (see Fig. 568). The visible portion of the aorta is then directed outward and downward and forms an obtuse angle with the diaphragm. The appearance may suggest a collapsed left lower lobe or a diaphragmatic hernia. The differentiation can be made from the left oblique or lateral views which demonstrate the course of the tortuous aorta quite clearly. If the aorta buckles sharply just above

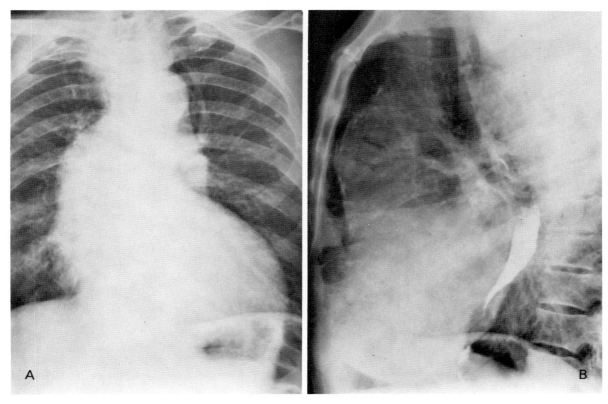

FIG. 506. ANEURYSM OF ASCENDING AORTA

A: The bulging of the right border of the mediastinum is due to widening of the ascending aorta. The apex of the heart is displaced downward and outward indicating dilatation of the left ventricle. The descending aorta appears normal. This combination is most commonly seen with Marfan's syndrome or luetic aortitis. Arteriosclerotic widening of the ascending aorta is practically always associated with tortuosity or widening of the descending aorta. *B:* Lateral View. The aortic aneurysm extends anteriorly and encroaches on the retrosternal space. Fine linear calcific plaques outline this portion of the aorta. This appearance is characteristic of syphilitic aortitis.

the diaphragm as it courses toward the midline, it may be projected on end in the lateral view to cast a sharply demarcated round shadow resembling a neoplasm.

When the tortuosity is confined to the midportion of the descending aorta, the vessel bulges into the pulmonary field at the level of the lung root and simulates a mediastinal tumor on the frontal view. Since the elongated aorta bows posteriorly as well as laterally, it lies in the paravertebral region well behind the pulmonary hilum. On the frontal view, the silhouette of the pulmonary vessels can be seen through the shadow, indicating that the mass is not related to the hilar structures. If the arch is also elongated, the aorta curves widely to the left, producing a large, sharply demarcated shadow extending from the aortic knob to the diaphragm, simulating an aneurysm.

Occasionally the junction of the arch and descending aorta is firmly fixed by the ligamentum arteriosum. As the aorta elongates, both the arch and descending portion bulge outward and backward on either side of the point of fixation. In the frontal view an indentation is seen on the lateral border of the aorta just below the knob where the two curves meet, simulating coarctation. The lateral or left oblique view usually reveals the sharp anterior angulation of the aorta at the level of the ligamentum and the exaggerated curves of the aorta above and below this point, typical of *pseudocoarctation.*

In rare instances, the descending aorta buckles to the right in front of the spine. It can then project beyond the right border of the heart either at the level of the hilum or just above the diaphragm. A similar shadow may be produced by tortuosity of an anomalous right-sided aorta. In either case, the shadow is easily confused with that of a neoplasm, especially when the film is not exposed sufficiently to show detail through the cardiac silhouette (Fig. 507).

There are several roentgen signs which help to identify a tortuous aorta. The tubular shape of

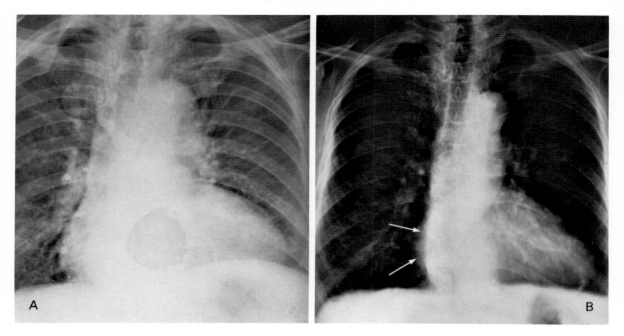

FIG. 507. BUCKLED AORTA

A: A hemispherical density is visible within the right cardiac silhouette on a routine chest film. This was thought to represent an epiphrenic diverticulum or a neurogenic tumor. *B*: An overpenetrated film made in full inspiration shows the descending aorta to be tortuous. Its lower portion (arrows) is buckled to the right and extends beyond the cardiac border. This created the impression of a mass on the ordinary film.

its shadow is usually revealed in the left oblique or lateral views although it may be evident on the frontal projection, particularly on Bucky films. Calcific plaques may be demonstrated along both borders of the shadow. If only the lateral border shows calcification, the possibility of an aneurysm remains. Since the esophagus is attached to the aorta, it follows the curve of the tortuous vessel. Barium studies will generally show the esophagus displaced toward the shadow of a tortuous descending aorta, while a neoplasm or an aneurysm pushes the esophagus to the opposite side. In some instances the esophagus is fixed at the level of the carina by adhesions from inflammatory disease of the subcarinal nodes. The esophagus then does not follow the tortuous aorta and the barium study may be misleading.

INNOMINATE ARTERY. The innominate artery is fixed at the root of the neck and at its origin from the ascending limb of the arch of the aorta. Therefore, it buckles between these two points as it elongates. The curve of the tortuous artery is often complex, but the main segment of the vessel bends to the right and projects from the upper mediastinum into the right pulmonary field. Only its outer border is outlined. The mesial portion of the shadow merges imperceptibly

with that of the superior mediastinum, while the upper border is lost in the shadow of the neck (Fig. 508). The lateral margin of a tortuous innominate artery is sharply delineated and presents a smooth curve similar to that of a substernal goiter. However, it differs in certain respects. There is no displacement of the trachea and the shadow does not rise on swallowing. Pulsations are visible fluoroscopically, but cannot be differentiated from transmitted pulsations which can occur in a thyroid tumor. Unless the walls of the vessel are calcified, it is impossible to distinguish a tortuous innominate from one which is aneurysmal, without the aid of angiography. However, tortuosity of the innominate artery is extremely common in older people while aneurysms of this vessel are very rare.

Aneurysms of the Aorta. These may be congenital in origin or result from weakening of the aortic wall as a result of infection, trauma or degenerative disease. They range from localized sacculations of varying size to diffuse fusiform dilatations.

The aneurysm is depicted on conventional roentgen films as a homogeneous, circumscribed density protruding from the mediastinum in relation to the course of the aorta. It is usually sharply demarcated, with a smooth, curved bor-

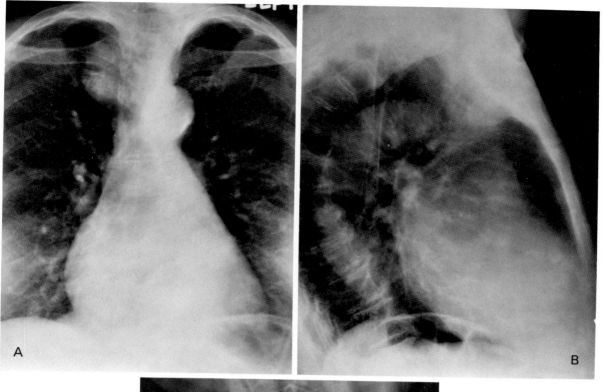

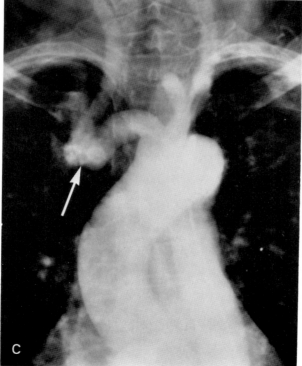

FIG. 508. TORTUOUS INNOMINATE ARTERY

A: A 65 year old woman was found to have a shadow projecting from the right side of the mediastinum on a routine x-ray examination. The mass is sharply outlined and semicircular in shape. Its upper border is lost in the shadow of the neck and it does not displace the trachea. *B*: On the lateral view the mass is seen anteriorly, abutting on the upper portion of the manubrium, extending upward into the neck. The trachea is not displaced posteriorly and the mass did not rise on swallowing, making a substernal goiter extremely unlikely. *C*: Aortography reveals a buckled innominate artery (arrow) which is responsible for the abnormal mediastinal shadow.

der. The border may appear undulated or scalloped when the aneurysmal dilatation is not uniform or when it is formed by multiple aneurysms. The border becomes hazy when blood seeps out through a small perforation, and it may be obscured when there is atelectasis of the adjacent lung.

Calcification in the rim of the shadow is helpful in the diagnosis of an aneurysm, but calcific deposits can also be present in the wall of a dermoid or within a thymoma. In an aneurysm, the calcification usually occurs in the form of multiple plaques which are seen on end as a series of short, curvilinear streaks along the border. The calcific deposits in a thymoma usually appear as irregular, dense masses within the substance of the shadow, as well as on the surface. The circumferential distribution of calcium in the wall of a dermoid is more similar to that of an aneurysm. However, the calcific deposits in a dermoid are more continuous and regular and not in the form of individual plaques. The demonstration of calcification in the ascending aorta in a patient with a mass that cannot be separated from the aortic shadow favors the diagnosis of an aneurysm.

Pulsations are frequently absent in an aortic aneurysm, especially when it is partially clotted. In large aneurysms, pulsations may not be demonstrable even in the absence of a mural thrombus. This is due simply to the small change in the diameter of the aneurysm in relation to the change in its volume with each heart beat. Since mediastinal masses frequently transmit pulsations from the great vessels, the observation of pulsation is not diagnostic of an aneurysm unless it is shown to be expansile. While this can often be determined by fluoroscopy, a more accurate evaluation can be made, and a permanent record obtained, by kymography or ciné recording.

The possibility of an aneurysm should be considered whenever there is a circumscribed, homogeneous mediastinal mass which cannot be separated from the aorta in any projection. At times it is impossible to differentiate between an aneurysm and a mediastinal neoplasm from conventional radiographic and fluoroscopic examinations even in conjunction with the clinical findings. The diagnosis then depends entirely upon angiography.

In addition to the shadow of the aneurysm, secondary changes may be evident on the films. These include erosion of adjacent bony structures, atelectasis due to bronchial compression, paralysis of the diaphragm from pressure on the phrenic nerve, and changes due to perforation of the aneurysm. Rupture into the mediastinum results in a hematoma which causes widening of the mediastinal shadow. Perforation into the pleura produces a hemothorax, and perforation into a bronchus results in pulmonary densities of varying extent from inundation of the lung.

SINUS OF VALSALVA. A sinus aneurysm most commonly involves the noncoronary or right coronary sinus. When small, the aneurysm cannot be seen on conventional films. Large ones project from the right side of the mediastinum at about the level of the insertion of the inferior pulmonary veins and obscure the cardiac border in this region. As the aneurysm increases in size it can extend to the diaphragm. The appearance can simulate either a parapericardial cyst or a thymoma on the frontal projection. However, in the lateral view, the border of a sinus aneurysm is usually poorly visualized or not seen at all, while most thymomas appear as well demarcated masses abutting on the sternum. When the aneurysm is large it can extend forward and cloud the retrosternal space. However, unlike a thymoma, the posterior border of a sinus aneurysm is not visible, as it blends with the shadow of the heart.

Aneurysms of the left coronary sinus are almost always completely contained within the mediastinal shadow. They produce a local increase in the density of the mediastinum and can mimic a large left atrium or a subcarinal bronchogenic cyst.

Aneurysms of the sinuses of Valsalva are frequently associated with enlargement of the left ventricle secondary to insufficiency of the aortic valve. Occasionally the aneurysm perforates into the right side of the heart. This produces a left-to-right shunt, manifested by an increase in the pulmonary vasculature and accentuated pulsations of the pulmonary arteries. A large aneurysm can erode the sternum.

ASCENDING AORTA. Fusiform aneurysms of the ascending aorta usually extend from the sinuses of Valsalva to the beginning of the aortic arch, and are frequently associated with aortic insufficiency. In most cases the lesion underlying the aneurysm is a diffuse necrosis of the media. Syphilis used to be the common cause of the necrosis, and is still encountered in older patients, but in the younger age group the lesion of the media is usually part of Marfan's syndrome.

On the frontal film, the right mediastinal border makes a sweeping curve from the cardiac silhouette to the level of the innominate artery. The convexity is more pronounced in the left oblique projection. On the lateral view, the widened aorta encroaches on the entire retrosternal space, obliterating its lower portion. Calcification occurs frequently in syphilitic aneurysms, but not so often in the others (Fig. 506).

Since the mesial and posterior borders of the ascending aorta are lost in the mediastinal shadow on the oblique and lateral projections, as well as on the frontal, it is difficult to differentiate between a fusiform aneurysm and tortuosity of the ascending aorta without angiography. Concomitant tortuosity of the descending aorta favors the latter. An exaggerated curve of the ascending aorta in the presence of a normal aortic knob and descending aorta, suggests aneurysmal dilatation. In the unusual instance in which the posterior or mesial wall of the ascending aorta is delineated by calcific deposits, the differential diagnosis is clear.

Saccular aneurysms of the ascending aorta almost always project outward from the right border of the mediastinum. In some instances the protuberance is more pronounced anteriorly and is then obvious on the left oblique or lateral view. Rarely the aneurysm arises from the mesial wall of the aorta and is entirely hidden within the mediastinal shadow. If such an aneurysm is large, it may project on the left border of the mediastinum (Fig. 509). Because the aneurysm is situated anteriorly, its shadow does not obscure the outline of the descending aorta. This is the exception to the rule that an anterior mediastinal mass on the left side is not an aneurysm.

A saccular aneurysm of the ascending aorta can produce paralysis of the right leaf of the diaphragm from pressure on the phrenic nerve. A large aneurysm can extend to the anterior chest wall and erode the sternum and the mesial ends of the upper ribs. Rupture of an aneurysm of the ascending aorta into the superior vena cava results in widening of the superior mediastinal shadow which may obscure the underlying aneurysm. The lungs show an increase in vascularity because of the left-to-right shunt. An aneurysm extending mesially can rupture into the

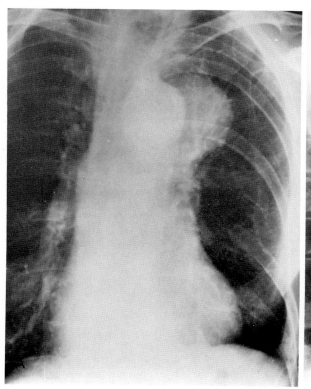 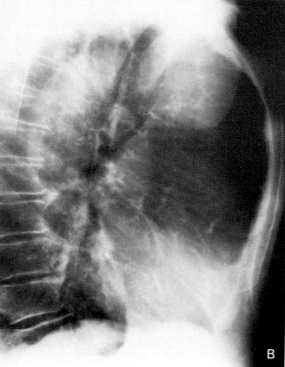

FIG. 509. ANEURYSM OF AORTIC ARCH

A: Frontal view. A large, round mass at the level of the distal aortic arch has the appearance of a bronchogenic carcinoma. The possibility of an aortic aneurysm was considered less likely because aneurysms at this level almost always arise from the uppermost portion of the descending aorta and therefore obscure the aortic knob. The aortic knob is clearly delineated within the shadow of the mass. *B*: Lateral view. The well-demarcated mass is situated anteriorly, overlying the ascending aorta. Because the mass could not be separated from the aorta in any projection, an angiogram was performed. The mass proved to be aneurysm arising from the mesial surface of the ascending portion of the aortic arch. It extended to the left in front of the aortic knob and therefore did not obliterate its contour.

adjacent pulmonary artery. If the aneurysm is small, a large pulmonary artery and plethora of the lungs may be the only roentgen manifestations.

AORTIC ARCH. The roentgen appearance of an aneurysm of the arch of the aorta depends on its size and location.

An aneurysm of the proximal portion of the arch usually extends upward and to the right, and obliterates the upper border of the ascending aorta. A large aneurysm in this region may displace the trachea posteriorly and to the left.

A small aneurysm arising from the superior aspect of the arch, between the great vessels, extends directly upwards. The upper border of the aneurysm may be visualized on the frontal projection, but more commonly the only sign in this view is an increase in the density of the upper mediastinal shadow. On the lateral view the aneurysm can usually be seen as a hump on the aortic arch, obscuring its superior border. As the aneurysm enlarges, it splays the innominate and left carotid arteries, widening the shadow of the superior mediastinum. A large aneurysm can project beyond the borders of the mediastinum. If, as is usually the case, it extends to the left side, the shadow overlies the aortic knob. Because the aortic knob represents the most distal portion of the arch, it lies posterior to the aneurysm and, therefore, its silhouette is usually not obliterated. Thus, visualization of a normal aortic knob does not exclude the possibility that a mass in this location represents an aneurysm of the aorta (Fig. 28).

An aneurysm originating from the undersurface of the arch gives rise to a sharply demarcated density projecting from either side of the mediastinum below the level of the aortic knob. On the frontal view this does not appear to be related to the aorta whose silhouette is maintained. However, the left oblique and lateral views disclose a rather characteristic appearance. In these projections, the aneurysm appears as a sharply demarcated bulge on the under aspect of the arch, encroaching on the aortic window above the pulmonary artery. The lower border of the arch is obliterated by the aneurysm.

An aneurysm of the distal portion of the arch is depicted as a sharply demarcated density which replaces the aortic knob. This usually extends upward as well as outward. Its border is generally smooth but may be wavy as a result of multiple outpouchings of the aneurysmal wall. When large, the aneurysm displaces the trachea and the esophagus to the right, and it may cause considerable tracheal compression. The pressure defect on the left side of the esophagus is much larger than that caused by the normal arch of the aorta.

Since the distal portion of the aortic arch crosses over the left main bronchus at its junction with the trachea, the aneurysm depresses the bronchus and displaces the lower part of the trachea and tracheobronchial angle to the right. This narrows the angle of the carina and produces a marked rounding of the left tracheobronchial angle. The resulting hook-shaped contour of the trachea and left main bronchus is similar to that produced by a large mass of tracheobronchial nodes (Fig. 421). The pressure of the aneurysm can cause marked narrowing of the left main bronchus, and may lead to obstructive emphysema, recurrent pulmonary infections and bronchiectasis. Complete obstruction of the left main bronchus or left upper lobe bronchus results in atelectasis.

The aneurysm is usually densely adherent to the trachea and left main bronchus. The upward pull of the trachea during swallowing is, therefore, transmitted to the aneurysm, which can be seen to rise with deglutition.

The diaphragm may be paralyzed because of pressure on the left phrenic nerve. The left recurrent laryngeal nerve, which loops under the arch of the aorta, can be similarly affected. Thus, a mass in the left tracheobronchial region associated with paralysis of the diaphragm or left vocal cord, together with evidences of bronchial obstruction, may represent an aneurysm of the distal aortic arch and does not necessarily indicate a bronchogenic neoplasm involving the mediastinum. Calcification at the border of the mediastinal shadow is indicative of an aneurysm. Similarly, calcification confined to the ascending aorta, widening of the ascending aorta, or evidence of aortic insufficiency favor the diagnosis of aneurysm.

DESCENDING AORTA. Aneurysms of the descending aorta are situated behind the heart. On the frontal film they may be projected entirely within the cardiac shadow (Fig. 510) or they may extend beyond the heart into the left pulmonary field. Because the aneurysm lies in a plane posterior to the heart, the left cardiac border remains sharply outlined. In arteriosclerotic or syphilitic aneurysms changes are usually visible in other parts of the aorta. When the remainder of the aorta appears entirely normal, the possibility of a congenital, traumatic, or mycotic aneurysm should be considered.

If the aortic wall is not calcified, it may be impossible to differentiate between a tortuous descending aorta and a fusiform aneurysm on the frontal film unless the esophagus is outlined

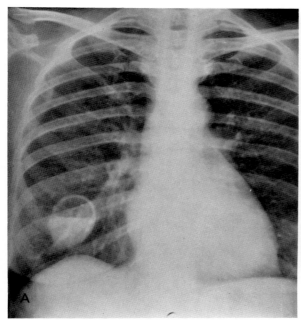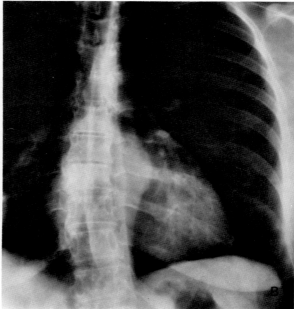

FIG. 510. ANEURYSM OF DESCENDING AORTA

A: The smooth-walled cavity in the right lower lobe was due to coccidioidomycosis. There is a suggestion of a faint increase in the paravertebral shadow behind the heart at the level of the eighth intercostal space. *B*: A Bucky film shows a protuberance on the shadow of the descending aorta. This proved to be a localized aneurysm.

with barium. Usually the esophagus is displaced together with the tortuous aorta, while an aneurysm deviates the esophagus toward the opposite side. A fusiform aneurysm can often be demonstrated on the lateral or left oblique view without the aid of barium because the opposing margins of the aorta can be delineated in these projections.

A saccular aneurysm of the descending aorta produces a localized bulge on the aortic contour. When the aneurysm is small or of moderate size, it may appear as a semicircular protuberance on the shadow of the aorta on the frontal view, and as a round, tumor-like density on the lateral projection. This may extend as far back as the posterior ribs. Even an aneurysm of moderate size can cause pressure erosion on the anterior and left aspects of the vertebral bodies. Larger ones may erode the paravertebral portions of the ribs as well. Very large aneurysms that extend to the diaphragm, can simulate a pleural effusion or a collapsed left lower lobe.

Dissecting Aneurysms of the Aorta. A dissecting aneurysm results from separation of the layers of the aortic wall by blood, with the formation of an intramural false channel. It is believed that many dissecting aneurysms begin with rupture of one of the vasa vasorum within the media, resulting in a hematoma within the

aortic wall. This often ruptures through the intima to establish a communication with the true lumen. On the other hand, the aneurysm possibly begins with an intimal tear which permits blood from the aorta to dissect into the media. In either instance, the dissection extends for a variable distance and may involve the entire length of the aorta. In some cases the distal part of the false channel ruptures back into the true lumen, allowing a free flow of blood within the aortic wall, resulting in what amounts to a double-barreled aorta.

Most dissecting aneurysms occur in association with hypertension. Some are secondary to trauma, and others are due to a congenital defect of the elastic tissue of the aorta, as in Marfan's syndrome. The latter is common enough to warrant a careful search for evidence of Marfan's syndrome whenever a dissecting aneurysm is suspected.

The aneurysm commonly begins in the arch of the aorta, just distal to the origin of the left subclavian artery, and causes enlargement of the aortic knob and widening of the descending aorta. An increase in the caliber of the descending aorta without any change in the size or contour of the aortic knob is rare. When the dissection begins immediately above the aortic valve, the ascending aorta becomes widened. The dissection usually extends further, causing enlargement of the aortic knob and widening of the descending aorta. Rarely the false channel reenters the aortic lumen proximal to the arch so that the aortic knob and descending aorta are not affected.

The widened aortic shadow caused by a dissecting aneurysm often has an irregular or wavy outer border. When the aneurysm begins just beyond the left subclavian artery, a localized hump may be seen on the superior aspect of the distal aortic knob, especially in the lateral or left oblique projection. However, in some cases the appearance of the aorta is normal or simply shows some nonspecific widening without any findings suggestive of a dissection (Fig. 511).

Differentiation between a fusiform or saccular aneurysm and a dissecting aneurysm is often difficult without angiography unless calcific plaques are visualized in the wall of the aorta. Since these plaques are situated on the intima the thickness of the aortic wall can be gauged by observing the distance between the plaques and the outer border of the aortic shadow. In a sac-

cular or fusiform aneurysm, the intima follows the contour of the aneurysmal pouch, and the distance between the intimal plaques and the outer border of the aorta measures no more than a few millimeters. In a dissecting aneurysm the accumulation of blood within the media displaces the intima inward, separating the calcific plaques from the aortic contour (Fig. 512). This sign is most valid in the descending aorta. It must be interpreted with caution in the arch, particularly on the frontal film, because the aorta is foreshortened in this view and the calcific plaques may lie in a different portion of the aorta from that which forms the border of the knob.

Dissecting aneurysms develop over a relatively short period of time. A sudden change in the configuration of the aorta is strongly suggestive of a dissection. When the aneurysm involves the ascending aorta, the aortic valve is frequently distorted so that it becomes insufficient. This causes dilation of the left ventricle together with the changes in the aorta.

A dissecting aneurysm can heal if the false channel becomes clotted and organization takes

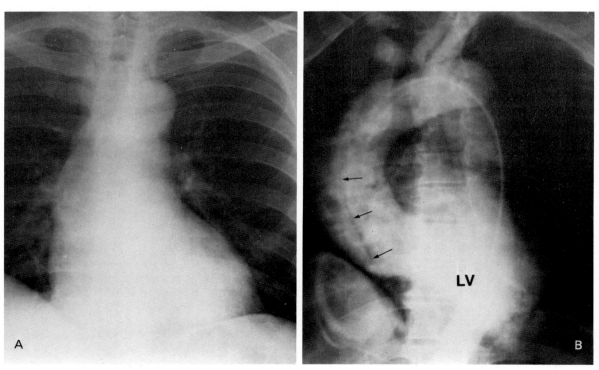

FIG. 511. DISSECTING ANEURYSM OF THE AORTA

A: The film of a 62 year old man shows moderate enlargement of the heart and tortuosity of the aorta. The appearance is compatible with the patient's history of long standing hypertension. However, because he had excruciating chest pain radiating to the back, a dissecting aneurysm was suspected. *B:* Supravalvular aortogram. The opacified aortic lumen is divided into two channels by the lucent line (arrows) representing the dissected intima. There is reflux of contrast material into the left ventricle (LV) because of insufficiency of the aortic valve.

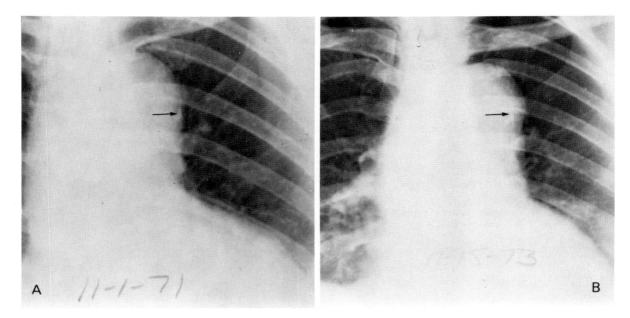

FIG. 512. DISSECTING ANEURYSM

A: 11-1-71. Routine chest film of a hypertensive patient. The aorta is widened. A calcific plaque (arrow) is seen on the outer contour of the descending aorta. *B*: 11-15-73. The patient was admitted with excruciating chest pain. The film now shows the calcific plaque (arrow) inside the contour of the aorta. The inward displacement of the intimal plaque is pathognomonic of a dissecting aneurysm.

place. When the false channel is obliterated, the width of the aortic shadow diminishes and the displaced calcific plaques revert toward their normal position in relation to the outer border of the aorta.

Dissecting aneurysms often rupture outward through the adventitia. This can produce a mediastinal hematoma which obscures the underlying aneurysm. Rupture into the pleural cavity occurs more commonly on the left side. The hemothorax may be small at first and may even resorb. Frequently, however, a massive hemothorax results. Rupture into the pericardium can also occur.

The definitive diagnosis of a dissecting aneurysm depends upon the demonstration of a second channel in the wall of the aorta. This is best done by angiography. However, if there is no free flow of blood within the false channel, the latter is not opacified, and the angiographic appearance is similar to that of a true aneurysm with a mural thrombus.

Dilatation of the Pulmonary Artery. Aneurysms of the pulmonary artery are exceedingly rare and it is often difficult, if not impossible, to differentiate them from simple dilatation of this vessel.

Dilatation of the pulmonary artery may be idiopathic but is generally due to either increased resistance in the pulmonary circulation or increased blood flow through the lungs. In pulmonary hypertension, the major pulmonary arteries are dilated while the peripheral vessels are narrow (Fig. 268). When there is increased blood flow, as in a left-to-right shunt, the peripheral vessels are also dilated (Fig. 117). In an uncomplicated aneurysm of the main pulmonary artery, none of the branches are widened.

True aneurysms of the pulmonary artery may be mycotic, luetic or congenital in origin, or may be part of a diffuse vasculitis. Radiologically, there is a well-demarcated bulge in the region of the pulmonary artery segment while the hilar vessels are of normal caliber. The bulge of the pulmonary artery is particularly notable in the right oblique view. Prominent pulsations are the rule and are seen in the lateral and right oblique views as well as in the frontal projection. Mediastinal tumors may transmit pulsations from the heart or pulmonary artery, but the pulsation is not apt to be seen in all projections. Such transmitted pulsations may disappear during deep inspiration as the heart drops away from the tumor, while pulsations of a dilated artery are unaffected.

Aneurysmal dilatation of the pulmonary artery frequently occurs distal to a stenotic pulmonic valve. However, as a rule, the poststenotic dilatation also involves the left pulmonary artery which can be recognized on the frontal view outside the bulge of the main artery. This combination is characteristic of pulmonic valvular stenosis.

Dilatation of the Great Veins. SUPERIOR VENA CAVA. The superior vena cava forms the right border of the superior mediastinum. If the vessel is of normal caliber, there is only a narrow band of opacity between the right wall of the trachea and the mediastinal border. When the superior vena cava is widened, the width of the right side of the mediastinal shadow is increased. This is best seen on the frontal projection.

The most common cause of widening of the superior vena cava is cardiac failure. In this condition the heart is usually enlarged and the pulmonary vessels are dilated.

The superior vena cava also becomes widened when it is obstructed by a mediastinal neoplasm, an aortic aneurysm, or as a result of mediastinitis or primary thrombosis. Except in the last instance, the pathologic process about the superior vena cava contributes to the widening of the mediastinal shadow. In simple thrombosis, the clot itself can cause some widening of the mediastinum. This may revert to normal as recanalization takes place and collateral channels form to relieve the obstruction. In some cases, however, numerous small new channels form in and about the wall of the obstructed vein, causing the formation of a cylindrical mass of spongy tissue (cavernous transformation) and result in permanent widening of the superior mediastinum.

AZYGOS SYSTEM. The azygos and hemiazygos veins represent the thoracic continuations of the lumbar veins and course upward immediately anterior to the vertebral bodies. The azygos vein lies slightly to the right of the midline. At the level of about the fifth thoracic vertebra, it arches forward and to the right, crossing over the right main bronchus at the tracheobronchial angle to enter the superior vena cava. The hemiazygos vein runs upward on the left between the aorta and the vertebral bodies and crosses the posterior mediastinum at the level of the eighth dorsal vertebra to empty into the azygos vein.

The esophageal, bronchial and mediastinal veins and the veins draining the chest wall enter the azygos system. The upper intercostal veins on the left side drain into the azygos by way of the accessory, or superior, hemiazygos vein. The latter crosses the spine at about the sixth or seventh dorsal vertebra.

Azygos Vein. The arch of the normal azygos vein can frequently be seen on the conventional frontal projection as a semielliptical shadow projecting from the right border of the mediastinum at the level of the tracheobronchial angle. It can always be demonstrated by tomography in this projection. Frequently the entire cross section of the vein can be delineated on the tomograms and it then appears as a perfectly round density. The entire circumference of the azygos vein can be visualized on conventional films only when the vein is separated from the mediastinum, as in the case of an azygos lobe (Fig. 213).

Dilatation of the azygos vein is almost always the result of increased flow of blood through the vessel or increased resistance to its emptying. The azygos system not only connects with the superior vena cava but also communicates with the portal system through the esophageal veins and with the inferior vena cava through the ascending lumbar veins. Thus, the azygos vein can act as a collateral channel when there is obstruction of any of these major pathways, and it often dilates because of the additional load. Increased resistance to emptying of the azygos vein and consequent dilatation of the vessel occurs when there is interference with the flow of blood through the right side of the heart. This is most commonly due to heart failure. Rarely, dilatation of the azygos vein occurs without known cause and it may be congenital.

A large azygos vein is readily visible on conventional frontal films. It appears as an oval or semicircular, homogeneous density with a smooth, regular border, projecting from the right side of the mediastinum at the level of the tracheobronchial angle. Simple enlargement of the vein can cast a shadow measuring as much as 2.5 cm in diameter. A larger shadow suggests the possibility of an aneurysm.

An enlarged azygos vein may not protrude beyond the border of the mediastinum. Sometimes it can be visualized through the shadow of the superior vena cava on adequately penetrated films, but more often tomography is required. Frontal sections should be made at the same plane as the trachea. A markedly dilated azygos vein can cause an indentation on the tracheal wall.

Radiologically, a dilated azygos vein can simulate an enlarged tracheobronchial lymph node. The long axis of the shadow of the azygos vein is characteristically oblique, extending downward and outward (Fig. 513) while the long axis of an enlarged tracheobronchial node tends to be more vertical. The azygos vein usually appears more prominent on films made in the recumbent position. In contradistinction to a large lymph node the vein becomes smaller during straining and it

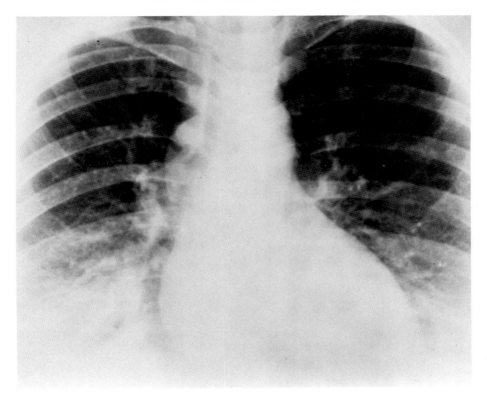

FIG. 513. PROMINENT AZYGOS VEIN

The long axis of the oval-shaped mass in the right tracheobronchial angle is oriented downward and to the right. This is characteristic of the azygos vein. The vein is dilated because the patient was in congestive failure and the systemic venous pressure was elevated.

may become larger during the Mueller maneuver.

A clear delineation of the vein can be obtained by azygography. In this procedure, a bone marrow needle is inserted into one of the lower ribs or a vertebral spinous process, and contrast material is injected. Since the marrow space drains freely into the azygos system, the veins are clearly visualized (Fig. 514).

The most common cause of dilatation of the azygos vein is cardiac failure. This is associated with enlargement of the heart and dilatation of the superior vena cava. If the failure is primarily left-sided, the pulmonary arteries and veins are also dilated. In heart failure secondary to lung disease or primary pulmonary hypertension, the major pulmonary arteries are widened, while the veins appear normal. In the case of pericardial tamponade or disease of the tricuspid valve, none of the pulmonary vessels are dilated. When the heart failure is relieved the azygos vein becomes smaller.

In the presence of obstructive portal hypertension, a prominent collateral pathway may be established through the coronary and short gastric veins. These anastomose with the esophageal venous plexus which drains into the azygos system. Thus, much of the blood which normally flows through the hepatic vein into the inferior vena cava, is diverted into the azygos system, resulting in dilatation of the azygos vein. Significant enlargement of the azygos vein from this cause is associated with esophageal varices. Therefore, when there is a density in the right tracheobronchial angle resembling a dilated azygos vein in the absence of cardiac failure, the esophagus should be examined for varices. In rare instances, collateral veins draining into the azygos system produce wavy shadows to the right of the spine just above the diaphragm. Since this region is generally hidden by the heart, overpenetrated films are required.

When the superior vena cava is obstructed below the entrance of the azygos vein, the azygos becomes dilated because it acts as a collateral pathway. The direction of flow within the azygos vein is reversed and blood from the superior vena cava is shunted into the inferior vena cava by way of the ascending lumbar veins or through the portal system. Intraosseous azygography will

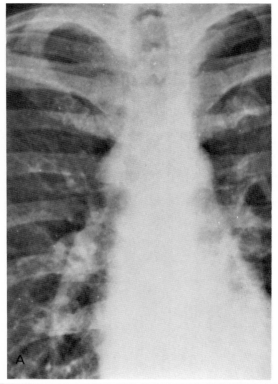

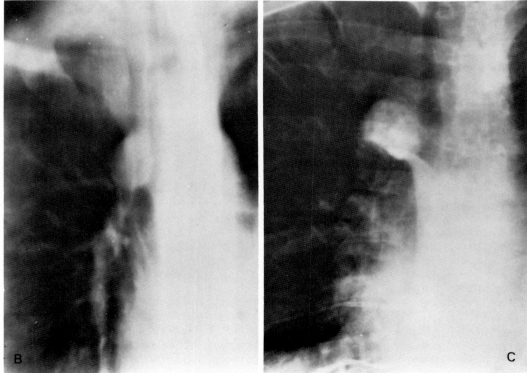

FIG. 514. DILATED AZYGOS VEIN

A: A middle-aged woman was referred because of a shadow in the right tracheobronchial angle thought to be an enlarged lymph node. However, the shadow appeared to diminish somewhat during the Valsalva maneuver. *B*: Tomography shows the mass to be sharply demarcated and oval in shape. Its long axis runs in an oblique direction outward and downward. This corresponds to the axis of the azygos vein. *C*: Azygography, by injection of contrast material into the marrow of the eighth rib, results in opacification of the mass confirming that it represents the azygos vein.

not demonstrate the proximal portion of the azygos vein because of the abnormal direction of flow, and can be misinterpreted to indicate obstruction of this vessel. Venography through a vein in the upper extremity is required to demonstrate the block in the superior vena cava and to outline the proximal portion of the azygos vein.

Marked dilatation of the azygos vein is a characteristic finding in congenital interruption of the inferior vena cava. Blood from the lower extremities then drains via the lumbar veins into the azygos system and reaches the heart through the superior vena cava. When the azygos vein appears dilated and no cause is apparent, venography should be performed through a vein in the lower extremity to determine whether or not an inferior vena cava is present. A similar, although less marked, dilatation of the azygos vein can occur following ligation or thrombosis of the inferior vena cava. A dilated azygos vein should

never be ligated before adequacy of the inferior vena caval system has been confirmed.

Cases of large azygos veins without demonstrable cause have been reported. Such instances have generally been considered as representing either localized aneurysms or idiopathic dilatation of the vein. In either case, azygos venography is required for a definitive diagnosis.

Hemiazygos Vein. The hemiazygos vein lies in front of the left side of the vertebral column, behind the aorta and crosses the spine to join the azygos vein at the level of the eighth or ninth dorsal vertebra. The normal hemiazygos vein is not visible without the aid of angiography. Even when considerably dilated, it may not produce any detectable change on ordinary films. In some cases the dilated hemiazygos vein causes a widening of the left paraspinal shadow. In rare instances, varicose or aneurysmal dilatation of the hemiazygos vein produces a wavy vertical shadow alongside the left border of the spine.

DISEASES OF THE PLEURA

The normal pleura cannot be visualized radiologically unless it is outlined by air on both sides. Even then, the pleura is so thin that it cannot be delineated if it does not lie in a plane parallel to the x-ray beam. The only portions of the pleura that meet these criteria are those that line the interlobar fissures. However, the visceral pleura covering the outer surface of the lung can be seen in the presence of a pneumothorax because it is outlined by air in the lung on one side and the air in the pleural cavity on the other.

Most abnormalities of the pleura are secondary to disease of the lung or of adjacent structures outside the pleural cavity: the mediastinum, chest wall or subphrenic region. Usually, evidences of the underlying process are visible radiologically, but in many instances the primary disease is obscured by the pleural changes, particularly when there is a large effusion. Less commonly, the disease originates in the pleura itself, or is secondary to a lesion so small or so situated, that the disease is not detectable.

Disease of the pleura is manifested radiologically either by shadows referable to the pleural abnormality itself or to the changes it produces in the surrounding structures.

Thickening of the pleura, whether by exudate, fibrosis or neoplasm, tends to cause a homogeneous shadow whose density is roughly proportional to the thickness of the diseased tissue traversed by the x-ray beam. Most large pleural effusions form a thick layer of fluid around the

lung, and regularly give rise to a dense, homogeneous shadow which obliterates the underlying pulmonary markings unless the film is overpenetrated. In the case of smaller effusions, the fluid layer is thinner and its shadow fainter, so that it casts a diffuse haze through which the vessels of the lung are easily visualized. However, even if the effusion is small, its shadow is extremely dense where it is viewed tangentially. Here it obscures the silhouette of the adjacent diaphragm, mediastinum or chest wall. Likewise, calcific plaques on the pleura, although radiopaque, cast only a faint shadow when viewed *en face,* but appear extremely dense and sharply demarcated when projected on end.

The main manifestation of pleural disease may be referable to its effect on adjacent structures. Shrinkage of the thoracic cavity with marked diminution in expansion of the lung during inspiration can be caused by thickening of the pleura so slight that it is hardly noticeable on the film. A dense shadow in the costophrenic or cardiophrenic angle or at the apex of the lung may result simply from retraction of the lung associated with pleural adhesions which themselves cast very little shadow. This can simulate marked thickening of the pleura. Elevation of the diaphragm and limitation of its motion may be the presenting signs of disease of the pleura.

Disease of the pleura may be overlooked or mistaken for an abnormality of the lung unless the lesion is projected tangentially. When the layer of involvement is thin, it may not be visible when viewed *en face*. When the lesion is thicker, it can cast a homogeneous density which is easily confused with intrapulmonary disease. However, the shadow of the diseased pleura causes an intensification of the vascular markings in the lung beneath it, while in pulmonary disease, the shadows of the vessels are either distorted or obscured.

The diagnosis of disease of the pleura cannot be confirmed without demonstrating that the lesion is broad-based against the pleural surface. This requires that it be projected tangentially. The frontal view suffices if the process is situated along the lateral border of the chest or against the short fissure. When the lesion is situated elsewhere on the pleura, lateral or oblique projections are required.

Because of the wide curve of the lateral border of the chest, the standard oblique projection may not provide a proper tangential view, especially in the case of small lesions. The optimum degree of obliquity is best determined by rotating the patient under fluoroscopic observation. The oblique view is also useful in disclosing small effusions or tumors in the posterior costophrenic sulcus, a region which is hidden by the subphrenic structures on the frontal projection.

Films made with the patient in the recumbent or decubitus positions often provide useful information in cases of pleural disease. Free fluid in the pleural cavity can be recognized by its shift into the dependent portion of the chest. Displacing the fluid in this way serves to uncover the underlying lung or a loculated effusion otherwise obscured by the free fluid.

In the supine position, free fluid flows away from the base of the pleural cavity, to be distributed over a large area in the posterior portion of the chest. The layer of fluid is then thin and may cast only a faint haze over a large part of the hemithorax. At the same time the border of the diaphragm becomes visible, contrasted against the lung which is no longer separated from it by the fluid. With the patient in the supine position, a small collection of free fluid on the left side tends to gravitate into the paravertebral gutter. It then displaces the paravertebral line laterally, often beyond the border of the descending aorta. These changes may be noted on films of the esophagus or dorsal spine and may be the first indication of a pleural effusion.

The lateral decubitus film is made with a horizontal x-ray beam and the patient lying on his side. The view is designated according to the dependent side. Thus, the term right lateral decubitus denotes that the patient is resting on his right side. The lateral decubitus position is particularly useful in disclosing small collections of fluid. Fluid at the base of the pleural cavity shifts its position to layer against the lateral portion of the chest upon which the patient lies. This produces a band of homogeneous density alongside the axillary border of the chest. When the film is made in the opposite decubitus position, this shadow disappears and the costophrenic sinus becomes clear as the fluid is displaced toward the mediastinum. The latter position is also useful in the case of a large effusion to permit study of the diaphragm and the lateral pleural surface. The lateral decubitus position is useful to differentiate between a loculated and a free effusion, to disclose the presence of an air-fluid level in doubtful cases, and to depict the upper limit of an empyema cavity.

Films made in expiration can disclose a small pleural effusion or a pneumothorax which is not visible or only suspected on films made in full inspiration (Fig. 32). Fluid in the lateral costophrenic sinus frequently simulates diaphragmatic adhesions, and a small effusion in the depths of a costophrenic sinus may not be visible on inspiration, even on oblique views. During expiration the diaphragm approximates the chest wall, obliterating the costophrenic sinus. This forces the fluid upward along the lateral chest wall where it is more easily recognized. In the case of a pneumothorax, elevation of the diaphragm during expiration decreases the height of the collection of air in the pleura. Since the volume of the pneumothorax remains unchanged, its width must increase. A tiny pneumothorax which is easily overlooked, therefore, becomes readily apparent during expiration. Furthermore, as air is expired, the lung becomes more opaque so that its edge, which is difficult to identify during inspiration, becomes strikingly clear against the lucency of the pneumothorax (Fig. 515).

Calcified plaques on the pleura can be differentiated from ordinary pleural thickening by means of Bucky films. Bucky films are also useful for the detection and delineation of lesions in the lung that are hidden by markedly thickened pleura. Tomograms, which reveal greater detail, are used for the same purpose when Bucky films do not provide sufficient information.

Fluoroscopy. Fluoroscopy is a useful adjunct in the study of pleural disease. It aids in determining the position in which the x-ray beam is tangential to the lesion in the pleura. The examination may disclose an unusual flutter of the heart, quite characteristic of pneumothorax. This is frequently present even when the collection of

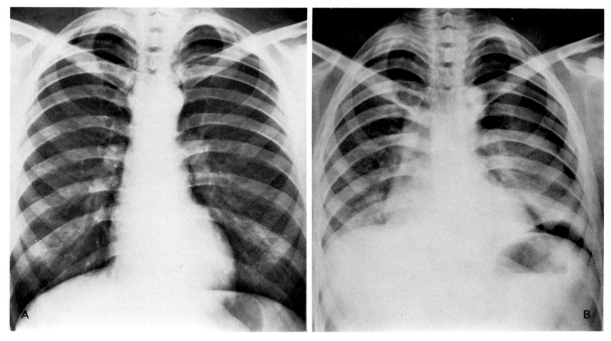

FIG. 515. PNEUMOTHORAX: INSPIRATION-EXPIRATION

A: Inspiration. With the lungs completely expanded it was almost impossible to detect the pneumothorax even on the original film. *B*: Expiration. The lungs are now clouded. The pneumothorax on the left side is now obvious. This is due to the increased contrast between the air in the pleura and the partly collapsed lung and because the pneumothorax space is wider. The pneumothorax appears larger because its volume has not changed while that of the hemithorax has diminished considerably.

air is so small that it is not readily seen on the films. Adequate localization for aspiration of a small loculation of fluid or for needle biopsy of a small tumor involving the pleura is best done under fluoroscopic control.

Fluoroscopic observation of relative movement between a density in the pulmonary field and the overlying ribs indicates that the lesion is situated either in the lung or visceral pleura, and that it is not adherent to the parietes. Conversely, lack of motion between the lesion and the ribs indicates either that the lesion is related to the parietal pleura or that the pleural surfaces are adherent to each other. To guard against contamination of the pleural cavity in performing a needle biopsy, it is important to determine whether the pleura is adherent over the lesion. Motion between the lesion and the ribs indicates that the pleural space is not obliterated. However, fluoroscopy in the erect position may be misleading. In some cases, motion between the lesion and the overlying ribs cannot be demonstrated during deep inspiration, even though the pleural cavity is free of adhesions. This is probably due to the weight of the lesion which limits its mobility when the patient is erect. Relative motion between the lesion and the ribs may be observed during the act of coughing or by examination of the patient in the recumbent position.

If the pleural cavity is free, differentiation between a lesion of the visceral pleura from one on the parietal side can be made by x-ray examination after induction of a pneumothorax (Fig. 25). A lesion on the visceral pleura retracts together with the lung, while one on the parietal side appears as a projection from the chest wall into the pneumothorax space. Nodules on the pleura that are hidden by an effusion are not always visible after the fluid is removed, but are frequently demonstrable when air is instilled into the pleural cavity (see Fig. 562). The nodules are most clearly delineated on films made in the decubitus position with the affected side uppermost.

Pleural Adhesions and Thickening

Pleural adhesions are an extremely common finding at postmortem examination. The degree of pleural thickening associated with these fibrotic adhesions is relatively minor and is insufficient to produce a shadow on the roentgen film unless the slightly thickened pleura is projected on end. Often adhesions in the pleural fissures cannot be differentiated from the linear shadows produced by the normal pleura lining the fissures. However, the adherent pleura is seen more consistently because it is dense enough to cast a shadow even when the x-ray beam is not exactly parallel to the fissure.

On the frontal projection, the short fissure, which divides the upper from the middle lobe, is seen as a horizontal, linear shadow crossing the anterior part of the fourth rib in the anterior axillary line (Fig. 122). The long fissure is best seen on the lateral view, extending downward and forward from the fourth or fifth dorsal vertebra. On the right side the fissure reaches the anterior extremity of the diaphragm, immediately behind the sternum, while on the left it makes contact with the diaphragm 3 or 4 cm behind this point (Fig. 53).

Normally the fissures are straight or show a gentle curve. On the lateral view, the upper portion of the long fissure may be bent slightly downward. When curved in this manner, the upper portion of the fissure can lie parallel to the x-ray beam in the posteroanterior projection, particularly if the tube is elevated. The fissure is then visualized, in this view as an oblique or curved line, running downward and outward from the mediastinum to the lateral chest wall. On the right side it either crosses or lies below the short fissure. If the long fissure has an S-shaped curve, the lower as well as the upper portion of the fissure may be parallel to the x-ray beam. This results in two linear shadows, suggesting multiple fissures.

An acquired pleural fissure can form in association with a focal area of atelectasis as the visceral pleura is drawn inward when the involved portion of lung collapses (Fig. 99). The infolded pleura produces a streak-like shadow when viewed on end (Fleischner line). This disappears when the lung reexpands. However, the linear shadow becomes permanent if adhesions develop within the newly formed fissure (Fig. 98).

Adhesions between the visceral and parietal pleura do not cast a shadow unless they are associated with marked pleural thickening. They are recognized only by their effects on adjacent structures. A dense shadow in the costophrenic sulcus is most commonly the result of adhesion of the diaphragm to the chest wall with comparatively little thickening of the pleura (Fig. 114). Similarly, blunting of the cardiophrenic angle is usually caused by adhesion between the mediastinal and diaphragmatic pleura, obliterating the normal recess in this region. Obliteration of the pleural recess between the anterior mediastinum and the chest wall by adhesions results in a straightening of the border of the mediastinum. The contours of the individual mediastinal structures, normally seen in the frontal projection, are effaced and the definition of the mediastinal border becomes exceedingly sharp (Fig. 75).

Dense, sharply pointed, triangular shadows extending into the pulmonary field from the diaphragm or the borders of the mediastinum (tenting) have been considered to result from traction by pleural adhesions. However, it is most probable that they are really caused by foci of atelectasis in the underlying lung, producing a fissure into which a portion of the parietal pleura and its subjacent tissues are drawn (Fig. 516). This is proved by disappearance of the pleural tent when the lung is separated from the diaphragm by a pneumothorax, and its reappearance when the pneumothorax is absorbed. If the lung is adherent to the diaphragm in this region, the tent-like shadow persists despite the pneumothorax.

Pleural adhesions which are not evident under ordinary circumstances may be demonstrated after induction of a pneumothorax (Fig. 293). If the adhesions involve the entire surface of the lung, the pleural space is completely obliterated and no air can enter it. However, if the adhesions are localized or scattered, only those portions of the lung that are adherent are prevented from collapsing. If the area of adhesion is small, almost the entire lung will collapse, stretching the fixed portion so that it casts a strand-like shadow extending across the pneumothorax space to the chest wall. When the area of adhesion is extensive, a considerable portion of the lung remains in contact with the chest. However, if the pneumothorax is not large, incomplete collapse of the lung does not necessarily signify pleural adhesions. Under these circumstances, it is possible for the pneumothorax to remain localized to the upper portion of the chest while the lower part of the lung remains fully expanded.

Thickening of the pleura beyond that associated with adhesions may be caused simply by fibrosis of the pleura. However, marked thickening, producing a dense roentgen shadow, is rarely due to fibrous tissue alone. It may be caused by fibrinous exudate, either fresh or in the process of organization, or by granulation tissue accompanied by exudate signifying the presence of active inflammation.

Diffuse fibrosis of the pleura unaccompanied by active inflammation usually causes no visible change in the general density of the pulmonary

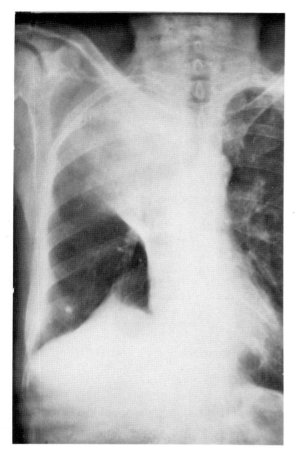

FIG. 516. DIAPHRAGMATIC TENTING

The right upper lobe is completely collapsed as a result of an obstructing bronchogenic carcinoma. The outer portion of the short fissue is displaced upward. The right leaf of the diaphragm is paralyzed. It is elevated and shows a triangular peak in its midportion. This is due to a focal area of atelectasis at the base of the lung, drawing the diaphragmatic pleura upward.

field, but occasionally it produces a faint haze over one side of the chest. The thickened pleura is best visualized along the border of the lung, where it appears as a sharply defined, narrow, opaque rim, paralleling the chest wall. When the process extends over the entire lung, the shadow extends from the apex down to the costophrenic sulcus, which is partially or completely obliterated. Often the thickened pleura is best seen in the oblique projection. In the case of simple fibrosis, the thickened pleura, viewed on end, rarely measures more than one or two millimeters in width. A thicker shadow indicates active inflammatory disease or a layer of fluid. When the causative agent is eliminated, the exudate is absorbed, the granulation tissue atrophies, and

only a thin layer of fibrous tissue remains. Active disease should be suspected even though the appearance remains unchanged for a long time.

When the lung is collapsed by a pneumothorax or a pleural effusion, even a thin layer of fibrous tissue deposited on the visceral pleura can prevent its complete reexpansion. Despite the partial atelectasis and the pleural thickening, the pulmonary field is only slightly clouded. The incomplete expansion of the lung results in a decrease in the volume of the affected hemithorax. The ribs are drawn together and their obliquity is increased, flattening the lateral chest wall and the dome of the thorax. The mediastinum usually shifts slightly toward the affected side, the costophrenic sinus is obliterated, and the diaphragm becomes elevated (Fig. 75).

Persistence of the source of irritation prolongs the inflammatory process in the pleura and increases the pleural thickening. Chronic infection in the underlying lung, as in tuberculosis, lung abscess or bronchiectasis, can result in thickening of the pleura extensive enough to obscure the pulmonary disease. Especially marked thickening occurs in certain fungous infections. Noninfectious irritants may also cause chronic pleural thickening, as in the case of some of the dust diseases (see Figs. 553 and 554) or following the instillation of talc or Lipiodol into the pleural space. A similar effect can be produced by the hemosiderin deposited in the pleura following a hemothorax. This acts as a chronic irritant and maintains the pleural thickening long after the hemothorax has been absorbed (Fig. 31).

Diffuse inflammatory thickening of the pleura is manifested chiefly by a homogeneous shadow over the lungs. The density of the shadow varies according to the thickness of the pleura and the radiographic technique employed. If the pleura is only moderately thickened, the markings of the lung are visible through the shadow, and a fairly well demarcated band of increased density separates the lung from the chest wall wherever the pleura is projected tangentially. Extreme thickening of the pleura produces a diffuse opacity, which obscures these details on standard films. Recognition of disease in the underlying lung then depends on films made with increased penetration or tomography.

The possibility that a dense shadow associated with a chronic pleuritis may be caused by a residual empyema should always be considered. Only a minor shadow of pleural thickening remains if an empyema has been adequately treated and the disease in the underlying lung has resolved. Persistence of a dense pleural shadow indicates persistence of the infection. If there is no evidence of continuing pulmonary disease, the shadow resembling marked pleural thickening must be attributed to a residual empyema (see Fig. 540).

Localized Pleural Thickening. Local thickenings of the pleura take on various forms depending upon their location and extent, and the type of disease they represent.

Thickening of the pleura at the apex of the lung is often characterized by a crescentic shadow, usually following the curve of the posterior part of the second rib. This may be unilateral or bilateral and is most often secondary to apical tuberculosis (Fig. 495). When it is confined to one side, evidences of the underlying tuberculous lesion are almost always visible in the form of active infiltrations, fibrous strands, or fibrous or calcified tubercles. In the absence of such changes, the possibility of an apical carcinoma involving the pleura must be considered if the lesion is unilateral. Bilateral pleural caps are not infrequently encountered without any shadows to indicate the presence of disease in the apex of the lung. These are mostly due to healed, hematogenous tuberculosis.

A dense shadow in a costophrenic sinus, simulating a small collection of fluid, can be caused by fibrinous exudate or fibrosis involving the pleura in this region. The shadow differs from that of fluid in that its upper border is apt to appear irregular and does not ascend along the lateral chest wall like the meniscus of an effusion. In addition, there is usually a deformity of the outer part of the diaphragm, caused by adhesions to the parietes (Fig. 75).

A dense, local thickening of the pleura by exudate in the anterior or posterior part of the chest may cast a faint homogeneous shadow on the frontal film, simulating disease in the underlying lung. The homogeneity of the shadow, the lack of distortion of the pulmonary vessels visualized through it, the gradually increasing opacity as the shadow approaches the lateral portion of the chest and its gradual fading into the remainder of the field, serve to differentiate this type of pleural thickening from a lesion of the lung.

An unusual, but characteristic, type of pleural thickening is depicted by a stellate shadow, broadbased against the chest wall. Sharply defined linear strands radiate from the area of pleural thickening into the pulmonary field. The ribs are drawn together over the lesion, and their motion is restricted. This bizarre appearance results from the absorption of a loculated effusion which had been present for a considerable length of time while fibrous tissue was being deposited over the portion of lung compressed by the fluid. This sequence of events can occur during the course of a pulmonary infarct, as well as with other conditions associated with a localized effusion. The radiating streaks represent adherent infoldings of the pleura associated with focal areas of atelectasis in the lung. Absorption of the fluid and contraction of the pleura by fibrosis account for the convergence of the streak-like shadows. Once formed, this picture persists indefinitely.

Certain localized thickenings of the pleura present an appearance easily confused with that of nodules situated within the lung. Small, nodular shadows, up to three or four millimeters in diameter, may suggest pulmonary metastases. They are few in number and bilateral in distribution. At operation or autopsy, they are seen to be situated within the visceral pleura and consist of fibrous tissue containing anthracotic deposits. Radiologically, the nodules are well demarcated and appear rather irregular in shape. Their nature may be suspected from their peripheral situation, as determined by oblique films or by rotating the patient during fluoroscopy.

Larger nodules can be caused by fibrin bodies in the pleura. These usually develop in association with a pneumothorax. They are easily recognized at that time because they lie in the free pleural cavity and are demarcated by the contrasting air (see Fig. 549). When the lung expands, the fibrin body may still be evident as a fairly well localized shadow, 1.5 to 2 cm in diameter. Several such shadows may be present in patients who have had pneumothorax treatment for tuberculosis, and may closely resemble tuberculous nodules within the lung. That they represent nonspecific fibrin bodies can be determined by review of films made while the pneumothorax was present or by making tangential films to show their relationship to the pleura.

A rare form of localized thickening of the pleura, of unknown cause, is characterized by the presence of hyaline fibrotic plaques confined to the parietal pleura. These have a smooth surface and are not adherent to the underlying lung. They produce oval or irregular, rather poorly demarcated densities, varying up to 3 to 4 cm in diameter. They may be single or multiple, and bilateral. They are rather flat and therefore usually can be differentiated from lesions in the lung by examination in a position in which the lesion is projected on end. Although calcific deposits may be present within the lesions, they are rarely dense enough to be demonstrated radiologically. This is in contrast to the pleural plaques of asbestosis in which calcification is a common and characteristic finding on the films.

In the absence of adhesions, fluoroscopic examination shows movement between the lung markings and the shadow. The latter maintains its relationship to the overlying ribs during respiration and coughing. An induced pneumothorax will separate the lung from the lesion which remains fixed to the chest wall. These observations serve to differentiate this type of hyaline plaque from one on the visceral pleura and from a lesion in the lung. However, it may be difficult, if not impossible, to differentiate it from a tumor of the parietal pleura. The latter is usually more dome-shaped when viewed in the proper projection, but it can be flat and present the same appearance as a hyaline pleural plaque.

Calcification of the Pleura. Although the causes of pleural calcification are varied, there are only a limited number of conditions in which the calcification is extensive enough to be recognized radiologically. Often the type and distribution of the calcific deposits is sufficiently characteristic to indicate a specific cause.

Calcification of the pleura may result from tuberculous pleurisy and also develops quite frequently following pneumothorax treatment for pulmonary tuberculosis. The deposition of calcium may be due to a complicating tuberculous pleurisy or it may result from bleeding in the pleura caused by the pneumothorax needle. Calcium is frequently deposited in the wall of a tuberculous empyema or around an oleothorax (see Fig. 541). The wall of a chronic empyema may also become calcified. Pleural calcification can occur in the wake of a hemothorax, either traumatic (Fig. 517) or secondary to a pulmonary infarct. Finally, asbestosis and talcosis are frequently accompanied by the formation of calcific plaques on the pleura (Figs. 330 and 333).

Perhaps the most common example of pleural calcification is that which occurs in association with the fibrotic apical pleural cap resulting from hematogenous pulmonary tuberculosis. The calcification is usually bilateral and is characterized by a thin, dense, sharply outlined, curvilinear shadow over the apex of the lung (Fig. 518). Its proximity to the dome of the thoracic cavity depends upon the degree to which the apex of the lung has retracted.

Calcific plaques of various sizes occur in association with sheet-like thickening of the pleura following tuberculous pleurisy, hemothorax or pneumothorax treatment. Unless the plaques are viewed on end, they produce rather faint, bizarre, irregular shadows, quite unlike those which occur in disease of the lung. When seen *en face*, the

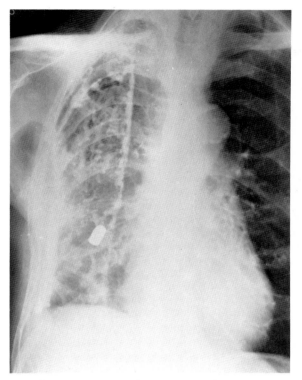

Fig. 517. Pleural Calcification Following Hemothorax

Many years previously the patient had a hemothorax as the result of a gunshot wound. At present the film shows shrinkage of the right hemithorax and generalized thickening of the pleura. The pleura is calcified. It casts a linear shadow where it is projected tangentially. The metallic density represents the bullet.

shadows appear lace-like because of the irregular manner in which the calcium is deposited within the thickened pleura. When the calcium deposit surrounds an area of noncalcified pleura, it can simulate a cavity within the lung (Fig. 133). In any case, a tangential projection will show the characteristic density of calcium and will demonstrate the position of the lesion in relation to the chest wall, proving that it is situated in the pleura rather than in the lung.

The calcium is usually deposited slowly so that the shadow of the thickened, calcified pleura increases in density and extent as the years go by. Often, there is marked thickening of the pleura peripheral to the layer of calcification, producing a relatively lucent zone of soft tissue density between the rim of calcified pleura and the thoracic cage. This occurs particularly in tuberculous pleurisy, an extensive hemothorax or a chronic empyema.

An irregular deposition of calcium can take place within a pleural fibrin body which can

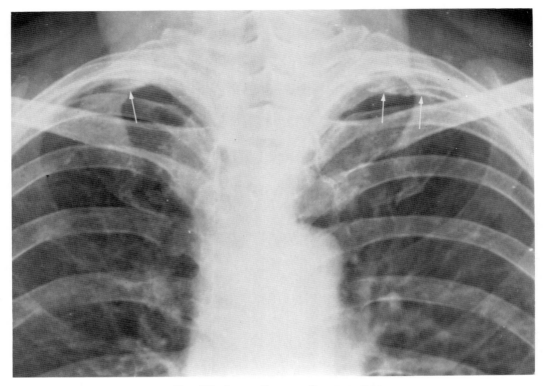

FIG. 518. APICAL PLEURAL CALCIFICATION

The dense, linear shadows (arrows) parallel to the dome of the thorax on each side, represent calcified pleural plaques. These are probably the residua of hematogenous tuberculosis.

retain its round appearance on all views, simulating a calcified lesion in the lung. The diagnosis should be suspected if there is a history of pneumothorax therapy or severe chest trauma, and can be proved by identifying the fibrin body in the free pleural space on films made at the time of the pneumothorax.

The dense shadow of a chronic empyema, either tuberculous or pyogenic, may be partly stippled or show a lace-like pattern as a result of calcium within its wall. Here again the calcification produces a sharply defined, dense, curvilinear shadow where it is viewed on end. The calcium is deposited in the lining of the empyema adjacent to the collection of pus. The rim of calcification is, therefore, separated from the ribs by a band of lesser density representing markedly thickened, indurated, fibrotic pleura. A similar rim of calcium is sometimes deposited in the wall of an oleothorax.

Calcific plaques on the pleura are frequently encountered in workers exposed to talc or asbestos dust, and in some cases of diatomaceous earth pneumoconiosis. Usually, the calcific deposits do not become apparent for a period of 10 or 15

years after the initial exposure. Their incidence and extent increase as the exposure continues, but the calcific deposits may first appear and progress years after exposure has ceased. Usually the plaques are rather small, measuring 2 to 3 cm in length, and are situated mainly in the lower half of the chest, most frequently over the dome of the diaphragm. Most of the plaques are thin and are either invisible or cast an extremely faint shadow when projected *en face* (Fig. 331). They are much more easily detected when viewed on end. A frontal film, therefore, is not sufficient to exclude the presence of these plaques. Oblique and lateral projections are required, but even when viewed tangentially, the calcification may not be recognizable without Bucky films. If searched for, the plaques can often be seen on both sides of the chest. In patients with prolonged exposure to talc or asbestos the pleural calcification can be very extensive and thick plaques can appear as bizarre shadows over a large part of the pulmonary field (Fig. 333).

Although some of the plaques involve the visceral pleura, the majority are confined to the parietal layer. In contrast to pleural calcification from other causes, pleural adhesions are often absent over the plaques. The fact that the pleural space is free, can be determined by fluoroscopy which will show relative movement between the plaque and the markings in the underlying lung during respiration or coughing.

The recognition of pleural plaques on the roentgen film should always suggest the possibility of silicatosis. At times, well-developed, calcified plaques are present even though the pulmonary fibrosis is barely visible or not seen at all. Discovery of even one plaque should lead to a careful inquiry regarding possible exposure to talc or asbestos. In other cases, when the pulmonary fibrosis is marked, the plaques may be overlooked. Since they have such great diagnostic significance, they should be searched for carefully in all persons with bilateral interstitial disease of the lungs, as well as in all cases where the possibility of asbestosis is suspected.

Pleural Effusion

A pleural effusion is generally caused by disease outside the pleura; only rarely is it a manifestation of a pathologic process originating in the pleura itself. The most common causes are congestive heart failure and disease of the underlying lung, although, not infrequently, the effusion is secondary to disease of the mediastinum, diaphragm or chest wall. Occasionally, the effusion is part of a more generalized disease, such as disseminated tuberculosis, some other systemic infection or one of the autoimmune states. A collection of fluid in the pleura can also occur in association with a benign or malignant tumor of one of the pelvic organs. Finally, the effusion may be secondary to conditions which affect the distribution of the body fluids, such as nephrosis, liver disease or myxedema.

The roentgen appearance of the effusion is the same whether the fluid is serous, sanguinous, chylous or purulent, and the density of the shadow is similar to that of the soft tissues in the body. The basic characteristics of the shadow are its homogeneity and the fact that the pulmonary markings are visible within it. The degree of opacity of the shadow depends upon the thickness of the layer of fluid traversed by the rays and by the presence of disease in the underlying lung.

If the pleural effusion is not loculated, it is distributed around the lung, forming a curved envelope of fluid. The shadow of the effusion is more dense where the x-ray beam is tangential to the curve because here the rays traverse the greatest depth of fluid. Conversely, where the fluid layer lies perpendicular to the x-ray beam, its shadow is fainter (Fig. 520).

Fluid in the pleural cavity displaces the lung from the chest wall. Because of this, no lung markings are seen in the portion of the chest where the fluid layer is projected tangentially. On the other hand, where the effusion is viewed *en face*, the displacement of the lung cannot be appreciated because it occurs in a direction perpendicular to the film. If the rays are sufficiently penetrating, the vascular markings of the lung can be visualized within the homogeneous shadow of the effusion. Conversely, in the case of consolidation of the lung, the vascular markings of the affected portion are obliterated on all views. In the rare instance where a pleural effusion is associated with complete atelectasis of the underlying lung, no pulmonary markings are visible.

The roentgen appearance of an effusion varies with the amount of fluid, its distribution, and whether it is free or loculated. These characteristics, together with abnormalities of the remainder of the pleura, the underlying lung and neighboring structures are often helpful in identifying the cause of the effusion.

Free Fluid

A free effusion is one which is not confined to any portion of the pleural cavity and is free to change its distribution with changes in the position of the patient. Although the lung may be adherent to the parietal pleura in one or more places, these adhesions do not prevent shifting of the fluid. The effusion may represent either a transudate or an exudate or consist of blood which is partly clotted, and still lie free within the pleural space. A free effusion which is purulent should be called a *pyothorax* rather than an empyema since the latter term indicates loculation of the pus.

The distribution of the fluid in the pleural cavity depends primarily on the influence of gravity, capillary attraction and the resistance of the lung to expansion. A small effusion tends to collect first in the posterior and lateral costophrenic sinuses. As the volume of the fluid increases, it spreads over the entire diaphragm, obscuring its dome and extending upward for a variable distance along the chest wall to surround the lower part of the lung. If the lung is normal, the collection of fluid diminishes in thickness as it extends upward. This pattern is altered when the lung is abnormal, one portion having a greater tendency to retract than the rest. The fluid will then tend to accumulate over the region where the lung is the least distensible. This accounts for most variations from the usual pattern of distribution of fluid in the pleural cavity.

Typical Pattern of Free Effusion. Small effusions usually cause blunting of the costophrenic sinus. Since the posterior costophrenic sinus is the most dependent, the fluid tends to collect here first. Fluid in the posterior costophrenic sinus is best visualized by examining the patient in the oblique projection, the right oblique for an effusion on the right side, and the opposite oblique for an effusion on the left. An effusion of this size often is not detectable on the frontal projection because only the lateral costophrenic sinus is visible, while the posterior sinus is hidden by the shadows of the diaphragm and abdominal viscera. Even smaller amounts of fluid can be demonstrated by examining the patient in the oblique view during expiration, because the costophrenic sinus is partially obliterated as the diaphragm rises, displacing the fluid upward.

A small collection of fluid in the lateral costophrenic sinus may not blunt or obliterate the sinus if the fluid extends upward along the lateral border of the chest. The costophrenic sinus appears sharp on the frontal projection, but its lateral border is abnormally thick and dense. This shadow, representing fluid is often overlooked because it is easily confused with that of the anterior axillary portion of one of the ribs which runs in the same direction. It may also be mistaken for thickening of the parietal pleura.

A small effusion must be differentiated from pleural adhesions, which also cause blunting or obliteration of the costophrenic sinus. An irregularity of the upper border of the obliterated sinus favors adhesions, while a smooth, concave meniscus is more indicative of fluid.

A definitive diagnosis of free fluid in the costophrenic sinus can be made by demonstrating a change in the shadow when the patient is examined in a tilted or decubitus position. Clouding of the lung above the costophrenic sinus when the patient is tilted toward that side proves the presence of fluid. Extremely small collections of fluid may be demonstrated in the lateral decubitus position with the patient lying on the involved side. A characteristic linear density appears along the lateral border of the chest, representing fluid which has gravitated to the dependent side. A film made in the opposite decubitus is of equal value. If the involved side is uppermost, the fluid flows away from the costophrenic sinus which then appears clear. The fluid

which layers alongside the mediastinum usually cannot be identified. If the blunting of the sinus is due to adhesions, its appearance does not change significantly regardless of the patient's position.

Larger effusions occupy the entire lower portion of the chest. The shadow of the fluid is most dense at the base and becomes progressively more lucent in its upper portion as the layer of fluid becomes thinner (Fig. 519). With the exception of infrapulmonary effusions, the shadow of the fluid is highest along the outer border of the chest, suggesting that it extends upward for a greater distance in this location. However, this is not actually the case. The layer of fluid around the lung extends to the same level across the entire hemithorax. This can be demonstrated by injecting a dilute solution of iodized oil into the effusion. The light, radiopaque material floats to the top of the fluid and forms a horizontal level, crossing the hemithorax at the same height as the upper limit of the shadow of the fluid along the chest wall (Fig. 520).

The curvilinear border of the effusion on the film results from the relation of the fluid collection around the lung to the x-ray beam. In the frontal projection, the shadow of the upper part of the fluid is dense in the axillary region because here the rays pass tangentially through the layer of fluid as it curves around the lung. More mesially the layer of fluid is viewed *en face*. Even though the rays pass through the fluid both in front of the lung and behind it, the layers are so thin that they cast little or no shadow. This is true in all erect positions—the fluid always appears to extend highest at the periphery of the pulmonary field (Fig. 88).

Whereas effusions of moderate or large size are immediately apparent on the frontal or oblique projection, they often are not so obvious on the lateral view. The fluid may not be visualized at all on this projection because of superimposition of the two lungs, the subphrenic organs, the heart and the spine. The presence of an effusion can be suspected from the appearance of the diaphragm. Normally, on the lateral projection, both leaves of the diaphragm are sharply outlined by the air in the adjacent lung. When fluid covers the dome of the diaphragm, it displaces the lung upward and obliterates the diaphragmatic silhouette. If the effusion is unilateral, only one leaf of the diaphragm is visible on the lateral film. If the effusion is bilateral, neither leaf can be identified.

Even with a small effusion, some of the fluid probably extends into the interlobar fissures, but this is often difficult to recognize radiologically.

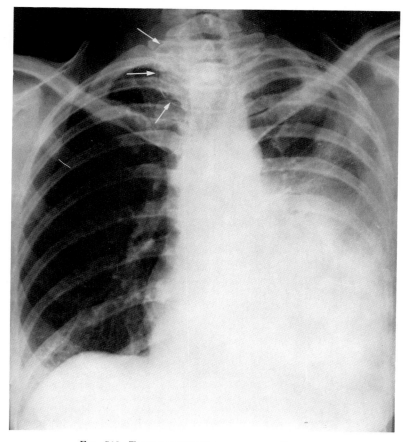

FIG. 519. TUBERCULOUS PLEURISY WITH EFFUSION

There is a moderate-sized effusion in the left pleural cavity. The upper border of the fluid is indistinct because of considerable thickening of the pleura. Infiltrations are present at the apex of each lung and there is an area of consolidation beneath the left clavicle. This was due to active tuberculosis. The lower cervical trachea is displaced to the left by a thyroid adenoma which is outlined by a rim of calcium (arrows).

If the effusion is of moderate size, its interlobar extension is usually visible. Fluid between the upper and middle lobes is clearly outlined because the short fissure is projected tangentially on films made in the erect position. When the interlobar collection is extremely small, it may cause only an accentuation of the fissure. As the amount of fluid increases, the fissure becomes widened. Fluid in the long fissure is best seen in the lateral view since the fissure is projected on end in this projection. On the frontal projection, fluid in the long fissure is often represented by a rather faint, oblique, band-like density which tapers as it runs upward and inward from the lower portion of the chest. The borders of the faint shadow are usually curved with the convexity upward, corresponding to the lines where the edges of the lobes are in contact with the chest wall.

Larger effusions extend upward over the apex of the lung, producing a curved shadow of variable width paralleling the dome of the thoracic cavity. When the effusion fills the hemithorax, the entire pulmonary field appears uniformly opaque on films made with ordinary exposure. However, with increased exposure, particularly on Bucky films, it is usually possible to penetrate the shadow of the fluid and visualize the pulmonary markings contrasted against the air in the underlying lung.

Atypical Distribution of Free Fluid. Variations in the distribution of free fluid in the pleural cavity are mainly due to variations in the compliance of different parts of the lung. The fluid tends to accumulate over the portion of the lung that is least expansile, i.e., where the compliance is the lowest. The diminished compliance is most frequently due to plugging of bronchi. Thus, most of the fluid may accumulate over an atelectatic lobe or it may extend into the pleural

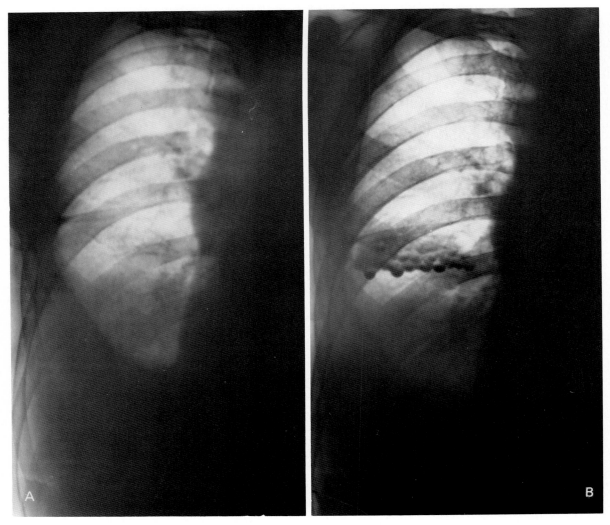

FIG. 520. TRUE LEVEL OF FREE PLEURAL EFFUSION

A: An erect film shows the usual meniscus configuration of a free pleural effusion. The horizontal line in the middle of the hemithorax represents a small amount of fluid in the short fissure. *B*: A small amount of dilute Lipiodol was injected into the effusion. The oil, which is lighter than the fluid, floats to its surface. The globules of oil outline the upper level of the fluid which is not visible on ordinary films. This portion of the fluid layer is too thin to cast a shadow when viewed *en face*. Its lateral portion can be seen because it is projected tangentially. (Courtesy of Dr. J. Kaunitz, New York, N. Y.)

cleft caused by obstruction of a subsegmental bronchus (Fig. 100). Atypical distribution of fluid may also be due to interstitial infiltrations which interfere with pulmonary expansion or to imprisonment of a portion of the lung by thickened pleura. In some instances the cause is not entirely clear.

INFRAPULMONARY EFFUSION. An infrapulmonary effusion is one in which the bulk, if not all, of the fluid is situated between the lung and the diaphragm. Actually, in the erect position, the lung floats on the fluid. Its occurrence in cardiac failure is probably due to lessened expan-

sibility of the lower lobes caused by interstitial edema together with obstruction of small bronchi resulting from congestion of the bronchial mucosa. However, its rather frequent occurrence in nephrosis and in hepatic insufficiency is not readily explained. Possible factors are decreased aeration of the lung bases because of restriction of diaphragmatic motion from concomitant ascites and perhaps diminished viscosity of the fluid because of its low protein content.

Because the fluid extends through the entire thickness of the chest from front to back, it casts a very dense, homogeneous shadow, comparable to that of the liver. Since the lung is displaced upward, pulmonary markings cannot be visualized within the shadow of the fluid even with the use of the most penetrating rays. When an appreciable portion of the fluid extends upward around the lung, the bulk of the effusion beneath the lung is not obvious. What appears to be a small or moderate-sized effusion may prove, on aspiration, to amount to 1000 cc or more.

In some cases, the upper limit of the fluid appears as a rather sharply defined, horizontal line. At first glance, this can be confused with an air-fluid level. However, on close inspection, the border of the fluid is seen to be slightly wavy, with a small meniscus at its outer extremity. This is in contrast to the sharply edged, straight, horizontal line that characterizes an air-fluid level.

More difficult to recognize is the infrapulmonary effusion whose upper border forms a sharply defined convexity without any upward extension along the chest wall. The shadow then simulates an elevated diaphragm. However, the contour of the upper border of the effusion differs somewhat from that of a high diaphragm. The shadow of an elevated diaphragm exhibits a uniform, sweeping curve whose highest point is situated at the junction of its mesial and middle thirds. On the other hand, the contour of an infrapulmonary effusion is generally made up of two components. The mesial half or two-thirds is more or less horizontal, while its outer portion

dips downward rather sharply to form an acute angle with the lateral chest wall, simulating a costophrenic sinus (Fig. 521). The mesial border of the "sinus" is formed by the fluid which abuts on the undersurface of the inferior lappet of the lower lobe.

On the lateral view, the posterior costophrenic sinus usually appears clouded or blunted, or reveals a well-outlined fluid meniscus. Here again, in contrast to the uniform curve of the diaphragm, the border of an infrapulmonary effusion often consists of two components: the posterior two-thirds presents a rather sharp, horizontal curve, cutting off the normally acute angle of the posterior costophrenic sinus, while anteriorly, where the fluid reaches the base of the long fissure, the border curves sharply downward to form an acute angle with the anterior chest wall. This angle is occupied by the inferior lappet of the middle lobe or the lingula. Its posterior border corresponds to the long fissure, against which the effusion abuts. Apparently, the lower lobe has a greater tendency to retract upward than the middle lobe. Therefore, most of the fluid is confined to the region beneath the lung behind the long fissure. Not uncommonly, a small amount of fluid extends upward into this fissure.

The position of the stomach bubble is most helpful in the recognition of an infrapulmonary effusion on the left side. Normally, in the erect position, a stomach bubble of fair size approxi-

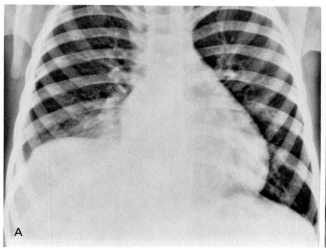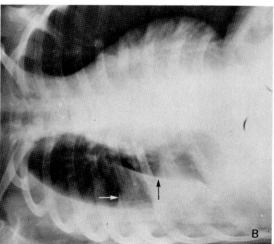

FIG. 521. INFRAPULMONARY EFFUSION

A: Erect film of a 7 year old boy following repair of an interatrial septal defect. At first glance, the right diaphragm appears elevated. However, the contour of the shadow is unlike that of the diaphragm. Its mesial two-thirds is horizontal with a sudden declivity of its outer portion. This is characteristic of a collection of fluid between the lung and diaphragm. *B*: Right lateral decubitus. The fluid has gravitated to the most dependent portion of the chest and also extends into the long fissure (black arrow) and the short fissure (white arrow). The black curved lines beneath the diaphragm are artifacts (pinch marks).

mates the diaphragm, and is separated from the lung by a distance of only a few millimeters (Figs. 131 and 237). In the presence of an infrapulmonary effusion the upper border of the collection of fluid which simulates an elevated diaphragm, is separated from the stomach bubble by a variable distance, depending upon the size of the effusion (Fig. 522). If the stomach bubble is small or not visible, the examination can be repeated after the administration of charged water or a Seidlitz powder.

While an increase in the space between the base of the lung and the stomach bubble is most frequently due to a collection of fluid between the diaphragm and the lung, a similar appearance can be caused by conditions below the diaphragm which depress the stomach bubble. Chief among these are ascites and subphrenic abscess. A large

spleen and, rarely, a large left lobe of the liver, may insinuate themselves between the stomach bubble and the diaphragm. Care must be taken in interpreting separation of the stomach bubble from the lung when the bubble is small, for this can occur under normal circumstances.

A striking and pathognomonic sign of infrapulmonary effusion, consisting of a fluid wave caused by the beating of the heart, is sometimes observed fluoroscopically. This is seen as a series of ripples extending outward from the heart to the lateral chest wall. It is more evident in the case of an effusion on the left side. The characteristic rippling should not be confused with transmission of the cardiac movement to the diaphragm by pleuropericardial adhesions. In the latter instance the movement of the diaphragm is entirely synchronous with the heart beat, with-

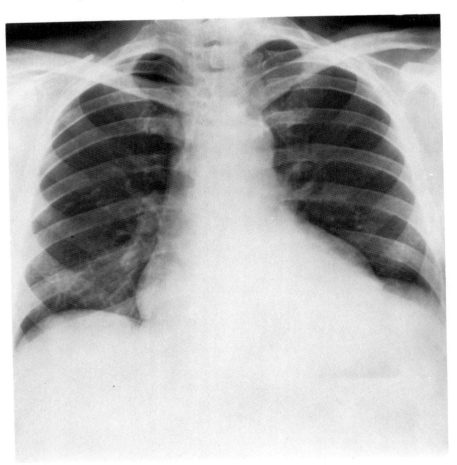

FIG. 522. INFRAPULMONARY EFFUSION

The erect film shows what appears to be an elevated left diaphragm. The stomach bubble is separated by a considerable distance from the base of the lung. This can occur with either a subphrenic abscess or an infrapulmonary effusion. However, there is a retrocardiac triangular shadow that is continuous with the contour of the "diaphragm." This indicates that both shadows are due to a single collection of fluid in the pleura. The retrocardiac component of the effusion lies behind the inferior pulmonary ligament in the posterior portion of the paramediastinal space.

out a propagated wave, and it is generally limited to the diaphragmatic segment adjacent to the heart.

Although the contour of an infrapulmonary effusion suggests loculation, the fluid is free to move with changes in the position of the patient. Tilting or placing him in the lateral decubitus position will cause the fluid to spill out of the infrapulmonary region and to gravitate along the dependent side of the chest (Fig. 521). This provides a definite method for confirming the diagnosis of infrapulmonary effusion.

MESIAL EFFUSIONS. A mesial or paramediastinal effusion refers to a collection of fluid in the pleural cavity between the lung and the mediastinum. In most free pleural effusions, with the exception of those that are quite small, some of the fluid ascends in the paramediastinal space for a variable distance. An especially large concentration of fluid in the mesial portion of the pleural cavity occurs particularly in association with an infrapulmonary effusion. The fluid in the paramediastinal region may extend to the level of the clavicle or even to the dome of the pleural cavity. When the collection of fluid is small, it may produce only a narrow band of density extending upward along the mediastinum. In the case of a large infrapulmonary effusion the paramediastinal component is usually more prominent. It may then appear on the film as a triangular shadow based on the diaphragm with the apex directed toward the root of the lung. The roentgen appearance is then easily confused with that of atelectasis of the lower lobe (Fig. 522).

The lower half of the mesial portion of the pleural cavity is divided into an anterior and a posterior component by the inferior pulmonary ligament. This is a sheet-like structure formed by the reflection of the visceral pleura covering the mesial portion of the lung onto the mediastinum. The ligament extends downward from the root of the lung. The mesial portion of the ligament is often attached to the diaphragm while the remainder of its lower border is usually free. The anterior and posterior pulmonary compartments communicate with each other under the free edge of the ligament and through the space between the undersurface of the lower lobe and the diaphragm, lateral to the ligament. A free mesial effusion occupies the anterior as well as the posterior compartment, and its shadow, therefore, blends with and obliterates the cardiac border. Because of this, the shadow of a mesial effusion can simulate that of a large heart.

If the compliance of the posterior part of the lower lobe is diminished, fluid tends to collect mainly in the posterior compartment. Since most of the effusion is situated behind the heart, the cardiac contour is not affected and the collection of fluid produces a triangular shadow suggesting a collapsed lower lobe. However, the lung root is not depressed and the short fissure, which is usually visible, is elevated. In addition, the angle between the outer border of the paramediastinal effusion and the infrapulmonary collection of fluid is more obtuse than the angle between the diaphragm and an atelectatic lower lobe.

PARIETAL EFFUSIONS. A free effusion does not always ascend along the parietal border of the chest in the usual tapering manner. It may be distributed in an atypical fashion over the outer part of the lung.

In some cases a broad band of density, representing a rather thick layer of fluid, extends from the diaphragm to the level of the short fissure. Here the band is partly cut off and only a thin layer of fluid ascends over the upper lobe. The shape of the shadow, with a ledge at the level of the short fissure, has given rise to the term, *middle lobe step* (Fig. 523). The reason for this pattern of fluid distribution most probably lies in a difference between the compliance of the upper lobe and the remainder of the lung. When the middle lobe or the middle and lower lobes are diseased, they tend to retract from the chest wall to a greater degree than does the upper lobe. This leads to accumulation of more of the fluid over these portions of the lung with a sharp change at the short fissure.

If there is diminished compliance of the upper lobe, the situation is reversed. There will then be a thin band of fluid over the lower lobe with a sudden step-like break at the short fissure from which a wider band of fluid ascends over the outer part of the upper lobe. If only part of the upper lobe is diseased, there may simply be an inward bulge of the border of the fluid at the level of the involved area without the formation of a step. In either case, the underlying mechanism is comparable to that of selective collapse of the lung in pneumothorax treatment of tuberculosis.

An unusual, but characteristic variation in the distribution of a free effusion, occurs in relation to a focal area of atelectasis (discoid atelectasis). The atelectatic area generally appears as a streak-like shadow on the film (Fleischner line). This is associated with an indrawing of the visceral pleura, producing a cleft over the atelectatic portion of lung. If the cleft is not obliterated by adhesions, a free effusion can extend into it. The fluid in the cleft produces a triangular density with its base on the parietes and its apex pointing in the direction of the hilum (Fig. 100).

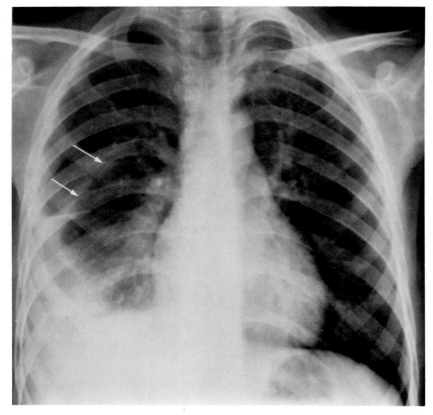

FIG. 523. PLEURAL EFFUSION: MIDDLE LOBE STEP

The pleural effusion over the outer part of the right lower lobe stops abruptly at the short fissure. The infiltrations in the right lower lobe have diminished its compliance and this is responsible for the atypical distribution of the fluid. The oblique linear shadow (arrows) extending above the short fissure, represents fluid tracking into the long fissure.

Effects of the Effusion on Neighboring Structures. As fluid accumulates within the pleural cavity, it exerts pressure on the lung, mediastinum, chest wall and diaphragm. This causes compression of the lung and tends to displace the surrounding structures away from the effusion. The degree of compression and displacement depends upon the volume of the fluid, the condition of the underlying lung, and the mobility of the other structures. Occasionally the adjacent structures are displaced to the side of the effusion. This can occur when fibrous tissue is deposited on the pleura while the lung is partially collapsed by an effusion or a hemothorax. The encased lung cannot reexpand completely as the fluid is resorbed. This causes an increase in the negativity of the pleural pressure so that the normal pressure in the opposite hemithorax pushes the structures towards the effusion.

LUNG. The lung is the structure most affected by a pleural effusion. It is compressed by the fluid. Usually the reduction in pulmonary volume takes place more or less uniformly throughout the lung. However, streak-like shadows representing focal areas of atelectasis occur quite frequently (Fig. 524), particularly in the basal segments. These are caused by stagnation of secretion in the small bronchi and interference with collateral respiration because of the limitation of respiratory motion of the lung due to the pressure of the fluid.

Even a huge effusion rarely produces complete atelectasis of the lung unless there are complicating factors. As the fluid increases, it displaces the mediastinum and diaphragm, thus limiting the pressure on the lung. The small amount of air that remains in the lung, even in extremely large effusions, permits the pulmonary vascular pattern to be recognized, provided that sufficient exposure is used. Inability to visualize the pulmonary vessels on well-penetrated films is generally indicative of consolidation or complete atelectasis. While complete atelectasis is gener-

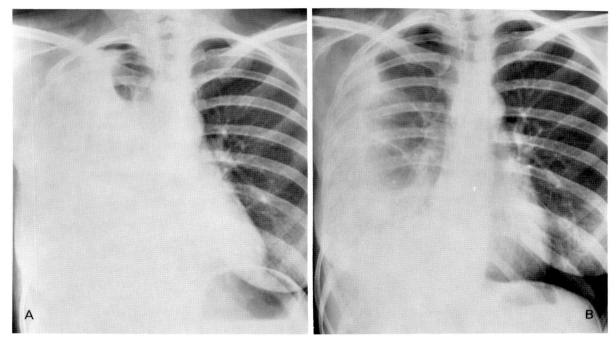

FIG. 524. FOCAL ATELECTASIS WITH PLEURAL EFFUSION

A: The fluid in the right chest was due to tuberculous pleurisy although it is most unusual to have an effusion of this size in tuberculosis. *B*: Three weeks later, after aspiration and partial absorption of the fluid, the lung that had been obscured by the fluid is visualized. It contains several streak-like shadows representing areas of focal atelectasis. These formed as a result of obstruction of small bronchi by secretion when the lung was compressed and immobilized by the effusion.

ally due to concomitant bronchial obstruction, it may be produced by the effusion alone if the diaphragm and mediastinum are fixed.

MEDIASTINUM. Although the normal mediastinum is not fixed and is therefore subject to lateral displacement by an imbalance of the pleural pressures between the two sides, it is usually not displaced by an effusion of small or moderate size. This is due to the fact that the pressure of the fluid is relieved by expulsion of some of the air from the lung and by downward displacement of the diaphragm, since these structures offer less resistance than the mediastinum. However, if the effusion is large, the mediastinum commonly shifts toward the opposite side. The degree of displacement depends on the size of the effusion and the mobility of the diaphragm as well as that of the mediastinum.

The condition of the underlying lung also affects the position of the mediastinum. If the lung cannot deflate because it is consolidated or is the seat of obstructive emphysema, a small effusion can cause displacement of the mediastinum. On the other hand, if the lung is shrunken as a result of previous disease, before the onset of the effusion, the mediastinum may not be displaced to the opposite side even if the effusion is very large. Most often, however, absence of displacement of the mediastinum to the opposite side in the presence of a large effusion is due to obstruction of a major bronchus.

Effusions of moderate or large size can produce pendular movement of the mediastinum during respiration in the absence of bronchial obstruction. Movement of the mediastinum towards the opposite side during expiration is caused by the inordinate increase in the intrapleural pressure on the side of the effusion. If the mediastinum is in its normal position during inspiration, it becomes displaced away from the effusion during expiration. When the mediastinum is already displaced to the opposite side in inspiration, the displacement is increased during expiration.

DIAPHRAGM. A free effusion affects the diaphragm primarily because of its weight. As the volume of fluid increases, the diaphragm is displaced progressively downward and its normal upward excursion during expiration is limited.

If the effusion is large enough to cover the dome of the diaphragm, its silhouette is obscured. However, the level of the left leaf of the diaphragm can be inferred from the position of the stomach bubble which is situated immediately beneath the dome. Determination of the position of the right hemidiaphragm is difficult because the only landmark is the lower border of the liver, and this may be low simply because the liver is large.

The motion of the diaphragm may be studied by observing the position of the stomach bubble or the height of the fluid in the chest during inspiration and expiration. However, the excursion of the fluid level in the chest is also affected by movement of the chest wall. As the ribs flare out during inspiration, the width of the base of the thoracic cavity increases, and since the volume of the fluid is unchanged, the effusion tends to diminish in height. The upper level of the fluid may then move downward during inspiration, even if the diaphragm remains immobile.

The diaphragm is normally arched during expiration when its muscle fibers are relaxed and at their greatest length. As the fibers contract during inspiration, the diaphragm becomes shortened in all diameters. It therefore tends to straighten out, approaching a flat plane in full inspiration.

Because of its weight, a large effusion often depresses the diaphragm so much that it is practically flat during expiration and therefore does not change in shape or position during inspiration. Diaphragmatic motion is then absent, even though the organ is not paralyzed.

Large effusions may even be heavy enough to bow the diaphragm downward so that its curve is inverted during expiration. The downward curve of the diaphragm may sometimes be observed through the stomach bubble. As the diaphragm contracts, it straightens and therefore moves upward during inspiration. This paradoxical motion mimics that of a paralyzed diaphragm. The phenomenon occurs only on the left side, apparently because inversion of the right hemidiaphragm is prevented by the liver. Since the upper border of the diaphragm is obscured by the fluid, its motion is determined by observing the movement of the stomach bubble or the level of the effusion, both of which move upward during inspiration if the diaphragm is inverted. In contrast to paralysis of the diaphragm in which the stomach bubble is higher than normal during both phases of respiration, the bubble is depressed, at least during expiration, when there is a large pleural effusion. Normal motion of the diaphragm is restored when the patient is placed in the supine or Trendelenburg position, as the weight of the fluid is shifted away from the diaphragm.

Inversion of the diaphragm disappears and the organ becomes flat as the effusion diminishes. The diaphragm then remains immobile during respiration. With a further decrease in the size of the effusion, the normal curve of the diaphragm, and its downward excursion during inspiration, are restored.

Because of the depression of the diaphragm by the effusion, a large collection of fluid may be present but not extend high in the chest. It is, therefore, difficult to judge the true size of an effusion from its height in the chest alone. The degree of downward displacement of the diaphragm must be taken into consideration. On the left side this is judged by displacement of the stomach bubble and on the right by the downward displacement of the hepatic flexure of the colon.

CHEST WALL. A free effusion which fills most of the pleural cavity tends to displace the chest wall outward, increasing the width of the thoracic cavity on that side. The anterior portion of the rib cage is shifted upward so that the ribs lie in a more horizontal plane. The diminution in the obliquity of the ribs results in a widening of the intercostal spaces.

These changes may also take place with smaller effusions if the mediastinum is fixed. On the other hand, even a large effusion may not displace the chest wall if the underlying lung is atelectatic as a result of bronchial obstruction. In fact the chest wall may be retracted if the total volume of the lung and the fluid is less than that of the normal thoracic cavity. Diminution in the width of the rib spaces and flattening of the chest wall on the side of an effusion, together with displacement of the trachea to the *opposite* side is indicative not only of bronchial obstruction but also of the presence of large paratracheal lymph nodes.

Diagnosis of Underlying Disease. Certain roentgen characteristics are often helpful in identifying the cause of a free effusion. Aspects which should be considered are the size of the effusion, the position of the mediastinum, the side on which the fluid is located, the association with enlargement of the heart and the presence of discoid atelectasis on the side opposite the effusion.

A huge effusion which fills the entire hemithorax occurs in pyogenic infections of the pleura in children. In adults, however, it almost always signifies the presence of an underlying neoplasm. In rare instances, such a huge effusion is associated with a traumatic hemothorax. It is extremely rare in tuberculosis and is never observed in pulmonary infarction.

It is to be expected that such a total effusion, if not complicated by other factors, would displace the mediastinum to the opposite side. Shift of the mediastinum toward the effusion indicates atelectasis of the underlying lung which is practically always due to bronchial obstruction. Retention of the mediastinum in its normal position despite a large effusion indicates either atelectasis of the lung or fixation of the mediastinum, which is generally due to neoplasm (Fig. 388). Flattening of the chest wall on the side of a large effusion with displacement of the trachea to the opposite side is indicative not only of bronchial obstruction, but also of large paratracheal lymph nodes.

A unilateral effusion due to cardiac failure is practically always on the right side. When the effusion is bilateral, it is greater on the right. In extremely rare instances the effusion is present only on the left side. This occurs when the right pleural cavity is entirely obliterated by adhesions. The presence of these adhesions may be indicated by obliteration of the costophrenic sinus. However, despite the presence of such extensive pleurodesis, at least a portion of one or both of the interlobar fissures usually remains free, permitting the formation of an interlobar effusion on the right side in conjunction with the free effusion on the left.

The effusion resulting from heart failure is most often associated with congestion of the lungs as well as enlargement of the heart. However, the pulmonary congestion may respond quite rapidly to treatment of the heart failure and the appearance of the lungs can return to normal before the effusion is absorbed. The cardiac enlargement generally persists and a return of the heart to normal size occurs slowly, if at all, so that it is quite unusual for a pleural effusion to be due to heart failure in the absence of cardiomegaly.

Although a pleural effusion together with a large heart usually signifies cardiac failure, it may occur as the result of pulmonary infarction in a patient with heart disease or in pleuropericarditis without heart failure. In addition, the possibility that the cardiac enlargement is purely coincidental and unrelated to the pleural effusion in any way, should also be considered.

A left-sided effusion in a patient with cardiac failure is most commonly due to pulmonary embolization and infarction. Pericarditis from any cause may be associated with an effusion confined to the left side. However, the contour of the enlarged heart shadow suggests the presence of pericardial fluid, and the lungs are usually not congested. Absence of pulmonary congestion in association with enlargement of the heart and a pleural effusion also occurs in myxedema, with or without a pericardial effusion. A pleural effu-

sion together with pulmonary congestion and edema, with or without fluid in the pericardium, may occur in acute nephritis because of increased blood volume and increased permeability of the blood vessels.

When the effusion is bilateral, it may be necessary to repeat the roentgen examination after thoracentesis to determine whether the heart is enlarged. We have seen bilateral effusions from heart failure with normal-sized hearts only in acute myocardial infarction associated with shock, or in the Kimmelstiel-Wilson syndrome. Pleural effusions in the nephrotic syndrome or cirrhosis of the liver are usually bilateral, even when small. If the effusion is confined to one side, the possibility of some other cause for the fluid must be considered. It should be borne in mind that hematogenous tuberculosis and tuberculous pleurisy are not uncommon in patients with hepatic cirrhosis.

A useful sign of pulmonary embolization as the cause of an effusion is the presence of Fleischner lines on the opposite side (Fig. 307). Whereas the streak-like shadows of focal areas of atelectasis are frequently present on the same side as the effusion in pleuritis from any cause, they are rarely found on the opposite side, except in the case of embolization.

A bilateral effusion is common in lymphomatous disease of the mediastinum. Failure to visualize the mass in the mediastinum does not exclude this possibility. In fully half of our cases of bilateral effusion secondary to lymphoma, the mediastinal shadow was not widened. On the other hand, a bilateral effusion is unusual in bronchogenic carcinoma. In the few cases that we have observed there was always roentgen evidence of mediastinal involvement.

Clearing of an effusion, either spontaneously or after antibiotic treatment in a patient with an obstructing carcinoma, indicates that the fluid was due to infection of the lung secondary to the obstruction rather than pleural metastasis. Clearing of an effusion after x-ray treatment of a mediastinal tumor indicates that the effusion was the result of obstruction to lymphatic drainage through the mediastinum instead of involvement of the pleura itself.

A pleural effusion, either unilateral or bilateral, can occur in association with a benign tumor of the uterus or ovary (Meigs' syndrome) (Fig. 525). This can also occur in a malignant tumor of the ovary without any evidence of pleural metastasis. In either instance, the effusion may be hemorrhagic and is frequently associated with ascites. In any case, the fluid disappears after the pelvic tumor is resected.

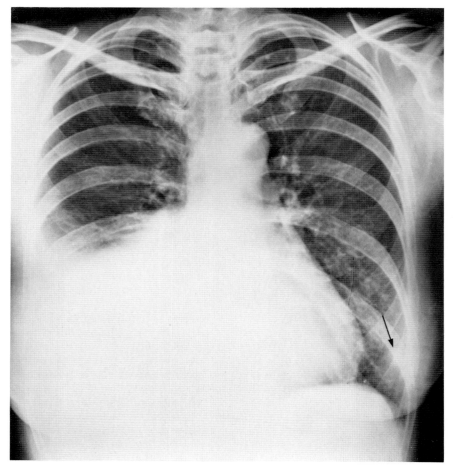

FIG. 525. MEIGS SYNDROME

A young woman with a large ovarian mass presented with ascites and a right pleural effusion. The nodule (arrow) projected over the left lower lung represents a nipple shadow and not a metastatic neoplasm. Thoracentesis revealed clear fluid without malignant cells. The ovarian mass proved to be a benign fibroma and the pleural fluid absorbed spontaneously following removal of the tumor.

Loculated Effusion

The sequence of events that leads to the development of a loculated effusion varies in different cases. Obliteration of most of the pleural cavity by adhesions may antedate the effusion and the fluid may collect in the space that is still free. On the other hand, the effusion may occur first and incite the development of pleural adhesions which wall off the fluid. In other instances, pleural adhesions and the effusion form concurrently. This occurs most frequently in relation to an inflammatory lesion in the lung. An exudate rich in fibrin is produced over the area of pulmonary involvement and entraps the fluid as it forms.

A loculated effusion may be situated anywhere in the pleural cavity but occurs most often in the posterolateral portion of the chest above the diaphragm. It is useful, from a radiologic as well as a clinical standpoint, to classify the effusions according to their location. The fluid may be localized between the lung and the chest wall, *parietal* effusion; it may be situated between the lobes of the lung, *interlobar* effusion; it may lie between the mediastinum or spine and the mesial surface of the lung, *mesial* or *paramediastinal* effusion, or may be confined between the lung and the diaphragm, *infrapulmonary* effusion. Finally, the collection of fluid may be situated between the apex of the lung and the dome of the pleural cavity, *apical* effusion.

Parietal Loculation. Characteristically, a loculated effusion between the lung and the chest wall appears as a homogeneous, semicircular or semielliptical density with its base against the parietes, demarcated from the lung by a sharply defined, curved mesial border. This configuration is seen only when the rays are tangential to the inner border of the loculation and when this border is not obscured by disease of the adjacent lung or a sympathetic effusion. A loculated effusion in the lateral portion of the chest will show the characteristic picture in the frontal projection, while oblique views are usually required if the effusion is loculated in the antero- or posterolateral portions of the thorax (Fig. 526). In unusual instances, the fluid is completely confined to the anterior or posterior part of the pleural space. The frontal film then shows only an ill-defined density which may suggest pulmonary consolidation. However, the sharply defined curved inner border of the effusion is visible on the lateral view. An effusion should be suspected if the vascular pattern of the lung can be seen within the shadow on the frontal projection.

A parietal effusion near the base of the pleural cavity is often associated with considerable elevation of the diaphragm, particularly in its outer portion, together with obliteration of the costophrenic sinus by adhesions. Frequently the elevated diaphragm is obscured by the effusion, especially on the right side. Under these circumstances, aspiration of the chest through the eighth or ninth intercostal space may fail to enter the collection of fluid which is loculated at a higher level. Most often, however, the mesial part of the diaphragm can be seen extending upward and outward to indicate that the outer portion of the diaphragm is elevated.

Occasionally, although the main body of fluid lies in the lateral part of the pleural cavity, some of it extends anteriorly and posteriorly in a thin layer which partially envelops the lung. Under such circumstances, the fluid, although loculated, does not produce the usual sharply demarcated, bulging shadow. Instead, there is a more diffuse density over the outer portion of the chest grad-

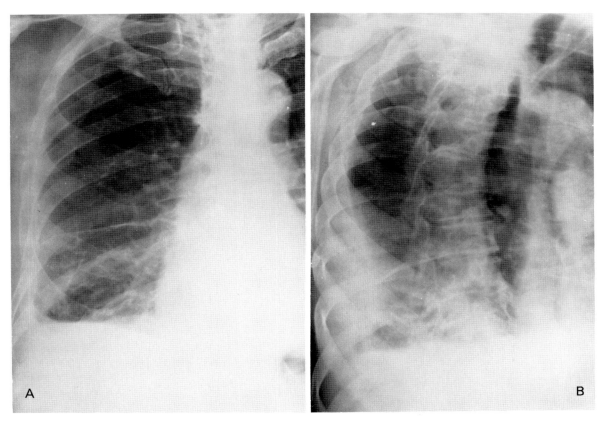

FIG. 526. LOCULATED EFFUSION

A: A 65 year old male with persistent low grade fever following pulmonary embolization. The right costophrenic sinus is obliterated and there is a narrow band-like density extending along the lateral chest wall. These findings, together with the faint haze over the lower half of the lung and the clinical history suggest thickening of the pleura by fibrinous exudate. *B*: The right oblique view demonstrates a well-defined loculation of fluid in the posterolateral portion of the right pleural cavity. Aspiration revaled foul pus, the empyema being the result of secondary infection of a pulmonary infarct.

ually fading as it extends mesially. This can mimic consolidation of the lung. However, in most cases the outer portion of the diaphragm is elevated. Adequately exposed Bucky films penetrate the anterior and posterior components of the fluid collection and disclose a broad, sharply demarcated band of increased density between the air-containing lung and the thoracic cage.

A parietal effusion loculated at a higher level is rather unusual, and can simulate a neoplasm of the pleura or a peripheral carcinoma of the lung. The differentiation usually cannot be made roentgenologically without recourse to previous films.

Occasionally, a parietal effusion is multiloculated. It may present radiologically as a lobulated, sharply demarcated density along the lateral border of the chest or in the form of individual bulging shadows (Fig. 527). Even when these appear to be separated, the loculations practically always communicate with each other.

Small scalloped shadows are occasionally observed along the border of the pulmonary field in cardiac failure. The appearance is identical with that of metastatic neoplasm of the pleura. However, the presence of a large heart together with pulmonary congestion should suggest the possibility of heart failure in a patient with ex-

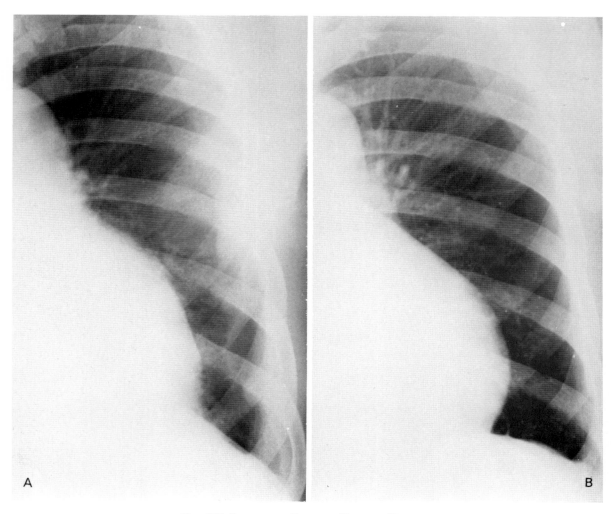

FIG. 527. LOCULATED PARIETAL PLEURAL EFFUSION

A: Multiple scalloped shadows are seen along the pleura on the left side in this patient with a nephrotic syndrome. No abnormality was seen in the right hemithorax. The appearance is most suggestive of neoplasm involving the pleura. *B*: Three days later, following treatment, the scalloped shadows have disappeared. They represented collections of fluid in the pleura associated with the nephrotic syndrome. The loculation was undoubtedly due to preexisting pleural adhesions. No fluid was present on the right, presumably because of complete obliteration of the pleural space on that side.

tensive pleural adhesions. The diagnosis is proved if the shadows become smaller or disappear after diuretic treatment.

Interlobar Loculation. Most often, fluid in an interlobar fissure represents an extension of an effusion in the free pleural cavity. It may also occur in a loculated parietal effusion if a fissure is included in the loculation. Neither case should be designated as an interlobar effusion because the fluid in the fissure is only part of a larger, more important collection in the main pleural space.

A true interlobar effusion is one which is confined to the space between the lobes. The interlobar effusion may be confined entirely within the depths of the fissure or it may extend peripherally, spreading the lobes apart as far as the chest wall.

True interlobar effusions are uncommon. Most often they occur in patients with heart failure in whom the main pleural space is obliterated by adhesions, while a portion of one or more of the fissures remains free so that fluid can collect within it. An interlobar effusion can also develop in association with inflammatory disease. In such instances the cause of the effusion is usually an abscess of the lung which has ruptured into the fissure (Fig. 528). The fluid is loculated because the adjacent pleural surfaces have been closed off by dense fibrinous exudate over the abscess before actual perforation took place.

The roentgen appearance of an interlobar effusion depends largely upon the projection in which the film is made. The collection of fluid almost always has a lenticular, biconvex shape, thickest in its midportion, and thinning toward the edges where the lobes are adherent. This characteristic shape is seen only when the x-ray beam is oriented parallel to the plane of the fissure. The effusion then casts a sharply circumscribed, spindle-shaped shadow of homogeneous density. On films made in other projections, the shadow of the fluid loses its spindle shape and is more poorly demarcated (Fig. 529). In rare instances, usually in perforated lung abscess, the effusion is spherical and casts a round shadow in all views.

SHORT FISSURE. Since the short fissure lies predominantly in a horizontal plane, the x-ray beam is parallel to it in all projections when the patient is erect. The characteristic shape of the effusion is therefore visible in the frontal as well as the lateral and oblique views. On the frontal projection, a thin line can usually be seen ex-

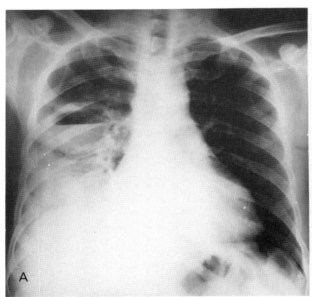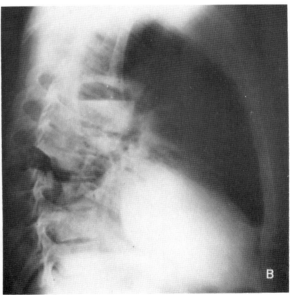

FIG. 528. INTERLOBAR PYOPNEUMOTHORAX

A: The oval cavity with an air-fluid level in the right side of the chest has the appearance of a pulmonary abscess. There is a rather homogeneous shadow over the lower part of the right lung. *B:* On the lateral view the cavity is seen to be situated in the region of the upper part of the long fissure. The lower part of the chest appears clouded and the border of the right leaf of the diaphragm is obliterated. Operation disclosed a foul pyopneumothorax, loculated in the upper part of the long fissure, and an empyema at the right base. While the location of the cavity suggests that it lies within the fissure, it cannot be differentiated from an abscess in the lung from the films alone. The fusiform shadow in the lower anterior portion of the chest is produced by the overlapping shadows of the heart and liver.

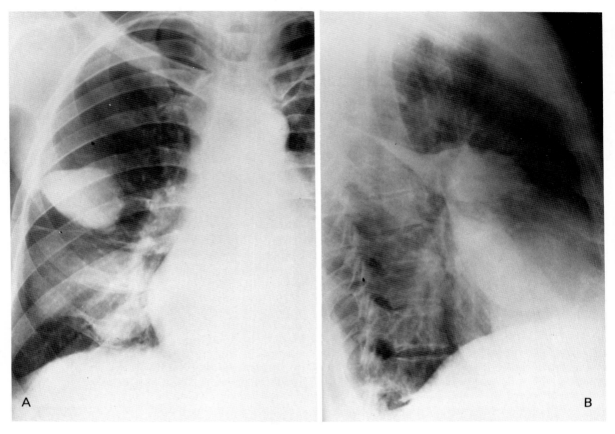

FIG. 529. INTERLOBAR EFFUSION

A: Frontal projection. The sharply defined, homogeneous shadow lies at the level of the short fissure. It is ovoid in shape and its long axis is directed horizontally. The horizontal streak below the shadow represents an accessory fissure between the superior segment and the basal segments of the lower lobe and not the short fissure. The hazy density over the lower part of the lung has a well-demarcated lower border and does not obscure the outlines of the pulmonary vessels. The costophrenic sinus is obliterated. These findings are indicative of effusions in both fissures but this diagnosis requires confirmation with an oblique or a lateral film. *B*: Lateral projection. Both fissures are now projected on end. The characteristic spindle-shaped shadow of the interlobar effusion in the lower part of the long fissure is projected over the cardiac silhouette. The effusion in the short fissure extends backward into the upper part of the long fissure.

tending mesially and laterally from the shadow of the effusion. This represents the thickened, adherent layers of pleura in the obliterated portion of the fissure. On the lateral and left anterior oblique views, the shadow is more triangular in shape if the fluid is loculated in the anterior portion of the fissure.

LONG FISSURE. The long fissure of each lung lies in a plane perpendicular to the lateral chest wall. Since the fissure is tilted downward and forward, it is projected on end only in the lateral view. The spindle shape of an effusion in this fissure is best demonstrated in this view (Fig. 529) although it may also be seen in a marked oblique projection. The long axis of the density runs downward and forward along the course of the fissure. It is continuous with a line repre-

senting thickened interlobar pleura adjacent to the loculated effusion (Fig. 530). This line is usually seen at both extremities of the collection of fluid, but is absent at one end when the effusion extends to the periphery. The shadow of the fluid then assumes a more triangular shape. This occurs more frequently when the lower part of the fissure is involved. The base of the triangle is then situated over the anterior portion of the diaphragm.

Unless the long fissure is displaced, it is not viewed on end in the frontal projection. For this reason, even when considerably thickened, the long fissure is not visible in this view, and an effusion within it does not present the characteristic, sharply demarcated shadow seen on the lateral film. Usually the effusion appears as a

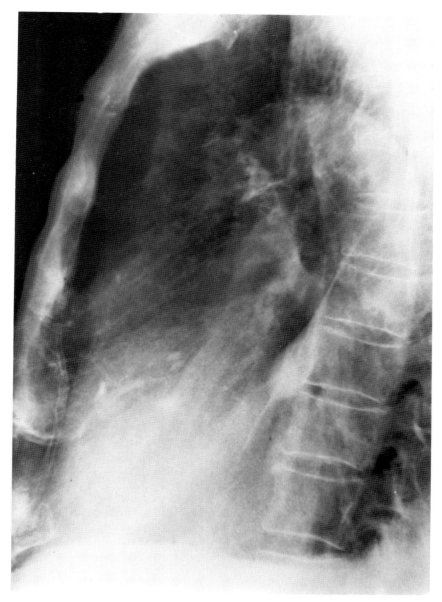

FIG. 530. INTERLOBAR EFFUSION

The lenticular-shaped shadow represents a collection of fluid within the long fissure on the left side. The remainder of the fissure is obliterated by adhesions. The thickened pleura casts a linear shadow extending from either end of the effusion.

hazy, poorly demarcated density through which undistorted pulmonary vessels in front and behind can be visualized.

Occasionally the shadow of an effusion in the long fissure is rather sharply demarcated on the frontal projection and simulates a tumor. When situated in the upper part of the fissure, the collection of fluid tends to assume an oval shape with the long axis running obliquely upward and inward. Even if the lower border is sharply outlined, the upper border is usually hazy (Fig. 531).

When the effusion is situated in the lower part of the long fissure, its shadow is generally rounder and is more suggestive of a neoplasm. However, here also, its upper border tends to be indistinct despite the sharp definition of its lower margin.

Since only the midportion of the outer edge of the long fissure reaches the lateral chest wall, the shadow of an effusion in the upper or lower part of the fissure is separated from the outer border of the chest on the frontal view (Fig. 532).

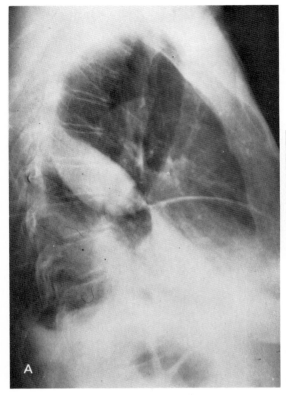
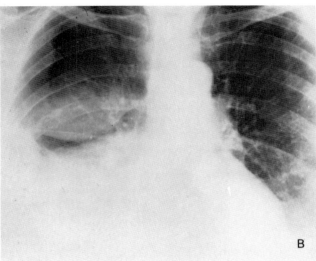

FIG. 531. INTERLOBAR EFFUSION

A: The lateral view discloses two spindle-shaped densities characteristic of a biloculated effusion in the long fissure. An additional density behind the long fissure is due to a parietal loculation of fluid. The posterior costophrenic sinus is obliterated by a small collection of free fluid. The short fissure is markedly thickened. *B*: Frontal view. The spindle-shaped shadow in the right midlung field is oriented horizontally and appears to be in the region of the short fissure. The haziness of its upper border excludes the possibility of an effusion in this fissure but is a common finding with fluid loculated in the upper portion of the long fissure.

When there are distinct loculations in the lower and upper part of the fissure, the components are usually connected by a narrow density in the axillary part of the chest. The shadow of the bilocular effusion then has a reniform configuration. Such an effusion on the right side is almost always associated with thickening of the short fissure. This is visualized as a horizontal line extending mesially from the junction of the two loculations. The line is thicker if fluid is present in the short fissure.

DIAGNOSIS. The roentgen diagnosis of interlobar effusion depends upon the demonstration of a characteristic spindle- or triangular-shaped shadow in the plane of the fissure together with a line of thickened interlobar pleura extending from at least one extremity of the shadow. This is clearly evident on the lateral view if either fissure is involved. When the effusion is confined to the short fissure, the diagnosis can also be made from the frontal projection, although lateral or oblique films are useful for confirmation.

Difficulty arises in the diagnosis of an effusion in the long fissure when only a frontal film is available. Such an effusion should be suspected if the frontal film discloses thickening of the short fissure in association with a round or oval shadow above or below it. An effusion in the long fissure should also be suspected when there is a hazy shadow in the midclavicular line through which normal pulmonary markings are visible and which is associated with a large heart, congestion of the lungs or obliteration of the costophrenic sinus on the side of the lesion.

A benign tumor of the interlobar pleura can also cast an oval shadow. This is easily confused with that of an interlobar effusion. However, the tumor is not apt to be associated with thickening of the adjoining part of the fissure and, therefore, the shadow does not have linear extensions (Fig. 533). An intercalated middle lobe, i.e., a collapsed middle lobe which has retracted toward the root of the lung, may be indistinguishable from a collection of fluid between the middle and lower lobes. An oblique line of thickened interlobar pleura is seen on the lateral view, extending from the shadow of the intercalated lobe downward and forward to the diaphragm. Here the line represents adhesion between the anterior portions of the upper and lower lobes which approximate each other when the middle lobe is retracted (Fig. 86). There is no line of thickened pleura extending upward from the superior border of the shadow. Moreover, the short fissure, which is usually visible when there is fluid in the long fissure (Fig. 534), is not evident.

Difficulty is frequently encountered in differentiating between an inflamed, collapsed middle lobe and an effusion in the lower part of the long fissure that extends to the diaphragm. In both instances, the lateral view discloses a triangular shadow directed downward and forward from the

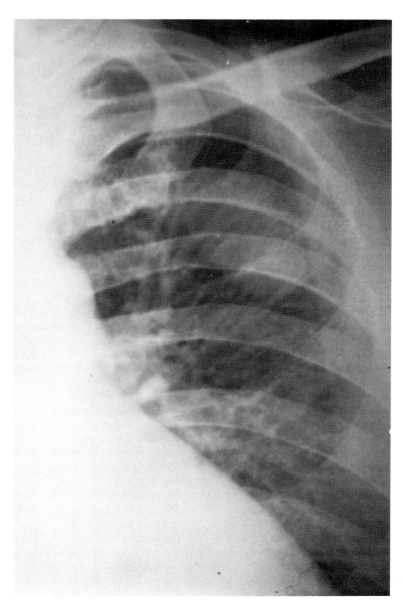

FIG. 532. INTERLOBAR EFFUSION

The faint, homogeneous density projected over the left upper lung represents a loculated collection of fluid in the uppermost portion of the long fissure. The fissure does not reach the lateral border of the chest in this area. The shadows of the pulmonary vessels are clearly seen crossing the density, indicating that it does not represent consolidation of lung. The diagnosis was obvious on the lateral projection.

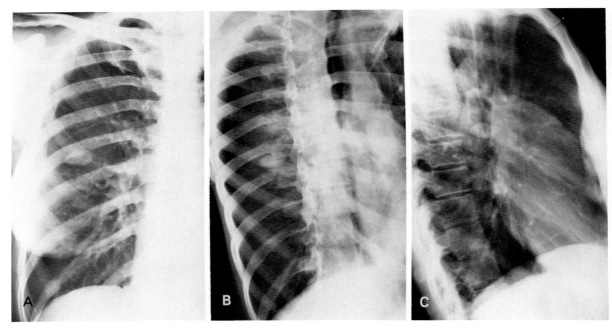

FIG. 533. INTERLOBAR FIBROMA OF THE PLEURA
Frontal (A), right oblique (B) and lateral (C) views show a spindle-shaped density at the juncture of the long and short fissures. The shadow is sharply defined and its long axis is horizontal so that it resembles an interlobar effusion. However, the adjacent part of the fissure is not thickened. The portion of the short fissure that is visible is considerably anterior to the lesion. At operation, a benign fibroma was found between the upper and middle lobes originating from the visceral pleura of the short fissure.

root of the lung. The distinction is easily made when a thickened short fissure is seen. Obviously, this will not be visualized if the middle lobe is collapsed, since the short fissure now forms the superior border of the atelectatic lobe (Fig. 12B). The location of the base of the triangular shadow is also helpful in the differential diagnosis. Normally, the long fissure on the right side ends at the anterior costophrenic angle. The posterior boundary of the shadow of a collapsed middle lobe corresponds to this fissure which remains in its normal position or is retracted upward. It cannot be displaced posteriorly. On the other hand, an interlobar effusion pushes the anterior segment of the lower lobe backward, so that the posterior border of the shadow intersects the diaphragm at a distance behind the anterior costophrenic sulcus.

Most interlobar effusions are due to congestive heart failure and are associated with evidences of engorgement of the lungs as well as enlargement of the heart. With restoration of cardiac compensation, the effusion tends to disappear. The evanescent nature of the shadow has given rise to the term "vanishing" or "phantom" tumor. Administration of a diuretic usually leads to a rapid diminution in size, or disappearance of the shadow, establishing the diagnosis of bland interlobar effusion. The congestive changes in the lungs often respond more rapidly to treatment of the cardiac failure than does the interlobar effusion. If the film is made within a few days after the administration of a diuretic, the pulmonary vessels may have returned to normal, while the effusion has not yet been absorbed. The absence of pulmonary congestion, therefore, does not exclude the possibility of an interlobar effusion secondary to cardiac failure. The presence of a large heart should suggest such an effusion and lead to appropriate studies.

Care must be taken not to confuse crossing shadows of the heart and liver with an interlobar effusion in the long fissure. This difficulty arises only in the right lateral projection. In this projection, particularly with the tube high, the right leaf of the diaphragm is at a considerably higher level than the left, so that the shadow overlies the lower posterior part of the heart (Fig. 59).

Mesial (Paramediastinal) Loculation. Effusions loculated in the mesial portion of the chest practically always lie, at least in part, adjacent to the mediastinum. Those situated posteriorly may be confined to the paravertebral region although, usually, they extend anteriorly to the paramediastinal region. The effusions are almost always secondary to suppurative disease in the lung, but occasionally they are associated with suppurative mediastinitis. Only rarely do they result from heart failure.

The mesial effusion usually lies in the posterior paramediastinal compartment and is limited anteriorly by the pulmonary ligament which runs from the root of the lung to the diaphragm. The fluid in this compartment practically always extends to the posterior chest wall and displaces the lung away from the spine. The effusion is limited laterally by adhesions between the posterior surface of the lung and the chest wall. The relationship of the collection of fluid to the chest wall is determined by these adhesions.

If the mesial surface of the lung is displaced laterally by the effusion before the adhesions to the chest wall are well developed, the fluid comes in contact with the posterior chest wall over a fairly wide area. A cross section of the fluid collection has the shape of a right angle triangle with one side against the posterior chest wall and the other against the spine and mediastinum.

The hypotenuse is formed by the border between the effusion and the lung. On the frontal view, therefore, the densest portion of the shadow lies adjacent to the spine. As the shadow of the fluid extends laterally, it gradually fades, so that its outer border is poorly demarcated.

When the lung is adherent to the chest wall close to the spine, the lateral extension of the fluid is limited and the effusion has only a small parietal representation. As it increases in size, the effusion bulges forward and outward, indenting the mesial surface of the lung and displacing it laterally. The film shows a rather sharply outlined density extending outward from the mediastinum for a considerable distance. It is important to bear in mind that despite the size of the shadow, the area of contact with the posterior chest wall is small. With an effusion of this type, a needle inserted at the center of the shadow will usually traverse the free pleural space and lung, before the fluid is reached. The puncture should be made close to the spine in order to enter the effusion directly without injuring the lung.

When the effusion does not extend as far down as the diaphragm, the shadow seen on the frontal projection is semielliptical in shape with the base

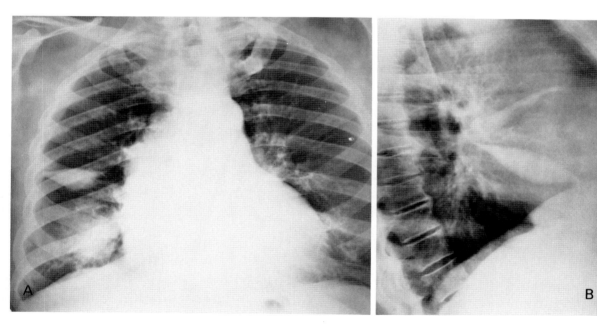

FIG. 534. INTERLOBAR EFFUSIONS

A: Two shadows are seen in the right lung. The upper is sharply outlined and fusiform in shape and is oriented horizontally. This is quite characteristic of a loculated effusion in the short fissure. The lower shadow could represent an area of pneumonia or an infarct. However, its association with fluid in the short fissure suggests that it is also an interlobar fluid collection. The heart is enlarged. *B*: The collection of fluid in each fissure is well demonstrated in the lateral view. The characteristic fusiform shape of the loculated fluid between the lower and middle lobes is apparent because the long fissure is projected on end in this view.

alongside the mediastinum. When it does reach the diaphragm, the shadow is either quadrantic or triangular. In the latter instance, the appearance suggests atelectasis of the lower lobe, but the lung root is not depressed.

The appearance on the lateral view varies. In some cases the anterior border curves forward and is quite well outlined. In others, the anterior border is hazy and indistinguishable, and the only evidences of an effusion are in increase in the density of the shadows of the vertebrae and a loss of the silhouette of the posterior part of the diaphragm.

A paramediastinal loculation which extends down to the diaphragm can continue forward beneath the lung so that it is partly infrapulmonary. It may also extend directly anteriorly between the mesial surface of the lung and the mediastinum, beneath the inferior edge of the pulmonary ligament, to enter the anterior paramediastinal compartment (Fig. 535). The loculated effusion is then dumbbell in shape, the two components being connected by a narrow neck. The anterior component is usually quite small.

Unless it contains air, this portion of the effusion is not recognizable on the lateral view because it lies over the heart and merges with the cardiac shadow.

A collection of fluid situated posteriorly does not obscure the cardiac border on the frontal view. On the other hand, an effusion in the anterior compartment lies adjacent to the heart and obliterates the cardiac silhouette. The anterior collection of fluid rarely reaches the anterior chest wall and the area of contact, if any, is small. The border of the fluid collection is therefore sharply defined and convex in the frontal view, simulating a large heart or a localized pericardial effusion. Because the pericardial reflection occurs over the midportion of the ascending aorta, these possibilities may be excluded if the shadow extends as high as the aortic arch. In any case, the anterior effusion can resemble a tumor of the mediastinum.

Infrapulmonary Loculation. Loculated collections of fluid between the base of the lung and the diaphragm are extremely rare. In most instances, effusions which appear confined to the

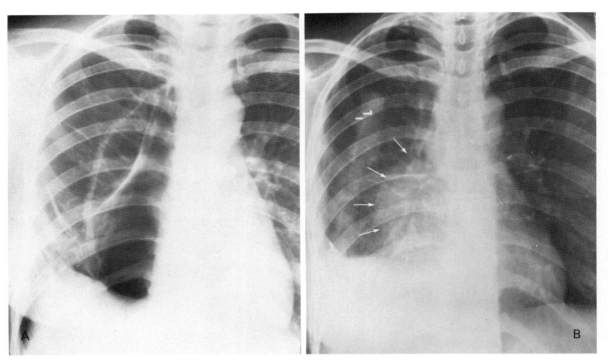

FIG. 535. PARAMEDIASTINAL EFFUSION

A: The film of a 39 year old woman who had sudden onset of right chest pain shows a pneumothorax limited to the mesial portion of the pleural cavity. The patient gave a history of repeated spontaneous pneumothoraces in the past. By this time most of the pleural cavity has been obliterated by adhesions, explaining the loculation of the current pneumothorax. *B*: Following thoracotomy, the previous pneumothorax space is now filled with fluid (arrows). This is loculated in the paramediastinal region and obscures the right border of the heart. The surgical clips and the broad, oblique shadow are the results of pleural biopsies. These disclosed endometrial implants on the pleura.

infrapulmonary space are not truly loculated but communicate freely with the general pleural cavity. In contradistinction to such free collections which are of a bland nature, loculated effusions in this location are of inflammatory origin and practically always represent localized empyemas secondary to pyogenic infection of the lung or subphrenic region. They are differentiated from free infrapulmonary effusions by the fact that they do not shift with change in the position of the patient.

The roentgen appearance of a loculated infrapulmonary effusion may simulate an elevated diaphragm (Fig. 536). However, the possibility of a collection of fluid should be considered if the costophrenic sinus is obliterated and the lower border of the lung remains fixed during respiration.

Not infrequently a loculated infrapulmonary effusion has a small lateral or posterior extension.

This is manifested by an opacity extending above the costophrenic sinus on either the frontal or lateral projection. Extension mesially produces a blunting of the angle between the spine and the diaphragm. If the mesial component is large, it casts a triangular paravertebral shadow whose lower portion is continuous with the infrapulmonary collection, while its hypotenuse frequently projects beyond the cardiac border. As in the case of free effusions, the posterior paramediastinal fluid may extend beneath the pulmonary ligament to enter the anterior compartment. This portion of the effusion is also loculated. Because of its anterior location it tends to obliterate the border of the cardiac shadow in the frontal view. It is not well visualized on the lateral view unless it contains air.

Apical Loculation. A collection of fluid confined to the apex of the pleural cavity is rare. Usually it is associated with a parietal compo-

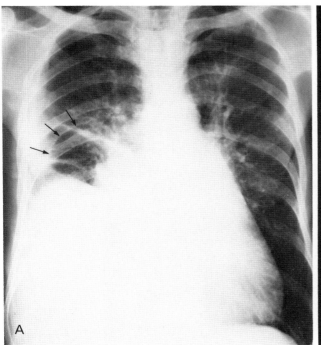 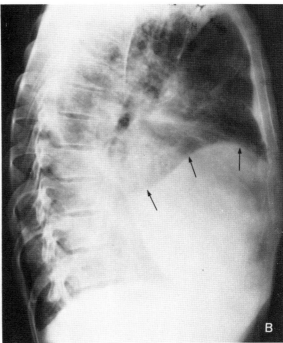

FIG. 536. INFRAPULMONARY EMPYEMA

A: The heart is displaced to the left and rotated to the right oblique position, apparently by an elevated diaphragm. However, the shadow of the thin layer of exudate ascending along the axillary portion of the right chest and its extension into the long fissure (arrows) suggest that the shadow at the base represents a collection of fluid. Thoracentesis disclosed an empyema between the diaphragm and the lower surface of the lung. The streak-like shadows above the loculated empyema represent focal areas of atelectasis (Fleischner lines). *B:* Right lateral view. The anterior part of the upper border of the infrapulmonary empyema (arrows) is sharply outlined. The posterior part is not demarcated because of the diffuse inflammatory reaction of the costal pleura above it. The oblique line that seems to constitute the posterior border of the empyema really represents the posterior border of the heart. Because the film was made with the patient's right side against the cassette, the left ribs extend further back and appear wider than those on the right. Only one leaf of the diaphragm is visualized, and since it extends to the ribs on the left side, it must represent the left diaphragm. The silhouette of the right diaphragm is obscured by the empyema.

nent. Radiologically the apical effusion appears as a dense, homogeneous shadow with a sharply defined, convex lower border over the apex of the lung (Fig. 537). On the frontal projection the border often extends to the mediastinum with which it forms an acute angle. As the collection of fluid becomes larger, its area of contact with the mediastinum increases, the acute angle disappears, and the shadow merges with that of the mediastinum. The fluid may extend downward in the paramediastinal space for a variable distance. The borders of both components of the effusion then form a continuous curve which blends with that of the normal mediastinum below. The lateral border of the apical effusion may form an acute angle with the chest wall, but the angle is usually blunted as a result of thickening of the pleura by exudate. The exudate may extend downward to form a band-like shadow along the periphery of the pulmonary field.

Special Types of Effusions

Empyema. An empyema is essentially a loculated collection of pus in the pleural cavity and, as such, should be differentiated from a pyothorax. In the latter, the pus lies free in the pleural space while an empyema, regardless of its size, is always shut off from some portion of the pleural cavity by adhesions.

The early stage of an empyema is usually manifested by a layer of thick, fibrinopurulent, plastic exudate over the pleura. This is characterized radiologically by a faint, diffuse shadow over the lung, gradually becoming denser toward the base. Where the collection of exudate is projected on end it is seen as a dense, broad stripe of opacity along the outer margin of the hemithorax. As the disease progresses, there is an accumulation of liquid purulent material which is walled off from the remainder of the pleural cavity by the exudate. Less commonly, the condition begins with a pyothorax characterized by a thin seropurulent exudate lying free in the pleural cavity. Within a few days, the exudate tends to become rich in fibrin and forms a thick pus which then is loculated by dense fibrinous adhesions. This sequence of events occurs most frequently in children.

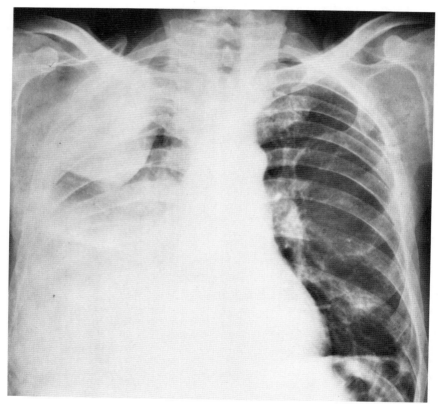

FIG. 537. APICAL EMPYEMA

The sharply circumscribed density at the right apex simulates a neoplasm. The lower part of the chest is clouded by what appears to be a free collection of fluid. However, both shadows proved to represent loculated empyemas. The left costophrenic sinus is obliterated by adhesions which bind the outer part of the diaphragm to the chest wall.

Radiologically, a very large empyema can present an appearance identical to that of a pyothorax. The entire hemithorax may be completely opacified, the mediastinum displaced to the opposite side and the rib spaces spread apart. Such an appearance occurs almost exclusively in children. However, even in large empyemas, the rib spaces have a tendency to become narrowed after a relatively short time as pleural thickening develops.

Films made earlier in the development of the empyema may show the upper portion of the hemithorax to be clear. The differentiation between a pyothorax and an empyema can be made at this stage by examining the patient in the recumbent position to determine whether the fluid shifts or is loculated. If a portion of the pulmonary field, either mesial or lateral to the collection of fluid, remains clear in both the erect and recumbent positions, it is obvious that the fluid is loculated.

Smaller empyemas are usually characterized by a homogeneous density with a sharply demarcated bulging border. However, the latter may not be evident on all projections because the empyema tends to taper at its periphery as it becomes continuous with the adjacent thickened pleura. The loculation appears well demarcated against the air-containing lung only when the x-ray beam is tangential to the interface and traverses the maximum thickness of the loculation (Fig. 538). To demonstrate this, lateral or oblique views are often required. The optimum projection may best be determined by fluoroscopy. In the rare instances in which a large empyema forms a concave shell about the lung,

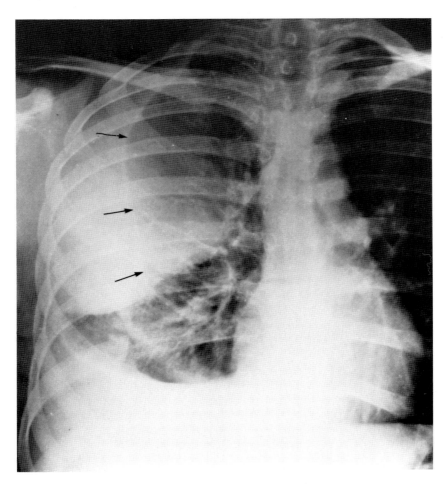

FIG. 538. EMPYEMA WITH SYMPATHETIC EFFUSION

The loculated collection of pus is wrapped around the upper part of the right lung. Where the empyema is viewed tangentially, it is sharply demarcated from the underlying lung (arrows). The indistinct mesial continuation of the shadow represents the anterior and posterior extension of the empyema that is viewed *en face*. There is also a free pleural effusion at the right base. Thoracentesis here revealed clear, sterile fluid, representing a sympathetic effusion.

the shadow fades off imperceptibly in all views and thus gives the impression of a free effusion (Fig. 537).

In the erect frontal projection, the shadow of an infrapulmonary empyema suggests an elevated diaphragm and is identical with that of a free infrapulmonary effusion. However, an empyema maintains its shape and position when the patient is examined in the decubitus position. Since an infrapulmonary empyema is encapsulated, it tends to displace the heart to the opposite side even though moderate in size (Fig. 536). An effusion which is not loculated is free to extend into the remainder of the pleural space and therefore does not displace the heart until it becomes large enough to fill a considerable part of the pleural cavity.

Infrapulmonary empyemas usually result from perforation of a lung abscess abutting on the diaphragm, or are secondary to a subphrenic or hepatic abscess. These empyemas rarely complicate a simple pneumonia, and when they do, practically always represent part of a larger parietal empyema (Fig. 539).

CHRONIC EMPYEMA. A chronic empyema results either from inadequate drainage of an acute empyema or from persistence of an infective focus adjacent to the pleura. The latter may consist of an abscess of the lung, a bronchial fistula, an abscess or fistulous tract extending from the subphrenic region or the mediastinum, or from an osteomyelitis of a rib. The disease of the rib may be the cause of the empyema or represent a secondary complication.

A chronic empyema is characterized by a dense shadow caused by marked thickening of the

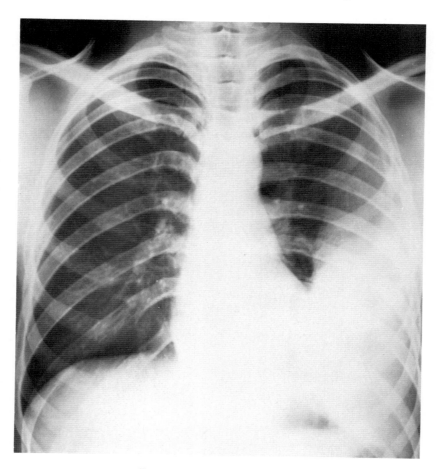

FIG. 539. LOCULATED EMPYEMA

The dense, homogeneous shadow in the outer portion of the left chest, bounded by a well-defined, smooth, regular border, represents a loculated collection of fluid in the pleural space. On thoracentesis this proved to be purulent. The major part of the empyema is situated posteriorly but there is an anterior loculation which is responsible for the obliteration of the cardiac apex. The stomach bubble is displaced downward by the diaphragm which is depressed by the infrapulmonary component of the empyema.

pleura as well as the collection of fluid itself. The amount of fluid may be quite small even when the shadow is most extensive. The ribs are drawn together flattening the hemithorax, and the diaphragm is elevated. Because of the marked thickening of the pleura and the common association with underlying pulmonary disease, the shadow of the empyema is usually poorly demarcated. A convex border of the shadow often cannot be demonstrated on any projection. In rare instances, calcium is deposited in the wall of a chronic pyogenic empyema, similar to a tuberculous empyema or a loculated hemothorax.

Development of a chronic empyema is prevented by eliminating the source of the infection and continuing treatment of the acute empyema until it has completely healed. The limits of the empyema can be delineated by filling it with radiopaque packing after it has been drained. X-ray examination may then disclose one or more undrained pockets. Injection of contrast material into an empyema sinus may reveal a poorly draining locule or a fistulous tract leading into a bronchus, the subphrenic region, or the mediastinum (Fig. 27). Bucky films may disclose the presence of osteomyelitis of a rib as the cause of persistent infection of the pleura. In the absence of a sinus tract, bronchography can be helpful in the identification of an underlying pulmonary lesion. Where there is a question as to whether the shadow on the chest film is due to pulmonary or pleural disease, bronchography may provide the answer by demonstrating inward displacement of the bronchi by a lesion outside the lung.

LATENT EMPYEMA. When an empyema is adequately treated, evidence of only minor pleural thickening remains. Little more should be seen on the film than obliteration of the costophrenic sinus and elevation of the outer portion of the diaphragm by adhesions. The persistence of any greater density after the empyema has presumably healed, strongly suggests the possibility of a residual empyema (Fig. 540).

The infection may remain dormant for many years, producing no symptoms, but eventually it spreads to the adjacent pleura and then becomes clinically manifest. If a latent empyema is not to be overlooked, periodic x-ray examinations should be made until the dense shadow of thickened pleura has cleared. Persistence of the shadow is an indication for aspiration to locate the suspected residual empyema.

Sympathetic Effusion. A sympathetic effusion is a collection of clear fluid uncontaminated by bacteria, which forms because of pleural irritation from adjacent disease. The causative lesion may be a pneumonia, lung abscess (Fig. 270),

osteomyelitis or osteochondritis of a rib, mediastinitis, subphrenic abscess, or a loculated empyema. Occasionally, a sympathetic effusion is secondary to a collection of bile beneath the diaphragm or a degenerating hematoma as may occur following splenectomy.

Frequently bacteria spread from the infected focus into the sympathetic effusion, converting it into a pyothorax or empyema. In other cases, the sympathetic effusion is absorbed as the infection is controlled. In either case, the sympathetic effusion rarely persists for any length of time as a collection of bland fluid.

Unless the fluid is contained by preexisting adhesions, a sympathetic effusion is not loculated and presents the same appearance on films as any other accumulation of free fluid in the pleural cavity (Fig. 538). Often the effusion overshadows and obscures the underlying disease. The possibility of a sympathetic effusion should be considered whenever clear fluid is aspirated from the chest of a patient with fever of unknown origin. Bucky films or tomograms may disclose a lung abscess or infection of a rib. Inordinate depression of the stomach bubble, fixation of the diaphragm or the presence of an extragastric air-fluid level beneath the diaphragm point to a subphrenic abscess. X-ray examination after thoracentesis may reveal an underlying pneumonia, pulmonary abscess or a loculated empyema. Because a sympathetic effusion shifts freely, the underlying lesion may be uncovered before thoracentesis by examining the patient in the recumbent position. The elevated diaphragm associated with a subphrenic abscess may also be visualized in this way.

Occasionally a sympathetic effusion develops secondary to pulmonary infection distal to an obstructing bronchogenic carcinoma (Fig. 424). Under these circumstances the presence of an effusion should not be assumed to indicate pleural metastasis. Frequently, the effusion clears after antibiotic treatment.

Hemothorax. Most often, bleeding in the pleural cavity is the result of trauma. Occasionally, a pure hemothorax results from ulceration of a neoplasm involving the pleura, or from perforation of an aneurysm. A few cases of hemothorax complicating hemoperitoneum have been described. Spontaneous hemothorax resulting from tear of a subpleural bulla is almost always associated with a pneumothorax. However, in rare instances, no air is visible and only the shadow of the blood in the pleural cavity is demonstrable.

Usually, a traumatic hemothorax is accompanied by one or more fractured ribs. However, it

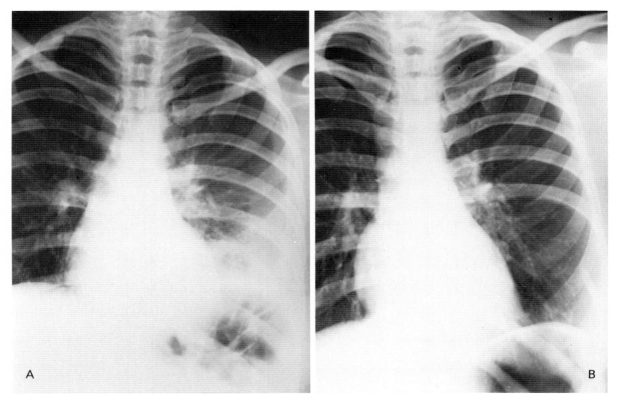

FIG. 540. CHRONIC EMPYEMA SIMULATING THICKENED PLEURA

A: An empyema on the left side had been drained 14 years previously. The residual shadow at the left base was considered to be due to thickened pleura. The patient felt well until a short time before the present admission when she developed high fever and pain in the chest. At operation an extremely thick-walled, chronic empyema was found. This undoubtedly had been present, but was latent throughout the years. Incidentally, there is a small cervical rib on the right side and a well developed one on the left. *B*: After unroofing and packing of the empyema, the chronic inflammation resolved. No residual shadow remains despite the long duration of the empyema and the marked induration of the pleura.

can also result from blunt trauma in the absence of a fracture. Penetrating wounds of the chest are most often associated with air as well as blood in the pleural cavity.

When blood fills the entire pleural cavity, the appearance is no different from that of any other massive pleural effusion. If the blood is partly coagulated, it frequently produces a characteristic roentgen appearance. The hemothorax appears as a dense shadow at the base, obscuring the dome of the diaphragm, while above this there are irregular, confluent shadows along the lateral chest border representing blood clots adherent to the pleura. The shadows are most dense in the axillary region and fade out towards the middle of the pulmonary field. Although this picture can occur with other conditions, such as neoplasms involving the pleura, it is characteristic enough to suggest very strongly the possibility of a hemothorax.

Even in the absence of rib fractures, the diag-

nosis of a hemopneumothorax can often be made radiologically. A wavy or irregular air-fluid level is characteristic. The appearance is produced by blood clots which project above the level of the fluid.

Following a hemothorax, the irritative action of the broken-down blood pigment may persist for many years producing a chronic, active, pleuritis, which is the cause of the persistent shadow over the lung (Fig. 31). The thickened pleura prevents complete reexpansion of the lung so that the hemithorax is contracted, the rib spaces are narrowed, the costophrenic sinus is obliterated and the dome of the chest flattened. When the hemothorax persists for a long time, calcium may be deposited over the pleura (Fig. 517).

Oleothorax. Various types of oil were used in the past in the collapse therapy of tuberculosis. The oil was instilled into the pleural cavity or into the extrapleural space. Usually an oleothorax was instituted when a therapeutic pneumothorax became loculated and began to shrink. The oil was introduced to maintain the collapse of the lung. It remained there permanently unless it was aspirated or, as happened occasionally, it was extruded through a bronchopleural fistula.

Although this method of treatment is no longer in use, cases of oleothorax in which the oil was instilled years ago are still encountered. The roentgen appearance is that of an encapsulated effusion. The encysted collection of oil is usually located in the upper outer portion of the chest. In some cases the oil remains encapsulated over the apex of the lung and produces a homogeneous shadow with a sharply demarcated, convex lower border (Fig. 541). After a number of years there is a tendency toward calcium deposition in the fibrous wall surrounding the collection of oil.

The possibility of oleothorax should be considered in all cases of a sharply demarcated, homogeneous density over the superior surface of the lung, especially when there is a rim of calcium in its border. The roentgen picture is pathognomonic of oleothorax when such shadows representing loculated collections of fluid, are bilateral and symmetrical.

Pneumothorax

The normal pleural cavity is only a potential space. The lung remains in approximation to the

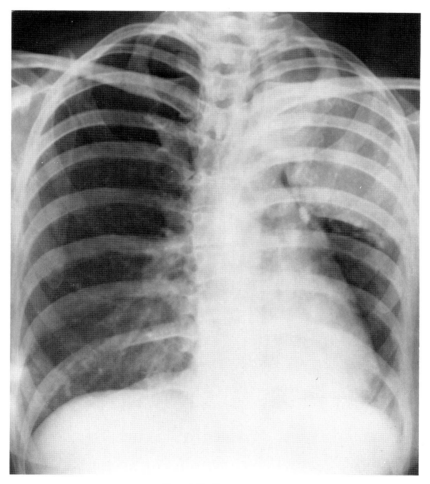

FIG. 541. OLEOTHORAX

The left hemithorax is somewhat shrunken, the heart and trachea are shifted to the left and the rib spaces on the left are narrowed. These changes were the result of previous pneumothorax treatment for tuberculosis. The upper half of the left chest is opacified. The shadow is homogeneous and its lower border is sharply outlined suggesting that it is due to a collection of fluid. Several calcific deposits are present at the border of the lesion. These findings are characteristic of oleothorax. Because the pneumothorax treatment failed, oil of gomenol was injected into the extrapleural space to obliterate a persistent cavity in the left upper lobe. The oil remains indefinitely and often results in deposition of calcium in the overlying pleura.

chest wall throughout its development and is drawn out with the chest wall as the thorax enlarges. This places the elastic tissue of the lung on the stretch. The inward pull of the tissue against the relatively rigid chest wall produces a negative pressure in the pleura during inspiration as well as expiration.

If air enters the pleural space, the lung is permitted to retract. As the volume of the lung diminishes, the tension of the elastic tissue is decreased and the degree of negative pressure in the pleura is lessened. As progressively more air enters the pleural space, a stage is reached in which the pleural pressure becomes positive during expiration. During inspiration, however, because of the increased volume of the thoracic cavity, the pleural pressure becomes negative.

When sufficient air has entered the pleura, the lung is completely collapsed. There is no longer any elastic recoil during ordinary inspiration, the pleural pressure equals atmospheric pressure, and there is no further ingress of air into the pleura. However, a forced inspiration can still result in a temporary decrease in the pleural pressure so that more air is drawn into the pleural cavity. If there is a check-valve mechanism preventing expulsion of air from the pleural space during expiration, the intrapleural pressure increases to exceed that of the atmosphere in both phases of ordinary respiration. This constitutes a tension pneumothorax.

A pneumothorax can be produced in several ways. Air may reach the pleural cavity directly from the outside through the parietal pleura either as the result of a wound of the chest wall, a thoracotomy, or insertion of a needle. Air can enter the pleural space from the lung when there is disruption of the visceral pleura. This may result from a puncture or tear of a normal lung or rupture of a bulla or cavity producing a communication between a bronchus and the pleural space. A pneumothorax can also result from rupture of alveoli into the interstitial tissues of the lung. This produces interstitial emphysema which extends to the visceral pleura and forms blebs which may rupture into the pleural cavity. The air in the interstitial tissues may also extend centrally to produce a pneumomediastinum (Fig. 356). The air can then rupture through the mediastinal pleura to produce a pneumothorax. A pneumomediastinum from any other cause may result in a pneumothorax in the same way.

Roentgen Appearance of Pneumothorax. As air accumulates in the pleural cavity, the lung retracts from the chest wall, creating a zone of radiolucency devoid of pulmonary markings in the periphery of the pulmonary field. The sharply defined border of the visceral pleura over the collapsed lung can always be recognized, (Fig. 358), though it may not be evident at first glance.

A small pneumothorax is easily overlooked if the visceral pleura is not significantly thickened. Most of the air tends to accumulate over the apex of the lung. The arcuate lucency of the pneumothorax may be difficult to distinguish from the lung because of the normal paucity of pulmonary markings in the apical regions and the fact that the border of the lung is often obscured by the overlapping shadows of the upper ribs. An unusual fluttering motion of the heart, seen during fluoroscopy, may be the first clue to the presence of a pneumothorax. This is due to absence of the steadying effect on the mediastinum by the adjacent lung.

Whenever a small pneumothorax is suspected and not clearly identified on the standard film of the chest, the examination should be repeated during expiration. During this phase the thoracic cavity becomes smaller and the volume of the lung decreases, but the amount of air in the pleura remains unchanged. As the diaphragm rises during expiration, the height of the thoracic cavity is decreased. The width of the pneumothorax must then become greater, increasing the separation of the lung from the chest wall (Fig. 32). Furthermore, as air is expelled during expiration, the lung becomes more dense, increasing its contrast with the air in the pleura so that the pneumothorax stands out more clearly (Fig. 515).

A larger pneumothorax is quite evident on films made in inspiration as well as in expiration. The lung, which is more collapsed in this case, is relatively denser and provides more contrast with the surrounding air in the pleura. The boundary of the lung is therefore more clearly outlined. Frequently the pneumothorax is complicated by a small collection of fluid at the base. This may be caused by inflammatory reaction to a tear in the pleura, seepage of a small amount of blood into the pleural cavity or the irritative effect of the air itself.

If the underlying lung is relatively normal, it retracts in a more or less uniform manner toward its root as the air in the pleural space increases. However, the pneumothorax appears greater in the upper portion of the chest. This is partly due to the inferior pulmonary ligament which holds the mesial portion of the lower lobe in place and limits its upward retraction. The peripheral portion of the lower lobe does become elevated and displaced from the lateral chest wall. This is evident on the frontal film. Oblique films are required to disclose the retraction of the anterior and posterior portions of the lung. In the absence of adhesions, the air has a tendency to extend into the fissures so that the individual lobes of the lung can frequently be identified.

As air accumulates in the pleura, the mediastinum tends to shift to the opposite side. This is not noticeable during inspiration if the pneumothorax is not very large, but it is quite evident during expiration even with a pneumothorax of moderate size (Fig. 542). The shift of the mediastinum is more apparent during fluoroscopy than on films made in inspiration and expiration, and is characterized by a pendular movement during breathing.

It is not necessary for the intrapleural pressure to be positive on the side of the pneumothorax in order to produce the mediastinal shift. If the mediastinum is not fixed, the diminished negative pressure produced by the pneumothorax creates an imbalance between the pleural pressures on the two sides of the chest, sufficient to cause displacement of the mediastinum during expiration. The pendular movement of the mediastinum thus produced is similar to that which occurs in obstructive emphysema.

When the pneumothorax is very large, the lung tends to collapse completely and the pressure in the pleural cavity becomes positive during both phases of respiration. If the lung is not adherent to the parietal pleura, it retracts toward its root, becoming separated from the diaphragm as well as from the chest wall. However, the degree of retraction of the mesial portion of the lower lobe depends upon the attachment of the inferior pulmonary ligament. If the ligament is not completely attached to the diaphragm, the mesial portion of the lower lobe can retract upward and expose the free falciform edge of the ligament.

If the mediastinum is not fixed, a tension pneumothorax displaces it to the opposite side during both inspiration and expiration (Fig. 543). However, it will still exhibit pendular motion because the displacement is greater during expiration. The diaphragm is depressed and the ribs are spread apart by the positive pressure in the pleural cavity.

When the lung is completely collapsed, it offers considerable resistance to the flow of blood. As a result, most of the blood from the main pulmonary artery is shunted to the opposite lung and the blood vessels on that side become more prominent. If, in addition, the mediastinum is displaced, the contralateral lung is compressed, less well aerated, and appears denser than normal. The prominent blood vessels together with the increased density of the lung often simulate interstitial infiltrations. However, the shadows

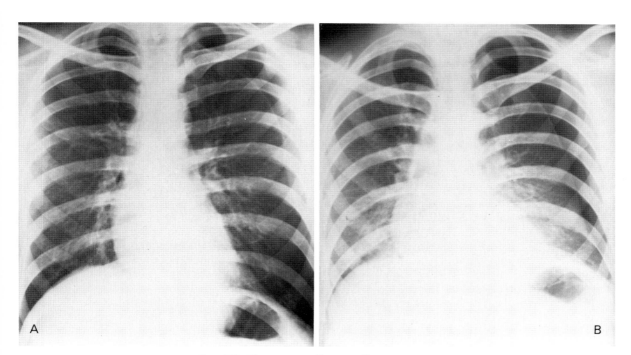

FIG. 542. MEDIASTINAL SHIFT IN PNEUMOTHORAX

A: Inspiration. There is a 20% pneumothorax on the left side. The heart and mediastinum are in their normal positions. *B*: Expiration. As the diaghragm elevates, the width of the pneumothorax increases and the mediatinum is displaced to the opposite side. Shift of the mediastinum only during expiration does not indicate a tension pneumothorax.

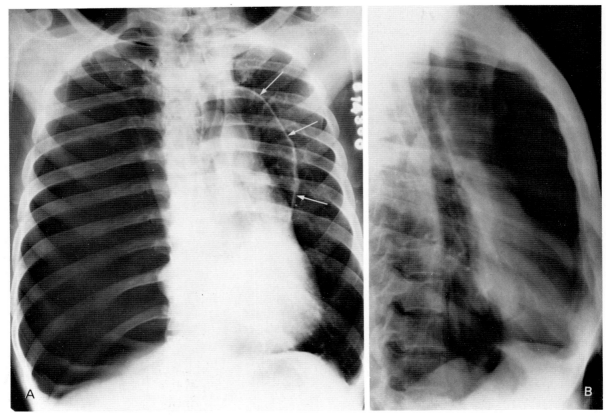

FIG. 543. TENSION PNEUMOTHORAX: MEDIASTINAL HERNIATION

A: The patient had a chronic bronchopleural fistula on the right side that produced a tension pneumothorax. The heart and mediastinum are displaced to the left. The curvilinear shadow (arrows) is the result of herniation of the right pleural cavity across the anterior mediastinum. It is formed by the two layers of mediastinal pleura and connective tissue between them, together with the visceral pleura of the left lung. The right lung is completely collapsed and is hidden by the heart. *B:* The lateral view shows an increased lucency of the retrocardiac space, indicating herniation through the posterior mediastinum as well.

disappear promptly when the pneumothorax is absorbed.

The distribution of the air in the pleural cavity is affected by pleural adhesions and by disease of the underlying lung. Retraction of the lung is prevented where the visceral and parietal pleura are adherent. Extensive adhesions may result in a loculated pneumothorax. Small adhesions produce strand-like shadows extending from the parietal pleura to the surface of the lung. These usually widen in tent-like fashion as they approach the lung. Although they appear like bands of fibrous tissue, they really represent thin, drawn out portions of the lung which are stretched as the rest of the lung retracts from the chest wall (Fig. 293). When lysing such an adhesion it is necessary to resect a small portion of the parietal pleura to avoid severing the lung and creating a bronchopleural fistula.

When the adhesions are more extensive, large portions of the lung are fixed to the chest wall and therefore remain more or less completely expanded. If the adhesions close off the lateral portion of the pleura, the air may accumulate in the paramediastinal portion of the thoracic cavity (Fig. 535). The border of the collapsed lung is then separated from the mediastinum but maintains its contact with the chest wall. The appearance is similar to that of a pneumomediastinum. However, continuation of the lucent collection of air over the apex of the lung identifies it as a pneumothorax. Air confined to the anterior or posterior portion of the pleural cavity may be impossible to detect on the frontal view but is clearly defined in the oblique or lateral projection.

If the underlying lung is diseased, the distribution of the air in the pleural cavity depends upon the tendency of the involved portion of lung to retract. Usually the diseased area tends to retract to a greater degree than does the normal lung adjacent to it. This occurs particularly where there is scarring of the lung or bronchial obstruction with secondary atelectasis. This fact was most important in the pneumothorax treatment of tuberculosis. It permitted the *selective* collapse and immobilization of the diseased area by a relatively small pneumothorax, allowing the remainder of the lung to function normally (Fig. 544).

Conversely, some diseases interfere with retraction of the lung and tend to keep it expanded. In these cases a pneumothorax will cause inordinate collapse of the normal portion of the lung. This is seen with obstructive emphysema or bullous disease, or when the lung is rigid because of consolidation, extensive interstitial infiltration or interstitial emphysema.

When the underlying lung is rigid and resists collapse, even a small amount of air results in a considerable increase in the intrapleural pressure with consequent displacement of the surrounding structures. A pneumothorax of moderate size may also cause an inordinate increase in the pleural pressure if most of the lung is adherent to the parietal pleura and is therefore unable to collapse. Because the lung is largely fixed in position, the heart and mediastinal structures are not displaced. However, a portion of the lung may herniate into the opposite hemithorax. This usually occurs through the upper anterior or lower posterior mediastinum where there is little support from the heart, trachea and blood vessels.

Resorption of Pneumothorax. Air does not remain indefinitely in the pleural cavity. Absorption takes place constantly, and once the opening in the pleura is sealed, the lung undergoes progressive reexpansion. Small pneumothoraces are usually absorbed within a matter of days and even large pneumothoraces can disappear within 2 to 4 weeks if they are not renewed. Absorption

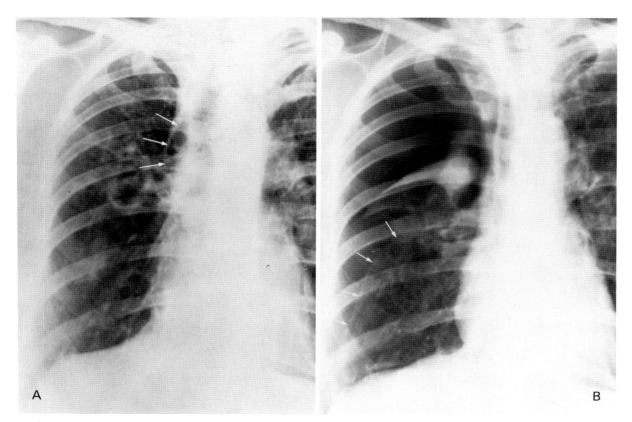

FIG. 544. PNEUMOTHORAX: SELECTIVE COLLAPSE

A: A patient with active tuberculosis. There are fine infiltrations in the partially collapsed right upper lobe. The short fissure is elevated, the trachea is displaced to the right and the anterior lappet of the left upper lobe (arrows) has herniated through the mediastinum. The cavity is situated in the superior segment of the lower lobe. *B*: After induction of a pneumothorax, the right upper lobe is completely collapsed. The lower lobe (arrows) remains almost completely expanded. The cavity is no longer evident.

proceeds more slowly if the pleura is thickened or if there is an especially high negative intrapleural pressure. Such high negative pressures occur during the absorption of air from the pleura when the underlying lung resists reexpansion because of fibrosis, bronchial obstruction or encasement by thickened visceral pleura. Absorption of the pneumothorax may then be delayed for many weeks.

In the absence of marked thickening of the pleura or pulmonary fibrosis, delayed absorption should suggest the possibility of bronchial obstruction. Not uncommonly this is the result of a mucus plug (Fig. 74). Removal of the obstruction by bronchoscopy results in rather rapid reexpansion of the lung because of release of the high negative pressure established in the pleura during the period of bronchial obstruction.

Failure of a pneumothorax to diminish with time usually indicates persistence of an opening in the pleura which permits replenishment of the air in the pleural cavity. Most often this is due to a bronchopleural fistula. However, in the case of a tension pneumothorax, the roentgen findings can be misleading. Routine films may show no significant change in the appearance of the pneumothorax even though air is being resorbed. The pressure in the pleural space steadily decreases once the opening in the pleura is closed. Nevertheless, for a number of days the pressure may be sufficiently high to keep the lung completely collapsed in both inspiration and expiration. Films made in inspiration may show no change in the position of the mediastinum in the early stages of resorption of a tense pneumothorax. However, films made during expiration reveal less displacement of the mediastinum to the opposite side.

Special Types of Pneumothorax

Hydropneumothorax. When the pleural cavity contains air as well as fluid, the upper border of the effusion lies in a horizontal plane. Therefore, on films made with a horizontal x-ray beam, the air-fluid interface is projected as a sharply demarcated, straight, horizontal border. The fluid level extends across the entire hemithorax unless the effusion is loculated. When the collection of fluid is small and confined to the costophrenic sinus, only that portion of the fluid level lateral to the diaphragm is visible on films made with ordinary exposure. On overpenetrated films, the fluid level can be seen through the shadow of the diaphragm, extending medially to the spine. Similarly, in somewhat larger effu-

sions, the mesial portion of the air-fluid level may be hidden by the heart.

Generally, the fluid level is quite distinct because of the contrast between the lucent air and the dense shadow of the fluid. When there is only a thin mantle of air and fluid, the fluid level is not so prominent and can be overlooked, especially on films made during inspiration (Fig. 32). However, the characteristic level is always present.

An air-fluid level always remains horizontal, no matter whether the patient is tilted or recumbent. However, the fluid level does change its position in relation to the chest wall. This has given rise to the term *shifting fluid level*. An air-fluid level shifts rapidly with a change in the position of the patient. On the other hand, the shift of a pleural effusion in the absence of a pneumothorax is relatively slow and lags behind the movement of the patient.

Oftentimes a horizontal fluid level is the only evidence of air in addition to the fluid in the pleural cavity. If the line is truly horizontal it should be parallel to the lower edge of the film, since the latter is always horizontal if the cassette holder has been properly installed.

The fluid level cannot be visualized unless it is projected tangentially, and this requires a horizontal x-ray beam. The presence of an air-fluid level in the stomach indicates that the beam was horizontal. If the beam is deviated even slightly from the horizontal, the sharp line of the fluid level may disappear. However, the portion of the pleural cavity that contains the fluid appears more dense than the region above it which contains the air. When the beam is directed vertically, as is frequently the case when the patient is recumbent, the air and fluid layers are superimposed on each other. The only manifestation of the hydropneumothorax may then be a faint uniform clouding of the hemithorax, as in a simple effusion of small or moderate size. In the case of a loculated pyopneumothorax, containing only a small or moderate amount of air, a film made with a vertical beam will produce a round solid density simulating either a neoplasm or a simple loculated effusion (Fig. 545).

The presence of air together with the pus is of great clinical significance. If the air was not introduced through the chest wall, it must be assumed that it entered the pleural cavity from a lesion connected with a bronchus or the esophagus. The presence of a pneumomediastinum would indicate that the pyopneumothorax is secondary to a dehiscence in the esophagus. In any case, persistence of a fistulous tract in the pleura

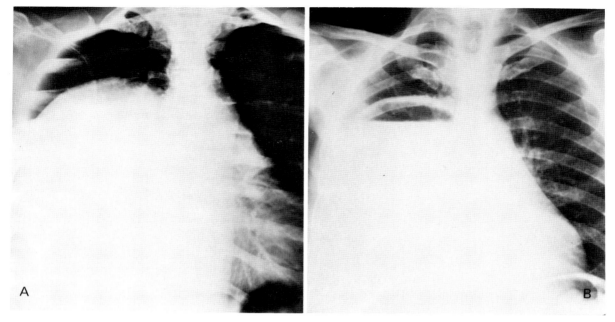

FIG. 545. LOCULATED PYOPNEUMOTHORAX

A: Supine position. The dense, homogeneous shadow with a sharply demarcated upper border occupies most of the right hemithorax. The displacement of the heart to the left suggests a huge neoplasm of the lung or pleura. *B*: Erect position. An air-fluid level is now seen excluding the possibility of a neoplasm. If the patient is too ill to maintain the erect position, a fluid level can be demonstrated in the lateral decubitus, using horizontal rays. Only a solid shadow is seen, regardless of the patient's position, if the x-ray beam is directed vertically.

is one of the causes of chronic empyema. The communication may be demonstrated radiologically by the introduction of radiopaque material into the bronchi, the esophagus or directly into the sinus tract.

During aspiration of the chest for diagnostic purposes, air may unknowingly be permitted to enter the pleural cavity, either through the needle or through a puncture of the lung. Subsequent roentgenograms showing a collection of air in the chest are then misleading. It is wise, therefore, never to omit a roentgen examination of the chest preliminary to the aspiration of fluid. It is only by this means that confusion and doubt can be eliminated in a consideration of the true cause of a collection of fluid and air.

Whenever a pleural effusion is suspected and the patient cannot be placed in the erect position, at least one film should be made with the x-ray beam directed horizontally. Regardless of whether the patient is semierect or recumbent, an air-fluid level can be demonstrated by this method. Although a lateral decubitus film is preferable, an across-the-table lateral view will suffice.

Pyopneumothorax. The most common cause of pus and air in the pleural cavity is rupture of an infected pulmonary focus that com-

municates with a bronchus. A pyopneumothorax can also result from rupture of the esophagus into the pleura, with or without an intervening mediastinal abscess. A penetrating wound of the chest may permit air to enter the pleural cavity from the outside, or from the lung if the visceral pleura is disrupted. Not uncommonly bacteria are introduced through the wound and a pyopneumothorax results.

It is frequently impossible to differentiate roentgenologically between a hydropneumothorax and a pyopneumothorax. Most often in the former, the pleura is thin but it is notably thickened when pus is present (Fig. 545*B*). The fibrinopurulent exudate causes a shaggy thickening of the parietal as well as the visceral pleura. In most cases a pyopneumothorax is loculated. Loculation is uncommon in a bland hydropneumothorax.

Differentiation between a loculated pyopneumothorax and a large abscess within the lung is sometimes difficult. The shell of lung separating such an abscess from the pleura may be very thin and the fluid level quite large. Even at thoracotomy it may be difficult to determine whether the collection of pus and air is situated in the lung or in the pleura. This is not an uncommon problem in staphylococcal infections, particularly in young children. Observation of the upper border of the cavity is often helpful in making the differentiation. In a pyopneumothorax the border forms a uniform sharp curve (Fig. 132), while in a large lung abscess it often appears irregular, scalloped or serrated because of the pulmonary septa which project into the abscess cavity (Fig. 275).

If the pyopneumothorax is not situated in an interlobar fissure, it always abuts on the parietes. This may not be evident on the frontal projection if the collection of pus and air does not lie against the lateral chest wall. However, it can always be demonstrated in the appropriate lateral or oblique view in which the lesion is projected tangentially. In this view, the curved border of the loculation facing the lung forms an obtuse angle where it meets the chest wall. In contradistinction, the border of a lung abscess tends to form an acute angle with the chest wall (Fig. 129). If the pyopneumothorax is situated at the base of the pleural cavity only the upper obtuse angle is visible, while if it involves the dome of the pleural cavity only the lower angle can be seen. A collection of fluid and air within an interlobar fissure is spindle-shaped, the pointed ends continuing with the line of the thickened fissure. On the other hand, an abscess which has perforated through the fissure into an adjacent lobe casts a round or oval shadow.

A pyopneumothorax loculated in the mesial portion of the chest must be differentiated from a mediastinal abscess that contains air. In the latter, the fluid level always crosses the shadow of the trachea in the frontal projection while the fluid level of a pyopneumothorax never crosses the border of the trachea (Fig. 546). A pyopneumothorax under pressure may cross the midline. It then displaces the trachea toward the opposite side but does not cross it.

Hemopneumothorax. Almost all cases of hemopneumothorax result from trauma to the chest. Sometimes the blood originates from an intercostal vessel injured by a penetrating wound of the chest wall, but most frequently the bleeding follows a tear of the lung. Occasionally a hemopneumothorax results from rupture of a bulla without any external injury (spontaneous hemopneumothorax).

If the blood does not clot, the roentgen appearance at first is similar to that of a hydropneumothorax. However, as the blood breaks down it causes pleural irritation and an inflammatory reaction, producing thickening of the pleura, most noticeable over the base of the lung. Frequently the blood clots, and the coagulum is

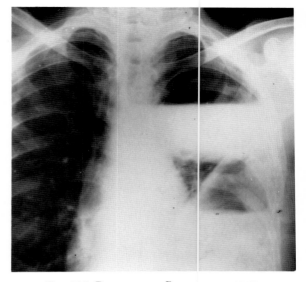

FIG. 546. BILOCULATED PYONEUMOTHORAX

There are two collections of fluid and air in the left pleural cavity. The upper fluid level seems to extend into the mediastinum because it crosses the border of the spine. It does not cross the shadow of the trachea which is displaced to the right. This is in contrast to the fluid level in an abscess of the mediastinum (see Fig. 444).

distributed in irregular fashion over the pleura. Both the visceral and parietal pleura may then present an irregular, shaggy outline. Blood clots projecting above the fluid produce an irregular, bumpy conformation to the air-fluid level. Such an irregular fluid level is quite characteristic of hemopneumothorax.

Underlying Causes of Pneumothorax

Frequently the cause of the pneumothorax can be inferred from the roentgen appearance of the chest. In some instances, particularly in traumatic or recurrent pneumothoraces, the clinical history is required for an evaluation of the underlying cause.

Trauma. In the presence of recent rib fractures it is justifiable to assume that the pneumothorax has been caused by a tear of the visceral pleura. A hemopneumothorax, indicated by the presence of irregular protrusions above a horizontal fluid level or an irregular thickening of the pleural layers, suggests a traumatic origin. However, similar changes are sometimes encountered in therapeutic pneumothorax where the irregularities are produced by masses of fibrin. Mediastinal emphysema may be associated with a pneumothorax caused by trauma to the chest wall or perforation of the esophagus. Air in both the pleural space and mediastinum may also occur in the absence of trauma in diseases complicated by interstitial emphysema of the lung.

When there is a sizeable defect in the chest wall, allowing free communication between the pleural space and the outside air (open pneumothorax), a characteristic type of mediastinal motion may occur. In contradistinction to a closed pneumothorax in which the mediastinum shifts *in the direction of the involved side* during inspiration, the movement of the mediastinum in the case of an open pneumothorax is toward the *opposite* side. If the opening in the chest wall is greater than the cross-sectional area of the glottis, the pressure in the pneumothorax tends to remain the same as that of the surrounding atmosphere during both phases of respiration. As the pleural pressure on the intact side becomes more negative during inspiration, the mediastinum is forced to that side by the atmospheric pressure of the pneumothorax.

The roentgenologist should be told of any instrumentation that might conceivably be the cause of the pneumothorax, such as aspiration of the chest, esophagoscopy or bronchoscopy, if he is not to be led astray in his interpretation. Perforation of the upper part of the esophagus is generally associated with mediastinal emphysema, usually without a complicating pneumothorax, while a perforation of the lower esophagus more frequently extends directly into the pleural cavity without a concomitant pneumomediastinum. Bronchoscopy is a rare cause of pneumothorax. This complication occurs particularly during the extraction of foreign bodies and the performance of deep biopsies.

Bullae. Rupture of a bulla is the most common cause of spontaneous pneumothorax. Most often the reason for the rupture is not known. In rare instances, it is caused by intermittent positive pressure breathing. The bulla, which is practically always situated at the apex of the lung, is rarely visualized on films even if it remains inflated while the lung is collapsed. Occasionally, however, the bulla can be seen as a sharply defined lucency bounded by a thin, annular shadow protruding from the surface of the lung. Films made before the pneumothorax may disclose one or more bullae, not visible when there is air in the pleura. Since most bullae are bilateral, visualization of a bulla on the opposite side should suggest rupture of a similar lesion as the cause of the pneumothorax.

Rupture of a bulla when the lungs otherwise appear normal, occurs most frequently in patients between the ages of 20 and 40. In older persons, the bullae are commonly part of generalized emphysema with bullous changes which are quite evident on the films. Among the pneumoconioses, extensive bullous changes complicated by pneumothorax occur characteristically in Shaver's disease.

A very large bulla can simulate a localized pneumothorax. The two are differentiated by the configuration of the lung adjacent to the collection of air. In a pneumothorax the border of the lung can always be visualized, on properly exposed films, as a well defined, smooth, convex line, while large bullae are usually poorly delineated from the adjacent emphysematous lung. When the border of the bulla is sharply demarcated from the lung, it casts a concave curvilinear shadow, usually forming an acute angle with the lateral chest wall below it. In the case of a tense, loculated pneumothorax, the border of the collapsed lung may also be concave but it makes an obtuse angle with the chest wall below the pneumothorax.

Tuberculosis. Rupture of a tuberculous cavity, common when pneumothorax treatment was in vogue, is now rare. Because extensive adhesions over the cavity are not the rule in this disease, the resulting pneumothorax is often generalized. Evidence of a pleural reaction may be lacking for a few days but soon an effusion of considerable size develops and the pleura becomes thickened by plastic exudate. This differs from the majority of cases of ruptured bulla in which the effusion, if present, is small, and the pleura shows little if any thickening.

Nowadays, a spontaneous pneumothorax in a patient with tuberculosis is usually due to rupture of a noninfected bulla even though a tuberculous cavity is present. The roentgen manifestations are the same as those of rupture of a simple bulla except for evidence of the underlying tuberculosis. The intact tuberculous cavity may become more clearly outlined by contrast with the surrounding lung which is collapsed by the pneumothorax. Extensive scarring at both apices, even though no bullae are visible on the film, indicates that the pneumothorax is most probably due to rupture of a bulla associated with an old tuberculous process.

Lung Abscess. The pneumothorax associated with perforation of a lung abscess is always accompanied by a collection of purulent exudate in the pleura. Unlike the tuberculous cavity, the pleural layers over a lung abscess are adherent so that the resultant pyopneumothorax is usually loculated. After a time it frequently perforates into the general pleural cavity to produce a large collection of fluid and air. Moreover, the tuberculous cavity has a wide communication with its entering bronchus, while the bronchial opening into a perforated lung abscess is small. Therefore, when an abscess ruptures, its walls tend to collapse and the cavity can no longer be visualized.

Croup and Tracheobronchitis. A pneumothorax that complicates partial obstruction of the larynx or bronchi in severe inflammatory disease in children is associated with interstitial emphysema of the lung and, not infrequently, with mediastinal emphysema (Fig. 547). Severe coughing causes rupture of the overdistended alveoli into the adjacent interlobular septa. The air then tracks through the interstitial tissues to the pleura and mediastinum. Rupture of a bleb through the visceral pleura or rupture of a large mediastinal air vesicle through the parietal pleura produces a pneumothorax.

Usually the pneumothorax is small because of the indirect communication with the bronchial tree. Frequently, mediastinal blebs rupture into both pleural cavities and produce a bilateral pneumothorax. The pneumomediastinum itself may not be visualized, but its presence can be inferred from the observation of air within the tissue planes at the root of the neck.

The interstitial emphysema produces rigidity of the lung, which resists collapse. A small, unilateral pneumothorax can therefore cause an inordinate shift of the mediastinum to the opposite side, particularly during expiration. Such mediastinal shift in the presence of a small pneumothorax should suggest either interstitial emphysema of the lung or a check valve bronchial obstruction.

Pneumothorax of the Newborn. Here again, the pneumothorax is the result of alveolar rupture, often in association with interstitial emphysema and pneumomediastinum. Also, the pneumothoraces are mostly small and frequently bilateral. When unilateral, there may be an inordinate shift of the mediastinum because of the interstitial emphysema.

Most cases of spontaneous pneumothorax of the newborn occur in mature or postmature infants, particularly following difficult or instrumental deliveries complicated by aspiration of meconium, or where positive pressure breathing has been employed. The spontaneous pneumo-

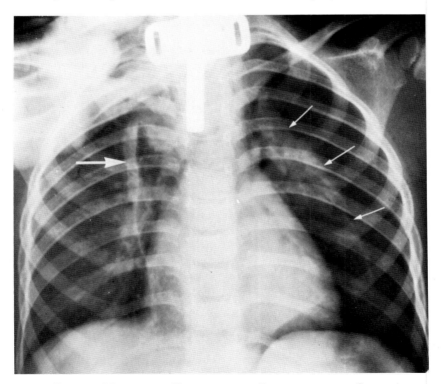

Fig. 547. Mediastinal Emphysema and Pneumothorax in Croup

The vertical streak on the right (arrow) represents the mesial part of the lung which has been displaced and compressed by the mediastinal emphysema. There is a large pneumothorax on the left side, probably due to rupture of a mediastinal air vesicle. The left lung is collapsed (arrows). The lucency between the left lung and the mediastinum represents either mediastinal emphysema or a portion of the pneumothorax. The complication followed a tracheotomy.

thorax may also be due to emphysema caused by partial bronchial obstruction by mucus or to hyaline membrane disease. In rare instances it may conceivably be due to the extremely high negative intrathoracic pressure which occurs with the infant's first breath.

Since small pneumothoraces are not apt to produce obvious symptoms, they often go unrecognized unless a roentgen examination is made for some other reason. The distribution of the pneumothorax is somewhat different from that in older children because films of the newborn are made in the supine position in which there is a tendency for the lung to retract upward. This permits the air to accumulate between the lung and the diaphragm. In fact, only the infrapulmonary collection of air may be visualized on the frontal projection. Although in some cases the pneumothorax is not detectable in this view, the collection of air is readily visualized over the anterior portion of the lung on a cross-the-table lateral projection.

Pneumomediastinum also occurs in the newborn as a result of alveolar rupture without a concomitant pneumothorax. It may be difficult to differentiate between a large collection of air in the mediastinum and a collection of air in the pleural cavity. Subcutaneous emphysema, of course, is indicative of pneumomediastinum, but is rather unusual in the newborn. Much more common is outward and upward displacement of the thymus gland by the air in the mediastinum (Fig. 440). Observation of air beneath the lung or delineation of the outer border of the partially collapsed lung indicates the presence of an associated pneumothorax. Oblique views may be required for the identification of both the pneumothorax and the mediastinal emphysema.

An erroneous diagnosis of pneumothorax is easily made in the newborn, especially in premature infants, whose skin is lax and thrown into folds. A vertical skin fold frequently forms on the back near the lateral portion of the chest when the infant lies in the supine position. Since this is the position in which the film is almost always made, the fold may be projected as a fine line paralleling the lateral chest wall, mimicking the lateral border of a partially collapsed lung. A similar appearance can be seen in patients who are emaciated (Fig. 65). The presence of an additional line, representing another fold or extension of the line beyond the bounds of the thoracic cavity is an indication of a skin fold rather than a pneumothorax. Either a prone or an oblique view will eliminate the fold and resolve the difficulty.

Neoplasms. Although rare, a significant number of cases of spontaneous pneumothorax associated with pulmonary neoplasms have been reported. Almost all have occurred in patients with metastases from a sarcoma, particularly of bone. Because of the age incidence of malignant osseous tumors, a large percentage of these pneumothoraces have been in children. Although a ball-valve mechanism in a small bronchus involved by tumor may account for some of the pneumothoraces, the pathologic descriptions indicate that the usual cause is rupture of a necrotic portion of the tumor, establishing a bronchopleural communication.

The pneumothoraces are usually large and persistent, and are frequently bilateral. An effusion may be absent. When the lung is completely collapsed, the metastatic nodules within it cannot be identified but their presence in the opposite lung makes the diagnosis quite clear. If both lungs are collapsed, the diagnosis of ruptured metastatic neoplasm may be suggested by a history of a sarcomatous growth elsewhere. The diagnosis can be proved by demonstrating nodules in the lung after aspiration of the pleural air.

Despite the fact that obstructive emphysema, necrosis of the tumor and incidental bullae are common in primary bronchogenic carcinoma, a complicating spontaneous pneumothorax is extremely rare. With only one exception, in the few cases that have been reported, the pneumothorax appears to have been caused by rupture of a bulla rather than by perforation of the neoplasm into the pleura. The presence of a pneumothorax, therefore, does not indicate that the pleura has been contaminated by tumor and that the neoplasm is inoperable.

Pulmonary Infarction. A pneumothorax can result from a broken-down pulmonary infarct which communicates with a bronchus and perforates through the pleura. This combination of events rarely takes place unless the infarct is infected or positive pressure breathing employed. In either case, the pneumothorax is always associated with a collection of fluid in the pleura. If the infarct is infected, the combination of fluid and air represents a pyopneumothorax, which may be loculated. The bloody fluid and air following perforation of a bland infarct are more apt to lie free in the pleural cavity.

There are three types of infected infarcts. A single infarct, originally bland, may become secondarily infected through the bronchial tree to produce what amounts to a lung abscess. The x-ray appearance is similar to that of an aspiration abscess though the wall of the necrotic infarct tends to be thicker. This may perforate into the pleura in the same way as a primary lung abscess.

Thrombosis of an artery within an area of pneumonia can produce a focus of aputrid necrosis which, in rare instances, perforates into the pleura to produce a pyothorax or a pyopneumothorax, depending on whether there is a bronchial communication.

A suppurative thrombophlebitis elsewhere in the body may give rise to infected emboli which produce multiple abscesses in the lungs. If these involve bronchi of fair size, cavities develop, and if one ruptures into the pleura, a pyopneumothorax results. The association of one or more cavities in the lungs, with or without a fluid level, together with a pneumothorax in a patient with bacteremia should suggest perforation of an embolic abscess. This should lead to a search for a primary focus outside the lungs, although, in rare instances, the same picture may be due simply to a staphylococcal bronchopneumonia. In the absence of multiple lesions, it is impossible without a clinical history or previous films which indicate the presence of pulmonary infarction, to determine that the pyopneumothorax is secondary to an infected infarct.

Recurrent Pneumothorax

Apical Bullae. By far the most common cause of recurrent pneumothorax is rupture of a bulla at the apex of the lung. About 25% of patients with spontaneous pneumothorax later develop one or more pneumothoraces, either on the same side or the opposite one.

As often as not, the bullae are bilateral even though they are not visualized as such radiologically. Usually no abnormality is noted, or there is simple a paucity of pulmonary markings at the apices. Occasionally, fine angular linear markings are seen, representing septa within or between the bullae. Only rarely are the round borders of the cyst-like structures visible. Sometimes they can be seen on the side of the pneumothorax when the lung is partly collapsed. In other cases the only indication that a ruptured bulla is the underlying cause of the pneumothorax is the presence of bullae in the apex of the opposite lung.

Honeycomb Lung. The diseases which produce the pathologic picture of honeycomb lung and which tend to be complicated by recurrent spontaneous pneumothoraces are histiocytosis X, systemic sclerosis (scleroderma) and tuberous sclerosis. In all of these, the pulmonary involvement is bilateral and tends to be symmetrical. The disease is, therefore, manifest on the opposite side even if it is completely obscured on the side of the pneumothorax when the lung is collapsed.

In systemic sclerosis the pulmonary manifestations are usually characterized by fine interstitial infiltrations, best seen in the lower half of the lungs, and the microcysts, even though present in great numbers are generally not visible. On the other hand, the lesions of histiocytosis X are distributed more or less evenly throughout the lungs and are composed of nodular densities (Fig. 358) or well defined, extremely thin-walled microcysts. In tuberous sclerosis, a coarse, reticular pattern is usually seen, and on careful examination, small cystic lucencies may be visualized within the network of shadows, particularly on the oblique projection. Most often, the pulmonary lesions are only part of these generalized diseases. Characteristic roentgen changes are often present in other organs.

Menstruation. Cases of pneumothorax with multiple recurrences during the first 2 days of menstruation have been reported. In all of them the pneumothorax occurred on the right side. In half of the cases there was evidence of pelvic endometriosis and in some the pleural surface of the right leaf of the diaphragm was involved (Fig. 535). Tiny perforations of the diaphragm were seen at thoracotomy in a few of the cases, with and without local endometriosis. All these observations indicate a direct relationship between the recurrent pneumothoraces and menstruation. It is interesting to note, in this connection, that in all 20 reported cases in which a pneumothorax complicated an induced pneumoperitoneum, the air in the pleura was always on the right side. This suggests that there may normally be openings in the right side of the diaphragm too small to be recognized grossly.

The pneumothoraces related to menstruation are almost always small and easily overlooked. The possibility of a pneumothorax should be considered whenever there is chest pain at the beginning of the menstrual period. Since the pneumothoraces are small and absorb rapidly, films should be made promptly and in full expiration.

Lipiodol Treatment of Recurrent Pneumothorax. Recurrent pneumothoraces can be prevented by producing a pleurodesis which obliterates the pleural cavity. Iodized oil causes a persistent mild pleural irritation when injected into the pleural cavity and has been used for this purpose. The opaque oil is usually visible on the chest film for years.

When first injected into the pneumothorax space, the oil shifts with change in the position of the patient. However, when the air is absorbed, the pleural layers become adherent, keeping the oil in place. The resultant roentgen appearance is similar to that of calcification of the pleura, with blotchy shadows over the pulmonary field and linear shadows along the chest wall or mediastinum. However, the shadow of the iodized oil is considerably denser than the usual type of pleural calcification, particularly at the base of the pleural cavity where the oil tends to accumulate. Moreover, a characteristic striated shadow may be present when a small quantity of the oil infiltrates between the bundles of the intercostal muscle at the time of the injection.

Therapeutic Pneumothorax

Before the advent of effective chemotherapy and the perfection of resective surgery, long term artifical pneumothorax was the treatment of choice for cavitary tuberculosis. It was used primarily to produce collapse of the cavity and to diminish the respiratory motion of the lung.

Selective Collapse. A small or moderate-sized pneumothorax is often effective in producing collapse of the diseased portion of lung. This is due to the diminished compliance of the affected part of the lung resulting from infiltration and fibrosis, and obstruction of small bronchi. The distribution of the pneumothorax is therefore uneven, the involved segments contracting more than the healthy portion. If the pneumothorax is too large, the entire lung tends to collapse more uniformly.

The amount of air that is introduced is insufficient to produce a positive pressure within the pleural cavity during both phases of respiration. The pressure remains negative, at least during inspiration, permitting air to enter the cavity as well as the partially collapsed lung. However, after a variable period of time, the retraction of the lung distorts the bronchi and tends to cause kinking of the bronchus leading to the cavity. When the bronchus is completely occluded, the air that is absorbed from the cavity is no longer replaced and the cavity collapses.

Preexisting Pleural Adhesions. Adhesions of the pleura over the diseased portion of the lung interfere with satisfactory collapse and may render the pneumothorax ineffective (Fig. 293). If the adhesions are broad, the diseased portion is fixed to the chest wall and the injected air collapses the healthy part of the lung. When the area of pleurodesis is small, the diseased part may collapse but remains attached to the chest wall by one or more strand-like structures which

cross the pneumothorax space. These resemble fibrous strands. However, most often, they represent attenuated lung tissue put on the stretch when the rest of the lung collapses (Fig. 549). It is important to bear this in mind when planning lysis of the adhesions.

Complications. Pneumothorax treatment for tuberculosis was frequently associated with various complications. These occurred particularly late in the course of treatment or in cases where the pneumothorax was administered in the presence of adhesions. The complications often resulted in changes which persisted indefinitely after the pneumothorax was discontinued.

BALLOON CAVITY. Closure of the cavity by the pneumothorax is produced by kinking and consequent complete obstruction of the entering bronchus. This is followed by absorption of the air within the cavity and formation of a permanent stricture of the bronchial opening. If the entering bronchus is only partially obstructed, a check valve may be formed and result in ballooning of the cavity.

TEAR OF THE CAVITY. A sudden increase in the pressure within the pneumothorax resulting from straining or coughing can cause a tear of the lung at the site of a pleural adhesion. Since the adhesion is usually situated directly over a pulmonary cavity, a portion of the roof of the cavity may be torn, resulting in contamination of the pleura and establishment of a bronchopleural fistula. The pneumothorax increases in size and within a matter of hours or days a pleural effusion appears. Bacteria entering the pleura from the cavity produce a diffuse pleuritis so that the lung soon becomes covered with fibrinous exudate. This causes an increase in the density of the margin of the collapsed lung and produces a shadow along the inner border of the chest wall.

If the lung is completely torn from its attachment to the chest wall, total collapse ensues. However, in most cases, the adhesions are not completely severed so that a portion of the lung remains fixed to the chest wall even in the presence of a tension pneumothorax.

WHITE LUNG. An extraordinary phenomenon occasionally encountered was the sudden appearance of an extremely dense, homogeneous shadow over the diseased portion of the lung. This "white lung," which is associated with a pneumothorax, results from obstruction of a large bronchus and consequent atelectasis (Fig. 72). Induration of the lung, produced by spread of the tuberculous infection, contributes to the extreme density of the atelectatic area.

PLEURAL EFFUSION. A very small pleural effusion confined to the costophrenic sinus occurs quite frequently in therapeutic pneumothorax, and, as in the case of spontaneous pneumothorax, is of no clinical significance. However, larger effusions are usually associated with fever and are generally caused by spread of the tuberculous infection to the pleura. The x-ray films usually disclose thickening of the pleura in addition to a free collection of fluid and air. Unlike the effusion that follows rupture of a tuberculous cavity, the fluid usually does not become purulent for a considerable length of time because the pleura is not as heavily contaminated with tubercle bacilli and there is no secondary infection. In most instances the fluid is absorbed when the pneumothorax is discontinued. However, there is a tendency for the production of a tuberculous empyema if the lung is not permitted to reexpand.

PLEURAL THICKENING. Even in the absence of a pleural effusion, thickening of the pleura of greater or lesser degree was a relatively common complication of pneumothorax treatment (Fig. 548). In many instances the thickening was undoubtedly due to spread of the tuberculosis to the pleura. Fibrinous exudate accumulating on the visceral and parietal pleura eventually became organized into dense adhesions wherever the two layers made contact. This occurred especially in the paramediastinal and infrapulmonary regions. Adhesions of the pleural layers would extend gradually over the lung, progressively obliterating the pleural cavity and diminishing the space available for the pneumothorax. The dense, fibrous coat deposited around the lung while it was partially collapsed interfered with its reexpansion when the pneumothorax was abandoned (restrictive atelectasis). Because of the encasement of the lung, absorption of only a small amount of air from the pleura produced a high negative intrapleural pressure. This, together with contraction of the parietal pleura from the organizing pleuritis, resulted in flattening of the chest wall, increased obliquity of the ribs and diminution in the size of the affected hemithorax (Fig. 75). In some cases, when abandoning the pneumothorax, the negative pleural pressure would become great enough to cause transudation of fluid into the pleural cavity.

FIBRIN BODIES. Occasionally, when the pneu-

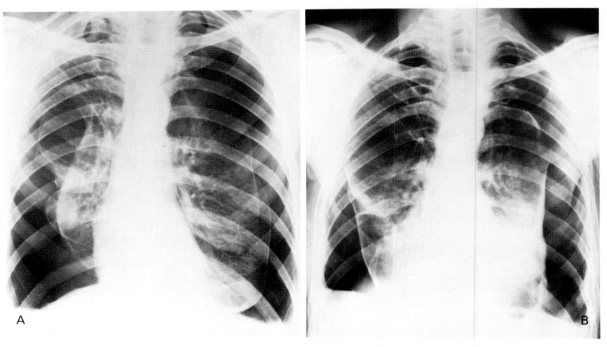

FIG. 548. PLEURAL THICKENING IN PROLONGED PNEUMOTHORAX

A: 1948. The patient had been receiving bilateral pneumothorax treatment for tuberculosis for the past 3 years. Both lungs are partially collapsed. The right upper lobe remains expanded because it is fixed to the chest wall by adhesions. The pleura over the apex of the left upper lobe is hardly visible because it is not thickened. The pleura over the remainder of both lungs is thickened and therefore is sharply outlined. *B:* 1955. Despite the rotengen findings, pneumothorax treatment was continued. The thickening of the pleura has progressed, imprisoning both lungs. The shadow obscuring the left cardiac border is probably due to a large fibrin body in the long fissure. Both costophrenic sinuses are obliterated by adhesions of the diaphragm to the chest wall.

mothorax was complicated by pleurisy with effusion, one or more sharply outlined, round, homogeneous opacities appeared in the pleural cavity as the fluid was absorbed. These represented masses of fibrin, precipitated in the effusion. The fibrin body is of moderate size, usually ranging from 2 to 4 cm in diameter (Fig. 549). A similar mass of fibrin can form within a hemothorax, but is not spherical in shape because it does not lie free within a pneumothorax space.

Once formed, most fibrin bodies remain unchanged for many years, but they may undergo calcification. If first seen on a film made after the lung has reexpanded, the fibrin body does not appear so sharply demarcated and simulates a lesion in the lung. However, when a fibrin body is present, there are almost always other signs of previous pleuritis and this should lead to an inquiry concerning pneumothorax treatment.

MEDIASTINAL HERNIATION. The persistently elevated pleural pressure within a long standing pneumothorax often results in herniation of the pleura across the midline (Fig. 543). This occurs through one of the unsupported areas of the mediastinum; either superiorly, in front of the ascending aorta, or inferiorly, behind the heart. When the collapsed lung cannot reexpand as the air is absorbed from the pleura, an extremely high negative intrapleural pressure develops on that side. The mediastinal herniation then occurs in a paradoxical direction, the normal lung herniating toward the pneumothorax (Fig. 550).

Postpneumothorax Lung. Although there may be no apparent residual changes in the lung after it has reexpanded, some evidence of the previous pneumothorax almost always remains. The abnormalities seen on the film are referable almost entirely to the thickening of the pleura that occurred at the time of the pneumothorax. The mildest change consists of a localized pleural thickening causing blunting of the costophrenic sinus, usually associated with widening of the

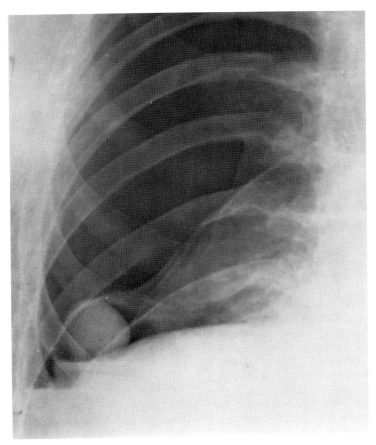

FIG. 549. FIBRIN BODY

The film made during pneumothorax treatment shows collapse of the right lung. The sharply demarcated, round, homogeneous density above the right costophrenic sinus followed slight bleeding which complicated an intrapleural pneumolysis. It changed little over a period of 2 years. The mass represents an old blood clot in the pleural cavity. The linear shadows crossing this fibrin body represent attenuated bands of lung fixed to the partietal pleura by adhesions.

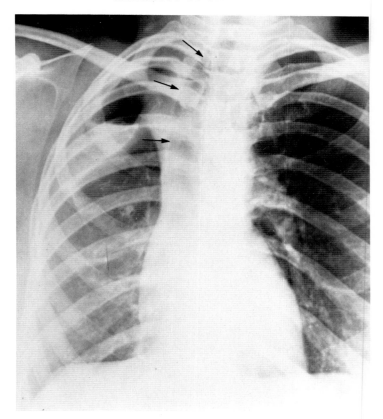

FIG. 550. PARADOXICAL MEDIASTINAL HERNIATION

Six months following cessation of pneumothorax treatment, a collection of air and fluid remains in the pleural space over the right upper lobe. The right lung appears clouded because of the thickened pleura that encases it. Because of the inability of the upper lobe to reexpand completely, as the air is absorbed from the pleura the negative pressure in the pleural space becomes greater than that on the left side. This has resulted in herniation of the left upper lobe (arrows) across the mediastinum to the side of the pneumothorax.

cardiophrenic angle and ironing out of the mediastinal contours.

Diffuse thickening of the pleura, even though slight in degree, is often sufficient to entrap the lung and prevent its complete reexpansion. As the pneumothorax is absorbed, the hemithorax becomes narrowed, partly by displacement of the mediastinum, but mostly by flattening of the chest wall. Since the thickening of the pleura is rather uniform, the slight increase in the opacity of the lung that it causes, is not easily recognized on the films (Fig. 75). However, in some cases a thin band of increased density is detectable along the lateral chest wall. Narrowing of the intercostal spaces and increased obliquity of the ribs can be slight and yet produce significant narrowing of the hemithorax. This may not be appreciated unless both sides of the chest are actually measured.

Narrowing of the lower half of the hemithorax together with evidences of old tuberculosis, such as fibrosis and calcification in the upper portion of the lung, with or without angulation of the trachea toward the involved side, should suggest the possibility of previous pneumothorax treatment. In some cases the pulmonary field is quite clear, and the only residuum of the previous tuberculous process in the lung is elevation of the hilum.

Unusual, poorly demarcated densities of moderate size at the base of the lung can represent fibrin bodies which lost their characteristic round shape and sharp demarcation when they were flattened by the reexpanding lung. Their situation on the pleura rather than within the lung can usually be suspected from tangential projections. A localized area of pleural calcification can represent calcium deposited within a fibrin body.

More diffuse calcification of the pleura occasionally develops over a period of years following reexpansion of the lung (Fig. 551). While this is usually associated with thickening of the pleura

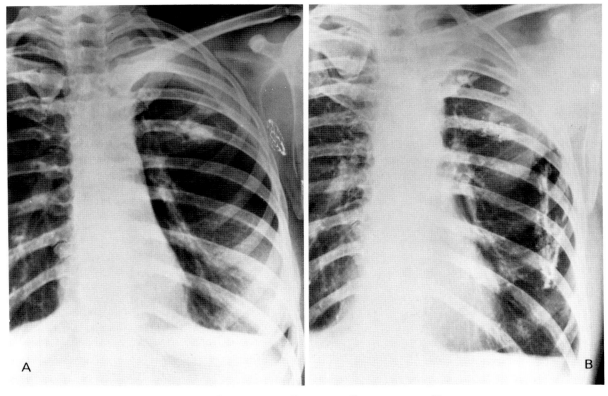

FIG. 551. PLEURAL CALCIFICATION FOLLOWING PNEUMOTHORAX TREATMENT

A: 1950. Pneumothorax treatment for tuberculosis was instituted in 1945 and discontinued 3 years later. As a result of fibrous thickening of the pleura, the heart is drawn to the left, the costophrenic sinus is obliterated by adhesions, the mediastinal contours are ironed out and there is a marked increase in the thickness of the pleura over the apex. The density in the left upper lobe represents a blocked tuberculous cavity. *B*: 1974. During the interveining years there has been progressive calcification of the pleura despite any evidence of active pleural disease. The blocked cavity disappeared as a result of chemotherapy and only a small cluster of calcific deposits remains.

from a dense fibrinous pleuritis secondary to the pneumothorax, evidence of pleurisy may be lacking preceding deposition of the calcium.

Transudate collecting in the pleural cavity during reexpansion of the lung generally becomes loculated over the outer portion of the upper lobe, since this is the last portion to expand. The transudate may be only partially absorbed and persist indefinitely as a bland, uninfected loculation of clear fluid which cannot be differentiated from a tuberculous empyema without aspiration (Fig. 552).

Specific Inflammatory Disease of the Pleura

Tuberculosis. Primary tuberculous infection of the lung is characterized by a localized area of pneumonia and caseation situated directly under the pleura. This is regularly associated with a local fibrinous pleuritis but the exudate is rarely

sufficient to produce a shadow on the roentgen film. Frequently, however, there is exudation of a small amount of fluid into the pleural cavity, detectable, as a rule, only by examination in the lateral decubitus position. In some instances the effusion is larger. The tiny effusions probably represent a sympathetic reaction to the infection in the lung. The larger ones are usually the result of actual infection of the pleura by the tubercle bacilli either from the primary lesion in the lung or from large caseous tuberculous lymph nodes which are part of the primary complex.

The common variety of tuberculous pleurisy results from lymphhematogenous dissemination of the primary infection. It is associated with an obvious effusion and usually occurs in adolescent or young adult life some time after establishment of the primary complex. Tubercle bacilli spreading to the blood stream via the thoracic duct cause the formation of small caseous foci in the lungs as well as in other organs of the body.

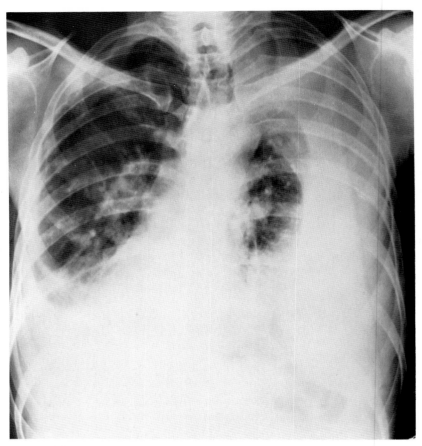

FIG. 552. PERSISTENT EFFUSION FOLLOWING PNEUMOTHORAX

The patient had bilateral pneumothorax treatment for tuberculosis many years previously. This was complicated by pleural effusions on both sides. The film shows a large loculated collection of fluid on the left side and a small one on the right. The heart is shifted to the right, as would be expected. However, there is a paradoxical shift of the trachea to the left, the side of the larger effusion. This indicates inability of the left upper lobe to expand. The fluid was aspirated and proved to be clear and noninfected.

Rupture of one of these foci through the pleura results in spread of the infection throughout the pleural cavity and the formation of numerous tubercles which, however, do not tend to caseate. The fluid is therefore usually clear but is associated with deposition of a considerable amount of fibrin which tends to loculate the effusion after one or more weeks.

Most often, the effusion is moderate in size and fills about a third of the pleural cavity. Occasionally, it is quite large (Fig. 519) but almost never fills the entire pleural cavity to the extreme apex. In this respect it differs from carcinomatous pleurisy and from some cases of pyogenic pleural infection. Occasionally tuberculous effusions are bilateral.

At first the effusion increases in size, but it usually becomes stablized after a week to 10 days and begins to absorb after a few weeks. Complete resorption of the fluid may require several months, during which time the pleura becomes quite thick. Where resorption occurs early there is little residual thickening of the pleura, but even when absorption is delayed, the thickening of the pleura gradually subsides. Eventually, all that remains in most cases is obliteration of the costophrenic sinus. In rare instances a dense thickening of the pleura persists indefinitely as an extremely firm, hyalinized mass of connective tissue partly encasing the base of the lung.

In young children, hilar or paratracheal densities, representing the lymph node component of the primary complex, are usually evident together with the effusion. The primary lesion in the lung may not be visible. However, when an effusion complicates primary tuberculosis in adolescents or young adults, it is rather unusual to visualize either the lesion in the lung or the lymph nodes (Fig. 300). Occasionally, numerous miliary or submiliary shadows are visible at the apices above the clavicles. These represent tubercles resulting from hematogenous dissemination of the disease, and indicate that the tuberculous pleurisy is hematogenous in origin. It is also justifiable to conclude that the tuberculous pleurisy is hematogenous when the effusion is bilateral or if a primary lesion is seen on the side opposite to the fluid.

If caseation takes place in the pleural tubercles and one or more rupture, a tuberculous empyema may form. This is characterized by a persistent dense shadow at the base of the lung. In its early stages the empyema cannot be differentiated radiologically from a simple tuberculous effusion which will eventually resorb.

The pulmonary lesion in the reinfection type of tuberculosis is also situated directly beneath the pleura. Although local pleuritis is extremely common at the onset of the infection, as evidenced by the occurrence of pain in the upper scapular region, it is rarely demonstrable radiologically at that time. The exudate is fibrinous and not infrequently results in the formation of pleural adhesions.

Dense thickening of the pleura by fibrosis and infiltration with cellular elements may occur later. This is manifested radiologically by a semilunar shadow over the apex of the lung (pleural cap), running parallel to the posterior portion of the second or third rib (Fig. 408) often extending for a short distance downward along the outer portion of the pulmonary field. Marked thickening of the pleura covering the upper portion of the upper lobe tends to obscure details of the underlying tuberculous lesion unless the film is heavily exposed. Occasionally calcium is deposited within the thickened pleura over the pulmonary lesion. This can result in the formation of a shell-like plaque over the apex of the lung, manifest on the roentgen film as a dense curvilinear shadow at the dome of the thoracic cavity (Fig. 518).

In contrast to the primary infection, a pleural effusion is rare in reinfection tuberculosis except as a complication of pneumothorax treatment. When it does occur, the effusion results either from ulceration of a tuberculous cavity into the pleura or from a spreading caseous pneumonia, particularly in old or debilitated patients. Occasionally, a tuberculous effusion occurs in the aged from reactivation and caseation of an old infection in the mediastinum.

TUBERCULOUS EMPYEMA. While pleural effusions occur most commonly in association with a primary tuberculous infection, they rarely lead to the formation of an empyema in these cases. Empyemas occur more frequently in the reinfection type of tuberculosis, especially as a complication of pneumothorax therapy. Since the introduction of efficacious chemotherapy, tuberculous empyemas have been a rare complication, but old empyemas, predating the chemotherapeutic era, are still encountered. In many of these cases the disease is dormant, producing few, if any, symptoms and can remain unsuspected for many years.

Characteristically, a tuberculous empyema is loculated by an extremely thick, irregular wall. Most often the main body of the empyema is situated in the lower, posterior part of the pleural cavity. A tract usually leads upward from the empyema to the posterior part of the upper lobe where there is often a bronchopleural fistula from a ruptured tuberculous cavity. When the empyema complicating pneumothorax treatment is not due to a tear of a pulmonary cavity, it is most often located over the upper part of the lung. This is due to the fact that the empyema develops slowly, and when the pneumothorax is abandoned, the lower lobe is the first to reexpand and make contact with the chest wall. The empyema then collects over the upper lobe. Loculation of a tuberculous empyema over this region also occurs as a complication of plombage.

A tuberculous empyema casts a dense, homogeneous shadow on the roentgen film. When situated in the lower part of the chest, its border is often poorly defined on the frontal projection, making it difficult to differentiate between a loculated collection of fluid and marked thickening of the pleura. The curved border which characterizes an empyema, in contradistinction to the straight border of the shadow of thickened pleura, is usually more clearly delineated in the lateral or oblique views. On the other hand, an empyema localized to the upper part of the chest, usually shows a sharply demarcated, convex mesial border in the frontal as well as other views. In either case, the diaphragm tends to be elevated and the chest wall over the empyema is contracted.

The presence of an air-fluid level within the shadow, when no air has been injected, or the persistence of such a level for a considerable length of time after pneumothorax treatment has been abandoned, is indicative of a pyopneumothorax associated with a bronchopleural fistula (Fig. 208). Marked thickening of the pleura may obscure the air-fluid level on films made with ordinary exposure. Overpenetrated or Bucky films are, therefore, required in all cases of suspected tuberculous empyema. It should be borne in mind that a fistula may be present even though no air can be demonstrated in the pleural cavity by any method. The fistulous tract may be tortuous or obstructed by caseating tissue or inspissated pus, preventing egress of the exudate from the pleura and ingress of air. In most instances of bronchopleural fistula, however, the tract eventually opens, at least temporarily, so that some of the pus empties through the bronchus, permitting air to enter the empyema cavity.

In the later stages, calcium is often deposited in the wall of the empyema. This takes the form of dense, irregular plaques of varying size, either separated from each other or joined to form a continuous shell about the collection of pus. Since the calcium is deposited primarily in the caseous tissue lining the empyema sac, the calcified plaques are separated from the rib cage by a thick layer of fibrous tissue which forms the remainder of the wall of the empyema.

A tuberculous empyema is usually an indolent type of infection and frequently remains unrecognized because it produces few or no symptoms. The diagnosis should be entertained whenever a tuberculous effusion fails to absorb completely within a few months, even though the patient looks and feels well. It should also be considered when the patient with a residual effusion after pneumothorax treatment develops fever without obvious cause or if he suddenly expectorates a quantity of pus. Calcific plaques or a rim of calcium on the border of a homogeneous density associated with thickening of the pleura is most suggestive of tuberculous empyema although it can occur in an old hemothorax or a nonspecific chronic suppurative infection. In the last instance there is practically always a history of an operation for a pyogenic empyema.

Shadows in an upper lobe indicative of old tuberculosis, with or without cavitation, should always suggest that an accompanying effusion represents a tuberculous empyema. Thick pleura may obscure the underlying disease but the latter can be disclosed on Bucky films or tomograms. The final diagnosis of tuberculous empyema, of course, depends upon aspiration and examination of the fluid.

Fungous Infections. Infection of the pleura by fungi almost always occurs as an extension from a focus in the underlying lung. By far the most common finding is thickening of the pleura. Occasionally the pleural disease takes the form of a clear effusion. An empyema or pyopneumothorax is unusual.

The pleural thickening is most marked directly over the pulmonary lesion, and is sometimes dense enough to obscure the disease in the lung.

An extremely thick pleura is present characteristically in actinomycosis and nocardiosis. In these diseases there is a tendency for the infection to spread directly through the pleura into the chest wall to produce peripleuritis, periostitis of the overlying ribs (Figs. 250 and 263) and swelling of the chest wall, often associated with one or more fistulous tracts. Radiologically, the pleural and peripleural involvement is manifested by contraction of the chest wall with narrowing of the intercostal spaces and increased obliquity of the ribs, thickening and erosion of the ribs whose borders are often poorly demarcated, and an increase in the thickness of the chest wall. Marked thickening of the pleura with contraction of the chest wall is also a common finding in aspergillosis (Fig. 350) even when the disease is manifested by a fungus ball of low grade virulence (mycetoma). Extension of the infection into the chest wall with changes in the ribs has also been reported in a few cases of North American blastomycosis.

Pleurisy is quite common in the early stage of coccidioidomycosis, even when the disease takes the form of a small pulmonary nodule. Small collections of free fluid occur occasionally but large ones are uncommon. Effusions are rarely encountered in the other fungous infections.

Because of the tendency to marked pleural thickening and extensive pleural adhesions which obliterate the pleural cavity over the lesion, empyema is a rare complication of fungous infection of the lungs. However, occasionally, an empyema does form from extension of a suppurative pulmonary focus in actinomycosis, and a pyopneumothorax occasionally results from rupture of a pulmonary cavity in coccidioidomycosis. More commonly, an empyema or pyopneumothorax is a complication of resective surgery for a fungous infection of the lung, and occurs particularly following segmental resection. The radiological appearance is indistinguishable from an empyema or pyopneumothorax from some other type of infection.

The finding of fungi, particularly actinomyces, aspergilli or monilia in pleural pus does not necessarily indicate a true fungal infection of the pleura. These organisms may act simply as saprophytes while the course of the infection is determined by other, more virulent organisms. This is the situation in some cases of putrid lung abscess in which fungi, commonly present in the mouth, are aspirated together with other organism, but are not responsible for the disease.

Protozoan and Parasitic Diseases. In this group of diseases, *amoebiasis* is the one most frequently associated with significant pleural manifestations. These may take the form of thickening of the pleura, a collection of free fluid representing a sympathetic effusion or a pyothorax, or a loculated empyema.

Most often, the pleural complication is secondary to an abscess in the liver, with or without an intervening subphrenic abscess. The right pleural cavity is therefore the one that is most frequently affected. The right leaf of the diaphragm is always raised, but sometimes in only one area.

The most common change is blurring of the border of the diaphragm because of thickening of the pleura at the base and obliteration of the costophrenic sinus by fibrinous exudate. A small or moderate-sized collection of free fluid, representing a sympathetic effusion, may also occur. A large effusion is generally indicative of infection of the pleura by the amoebae, resulting from perforation through the diaphragm of an abscess in the liver or subphrenic space. The fluid may fill the entire hemithorax and cause marked displacement of the mediastinum to the opposite side.

Less commonly the pleural involvement is secondary to amoebic infection of the lung. The pulmonary focus is in the right middle or lower lobe when it results from extension of the disease through the diaphragm (Fig. 264), but it may be situated in any part of either lung when it results from hematogenous dissemination of the amoebae. In either instance, the effusion may take the form of an empyema or pyopneumothorax. In the case of perforation of a hematogenous focus, one or more additional lesions may be visible in the same lung or on the opposite side.

In *echinococcus disease* of the lung, local rupture of a cyst into the adjacent pulmonary tissue results in an inflammatory reaction with thickening of the pleura over the lesion. Perforation of the cyst into the pleural cavity, either spontaneously, at operation or needle aspiration, results in a large effusion and the formation of numerous daughter cysts on the pleura. The cysts may be large enough to be visualized radiologically. They are best seen after thoracentesis, particularly if the fluid is replaced by air. They cannot be differentiated radiologically from metastatic neoplasms.

In *paragonimiasis* the pleura becomes involved when the larvae penetrate the diaphragm to pass from the peritoneal cavity into the lung. This may result in the formation of plastic exudate on the pleura or a small effusion. A small pneumothorax may also develop as the larvae perforate the visceral pleura. The pleural involvement may be bilateral.

Tropical eosinophilia may be associated with pleural thickening, most evident in the fissures. Free pleural effusions can occur but they are rare.

Radiation Pleuritis. Inflammation of the pleura is a common accompaniment of radiation pneumonitis. In most cases the roentgen picture is dominated by the reaction in the lung. In some, however, particularly when the radiation has been directed tangential to the chest wall, the reaction may be most marked in the pleura and peripleural tissues. Generally, by the time the pleural changes become manifest, there is already evidence of injury to the lung. In addition to the changes due to pulmonary inflammation, there is practically always shrinkage of the lung, due in part to contraction of the pleura. While the reaction in the lung is more or less localized to the field of treatment, the reaction in the pleura usually extends much further.

The most common finding is thickening of the pleura associated with shrinkage of the hemithorax. The pleural thickening produces a homogeneous haze over the affected portion of the pulmonary field, frequently with a band of increased density over the periphery, parallel to the chest wall. The thickening may extend to the base even though the radiation was limited to the upper portion of the pulmonary field. The pleural reaction causes straightening of the border of the mediastinum, obliterating the normal angles and curves made by the mediastinal structures. The cardiophrenic angle may become obtuse and the costophrenic sinus obliterated by adhesions. The chest wall is flattened, the mediastinum is drawn to the affected side and the diaphragm is elevated.

Frequently a pleural effusion develops 2 or 3 months after completion of the treatment. The fluid is usually small in amount and confined to the costophrenic sinus, although it may collect between the lung and diaphragm, producing a triangular shadow simulating a large diaphragmatic tent. This is quite characteristic of radiation reaction. Why the fluid collects in this fashion is not entirely clear but it is probably due to indrawing of a portion of the base of the lung because of an area of focal atelectasis.

The effusion usually resorbs slowly over a period of several months. It can persist for years, but does not tend to increase after the first few months. A large effusion is unusual. Effusions which first appear more than 6 months after radiotherapy, massive effusions, and those which continue to increase in size, are much more likely to be caused by spread of the neoplasm than by the irradiation.

The pleural effusion is always associated with

marked thickening of the pleura, and therefore tends to be loculated. The border of the loculated fluid is usually not sharply demarcated because it blends with the shadow of the diffusely thickened pleura around it. The pleural thickening and contraction of the chest remain indefinitely after the effusion has absorbed.

Inflammation and fibrosis of the peripleural tissues frequently accompany the pleural reaction. Occasionally the ribs are affected and weakened so that fractures can occur simply from the strain of coughing (Fig. 165). As in the case of other cough fractures, these occur at the bends of the ribs, particularly in the anterior axillary line. They tend to be multiple, involving corresponding portions of adjacent ribs.

Pneumoconiosis. Pleural involvement in the dust diseases is seen primarily in those caused by asbestos or talc (particularly tremolite talc) and,

less commonly, diatomaceous earth and mica. In these pneumoconioses there is a tendency to formation of hyaline plaques on the parietal pleura (Fig. 553). Calcium is frequently deposited within the plaques. The incidence of pleural calcification increases with the length of time elapsed after the original exposure and continues to increase even after cessation of exposure to the offending dust.

The calcific plaques are situated most frequently on the diaphragm and along the lower portion of the costal and mediastinal borders. They are most easily recognized when projected tangentially, appearing as sharply defined, linear densities which vary up to several centimeters in length. When seen *en face* they produce much fainter densities, often irregular and geographic in outline (Fig. 331). Although only a single calcific plaque may be evident, often they are mul-

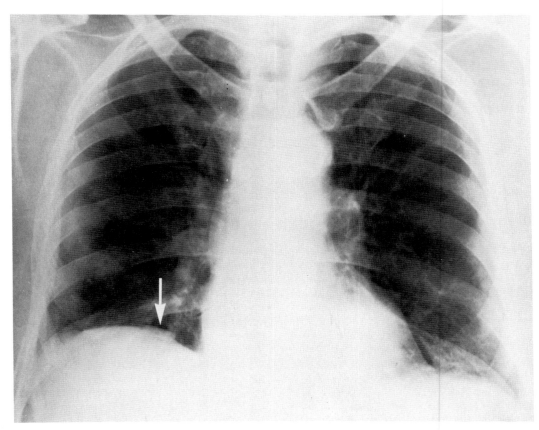

FIG. 553. HYALINE PLEURAL PLAQUES IN ASBESTOSIS

There is a sharply demarcated band-like density along the outer border of the right lung representing thickened pleura seen tangentially. The hazy shadows mesial to this are caused by the thick pleura in the posterior and anterior axillary region which is projected obliquely and *en face*. Similar hazy densities are present along the lateral border of the left lung. A dense, sharply demarcated plaque is present over the right leaf of the diaphragm (arrow). The indistinctness of the left diaphragm is due to interstitial infiltrations in the lung. The roentgen appearance is characteristic of asbestosis, predominently involving the pleura. The patient had been exposed to asbestos dust while working in a shipyard 30 years previously.

tiple and bilateral. The additional calcific densities may be brought to view by films made in the oblique and lateral projections.

The pleural calcification in pneumoconiosis differs from the calcification in tuberculosis, chronic empyema and hemothorax. In tuberculosis the deposits occur most frequently over the apex of the lung, an area which is spared in asbestosis and talcosis except when the pleura is most extensively involved. Calcification of the pleura near the base of the lung resulting from tuberculous pleurisy, chronic empyema or a hemothorax is unilateral and takes the form of a single, large, irregular deposit, associated with considerable pleural thickening and shrinkage of the hemithorax.

The noncalcified plaques are more difficult to recognize, and most commonly are found only on direct inspection of the pleura at thoracotomy or autopsy. If demonstrable radiologically, they are best visualized when projected on end, appearing as shallow protuberances on the inner border of the chest wall like pleural metastases. They sometimes can be seen when viewed *en face* and

appear as poorly defined, irregular densities of moderate size. Small areas of calcification occasionally are visualized within the plaque, indicating that the plaques are due to pneumoconiosis rather than neoplastic disease.

In asbestosis and talcosis the involvement of the pleura is often manifested radiologically by diffuse thickening without calcification. The thick pleura is more noticeable over the lower half of the lungs and presents as a sharply defined, smooth, vertical, strip-like density along the outer border of the chest (Fig. 554). Frequently it is visible only on the oblique view.

A very dense, irregular, sharply demarcated shadow on the pleura suggests the possibility of mesothelioma, a not infrequent complication of asbestosis. However, the mesothelioma may be masked by a pleural effusion. Pleural effusions also result from carcinoma of the lung, another common complication of asbestosis. Asbestosis itself is an uncommon cause of pleural effusion.

Thickening of the pleura is occasionally observed in cases of silicosis and is probably due to secondary infection rather than to the silicosis

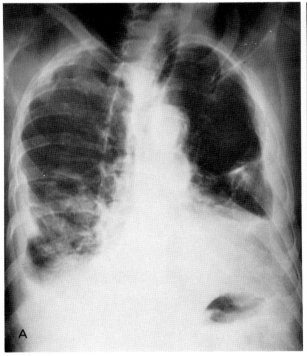 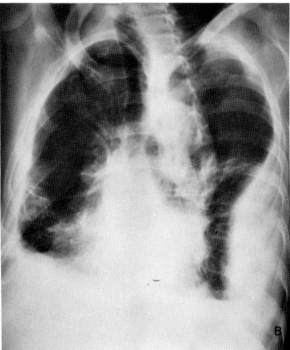

FIG. 554. ASBESTOSIS: BENIGN PLEURAL THICKENING

A: The patient had been exposed to asbestos dust for many years. The right oblique view shows a broad, band-like density along the borders of the ribs on both sides, cast by markedly thickened pleura. Diffuse interstitial infiltrations are present in the lower half of the right lung and there is a small area of atelectasis and fibrosis in the lower part of the anterior portion of the left upper lobe. *B*: In the left oblique view, a dense, sharply demarcated shadow is seen on the left side, suggesting either a loculated pleural effusion or a mesothelioma. Thoracotomy, however, disclosed only extensive fibrosis of the pleura.

itself. The most marked thickening occurs over the massive fibrotic lesions. Thickening of the pleura at the bases, with obliteration of the costophrenic sinuses, occurs frequently in association with the emphysema and chronic interstitial pneumonitis that is secondary to bronchial infections in the later stages of silicosis. A pleural effusion may be due to tuberculosis to which silicotics are predisposed.

The benign pneumoconioses, such as siderosis, stannosis, baritosis, etc., are not associated with pleural complications.

Autoimmune Diseases. LUPUS ERYTHEMATOSUS. Pleurisy is a common accompaniment of lupus erythematosus and may be the first manifestation of this disease. Most frequently it is associated with a pleural effusion containing little fibrinous exudate so that the fluid lies free in the pleural cavity and does not become loculated. The effusions usually are small but may fill the lower half of the thorax. Not infrequently they are bilateral, and are sometimes accompanied by a pericardial effusion of small or moderate size. The lungs are not congested and, when not sec-

ondarily infected, are free of visible infiltrations. In some cases there is deposition of fibrinous exudate over the base of the lung, producing a dense shadow which obscures the diaphragm and simulates a pleural effusion. In these instances of dry pleurisy the diaphragm is apt to be elevated and its motion markedly limited.

The pleural changes occur particularly in the acute stage of the disease and are most commonly encountered in young adult females. There is a tendency to spontaneous regression as the patient's condition improves. Resorption of the exudate proceeds rapidly under steroid treatment as in the other autoimmune diseases.

EOSINOPHILIC PNEUMONIA (LÖFFLER'S SYNDROME AND DIFFUSE VASCULITIS). Pleural effusions are encountered occasionally in these diseases. Generally the fluid collections are small and not loculated. The pulmonary lesions are clearly visible in eosinophilic pneumonia (Fig. 555) but may not be evident in some of the other forms of diffuse vascular disease.

RHEUMATOID DISEASE. The pleura is frequently involved in rheumatoid disease. This is

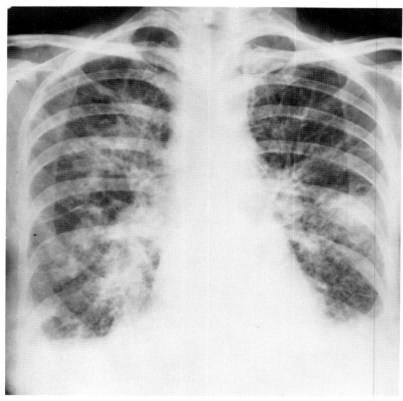

FIG. 555. BILATERAL EFFUSION IN EOSINOPHILIC PNEUMONIA

A small effusion is present at the base of each pleural cavity. Fine and coarse interstitial infiltrations are scattered throughout the lungs. The absence of cardiac enlargement makes it unlikely that congestive failure is the cause of these changes. The patient proved to have eosinophilic penumonia.

manifested by symptoms of pleurisy and by the finding of characteristic rheumatoid lesions on pathologic examination. However, the roentgen examination often fails to disclose any abnormality in either the lungs or pleura. Occasionally, thickening of the pleura is recognizable on the roentgen film.

Pleural effusions have been reported in 2 to 5% of cases of rheumatoid disease. They are usually small or moderate in size and are bilateral in about one-fourth of the cases. Apparently they occur far more frequently in males. In about two-thirds of the cases, there are no visible pulmonary lesions. In some instances the pleurisy antedates the joint symptoms, but most often it occurs in relation either to the onset or to an exacerbation of the arthritis. Without steroid treatment, the effusion absorbs rather slowly, usually disappearing completely within a few months, but it may recur. Occasionally the fluid persists for a year or more, leaving residual thickening of the pleura.

A few cases of spontaneous pneumothorax have been reported as a direct complication of rheumatoid disease. The pneumothorax results from rupture of a subpleural pulmonary nodule which has undergone cavitation.

RHEUMATIC FEVER. Pleurisy is rather common during the acute phase of rheumatic fever. Often it is associated with evidences of pericarditis and, sometimes, with patchy shadows in the lungs, probably representing areas of rheumatic pneumonia. Frequently the lungs are congested, a finding absent in rheumatoid arthritis.

The pleurisy is manifested by considerable thickening of the pleura with plastic exudate, or by an effusion. The latter may be bilateral. When unilateral the effusion is usually associated with evidence of pericarditis and is situated on the left side. In many cases, pleurisy or pericarditis is the main manifestation of the disease, while the joint symptoms are either absent or relatively minor.

In a patient with rheumatic fever it is often difficult to differentiate an effusion due to rheumatic pleurisy from that caused by heart failure. Congestive failure is rarely the cause of an effusion confined to the left side.

Neoplasms of the Pleura

Primary Pleural Tumors

Although primary neoplasms of the pleura are comparatively rare, they occur frequently enough to warrant consideration in the differential diagnosis of pleural effusions and of circum-

scribed shadows on the border of the pulmonary field. Several varieties of neoplasm can originate in the pleura, differing in their gross as well as microscopic appearance. The type of tumor depends on the particular layer of the pleura from which it arises.

Essentially the pleura is composed of two layers: a superficial layer of flat cells, the mesothelium, and a layer of connective tissue which binds the mesothelium to the lung, chest wall and mediastinum. The mesothelium, which is derived from the mesenchyme, has the potentiality of developing in the direction of both epithelial and connective tissues when it undergoes neoplastic change.

The connective tissue underlying the mesothelium lining the parietes does not appear to be any different from the connective tissue elsewhere in the body, and the tumors to which it gives rise may be benign or malignant. They are discussed under the heading Extrapleural Neoplasms (p. 703). On the other hand, the connective tissue component of the visceral pleura appears to be somewhat different. It has a loose reticular structure which, in some areas, has a more or less gelatinous appearance similar to the mesenchymatous connective tissue of the umbilical cord. This, apparently, is a special type of connective tissue. It can give rise to a variety of neoplasms, fibromas, fibrosarcomas, chondromas and hemangiomas. The most common are the fibromas and the fibrosarcomas. It is a peculiar fact that the latter, which in the parietal pleura, as well as in other parts of the body are malignant, when situated in the visceral pleura, act as benign tumors. In the many cases we have studied, only one developed metastases (Klemperer and Rabin). Because of their multiple potentialities on tissue culture, these tumors have been considered as localized forms of mesothelioma (Stout and Murray), and apparently most pathologists have accepted them as such. However, we feel that they really originate from the submesothelial connective tissue because they are regularly covered by a smooth mesothelial layer composed of cells which appear to be different from those which make up the body of the tumor.

Benign Tumors. The benign neoplasms arising from the visceral pleura grow very slowly. Generally the chondromas, hemangiomas and myomas remain quite small, while the fibromas and lipomas may reach huge proportions. Most of the tumors are pedunculated, but the pedicle may not be obvious because the tumor alongside the pedicle has become secondarily adherent to the lung. The neoplasms may be situated anywhere along the visceral pleura, in the interlobar regions as well as on the surface of the lung.

The most common types have the microscopic appearance of fibromas and fibrosarcomas. Of the two, the fibromas are less cellular and more fibrous, and often have a histologic pattern suggestive of a neurinoma with which they may be confused. The more cellular tumors have regular nuclei and the cells appear uniform. Although they behave in a benign fashion, they have the same microscopic appearance as some of the malignant fibrosarcomas that occur elsewhere in the body.

When the pleural tumor is situated on the costal surface of the lung, its location is demonstrable when viewed tangentially, i.e., with the x-ray beam parallel to the plane of contact between the tumor and the chest wall. When the tumor is situated in the midaxillary line the tangential film is the one made in the frontal projection. Tumors on the anterior or posterior surface of the lung are projected tangentially in the lateral view, while those situated at the anterior or posterior bends of the ribs require the proper oblique view. It may be necessary to fluoroscope the patient to determine the optimum degree of obliquity.

On the tangential view, the tumor is seen to be in contact with the chest wall. It appears as a homogeneous density with an exquisitely sharp border except where its shadow merges with the parietal structures. When the tumor is small, only a minor portion of its circumference may be in contact with the chest wall, and the shadow is almost completely circular in outline. As the tumor increases in size, it has a tendency to flatten against the chest wall, but its visible circumference still comprises the greater part of a circle. As a result, the border of the tumor forms an acute angle where it meets the chest wall. The larger tumors often show some lobulation, but their borders remain sharp.

When the x-rays are directed perpendicular to the tangential plane, the tumor is visualized *en face* and the shadow of the growth is surrounded by the lucent air-containing lung. Since the tumor is well circumscribed and roughly spherical in shape, it is represented on the film by a round density with an extremely well demarcated, regular border (Fig. 556). Although the shadow of the tumor itself is homogeneous, the vessels of the underlying lung are visualized within it. As in the case of other pleural lesions, the vessels do not appear displaced or distorted.

When the pleural tumor is situated in the anterior or posterior axillary line, it is not projected tangentially on either the frontal or lateral view and therefore often appears to be separated from the chest wall in these projections. Moreover, it is not visualized *en face* so that the entire border of the mass is not well outlined in these views. The mesial surface of the tumor lies against the lung and therefore displays a sharp border. However, the outer surface of the tumor is in contact with the chest wall and its shadow fades out gradually. This characteristic, namely a sharp definition of the mesial portion of the shadow and indistinctness or lack of visualization of the lateral border, is not specific for a primary tumor of the pleura. A similar type of shadow can be produced by other localized lesions abutting on the chest wall at the bends of the ribs, such as metastatic tumors of the pleura or tumors of the extrapleural tissues.

Since a benign neoplasm arising from the visceral pleura is covered by a layer of smooth mesothelium, it usually does not adhere to the parietal pleura and moves with the lung during respiration. Motion between the tumor and the rib cage during breathing, observed on fluoroscopy or on films made in inspiration and expiration, differentiates the tumor from one that originates beneath the parietal pleura. However, the weight of a tumor of the visceral pleura may prevent its upward motion during expiration when the patient is erect. Motion of the tumor during respiration can be demonstrated if the patient is examined in the recumbent position.

The relation of the tumor to the visceral rather than the parietal pleura can also be demonstrated by examination after the induction of a pneumothorax (Fig. 25). In the absence of adhesions, this will separate the mass from the chest wall. If the tumor is pedunculated, it will lie unsupported in the pleural cavity and will show a wide range of motion when the patient is moved from the erect to the Trendelenburg position. However, we do not recommend induction of a pneumothorax for this purpose because the tumor may twist on its pedicle and become strangulated.

Tumors which originate from the pleura on the undersurface of the lung appear as more or less semicircular densities based on the diaphragm. They move with the diaphragm and usually cannot be differentiated from diaphragmatic tumors without induction of a pneumothorax. This will separate the tumor from the diaphragm when the patient is placed in the Trendelenburg position. When situated posteriorly, a pleural tumor at the base of the lung simulates a hernia of the foramen of Bochdalek. A tumor situated on the mediastinal surface of the lung must be differentiated from a mass arising from the mediastinum or the paravertebral tissues. The latter maintains a constant relationship to

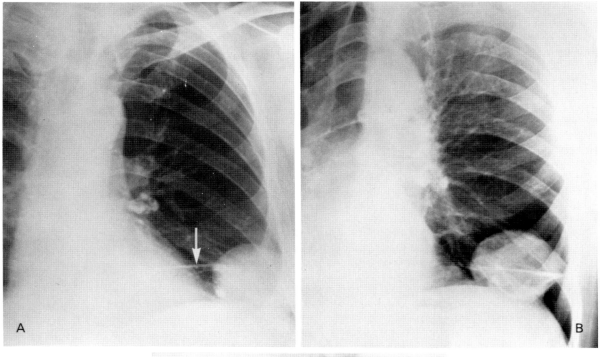

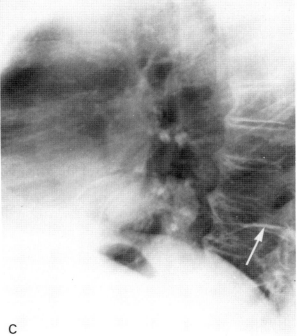

FIG. 556. FIBROMA OF VISCERAL PLEURA

A: Frontal projection. The mesial and upper border of the round mass at the base of the lung is extremely well demarcated and smooth. The lateral border merges with the shadow of the chest wall. The Fleischner line (arrow) representing an area of discoid atelectasis, appears to be connected with the mass. However, it does not extend peripherally as would be expected with a bronchogenic carcinoma. *B*: Left oblique view. The entire border of the mass, with the exception of the small portion adjacent to the diaphragm, is now clearly visualized. Its sharp demarcation is unlike that of a bronchogenic carcinoma. The lung around the mass is hyperlucent. *C*: Lateral view. The Fleischner line can now be localized in the posterior portion of the lung, not related to the mass (arrow). The curvilinear shadows anterior to the mass represent the walls of bullae. Operation disclosed a pedunculated fibroma hanging from the visceral pleura by a narrow stalk.

the vertebral bodies, whereas a visceral pleural tumor shifts during respiration or on change from the erect to the recumbent position.

When the tumor originates from the interlobar pleura, it is either oval or spherical in shape and is easily confused with an interlobar effusion (Fig. 533). However, the latter is almost always associated with thickening of the remainder of the interlobar fissure, extending from one or both ends of the shadow of the loculated effusion. Absence of such a line of thickened pleura should suggest the possibility of a neoplasm.

Fibromas, fibrosarcomas and lipomas of the visceral pleura may attain huge proportions. The area of contact with the chest wall or diaphragm is then extensive and the tumor loses its circular shape. It presents as a large homogeneous density with a broad base against the parietes, and a sharply demarcated, convex border which may be lobulated, against the aerated lung (Fig. 557). The tumor can become so large that it extends from the front of the chest to the back. The pulmonary vessels, then, are not visualized within the shadow of the growth except at its borders. Large tumors situated at the base of the hemithorax depress the diaphragm for a considerable distance and, when on the left side, displace the stomach bubble. Those that fill a large portion of the pleural cavity displace the mediastinum to the opposite side, particularly during expiration. The ribs are usually not spread apart unless the tumor fills most of the hemithorax. Because of their size and weight, these tumors may not move with respiration.

Because of the relative radiolucency of fatty tissue, lipomas of the pleura may show a characteristic roentgen picture, especially when large. Although the smaller lipomas cast shadows of less density than other pleural tumors of comparable size, this may be difficult to appreciate. The large tumors, which are often lobulated, appear quite dense, simply because of their thickness. However, the shadow becomes fainter in its upper portion where the tumor tends to thin out. Linear opaque streaks, representing fibrous septa, can often be seen within the more lucent portion of the growth. This finding is rather unique for a lipoma of the pleura.

On rare occasions, a pleural effusion occurs in association with a benign pleural tumor. We have observed two cases of pleural fibroma in which the fluid was bloody. This was probably due to rupture of a blood vessel in the capsule of the tumor.

Malignant Tumors. For the purpose of this discussion, the only neoplasm that will be considered is the diffuse mesothelioma. The tumors that have been classified as localized forms of mesothelioma probably arise from the connective tissue component of the visceral pleura and not from the mesothelial layer. Although they may have the histologic appearance of a fibrosarcoma, they are benign lesions and form a single, circumscribed mass which does not spread along the surface of the pleura. On the other hand, the fibrosarcomas that arise from the connective tissue component of the parietal pleura are malignant.

In the early stage, a diffuse mesothelioma appears as a localized area of pleural thickening. It usually involves the pleura over the lower part of the lung and extends to the diaphragm, obliterating the costophrenic sinus (Fig. 558). As the neoplasm grows, it spreads over the pleura and forms a series of scalloped densities along the inner border of the chest wall, eventually extending from the diaphragm to the dome of the thorax. Further growth of the tumor results in fusion of the individual scallops to form an elongated lobulated density which is usually sharply demarcated from the lung (Fig. 559). Where the tumor extends around the bend of the ribs, its borders may appear hazy. The tumor involving the anterior or posterior portion of the pleura is projected *en face* in the frontal view and may appear to be within the lung. However, the pleural location of the tumor becomes obvious on lateral or oblique films.

A mesothelioma can grow slowly over a period of years without causing a pleural effusion. The spreading neoplasm tends to encase the lung and produce a dense, homogeneous shadow over the entire hemithorax. The underlying lung is compressed, the mediastinum can be displaced to the opposite side and the diaphragm depressed in the same way as with an enormous pleural effusion. The ribs may be spread apart but, in other cases, they are drawn together and the dome of the thorax is flattened. In rare instances, the tumor extends between the ribs into the chest wall.

Invasion of the mediastinum is not rare and diaphragmatic paralysis can result from involvement of the phrenic nerve. A pericardial effusion indicates direct spread of the tumor to the pericardium. Despite extensive invasion of the mediastinal pleura, the lymph nodes are often spared. Even when they are involved, the enlarged nodes usually cannot be recognized on films because they are obscured by the tumor covering the mediastinal surface of the lung.

In about half of the cases of mesothelioma, there is an associated pleural effusion. If the fluid collection is small, the irregular pleural thicken-

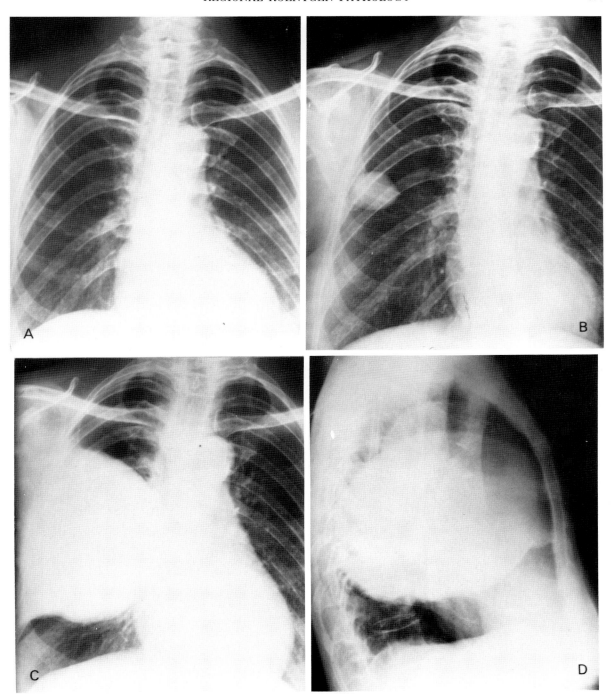

FIG. 557. PLEURAL FIBROMA

A: 1950. The small, spindle-shaped, sharply demarcated shadow in the right midlung was discovered at a routine examination. The conformation of the shadow is indicative either of an effusion or a neoplasm within the short fissure. The patient refused surgery. *B*: 1964. The mass grew very slowly. It appears more rounded but still retains its sharply outlined border. *C*: 1972. Because of the marked increase in the size of the lesion, the possibility of malignant change was considered. The mass now extends to the lateral chest wall. *D*: 1972. The lateral view shows that the mass has retained its sharp outline although it is somewhat lobulated. At thoracotomy a benign fibroma was removed.

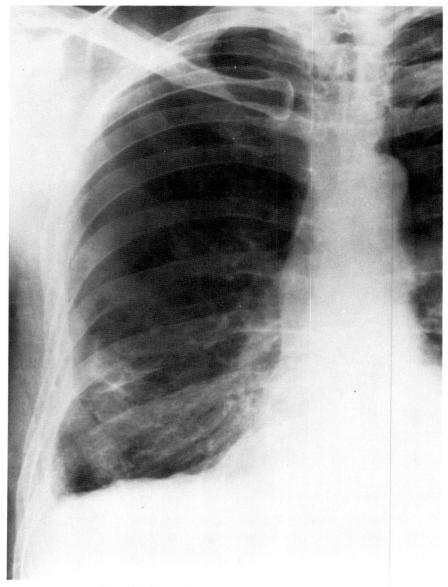

FIG. 558. EARLY MESOTHELIOMA OF THE PLEURA

The patient had been exposed to asbestos dust many years previously. The pleura over the lower part of the right lung is thickened. The right costophrenic sulcus and the cardiophrenic angle are obliterated. Although pleural thickening is not uncommon in simple asbestosis, obliteration of the costophrenic sulcus by thickened pleura is a rare occurrence. In addition, the pleura over the diaphragm has an irregular, nodular appearance. This is diagnostic of mesothelioma. Fine interstitial infiltrations are present throughout the lower portions of the lungs, obscuring the shadows of the peripheral pulmonary vessels and producing a ground-glass appearance.

ing caused by the tumor may be visible above it (Fig. 560). However, a large effusion can completely obscure the underlying neoplasm (Fig. 561). The latter is almost always visualized on films made after thoracentesis if some of the fluid that was withdrawn is replaced with air (Fig. 562). This is especially important in those cases in which a large effusion occurs early and is the only sign of the disease. Occasionally, there are multiple loculations of fluid, closed off by surrounding tumor tissue.

Most often, it is not possible to differentiate a mesothelioma of the pleura from metastatic disease (Fig. 563). The latter is considerably more

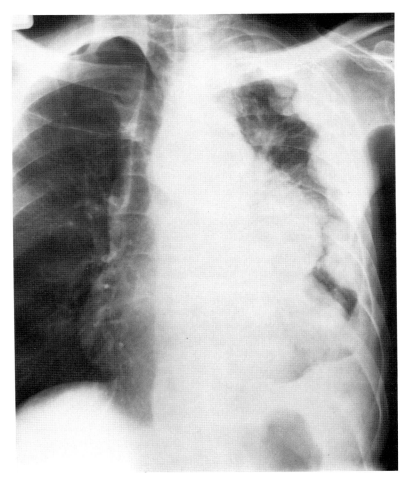

FIG. 559. MESOTHELIOMA OF THE PLEURA

Almost the entire pleura over the mediastinum and chest wall shows sharply defined, confluent, scalloped shadows. There is little, if any, fluid in the left pleural space. The trachea is deviated to the right by a large mass on the mediastinal pleura. There is no evidence of tumor on the right side. Fibrosis cannot be seen in the lung nor are there any clacified pleural plaques. The patient had worked in a shipyard many years previously and was exposed to asbestos dust.

common than the mesothelioma, which is a rare tumor. Bilateral pleural involvement indicates metastatic disease as does the presence of nodular lesions within the lungs. Single or discrete scalloped shadows on the pleura are more characteristic of metastatic tumors, whereas a continuous, lobulated density is more suggestive of a mesothelioma.

The great majority of mesotheliomas occur in patients who have been exposed to asbestos dust. The tumor appears many years after the exposure which may have been only to a moderate concentration of the dust and of relatively short duration. Nevertheless, large numbers of asbestos bodies can usually be demonstrated in the lungs of patients with a pleural mesothelioma. Interstitial pulmonary fibrosis can be identified on films in only about half of the cases. The combination of a pleural tumor on one side with interstitial infiltrations in the lungs is indicative of mesothelioma with asbestosis. The finding of one or more calcific plaques on the pleura has the same significance even if the lungs appear normal. It is notable that the benign, circumscribed tumor of the visceral pleura has rarely, if ever, been found in patients with asbestosis.

Inflammatory thickening of the pleura is a common finding in asbestosis. However, the thickening is usually regular and not scalloped and involves both sides more or less symmetrically. On the other hand, localized fibrotic, collagenous plaques, which also occur in asbestosis, may cast a scalloped shadow and are indistinguishable from a mesothelioma. Similarly,

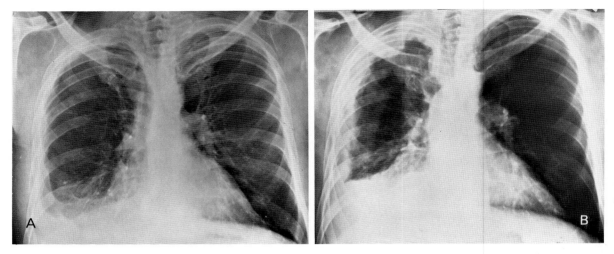

FIG. 560. MESOTHELIOMA OF THE PLEURA

A: 5-21-69. The annual film of an asbestos worker showed a moderate-sized right pleural effusion with thickening of the pleura above the fluid. Pleural thickening and a small effusion can occur in uncomplicated asbestosis. However, in this case the irregularity of the pleural thickening, the inordinate involvement of the pleura over the apex and the flattening of the dome of the thorax favor a diagnosis of mesothelioma. *B*: 4-21-70. The pleural thickening has progressed and now extends around the entire lung including its mediastinal surface. The marked nodularity of the pleura is characteristic of mesothelioma.

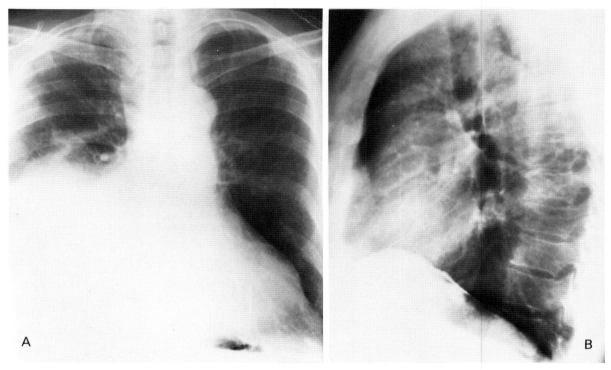

FIG. 561. MESOTHELIOMA OF THE PLEURA

A: Frontal view. There is a large pleural effusion on the right side with extension of the fluid into the long fissure. A small calcific density is seen over the outer part of the left diaphragm. The left costophrenic sinus is not obliterated. No infiltrations can be detected in the lungs. *B*: Left lateral view. The flat calcific plaque on the left diaphragm is diagnostic of asbestosis. Although an inflammatory effusion can occur in asbestosis, a collection of fluid of this size is most often due to an underlying mesothelioma.

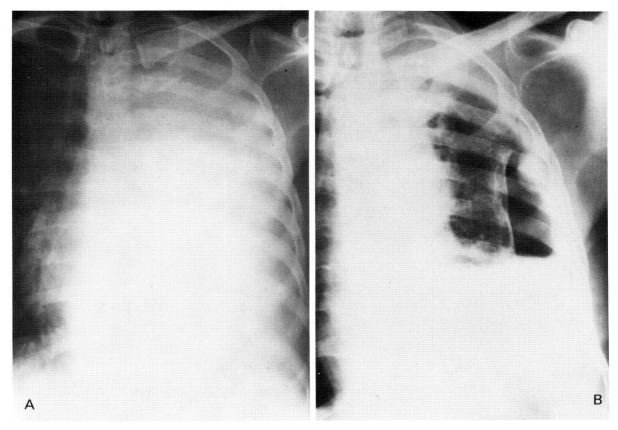

FIG. 562. DIAGNOSTIC PNEUMOTHORAX

A: The entire left hemithorax is obscured by a massive pleural effusion. The heart and trachea are displaced to the right. *B*: Air injected into the pleural space after thoracentesis reveals a scalloped thickening of the parietal pleura indicative of neoplasm. This proved to be secondary to a primary bronchogenic carcinoma.

pleural effusions, sometimes loculated, can occur in asbestosis in the absence of neoplasm. These effusions usually absorb spontaneously after a short period of time leaving only a residuum of thickened pleura.

Metastatic Tumors of the Pleura

The most common roentgen manifestation of metastatic neoplasms of the pleura is an effusion. The pleura is usually diffusely involved by tumor tissue, but the individual lesions are so tiny that, as a rule, they cannot be visualized on the film even when the effusion is small. Larger tumor implants may be seen above the level of the fluid, but are hidden when the effusion is large. The effusion is rarely loculated. In the adult, extremely large collections of fluid, especially those filling the entire hemithorax, are almost always due to metastatic neoplasm. Rapid recurrence of

the fluid after thoracentesis strongly suggests neoplastic involvement of the pleura.

In some cases, pleural nodules indicative of neoplasm become apparent after the fluid is aspirated. They are best seen on films made in the lateral and oblique decubitus positions, in which the remaining fluid shifts away from the diaphragm and chest wall. Better visualization of the pleural masses is obtained by injecting air into the pleural cavity after the fluid is withdrawn (Fig. 562). However, even this method frequently fails to disclose the pleural lesions because they are so small.

When they can be visualized, the pleural nodules are best demonstrated on the tangential projection, appearing as discrete, scalloped shadows projecting into the pulmonary field from the border of the hemithorax (Fig. 563). When viewed *en face*, the shadows are either very faint and ill-defined or completely invisible. When pro-

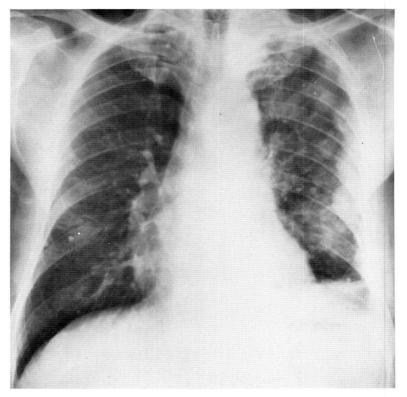

FIG. 563. METASTATIC CARCINOMA OF THE PLEURA

The scalloped shadows along the outer border of the left lung represent nodular pleural metastases. The appearance is indistinguishable from that of a mesothelioma. However, no pulmonary markings can be seen through the left side of the cardiac silhouette, the root of the left lung is low and the diaphragm is elevated, indicating atelectasis of the left lower lobe. Bronchoscopy revealed a carcinoma obstructing the left lower lobe bronchus.

jected obliquely, the mesial border of the mass may be clearly defined, while the lateral margin of the shadow fades into the surrounding lung.

Sharply defined scalloped shadows along the border of the chest often represent tumors arising from the tissues outside the parietal pleura rather than from the pleura itself. Most commonly they represent metastases to the ribs bulging into the thoracic cavity. If the ribs in the region of the scalloped shadow are not clearly visualized, special films for rib detail should be obtained.

Pleural metastases from a primary tumor of the lung are generally confined to the side of the original neoplasm (Fig. 393). In the unusual instance when there are bilateral pleural effusions because of metastatic tumors, there is generally evidence of extensive involvement of the mediastinum (Fig. 423). The tumor of the lung can usually be visualized after thoracentesis. However, the primary growth may be so small that it cannot be identified even though all of the fluid is removed. Shift of the mediastinum to the side

of an effusion should suggest the possibility of an underlying obstructing bronchogenic carcinoma. In any case, the presence of an effusion does not necessarily indicate involvement of the pleura by tumor. It may simply be due to infection distal to the bronchial obstruction (Fig. 424).

Pleural metastases from carcinoma of the breast occur most frequently on the same side as the primary tumor. However, bilateral effusions are rather common and, in rare instances, the effusion may occur only on the opposite side. When the fluid appears on the same side as the breast tumor within 4 or 5 months after radiotherapy, the possibility that it is due to irradiation rather than to metastasis must be considered.

Pleural involvement in the lymphomatous diseases is most commonly manifested by an effusion, often bilateral. Only rarely can the tumor plaques on the pleura be visualized. Because of this it is usually impossible to determine from the films whether the effusion is due to implants on the pleura or to blockage of the lymphatics in the mediastinum. In the latter instance the effusion often disappears following irradiation of the mediastinum alone.

Thymic tumors, even those which appear benign histologically, not infrequently give rise to pleural implants, which may be bilateral. They appear as local pleural thickenings or scalloped shadows when projected tangentially (Fig. 486). Because they are generally quite flat, they produce very faint shadows, if any, when viewed *en face*. Even on the tangential projection, the shadows may be easily overlooked. Not infrequently they are situated on the diaphragm, and are then best visualized on the lateral view, appearing as local protrusions on the diaphragmatic contour. As a rule, pleural effusions occur late, and extensive involvement of the pleura may exist even in the absence of fluid.

Extrapleural Neoplasms

The extrapleural tumors that arise from the connective tissue binding the parietal mesothelial lining to the chest wall, diaphragm and mediastinum, are mostly fibromas or fibrosarcomas. Lipomas are encountered occasionally.

The extrapleural connective tissue differs from the connective tissue that binds the visceral mesothelial layer to the lung. It does not appear to have any special characteristics and does not behave differently from connective tissues elsewhere in the body. Although some of the extrapleural connective tissue tumors are benign, malignant tumors, such as fibrosarcomas and spindle cell sarcomas, are more common. Cellular tumors, which are benign when they originate beneath the visceral mesothelial layer, generally prove to be malignant when they arise outside the parietal pleural lining.

The extrapleural tumors characteristically bulge into the thoracic cavity and produce a sharply demarcated, semicircular or elongated, scallop-like shadow with a broad base against the chest wall. Those situated over the diaphragm and over the mediastinum cannot be differentiated from tumors arising from other tissues in these regions.

The shadow of an extrapleural tumor is generally elongated and tapers at both ends in spindle-shaped fashion. Not infrequently the angle formed by the junction of the tumor and the chest wall is blunted (extrapleural sign of Fel-

son). This results from elevation of the pleura by the tumor. A similar contour may be observed in malignant tumors on the mesothelial surface of the parietal pleura. Here the conformation is due to local extension of the growth. As in the case of other pleural tumors, the shadow is most dense and best demarcated on the tangential view. It may be quite faint and ill-defined when viewed *en face*, and only the mesial border may be outlined when seen obliquely.

The nature of a tumor which involves the extrapleural tissues can usually be determined by percutaneous needle biopsy. Unless a mass can be felt on the chest wall, this should be performed under fluoroscopic control.

Fibromas and Fibrosarcomas. The fibromas are generally quite small and present a homogeneous density with a smooth, regular, sharply defined border on the tangential view. Usually the shadow is hemispherical in shape.

The fibrosarcomas and spindle cell sarcomas are usually larger and grow more rapidly. They are often lobulated. In advanced cases and, particularly, when there is recurrence after resection, the tumor may appear as a series of scalloped shadows similar to a mesothelioma. The tumor may invade the lung and the structures of the chest wall. When it extends into the lung, part of its margin may be irregular and indistinct. Large extrapleural sarcomas invading the chest wall tend to obscure the demarcation of the fascial planes and produce a bulge on the external contour of the chest. Because they grow by infiltration, there may be extensive involvement of the parietes without splaying of the ribs. Rib destruction is much less common than in peripherally infiltrating bronchogenic carcinomas.

Lipomas. Because of the relative radiolucency of adipose tissue, extrapleural lipomas cast a fainter shadow than other tumors of similar size (Fig. 564). The growths are sometimes lobulated. This may produce overlapping shadows which give the tumor a double contour. Occasionally the capsule is partially calcified, casting an extremely fine, curvilinear density on the border of the tumor. Because of the lobulation, the calcified rim may be projected within the shadow of the growth.

The lipoma can extend through the intercostal space into the chest wall in dumbbell fashion. It may then cause pressure atrophy and splaying of the ribs.

THE DIAPHRAGM

Abnormalities in the position of the diaphragm and disturbances in its movement have been discussed in the section on Fluoroscopy, because more information can be obtained in this manner

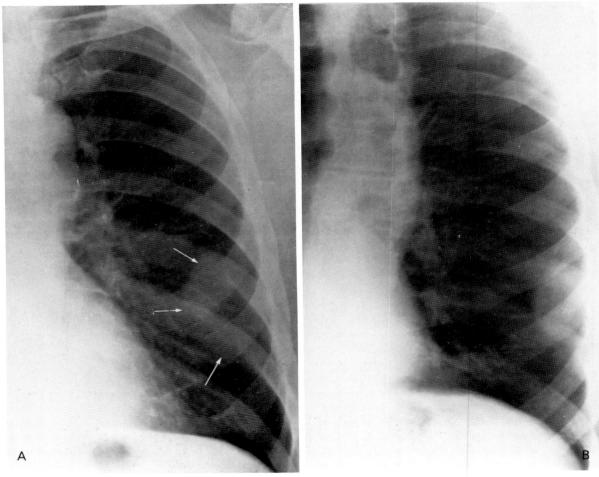

FIG. 564. EXTRAPLEURAL LIPOMA

A: The frontal view shows an extremely faint, rather poorly demarcated density at the level of the eighth intercostal space, posteriorly (arrows). B: In the left oblique projection, the lesion is more distinct because it is visualized tangentially. It has an elongated shape and is broad-based against the chest wall. The lesion appears much less dense than would be expected with a tumor of this size. This is characteristic of a lipoma. The diagnosis was proved at operation.

than from study of films. Certain abnormalities, such as diaphragmatic hernias, subphrenic abscesses, and neoplasms are more clearly depicted on the roentgen films since they show more detail. In many instances, fluoroscopy is required in addition to roentgenograms for a final diagnosis.

Subphrenic Abscess. The roentgen manifestations of subphrenic abscess are varied. They consist of immobilization of the diaphragm, the elevation by pressure of the exudate beneath it, abnormal shadows beneath the diaphragm, and inflammation of the pleura and sometimes of the adjacent lung. In addition to affording information from which the diagnosis of a subphrenic abscess can be made, the roentgen examination is required for localization of the lesion. This is

essential for a proper approach to its drainage. If symptoms of infection persist after surgical evacuation of the subphrenic abscess, x-ray examination with the aid of a contrast medium is helpful in the location of incompletely drained foci and in the demonstration of fistulas that may require surgical treatment.

FIXATION OF THE DIAPHRAGM. Of all the roentgen signs of subphrenic abscess, fixation of the diaphragm is the only one constantly present on examinations made in the erect position. Diaphragmatic fixation is a most helpful sign because if absent, the possibility of a subphrenic abscess can practically always be excluded from consideration. Rarely, some motion of the diaphragm can be detected when the patient is recumbent. To avoid error, the diaphragm should be observed fluoroscopically in every patient before operation for a subphrenic abscess.

ELEVATION OF THE DIAPHRAGM. Because of its attachment, there is resistance to downward displacement of the liver by a subphrenic abscess. A collection of pus on the right side, therefore, tends to elevate the diaphragm as well as to depress the liver (Fig. 565). On the left side, however, the abscess can expand downward with little hindrance because the stomach and bowel are easily displaced. Thus, the left leaf of the diaphragm is not always elevated by a subphrenic collection of pus, and the diagnosis then depends on other changes.

SUBPHRENIC SHADOWS. A pathognomonic sign of subphrenic abscess is the demonstration of a collection of fluid and air immediately beneath the diaphragm but situated outside the stomach or intestine. It is manifested by an area of radiolucency whose lower border is demarcated by a horizontal fluid level, visualized on films made with horizontal rays. The films may be made with the patient in either the erect or recumbent position. In the latter instance, it is better to make the exposure with the patient lying on his side (Fig. 566). Sometimes it is necessary to utilize both positions to make certain that the horizontal line really represents a fluid level.

The presence of an air-fluid level between the diaphragm and the liver is practically always due to a subphrenic abscess (Fig. 565). However, in a patient with interposition of the colon, a fluid level can occur in this location when the large bowel is obstructed or shortly after the administration of an enema. The fluid level of a subphrenic abscess on the left side should not be confused with the level usually present in the stomach. The two can be differentiated in several ways. If the fluid level rises after drinking water or if it becomes more sharply outlined and surmounted by a large gas bubble, after the administration of charged water or a Seidlitz powder, it is obvious that it is in the stomach. This can also be accomplished by observing the patient in the upright position after the ingestion of a capsule filled with barium. The capsule will float on the surface of the fluid if the fluid level is in the stomach. In our experience, this method is more helpful than a barium swallow in recognizing the fluid level of subphrenic abscess.

Occasionally the air in a subphrenic abscess can be recognized on films made with a vertical or inclined x-ray beam. A fluid level is not visible but the air may be visualized in the form of multiple, small lucencies, representing air bubbles, or a larger lucency which does not conform

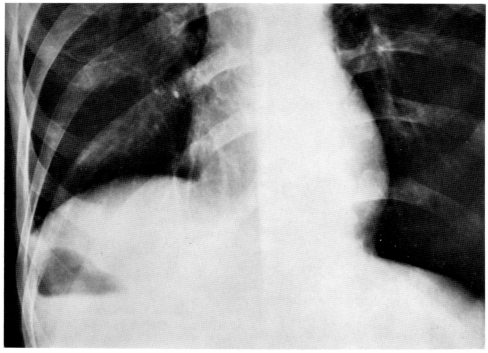

FIG. 565. SUBPHRENIC ABSCESS

The right leaf of the diaphragm is considerably elevated and there is a fluid level beneath its outer portion, indicating the presence of a subphrenic abscess containing air.

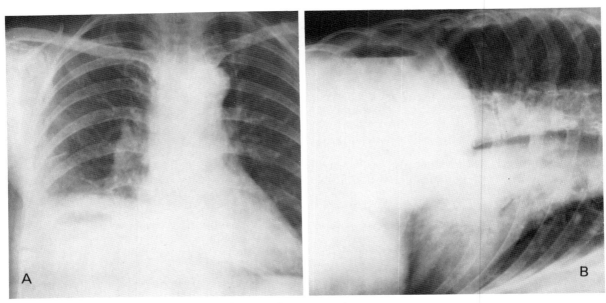

FIG. 566. SUBPHRENIC ABSCESS

A: There is an air-fluid level beneath the right diaphragm. This represents a subphrenic abscess which is responsible for the elevation of this leaf of the diaphragm. The outer border of the chest is hazy because of exudate on the pleura secondary to the subphrenic inflammation. *B:* Oblique decubitus position. The patient was placed on his left side and tilted forward toward the right oblique position. Fluid in the abscess has shifted to the most dependent position and the air outlines the portion of the abscess closest to the chest wall. This indicates that the abscess should be approached through the posterior axillary line.

to the shape of one of the hollow viscera. Gas in the abscess is more easily recognized on the right side.

In the absence of a fluid level, the diagnosis of a subphrenic abscess on the right side depends largely on elevation and fixation of the right leaf of the diaphragm. These changes also occur in paralysis of the diaphragm. The differentiation is made by observing the position of the lower border of the liver. If it is displaced upward, the diagnosis of a subphrenic abscess is untenable. The position of the lower border of the liver cannot always be seen, but it may be inferred from the position of the hepatic flexure or transverse colon.

An apparent elevation of the right leaf of the diaphragm can be caused by an infrapulmonary empyema. That the pus is located above the diaphragm may be determined by induction of a pneumoperitoneum. This will show the space between the diaphragm and the liver to be clear.

An abscess beneath the left leaf of the diaphragm without a fluid level is depicted as a homogeneous shadow whose lower border is usually outlined by gas within the stomach and splenic flexure. The latter is depressed, while the stomach bubble, which normally is situated adjacent to the diaphragm, is displaced downward and mesially by the collection of pus. The shadow

of the subphrenic abscess is usually crescentic in shape. If there is no air in the stomach at the time of the examination, the lower border of the abscess in not outlined, but its relationship to the stomach and the separation of the latter from the diaphragm, can be demonstrated by the administration of charged water or a Seidlitz powder.

PLEURITIS. In most cases of subphrenic abscess, there is some degree of inflammation of the pleura over the diaphragm. This usually occurs early in the development of the abscess, and is manifested by obliteration of the costophrenic sinus by exudate. If the pleura is more severely inflamed, the shadow of the exudate may be seen as a narrow strip of density extending upward along the outer border of the pulmonary field for a variable distance (Fig. 566). The interlobar fissue may also be outlined by exudate. (Fig. 567*A*). A more severe reaction of the pleura results in an effusion. This is usually small or moderate in size. At first, it is of the sympathetic variety and then has the characterstics of a free effusion.

A pleural effusion tends to obscure the diaphragm. When the left side is involved, absence of movement of the stomach bubble or of gas in the splenic flexure during respiration may be relied upon to indicate that the diaphragm is

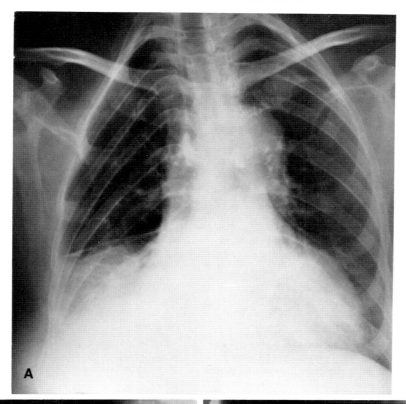

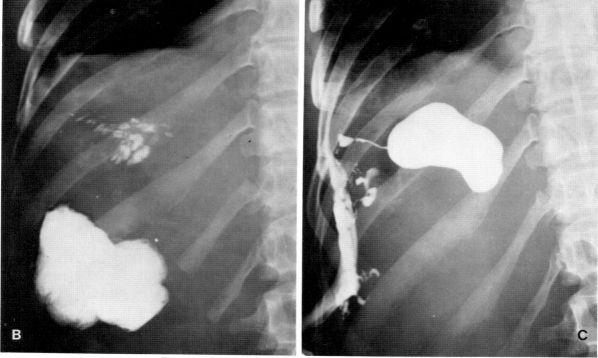

FIG. 567. SUBPHRENIC ABSCESS: INADEQUATE DRAINAGE

A: Despite drainage of the subphrenic abscess, a sympathetic effusion persists at the base of the right pleural cavity. It obscures the diaphragm and extends to the level of the short fissure which is outlined by adhesions. Persistence of the sympathetic effusion indicates that the subphrenic abscess has been incompletely drained. *B*: On a supine film, the right diaphragm is visualized because the free sympathetic effusion has gravitated posteriorly. The drained part of the subphrenic abscess has been filled with radiopaque packing. The wide separation between the packing and the dome of the diaphragm indicates that an additional loculation of pus is present. The irregular density above the packing is caused by Lipiodol injected into the chest wall to indicate the site for additional drainage. *C*: The radiopaque packing has been removed. Iodized oil was injected into the sinus tract in the upper portion of the wound. The oil outlines a large, kidney-shaped pocket which had been draining poorly because of the narrow caliber of the sinus.

fixed. Because the pleural fluid gravitates to the most dependent part of the thorax, the superior surface of the diaphragm can often be disclosed by fluoroscopy in the supine or lateral recumbent position.

If the subphrenic abscess is neglected, a sympathetic effusion in the pleural cavity often becomes infected to produce an empyema. This is practically always loculated, and in patients first examined at this time, it may be extremely difficult or impossible to diagnose a subphrenic abscess from the roentgen findings. Elevation and immobility of the diaphragm are then of little significance in the differential diagnosis. If a subphrenic fluid level cannot be detected, the diagnosis of a subphrenic abscess as the cause of the empyema rests entirely on clinical grounds.

PERFORATION INTO THE LUNG. Perforation of a subphrenic abscess through the diaphragm into the pleural cavity produces an empyema or a pyopneumothorax. If, as is frequently the case, the base of the pleural cavity has been obliterated by adhesions, the abscess can perforate directly into the lung without contaminating the pleural cavity. No case has come under our observation in which the connection with the lung occurred through an intervening empyema.

Perforation of a subphrenic abscess into the lung is often heralded by the sudden expectoration of large quantities of pus. The roentgen film at this time may show diffuse clouding of the lower part of the chest as the result of elevation of the diaphragm, inflammation of the lung and plastic exudate on the pleura. This picture may suggest an empyema in addition to the perforated subphrenic abscess. If it is realized that an empyema is not part of the pathologic process, needless aspiration of the chest and unnecessary surgical exploration of the pleura are avoided.

Occasionally, when a lung abscess is found to communicate with a subphrenic abscess, the question arises whether the primary lesion is in the lung and has perforated through the diaphragm to produce the subphrenic abscess or whether the reverse is the case. It may be stated with considerable certainty that an abscess in the lung does not perforate through the diaphragm and that the subphrenic abscess is the primary lesion in such instances. Surgical drainage, therefore, should be performed through the subphrenic abscess rather than through the lung.

LOCALIZATION. As in the case of abscess of the lung, it has been found that the best approach to the surgical drainage of a subphrenic abscess is at the place where it is most superficial. The position of the abscess is determined by taking into consideration the following: (1) the location of a protuberance on a portion of the diaphragm or of a fluid level beneath it. If the protuberance of the diaphragm cannot be seen because of the presence of a pleural effusion, the obscuring fluid should be removed before the examination. (2) The location of an impression on the contour of the stomach or splenic flexure by the abscess. (3) If there is no localized indentation on the stomach or colon, the position of the abscess may be determined by the direction in which these organs are displaced.

CONTRAST MEDIA. Contrast media are useful in the demonstration of undrained or poorly drained loculations and of fistulous tracts following evacuation of a subphrenic abscess. When a patient continues to have fever after a subphrenic abscess has been drained, it is advisable to reexamine him after filling the drained abscess cavity with radiopaque packing (Fig. 567B) Iodoform gauze is well suited for this purpose. Films should then be made in multiple projections to determine the relationship of the packing to the dome of the diaphragm. If there is a space between the two in all projections, it should be concluded that an undrained focus is present.

If a sinus tract persists during the healing of a subphrenic abscess, it should be injected with a radiopaque solution and the roentgen examinations repeated. Puddling of the contrast material at the end of a narrow, tortuous sinus tract indicates the presence of a poorly drained pocket (Fig. 567C). If the cavity is filled with pus under tension, only a small quantity of the opaque substance may enter a large residual abscess cavity. This should be suspected if oily contrast material is used and collects in globules at the end of the tract.

Persistence of the sinus may be due to a fistulous communication with one of the hollow viscera in the abdomen or with a bronchus. Such fistulas are easily detected after injection of the tract with radiopaque material.

Diaphragmatic Hernias. The possibility of a diaphragmatic hernia should be considered in the interpretation of shadows in the lowermost part of the chest. A hernia of the diaphragm may simulate a pulmonary or mediastinal neoplasm, cystic disease of the lung, an aneurysm of the descending aorta, or a collection of fluid and air in the pleural cavity. We have observed several cases in which the chest was mistakenly aspirated for a pyopneumothorax when the patient really had a diaphragmatic hernia.

The most common diaphragmatic hernias are those involving the esophageal hiatus. Hernias through the foramen of Morgagni or the foramen of Bochdalek are not infrequent. Traumatic her-

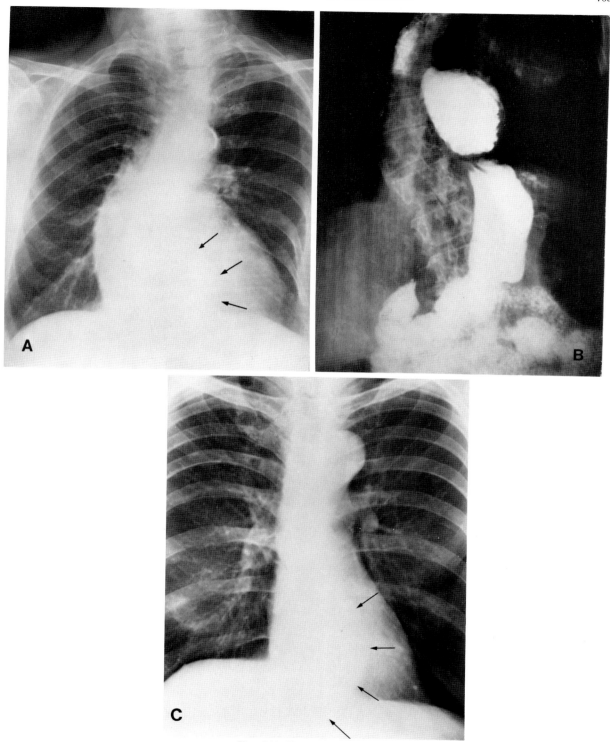

FIG. 568. HIATUS HERNIA

A: The sharply circumscribed mass (arrows) seen through the heart could represent a hiatus hernia or a tortuous aorta. However, the fact that its shadow ends at the diaphragm indicates that the mass lies at the dome of the diaphragm which is anterior to the position of the aorta. The shadow on the right side of the mediastinum is due to scoliosis. *B*: Barium swallow shows a large hiatus hernia. *C*: The film of a different patient shows a similar shadow, but its lower border (arrows) can be seen below the diaphragm. This represents a tortuous aorta.

nias in the diaphragm are much less common, and other diaphragmatic hernias are quite rare.

HIATUS HERNIA. Small hernias through the esophageal hiatus are especially common, but are usually not seen on the roentgen film of the chest. Even large ones are not visible if they reduce themselves when the patient is in the erect position. Because they are usually situated in the posterior mediastinum, hiatal hernias may be obscured by the heart on the frontal projection but often can be seen within the cardiac shadow if the film is properly exposed (Fig. 568).

Most often the hiatal hernia contains a portion of the stomach. If this is filled with air, only an annular shadow is visible. If both fluid and air are present, a fluid level can be seen, but if the stomach is filled with food or fluid, the hernia casts a solid shadow which can simulate a neoplasm. The location of the shadow in the posterior mediastinum is determined by examination in either the oblique or lateral view. The hernia may be demonstrated by examination in the erect position following the administration of charged water or a Seidlitz powder, or in the recumbent position after a barium meal. Most round shadows, extending to both sides of the midline in the lowermost part of the chest represent hiatus hernias.

The shadow of a large hiatus hernia extending beyond the cardiac border can simulate an enlarged heart when the stomach is full. However, on an adequately penetrated film, the border of the cardiac silhouette can be visualized within the shadow of the hernia, which is situated behind the heart (Fig. 569).

FORAMEN OF MORGAGNI. A hernia of the foramen of Morgagni protrudes through a poorly developed portion of the diaphragm behind the sternum. The hernia is practically always situated on the right side because the anterior part of the diaphragm on the left is protected by the heart.

Most of the hernias are small and contain properitoneal fat which extends anterior to the right border of the heart and into the pulmonary field in the region of the right cardiophrenic angle. This produces a homogeneous shadow which is quadrantal in shape and has a convex, sharply outlined, rather regular border which demarcates it from the lung (Fig. 570). Below, the shadow merges with the diaphragm and liver. Mesially, it is continuous with the shadow of the lower part of the heart.

The anterior location of the lesion is easily determined on films made in the lateral or partial left oblique position. On the lateral view, the

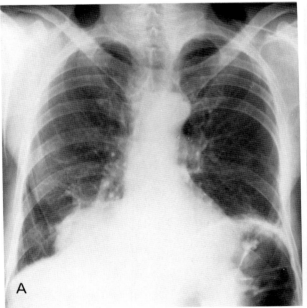
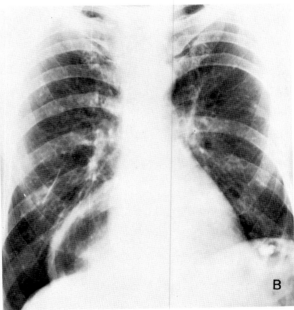

FIG. 569. HIATUS HERNIA

A: The homogeneous quadrantic density in the region of the right cardiophrenic angle does not obliterate the border of the heart and is therefore situated posteriorly. The shadow of the mass also projects slightly to the left of the spine. The extension to both sides of the spine suggests a hiatus hernia. The posterior part of the seventh rib on the left side has previously been resected. B: A film made after administration of a carbonated beverage shows the mass to be filled with air, confirming the diagnosis of a hiatus hernia.

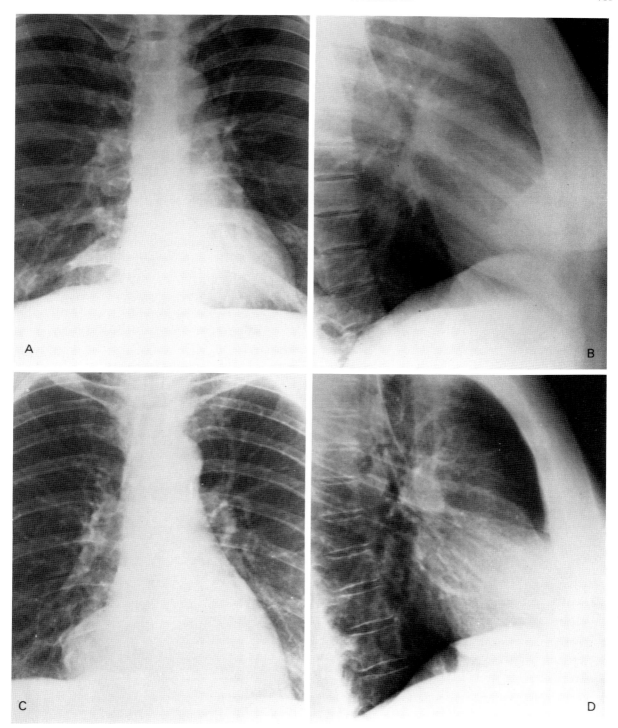

FIG. 570. HERNIA OF THE FORAMEN OF MORGAGNI

A: The lucency of the mass in the right cardiophrenic angle suggests that it is composed of fat. The differential diagnosis of such a mass lies between properitoneal fat herniated through the foramen of Morgagni and an epicardial fat pad. *B*: The lateral view shows the mass to be located far anteriorly, immediately behind the sternum. The upper portion of its posterior border is sharply outlined. This excludes an epicardial fat pad from consideration. *C*: Another patient with a mass in the right cardiophrenic angle. In this case, the mass is denser and more rounded than in the previous one. *D*: Lateral view. The mass is situated anteriorly. However, unlike the collection of herniated properitoneal fat, its posterior border is poorly demarcated and it merges with the shadow of the heart. The mass proved to be a pericardial cyst.

shadow is also quadrantal in shape, and occupies the anteroinferior angle of the pulmonary field. The superior and posterior surfaces in this projection are fairly well outlined by a convex border. Occasionally, when the shadow is most dense anteriorly, its posterior border is poorly delineated. The lower border of the mass is continuous with the shadow of the diaphragm and liver and cannot be delineated from these structures.

A small hernia containing properitoneal fat usually cannot be differentiated from a mediastinal lipoma that protrudes into the pulmonary field. However, the latter is quite rare and is generally not so sharply outlined. An epicardial fat pad which also presents in the cardiophrenic angle, is generally more triangular in shape and when one is present on the right side, a second can usually be seen on the left, at the cardiac apex.

Larger hernias of the foramen of Morgagni may contain stomach and omentum, or a portion of the intestine. The presence of air or an airfluid level within the shadow is indicative of a hernia. In the absence of air, the diagnosis can be made by means of barium studies.

FORAMEN OF BOCHDALEK. A hernia through the foramen of Bochdalek results from incomplete fusion of the paravertebral and lateral portions of the diaphragm. The defect may involve only the muscular part of the diaphragm, resulting in the formation of a hernial sac composed of peritoneum and pleura that projects into the thorax. If these layers are lacking, there is a free communication between the peritoneal and pleural cavities. A dehiscence in the diaphragm may be blocked by one of the solid viscera. Thus, the spleen, kidney, or liver may effectively prevent the stomach and intestines from entering the pleural cavity (Fig. 571).

When there is no dehiscence, a hernia through the foramen of Bochdalek is usually small. It is situated over the posterior part of the diaphragm, somewhat lateral to the spine, and is usually represented by a homogeneous shadow with a sharply demarcated, round upper border. The lower border merges with the shadows of the

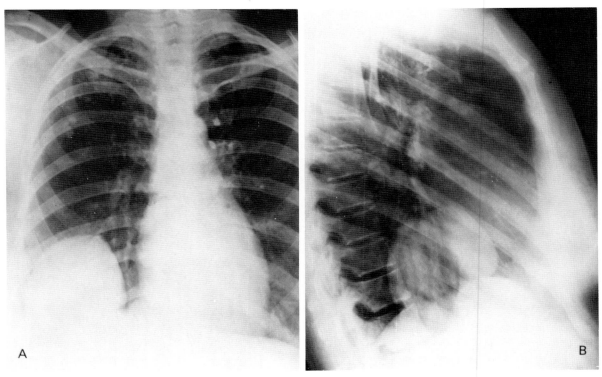

FIG. 571. DEHISCENCE OF THE DIAPHRAGM

A: The unusual, sharply demarcated, dome-like shadow at the base of the right lung represents a portion of the liver which has herniated into the thoracic cavity through a congenital defect in the central portion of the diaphragm. *B:* Lateral view. The herniated portion of the liver is projected over the central part of the diaphragm. The liver has been constricted by the edges of the diaphragmatic defect causing acute angles where the mass meets the diaphragm. The impaction of the liver has prevented other viscera from herniating into the chest. The increased density of the anterior and posterior portions of the shadow is due to superimposition of the posterior part of the heart and the spine on the mass.

abdominal contents. Such a hernia is more common on the left side where it is often visible within the cardiac silhouette. Although it may be mistaken for a neoplasm of the lung, the characteristic location and the semicircular shape of the shadow should suggest a Bochdalek hernia. Most often, the respiratory excursion of the hernia is less than that of the rest of the diaphragm and not infrequently it doesn't move at all. Paradoxical motion of the mass on sniffing confirms the diagnosis of hernia. A tumor of the diaphragm or one at the base of the lung will follow the motion of the diaphragm during sniffing as well as during ordinary respiration.

Usually these hernias are best visualized on the oblique or lateral views, because they are situated posteriorly behind the dome of the diaphragm and are partly hidden by the liver or the heart. Because of its posterior location, the hernia generally does not contain stomach or bowel and therefore casts an opaque shadow. Not infrequently, the upper pole of the kidney projects into the hernia, particularly when it is situated on the left side (Fig. 572). The nature of the shadow can then be determined by intravenous urography. Occasionally a portion of the spleen lies within the hernia and can be demonstrated by a radioisotope scan. Difficulty in differentiating a hernia of the foramen of Bochdalek from a cyst or neoplasm of the diaphragm or of the lung may be resolved following induction of a pneumoperitoneum or by angiography. On films made in the erect position following pneumoperitoneum, the hernial sac is usually clearly outlined.

When there is free communication between the peritoneal and pleural cavities, the stomach

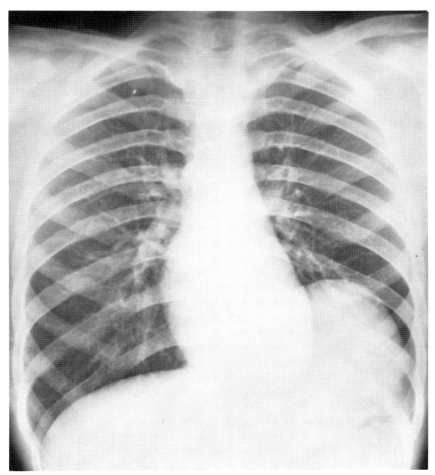

FIG. 572. HERNIA OF FORAMEN OF BOCHDALEK

The smoothly outlined, homogeneous density at the left base merges with the diaphragm. The left cardiac border is clearly visible, indicating that the lesion is situated posteriorly. The differential diagnosis lies between a benign tumor of the visceral pleura and a hernia of the foramen of Bochdalek. An intravenous pyelogram showed part of the kidney within the shadow indicating that it represents a hernia.

and a considerable portion of the intestines can enter the pleural cavity. Because they are not confined by a hernial sac, these structures can ascend to the dome of the thorax. The distended intestinal coils frequently simulate a cystic lung. Fluid levels in the stomach or intestine may lead to an erroneous diagnosis of lung abscess or pyopneumothorax, especially if the abnormality is first found on a chest film made because of a febrile illness of unknown cause.

When the dehiscence is small or moderate in size, the liver may become tightly wedged within the opening. The diaphragmatic rim constricts the liver and divides it into a thoracic and an abdominal portion. Under these circumstances, air injected into the abdomen may be prevented from passing into the thorax. A neoplasm of the liver growing through the diaphragm can produce a similar picture. The two can be differentiated on a liver scan which shows normally functioning liver tissue in the thorax in the case of a hernia.

Absence of the Diaphragm. One leaf of the diaphragm may be entirely absent, or only a small vestige may be present forming a rim of muscular tissue about the base of the thoracic cavity. In such cases, more than one of the abdominal organs is situated in the chest. The solid shadows of the liver or spleen, kidney and omentum mingle with the radiolucent air in the gastrointestinal tract and produce a bizzare appearance (Fig. 573). The mediastinum is usually displaced to the opposite side. Dyspnea is usually severe and calls attention to the abnormality in early infancy. A similar picture can be produced by a moderately large dehiscence of the diaphragm. This can often be recognized after ingestion of barium. If a sizable portion of the diaphragm is present, it produces a shelf partially separating the abdominal from the intrathoracic portion of the gastrointestinal tract.

Rupture of the Diaphragm. Disruption of the diaphragm can result from severe blunt trauma to the chest or abdomen, as well as from

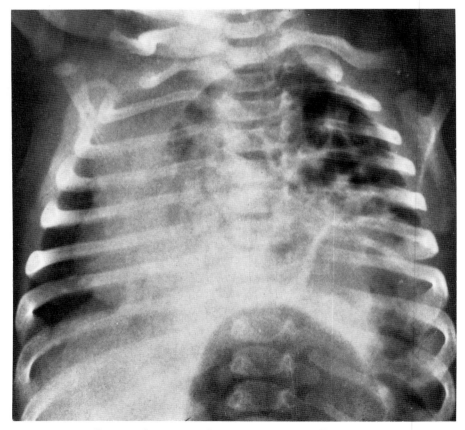

FIG. 573. INCOMPLETE DEVELOPMENT OF THE DIAPHRAGM

The roentgen appearance which simulates a huge cystic lung, is due to the presence of a large part of the intestinal tract within the left chest. The extreme displacement of the mediastinum to the right without concomitant downward displacement of the stomach bubble and splenic flexure, excludes a cystic lung from consideration.

a penetrating injury. The trauma may cause through and through rupture of the diaphragm or only a tear of its muscular layer. The latter results in a diaphragmatic hernia. The lateral portion of the diaphragm is most frequently affected (Fig. 574). This differs from a congenital hernia which usually involves the anterior or posterior portion of the diaphragm. In addition, the patient will practically always recall the injury, if questioned. A complete tear of the diaphragm is almost always a catastrophic event and is recognized immediately after the injury.

Eventration of the Diaphragm. The term eventration denotes an absence of musculature in a part or all of a hemidiaphragm. The involved portion of the diaphragm cannot contract and therefore responds passively to differences between the abdominal and intrathoracic pressures. The eventrated portion of the diaphragm is always elevated and moves paradoxically on sudden inspiration.

Complete eventration most often involves the left hemidiaphragm which is elevated and thin. When the elevation is marked it causes the heart to tilt toward the opposite side. Significant elevation of the right hemidiaphragm is uncommon because of the weight of the liver. It is not possible to distinguish radiologically between congenital eventration and eventration due to muscle atrophy secondary to paralysis from injury or disease of the phrenic nerve.

Partial eventration most often occurs on the right side and involves the anteromedial portion of the diaphragm. Radiologically, a right-sided eventration appears as a solid mass because of the upward displacement of the liver (Fig. 575). On the left side, the elevated portion of the diaphragm usually contains a part of the stomach or colon. Local eventration of the diaphragm can be distinguished from a diaphragmatic hernia by its location. In addition, an eventration will practically always move paradoxically with sniffing. This is often not true of a hernia. Because the hernial ring is generally small in comparison to the size of the hernia, paradoxical motion often is absent.

Tumors of the Diaphragm. Diaphragmatic tumors are extremely rare and difficult to differ-

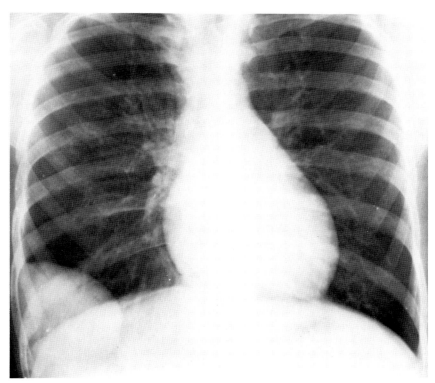

FIG. 574. TRAUMATIC DIAPHRAGMATIC HERNIA

The sharply outlined, rounded density in the region of the right costophrenic sulcus represents a portion of the liver which had herniated into the chest following an automobile accident. The tear occurred in the anterior portion of the diaphragm. Therefore, the diaphragmatic contour, which is formed by its dome, can be seen through the mass while the mesial border of the mass, which lies in front of the dome of the diaphragm, is also visualized.

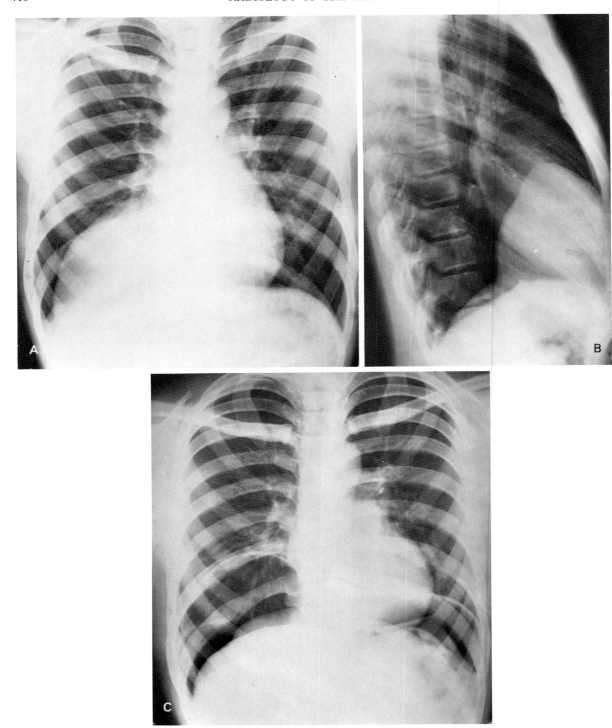

FIG. 575. EVENTRATION OF THE DIAPHRAGM

A: The frontal film of this asymptomatic patient shows a large mass in the lower right chest. The right cardiac border is obliterated. It is not possible from this single film to determine the position of the right leaf of the diaphragm. The mass could represent a large pericardial cyst, but if its upper margin is formed by the diaphragm, then the mass most likely arises from the liver. *B*: In the lateral view, the cone-shaped mass is sharply outlined and broad-based inferiorly. This excludes a pericardial cyst from consideration. The position of the diaphragm still can not be determined with certainty. *C*: Following induction of a pneumoperitoneum, the normal diaphragmatic leaves are visualized as thin, arcuate shadows. The anterior portion of the right diaphragm is markedly elevated. The liver, which caused the shadow on the routine chest films, has dropped down to merge with the other abdominal viscera.

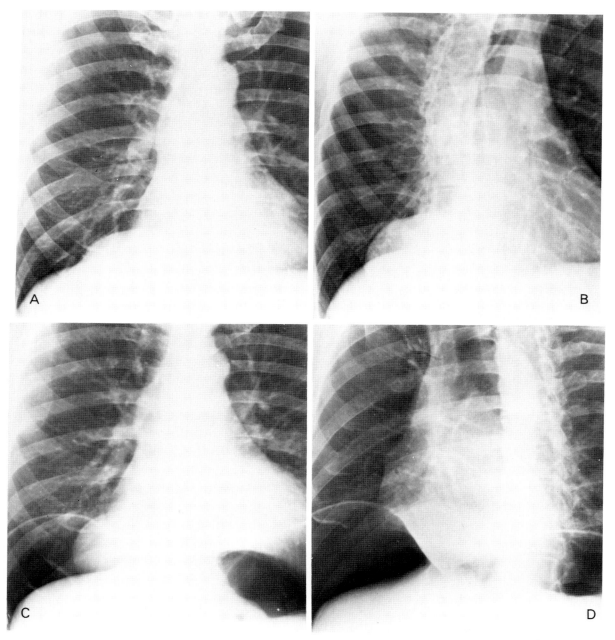

FIG. 576. DIAPHRAGMATIC CYST

A: Routine examination of a 53 year old man revealed a sharply circumscribed density in the right cardiophrenic angle. The appearance is identical with that of a partial eventration of the right hemidiaphragm. *B*: In the right oblique view, the mass is seen to be situated posteriorly. This differs from a localized eventration which almost always involves the anterior portion of the diaphragm. *C*: Frontal film following induction of a pneumoperitoneum. The diaphragm is outlined by air. No air has entered the mass, making the possibility of an eventration or a diaphragmatic hernia extremely unlikely. In addition, the mass appears to be separated from the liver. *D*: Left oblique view. The mass bulges both above and below the diaphragm. This is indicative of either a cyst or neoplasm of the diaphragm. At surgery, a diaphragmatic cyst filled with clear fluid was removed.

entiate radiologically from diaphragmatic hernias, partial eventrations and tumors originating in the base of the lung or in the liver. Most primary tumors of the diaphragm are benign and represent either congenital cysts or neoplasms of mesodermal origin. Sacromas occur, but are exceedingly rare. Metastatic neoplasms of the diaphragm are practically always small and most often cannot be visualized radiologically. They may cause a slight irregularity of the diaphragm, but this usually is insufficient for diagnosis. However, fairly large masses can result from extension of a neoplasm of the liver or stomach through the diaphragm, or from implantation of malignant cells on its pleural surface.

A diaphragmatic tumor produces a sharply outlined, dome-shaped, homogeneous protuberance on the upper contour of the diaphragm (Fig. 576). Special studies are required to differentiate it from other lesions in this region. If adhesions are absent, a tumor of the diaphragm can be recognized by examination after induction of a pneumothorax and pneumoperitoneum. Both

surfaces of the diaphragm are then outlined, and the shadow of the tumor is seen to be continuous with the diaphragm, separated from the viscera above and below by the injected air.

Extension of a hepatic tumor should be suspected if the pneumoperitoneum fails to separate the liver from the diaphragm in the region of the mass. The diagnosis can be confirmed by arteriography. The mass formed by extension of a carcinoma of the stomach is soon obscured by a pleural effusion. A malignant tumor of the diaphragm may be as sharply defined as a benign tumor, but its border becomes indistinct when it infiltrates the lung and is obscured when a pleural effusion develops.

APPENDIX: COMPUTED TOMOGRAPHY OF THE CHEST

In the few years since its introduction, computed tomography (CT) has become almost indispensable for the practice of neuroradiology and has proven to be of considerable value for the study of the abdomen and pelvis. Its impact on diagnosis of chest diseases has not been as great because most of the thoracic structures can be well visualized by standard radiographic techniques. Nevertheless, the ability of the CT scanner to produce a highly detailed picture of the thorax in cross section has considerably broadened the scope of chest radiology.

As with other radiographic pictures, the images on a CT scan reflect differing degrees of absorption of an x-ray beam by the tissues that lie in its path. Basically, the scanner consists of an x-ray tube that emits a highly collimated, slit-like beam of radiation on one side of the patient, and a system of detectors on the opposite side. The detectors measure the intensity of the emergent x-ray beam at multiple points as the tube rotates around the patient during the scan. Utilizing these measurements, the computer then calculates the absorption values for thousands of points within the section and generates the final image on a television monitor. Each CT image represents a "slice" of the patient, usually 13 mm in thickness, although thinner sections can be obtained. In order to completely study the chest, about 30 sections are required.

Most CT scanners arbitrarily divide the range of relative absorption values that they encompass into 2000 increments, ranging from air, the most radiolucent, to dense bone, the most radiopaque. Water, whose density is in the middle of this range, is assigned a CT value of zero. Various CT values are represented on the final image as different shades of gray. Although all the data

from a scan are stored in the computer, because the gray scale that can be reproduced by a television monitor or appreciated by the human eye is limited, only a segment of the range of CT numbers is displayed on any single picture. The choice of which segment of numbers is to be displayed and the width of the segment determines which structures will be seen and the character of the picture. A window level centered on the higher CT numbers will show the soft tissues and bones of the chest wall, while a setting considerably below zero is required to picture details of the smaller pulmonary vessels within the air-filled lungs (Fig. 577). By using a narrow window, the contrast of the image is increased and it is easier to distinguish one type of tissue from another (Fig. 583).

The CT scanner can distinguish differences in absorption values 6 to 10 times smaller than the linear tomogram. As a result, many tissues that cast identical shadows on radiographs can be differentiated from one another on the CT image. In addition, because the relative CT number of any segment of the image can be determined, it is often possible to identify a specific type of tissue or substance.

Lungs

Because of the high resolution of CT, pulmonary nodules as small as 3 mm in diameter are routinely demonstrable on CT scans although they often are not visible on standard tomograms. However, the clinical significance of these small nodules is not always certain because many of them simply represent granulomas. Unless calcium is demonstrated within the nodules, it is not possible to distinguish them from neoplastic

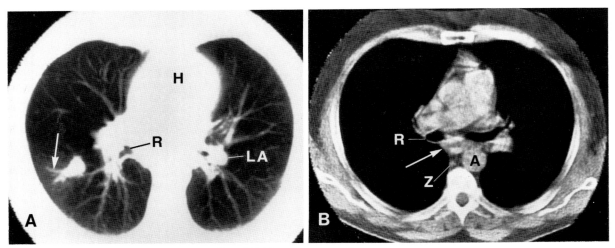

FIG. 577. BRONCHOGENIC CARCINOMA

A: Section through the lower portion of the pulmonary hila. The neoplasm is seen as an irregular nodule in the right lower lobe with a Fleischner line (arrow) extending peripherally. The window setting was adjusted for the lungs and therefore no detail can be seen within the cardiac silhouette (H) or the chest wall. Right lower lobe bronchus (R), left pulmonary artery (LA). *B*: Section immediately below the carina. Window adjusted for mediastinal detail. The soft tissue mass (arrow) immediately posterior to the intermediate bronchus (R), partially filling in the azygoesophageal recess represents enlarged subcarinal nodes. The azygos vein is seen as a small, round shadow (Z) surrounded by mediastinal fat. Descending aorta (A).

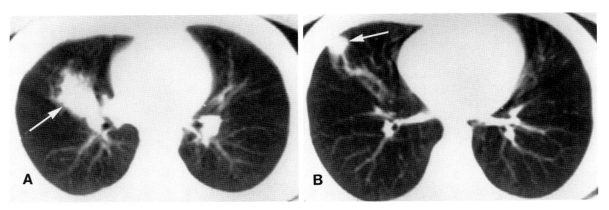

FIG. 578. PULMONARY ARTERIOVENOUS (A-V) MALFORMATION, CONTRAST-ENHANCED SCAN

A: Section through the lower portion of the hila. The irregular mass in the right lung (arrow) represents a racemose collection of abnormal vessels. *B*: Section through the lower lobe. A second A-V malformation is seen in the right lower lobe (arrow). The paired vessels extending toward the hilum represent the feeding pulmonary artery and the draining vein.

foci. Therefore, it is doubtful that resection of a primary malignancy should be withheld simply because a small number of these nodules are found in the lungs.

The CT appearance of a peripheral bronchogenic carcinoma is essentially the same as on routine films—an irregular or indistinctly margined mass, often with one or more Fleischner lines extending peripherally (Fig. 577*A*). In the majority of cases, CT does not add any significant diagnostic information. Small areas of calcification may be detected within the lesion on a CT scan but it is often difficult, because of the thinness of the section, to determine their distribution. If the pattern of calcification cannot be clearly demonstrated, it is of little use for distinguishing between a benign and a malignant lesion (p. 176).

CT of the chest is indicated in the patient with positive sputum cytology when a pulmonary lesion is not visible on routine studies. In an occasional case, a primary carcinoma, which is hidden by the mediastinum or the diaphragm, will be visible when the chest is viewed in cross section.

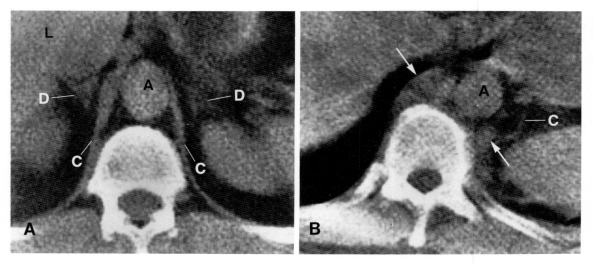

FIG. 579. RETROCRURAL SPACE

A: Normal. Magnified section at the level of D-12. The descending aorta (A) is outlined by fat in the space bounded by the fibrous diaphragmatic crura (C). Liver (L), adrenal gland (D). *B*: Adenopathy in a patient with lymphoma. The masses (arrows) on either side of the aorta in the retrocrural space represent enlarged lymph nodes. No widening of the paraspinal line could be appreciated on plain films.

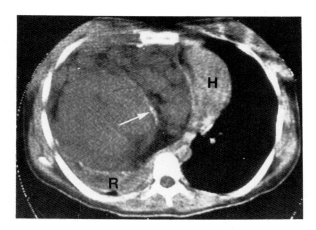

FIG. 580. MEDIASTINAL TERATOMA

Plain films of the chest showed a large, homogeneous mass filling the lower two-thirds of the right hemithorax. On linear tomograms, a faint rim of calcification was seen at its upper border. The mediastinum was shifted to the left. The contrast enhanced CT scan shows the large mass compressing and displacing the heart (H) and the right lung (R). The mass is not homogeneous and is composed of fat (darker areas) interspersed with other soft tissues. A portion of the calcific rim (arrow) can be seen. The multiple types of tissue indicate a mass of developmental origin. The irregularity and lack of encapsulation signify malignancy.

CT is extremely useful for the preoperative study of the patient with a known bronchogenic carcinoma because spread of the tumor to the mediastinum or pleura can be detected even though other studies are negative.

If an intravenous infusion of contrast material is administered during the CT scan, shadows of the pulmonary and systemic vessels, as well as highly vascular lesions, will show a significant increase in density. This provides an effective noninvasive means for establishing the diagnosis of a pulmonary arteriovenous malformation (Fig. 578). Failure of a mass in the lung to "light up" on a contrast-enhanced study excludes such a malformation from consideration. If the scan is positive, pulmonary arteriography is usually required in order to map out the relevant vascular anatomy prior to surgery.

With the appropriate window setting, the pulmonary interstitium and the smaller vessels can be clearly delineated and infiltrations or pulmonary fibrosis may be detected before they become manifest on standard radiographs. Small bullae, not otherwise visible, may be very apparent on the CT image. This suggests the use of CT for preoperative evaluation of the patient with respiratory difficulty because of compression of the lung by one or more large bullae. Evidence of diffuse emphysematous involvement of the lungs may serve as a contraindication for bullectomy (p. 390).

Mediastinum

Masses in the mediastinum that do not displace the trachea or bronchi are difficult to detect unless they protrude beyond the normal mediastinal border and are outlined against the adjacent

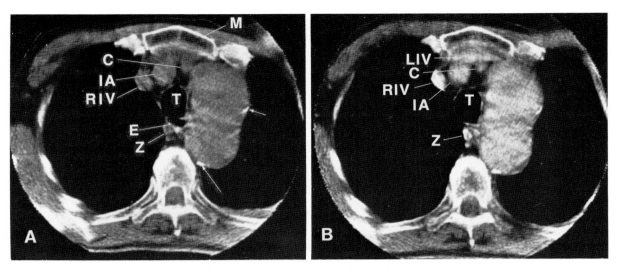

FIG. 581. ANEURYSM OF THE AORTIC ARCH

A: Preliminary scan. The large, fusiform mass to the left of the trachea (T) contains several calcific plaques (arrows) in its wall suggesting that it represents an aneurysm of aortic arch. Manubrium (M), right innominate vein (RIV), left innominate vein (LIV), innominate artery (IA), left carotid artery (C), esophagus (E), azygos vein (Z). *B*: Repeat scan during intravenous infusion of contrast material. The great arteries and veins are opacified. The density of the mass is considerably greater than on the preliminary scan and its CT number is comparable to the other vascular structures. On this basis a diagnosis of aneurysm of the aortic arch was made. This was confirmed by aortography.

lung. Because the mediastinum is not a smooth, regular structure, all of its contours cannot be visualized on standard films, even with oblique projections and tomograms. However, the entire mediastinum-lung interface is clearly outlined in the cross sectional view, and, therefore, full chest CT scans are the most accurate method for detecting such lesions. This is particularly true when searching for enlarged nodes or neoplastic infiltration.

Adenopathy in the subcarinal region can be recognized on plain films only when the nodes are large enough to splay the carina and displace the major bronchi. However, lesser degrees of nodal enlargement are usually obvious on a CT scan at the level of the right main bronchus. A tongue of the right lower lobe normally extends medially behind the right bronchus and abuts against the esophagus and the azygos vein. Enlarged subcarinal nodes present as a soft tissue mass that fills in this recess and displaces the lung outward (Fig. 577*B*). Large esophageal nodes usually are seen as a mass on the left side of the posterior mediastinum, blending in with the shadow of the descending aorta. Nodes in the region of the aortopulmonary window efface the normal lung-filled recess between the left pulmonary artery and the descending aorta.

On a section through the upper abdomen, just below the dome of the diaphragm, the tendinous insertions of the diaphragm are visualized, delimiting the aortic hiatus. The space between the diaphragmatic crura contains the descending aorta and a fair amount of fat (Fig. 579*A*). Occasionally, the azygos and hemiazygos veins are seen as small round densities immediately in front of the vertebral body. One or two small lymph nodes may also be visualized in the same area. When the nodes are enlarged, they fill in the retrocrural space (Fig. 579*B*). Abnormal nodes can be detected before they are large enough to produce recognizable displacement of the paraspinal line on the frontal chest film.

Large internal mammary nodes can sometimes be recognized as a retrosternal density on the lateral chest film but are more easily visualized on a CT scan. Hilar adenopathy can also be detected by CT but linear tomography, with the patient in a 55° posterior oblique position, is more accurate for this purpose.

A tumor of the thymus, or hyperplasia of the gland, cannot always be demonstrated on plain films because their shadows are not very dense. We have encountered several patients with myasthenia gravis in whom a thymoma could be detected only on lateral tomograms of the anterior mediastinum. As this region is pictured in considerably greater detail by CT, a CT scan should be performed if other studies are negative before concluding that there is no tumor or enlargement of the thymus.

It is often possible to determine the specific

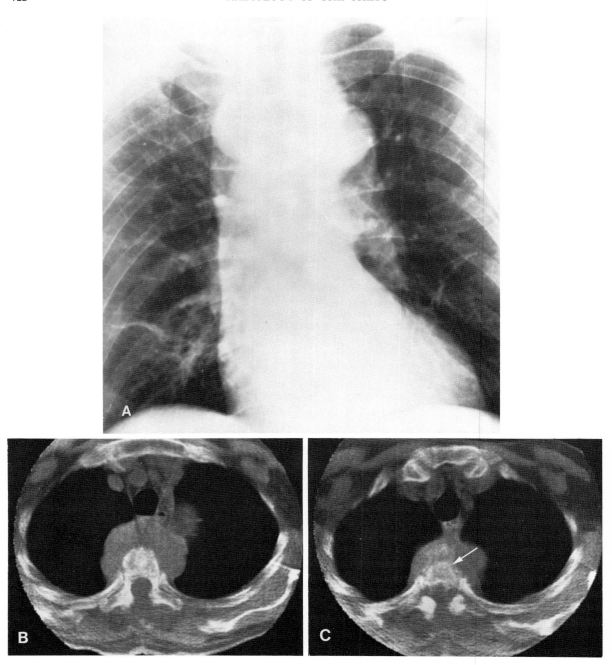

FIG. 582. METASTATIC SCHWANNOMA

A 62-year-old male had a malignant schwannoma removed from the lumbar region several years ago. He experienced the recent onset of severe upper back pain and was studied at another hospital where a dorsal laminectomy was performed. Because the pain became worse a CT examination was requested. *A*: The frontal film of the chest shows well demarcated masses bulging from either side of the mediastinum above the level of the aortic arch. Films of the dorsal spine suggested some destruction of the vertebral bodies in this region but were not conclusive. *B*: CT section at the level of the upper portion of the manubrium. When the thorax is viewed in cross section, it is obvious that there is only a single continuous mass surrounding the vertebral body and extending into the posterior mediastinum. The laminae and spinous process are absent because of the previous surgery. *C*: Section at the sternomanubrial junction shows extensive destruction of the vertebral body (arrow).

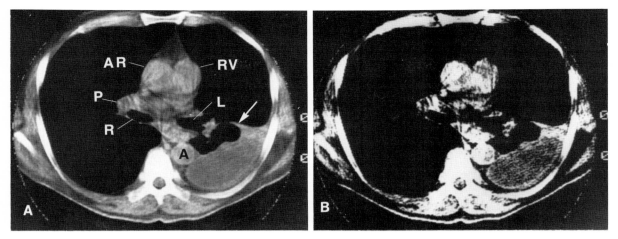

FIG. 583. CHRONIC EMPYEMA

The patient, who was a shipyard worker and had a long history of exposure to asbestos dust, complained of severe pleuritic left chest pain. Plain films showed marked thickening of the posterior pleura on the left involving the lower half of the hemithorax. A mesothelioma was suspected. *A*: A section just below the carina shows a large mass in the posterior left hemithorax which is continuous with an area of pleural thickening in the long fissure (arrow). Becaue the mass is not homogeneous but appears to have a dense rim around it, an empyema was considered most likely. Descending aorta (A), aortic root (AR), outflow tract of right ventricle (RV), right main bronchus (R), left main bronchus (L), right pulmonary artery (P). *B*: The same section, utilizing a narrower window to increase contrast, clearly demonstrates the denser rim around the fluid collection. The diagnosis of a chronic empyema was confirmed surgically.

nature of a mediastinal mass from the CT scan. The position of the mass in the chest and its relationship to the normal structures is clearly demonstrated and, at times, the tissues composing the mass can be identified (Fig. 580). Fat is easily recognized because of its low CT number. Herniated properitoneal fat or an epicardial fat pad can be unequivocally recognized on the CT image and no further diagnostic studies are required. Similarly, differentiation between a fat pad and an enlarged cardiophrenic node is easily accomplished. Although diffuse widening of the mediastinum due to lipomatosis can sometimes be recognized on plain films (p. 571), in many instances the mediastinal shadow is not particularly radiolucent and neoplastic infiltration cannot be excluded. On the CT scan, the lesser density of the fat-filled mediastinum is obvious and the great vessels stand out in sharp contrast to their more lucent surroundings.

A pericardial cyst, which appears as a soft tissue mass on plain films, can usually be recognized on the CT scan because of the water density of its fluid content. This is also true of some bronchogenic cysts, although in others, the cyst contents are so viscid that the cyst cannot be distinguished from a solid mass.

When a mediastinal mass cannot be separated from the aorta in at least one view, aortography is often required in order to exclude an aneurysm from consideration. A fine rim of calcification can be demonstrated on the CT scan in the wall of most aneurysms, even though none is seen on routine studies. In the absence of calcification, the aneurysm can still be identified because the density of its image increases when contrast material is infused during the scan (Fig. 581). Differentiation between a fusiform aneurysm and a dissecting aneurysm is often not possible by computed tomography because of blurring due to motion. However, with 2- to 3-second scanners, especially when the exposure is gated by the electrocardiogram, it is possible to visualize the dissected intima as a linear band separating the two aortic channels.

Extension of a mediastinal mass into the chest wall, or origin of the mass in the chest wall, is often not obvious on plain films, because the shadows of the soft tissues and cartilage blend imperceptibly with one another. The CT scan provides a detailed picture of these structures so that infiltration and interruption of the normal tissue planes can be identified. In other cases, bone destruction, not visible even on films exposed for bone detail is detectable (Fig. 582). All the different tissues are included on each CT scan, and can be evaluated without restudying the patient by simply manipulating the image when interpreting the examination.

Pleura

Many lesions of the pleura are difficult to see on plain chest films or tomograms because they are relatively flat and cast a faint, indistinct shadow when viewed *en face*. Unless that portion of the pleura is projected tangentially, a localized thickening often escapes notice. On the CT scan, the entire pleura, except for the portions that cover the diaphragm and extend over the apex of the lung, is viewed on end.

Multiple pleural nodules, none of which may be visible on plain films, almost always indicate metastatic neoplastic involvement. However, in the majority of instances, it is not possible to determine whether a localized pleural lesion is benign or malignant. Although the CT scan can detect pleural thickening in asbestosis at a relatively early stage, it cannot distinguish between a benign fibrous pleural plaque and a mesothe-lioma. If the lesion is more extensive or has an irregular contour, the latter diagnosis is more likely. One lesion that can be expected to present a pathognomonic CT appearance is the extra-pleural lipoma because the mass arising in the chest wall will have a CT number characteristic of fat.

A free pleural effusion appears as a band of density against the chest wall. Small effusions can be distinguished from pleural thickening by repeating the CT scan with the patient in the decubitus position. A shift of the abnormal shadow to the dependent portion of the chest confirms the presence of free fluid.

Recognition of a loculated collection of fluid or pus is often difficult on plain films because its appearance can mimic that of a solid tumor. It is often possible to recognize clear pleural fluid by CT scan because its CT number approximates that of water. In other cases, demonstration of a rim of denser tissue around the fluid collection identifies it as an encapsulated effusion or an empyema (Fig. 583).

Bibliography

REFERENCE TEXTS

Assmann, H.: *Die klinische Röntgendiagnostik der inneren Erkrankungen*, Ed. 5. F. C. W. Vogel, Leipzig, 1932.

Baum, G. L. (Ed.): *Textbook of Pulmonary Diseases*. Little, Brown, Boston, 1974.

Brednow, W., and Hofmann, E.: *Roentgenatlas der Lungenerkrankungen*, Ed. 2. Urban & Schwarzenberg, Berlin, 1933.

Felson, B.: *Fundamentals of Chest Roentgenology*. W. B. Saunders, Philadelphia, 1960.

Felson, B., Weinstein, A. S., and Spitz, H. B.: *Principles of Chest Roentgenology*. W. B. Saunders, Philadelphia, 1965.

Felson, B.: *Chest Roentgenology*. W. B. Saunders, Philadelphia, 1973.

Fraser, R. G., and Paré, J. A. P. *Diagnosis of Diseases of the Chest*. W. B. Saunders, Philadelphia, 1977.

Graham, E. A., Singer, J. J., and Ballon, H.: *Surgical Diseases of the Chest*. Lea & Febiger, Philadelphia, 1935.

Heitzman, E. R. The Lung: *Radiologic-Pathologic Correlation*. C. V. Mosby, St. Louis, 1973.

Hinshaw, H. C., and Garland, L. H. *Diseases of the Chest*, Ed. 2 W. B. Saunders, Philadelphia, 1963.

Liebow, A. A., and Smith, D. D. (Eds.): *The Lung*. Williams & Wilkins, Baltimore, 1968.

Lillington, G. A., and Jamplis, R. W.: *A Diagnostic Approach to Chest Diseases*. Williams & Wilkins, Baltimore, 1965.

Miller, W. S.: *The Lung*. Charles C Thomas, Springfield, Ill., 1937.

Perry, K. M. A., and Holmes Sellors, T.: *Chest Diseases*. Butterworth, London, 1963.

Rigler, L. G.: *The Chest*. Year Book, Chicago, 1946.

Ritvo, M.: *Chest X-ray Diagnosis*, Ed. 2. Lea & Febiger, Philadelphia, 1956.

Rubin, E. H., and Siegelman, S. S.: *The Lungs in Systemic Disease*. Charles C Thomas, Springfield, Ill., 1969.

Sergent, E., et al.: *Exploration radiologique de Pappareil respiratoire*. Masson, Paris, 1931.

Shanks, S. C., and Kerley, P. (Eds.): *A Textbook of X-ray Diagnosis, Vol. 3: Respiratory System*, Ed. 4. W. B. Saunders. Philadelphia, 1970.

Simon, G.: *Principles of Chest X-ray Diagnosis*, Ed. 4. Butterworth, London, 1978.

Snow, W.: *Principles in Roentgen Study of the Chest*. Charles C Thomas, Springfield, Ill., 1946.

Spencer, H.: *Pathology of the Lung*. Pergamon Press, Elmsford, N. Y., 1977.

Wessler, H., and Jaches, L.: *Clinical Roentgenology of Diseases of the Chest*. Southworth, Troy, N. Y., 1923.

Westermark, N.: *Roentgen Studies of the Lungs and Heart*. University of Minnesota Press, Minneapolis, 1948.

Part I: General Considerations

USES AND LIMITATIONS

Beilin, D. S., Fink, J. P., and Leslie, L. W.: Correlation and postmortem pathological observations with chest roentgenograms. Radiology, *57:* 361, 1951.

Berkson, J., Good, C. A., Carr, D. T., and Bruwer, A. J.: Identification of "positives" in roentgenographic readings. Am. Rev. Respir. Dis. *81:* 660, 1960.

Birkelo, C. C., et al.: Tuberculosis case finding; a comparison of the effectiveness of various roentgenographic and photofluorographic methods. J.A.M.A. *133:* 359, 1947.

Christie, A. C.: Some medical and roentgenological aspects of mass chest surveys. A.J.R. *61:* 147, 1949.

Cochrane, A. L., Campbell, H. W., and Stein, S. C.: The value of roentgenology in the prognosis of minimal tuberculosis. A.J.R. *61:* 153, 1949.

Garland, L. H.: On the reliability of roentgen survey procedures. A.J.R. *64:* 32, 1950.

Garland, L. H.: Studies on the accuracy of diagnostic procedures. A.J.R. *82:* 25, 1959.

Greening, R. R., and Pendergrass, E. P.: Postmortem roentgenography with particular emphasis upon the lung. Radiology *62:* 720, 1954.

Hessel, S. J., Herman, P. G., and Swenson, R. G.: Improving performance by multiple interpretations of chest radiographs. Radiology *127:* 589, 1978.

Cola, G., and Lo Monaco, G.: Saggi di radiochimografia polmonare. Radiol. Med. *22:* 297, 1935.

Crombie, D. W., and Andrus, P. M.: Vertical tomography of the thorax. Am. Rev. Tuberc. *62:* 170, 1950.

Dack, S., and Paley, D. H.: Electrokymography; I. The ventricular electrokymogram, II. The great vessel and auricular electrokymograms. Am. J. Med. *12:* 331, 447, 1952.

Ellison, R. T.: Oblique films for study of adhesions in artificial pneumothorax. A.J.R. *34:* 592, 1935.

Favez, G., and Soliman, O.: *Radiological Examination of the Lung & Mediastinum with the Aid of Posterior Oblique Tomography at an Angle of 55 Degrees*. Hafner, Riverside, N. J., 1966.

Favis, E. A.: Planigraphy (body section radiography) in detecting tuberculous pulmonary cavitation. Dis. Chest *27:* 668, 1955.

Fredzell, G., et al.: Direct serial roentgenography in two planes simultaneously at 0.08 second intervals. A.J.R. *65:* 548, 1950.

Frimann-Dahl, J.: Value of planigraphy in bronchial cancer. Radiology *27:* 99, 1946.

Goldenthal, S., Armstrong, B. W., and Lowman, R. M.: Roentgen studies of ventilatory dysfunction: an analysis of diaphragmatic movement in obstructive emphysema. A.J.R. *79:* 279, 1958.

Hallenbeck, G. S.: Clinical evaluation of the 350-KV chest radiography system. Radiology *117:* 1, 1975.

Husen, L., Fulkerson, L. L., Del Vecchio, E., Zack, M. B., and Stein, E.: Pulmonary tuberculosis with negative findings on chest x-ray films: a study of 40 cases. Chest *60:* 540, 1971.

Newell, R. R., and Garneau, R.: The threshold visibility of pulmonary shadows. Radiology *57:* 409, 1951.

Rigler, L. G.: The possibilities and limitations of x-ray diagnosis in diseases of the chest. In *Roentgenology of the Chest*, edited by C. B. Rabin. Charles C Thomas, Springfield, Ill., 1958.

Stein, G. H.: Pneumonic densities obscured by cardiac shadow. Radiology *41:* 576, 1943.

Tuddenham, W. J.: Problems of perception in chest roentgenology: facts and fallacies. Radiol. Clin. North Am. *1:* 282, 1963.

Twining, E. W.: Radiology of the chest; an introduction to the study of radiograms of the chest. Br. J. Radiol. *4:* 658, 1931.

TECHNIQUE

Bonorino Udaondo, C., Maissa, P. A., and Vadone, V.: La radiografiá lateral en las lesiones lobulares totales. Bol. Acad. Nac. Med. Buenos Aires, p. 148, 1933.

Capitanio, M. A., and Kirkpatrick, J. A.: The lateral decubitus film. An aid in determining air-trapping in children. Radiology 103: 460, 1972.

Hodes, P. J., De Moor, J., and Ernst, R.: Body-section radiography: fundamentals. Radiol. Clin. North Am. 1: 229, 1963.

Jackson, F. I.: The air-gap technique; and an improvement by anteroposterior positioning for chest roentgenography. A.J.R. 92: 688, 1964.

Jacobson, G., and Sargent, E. N.: Apical roentgenographic views of the chest. A.J.R. 104: 822, 1968.

Jacobson, G., Bohlig, H., and Kiviluoto, R.: Essentials of chest radiography. Radiology 95: 445, 1970.

Korol, E., and Scott, H. A.: Use of chest roentgenograms taken with breath held in expiration. A.J.R. 31: 267, 1934.

Lasser, E. C.: Some aspects of pulmonary dynamics revealed by concurrent roentgen kymography of spirometric movements and diaphragmatic excursions. Radiology 77: 434, 1961.

Littleton, J. T.: Tomography: Physical Principles and Clinical Applications. Williams & Wilkins, Baltimore, 1976.

Lynch, P. A.: A different approach to chest roentgenography: triad technique (high kilo-voltage, grid, wedge filter). A.J.R. 93: 965, 1965.

Manges, W. F.: Roentgen diagnosis and localization of opaque foreign bodies in air passages. A.J.R. 29: 368, 1933.

McCleod, R. A., Brown, L. R., Miller, W. E., and DeRemee, R. A.: Evaluation of the pulmonary hila by tomography. Radiol. Clin. North Am. 14: 51, 1976.

Miller, W. E., Crowe, J. K., and Muhm, J. R.: The evaluation of pulmonary parenchymal abnormalities by tomography. Radiol. Clin. North Am. 14: 85, 1976.

Morgenstern, P., and Pine, I.: Pulmonary cavities "below the diaphragm." A.J.R. 59: 677, 1948.

Morgenstern, P., Carr, C. E., and Nalls, W. L.: Evaluation of planigrams in pulmonary tuberculosis. A.J.R. 62: 402, 1949.

Polga, J. P., and Watnick, M.: Whole lung tomography in metastatic disease. Clin. Radiol. 27: 53, 1976.

Poznanski, A. K.: Practical Approaches to Pediatric Radiology. Year Book, Chicago, 1976.

Rigler, L. G., and Merner, T. B.: Planigraphy in diagnosis of bronchogenic carcinoma. A.J.R. 58: 267, 1947.

Rundle, F. F., DeLambert, R. M., and Epps, R. G.: Cervicothoracic tumors: a technical aid to their roentgenologic localization. A.J.R. 81: 316, 1959.

Scott, W. G., and Moore, S.: Roentgen kymography of respiratory movements of thorax, diaphragm, lungs, bronchi and mediastinal structures. A.J.R. 37: 721, 1937.

Simonds, B., Friedman, P. J., and Sokoloff, J.: The prone chest film. Radiology 116: 11, 1975.

Tager, S. N.: Use of overpenetrated film technic in diagnosis of cavities. Radiology 39: 389, 1942.

Vix, V. A., and Klatte, E. C.: The lateral chest radiography in the diagnosis of hilar and mediastinal masses. Radiology 96: 307, 1970.

Wasson, W. W.: The evaluation of the lesser circulation as portrayed by the roentgenogram. A.J.R. 61: 30, 1949.

Westermark, N.: The influence of the intra-alveolar pressure upon the roentgen appearance of the chest, with particular reference to the Valsalva and Muller maneuver and cough. In Roentgenology of the Chest, edited by C. B. Rabin. Charles C Thomas, Springfield, Ill., 1958.

Zanca, P.: Roentgenographic measurements of diaphragmatic motion-respiratory compliance. A.J.R. 110: 717, 1970.

Zinn, B., and Monroe, J.: The lordotic position in fluoroscopy and roentgenography of the chest. A.J.R. 75: 682, 1956.

USE OF CONTRAST MEDIA

Baron, M. G.: Dissecting aneurysm. Circulation 44: 475, 1971.

Berne, A. S., Itkins, P. M., and Bueden, W. F.: CO_2-O_2 pneumomediastinography with polytomography for the preoperative evaluation of bronchogenic carcinoma. Radiology 88: 519, 1967.

Boijsen, E., and Zsigmond, M.: Selective angiography of bronchial and intercostal arteries. Acta Radiol. 3: 513, 1965.

Boushy, S. F., North, L. B., and Trice, J. A.: The bronchial arteries in chronic obstructive pulmonary disease. Am. J. Med. 46: 506, 1969.

Celis, A., Pacheco, C. R., and Del Castillo, H.: Angiocardiographic diagnosis of mediastinal tumors, with special reference to aortic aneurysms. Radiology 56: 31, 1951.

DiRienzo, S.: Radiologic Exploration of the Bronchus. Charles C Thomas, Springfield, Ill., 1949.

Disenberg, C. E., and Arismendi, L.: The angiographic demonstration of pulmonary arteriovenous fistula. Radiology 53: 66, 1949.

Dunbar, J. S., Skinner, G. B., Wortzman, G., and Stuart, J. R.: An investigation of effects of opaque media on the lungs with comparison of barium sulfate, lipiodol and Dionosil. A.J.R. 82: 902, 1959.

Fariñas, P. L.: Bronchography by atomization. Radiology 51: 491, 1948.

Feist, J. H.: Selective cinebronchography in obstructive and restrictive pulmonary disease. A.J.R. 99: 543, 1967.

Fennessy, J. J.: A technique for the selective catheterization of segmental bronchi using arterial catheters. A.J.R. 90: 936, 1966.

Fennessy, J. J.: Bronchographic criteria of inflammatory disease and radiologic lung biopsy techniques. Radiol. Clin. North Am. 11: 371, 1973.

Ferris, E. J., Stanzler, R. M., Rourke, J. A., Blumenthal, J., and Messer, J. V.: Pulmonary angiography in pulmonary embolic disease. A.J.R. 100: 355, 1967.

Franklin, P., and Orley, A.: Simple technique for introducing lipiodol into lungs. Br. Med. J. 2: 847, 1931.

Greenspan, R. H., and Capps, J. H.: Pulmonary angiography: its use in diagnosis and as a guide to therapy in lesions of the chest. Radiol. Clin. North Am. 1: 215, 1963.

Heitzman, E. R., and McAfee, J. G.: Aneurysms of the thoracic aorta and its branches. In Angiography, edited by H. L. Abrams. Little, Brown, Boston, 1971.

Holden, W. S., and Marshall, R.: Variation in bronchial movement. Clin. Radiol. 26: 439, 1975.

Hsu, J. T., Bennett, G. M., and Wolff, E.: Radiologic assessment of bronchopleural fistula with emphysema. Radiology 103: 41, 1972.

Kärcher, K. H., and Schenk, P.: Phlebographische und szintigraphische Untersuchung des Retrosternalraumes. Fortschr. Geb. Röntgenstrahl. 106: 343, 1967.

Kreel, L., Blendis, L. M., and Piercy, J. E.: Pneumo-mediastinography by the trans-sternal method. Clin. Radiol. 15: 219, 1964.

Low, L. R., Keyting, W. S., and Daywitt, A. L.: Azygography in management of carcinoma of the lung. Radiology 81: 96, 1963.

Nelson, S. W., and Christoforidis, A. J.: Bronchography in diseases of the adult chest. Radiol. Clin. North Am. 11: 125, 1973.

Nadel, J. A., Wolfe, W. G., and Graf, P. D.: Powdered tantalum as a medium for bronchography in canine and human lungs. Invest. Radiol. 3: 229, 1968.

Neuhof, H.: Bronchography in amplification of roentgen film in chronic pulmonary tuberculosis. A.J.R. 31: 289, 1934.

Nordenström, B.: Selective catheterization and angiography of bronchial and mediastinal arteries in man. Acta Radiol. *6:* 13, 1967.

Nordenström, B. E. W., and Norlin, U. A. T.: Bronchography with Metras catheters. Acta Radiol. *35:* 246, 1951.

Poppe, J. K.: A simple and practical method of obtaining complete bronchograms. Am. Rev. Tuberc. *54:* 104, 1946.

Rivero, E.: Bronchography in children. A.J.R. *65:* 173, 1951.

Roodvoets, A. P., Swierenga, J., and Oefner, A. P.: Transient pulmonary densities around retained Lipiodol. Thorax *21:* 473, 1966.

Sanders, D. E., Delarue, N. C., and Lau, G.: Angiography as a means of determining resectability of primary lung cancer. A.J.R. *87:* 884, 1962.

Sargent, E. N., and Turner, A. F.: Percutaneous transcricothyroid membrane selective bronchography. A.J.R. *104:* 792, 1968.

Schwartz, S., Handel, J., and Candel, S.: Azygography. Radiology *72:* 338, 1959.

Skinner, D. B., Dreyfuss, J. R., and Nardi, G. L.: Azygography in the evaluation of operability of pulmonary carcinoma. N. Engl. J. Med. *267:* 232, 1962.

Steinberg, I., and Robb, G. P.: Mediastinal and hilar angiography in pulmonary diseases. Am. Rev. Tuberc. *38:* 557, 1938.

Sussman, M. L.: The differentiation of mediastinal tumor and aneurysm by angiocardiography. A.J.R. *58:* 584, 1947.

Summerling, M. D., and Irvine, W. J.: Pneumomediastinography. A.J.R. *98:* 541, 1966.

Takaro, T.: Angiography of the minute vessels of the lung. Dis. Chest *45:* 28, 1964.

Templeton, A. W., and Fendley, C. E.: Selective transtracheal bronchography using a radiopaque catheter. A.J.R. *92:* 591, 1964.

Trapnell, D. H., and Gregg, I.: Some principles of interpretation of bronchograms. Br. J. Radiol. *42:* 125, 1969.

Williams, J. R., and Wilcox, W. C.: Pulmonary embolism: roentgenographic and angiographic considerations. A.J.R. *89:* 333, 1963.

Wilson, J. F., Peters, G. N., and Fleshman, K.: A technique for bronchography in children. An experience with 575 patients using topical anesthesia. Am. Rev. Respir. Dis. *105:* 564, 1972.

Wishart, D. E. S.: Bronchography in bronchiectasis in children. Ann. Otol. Rhinol. Laryngol. *56:* 404, 1947.

Kirklin, B. R., and Gilbertson, E. L.: Roentgenograms of thorax that suggest carcinoma of the stomach. J.A.M.A. *134:* 1228, 1947.

Kourilsky, R., Marchal, M., and Marchal, M. T.: Recording respiratory function by x-rays: basic principles. Thorax *20:* 428, 1965.

Laws, J. W., and Steiner, R. E.: X-ray densitometry in the study of pulmonary ventilation and the pulmonary circulation. Br. J. Radiol. *38:* 512, 1965.

Lenk, R.: Das "Mediastinalschnellen" ein funktionelles Symptom bei Bronchostenosen geringen Grades. Fortschr. Geb. Röntgenstr. *47:* 90, 1933.

Oderr, C.: Air trapping, pulmonary insufficiency and fluorodensitometry. A.J.R. *92:* 501, 1964.

Polgar, F.: Studies of respiratory mechanics. A.J.R. *61:* 637, 1949.

Potchen, E. J., Evens, R. G., Hill, R., Adatepe, M., Holman, L., Lindeman, J., and Markham, J.: Regional pulmonary function in man. Quantitative transmission radiography as an adjunct to lung scintiscanning. A.J.R. *108:* 724, 1970.

Reinke, R. T., Silverman, N. R., Rosen, L., and Helland, D. H.: Pulmonary videodensitometry in the diagnosis of carcinoma of the lung. Radiology *118:* 521, 1976.

Riley, T. R.: The importance of fluoroscopy in the investigation of sinus tracts of the thorax. Br. J. Radiol. *20:* 483, 1947.

Robinson, A.: Physical aspects of x-ray pulmonary densitometry. Br. J. Radiol. *40:* 905, 1967.

Silverman, N. R.: Clinical video-densitometry. Pulmonary ventilation analysis. Radiology *103:* 263, 1972.

Snider, G. L., and Doctor, L.: Shift of the mediastinum with respiration. A bronchospirometric study in pulmonary tuberculosis. Dis. Chest *47:* 264, 1965.

Storch, C. B.: *Fundamentals of Clinical Fluoroscopy.* Grune & Stratton, New York, 1951.

Sutherland, G. R., Hume, R., Davison, M., and Kennedy, J.: The use of pulmonary x-ray densitometry in evaluating regional bronchospasm in patients with bronchial asthma. Br. J. Radiol. *45:* 432, 1972.

Welin, S.: Parallactic fluoroscopy as an aid in the bronchoscopic extraction of foreign bodies. Acta Radiol. *28:* 313, 1947.

Zimmer, E. A.: *Technique and Results of Fluoroscopy of the Chest.* Charles C Thomas, Springfield, Ill., 1954.

Bronchovascular Segments. Charles C Thomas, Springfield, Ill., 1960.

Boyden, E. A.: *Segmental Anatomy of the Lung.* McGraw-Hill, New York, 1955.

Boyden, E. A., and Hamre, C. J.: An analysis of variations in the bronchovascular patterns of the middle lobe in fifty dissected and twenty injected lungs. J. Thorac. Surg. *21:* 172, 1951.

Boyden, E. A., and Hartmann, J. F.: An analysis of variations in the bronchopulmonary segments of the left upper lobes of fifty lungs. Am. J. Anat. *79:* 321, 1946.

Boyden, E. A., and Scannell, J. G.: An analysis of variations in the bronchovascular pattern of the right upper lobe of fifty lungs. Am. J. Anat. *82:* 27, 1948.

Brock, R. C.: The nomenclature of broncho-pulmonary anatomy. An international nomenclature accepted by the Thoracic Society. Thorax *5:* 222, 1950.

Brock, R. C.: *The Anatomy of the Bronchial Tree,* Ed. 2. Oxford University Press, London, 1954.

Davis, L. A.: The vertical fissure line. A.J.R. *84:* 451, 1960.

Dotter, C. T.: The normal pulmonary arteriogram. In *Angiography,* edited by H. L. Abrams. Little Brown, Boston, 1971.

Ferry, R. M., and Boyden, E. A.: Variations in the bronchovascular patterns of the right lower lobe of fifty lungs. J. Thorac. Surg. *22:* 18, 1951.

Foster-Carter, A. F.: The anatomy of the bronchial tree. Br. J. Tuberc. *36:* 19, 1942.

Foster-Carter, A. F.: Broncho-pulmonary abnormalities. Br. J. Tuberc. *40:* 111, 1946.

Foster-Carter, A. F., and Hoyle, C.: The segments of the lungs. A commentary on their investigation and morbid radiology. Dis. Chest *11:* 511, 1945.

Friedman, E.: Further observations on the vertical fissure line. A.J.R. *97:* 171, 1966.

Glass, A.: Bronchopulmonary segment with special reference to putrid lung abscess. A.J.R. *31:* 328, 1934.

Huizinga, E., and Smelt, G. J.: *Bronchography.* Van Gorcum, Assen, Netherlands, 1949.

Jackson, C. L., and Huber, J. F.: Correlated applied anatomy of the bronchial tree and lungs with a system of nomenclature. Dis. Chest *9:* 319, 1943.

Kane, I. J.: Segmental localization of pulmonary disease on the posteroanterior roentgenogram. Radiology *59:* 229, 1952.

Kováts, F., Jr., and Zsebök, Z.: *Röntgenanatomische Grundlagen der Lungenuntersuchung.* Akadémiai Kiadó, Budapest, 1959.

Krause, G. R., and Lubert, M.: The anatomy of the bronchopulmonary seg-

FLUOROSCOPY

DiRienzo, S.: Bronchial dynamism. Radiology *53:* 168, 1949.

ANATOMY OF THE LUNGS

Bloomer, W. E., Liebow, A. A., and Hales, M. R.: *Surgical Anatomy of the*

ments: clinical applications. Radiology *56:* 333, 1951.

LeRoux, B. T.: The bronchial anatomy of the left upper lobe. J. Thorac. Cardiovasc. Surg. *44:* 216, 1962.

Levitin, J., and Brunn, H.: Study of roentgenologic appearance of lobes of lung and interlobar fissures. Radiology *25:* 651, 1935.

Medlar, E. M.: Variations in interlobar fissures. A.J.R. *57:* 723, 1947.

Meschan, I.: *An Atlas of Anatomy Basic to Radiology.* W. B. Saunders, Philadelphia, 1975.

Michelson, E., and Salik, J. O.: The vascular pattern of the lung as seen on routine and tomographic studies. Radiology *73:* 511, 1959.

Neil, J. H., Gilmour, W., and Gwynne, F. J.: Broncho-pulmonary segments: radiological, pathological and bronchoscopic considerations, with special reference to sub-apical broncho-pulmonary segment. M. J. Aust. *2:* 165, 1937.

Potchen, E. J.: Some newer anatomic considerations in the lung. In *Frontiers of Pulmonary Radiology*, edited by M. Simon, E. J. Potchen, and M. Lemay. Grune & Stratton, New York, 1969.

Pump, K. K.: The morphology of the finer branches of the bronchial tree of the human lung. Dis. Chest *46:* 379, 1964.

Pump, K. K.: The circulation in the peripheral parts of the human lung. Dis. Chest *49:* 119, 1966.

Pump, K. K.: Morphology of the acinus of the human lung. Chest *56:* 126, 1969.

Pump, K. K.: Distribution of bronchial arteries in the human lung. Chest *62:* 447, 1972.

Sante, L. R.: The anatomy and physiology of the lesser circulation. A.J.R. *61:* 1, 1949.

Scannell, J. G.: A study of variations of the bronchopulmonary segments in the left upper lobe. J. Thorac. Surg. *16:* 530, 1947.

Scannell, J. G.: An anatomic approach to segmental resection. J. Thorac. Surg. *18:* 64, 1949.

Scannell, J. G., and Boyden, E. A.: A study of variations of the bronchopulmonary segments of the right upper lobe. J. Thorac. Surg. *17:* 232, 1948.

Smith, F. R., and Boyden, E. A.: An analysis of variations of the segmental bronchi of the right lower lobe of fifty injected lungs. J. Thorac. Surg. *18:* 195, 1949.

Temple, H. L., and Evans, J. A.: The bronchopulmonary segments. A.J.R. *63:* 26, 1950.

Van Allen, C. M., and Lindskof, G. E.: Collateral respiration in lung. Surg. Gynecol. Obstet. *53:* 16, 1931.

Part II: General Roentgen Pathology

NORMAL CHEST

Bachman, A. L., and Teixidor, H. S.: The posterior tracheal band: a reflector of local superior mediastinal abnormality. Br. J. Radiol. *48:* 352, 1975.

Christensen, E. E., and Dietz, G. W.: The supraclavicular fossa. Radiology *118:* 37, 1976.

Cimmino, C. V.: Contacts of the left lung with the mediastinum. Sources of diagnostic error. A.J.R. *124:* 412, 1975.

Farrell, J. T., Jr.: Roentgen appearance of chest of new-born infant. A.J.R. *24:* 140, 1930.

Fleischner, F.: Lungenspitzenbefunde im Röntgenbild. Fortschr. Geb. Röntgenstr. *35:* 749, 1927.

Gluck, M. C., Twigg, H. L., Ball, M. F., and Rhodes, P. G.: Shadows bordering the lung on radiographs of normal and obese persons. Thorax *27:* 232, 1972.

Groshey, R.: *Atlas typischer Röntgenbilder vom normalen Menschen.* J. F. Lehmann, Munich, 1928.

Hampton, A. O., and King, D. S.: Middle lobe of right lungs; its roentgen appearance in health and disease. A.J.R. *45:* 721, 1936.

Heitzman, E. R., Markarian, B., Berger, I., and Dailey, E.: The secondary pulmonary lobule: a practical concept for interpretation of chest radiographs; I. Roentgen anatomy of the normal secondary pulmonary lobule. Radiology *93:* 507, 1969.

Heitzman, E. R., Markarian, B., Berger, I., and Dailey, E.: The secondary pulmonary lobule: a practical concept for interpretation of chest radiographs; II. Application of the anatomic concept to an understanding of roentgen pattern in disease states. Radiology *93:* 513, 1969.

Heitzman, E. R., Lane, E. J., Hammack, D. B., and Rimmler, L. J.: Radiological evaluation of the aortic-pulmonary window. Radiology *116:* 513, 1975.

Keats, T. E.: *An Atlas of Normal Roentgen Variants That May Simulate Disease.* Year Book, Chicago, 1973.

Köhler, A.: *Borderlands of Normal and Early Pathologic in Skeletal Roentgenology*, Ed. 11, edited by E. A. Zinner (tr. S. P. Wilk). Grune & Stratton, New York, 1968.

Lennon, A. E., and Simon, G.: The height of the diaphragm in the chest radiograph of normal adults. Br. J. Radiol. *38:* 937, 1965.

Ominsky, S., and Berinson, H. S.: The suprasternal fossa. Radiology *122:* 311, 1977.

Peirce, C. B., and Stocking, B. W.: Oblique projection of thorax, anatomic and roentgenologic study. A.J.R. *38:* 245, 1937.

Pendergrass, E. P., and Hodes, P. J.: Healthy chest. A.J.R. *38:* 15, 1937.

Riggs, W., Jr., and Parvey, L.: Differences between right and left lateral chest radiographs. A.J.R. *127:* 997, 1976.

Savoca, C. J., Austin, J. H. M., and Goldberg, H. I.: The right paratracheal stripe. Radiology *122:* 295, 1977.

Shields, J. B., and Holtz, S.: The retrotracheal space. Radiology *120:* 19, 1976.

Simon, G.: The anterior view chest radiograph—criteria for normality derived from a basic analysis of the shadows. Clin. Radiol. *26:* 429, 1975.

ATELECTASIS

Baron, M. G.: Fleischner lines and pulmonary emboli. Circulation *45:* 171, 1972.

Cohen, A. G.: Atelectasis of the right middle lobe resulting from perforation of tuberculous lymph node into bronchi in adults. Ann. Intern. Med. *35:* 821, 1951.

Cranz, H. J., and Pribram, H. F. W.: The pulmonary vessels in the diagnosis of lobar collapse. A.J.R. *94:* 665, 1965.

Culiner, M. M.: The right middle lobe syndrome, a non-obstructive complex. Dis. Chest *50:* 57, 1966.

Fleischner, F. G.: Über das Wesen der basalen horizontalen Schattenstreifen im Lungenfeld. Wien. Arch. Inn. Med. *28:* 461, 1936.

Fleischner, F., Hampton, A. O., and Castleman, B.: Linear shadows in the lungs (interlobar pleuritis, atelectasis and healed infarction). A.J.R. *46:* 610, 1941.

Graham, E. V., Burford, T. H., and Mayer, J. H.: Middle lobe syndrome. Postgrad. Med. *4:* 29, 1948.

Hurst, A., and Millner, T.: Segmental collapse in therapeutic pneumothorax. Radiology *55:* 228, 1950.

Kent, E. N.: Bronchial obstruction and pulmonary atelectasis. Am. Rev. Tuberc. *46:* 524, 1942.

Krause, G. R., and Lubert, M.: Gross anatomico-spatial changes occurring in lobar collapse: a demonstration by means of three-dimensional plastic models. A.J.R. *79:* 258, 1958.

Lodin, H.: Mediastinal herniation and displacement studied by transversal tomography. Acta Radiol. *48:* 337, 1957.

Lubert, M., and Krause, G. R.: Patterns of lobar collapse as observed radiographically. Radiology *56:* 165, 1951.

Lubert, M., and Krause, G. R.: Total unilateral pulmonary collapse: a study of the roentgen appearance in the lateral view. Radiology *67:* 175, 1956.

Lubert, M., and Krause, G. R.: Further observations on lobar collapse. Radiol. Clin. North Am. *1:* 331, 1963.

Manges, W. F., and Farrell, J. T., Jr.: Significance of roentgenologic changes in differential diagnosis of atelectasis. A.J.R. *30:* 429, 1933.

Pinck, R. L., Burbank, B., Cutler, S. S., Sbar, S., and Mangier, I. M.: Nonobstructive atelectasis. Am. Rev. Respir. Dis. *91:* 909, 1965.

Rivkin, M., Read, R. C., Lillehei, C. W., and Varco, R. L.: Massive atelectasis of the left lung in children with congenital heart disease. J. Thorac. Surg. *34:* 116, 1957.

Robbins, L. L., and Hale, C. H.: The roentgen appearance of lobar and segmental collapse of the lung: I. Technic of examination. Radiology *44:* 471, 1945; II. The normal chest as it pertains to collapse. Radiology *44:* 543, 1945; III. Collapse of an entire lung or a major part thereof. Radiology *45:* 23, 1945; IV. Collapse of the lower lobes. Radiology *45:* 120, 1945; V. Collapse of the right middle lobe. Radiology *45:* 260, 1945; VI. Collapse of the upper lobes. Radiology *45:* 347, 1945.

Rubin, E. H., and Rubin, M.: The shrunken right middle lobe with reference to the so-called "middle lobe syndrome." Dis. Chest *18:* 127, 1950.

Salinger, H.: The roentgen examination of the mediastinal lung hernia with reference to tomography. Acta Radiol. *29:* 130, 1948.

Simon, G.: The x-ray appearance of acquired atelectasis of the upper lobes. J. Fac. Radiol. *1:* 223, 1950.

Strickland, B.: "Sentinel lines"—an unusual sign of lower lobe contraction. Thorax *31:* 517, 1976.

Warner, W. P., and Graham, D.: Lobar atelectasis as cause of triangular roentgen shadows in bronchiectasis. Arch. Intern. Med. *52:* 888, 1933.

HYPERINFLATION

Barsby, B.: Tuberculous obstructive emphysema in children. Lancet *1:* 627, 1941.

Capitanio, M. A., and Kirkpatrick, J. A.: Obstructions of the upper airway in children as reflected on the chest radiograph. Radiology *107:* 159, 1973.

Edge, J. R., Millard, F. J. C., Reid, L., and Simon, G.: The radiographic appearances of the chest in persons of advanced age. Br. J. Radiol. *37:* 769, 1964.

Hernandez, J. A., Anderson, A. E., Holmes, B. S., and Foraker, A. G.: Macroscopic relations in emphysematous and aging lungs. Geriatrics *21:* 155, 1966.

Milne, E. N. C., and Bass, H.: The roentgenologic diagnosis of early chronic obstructive pulmonary disease. J. Can. Assoc. Radiol. *20:* 3, 1969.

Mori, P., Anderson, A. E., and Eckert, P.: The radiological spectrum of aging and emphysematous lungs. Radiology *83:* 48, 1964.

Pump, K. K.: The aged lung. Chest *60:* 571, 1971.

Rigler, L. G., and Kelby, G. M.: Emphysema; an early roentgen sign of bronchogenic carcinoma. Radiology *49:* 578, 1947.

Schorr, S., and Aschner, M.: Intercostal lung bulging, a roentgen sign of emphysema in adults. Dis. Chest *44:* 475, 1963.

Simon, G.: The appearance of the chest radiograph in old persons. Radiol. Clin. North Am. *3:* 293, 1965.

Snow, W., and Cassasa, C. S. B.: Obstructive emphysema and atelectasis in acute respiratory diseases in infants. A.J.R. *37:* 217, 1937.

Spivek, M. L.: Obstructive pulmonary emphysema due to partial obstruction of bronchi by tuberculous lesions. Am. J. Dis. Child. *51:* 69, 1936.

INFILTRATION

Conte, P., Heitzman, E. R., and Markarian, B.: Viral pneumonia. Roentgen pathological correlation. Radiology *95:* 267, 1970.

Felson, B.: Disseminated interstitial diseases of the lung. In *Frontiers of Pulmonary Radiology*, edited by M. Simon, E. J. Potchen, and M. Lemay. Grune & Stratton, New York, 1969.

Itoh, H., Tokunaga, S., Asamoto, H., Furuta, M., Funamoto, Y., Kitaichi, M., and Torizuka, K.: Radiologic-pathologic correlations of small lung nodules with special reference to peribronchiolar nodules. A.J.R. *130:* 223, 1978.

Johnson, T. H., Jr., Gajaraj, A., and Feist, J. H.: Patterns of pulmonary interstitial disease. A.J.R. *109:* 516, 1970.

Legge, D. A., Good, C. A., and Ludwig, J.: Roentgenologic features of pulmonary carcinomatosis from carcinoma of the prostate. A.J.R. *111:* 360, 1971.

Liebow, A. A., and Carrington, C. B.: The interstitial pneumonias. In *Frontiers of Pulmonary Radiology*, edited by M. Simon, E. J. Potchen, and M. Lemay. Grune & Stratton, New York, 1969.

Stolberg, H. O., Patt, N. L., Macewen, K. F., Warwick, O. H., and Brown, T. C.: Hodgkin's disease of the lung: roentgenologic-pathologic correlation. A.J.R. *92:* 115, 1964.

CONSOLIDATION

Dornhorst, A. C., and Pierce, J. W.: Pulmonary collapse and consolidation: The role of collapse in the production of lung field shadows and the significance of segments in inflammatory lung disease. J. Fac. Radiol. *5:* 276, 1954.

Felson, B.: The roentgen diagnosis of disseminated pulmonary alveolar diseases. Semin. Roentgenol. *2:* 3, 1967.

Fleischner, F. G.: Der sichtbare Bronchialbaum, ein differentialdiagnostiches Symptom im Röntgenbild der Pneumonia. Fortschr. Geb. Röntgenstr. *36:* 319, 1927.

Fleischner, F. G.: The visible bronchial tree: a roentgen sign in pneumonic and other pulmonary consolidations. Radiology *50:* 184, 1948.

Recavarren, S., Benton, C., and Gall, E. A.: The pathology of acute alveolar diseases of the lung. Semin. Roentgenol. *2:* 22, 1967.

Reed, J. C., and Madewell, J. E.: The air bronchogram in interstitial disease of the lungs. Radiology *116:* 1, 1975.

Ziskind, M. M., Weill, H., and Payzant, A. R.: The recognition and significance of acinus filling processes of the lungs. Am. Rev. Respir. Dis. *87:* 551, 1963.

CIRCULATORY DISTURBANCES

Chen, J. T. T., Capp, M. P., Johnsrude, I. S., Goodrich, J. K., and Lester, R. G.: Roentgen appearance of pulmonary vascularity in the diagnosis of heart disease. A.J.R. *112:* 559, 1971.

Doyle, A. E., Goodwin, J. F., Harrison, C. V., and Steiner, R. E.: Pulmonary vascular patterns in pulmonary hypertension. Br. Heart J. *19:* 353, 1957.

Harley, H. R. S.: The radiological changes in pulmonary venous hypertension, with special reference to the root shadows and lobular pattern. Br. Heart J. 23: 75, 1961.

Lieber, A., Rosenbaum, H. D., Hanson, D. J., and Kwaan, H. M.: Accuracy of predicting pulmonary blood flow, pulmonary arteriolar resistance and pulmonary venous pressure from chest roentgenograms. A.J.R. 103: 577, 1968.

Milne, E. C.: Correlation of physiologic findings with chest roentgenology. Radiol. Clin. North Am. 11: 17, 1973.

Rees, S.: The chest radiograph in pulmonary hypertension with central shunt. Br. J. Radiol. 41: 172, 1968.

Simon, M.: The pulmonary vessels: their hemodynamic evaluation using routine radiographs. Radiol. Clin. North Am. 1: 363, 1963.

Simon, M.: The pulmonary vasculature in congential heart disease. Radiol. Clin. North Am. 6: 303, 1968.

Steiner, R. E.: Radiology of pulmonary circulation. Chamberlain lecture—1963. A.J.R. 91: 249, 1964.

Swischuk, L. E.: Plain Film Interpretation in Congenital Heart Disease. Lea & Febiger, Philadelphia, 1970.

PULMONARY EDEMA

Barden, R. P., and Cooper, D. A.: The roentgen appearance of the chest in diseases affecting the peripheral vascular system of the lungs. Radiology 51: 44, 1948.

Barden, R. P., and Cooper, D. A.: Peripheral vascular disease in the lungs. A. J.R. 61: 17, 1949.

Calenoff, L., Kruglik, G. D., and Woodruff, A.: Unilateral pulmonary edema. Radiology 126: 19, 1978.

Coe, F. O., and Otell, L. S.: Acute pulmonary edema. A.J.R. 27: 101, 1931.

Domiach, I.: Uremic edema of the lungs. A.J.R. 58: 620, 1947.

Don, C., and Johnson, R.: The nature and significance of peribronchial cuffing in pulmonary edema. Radiology 125: 577, 1977.

Fishman, A. P.: Pulmonary edema. The water-exchanging function of the lung. Circulation 46: 390, 1972.

Fleischner, F. G.: The butterfly pattern of acute pulmonary edema. In Frontiers of Pulmonary Radiology, edited by M. Simon, E. J. Potchen, and M. Lemay. Grune & Stratton, New York, 1969.

Fleischner, F. G., and Reiner, L.: Linear x-ray shadows in acquired pulmonary hemosiderosis and congestion. N. Engl. J. Med. 250: 900, 1954.

Gleason, D. C., and Steiner, R. C.: The lateral roentgenogram in pulmonary edema. A.J.R. 98: 279, 1966.

Gould, D. M., and Torrance, D. J.: Pulmonary edema. A.J.R. 73: 336, 1955.

Grainger, R. G.: Interstitial pulmonary oedema and its radiological diagnosis: sign of pulmonary venous and capillary hypertension. Br. J. Radiol. 31: 201, 1958.

Grainger, R. G., and Hearn, J. B.: Intrapulmonary septal lymphatic lines (B lines of Kerley). Their significance and their prognostic evaluation before mitral valvulotomy. J. Fac. Radiol. 7: 66, 1955.

Greene, D. G.: Newer concepts of pulmonary edema. In Frontiers of Pulmonary Radiology, edited by M. Simon; E. J. Potchen and M. Lemay. Grune & Stratton, New York, 1969.

Harrison, M. O., Conte, P. J., and Heitzman, E. R.: Radiological detection of clinically occult cardiac failure following myocardial infarction. Br. J. Radiol. 44: 265, 1971.

Heard, B. E., Steiner, R. E., Herdan, A., and Gleason, D.: Oedema and fibrosis of the lungs in left ventricular failure. Br. J. Radiol. 41: 161, 1968.

Heitzman, E. R., and Zitter, F. M., Jr.: Acute interstitial pulmonary edema. A.J.R. 98: 291, 1966.

Heitzman, E. R., Ziter, F. M., Jr., Markarian, B., McClennan, B., and Sherry, H. S.: Kerley's interlobular septal lines: Roentgen pathologic correlation. A.J.R. 100: 578, 1967.

Herrnheiser, G., and Hinson, K. F. W.: An anatomical explanation of the formation of butterfly shadows. Thorax 9: 198, 1954.

Hodes, P. J., and Griffith, J. Q.: Chest roentgenograms in polycythemia vera and polycythemia secondary to pulmonary arteriosclerosis. A.J.R. 46: 52, 1941.

Hublitz, U., and Shapiro, J. H.: Atypical pulmonary patterns of congestive failure in chronic lung disease. Radiology 93: 995, 1969.

Kerley, P.: Radiology in heart disease. Br. Med. J. 2: 594, 1933.

Kreel, L., Slavin, G., Herbert, A., and Sandin, B.: Intralobar septal oedema: "D" lines. Clin. Radiol. 26: 209, 1975.

Logue, B., Rogers, J. V., Jr., and Gay, B. B., Jr.: Subtle roentgenographic signs of left heart failure. Am. Heart J. 65: 464, 1963.

Meszaros, W. T.: Lung changes in left heart failure. Circulation 47: 859, 1973.

Nessa, B., and Rigler, L. G.: Roentgenological manifestations of pulmonary edema. Radiology 37: 35, 1941.

Penaloza, D., and Sime, F.: Circulatory dynamics during high altitude pulmonary edema. Am. J. Cardiol. 23: 369, 1969.

Rendich, R. A., Levy, A. H., and Cove, A. M.: Pulmonary manifestations of azotemia. A.J.R. 46: 802, 1941.

Rigler, L., and Suprenant, E. L.: Pulmonary edema. Semin. Roentgenol. 2: 33, 1967.

Waqruddin, M., and Bernstein, A.: Reexpansion pulmonary oedema. Thorax 30: 54, 1975.

CAVITATION

Beatty, O. A., Saliba, A., and Levene, N.: A study of cavities and bronchi in pulmonary fungus diseases. Dis. Chest 47: 409, 1965.

Caffey, J.: Regional obstructive pulmonary emphysema in infants and children; emphysematous cavities and their similarity to necrotic cavities, congenital pulmonary cysts, and loculated pneumothorax. Am. J. Dis. Child. 60: 586, 1940.

Felson, B., Fleischner, F. G., McDonald, J. R., and Rabin, C. B.: Some basic principles in the diagnosis of chest diseases. Radiology 73: 740, 1959.

Hennell, H.: Cystic disease of lung. Arch. Intern. Med. 57: 1, 1936.

Laforet, E. G., and Laforet, M. T.: Nontuberculous cavitary disease of the lungs. Dis. Chest 31: 665, 1957.

Moolten, S. E.: Mechanical production of cavities in isolated lungs. Arch. Pathol. 19: 825, 1935.

Peirce, C. B.: "Cystic" disease of the lung. A.J.R. 40: 848, 1940.

Peirce, C. B., and Dirkse, P. R.: Pulmonary pneumatocele; certain considerations in cystic disease of lung. Radiology 28: 651, 1937.

Pinner, M., and Perker, M. E.: Cavity in pulmonary tuberculosis. A.J.R. 25: 455, 1931.

Salkin, D., Cadden, A. V., and McIndoe, R. B.: Blocked pulmonary cavity; anatomical, roentgenological, and clinical study. Am. Rev. Tuberc. 34: 634, 1936.

Weens, H. S., and Thompson, E. A.: The pulmonary air meniscus. Radiology 54: 700, 1950.

CALCIFICATION

Bloch, R. G.: Tuberculous calcification. A.J.R. 59: 853, 1948.

Christie, A., and Peterson, J. C.: Pulmonary calcification in negative reactors to tuberculin. Am. J. Public Health 35: 1131, 1945.

Doub, H. P.: Miliary calcification of the lung: etiologic aspect. Radiology 51: 480, 1948.

Felson, B.: Thoracic calcifications. Chest 56: 330, 1969.

Freedman, E., and Billings, J. H.: Active bronchopulmonary lithiasis. Radiology 53: 203, 1949.

Galloway, R. W., Epstein, E. J., and Coulshed, N.: Pulmonary ossific nodules in mitral valve disease. Br. Heart J. *23:* 297, 1951.

Grayson, C. E., and Blumenfeld, H.: "Eggshell" calcifications in silicosis. Radiology *53:* 216, 1949.

McLachlan, M. S. F., Wallace, M., and Seneviratne, C.: Pulmonary calcification in renal failure. Report of three cases. Br. J. Radiol. *41:* 99, 1968.

Mootz, J. R., Sagel, S. S., and Roberts,

T. H.: Roentgenographic manifestations of pulmonary calcifications. Radiology *107:* 55, 1973.

Raider, L.: Calcification in chickenpox pneumonia. Chest *60:* 504, 1971.

Salzman, E.: *Lung Calcifications in X-ray Diagnosis.* Charles C Thomas, Springfield, Ill., 1968.

Silverman, F. N.: Pulmonary calcification—tuberculosis? histoplasmosis?

A.J.R. *64:* 747, 1950.

Stead, E. A., and Castleman, B.: Sarcoidosis with calcified nodes. N. Engl. J. Med. *281:* 375, 1969.

White, F. C., and Hill, H. E.: Disseminated pulmonary calcification. A report of 114 cases with observations of an antecedent pulmonary disease in 15 individuals. Am. Rev. Tuberc. *62:* 1, 1950.

Part III: *Regional Roentgen Pathology*

DISEASES OF THE CHEST WALL

Bernstein, C., Loeser, W. D., and Manning, L. G.: Erosive rib lesions in paralytic poliomyelitis. Radiology *70:* 368, 1958.

Boone, M. L., Swenson, B. E., and Felson, B.: Rib notching: its many causes. A.J.R. *91:* 1075, 1964.

Drexler, C. J., Stewart, J. R., and Kincaid, O. W.: Diagnostic implications of rib notching. A.J.R. *91:* 1064, 1964.

Fichardt, T., Van Rhyn, J. L., and Van Selm, G. W.: A case of fluorosis. J. Fac. Radiol. *7:* 130, 1955.

Fulton, H.: The roentgenologic significance of funnel chest. A.J.R. *71:* 524, 1954.

Gayler, B. W., and Donner, M. W.: Radiographic changes of the ribs. Am. J. Med. Sci. *253:* 586, 1967.

Goldenberg, D. B., and Brogdon, B. G.: Congenital anomalies of the pectoral girdle demonstrated by chest radiography. J. Can. Assoc. Radiol. *18:* 472, 1967.

Gramiak, R., and Koerner, H. J.: A roentgen diagnostic observation in subpleural lipoma. A.J.R. *98:* 465, 1966.

Groff, D. B., and Adkins, P. C.: Chest wall tumors. Collective review. Ann. Thorac. Surg. *4:* 260, 1967.

Jones, C.: Rib defects simulating pulmonary cavitation. Radiology *25:* 533, 1935.

Kelleher, J., O'Connell, D. J., and MacMahon, H.: Intrathoracic rib: radiographic features of two cases. Br. J. Radiol. *52:* 181, 1979.

Ochsner, A., Jr., Lucas, G. L., and McFarland, G. B., Jr.: Tumors of the thoracic skeleton. Review of 134 cases. J. Thorac. Cardiovasc. Surg. *52:* 311, 1966.

Omell, G. H., Anderson, L. S., and Bramson, R. T.: Chest wall tumors. Radiol. Clin. North Am. *11:* 197, 1973.

Paul, L. A., and Pohle, E. A.: Radiation osteitis of the ribs. Radiology *38:* 543, 1942.

Pirnar, T., and Neuhauser, E. B. D.: As-

phyxiating thoracic dystrophy of the newborn. A.J.R. *98:* 358, 1966.

Rabushka, S. E., Love, L., and Kadison, H. I.: Isolated thoracic dysostosis. Radiology *106:* 161, 1973.

Ritvo, M., and Ritvo, M.: Roentgen study of the sternoclavicular region. A.J.R. *58:* 644, 1947.

Seltzer, R. A.: Subpleural lipoma. Lancet *84:* 100, 1964.

Stein, H. L.: Roentgen diagnosis of congenital absence of pectoralis muscles. Radiology *83:* 63, 1964.

Sweany, H. C.: Note on shadows of fenestrated ribs in roentgenograms. A.J.R. *28:* 541, 1932.

Toye, D. K. M.: The thoracic cage. Prog. Pediatr. Radiol. *1:* 201, 1967.

Wynn-Williams, N., and Young, R. D.: "Cough" fracture of the ribs. Including one complicated by pneumothorax. Tubercle *40:* 47, 1959.

THE TRACHEOBRONCHIAL TREE

Antunes, M. L., and Vieira da Luz, J. M.: Primary diffuse tracheo-bronchial amyloidosis. Thorax *24:* 307, 1969.

Ashley, D. J. B., Danino, E. A., and Davies, H. D.: Bronchial polyps. Thorax *18:* 45, 1963.

Bateson, E. M., and Woo-Ming, M.: Tracheobronchomegaly. Clin. Radiol. *24:* 354, 1973.

Battersby, J. S., and Kilman, J. W.: Traumatic injuries of the tracheobronchial tree. Arch. Surg. *88:* 644, 1964.

Baum, G. L., Vernstein, I. L., and Schwarz, J.: Broncholithiasis produced by histoplasmosis. Am. Rev. Tuberc. *77:* 162, 1958.

Bower, G.: Bronchial adenoma. A review of twenty-eight cases. Am. Rev. Respir. Dis. *92:* 558, 1965.

Braimbridge, M. V., and Keith, H. I.: Oesophago-bronchial fistula in the adult. Thorax *20:* 226, 1965.

Burke, J. F.: Early diagnosis of traumatic rupture of the bronchus. J.A.M.A. *181:* 682, 1962.

Butchart, E. G., Urquhart, W., Porteous,

I. B., and Barnsley, W. C.: Granular cell myoblastoma of the bronchus. Br. J. Radiol. *49:* 87, 1976.

Capitanio, M. A., and Kirkpatrick, J. A.: Obstructions of the upper airway in children as reflected on the chest radiograph. Radiology *107:* 159, 1973.

Carter, R., Wareham, E. E., and Brewer, L. A.: Rupture of the bronchus following closed chest trauma. Am. J. Surg. *104:* 177, 1962.

Chang, L. W. M. Lee, F. A., and Gwinn, J. L.: Normal lateral deviation of the trachea in infants and children. A.J.R. *109:* 247, 1970.

Chesterman, J. T., and Satsangi, P. N.: Rupture of the trachea and bronchi by closed injury. Thorax *21:* 21, 1966.

Cleveland, R. H., Nice, C. M., Jr., and Ziskind, J.: Primary adenoid cystic carcinoma (cylindroma) of the trachea. Radiology *122:* 597, 1977.

Comer, J. V., and Farrell, J. T.: Complete rupture of the left main bronchus with successful repair. J.A.M.A. *196:* 184, 1966.

Cook, A. J., Weinstein, M., and Powell, R. D.: Diffuse amyloidosis of the tracheobronchial tree. Bronchographic manifestations. Radiology *107:* 303, 1973.

Davis, C. M.: Inhaled foreign bodies in children. Arch. Dis. Child. *41:* 402, 1966.

Domm, B. M., Vassallo, C. L., and Adams, C. L.: Amyloid deposition localized to the lower respiratory tract. Am. J. Med. *38:* 151, 1965.

Dowling, E. A., Miller, R. E., Johnson, I. M., and Collier, F. C. D.: Mucoepidermoid tumors of the bronchi. Surgery *52:* 600, 1962.

Dunbar, J. S.: Upper respiratory tract obstruction in infants and children. Caldwell Lecture. A.J.R. *109:* 227, 1970.

Eijgelaar, A., and Homan van der Heide, J. N.: A reliable early symptom of bronchial or tracheal rupture. Thorax *25:* 120, 1970.

Feist, J. H., Johnson, T. H., and Wilson, R. J.: Acquired tracheomalacia: etiology and differential diagnosis. Chest *68:* 340, 1975.

Fiser, F., Tomanek, A., Rimanova, V., and Sedivy, V.: Tracheobronchomegaly. Scand. J. Respir. Dis. *50:* 147, 1969.

Fleischner, F. G.: The pathogenesis of bronchiectasis. A roentgen contribution. Radiology 53: 818, 1949.

Fraser, R. G., Fraser, R. S., Renner, J. W., Bernard, C., and Fitzgerald, P. J.: The roentgenologic diagnosis of chronic bronchitis: a reassessment with emphasis on parahilar bronchi seen end-on. Radiology *120:* 1, 1976.

Friedman, P. J., and Hellekant, C. A. G.: Radiologic recognition of bronchopleural fistula. Radiology *124:* 289, 1977.

Giovanniello, J., Grieco, R. V., and Bartone, N. F.: Laryngocele. A.J.R. *108:* 825, 1970.

Giustra, P. E., and Stassa, G.: The multiple presentations of bronchial adenomas. Radiology *93:* 1013, 1969.

Gosink, B., Friedman, P. J., and Liebow, A. A.: Bronchiolitis obliterans. A.J.R. *117:* 816, 1973.

Gregg, I., and Trapnell, D. H.: The bronchographic appearances of early chronic bronchitis. Br. J. Radiol. *42:* 132, 1969.

Harris, J. H., Jr.: The clinical significance of the tracheal bronchus. A.J.R. *79:* 228, 1958.

Hodson, M. E., Simon, G., and Batten, J. C.: Radiology of uncomplicated asthma. Thorax *29:* 296, 1974.

Holt, J. F., Haight, C., and Hodges, F. J.: Congenital atresia of the esophagus and tracheo-esophageal fistula. Radiology *47:* 457, 1946.

Howland, W. J., and Good, C. A.: The radiographic features of tracheopathia osteoplastica. Radiology *71:* 847, 1958.

Hungerford, G. D., Williams, H. B. L., and Gandevia, B.: Bronchial walls in the radiological diagnosis of asthma. Br. J. Radiol. *50:* 783, 1977.

Hutchin, P., and Lindskog, G. E.: Acquired esophagobronchial fistula of infectious origin. J. Thorac. Cardiovasc. Surg. *48:* 1, 1964.

Janower, M. L., Grillo, H. C., MacMillan, A. S., Jr., and James, A. E., Jr.: The radiological appearance of carcinoma of the trachea. Radiology *96:* 39, 1970.

Johnston, R. F., and Green, R. A.: Tracheobronchiomegaly. Am. Rev. Respir. Dis. *91:* 35, 1965.

Kamberg, S., Loitman, B. S., and Holtz, S.: Amyloidosis of the tracheobronchial tree. N. Engl. J. Med. *266:* 587, 1962.

Katz, I., Levine, M., and Herman, P.: Tracheobronchiomegaly. The Mounier-Kuhn syndrome. A.J.R. *88:* 1084, 1962.

Kaufman, G., and Klopstock, R.: Papillomatosis of the respiratory tract. Am.

Rev. Respir. Dis. *88:* 839, 1963.

Kushner, D. C., and Harris, G. B. C.: Obstructing lesions of the larynx and trachea in infants and children. Radiol. Clin. North Am. *16:* 181, 1978.

Landing, B. H., Lawrence, T-Y. K., Payne, V. C., and Wells, T. R.: Bronchial anatomy in syndromes with abnormal visceral situs, abnormal spleen and congenital heart disease. Am. J. Cardiol. *28:* 457, 1971.

Lemire, P., Trepanier, A., and Herbert, G.: Bronchocele and blocked bronchiectasis. A.J.R. *110:* 687, 1970.

Liebow, A.: Tumors of the lower respiratory tract. In *Atlas of Tumor Pathology*, Sect. 5, Fascicle 17. Armed Forces Institute of Pathology, Washington, D. C., 1952.

Linton, J. S. A.: Long-standing intrabronchial foreign bodies. Thorax *12:* 164, 1957.

Mangiulea, V. G., and Stinghe, R. V.: The accessory cardiac bronchus. Dis. Chest *54:* 35, 1968.

Margolin, H. N., Rosenberg, L. S., Felson, B., and Baum, G.: Idiopathic unilateral hyperlucent lung: a roentgenologic syndrome. A.J.R. *82:* 63, 1959.

Meckstroth, C. V., Davidson, H, B., and Kress, G. O.: Muco-epidermoid tumor of the bronchus. Dis. Chest *40:* 652, 1961.

Morgan, A. D., and Bogomoletz, W.: Mucoid impaction of the bronchi in relation to asthma and plastic bronchitis. Thorax *23:* 356, 1968.

Neuhauser, E. B. D.: Tracheoesophageal constriction produced by right aortic arch and left ligamentum arteriosum. A.J.R. *62:* 493, 1949.

Ogilvie, A. G.: Bronchography in chronic bronchitis. Thorax *30:* 631, 1975.

Ozlu, C., Christopherson, W. M., and Allen, J. D., Jr.: Muco-epidermoid tumor of the bronchus. J. Thorac. Surg. *42:* 24, 1958.

Papamichael, E. E., and Fotiou, G.: Rupture of the thoracic trachea with avulsion of the apex of the right upper lobe. J. Thorac. Cardiovasc. Surg. *50:* 742, 1965.

Partridge, J. B., Scott, O., Deverall, P. B., and Macartney, F. J.: Visualization and measurement of the main bronchi by tomography as an objective indicator of thoracic situs in congenital heart disease. Circulation *51:* 189, 1975.

Polin, S. G., and Spiegel, P.: Rupture of a segmental bronchus. Ann. Thorac. Surg. *6:* 384, 1968.

Prowse, C. B., and Elliott, R. I. K.: Diffuse tracheo-bronchial amyloidosis: a rare variant of a protean disease. Thorax *18:* 326, 1963.

Rees, D. O., and Ruttley, M. S. T.: The bronchocele in bronchial neoplasm.

Clin. Radiol. *21:* 62, 1970.

Reichle, F. A., and Rosemond, G. P.: Mucoepidermoid tumors of the bronchus. J. Thorac. Cardiovasc. Surg. *51:* 443, 1966.

Reid, L., and Simon, G.: Pathological findings and radiological changes in chronic bronchitis and emphysema. Br. J. Radiol. *32:* 291, 1959.

Riggs, W., Jr.: Congenital tracheoesophageal fistula without esophageal atresia. South. Med. J. *62:* 135, 1969.

Robinson, A. E., and Campbell, J. B.: Bronchography in childhood asthma. A.J.R. *116:* 559, 1972.

Rowlands, D. T.: Fibroepithelial polyps of the bronchus. Dis. Chest *37:* 199, 1960.

Sakula, A.: Tracheobronchopathia osteoplastica. Its relationship to primary tracheobronchial amyloidosis. Thorax *23:* 105, 1968.

Samuels, M. L., Howe, C. D., Dodd, G. D., Jr., Fuller, L. M., Shullenberger, C. C., and Leary, W. L.: Endobronchial malignant lymphoma. A.J.R. *85:* 87, 1961.

Secrest, P. G., Kendig, T. A., and Beland, A. J.: Tracheobronchopathia osteochondroplastica. Am. J. Med. *36:* 815, 1964.

Sibala, J.: Endobronchial hamartoma. Chest *62:* 631, 1972.

Simon, G., Connolly, N., Littlejohns, D. W., and McAllen, M.: Radiological abnormalities in children with asthma and their relation to the clinical findings and some respiratory function tests. Thorax *28:* 115, 1973.

Slovis, T. L., Haller, J. O., Berdon, W. E., Baker, D. H., and Joseph, P. M.: Noninvasive visualization of the pediatric airway. Curr. Probl. Diagn. Radiol. *8:* 6, 1979.

Smith, W. G., and Clark, F. J.: Mucoid impaction of the bronchi. Australas. Ann. Med. *13:* 40, 1964.

Symgas, P. N., Logan, W. D., Jr., and Vakil, H. C.: Granular cell myoblastoma of the bronchus. Ann. Thorac. Surg. *9:* 136, 1970.

Talner, L. B., Gmelich, J. T., Liebow, A. A., and Greenspan, R. H.: The syndrome of bronchial mucocele and regional hyperinflation of the lung. A.J.R. *110:* 675, 1970.

Templeton, A. W., Moffat, R., and Nelson, D.: Bronchography and bronchial adenoma. Chest *59:* 59, 1971.

Urschel, H. C., Jr., Paulson, D. L., and Shaw, R. R.: Mucoid impaction of the bronchi. Ann. Thorac. Surg. *2:* 1, 1966.

Way, S. P. B.: Tracheopathia osteoplastica. J. Clin. Pathol. *20:* 814, 1967.

Webb, W. R., and Hare, W. V.: Primary fibrosarcoma of the bronchus. Am. Rev. Respir. Dis. *84:* 881, 1961.

Weber, A. L., and Grillo, H. C.: Tracheal

tumors. A radiological, clinical and pathological evaluation of 84 cases, Radiol. Clin. North Am. *16:* 227, 1978.

Wilson, W.: Mucoid impaction of the bronchi. Br. J. Radiol. *37:* 590, 1964.

Zack, B. J., and Owens, M. P.: Congenital tracheoesophageal fistula in adult. Arch. Surg. *95:* 674, 1967.

DISEASES OF THE LUNGS

Felson, B.: Acute miliary diseases of the lung. Radiology *59:* 32, 1952.

Felson, B.: Some special signs in chest roentgenology. In *Roentgenology of the Chest,* edited by C. B. Rabin. Charles C Thomas, Springfield, Ill., 1958.

Felson, B., and Felson, H.: Localization of intrathoracic lesions by means of the posteroanterior roentgenogram. Radiology *55:* 363, 1950.

Felson, H., and Heublein, G. W.: Some observations on diffuse pulmonary lesions. A.J.R. *59:* 59, 1948.

Fleischner, F.: Uber das Wesen der basalen horizontalen Schattenstreifen im Lungenfeld. Wien. Arch. Inn. Med. *28:* 461, 1936.

Jacobaeus. H. C., and Westermark, N.: Contribution to interpretation of localized roentgen opacities in neighborhood of interlobar fissures of lung. Acta Chir. Scand. *71:* 494, 1932.

Leigh, T. F., and Hopkins, W. A.: Roentgenographic findings in lesions of the lingula. Radiology *57:* 293, 1951.

Longuet, R., Phelan, J., Tanous, H., and Bushong, S.: Criteria of the silhouette sign. Radiology *122:* 581, 1977.

Marks, J. L., and Nathan, A.: The linear atelectasis sign in intra-abdominal lesions. Radiology *52:* 363, 1949.

Nemec, S. S.: Differential diagnosis of retrocardiac shadows. Radiology *50:* 174, 1948.

Richards, G. E.: Interpretation of triangular basal shadows in roentgenograms of chest. A.J.R. *30:* 289, 1933.

Rigler, L. G.: The density of the central shadow in the diagnosis of intrathoracic lesions. Radiology *32:* 316, 1939.

Webb, W. R.: The pleural tail sign. Radiology *127:* 309, 1979.

Westfall, R. E.: Obliteration of segmental pulmonary artery borders: a method of localizing right lower lobe infiltrates. Chest *56:* 305, 1969.

Anomalies

Apthorp, G. H., and Bates, D. V.: Report of a case of pulmonary telangiectasia. Thorax *12:* 65, 1957.

Atwell, S. W.: Major anomalies of the tracheobronchial tree. Dis. Chest *52:* 611, 1967.

Bartram, C., and Strickland, B.: Pulmonary varices. Br. J. Radiol. *44:* 927, 1971.

Bateson, E. M.: Relationship between intrapulmonary and endobronchial cartilage-containing tumours (so-called hamartomata). Thorax *20:* 447, 1965.

Bateson, E. M.: An analysis of 155 solitary lung lesions illustrating the differential diagnosis of mixed tumours of the lung. Clin. Radiol. *41:* 51, 1965.

Bateson, E. M., and Abbott, E. K.: mixed tumors of the lung, or hamartochondromas. Clin Radiol. *11:* 232, 1960.

Benfield, J. R., Gots, R. E., and Mills, D.: Anomalous single left pulmonary vein mimicking a parenchymal nodule. Chest *59:* 101, 1971.

Berman, E. J.: Extralobar (diaphragmatic) sequestration of the lung. Arch. Surg. *76:* 724, 1958.

Bleyer, J. M., and Marks, J. H.: Tuberculomas and hamartomas of the lung. Comparative study of 66 proved cases. A.J.R. *77:* 1013, 1957.

Booth, J. B., and Berry, C. L.: Unilateral pulmonary agenesis. Arch. Dis. Child. *42:* 361, 1967.

Borrie, J., Lichter, I., and Rodda, R. A.: Interlobar pulmonary sequestration. Br. J. Surg. *50:* 623, 1963.

Bragg, E. A., and Levene, G.: Hamartoma of the lung. Radiology *54:* 227, 1950.

Bronsther, B., Coryllos, E., Epstein, B., and Abrams, M. W.: Lung hernias in children. Pediatr. Surg. *3:* 544, 1968.

Bruwer, A. J.: Posteroanterior chest roentgenogram in two types of anomalous pulmonary venous connection. J. Thorac. Surg. *32:* 119, 1956.

Bruwer, A. J., Clagett. O. T., and McDonald, J. R.: Intralobar pulmonary sequestration. A.J.R. *71:* 751, 1954.

Butler, C., II, and Kleinerman, J.: Pulmonary hamartoma. Arch. Pathol. *88:* 584, 1969.

Capitanio, M. A., Ramos, R., and Kirkpatrick, J. A.: Pulmonary sling. Roentgen observations. A.J.R. *112:* 28, 1971.

Carter, R.: Pulmonary sequestration. Collective review. Ann. Thorac. Surg. *7:* 68, 1969.

Dawson, J.: Pulmonary tuberous sclerosis. Q. J. Med. *23:* 113, 1954.

Ellis, F. H., Jr., McGoon, D. C., and Kincaid, O. W.: Congenital vascular malformations of the lungs. Med. Clin. North Am. *48:* 1069, 1964.

Field, C. E.: Pulmonary agenesis and hypoplasia. Arch. Dis. Child. *21:* 61, 1946.

Gerle, R. D., Jaretzki, A., III, Ashley, C. A., and Berne, A. S.: Congenital bronchopulmonary-foregut malformation. Pulmonary sequestration communicating with the gastrointestinal tract. N. Engl. J. Med. *278:* 1413, 1968.

Gomes, M. R., Bernatz, P. E., and Dines, D. E.: Pulmonary arteriovenous fistulas. Ann. Thorac. Surg. *7:* 582, 1969.

Green, G. J.: The radiology of tuberose sclerosis. Clin. Radiol. *19:* 135, 1968.

Gruenfeld, G. E., and Gray, S. H.: Malformations of the lung. Arch. Pathol. *31:* 392, 1941.

Gudjberg, C. E.: Pulmonary hamartoma. A.J.R. *86:* 842, 1961.

Jaffe, R. B., and Condon, V. R.: Mycotic aneurysms of the pulmonary artery and aorta. Radiology *116:* 291, 1975.

Jensen, K. G., and Schidt, T.: Growth conditions of hamartoma of the lung: a study based on 22 cases operated on after radiographic observation for from one to 18 years. Thorax *13:* 233, 1958.

Jue, K. L., Ragh, B. G., Amplatz, K., Adams, P., Jr., and Edwards, J. E.: Anomalous origin of the left pulmonary artery from the right pulmonary artery. A.J.R. *95:* 598, 1965.

Kiely, B., Filler, J., Stone, S., and Doyle, E. F.: Syndrome of anomalous venous drainage of the right lung to the inferior vena cava. A review of 67 reported cases and three new cases in children. Am. J. Cardiol. *20:* 102, 1967.

Kilman, J. W., Battersby, J. S., Taybi, H., and Vellios, F.: Pulmonary sequestration. Arch. Surg. *90:* 648, 1965.

Levin, B., and White, H.: Total anomalous pulmonary venous drainage into the portal system. Radiology *76:* 894, 1961.

LeRoux, B. T.: Intralobar pulmonary sequestration. Thorax *17:* 77, 1962.

Lindgren, E.: Roentgen diagnosis of arteriovenous aneurysm of the lung. Acta Radiol. *27:* 585, 1946.

MacDonald, J. R., Harrington, S. W., and Clagett, O. T.: Hamartoma of the lung. J. Thorac. Surg. *14:* 128, 1945.

Madani, M. A., Dafoe, C. S., and Ross, C. A.: Multiple hamartomata of the lung. Thorax *21:* 468, 1966.

Mathey, J., Galey, J. J., Logeais, Y., Santoro, E., Vanetti, A., Maurel, A., and Wurflein, R.: Anomalous pulmonary venous return into inferior vena cava and associated bronchovascular anomalies (the scimitar syndrome). Thorax *23:* 398, 1968.

Milledge, R. D., Gerald, B. E., and Carter, W. J.: Pulmonary manifestations of tuberous sclerosis. A.J.R. *98:* 734, 1966.

Miller, R. D., and Divertie, M. B.: Kartagener's syndrome. Chest *62:* 130, 1972.

Newman, R. W., Tarasidis, G., and Chai, H. C.: Congenital absence or hypoplasia of pulmonary artery. J. Thorac. Cardiovasc. Surg. *47:* 740, 1964.

Nielsen, P. B.: Intralobar bronchopulmonary sequestration. A.J.R. *92:* 547,

1964.

Philip. T., Sumerling, M. D., Fleming, J., and Grainger, R. G.: Aberrant left pulmonary artery. Clin. Radiol. 23: 153, 1972.

Poirier, T. J., and Van Ordstrand, H. S.: Pulmonary chondromatous hamartomas. Report of seventeen cases and review of the literature. Chest 59: 50, 1971.

Ranniger, K., and Valvasorri, G. E.: Angiographic diagnosis of intralobar pulmonary sequestration. A.J.R. 92: 540, 1964.

Remy, J., Marache, P., Duplouy, E., and Dupuis, C.: Agenesies aplasies et hypoplasies lobaires. A propos de cinq observations. J. Radiol. Electrol. 57: 197, 1976.

Roehm, J. O. F., Jr., Jue, K. L., and Amplatz, K.: Radiographic features of the scimitar syndrome. Radiology 86: 856, 1966.

Rowen, M., Thompson, J. R., Williamson, R. A., and Wood, B. J.: Diffuse pulmonary hemangiomatosis. Radiology 127: 445, 1978.

Saegesser, F., and Besson, A.: Extralobar and intralobar pulmonary sequestrations of the upper and lower lobes. Chest 63: 69, 1973.

Sammons, B. P.: Arteriovenous fistula of the lung. Radiology 72: 710, 1959.

Sanger, P. W., Taylor, F. H., and Robicsek, F.: The "scimitar syndrome." Diagnosis and treatment. Arch. Surg. 86: 580, 1963.

Sargent, E. N., Barnes, R. A., and Schwinn, C. P.: Multiple pulmonary fibroleiomyomatous hamartomas. A.J.R. 110: 694, 1970.

Savic, B., Birtel, F. J., Tholen, W., Funke, H. D., and Knoche, R.: Lung sequestration: report of seven cases and review of 540 published cases. Thorax 34: 96, 1979.

Sluiter-Eringa, H., Orie, N. G. M., and Sluiter, H. J.: Pulmonary arteriovenous fistula. Am. Rev. Respir. Dis. 100: 177, 1969.

Smith, R. A.: A theory of the origin of intralobar sequestration of lung. Thorax 11: 10, 1956.

Smith, R. A., and Beck, A. O.: Agenesis of the lung. Thorax 13: 38, 1958.

Soulen, R. L., and Cohen, R. V.: Plain film recognition of pulmonary agenesis in the adult. Chest 60: 185, 1971.

Stork, W. J.: Pulmonary arteriovenous fistulas. A.J.R. 74: 441, 1955.

Stovin, P. G. I., Lum, L. C., Flower, C. D. R., Darke, C. S., and Beeley, M.: The lungs in lymphangiomyomatosis and in tuberous sclerosis. Thorax 30: 497, 1975.

Symbas, P. N., Hatcher, C. R. Jr., Abbot, O. A., and Logan, W. D., Jr.: An appraisal of pulmonary sequestration: special emphasis on unusual manifestations. Am. Rev. Respir. Dis. 99: 406, 1969.

Wagenvoort, C. A.: Pulmonary veno-occlusive disease. Entity or syndrome? Chest 69: 82, 1976.

Zelefsky, M. N., Janis, M., Bernstein, R., Blatt, C., Lin, A., and Meng, C-H.: Intralobar bronchopulmonary sequestration with bronchial communication. Chest 59: 266, 1971.

Pneumonia

Bell, R. S.: The radiographic manifestations of α_1-antitrypsin deficiency. Radiology 95: 19, 1970.

Benjamin, B., and Childe, A. E.: Localized bullous emphysema associated with pneumonia in children. J. Pediatr. 15: 621, 1939.

Blank, N., and Castellino, R. A.: The diagnosis of pulmonary infection in patients with altered immunity. Semin. Roentgenol. 10: 63, 1975.

Bragg, D. G., and Janis, B.: The roentgenographic manifestations of pulmonary opportunistic infections. A.J.R. 117: 798, 1973.

Felson, B., Jones, G. F., and Ulrich, R. P.: Roentgenologic aspects of diffuse miliary granulomatous pneumonitis of unknown etiology. A.J.R. 64: 740, 1950.

Ferguson, T. B., and Burford, T. H.: The changing pattern of pulmonary suppuration: surgical implications. Dis. Chest 55: 396, 1968.

Goodwin, T. C.: Lipoid cell pneumonia. Am. J. Dis. Child. 48: 309, 1934.

Graeser, J. B., Wu, C., and Robertson, O. H.: Physical signs and roentgenographic findings in lobar pneumonia in adults. Arch. Intern. Med. 53: 249, 1934.

Neuhof, H., and Thomas, A.: Acute suppurative bronchopneumonia. Arch. Intern. Med. 75: 45, 1945.

Neuhof, H., and Touroff, A. S.: Acute aerobic (nonputrid) abscess of lung. Surgery 4: 728, 1938.

Rabin, C. B.: Roentgen features of suppurative bronchopneumonia. J. Mt. Sinai Hosp. 8: 32, 1941.

Robbins, L. L., and Sniffen, R. C.: Correlation between the roentgenologic and pathologic findings in chronic pneumonitis of the cholesterol type. Radiology 53: 187, 1949.

Sodeman, W. A., and Stuart, B. M.: Lipoid pneumonia in adults. Ann. Intern. Med. 24: 241, 1946.

Sutcliffe, J., and Chrispin, A. R.: Chronic granulomatous disease. Br. J. Radiol. 43: 110, 1970.

Townley, R. G., Ryning, F., Lynch, H., and Brody, A. W.: Obstructive lung disease in hereditary α_1-antitrypsin deficiency. J.A.M.A. 214: 325, 1970.

Ude, W. H.: Roentogenologic studies in early lobar pneumonia. A.J.R. 26: 691, 1931.

Specific Infections of the Lungs

Baar, H. S., and Galindo, J.: Ossifying pulmonary granulomatosis due to larvae of ascaris. J. Clin. Pathol. 18: 737, 1965.

Bakir, F.: Serious complications of hydatid cyst of the lung. Am. Rev. Respir. Dis. 96: 483, 1967.

Balikian, J. P., Herman, P. G., and Kopit, S.: Pulmonary nocardiosis. Radiology 126: 569, 1978.

Bank, Y. W.: Pulmonary paragonimiasis as a cause of Loeffler's syndrome. Radiology 78: 598, 1962.

Barnhard, H. J., and Kniker, W. J.: Roentgenologic findings in pertussis with particular emphasis on the "shaggy heart" sign. A.J.R. 84: 445, 1960.

Bartrum, R. J., Jr., Watnick, M., and Herman, P. G.: Roentgenographic findings in pulmonary mucormycosis. A.J.R. 117: 810, 1973.

Bass, H. E., Schomer, A., and Berke, R.: Coccidioidomycosis; persistence of residual pulmonary lesions. Arch. Intern. Med. 82: 519, 1948.

Bates, M., and Cruickshank, G.: Thoracic actinomycosis. Thorax 12: 99, 1957.

Baum, G. L., and Schwartz, J.: North American blastomycosis. Am. J. Med. Sci. 238: 661, 1959.

Berk, J. E., Woodruff, M. T., and Frediani, A. W.: Pulmonary and intestinal changes in strongyloidiasis. Gastroenterology 1: 1100, 1943.

de Bernardi, E.: Pulmonary hydatid disease in man. Acta Radiol. 36: 236, 1951.

Bihss, F. E., and Berland, H. I.: Roentgenological manifestations of pleuropulmonary involvement in tularemia. Radiology 41: 431, 1943.

Bonakdarpour, A.: Echinococcus disease. Report of 112 cases from Iran and a review of 611 cases from the United States. A.J.R. 99: 660, 1967.

Bonmati, J., Rogers, J. V., Jr., and Hopkins, W. A.: Pulmonary cryptococcosis. Radiology 66: 188, 1956.

Bonoff, C. P.: Acute primary pulmonary blastomycosis. Radiology 54: 157, 1950.

Bothen, N. F.: The roentgen picture in cases of lung mycosis. Acta Radiol. 36: 35, 1951.

Braatelien, N. T., and Perlmutter, H. M.: Aspergillosis of the lung. Dis. Chest 39: 425, 1961.

Cameron, D. C., Borthwick, R. N., and Philp, T.: The radiographic patterns of acute mycoplasma pneumonitis. Clin. Radiol. 28: 173, 1977.

Castellino, R. A., and Blank, N.: Pulmonary coccidioidomycosis. The wide spectrum of roentgenographic manifestations. Calif. Med. *109:* 41, 1968.

Chartres, J. C.: Radiological manifestations of parasitism by the tongue worms, flat worms and the round worms more commonly seen in the tropics. Br. J. Radiol. *38:* 503, 1965.

Christoforidis, A. J.: Radiologic manifestations of histoplasmosis. A.J.R. *109:* 478, 1970.

Clark, D., and Gilmore, J. H.: Study of 100 cases with positive coccidioidin skin test. Ann. Intern. Med. *24:* 40, 1946.

Cohen, A. A., Davis, A., and Finegold, S. M.: Chronic pulmonary cryptococcosis. Am. Rev. Respir. Dis. *91:* 414, 1965.

Colburn, J. R.: Roentgenological types of pulmonary lesions in primary coccidioidomycosis. A.J.R. *51:* 1, 1944.

Comstock, C., and Wolfson, A. H.: Roentgenology of sporotrichosis. A.J.R. *125:* 651, 1975.

Connell, J. F., Jr., and Muhm, J. R.: Radiographic manifestations of pulmonary histoplasmosis: a 10 year review. Radiology *121:* 281, 1976.

Cush, R., Light, R. W., and George, R. B.: Clinical and roentgenographic manifestations of acute and chronic blastomycosis. Chest *69:* 345, 1976.

Danaraj, T. J.: Pathologic studies in eosinophilic lung (tropical eosinophilia). Arch. Pathol. *67:* 515, 1959.

Dennis, J. M., and Boudreau, J. P.: Pleuropulmonary tularemia: its roentgen manifestations. Radiology *68:* 25, 1957.

Druckmann, A.: X-ray study of development of pulmonary echinococcus. Radiology *14:* 209, 1945.

Dziadiw, R., Kinkhabwala, M., and Rabinowitz, J. G.: Pulmonary gumma. Radiology *103:* 59, 1972.

Edge, J. R., Stansfield, D., and Fletcher, D. E.: Pulmonary aspergillosis in an unselected hospital population. Chest *59:* 407, 1971.

Endress, Z. F., and Schnell, F. R.: Varicella pneumonitis. Radiology *66:* 723, 1956.

Evers, R. H., and Whereatt, R. R.: Pulmonary sporotrichosis. Chest *66:* 91, 1974.

Falkenbach, K. H., Bachmann, K. D., and O'Loughlin, B. J.: *Pneumocystis carinii* pneumonia. A.J.R. *85:* 706, 1961.

Fawcitt, J., and Parry, H. E.: Lung changes in pertussis and measles in childhood. A review of 1894 cases with a follow-up study of the pulmonary complications. Br. J. Radiol. *30:* 76, 1957.

Felson, B., Rosenberg, L. S., and Hamburger, M., Jr.: Roentgen findings in acute Friedlander's pneumonia. Radiology *53:* 559, 1949.

Flynn, M. W., and Felson, B.: The roentgen manifestations of thoracic actinomycosis. A.J.R. *110:* 707, 1970.

Forrest, J. V.: Radiographic findings in pneumocystis carinii pneumonia. Radiology *103:* 539, 1972.

Freedman, E., and Higley, C. S.: Syphilitic gumma of lung. A.J.R. *31:* 333, 1934.

Gershwin, L. J., Gershwin, M. E., and Kritzman, J.: Human pulmonary dirofilariasis. Chest *66:* 92, 1974.

Goodwin, R. A., Jr., and Des Prez, R. M.: Histoplasmosis. Am. Rev. Respir. Dis. *117:* 929, 1978.

Goodwin, R. A., Jr., Snell, J. D., Hubbard, W. W., and Terry, R. T.: Early chronic pulmonary histoplasmosis. Am. Rev. Respir. Dis. *93:* 47, 1966.

Goodwin, R. A., Jr., and Snell, J. D., Jr.: The enlarging histoplasmoma. Am. Rev. Respir. Dis. *100:* 1, 1969.

Greendyke, W. H., Resnick, D. L., and Harvey, W. C.: The varied roentgen manifestations of pulmonary coccidioidomycosis. A.J.R. *109:* 491, 1970.

Greening, R. R., and Menville, L. J.: Roentgen findings in torulosis. Radiology *48:* 381, 1947.

Grossman, C. B., Bragg, D. G., and Armstrong, D.: Roentgen manifestations of pulmonary nocardiosis. Radiology *96:* 325, 1970.

Guha, P. K., and Thompson, J. R.: Acute pulmonary blastomycosis. A diagnostic challenge in a tuberculosis sanitorium. Am. Rev. Respir. Dis. *86:* 640, 1962.

Hammer, H.: Ueber Lungensyphilis. Röntgenpraxis *3:* 301, 1931.

Harrison, B. B.: Influenza pneumonia—recent experiences. Br. J. Radiol. *34:* 392, 1951.

Harrison, E. G., Jr., and Thompson, J. H., Jr.: Dirofilariasis of the human lung. Am. J. Clin. Pathol. *43:* 224, 1965.

Hawley, C., and Felson, B.: Roentgen aspects of intrathoracic blastomycosis. A.J.R. *75:* 751, 1956.

Hawkins, J. A.: Cavitary pulmonary cryptococcosis. Am. Rev. Respir. Dis. *84:* 579, 1961.

Hebert, D. H.: The roentgen features of Eaton agent pneumonia. A.J.R. *98:* 300, 1966.

Herlinger, H.: Pulmonary changes in tropical eosinophilia. Br. J. Radiol. *36:* 889, 1963.

Herrera-Llerandi, R.: Thoracic repercussions of amebiasis. J. Thorac. Cardiovasc. Surg. *52:* 361, 1966.

Hodes, P. J., and Wood, F. C.: Eosinophilic lung (tropical eosinophilia). Am. J. Med. Sci. *210:* 288, 1945.

Hoeprich, P. D., Ward, J. R., and Schmidt, A. M.: Report of serologically proved case of Q fever in Utah. J.A.M.A. *170:* 180, 1959.

Holmes, R. B.: Friedlander's pneumonia. A.J.R. *75:* 728, 1956.

Holt, J. F.: Roentgenologic pulmonary manifestations of fatal histoplasmosis. A.J.R. *58:* 717, 1947.

Houk, V. N., and Moser, K. M.: Pulmonary cryptococcosis. Ann. Intern. Med. *63:* 583, 1965.

Ivie, J. McK.: Roentgenological observations on pleuropulmonary tularemia. A.J.R. *74:* 466, 1955.

Jacobs, L. G.: Pulmonary torulosis. Radiology *71:* 398, 1958.

Jacobson, G., Denlinger, R. B., and Carter, R. A.: Roentgen manifestations of Q fever. Radiology *53:* 739, 1949.

James, A. E., Dixon, G. D., and Johnson. H. F.: Melioidosis: a correlation of the radiologic and pathologic findings. Radiology *89:* 230, 1967.

Jamison, H. W., and Carter, R. A.: The roentgen findings in early coccidioidomycosis. Radiology *48:* 323, 1947.

Kegel, R. F. C., and Fatemi, A.: The ruptured pulmonary hydatid cyst. Radiology *76:* 60, 1961.

Kennedy, W. P. U., Malone, D. N., and Blyth, W.: Necrotizing pulmonary aspergillosis. Thorax *25:* 691, 1970.

Kevy, S. V., and Lowe, B. A.: Streptococcal pneumonia and empyema in childhood. N. Engl. J. Med. *264:* 738, 1961.

Laskey, W., and Sarosi, G. A.: The radiological appearance of pulmonary blastomycosis. Radiology *126:* 351, 1978.

Levin, E. J.: Pulmonary intracavitary fungus ball. Radiology *66:* 9, 1956.

Louria, D. B., Blumenfeld, H. L., Ellis, J. T., Kilbourne, E. D., and Rogers, D. E.: Studies on influenza in pandemic of 1956–58; II. Pulmonary complications of influenza. J. Clin. Invest. *38:* 213, 1959.

Mainzer, F.: On latent pulmonary disease revealed by x-ray in intestinal bilharziasis (*Schistosoma mansoni*). Puerto Rico J. Public Health Trop. Med. *15:* 111, 1939.

Malo, J. L., Pepys, J., and Simon, G.: Studies in chronic allergic bronchopulmonary aspergillosis; 2. Radiological findings. Thorax *32:* 262, 1977.

McBride, R., Corson, J., and Dammin, G.: Mucormycosis. Am. J. Med. *28:* 832, 1960.

McCarthy, D. S., Simon, G., and Hargreave, F. F.: The radiological appearances in allergic bronchopulmonary aspergillosis. Clin. Radiol. *21:* 366, 1970.

McIntyre, M. D.: Pulmonary syphilis. Arch. Pathol. *11:* 258, 1931.

Menon, N. K.: Roentgenographic appearances in hepatopulmonary amebiasis. Dis. Chest *46:* 219, 1964.

Meyers, H. I., and Jacobson, G.: Staphylococcal pneumonia in children and adults. Radiology 72: 665, 1959.

Miller, F. L., and Walker, R.: The roentgen characteristics of pulmonary paragonimiasis. Radiology 65: 231, 1955.

Mintzer, R. A., Rogers, L. F., Kruglik, G. D., Rosenberg, M., Neiman, H. L., and Patterson, R.: The spectrum of radiologic findings in allergic bronchopulmonary aspergillosis. Radiology 127: 301, 1978.

Navarette, A. R.: Pulmonary dirofilariasis. Chest 61: 51, 1972.

Newcombe, C. P., Nixon, P. G. F., and Thompson, H.: Influenzal pneumonia in mitral stenosis. Acta Med. Scand. 162: 441, 1958.

Ogakwu, M., and Nwokolo, C.: Radiological findings in pulmonary paragonimiasis as seen in Nigeria: a review based on one hundred cases. Br. J. Radiol. 46: 699, 1973.

O'Neill, R. P., and Penman, R. W. B.: Clinical aspects of blastomycosis. Thorax 25: 708, 1970.

Osborne, D.: Radiologic appearance of viral disease of the lower respiratory tract in infants and children. A.J.R. 130: 29, 1978.

Overholt, E. L., and Tigertt, W. D.: Roentgenographic manifestations of pulmonary tularemia. Radiology 74: 758, 1960.

Peterson, E., Spalding, O. B., and Wildman, O.: Psittacosis, clinical and roentgenological study of seven cases, with postmortem observations in one case. J.A.M.A. 95: 171, 1930.

Poh, S. C., and Soh, C. S.: Lung manifestations in leptospirosis. Thorax 25: 751, 1970.

Prioleau, W. H., Parker, E. F., Bradham, R. R., and Gregorie, H. B., Jr.: Dirofilaria immitis (dog heartworm) as a pulmonary lesion in humans. Ann. Thorac. Surg. 21: 382, 1976.

Rabin, C. B., and Janowitz, H. D.: Actinomyces in putrid empyema. J. Thorac. Surg. 19: 335, 1950.

Rabinowitz, J. G., Busch, J., and Buttram, W. R.: Pulmonary manifestations of blastomycosis. Radiology 120: 25, 1976.

Raider, L.: Calcification in chicken pox pneumonia. Chest 60: 504, 1971.

Ramah, S. J., Chomet, B., McLean, J., and Lemke, C.: Pulmonary granuloma due to brucellosis. J.A.M.A. 170: 1665, 1959.

Ramos, L., Hernandez-Mora, M., Illanas, M., Llorente, M. T., and Marcos, J.: Radiological characteristics of perforated pulmonary hydatid cysts. Radiology 116: 539, 1975.

Ramsay, G. C., and Meyer, R. D.: Cavitary fungus disease of the lungs. Radiology 109: 29, 1973.

Renner, R., Coccaro, A. P., Heitzman, E. R., Dailey, E. T., and Markarian, B.:

Pseudomonas pneumonia: a prototype of hospital-based infection. Radiology 105: 555, 1972.

Ritvo, M., and Martin, F.: The clinical and roentgen manifestations of pneumonia due to Bacillus mucosus capsularus (primary Friedlander pneumonia). A.J.R. 62: 211, 1949.

Robbins, J. B.: Pneumocystis carinii pneumonitis: a review. Pediatr. Res. 1: 131, 1967.

Rodriguez, H. F., Fernandez-Duran, A., Garcia-Moliner, L., and Rivera, E.: Cardiopulmonary schistosomiasis. Am. Heart J. 65: 253, 1963.

Rosen, B.: Ornithosis as an occupational hazard. Radiology 65: 373, 1955.

Rubin, H., Furcolow, M. L., Yates, J. L., and Brasher, C. A.: The course and prognosis of histoplasmosis. Am. J. Med. 27: 278, 1959.

Sagel, S. S.: Common fungal diseases of the lungs; I. Coccidioidomycosis. Radiol. Clin. North Am. 11: 153, 1973.

Salmon, M. A.: Pulmonary hydatidosis. Dis. Chest 40: 61, 1961.

Sante, L. R.: Pulmonary infection in tularemia. A.J.R. 25: 241, 1931.

Sante, L. R.: Roentgen manifestations of adult toxoplasmosis. A.J.R. 47: 825, 1942.

Sargent, E. N., Larson, M. J., and Reilly, M. D.: Roentgenographic manifestations of varicella pneumonia with postmortem correlation. A.J.R. 98: 305, 1966.

Scanlon, G. T., and Unger, J. D.: The radiology of bacterial and viral pneumonias. Radiol. Clin. North Am. 11: 317, 1973.

Schlanger, P. M., and Schlanger, H.: Hydatid disease and its roentgen picture. A.J.R. 60: 331, 1948.

Shaw, R. R.: Thoracic complications of amebiasis. Surg. Gynecol. Obstet. 88: 753, 1949.

Slade, P. R., Slesser, B. V., and Southgate, J.: Thoracic actinomycosis. Thorax 28: 73, 1973.

Small, M. J.: Late progression of pulmonary coccidioidomycosis. Arch. Intern. Med. 104: 730, 1959.

Spivey, C. G., Jr., Jones, F. L., and Bopp, R. K.: Cavitary coccidioidomycosis: experience in a tuberculosis hospital outside the endemic area. Chest 56: 13, 1969.

Stone, D. J., Colp, C., and Howard, E. J.: Staphylococcal pneumonia in the adult. Dis. Chest 42: 157, 1962.

Stuart, B. M., and Pullen, R. L.: Tularemic pneumonia: review of American literature and report of 15 additional cases. Am. J. Med. Sci. 210: 233, 1945.

Sweany, H. C., Gorelick, D., Coller, F. C., and Jones, J. L.: Pathologic and some diagnostic features of histoplasmosis in patients entering a Missouri hospital. Dis. Chest 42: 1, 1968.

Tan, D. Y. M., Kaufman, S. A., and Levene, G.: Primary chickenpox pneumonia. A.J.R. 76: 527, 1956.

Taylor, A. B., and Briney, A. K.: Observations on primary coccidioidomycosis. Ann. Intern. Med. 30: 1224, 1949.

Tew, J., Calenoff, L. A., and Berlin, B. S.: Bacterial or nonbacterial pneumonia: accuracy of radiographic diagnosis. Radiology 124: 607, 1977.

Tillotson, J. R., and Lerner, A. M.: Hemophilus influenzae bronchopneumonia in adults. Arch. Intern. Med. 121: 428, 1968.

Triebwasser, J. H., Harris, R. E., Bryant, R. E., and Rhoades, E. R.: Varicella pneumonia in adults. Report of seven cases and review of the literature. Medicine 46: 409, 1967.

Tucker, A. K., Pemberton, J., and Guyer, P. B.: Pulmonary fungal infection complicating treated malignant disease. Clin. Radiol. 26: 129, 1975.

Turner, P. P.: Schistosomal pulmonary arterial hypertension in East Africa. Br. Heart J. 26: 821, 1964.

Unger, J. D., Rose, H. D., and Unger, G. F.: Gram-negative pneumonia. Radiology 107: 283, 1973.

Vessal, K., Yeganehdoust, J., Dutz, W., and Kohout, E.: Radiological changes in inhalation anthrax. Clin. Radiol. 26: 471, 1975.

Vinik, M., Altman, D. H., and Parks, R. E.: Experience with Hemophilus influenzae pneumonia. Radiology 86: 701, 1966.

Warren, W-P., and Rose, B.: Hypersensitivity bronchopulmonary aspergillosis. Dis. Chest 55: 415, 1969.

Webster, B. H.: Pulmonary geotrichosis. Am. Rev. Tuberc. 76: 286, 1957.

Weller, M. H., and Katzenstein, A. A.: Radiologic findings in group B streptococcal sepsis. Radiology 118: 385, 1976.

Whitehouse, W. M., Davey, W. N., Engelke, O., and Holt, J. F.: Roentgen findings in histoplasmin-positive school children. J. Mich. Med. Soc. 58: 1266, 1959.

Wilson, E. S.: Pleuropulmonary amebiasis. A.J.R. 111: 518, 1971.

Winn, W. A., and Johnson, G. H.: Primary coccidioidomycosis. Ann. Intern. Med. 17: 407, 1942.

Witorsch, P., and Utz, J. P.: North American blastomycosis: a study of 40 patients. Medicine 47: 169, 1968.

Wolfe, J. N., and Jacobson, G.: Roentgen manifestations of torulosis (cryptococcosis). A.J.R. 79: 216, 1958.

Xanthakis, D., Efthimiadis, M., Papadakis, G., et al.: Hydatid disease of the chest. Report of 91 patients surgically treated. Thorax 27: 517, 1972.

Yang, S-P., Huang, C-T., Cheng, C-S., and Chiang, L-C.: The clinical and roentgenological courses of pulmonary paragonimiasis. Dis. Chest *36:* 494, 1959.

Young, L. W., Smith, D. I., and Glasgow, L. A.: Pneumonia of atypical measles. Residual nodular lesions. A.J.R. *110:* 439, 1970.

Young, R. C., Vogel, C. L., and DeVita, V. T.: Aspergillus lobar pneumonia. J.A.M.A. *208:* 1156, 1969.

Zimmerman, R. A., and Miller, W. T.: Pulmonary aspergillosis. A.J.R. *109:* 505, 1970.

Zornoza, J., Goldman, A. M., Valdivieso, M., and Bodey, G. P.: Radiologic features of gram-negative pneumonias in the neutropenic patient. A.J.R. *127:* 989, 1976.

Putrid Lung Abscess

Kramer, R., and Glass, A.: Bronchoscopic localization of lung abscess. Ann. Otol. Rhinol. Laryngol. *41:* 1210, 1932.

Neuhof, H., and Hirschfield, S.: Putrid empyema; ruptured putrid abscess of lung. Ann. Surg. *100:* 1105, 1934.

Neuhof, H., and Touroff, A. S. W.: Acute putrid abscess of the lung. J. Thorac. Surg. *1:* 637, 1932.

O'Reilly, G. V., Dee, P. M., and Otteni, G. V.: Gangrene of the lung: Successful medical management of three patients. Radiology *126:* 576, 1978.

Rabin, C. B.: Technique for more precise localization of pulmonary abscess. A.J.R. *46:* 130, 1941.

Wessler, H.: Lung abscess and bronchiectasis. A.J.R. *6:* 161, 1919.

Tuberculosis

Allison, R. G., and Medelman, J. P.: Pulmonary tuberculosis in childhood. A.J.R. *31:* 16, 1934.

Anderson, D. H., Grech, P., Township, R. H., and Jephcott, A. E.: Pulmonary lesions due to opportunistic mycobacteria. Clin. Radiol. *126:* 461, 1975.

Assmann, H.: Fruhinfiltrat. Ergeb. Ges. Tuberk. *1:* 115, 1930.

Banyai, A. L.: Diabetes and tuberculosis. Dis. Chest *36:* 238, 1959.

Berger, H. W., and Samortin, T. G.: Miliary tuberculosis: Diagnostic methods with emphasis on the chest roentgenogram. Chest *58:* 586, 1970.

Birkelo, C. C., and Rogue, P. O.: Accuracy of roentgen determination of activity of minimal pulmonary tuberculosis. A.J.R. *60:* 303, 1948.

Bloch, G.: Ghon's tubercle: re-evaluation of concept. A.J.R. *49:* 463, 1943.

Bobrowitz, I. D., and Hurst, A.: Minimal tuberculosis. Problems in roentgenologic interpretation. Radiology *52:* 519, 1949.

Braeuning, H., and Redeker, F.: *Die ha-*

matogene Lungentuberkulose des Erwachsenen. J. A. Barth, Leipzig, 1931.

Bruck, S.: Round foci type of pulmonary tuberculosis. A.J.R. *31:* 319, 1934.

Chadwick, H. D.: Evolution of pulmonary tuberculosis in children as revealed by roentgenogram. A.J.R. *27:* 47, 1932.

Cohen, S.: Lymphohematogenous tuberculosis. Am. Rev. Tuberc. *43:* 612, 1941.

Eloesser, L.: Bronchial stenosis in pulmonary tuberculosis. Am. Rev. Tuberc. *30:* 123, 1934.

Giammona, S. T., Poole, C. A., Zelkowitz, P., and Skrovan, C.: Massive lymphadenopathy in primary pulmonary tuberculosis in children. Am. Rev. Respir. Dis. *100:* 480, 1969.

Guggenheim, A.: Pulmonary emphysema and tuberculosis. A.J.R. *58:* 64, 1947.

Hennell, H.: Atelectasis as a factor in the evolution of chronic fibroid pulmonary tuberculosis. Am. Rev. Tuberc. *23:* 461, 1931.

Jacobson, H. G., and Shapiro, J. H.: Pulmonary tuberculosis. Radiol. Clin. North Am. *1:* 411, 1963.

Joffe, N.: Cavitating primary tuberculosis in infancy. Br. J. Radiol. *33:* 430, 1960.

Jones, E. M., Rafferty, T. N., and Willis, H. S.: Primary tuberculosis complicated by bronchial tuberculosis with atelectasis (epituberculosis). Am. Rev. Tuberc. *46:* 392, 1942.

Keller, R. H., and Runyon, E. H.: Mycobacterial diseases. A.J.R. *92:* 528, 1964.

Lewis, A. G., Dunbar, F. P., McAlister, E., and Cacciatore, R.: Chronic pulmonary disease due to atypical acid-fast bacilli. South. Med. J. *51:* 1241, 1958.

Lincoln, E. M.: Hematogenous tuberculosis in children. Am. J. Dis. Child. *50:* 84, 1935.

Medlar, E. M.: The behavior of pulmonary tuberculous lesions: a pathological study. Am. Rev. Tuberc. *71:* 1, 1955.

Miller, W. T., and MacGregor, R. R.: Tuberculosis: frequency of unusual radiographic findings. A.J.R. *130:* 867, 1978.

National Tuberculosis Association: *Diagnostic Standards and Classification of Tuberculosis.* National Tuberculosis Association, New York, 1961.

Ostrum, H. W., and Serber, W.: Early roentgen recognition of lower-lobe tuberculosis. Radiology *53:* 42, 1949.

Peirce, C. B., and Curtzwiler, F. C.: Tuberculous tracheobronchitis. A.J.R. *43:* 153, 1940.

Pinner, M.: Hematogenous (nonmiliary) pulmonary tuberculosis. A.J.R. *31:* 442, 1934.

Reisner, D.: Pulmonary tuberculosis of

lower lobe. Arch. Intern. Med. *56:* 258, 1935.

Rich, A. R.: The pathogenesis of tuberculosis. Springfield, Ill., Charles C Thomas, 1944.

Riley, R. L.: Apical localization of pulmonary tuberculosis. Bull. Johns Hopkins Hosp. *106:* 232, 1960.

Rubin, E. H.: Initial lobar tuberculosis. A.J.R. *34:* 175, 1935.

Scheidegger, S.: Zur rontgenologischen Differentialdiagnose der Miliartuberkulose. Fortschr. Geb. Rontgenstr. *51:* 209, 1935.

Sproull, J.: Collapse of lung occurring in pulmonary tuberculosis. A.J.R. *20:* 419, 1928.

Sweany, H. C., Cook, E., and Kegerreis, R.: Study of position of primary cavities in pulmonary tuberculosis. Am. Rev. Tuberc. *23:* 558, 1931.

Weber, A. L., Bird, K. T., and Janower, M. L.: Primary tuberculosis in childhood with particular emphasis on changes affecting the tracheobronchial tree. A.J.R. *103:* 123, 1968.

Wessler, H.: *Army X-ray Manual.* P. B. Hoeber, New York, 1918.

Westermark, N.: Entwicklung und Vorkommen von Atelektase bei Lungentuberkulose. Acta Radiol. *16:* 531, 1935.

Wiot, J. F., and Spitz, H. B.: Atypical pulmonary tuberculosis. Radiol. Clin. North Am. *11:* 191, 1973.

Wu, C., and Tang, B. H. Y.: Contralateral bronchial infection in pulmonary tuberculosis. A.J.R. *37:* 180, 1937.

Thromboembolic Disease

Alpert, J. S., Godtfredsen, J., Ockene, I. S., Anas, J., and Dalen, J. D.: Pulmonary hypertension secondary to minor pulmonary embolism. Chest *73:* 795, 1978.

Anderson, G., Reid, L., and Simon, G.: The radiographic appearances in primary and in thromboembolic pulmonary hypertension. Clin. Radiol. *24:* 113, 1973.

Arora, Y. C., Lyons, H. A., and Cantor, P. A.: Unusual clinical and roentgenographic features of pulmonary infarction. Am. Rev. Respir. Dis. *82:* 232, 1960.

Baron, M. G.: Fleischner lines and pulmonary emboli. Circulation *45:* 171, 1972.

Bjork, L., and Ansusinha, T.: Angiographic diagnosis of acute pulmonary embolism. Acta Radiol. *3:* 129, 1965.

Bookstein, J. J., and Silver, T. M.: The angiographic differential diagnosis of acute pulmonary embolism. Radiology *110:* 25, 1974.

Chait, A., Summers, D., Krasnow, N., and Wechsler, B. M.: Observations on the fate of large pulmonary emboli. A.J.R. *100:* 364, 1967.

Chang, C. H., and Davis, W. C.: A roentgen sign of pulmonary infarction. Clin. Radiol. *41:* 141, 1965.

Dalen, J. E., Banas, J. S., Brooks, H. L., Evans, G. L., Paraskos, J. A., and Dexter, L.: Resolution rate of acute pulmonary embolism in man. N. Engl. J. Med. *280:* 1194, 1969.

Ferris, E. J., Stanzler, R. M., Rourke, J. A., Blumenthal, J., and Messer, J. V.: Pulmonary angiography in pulmonary embolic disease. A.J.R. *100:* 355, 1967.

Fleischner, F. G.: Unilateral pulmonary embolism with increased compensatory circulation through the unoccluded lung. Roentgen observations. Radiology *73:* 591, 1959.

Fleischner, F. G.: Pulmonary embolism. Clin. Radiol. *13:* 169, 1962.

Fleischner, F. G.: Recurrent pulmonary embolism and cor pulmonale. N. Engl. J. Med. *270:* 1213, 1967.

Gomes, A. S., Grollman, J. H., Jr., and Mink, J.: Pulmonary angiography for pulmonary emboli: rational selection of oblique views. A.J.R. *129:* 1019, 1977.

Greenspan, R. H., and Steiner, R. E.: The radiologic diagnosis of pulmonary thromboembolism. In *Frontiers of Pulmonary Radiology*, edited by M. Simon, E. J. Potchen, and M. LeMay. Grune & Stratton, New York, 1969.

Grieco, M. H., and Ryan, S. F.: Aseptic pulmonary infarction. Am. J. Med. *45:* 811, 1968.

Hampton, A. O., and Castleman, B.: Correlation of postmortem chest teleroentgenograms with autopsy findings. With special reference to pulmonary embolism and infarction. A.J.R. *43:* 305, 1940.

Heitzman, E. R., Markarian, B., and Dailey, E. T.: Pulmonary thromboembolic disease. A lobular concept. Radiology *103:* 529, 1972.

Johnson, B. A., James, A. E., Jr., and White, R. L., Jr.: Oblique and selective pulmonary angiography in diagnosis of pulmonary embolism. A.J.R. *118:* 801, 1973.

Kaye, J., and Cohen, G.: Massive pulmonary embolism without infarction. Br. J. Radiol. *3:* 326, 1958.

Kerr, I. H., Simon, G., and Sutton, G. C.: The value of the plain radiograph in acute massive pulmonary embolism. Br. J. Radiol. *44:* 751, 1971.

Kjellberg, S. R., and Olsson, S. E.: Roentgenographical studies of experimental pulmonary embolism without complicating infarction in dog. Acta Radiol. *33:* 507, 1950.

Magidson, O., and Jacobson, G.: Thrombosis of main pulmonary arteries. Br. Heart J. *17:* 207, 1955.

Moses, D. C., Silver, T. M., and Book-stein, J. J.: The complementary roles of chest radiography, lung scanning, and selective pulmonary angiography in the diagnosis of pulmonary embolism. Circulation *49:* 179, 1974.

Novelline, R. A., Baltarowich, O. H., Athanosoulis, C. A., Waltman, A. C., Greenfield, A. J., and McKusick, K. A.: The clinical course of patients with suspected pulmonary embolism and a negative pulmonary arteriogram. Radiology *126:* 561, 1978.

Peterson, K. L., Fred, H. L., and Alexander, J. K.: Pulmonary arterial webs: A new angiographic sign of previous thromboembolism. N. Engl. J. Med. *277:* 33, 1967.

Simon, G.: Further observations on the long line shadow across a lower zone of the lung. Br. J. Radiol. *43:* 327, 1970.

Sisk, P. B.: Pulmonary thromboembolism. Atypical clinical and roentgen manifestations. Dis. Chest *47:* 539, 1965.

Starzl, T. E., Brittain, R. S., Hermann, G., Marchioro, T. L., and Waddell, W. R.: Pseudotumors due to pulmonary infarction. Am. J. Surg. *106:* 619, 1963.

Stein, P., Onnor, J. F., Dalen, J. E., Pur-Shahriari, A. A., Hoppin, F. G., Jr., Hammond, D. T., Haynes, F. W., Fleischner, F. G., and Dexter, L.: The angiographic diagnosis of acute pulmonary embolism: evauation of criteria. Am. Heart J. *73:* 730, 1967.

Stein, P. D.: Wedge arteriography for the identification of pulmonary emboli in small vessels. Am. Heart J. *82:* 618, 1971.

Symbas, P. N., Jacobs, W. F., and Schlant, R. C.: Chronic pulmonary arterial embolization or thrombosis. Am. J. Cardiol. *28:* 342, 1971.

Talbot, S., Worthington, B. S., and Roebuck, E. J.: Radiographic signs of pulmonary embolism and pulmonary infarction. Thorax *28:* 198, 1973.

Uehlinger, E.: Die pathologische Anatomie des hamorrhagischen Lungeninfarktes. Beitr. Klin. Erforsch. Tuberk. *137:* 245, 1968.

Weidner, W., Swanson, L., and Wilson, G.: Roentgen techniques in the diagnosis of pulmonary thromboembolism. A.J.R. *100:* 397, 1967.

White, R. I., Jr., James, A. E., Jr., and Wagner, H. N., Jr.: The significance of unilateral absence of pulmonary artery perfusion by lung scanning. A.J.R. *111:* 501, 1971.

Wiener, S. N., Edelstein, J., and Charms, B. L.: Observations on pulmonary embolism and the pulmonary angiogram. A.J.R. *98:* 859, 1966.

Woesner, M. E., Sanders, I., and White, G. W.: The melting sign in resolving transient pulmonary infarction. A.J.R. *111:* 782, 1971.

Emphysema

American Thoracic Society, Committee on Diagnostic Standards for Nontuberculous Respiratory Diseases: Definitions and classification of chronic bronchitis, asthma and pulmonary emphysema. Am. Rev. Respir. Dis. *85:* 762, 1962.

Anderson, W. F., Anderson, A. E., Jr., Hernandez, J. A., and Foraker, A. G.: Topography of aging and emphysematous lungs. Am. Rev. Respir. Dis. *90:* 411, 1964.

Bignon, J., Khoury, F., Even, P., Andre, J., and Brouet, G.: Morphometric study in chronic obstructive bronchopulmonary disease. Am. Rev. Respir. Dis. *99:* 669, 1969.

Boushy, S. F., Kohen, R., Billie, D. M., and Heiman, M. J.: Bullous emphysema: clinical, roentgenologic and physiologic study of 49 patients. Dis. Chest *54:* 17, 1968.

Boushy, S. F., North, L. B., and Trice, J. A.: The bronchial arteries in chronic obstructive pulmonary disease. Am. J. Med. *46:* 506, 1969.

Brewer, L. L., Moskowitz, P. S., Carrington, C. B., and Bensch, K. G.: Pneumatosis pulmonalis. A complication of idiopathic respiratory distress syndrome. Am. J. Pathol. *95:* 171, 1979.

Cremin, B. J., and Movsowitz, H.: Lobar emphysema in infants. Br. J. Radiol. *44:* 692, 1971.

Culiner, M. M.: The hyperlucent lung, a problem in differential diagnosis. Dis. Chest *49:* 578, 1966.

Fleischner, F. G.: Pathogenesis of chronic substantial (hypertrophic) emphysema. Am. Rev. Tuberc. *62:* 45, 1950.

Fouché, R. F., and D'Silva, J. L.: Hypertransradiancy of one lung field and its experimental production by unilateral miliary embolisation of pulmonary arteries in cats. Clin. Radiol. *11:* 100, 1960.

Fraser, R. G., and Bates, D. V.: Body section roentgenography in the evaluation and differentiation of chronic hypertrophic emphysema and asthma. A.J.R. *82:* 39, 1959.

Freedman, E.: Emphysematous blebs and bullae. A.J.R. *35:* 324, 1936.

Golden, R.: Abnormally wide respiratory movement of the lower lung structures. A.J.R. *44:* 325, 1940.

Gottlieb, L. S., and Turner, A. F.: Swyer-James (Macleod's) syndrome. Variations in pulmonary-bronchial arterial blood flow. Chest *69:* 62, 1976.

Gough, J.: The pathology of emphysema. Postgrad. Med. J. *41:* 392, 1965.

Heitzman, E. R., Markarian, B., and Solomon, J.: Chronic obstructive pulmonary disease. Radiol. Clin. North Am. *11:* 49, 1973.

Hogg, J. C., Macklem, P. T., and Thurlbeck, W. M.: Site and nature of airway obstruction in chronic obstructive lung disease. N. Engl. J. Med. 278: 1355, 1968.

Jacobson, G., Turner, A. F., Balchum, O. J., and Jung. R.: Vascular changes in pulmonary emphysema. The radiologic evaluation by selective and peripheral pulmonary wedge angiography. A.J.R. 100: 374, 1967.

Jones, J. C., Almond, C. H., Snyder, H. M., and Meyer, B. W.: Congenital pulmonary cysts in infants and children. Ann. Thorac. Surg. 3: 297, 1967.

Laws, J. W., and Heard, B. E.: Emphysema and the chest film: a retrospective radiological and pathological study. Br. J. Radiol. 35: 750, 1962.

Leopold, J. G., and Gough, J.: The centrilobar form of hypertrophic emphysema and its relation to chronic bronchitis. Thorax 12: 219, 1957.

Macklem, P. T., Fraser, R. G., and Brown, W. G.: Bronchial pressure measurements in emphysema and bronchitis. J. Clin. Invest. 44: 897, 1965.

Macleod, W. M.: Abnormal transradiancy of one lung. Thorax 9: 147, 1954.

Mayer, E., Blazsik, C., and Rappaport, I.: Emphysema and the lungs of the aged: a clinical study. Dis. Chest 34: 247, 1958.

McLean, K. H.: The pathogenesis of pulmonary emphysema. Am. J. Med. 25: 62, 1958.

Miller, W. S.: Human pleura pulmonalis; its relation to blebs and bullae of emphysema. A.J.R. 15: 599, 1926; 18: 42, 1927.

Milne, E. N. C., and Bass, H.: The roentgenologic diagnosis of early chronic obstructive pulmonary disease. J. Can. Assoc. Radiol. 20: 3, 1969.

Musk, A. W., Gandevia, B., and Palmer, F. J.: Peripheral pooling of bronchographic contrast material: evidence of its relationship to smoking and emphysema. Thorax 33: 193, 1978.

Nicklaus, T. M., Stowell, D. W., Christiansen, W. R., and Renzetti, A. D., Jr.: The accuracy of the roentgenologic diagnosis of chronic pulmonary emphysema. Am. Rev. Respir. Dis. 93: 889, 1966.

Rainer, W. G., Mitchell, R. S., Filley, G. F., and Eiseman, B.: Significance of tracheal collapse in pulmonary emphysema—cinefluorographic observations. Surg. Forum 12: 70, 1961.

Raynor, A. C., Capp, M. P., and Sealy, W. C.: Lobar emphysema of infancy. Collective review. Ann. Thorac. Surg. 4: 374, 1967.

Reid, L.: Emphysema: classification and clinical significance, Br. J. Dis. Chest. 60: 57, 1966.

Reid, L.: The Pathology of Emphysema. Lloyd-Luke (Medical Books) Ltd. London, 1967.

Reid, L., and Millard, F. J. C.: Correlation between radiological diagnosis and structural lung changes in emphysema. Clin. Radiol. 40: 293, 1964.

Rothstein, E., and Harley, B. F.: Fluid levels in emphysematous bullae. Dis. Chest 42: 620, 1962.

Rubin, E. H., and Buchberg, A. S.: Capricious behavior of pulmonary bullae developing fluid. Chest 54: 60, 1968.

Scarrow, G. D.: The pulmonary angiogram in chronic bronchitis and emphysema. Clin. Radiol. 17: 54, 1966.

Simon, G.: Radiology and emphysema. Clin. Radiol. 15: 293, 1964.

Simon, G.: Complexities of emphysema. In Frontiers of Pulmonary Radiology, edited by M. Simon, E. J. Potchen, and M. Lemay. Grune & Stratton, New York, 1969.

Sutinen, S., Christoforidis, A. J., Klugh, G. A., and Pratt, P. C.: Roentgenologic criteria for the recognition of nonsymptomatic pulmonary emphysema. Correlation between roentgenologic findings and pulmonary pathology. Am. Rev. Respir. Dis. 91: 69, 1965.

Swyer, P. R., and James, G. C. W.: A case of unilateral pulmonary emphysema. Thorax 8: 133, 1953.

Thurlbeck, W. M.: Aspects of chronic airflow obstruction. Chest 72: 341, 1977.

Thurlbeck, W. M., and Simon, G.: Radiographic appearance of the chest in emphysema. A.J.R. 130: 429, 1978.

Tomashefski, J. F., and Pratt, P. C.: Pulmonary emphysema: pathology and pathogenesis. Med. Clin. North Am. 51: 269, 1967.

Virtama, P., and Toivonen, S.: Roentgen diagnosis of pulmonary emphysema. Ann. Med. Intern. Fenn. 54: 59, 1965.

Wright, G. W., and Kleinerman, J. A.: Consideration of the etiology of emphysema in terms of contemporary knowledge. Am. Rev. Respir. Dis. 88: 605, 1963.

Wyatt, J. P., Fischer, V. W., and Sweet, H. C.: The pathomorphology of the emphysema complex. Part I. Am. Rev. Respir. Dis. 89: 533, 1964.

Inhalation Diseases

Aslett, E. A., Davies, T. W., and Jenkins, T. I.: Radiologic appearances in development of coal miners' pneumokoniosis. Br. J. Radiol. 16: 308, 1943.

Awe, W. C., Fletcher, W. S., and Jacob, S. W.: The pathophysiology of aspiration pneumonitis. Surgery 60: 232, 1966.

Bader, M. E., Bader, R. A., Teirstein, A. S., Miller, A., and Selikoff, I. J.: Pulmonary function and radiographic changes in 598 workers with varying duration of exposure to asbestos. Mt. Sinai J. Med. 37: 492, 1970.

Borrie, J. O., and Gwynne, J. F.: Paraffinoma of lung: lipoid pneumonia. Thorax 28: 214, 1973.

Bouhuys, A., Barbero, A., Schilling, R. S. F., and Van de Woestijne, K.: Chronic respiratory disease in hemp workers. Am. J. Med. 46: 526, 1969.

Brink, G. C., Grzybowski, S., and Lane, G. B.: Silicotuberculosis. Can. Med. Assoc. J. 19: 959, 1960.

Bristol, L. J.: Pneumoconioses caused by asbestos and other siliceous and non-siliceous dusts. Semin. Roentgenol. 2: 283, 1967.

Buechner, H. A., and Ansari, A.: Acute silico-proteinosis. A new pathologic variant of acute silicosis in sandblasters, characterized by histologic features resembling alveolar proteinosis. Dis. Chest 55: 274, 1969.

Buechner, H. A., Prevatt, A. L., Thompson, J., and Blitz, O.: Bagassosis: review with further historical data, studies of pulmonary function and results of steroid therapy. Am. J. Med. 25: 234, 1958.

Camiel, M. R., and Berkan, H. S.: Inhalation pneumonia from nitric fumes. Radiology 42: 175, 1944.

Caplan, A., Payne, R. B., and Withey, J. C.: A broader concept of Caplan's syndrome related to rheumatoid factors. Thorax 17: 205, 1962.

Cochrane, A. L., Moore, F., and Thomas, J.: The radiographic progression of progressive massive fibrosis. Tubercle 42: 72, 1961.

Cooper, D. A., Pendergrass, E. P., Vorwald, A. J., Maycock, R. L., and Brieger, H.: Pneumoconiosis among workers in an antimony industry. A.J.R. 103: 495, 1968.

Cornelius, E. A., and Betlach, E. H.: Silo-filler's disease. Radiology 74: 232, 1960.

Dee, P., Suratt, P., and Winn, W.: The radiographic findings in acute silicosis. Radiology 126: 539, 1978.

Dickie, H. A., and Rankin, P.: Farmer's lung: an acute granulomatous pneumonitis occurring in agricultural workers. J.A.M.A. 167: 1069, 1958.

Doig, A. T.: Baritosis: a benign pneumoconiosis. Thorax 31: 30, 1976.

Dundon, C. C., and Hughes, J. P.: Stannic oxide pneumoconiosis. A.J.R. 65: 797, 1950.

Dunner, L.: Occupational disease of lungs in boiler scalers. Br. J. Radiol. 16: 387, 1943.

Dunner, L., and Bagnall, D. J. T.: Pneumoconiosis in graphite workers. Br. J. Radiol. 22: 573, 1949.

Ehrhardt, D. R., Ahn, C., and Sawyers, T. M.: Pulmonary disease associated with the inhalation of cosmetic aerosols. Chest 64: 251, 1973.

Emanuel, D. A., Wenzel, F. J., Bowerman, C. I., and Lawton, B. R.: Farmer's lung. Am. J. Med. 37: 392, 1964.

Fletcher, C. M.: Classification of roentgenograms in pneumoconiosis. Arch. Indust. Health 11: 17, 1955.

Fletcher, D. E., and Edge, J. R.: The early radiological changes in pulmonary and pleural asbestosis. Clin. Radiol. 21: 355, 1970.

Foley, F. D., Moncrief, J. A., and Mason, A. D., Jr.: Pathology of the lungs in fatally burned patients. Ann. Surg. 167: 251, 1968.

Fraser, R. G., and Paré, J. A. P.: Extrinsic allergic alveolitis. Semin. Roentgenol. 10: 31, 1975.

Gaensler, E. A., Cadigan, J. B., Sasahara, A. A., Fox, E. O., and MacMahon, H. E.: Graphite pneumoconiosis of electrotypers. Am. J. Med. 41: 864, 1966.

Gardner, L. U.: Diagnosis of silicosis, with special reference to roentgenological manifestations. Ann. Intern. Med. 10: 166, 1936.

Garland, L. H.: X-ray aspects of pneumoconiosis. Radiology 27: 21, 1936.

Gernez-Rieux, C., Balgairies, E., Fournier, P., and Voisin, C.: Une manifestation souvent méconnue de la pneumoconiose des mineurs: la liquefaction aseptique des formations pseudo-tumorales. Semin. Hop. Paris 34: 1081, 1958.

Gilson, J. C.: Pathology, radiology and epidemiology of coal workers' pneumoconiosis in Wales. Arch. Indust. Health 15: 468, 1957.

Goldman, K. P.: The diagnosis of lung cancer in coal miners with pneumoconiosis. Br. J. Dis. Chest 59: 141, 1965.

Grayson, R. R.: Silage gas poisoning: nitrogen dioxide pneumonia, a new disease in agricultural workers. Ann. Intern. Med. 45: 393, 1956.

Greening, R. R., and Heslep, J. H.: The roentgenology of silicosis. Semin. Roentgenol. 2: 265, 1967.

Gross, P., Ronehart, W. E., and deTreville, R. T. P.: The pulmonary reactions to toxic gases. Am. Indust. Hyg. Assoc. J. 28: 315, 1967.

Hallee, T. J.: Diffuse lung disease caused by inhalation of mercury vapor. Am. Rev. Respir. Dis. 99: 430, 1969.

Hapke, E. J., Seal, M. E., Thomas, G. O., Hayes, M., and Meek, J. C.: Farmer's lung. A clinical, radiological, functional and serological correlation of acute and chronic stages. Thorax 23: 451, 1968.

Hargreave, F., Hinson, K. F., Reid, L., Simon, G., and McCarthy, D. S.: The radiological appearances of allergic alveolitis due to bird sensitivity (bird fancier's lung). Clin. Radiol. 23: 1, 1972.

Heacock, C. H.: Pneumonia in children

following the injection of petroleum products. Radiology 53: 793, 1949.

Hearn, C. E. D.: Bagassosis: an epidemiological, environmental and clinical survey. Br. J. Indust. Med. 25: 267, 1968.

Heuck, F., and Hoschek, R.: Cer-pneumoconiosis. A.J.R. 104: 177, 1968.

Hobbs, A. A., Jr.: A type of pneumoconiosis. A.J.R. 63: 488, 1950.

Hunt, A. C.: Massive pulmonary fibrosis from the inhalation of talc. Thorax 11: 287, 1956.

I.L.O. radiologic classification of the pneumoconiosis. Arch. Environ. Health 12: 314, 1966.

Jackson, E., and Welch, K. M. A.: Mushroom worker's lung. Thorax 25: 25, 1970.

Jiminez, J. P., and Lester, R. G.: Pulmonary complications following furniture polish ingestion. A.J.R. 98: 323, 1966.

Kleinfeld, M., Messite, J., Kooyman, O., and Shapiro, J.: Welder's siderosis. Arch. Environ. Health 19: 70, 1969.

Lanza, A. J. (Ed.): The Pneumoconioses. Grune & Stratton, 1963.

Lemone, D. V., et al.: Bagasse disease of the lungs. Radiology 49: 556, 1947.

Lesser, L. I., Weens, H. S., and McKey, J. D.: Pulmonary manifestations following ingestion of kerosene. J. Pediatr. 23: 352, 1943.

Mendelson, C. L.: The aspiration of stomach contents into the lungs during obstetric anaesthesia. Am. J. Obstet. Gynecol. 52: 191, 1946.

Meyer, E. C., Kratzinger, S. F., and Miller, W. H.: Pulmonary fibrosis in an arc welder. Arch. Environ. Health 15: 462, 1967.

Mindell, H. J.: Roentgen findings in farmer's lung. Radiology 97: 341, 1970.

Mitchell, J., Manning, G. B., Molyneux, M., and Lane, R. E.: Pulmonary fibrosis in workers exposed to finely powdered aluminum. Br. J. Indust. Med. 18: 10, 1967.

Naeye, R. L., and Dellinger, W. S.: Coal workers' pneumoconiosis. Correlation of roentgenographic and postmortem findings. J.A.M.A. 220: 223, 1972.

Nicholson, D. P.: Bagasse worker's lung. Am. Rev. Respir. Dis. 97: 546, 1968.

Pascucci, L. M.: Pulmonary disease in workers exposed to beryllium compounds: its roentgen characteristics. Radiology 50: 23, 1948.

Pendergrass, E. P., and Pryde, A. W.: Benign pneumoconiosis due to tin oxide. J. Indust. Hyg. Toxicol. 30: 119, 1948.

Pendergrass, E. P., and Robert, A. G.: Some considerations of the roentgen diagnosis of silicosis and conditions that may simulate it. Radiology 50: 725, 1948.

Pimentel, J. C., and Avila, R.: Respira-

tory disease in cork workers ("suberosis"). Thorax 28: 409, 1973.

Pump, K. K.: Studies in silicosis of the human lung. Dis. Chest 53: 237, 1968.

Putman, C. E., Loke, J., Matthay, R. A., and Ravin, C. E.: Radiographic manifestations of acute smoke inhalation. A.J.R. 129: 865, 1977.

Putman, C. E., Tummillo, A. M., Myerson, D. A., and Myerson, P. J.: Drowning: another plunge. A.J.R. 125: 543, 1975.

Ramirez-R. J., Lopez-Majano, V., and Schultze, G.: Caplan's syndrome. Am. J. Med. 37: 643, 1964.

Rankin, J., Kobayashi, M., Barbee, R. A., and Dickie, H. A.: Pulmonary granulomatoses due to inhaled organic antigens. Med. Clin. North Am. 51: 459, 1967.

Reed, E. S., Leikin, S., and Kerman, H. D.: Kerosene intoxication. Ann. J. Dis. Child. 79: 623, 1950.

Reed, E. S., Wells, P. O., and Wicker, E. H.: Coal miners' pneumoconiosis. Radiology 71: 661, 1958.

Robert, A. G.: A consideration of the roentgen diagnosis of chronic pulmonary granulomatosis of beryllium workers. A.J.R. 65: 467, 1950.

Sage, H. H.: Acute phosgene poisoning. A.J.R. 51: 9, 1944.

Sander, O. A.: Benign pneumoconiosis due to metal fumes and dust. A.J.R. 58: 277, 1947.

Scadding, J. G.: Diffuse pulmonary alveolar fibrosis. Thorax 29: 271, 1974.

Seal, R. M. E., Hapke, E. J., Thomas, G. O., Meek, J. C., and Hayes, M.: The pathology of the acute and chronic stages of farmer's lung. Thorax 23: 469, 1968.

Selikoff, I. J., Bader, R. A., Bader, M. E., Churg, J., and Hammond, E. C.: Editorial: asbestosis and neoplasia. Am. J. Med. 42: 487, 1967.

Shaver, C. G.: Further observations of lung changes associated with the manufacture of alumina abrasives. Radiology 50: 760, 1948.

Shull, J. R.: Asbestosis: roentgenologic review of 71 cases. Radiology 27: 279, 1936.

Siegal, W., Smith, A. R., and Greenburg, L.: The dust hazard in tremolite talc mining, including roentgenological findings in talc workers. A.J.R. 49: 11, 1943.

Stoeckle, J. D., Hardy, H. L., and Weber, A. L.: Chronic beryllium disease. Long-term follow-up of sixty cases and selective review of the literature. Am. J. Med. 46: 545, 1969.

Sunderman, F. W., Jr.: Nickel carcinogenesis. Dis. Chest 54: 41, 1968.

Tellesson, W. G.: Rheumatoid pneumoconiosis (Caplan's syndrome) in an asbestos worker. Thorax 16: 372, 1961.

Teng, C. T., and Brennan, J. C.: Acute

mercury vapor poisoning. Radiology 73: 354, 1959.

Thompson, C. M.: Pulmonary changes in carbon tetrachloride poisoning. A.J.R. 55: 16, 1946.

Unger, J. D., Fink, J. N., and Unger, G. F.: Pigeon breeder's disease. A review of the roentgenographic pulmonary findings. Radiology 90: 683, 1968.

Wall, N. M.: Anthracosilicosis with special reference to pulmonary cavitation. Am. Rev. Tuberc. 71: 544, 1971.

Weber, A. L., Stoeckle, J. D., and Hardy, H. L.: Roentgenologic patterns in long-standing beryllium disease. A.J.R. 93: 879, 1965.

Weill, H., Ferrans, V. J., Gay, R. M., and Ziskind, M. M.: Early lipoid pneumonia. Am. J. Med. 36: 370, 1964.

Wilkins, R. A., DeLacey, G. J., Flor, R., and Taylor, S.: Radiology in Mendelson's syndrome. Clin. Radiol. 27: 81, 1976.

Williams, J. L., and Moller, G. A.: Solitary mass in the lungs of coal miners. A.J.R. 117: 765, 1973.

Wright, K. W. (Ed.): Farmer's lung. Symposium. N. Y. State J. Med. 65: 3013, 1965.

Fibrosing Diseases

Addington, W. W., Cugell, D. W., Zelkowitz, P. S., O'Flynn, M. E., and Embry, S.: Cystic fibrosis of the pancreas—a comparison of the pulmonary manifestations in children and young adults. Chest 59: 306, 1971.

Arnett, N. L., and Schultz, D. M.: Primary pulmonary eosinophilic granuloma. Radiology 69: 224, 1959.

Auld, D.: Pathology of eosinophilic granuloma of the lungs. Arch. Pathol. 63: 113, 1957.

Bachman, A. L., and Macken, K.: Pleural effusions following supervoltage radiation for breast carcinoma. Radiology 72: 699, 1959.

Bernstein, S. S., and Sussman, M. L.: Thoracic manifestations of sarcoidosis. Radiology 44: 37, 1945.

Christoforidis, A. J., Nelson, S. W., and Pratt, P. C.: Bronchiolar dilatation associated with muscular hyperplasia: polycystic lung. A.J.R. 92: 513, 1964.

Cooper, G., Jr., Guerrant, J. L., Harden, A. G., and Teates, D.: Some consequences of pulmonary irradiation. A.J.R. 85: 865, 1961.

Deeley, T. J.: The effect of radiation on the lungs in the treatment of carcinoma of the bronchus. Clin. Radiol. 11: 33, 1960.

DiSant'Agnese, P. A., and Talamo, R. C.: Pathogenesis and physiopathology of cystic fibrosis of the pancreas. N. Engl. J. Med. 277: 1287, 1343, 1399, 1967.

Ellis, K., and Renthal, G.: Pulmonary sarcoidosis: roentgenographic observations on course of disease. A.J.R. 88: 1070, 1962.

Felson, B.: Uncommon roentgen patterns of pulmonary sarcoidosis. Dis. Chest 34: 357, 1958.

Fifer, W. R.: Atypical pulmonary histiocytosis-X. Am. Rev. Respir. Dis. 87: 568, 1963.

Fike, R. H.: Occurrence of roentgen pleuropneumonitis in treatment of breast cancer. A.J.R. 27: 509, 1932.

Freundlich, I. M., Libshitz, H. I., Glassman, L. M., and Israel, H. L.: Sarcoidosis. Typical and atypical thoracic manifestations and complications. Clin. Radiol. 21: 376, 1970.

Garland, L. H.: Pulmonary sarcoidosis: the early roentgen findings. Radiology 48: 333, 1947.

Genereux, G. P.: The end-stage lung. Radiology 116: 279, 1975.

Goin, L. S.: Fibrocystic disease of the pancreas. Radiology 51: 36, 1948.

Goldenberg, G. J., and Greenspan, R. H.: Middle lobe atelectasis due to endobronchial sarcoidosis, with hypercalcemia and renal impairment. N. Engl. J. Med. 262: 1112, 1960.

Gorske, K. J., and Fleming, R. J.: Mycetoma formation in cavitary pulmonary sarcoidosis. Radiology 95: 279, 1970.

Hamman, L., and Rich, A. R.: Acute interstitial fibrosis of the lungs. Bull. Hopkins Hosp. 74: 177, 1944.

Hoffman, L., Cohn, J. E., and Gaensler, E. A.: Respiratory abnormalities in eosinophilic granuloma of the lung. N. Engl. J. Med. 267: 577, 1962.

Holsti, L. B., and Vuorinen, P.: Radiation reaction in the lung after continuous and split-course megavoltage radiotherapy of bronchial carcinoma. Br. J. Radiol. 40: 280, 1967.

Holt, J. A. G.: The acute radiation pneumonitis syndrome. J. Coll. Radiol. Austral. 8: 40, 1964.

Johnson, T. H., Jr.: Radiology and honeycomb lung disease. A.J.R. 104: 810, 1968.

Katznelsen, D., Vawter, G. F., Foley, G. E., and Schwachman, H.: Botryomycosis, a complication in cystic fibrosis. J. Pediatr. 65: 525, 1964.

Kirks, D. R., McCormick, V. D., and Greenspan, R. H.: Pulmonary sarcoidosis. Roentgenologic analysis of 150 patients. A.J.R. 117: 777, 1973.

Kirks, D. R., and Greenspan, R. H.: Sarcoid. Radiol. Clin. North Am. 11: 279, 1973.

Libshitz, H. I., and Southard, M. E.: Complications of radiation therapy: the thorax. Semin. Roentgenol. 9: 41, 1974.

Lichtenstein, L.: Histiocytosis-X: Integration of eosinophilic granuloma of bone, Letterer-Siwe disease and Schuller-Christian disease as related manifestations of a single nosologic entity. Arch. Pathol. 56: 84, 1953.

Mandi, L.: Thoracic sarcoidosis in children. Acta Tuberc. Scand. 45: 256, 1964.

McCort, J. J., and Pare, P. J.: Pulmonary fibrosis and cor pulmonale in sarcoidosis. Radiology 62: 496, 1954.

Nadeau, P. J., Ellis, F. H., Jr., Harrison, E. G., Jr., and Fontana, R. S.: Primary pulmonary histiocytosis-X. Dis. Chest 37: 325, 1960.

Reisner, D.: Observations on the course and prognosis of sarcoidosis. With special consideration of its intrathoracic manifestations. Am. Rev. Respir. Dis. 96: 361, 1967.

Roswit, B., and White, D. C.: Severe radiation injuries of the lung. A.J.R. 129: 127, 1977.

Scadding, J. G.: Prognosis of intrathoracic sarcoidosis in England. A review of 136 cases after five years' observation. Br. Med. J. 2: 1165, 1961.

Scadding, J. G., and Hinson, K. F. W.: Diffuse fibrosing alveolitis (diffuse interstitial fibrosis of the lungs): correlation of histology at biopsy with prognosis. Thorax 22: 29, 1967.

Schmitt, E., Appelman, H., and Threatt, B.: Sarcoidosis in children. Radiology 106: 621, 1973.

Sharma, O. P., Hewlett, R., and Gordonson, J.: Nodular sarcoidosis: an unusual radiographic appearance. Chest 64: 189, 1973.

Sheft, D. J., and Moskowitz, H.: Pulmonary muscular hyperplasia. A.J.R. 93: 836, 1965.

Siltzbach, L. E.: Pulmonary sarcoidosis. Am. J. Surg. 89: 556, 1955.

Siltzbach, L. E.: The enigma of sarcoidosis. Hosp. Pract. 3: 80, 1968.

Smith, M., McCormack, L. J., Van Ordstrand, H. S., and Mercer, R. D.: "Primary" pulmonary histiocytosis-X. Chest 65: 176, 1974.

Spann, R. W., Rosenow, E. C., III, DeRemee, R. A., and Miller, W. E.: Unilateral hilar or paratracheal adenopathy in sarcoidosis: a study of 38 cases. Thorax 26: 296, 1971.

Swaye, P., Van Ordstrand, H. S., McCormack, L. J., and Wolpaw, S. E.: Familial Hamman-Rich syndrome. Dis. Chest 7, 1969.

Teirstein, A. S., and Siltzbach, L. E.: Sarcoidosis of the upper lung fields simulating pulmonary tuberculosis. Chest 64: 303, 1973.

Thompson, J. R., and Langer, S.: Eosinophilic granuloma of the lungs. Roentgenologic and pathologic features. Dis. Chest 46: 553, 1964.

Tomashefski, J. F., Christoforidis, A. J., and Abdullah, A. K.: Cystic fibrosis in young adults. An overlooked diagnosis, with emphasis on pulmonary function and radiological patterns. Chest *57:* 28, 1971.

Wentworth, P., Gough, J., and Wentworth, J. E.: Pulmonary changes and cor pulmonale in mucoviscidosis. Thorax *23:* 582, 1968.

White, H.: Fibrocystic disease of the pancreas: roentgen manifestations. Radiology *71:* 816, 1958.

Whitfield, A. G. W., Bond, W. H., and Kunkler, P. B.: Radiation damage to thoracic tissues. Thorax *18:* 371, 1963.

Autoimmune Diseases

Benoit, F. L., Rulon, D. B., Theil, G. B., Doolan, P. D., and Watten, R. H.: Goodpasture's syndrome. A clinicopathologic entity. Am. J. Med. *37:* 424, 1964.

Bischoff, M. E.: Noninfectious necrotizing granulomatosis: Pulmonary roentgen signs. Radiology *75:* 752, 1960.

Bulgrin, J. G., Dubois, E. L., and Jacobson, G.: Chest roentgenographic changes in systemic lupus erythematosus. Radiology *74:* 42, 1960.

Burrows, F. G. O.: Pulmonary nodules in rheumatoid disease: a report of two cases. Br. J. Radiol. *40:* 256, 1967.

Caplan, A.: Certain unusual radiological appearance in the chest of coal miners suffering from rheumatoid arthritis. Thorax *8:* 29, 1953.

Caplan, A., Payne, R. B., and Withey, J. L.: A broader concept of Caplan's syndrome related to rheumatoid factors. Thorax *17:* 205, 1962.

Carrington, C. B., and Liebow, A. A.: Limited forms of angiitis and granulomatosis of Wegener's type. Am. J. Med. *41:* 497, 1966.

Churg, J.: Allergic granulomatosis and granulomatous-vascular syndromes. Ann. Allergy *21:* 619, 1963.

Churg, J., and Strauss, L.: Allergic granulomatosis, allergic angiitis and periarteritis nodosa. Am. J. Pathol. *27:* 277, 1951.

Citro, L. A., Gordon, M. E., and Miller, W. T.: Eosinophilic lung disease. A.J.R. *117:* 787, 1973.

Crofton, J., Livingstone, J. L., Oswald, N. C., and Roberts, A. T. M.: Pulmonary eosinophilia. Thorax *7:* 1, 1952.

DeMuth, G. R., Furstenberg, N. A., Dabich, L., and Zarafonetis, C. J. D.: Pulmonary manifestations of progressive systemic sclerosis. Am. J. Med. Sci. *255:* 94, 1968.

Divertie, M. B., and Johnson, W. J.: Pulmonary involvement in renal disease. Med. Clin. North Am. *50:* 1055, 1966.

Divertie, M. B., and Olsen, A. M.: Pulmonary infiltration associated with blood eosinophilia (P.I.E.): A clinical study of Loeffler's syndrome and of periarteritis with P.I.E. syndrome. Dis. Chest *37:* 340, 1960.

Elkeles, A., and Glynn, L. E.: Serial roentgenograms of the chest in periarteritis nodosa as an aid to diagnosis, with notes on the pathology of the pulmonary lesions. Br. J. Radiol. *17:* 368, 1944.

Felson, B., and Braunstein, H.: Noninfectious necrotizing granulomatosis. Wegener's syndrome, lethal granuloma and allergic angiitis and granulomatosis. Radiology *70:* 326, 1958.

Frazier, A. R., and Miller, R. D.: Interstitial pneumonitis in association with polymyositis and dermatomyositis. Chest *65:* 403, 1974.

Gaensler, E. A., and Carrington, C. B.: Peripheral opacities in chronic eosinophilic pneumonia: the photographic negative of pulmonary edema. A.J.R. *128:* 1, 1977.

Getzowa, S.: Cystic and compact pulmonary sclerosis in progressive scleroderma. Arch. Pathol. *40:* 99, 1945.

Godman, G. C., and Churg, J.: Wegener's granulomatosis. Pathology and review of the literature. Arch. Pathol. *58:* 533, 1959.

Gohel, V. K., Dalinka, M. K., and Israel, H. L.: The radiological manifestations of Wegener's granulomatosis. Br. J. Radiol. *46:* 427, 1973.

Goldring, D., Behrer, M. R., Thomas, W., Elliott, G., and Brown, G.: Rheumatic pneumonia in children. Postgrad. Med. *26:* 739, 1959.

Gondos, B.: Roentgen manifestations in progressive systemic sclerosis (diffuse scleroderma). A.J.R. *84:* 235, 1960.

Goodpasture, E. W.: Significance of certain pulmonary lesions in relation to etiology of influenza. Am. J. Sci. *158:* 863, 1919.

Ham, J. C., and Zimdahl, W. T.: Loeffler's syndrome and pulmonary infiltrations accompanied by peripheral eosinophilia. Ann. Intern. Med. *29:* 488, 1948.

Harkavy, J.: Vascular allergy. Arch. Intern. Med. *67:* 709, 1941.

Harkavy, J.: Vascular allergy. J. Allergy *14:* 507, 1943.

Henderson, A. T., and Peirce, C. B.: Transitory focal pulmonary edema and eosinophilia (Loeffler's syndrome). A.J.R. *58:* 391, 1947.

Hennell, H., and Sussman, M. L.: Roentgen features of eosinophilic infiltrations in lungs. Radiology *44:* 328, 1945.

Hepper, N. G. G., Ferguson, R. H., and Howard, F. M., Jr.: Three types of pulmonary involvement in polymyositis. Med. Clin. North Am. *48:* 1031, 1964.

Herman, P. G., Balikian, J. P., Seltzer, S. E., and Ehrie, M.: The pulmonary-renal syndrome. A.J.R. *130:* 1141, 1978.

Hyun, B. H., Diggs, C. L., and Toone, E. C., Jr.: Dermatomyositis with cystic

fibrosis (honeycombing) of the lung. Dis. Chest *42:* 449, 1962.

Jordan, J. D., and Snyder, C. H.: Rheumatoid disease of the lung and cor pulmonale. Observations in a child. Am. J. Dis. Child. *108:* 74, 1964.

Kemp Harper, R. A., and Jackson, D. C.: Progressive systemic sclerosis. Br. J. Radiol. *38:* 825, 1965.

Kirkpatrick, J. A., Jr., and Fleisher, D. S.: The roentgen appearance of the chest in acute glomerulonephritis in children. J. Pediatr. *64:* 492, 1964.

Leggat, P. O., and Walton, E. W.: Wegener's granulomatosis. Thorax *11:* 94, 1956.

Levin, D. C.: Proper interpretation of pulmonary roentgen changes in systemic lupus erythematosus. A.J.R. *111:* 510, 1971.

Locke, G. B.: Rheumatoid lung. Clin. Radiol. *14:* 43, 1963.

Loffler, W.: Zur Differential-diagnose der Lungen Infiltrierungen; II Uber fluchtize Succedan-infiltrate (mit Eosinophilie). Beitr. Klin. Tuberk. *79:* 368, 1932.

Loffler, W.: Die fluchtigen Lungeninfiltrate mit eosinophilie. Schweiz. Med. Wochenschr. *66:* 1069, 1936.

Lustok, M. J., and Kuzma, J. F.: Rheumatic fever pneumonitis: a clinical and pathologic study of 35 cases. Ann. Intern. Med. *44:* 337, 1966.

Lynch, E. C., Fred, H. L., and Greenberg, S. D.: Pulmonary cavitation in Wegener's granulomatosis. A.J.R. *92:* 521, 1964.

Martel, W., Abell, M. R., Mikkelsen, W. M., and Whitehouse, W. M.: Pulmonary and pleural lesions in rheumatoid disease. Radiology *90:* 641, 1968.

Moersch, H., Purnell, D. C., and Good, C. A.: Pulmonary changes occurring in disseminated lupus erythematosus. Dis. Chest *29:* 166, 1956.

Montgomery, R. D., Stirling, G. A., and Hamer, N. A. J.: Bronchiolar carcinoma in progressive systemic sclerosis. Lancet *1:* 586, 1964.

Morgan, W. K. C., and Wolfel, D. A.: The lungs and pleura in rheumatoid arthritis. A.J.R. *98:* 334, 1966.

Mortensson, W., Larsson, L. E., and Lindqvist, B.: Pulmonary haemorrhage in renal disease. Acta Radiol. *7:* 457, 1968.

Naeye, R. L.: Pulmonary vascular lesions in systemic scleroderma. Dis. Chest *44:* 374, 1963.

Noonan, C. D., Taylor, F. B., Jr., and Engleman, E. P.: Nodular rheumatoid disease of the lungs with cavitation. Arthritis Rheum. *6:* 232, 1963.

Overholt, E. L.: Acute pulmonary-renal syndromes. Dis. Chest *48:* 68, 1965.

Parkin, T. W., Rusted, I. E., Burchell, H. B., and Edwards, J. E.: Hemorrhagic and interstitial pneumonitis with nephritis. Am. J. Med. *18:* 220, 1955.

Pierce, J. A.: Rheumatology and the lungs. J. Am. Geriatr. Soc. *16:* 514, 1968.

Popper, M. S., Bogdonoff, M. L., and Hughes, R. L.: Interstitial rheumatoid lung disease. A reassessment and review of the literature. Chest *62:* 243, 1972.

Portner, M. M., and Gracie, M. A., Jr.: Rheumatoid lung disease with cavitary nodules, pneumothorax and eosinophilia. N. Engl. J. Med. *275:* 697, 1966.

Purnell, D. C., Baggenstoss, A. H., and Olsen, A. M.: Pulmonary lesions in disseminated lupus erythematosus. Ann. Intern. Med. *42:* 619, 1955.

Richards, R. L., and Milne, J. A.: Cancer of the lung in progressive systemic sclerosis. Thorax *13:* 238, 1958.

Roberts, S. R., Jr.: Immunology and the lung: and overview. Semin. Roentgenol. *10:* 7, 1975.

Robertson, C. L., Shackelford, G. D., and Armstrong, J. D.: Chronic eosinophilic pneumonia. Radiology *101:* 57, 1971.

Rose, G. A., and Spencer, H.: Polyarteritis nodosa. Q. J. Med. *26:* 43, 1957.

Rubin, E. H., Gordon, M., and Thelmo, W. L.: Nodular pleuropulmonary rheumatoid disease. Am. J. Med. *42:* 567, 1967.

Schwartz, E. E., Teplick, J. G., Onesti, G., and Schwartz, A. B.: Pulmonary hemorrhage in renal disease: Goodpasture's syndrome and other causes. Radiology *122:* 39, 1977.

Seldin, B. W., Kaplan, H. S., and Bunting, H.: Rheumatic pneumonia. Ann. Intern. Med. *26:* 496, 1946.

Shapiro, H., and Lowman, R. M.: Roentgen manifestations of erythema exudativum multiforme (Stevens-Johnson syndrome) Dis. Chest *32:* 329, 1957.

Spiegel, R.: Clinical aspects of periarteritis nodosa. Arch. Intern. Med. *58:* 993, 1936.

Strimlan, C. V., Rosenow, E. C., III, Divertie, M. B., and Harrison, E. G.: Pulmonary manifestations of Sjogren's syndrome. Chest *70:* 354, 1976.

Svanberg, T.: Roentgenographical pulmonary changes in periarteritis nodosa. Acta Radiol. *26:* 307, 1945.

Sweeney, A. R., Jr., and Baggenstoss, A.: Pulmonary lesions of periarteritis nodosa. Proc. Mayo Clin. *24:* 35, 1949.

Sybers, R. G., Sybers, J. L., Dickie, H. A., and Paul, L. W.: Roentgenographic aspects of hemorrhagic pulmonary-renal disease (Goodpasture's syndrome). A.J.R. *94:* 674, 1965.

Taylor, T. L., and Ostrum, H.: The roentgenologic evaluation of systemic lupus erythematosus. A.J.R. *82:* 95, 1959.

Twersky, J., Twersky, N., and Lehr, C.: Scleroderma and carcinoma of the lung. Clin. Radiol. *27:* 203, 1976.

Walker, W. C., and Wright, V.: Diffuse interstitial pulmonary fibrosis and rheumatoid arthritis. Ann. Rheum. Dis. *28:* 252, 1969.

Walton, E. W.: Giant-cell granuloma of respiratory tract (Wegener's granulomatosis). Br. Med. J. *2:* 265, 1958.

Wanke, M.: Isolierte Periarteritis Nodosa der Lungen nebst Bemerleungen zur sogenannten entzundlichen Arteriosklerose. Z. Kreislaufforsch. *54:* 235, 1965.

Weaver, A. L., Divertie, M. D., and Titus, J. L.: Pulmonary scleroderma. Dis. Chest *54:* 4, 1968.

Wegener, F.: Uber ein eigenartige rhinogene Granulomatose mit besonderer Beteilung des Arteriensystems und der Nieren. Beitr. Pathol. Anat. *102:* 36, 1939.

Wolff, S. M., Fauci, A. S., Horn, R. G., and Dale, D. C.: Wegener's granulomatosis. Ann. Intern. Med. *81:* 513, 1974.

Miscellaneous Pulmonary Conditions

Adams, F. G., and Ledingham, I. McA.: The pulmonary manifestations of septic shock. Clin. Radiol. *28:* 215, 1977.

Andriole, V. T., Ballas, M., and Wilson, G. L.: The association of nocardiosis and pulmonary alveolar proteinosis. Ann. Intern. Med. *60:* 266, 1964.

Auerbach, R. C., Snyder, N. E., and Bragg, D. G.: The chest roentgenographic manifestations of pronestyl-induced lupus erythematosus. Radiology *109:* 287, 1973.

Avery, M. D.: *The Lung and its Disorders in the Newborn Infant.* W. B. Saunders, Philadelphia, 1964.

Baghdassarian, O., Avery, M. E., and Neuhauser, E. B. D.: A form of pulmonary insufficiency in premature infants. Pulmonary dysmaturity? A.J.R. *89:* 1020, 1963.

Belanger, R., LaFleche, L. R., and Picard, J-L.: Cystic adenomatoid malformation of the lung. Thorax *19:* 1, 1964.

Bergman, F., and Linder, E.: Tumor-forming amyloidosis of the lung. J. Thorac. Surg. *35:* 628, 1958.

Brown, J.: Primary amyloidosis. Clin. Radiol. *15:* 38, 1964.

Brown, W. G., Hasan, F. M., and Barbee, R. A.: Reversibility of severe bleomycin-induced pneumonia. J.A.M.A. *239:* 2012, 1978.

Bruwer, A. J., Kennedy, R. L. J., and Edwards, J. E.: Recurrent pulmonary hemorrhage with hemosiderosis: so-called idiopathic pulmonary hemosiderosis. A.J.R. *76:* 98, 1956.

Burrows, F. G. O., and Edwards, J. M.: A pulmonary disease in patients ventilated with high oxygen concentrations. Br. J. Radiol. *43:* 848, 1970.

Bush, J. K., McLean, R. L., and Sieker, H. O.: Diffuse lung disease due to lymphangiomyoma. Am. J. Med. *46:* 645, 1969.

Caffey, J.: *Pediatric X-ray Diagnosis*, Ed. 6. Year Book, Chicago, 1972.

Campbell, R. E.: Intrapulmonary interstitial emphysema: a complication of hyaline membrane disease. A.J.R. *110:* 449, 1970.

Celli, B. R., Rubinow, A., Cohen, A. S., and Brody, J. S.: Patterns of pulmonary involvement in systemic amyloidosis. Chest *74:* 543, 1978.

Clarysse, A. M., Cathey, W. J., Cartwright, G. E., and Wintrobe, M. M.: Pulmonary disease complicating intermittent therapy with methotrexate. J.A.M.A. *22:* 1861, 1969.

Craig, J. M., Kirkpatrick, J., and Neuhauser, E. B. D.: Congenital cystic adenomatoid malformation of the lung in infants. A.J.R. *76:* 516, 1956.

Craver, W. L.: Solitary amyloid tumor of the lung. J. Thorac. Cardiovasc. Surg. *49:* 860, 1965.

Crawford, W. O., Jr.: Pulmonary injury in thoracic and non-thoracic trauma. Radiol. Clin. North Am. *11:* 527, 1973.

Cremin, B. J.: Infantile thoracic dystrophy. Br. J. Radiol. *43:* 199, 1970.

Daughtry, D. C.: Traumatic torsion of the lung. N. Engl. J. Med. *256:* 385, 1957.

Davidson, J. K., and Macpherson, P.: Pulmonary changes in paraquat poisoning. Clin. Radiol. *23:* 18, 1972.

Dyck, D. R., and Zylak, C. J.: Acute respiratory distress in adults. Radiology *106:* 497, 1973.

Edwards, D. K., Wayne, M. D., and Northway, W. H.: Twelve years' experience with bronchopulmonary dysplasia. Pediatrics *59:* 839, 1977.

Everts, C. S., Westcott, J. L., and Bragg, D. G.: Methotrexate therapy and pulmonary disease. Radiology *107:* 539, 1973.

Fagan, C. J., and Swischuk, L. E.: Traumatic lung and paramediastinal pneumatoceles. Radiology *120:* 11, 1976.

Felman, A. H., Rhatigan, R. M., and Pierson, K. K.: Pulmonary lymphangiectasia. A.J.R. *116:* 548, 1972.

Firestone, F. N., and Joison, J.: Amyloidosis. J. Thorac. Cardiovasc. Surg. *51:* 292, 1966.

Foote, G. A., and Stewart, J. H.: The coexistence of pneumonia and the idiopathic respiratory distress syndrome in neonates. Br. J. Radiol. *46:* 504, 1973.

Gaensler, E. A., Goff, A. M., and Prowse, C. M.: Desquamative interstitial pneumonia. N. Engl. J. Med. *274:* 113, 1966.

Gibbs, A. R., and Seal, R. M. E.: Primary

lymphoproliferative conditions of lung. Thorax 33: 140, 1978.

Giedion, A., Muller, W. A., and Molz, G.: Angeborene lymphangiektasie der lungen. Helv. Paediatr. Acta 22: 170, 1967.

Gooding, C. A., and Gregory, G. A.: Roentgenographic analysis of meconium aspiration of the newborn. Radiology 100: 131, 1971.

Greening, R., Kynette, A., and Hodes, P. J.: Unusual pulmonary changes secondary to chest trauma. A.J.R. 77: 1059, 1957.

Grossman, H., Berdon, W. E., Mizrahi, A., and Baker, D. H.: Neonatal focal hyperaeration of the lungs (Wilson-Mikity syndrome). Radiology 85: 409, 1965.

Hall, R. M., and Margolin, F. R.: Oxygen alveolopathy in adults. Clin. Radiol. 23: 11, 1972.

Halprin, G. M., Ramirez, R. J., and Pratt, P. C.: Lymphoid interstitial pneumonia. Chest 62: 418, 1972.

Hanford, R. B., Schneider, G. F., and MacCarthy, J. D.: Massive thoracic extramedullary hemopoesis. N. Engl. J. Med. 263: 120, 1960.

Harris, G. B. C.: The newborn with respiratory distress: some roentgenographic features. Radiol. Clin. North Am. 1: 497, 1963.

Heitzman, E. R., Markarian, B., and Delise, C. T.: Lymphoproliferative disorders of the thorax. Semin. Roentgenol. 10: 73, 1975.

Hopewell, P. C., and Murray, J. F.: The adult respiratory distress syndrome. Ann. Rev. Med. 27: 343, 1976.

Israel, H. L., and Diamond, P.: Recurrent pulmonary infiltration and pleural effusion due to nitroforantoin sensitivity. N. Engl. J. Med. 266: 1024, 1962.

Joffe, N.: Roentgenologic findings in post-shock and postoperative pulmonary insufficiency. Radiology 94: 369, 1970.

Joffe, N., and Simon, M.: Pulmonary oxygen toxicity in the adult. Radiology 92: 460, 1969.

Julsrud, P. R., Brown, L. R., Ll, C.-Y., Rosenow, E. C., III, and Crowe, J. K.: Pulmonary processes of mature-appearing lymphocytes: pseudolymphoma, lymphocytic lymphoma, and lymphocytic interstitial pneumonitis. Radiology 127: 289, 1978.

Kapanci, Y., Tosco, R., Eggermann, J., and Gould, V. E.: Oxygen pneumonitis in man. Light and electron-microscopic morphometric studies. Chest 62: 161, 1972.

Kaye, M. D.: Pleuropulmonary complications of pancreatitis. Thorax 23: 297, 1968.

Knoblich, R.: Extramedullary hematopoesis presenting as intrathoracic tumors. Report of a case in a patient with thalassemia minor. Cancer 13: 462, 1960.

Korsten, J., Grossman, H., Winchester, P. H., and Canale, V. C.: Extramedullary hematopoesis in patients with thalassemia anemia. Radiology 95: 257, 1970.

Kwittken, J., and Reiner, L.: Congenital cystic adenomatoid malformation of the lung. Pediatrics 30: 759, 1962.

Lawrence, K. M.: Congenital pulmonary lymphangiectasis. J. Clin. Pathol. 12: 69, 1959.

Lee, S.-C., and Johnson, H. A.: Multiple nodular pulmonary amyloidosis. Thorax 30: 178, 1975.

Liebow, A. A., Carrington, C. B., and Friedman, P. J.: Lymphomatoid granulomatosis. Hum. Pathol. 3: 457, 1972.

Liebow, A. A., Steer, A., and Billingsley, J. G.: Desquamative interstitial pneumonia. Am. J. Med. 39: 369, 1965.

Lemire, P., Bettez, P., Gelinas, M., and Raymond, G.: Patterns of desquamative interstitial pneumonia (D.I.P.) and diffuse interstitial pulmonary fibrosis (D.I.P.F.). A.J.R. 115: 479, 1972.

Lowman, R. M., Bloor, C. M., and Newcomb, A. W.: Roentgen manifestations of thoracic extra-medullary hematopoesis. Dis. Chest 44: 154, 1963.

Macfarlane, A., and Davies, D.: Diffuse lymphoid interstitial pneumonia. Thorax 28: 768, 1973.

Madewell, J. E., Stocker, J. T., and Korsower, J. M.: Cystic adenomatoid malformation of the lung. A.J.R. 124: 436, 1975.

Milne, E., and Dick, A.: Circumscribed intrapulmonary hematoma. Br. J. Radiol. 34: 587, 1961.

Moncrieff, M. W., Cameron, A. H., Astley, R., Roberts, K. D., Abrams, L. D., and Mann, J. R.: Congenital cystic adenomatoid malformation of the lung. Thorax 24: 276, 1969.

Morrison, W. J., Wetherill, S., and Zyroff, I.: The acute pulmonary edema of heroin intoxication. Radiology 97: 347, 1970.

Munk, J.: The radiological differentiation between acute diffuse interstitial pneumonia and pulmonary interstitial oedema in infancy and early childhood. Br. J. Radiol. 47: 752, 1974.

Noonan, J. A., Walters, L. R., and Reeves, J. T.: Congenital pulmonary lymphangiectasis. Am. J. Dis. Child. 120: 314, 1970.

Patchefsky, A. S., Israel, H. L., Hoch, W. S., and Gordon, G.: Desquamative interstitial pneumonia: relationship to interstitial fibrosis. Thorax 28: 680, 1973.

Plenk, H. P., Swift, S. A., Chambers, W. L., and Peltzer, W. E.: Pulmonary alveolar proteinosis—a new disease? Radiology 74: 928, 1960.

Podoll, L. N., and Winkler, S. S.: Busul-

fan lung. Report of two cases and review of the literature. A.J.R. 120: 151, 1974.

Prowse, C. B.: Amyloidosis of the lower respiratory tract. Thorax 13: 308, 1958.

Ramirez-R. J.: Pulmonary alveolar proteinosis. A.J.R. 92: 571, 1964.

Ramirez-R. J., Nyka, W., and McLaughlin, J.: Pulmonary alveolar proteinosis. Diagnostic technics and observations. N. Engl. J. Med. 268: 165, 1963.

Reddy, P. A., Gorelick, D. F., and Christianson, C. S.: Giant cell interstitial pneumonia (G.I.P.). Chest 58: 319, 1970.

Reynolds, J., and Davis, J. T.: Injuries of the chest wall, pleura pericardium, lungs, bronchi and esophagus. Radiol. Clin. North Am. 4: 383, 1966.

Rohlfing, B. M.: Drug-induced lung disease. In Diagnostic Radiology 1977, edited by A. R. Margulis and C. A. Gooding. C. V. Mosby, St. Louis, 1977.

Rosen, S. H., Castelman, B., and Liebow, A. A.: Pulmonary alveolar proteinosis. N. Engl. J. Med. 258: 1123, 1958.

Rosenow, E. C., III: Drug-induced hypersensitivity disease of the lung. In Immunologic and Infectious Reactions in the Lung, edited by C. H. Kirkpatrick and H. Y. Reynolds. Marcel Dekker, New York, 1976.

Rudders, R. A., and Hensley, G. T.: Bleomycin pulmonary toxicity. Chest 63: 626, 1973.

Samuels, M. L., Johnson, D. E., Holoye, P. Y., and Lanzotti, V. J.: Large-dose bleomycin therapy and pulmonary toxicity. A possible role of prior radiotherapy. J.A.M.A. 235: 1117, 1976.

Schoeniger, E. L., Tucker, A. S., and Bolande, R. P.: Idiopathic pulmonary hemorrhage with hemosiderosis and microcystic anemia. Radiology 70: 191, 1958.

Schuller, H., Bolin, H., Linder, E., and Stenram, U.: Tumor-forming amyloidosis of the lower respiratory system. Report of a case in the lung and a short review of the literature. Dis. Chest 42: 58, 1962.

Schultze, G.: Chest film findings in neonatal respiratory distress. Radiology 70: 230, 1958.

Sears, M. R., Chang, A. R., and Taylor, A. J.: Pulmonary alveolar microlithiasis. Thorax 26: 704, 1971.

Sickles, E. A., and Gooding, C. A.: Asymmetric lung involvement in bronchopulmonary dysplasia. Radiology 118: 379, 1976.

Soergel, K. H., and Sommers, S. C.: Idiopathic pulmonary hemosiderosis and related syndromes. Am. J. Med. 32: 499, 1962.

Solliday, N. H., Shapiro, B. A., and Gracey, D. R.: Adult respiratory distress syndrome. Chest 69: 207, 1976.

Sorsdahl, O. A., and Powell, J. W.: Cavitary pulmonary lesions following nonpenetrating chest trauma in children. A.J.R. *95:* 118, 1965.

Sosman, M. C., Dodd, G. D., Jones, W. D., and Pillmore, G. U.: The familial occurrence of pulmonary microlithiasis. A.J.R. *77:* 947, 1957.

Sostman, H. D., Matthay, R. A., and Putman, C. E.: Cytotoxic drug-induced lung disease. Am. J. Med. *62:* 608, 1977.

Stern, W. Z., Spear, P. W., and Jacobson, H. W.: The roentgen findings in acute heroin intoxication. A.J.R. *103:* 522, 1968.

Summers, J. E.: Pulmonary alveolar proteinosis. Review of the literature with follow-up studies, a report of two cases. Calif. Med. *104:* 428, 1966.

Swischuk, L. E.: *Radiology of the Newborn and Young Infant.* Williams & Wilkins, Baltimore, 1973.

Swischuk, L. E.: Bubbles in hyaline membrane disease. Differentiation of three types. Radiology *122:* 417, 1977.

Swyer, P. R., Delivoria-Papadopoulous, M., Levison, H., Reilly, B. J., and Balis, J. U.: The pulmonary syndrome of Wilson and Mikity. Pediatrics *36:* 374, 1965.

Teixidor, H. S., and Bachman, A. L.: Multiple amyloid tumors of the lung. A case report. A.J.R. *111:* 525, 1971.

Ting, Y. M.: Pulmonary parenchymal findings in blunt trauma to the chest. A.J.R. *98:* 343, 1966.

Tudor, J., Young, L., Wigglesworth, J. S., and Steiner, R. E.: The value of radiology in the idiopathic respiratory distress syndrome: a radiological and pathological correlation study. Clin. Radiol. *27:* 65, 1976.

Veneziale, C. M., Sheridan, L. A., Payne, W. S., and Harrison, E. G., Jr.: Angiofollicular lymph-node hyperplasia of the mediastinum. J. Thorac. Cardiovasc. Surg. *47:* 111, 1964.

Wagenaar, S. S., Swierenga, J., and Wagenvoort, C. A.: Late presentation of primary pulmonary lymphangiectasis. Thorax *33:* 791, 1978.

Wentworth, P., Lynch, M. J., Fallis, J. C., Turner, J. A. P., Lowden, J. A., and Cohen, P. E.: Xanthomatous pseudotumor of lung. A case report with electron microscope and lipid studies. Cancer *22:* 345, 1968.

Wesenberg, R. L., Graven, S. N., and McCabe, E. B.: Radiological findings in wet-lung disease. Radiology *98:* 69, 1971.

Whitcomb, M. E.: Drug-induced disease. Critical review. Chest *63:* 418, 1973.

Williams, J. R.: The vanishing lung tumor—pulmonary hematoma. A.J.R. *81:* 296, 1959.

Williams, J. R., and Bonte, F. J.: *The Roentgenological Aspect of Nonpen-*

etrating Chest Injuries. Charles C Thomas, Springfield, Ill., 1961.

Williams, J. R., and Stembridge, V. A.: Pulmonary contusion secondary to nonpenetrating chest trauma. A.J.R. *91:* 284, 1964.

Wilson, J. M., Thomas, A. N., Goodman, P. C., and Lewis, F. R.: Severe chest trauma. Morbidity implication of first and second rib fracture in 120 patients. Arch. Surg. *113:* 846, 1978.

Wilson, M. G., and Mikity, V. G.: A new form of respiratory distress in premature infants. J. Dis. Child. *99:* 489, 1960.

Wilson, S. R., Sanders, D. E., and Delarue, N. C.: Intrathoracic manifestations of amyloid disease. Radiology *120:* 283, 1976.

Wynn-Williams, N., and Young, R. D.: Idiopathic pulmonary hemosiderosis in an adult. Thorax *11:* 101, 1956.

Pulmonary Neoplasms

Adamson, J. S., Senior, R. M., and Merrill, T.: Alveolar cell carcinoma. An electron microscopic study. Am. Rev. Respir. Dis. *100:* 550, 1969.

Anderson, H. J., and Pierce, J. W.: Carcinoma of the bronchus presenting as thin-walled cysts. Thorax *9:* 100, 1954.

Aufses, A. H., and Aufses, B. H.: Hypertrophic osteoarthropathy in association with pulmonary metastases from extra thoracic malignancies. Dis. Chest *38:* 399, 1960.

Bagshawe, K. D., and Garnett E. S.: Radiological changes in the lungs of patients with trophoblastic tumours. Br. J. Radiol. *36:* 673, 1963.

Baron, M. G., and Whitehouse, W. M.: Primary lymphosarcoma of the lung A.J.R. *85:* 294, 1961.

Barson, A. J., Jones, A. W., and Lodge, K. V.: Pulmonary blastoma. J. Clin. Pathol. *21:* 480, 1968.

Bartley, T. D., and Arean, V. M.: Intrapulmonary neurogenic tumors. J. Thorac. Cardiovasc. Surg. *50:* 114, 1965.

Bateson, E. M.: The solitary circumscribed bronchogenic carcinoma: a radiological study of 100 cases. Br. J. Radiol. *37:* 598, 1964.

Belgrad, R., Good, C. A., and Woolner, L. B.: Alveolar cell carcinoma (terminal bronchiolar carcinoma). A study of surgically excised tumors with special emphasis on localized lesions. Radiology *79:* 789, 1962.

Benfield, J. R., Bonney, H., Crummy, A. B., and Cleveland, R. J.: Azygograms and pulmonary arteriograms in bronchogenic carcinoma. Arch. Surg. *99:* 406, 1969.

Berkmen, Y.: The many facets of alveolar-cell carcinoma of the lung. Radiology *92:* 793, 1969.

Bodey, G. P., Powell, R. D., Jr., Hersh, E. M., Yeterian, A., and Freireich, E. J.: Pulmonary complications of acute leukemia. Cancer *19:* 781, 1966.

Brinkman, G. L.: The significance of pleural effusion complicating otherwise operable bronchogenic carcinoma. Dis. Chest *36:* 152, 1959.

Chaudhuri, M. R.: Cavitary pulmonary metastases. Thorax *25:* 375, 1970.

Chaudhuri, M. R.: Primary pulmonary cavitating carcinomas. Thorax *28:* 354, 1973.

Coussement, A. M., and Gooding, C. A.: Cavitating pulmonary metastatic disease in children. A.J.R. *117:* 833, 1973.

Deck, F. W., and Sherman, R. S.: Excavation of metastatic nodules in lung. Roentgenographic considerations. Radiology *72:* 30, 1959.

Decker, D. A., Dines, D. E., Payne, W. S., Bernatz, P. E., and Pairolero, P. C.: The significance of a cytologically negative pleural effusion in bronchogenic carcinoma. Chest *74:* 640, 1978.

Delarue, N. C., and Strasberg, S. M.: The rationale of intensive preoperative investigation in bronchogenic carcinoma. J. Thorac. Cardiovasc. Surg. *51:* 391, 1966.

Ellman, P., and Bowdler, A. J.: Pulmonary manifestations of Hodgkin's disease. Br. J. Dis. Chest *54:* 59, 1960.

Engelman, R. M.: Pulmonary fibroma: a rare benign tumor. Am. Rev. Respir. Dis. *96:* 1242, 1967.

Engelman, R. F., Shafer, P. W., and Higgins, G. A., Jr.: Pulmonary angiography in lung cancer suspects. J. Thorac. Cardiovasc. Surg. *57:* 356, 1969.

Fayos, J.: Extrapulmonary intrathoracic manifestations of Hodgkin's disease, Radiol. Clin. North Am. *6:* 131, 1968.

Feigin, D. S., Siegelman, S. S., Theros, E. G., and King, F. M.: Nonmalignant lymphoid disorders of the chest. A.J.R. *129:* 221, 1977.

Felson, B., and Wiot, J. F.: Some less familiar manifestations of carcinoma of the lung. Semin. Roentgenol. *12:* 187, 1977.

Fleischner, F. G.: The esophagus and mediastinal lymphadenopathy in bronchial carcinoma. Radiology *58:* 48, 1952.

Gajaraj, A., Johnson, T. H., Jr., and Feist, J. H.: Roentgen features of giant cell carcinoma of the lung. A.J.R. *111:* 486, 1971.

Garland, L. H., Coulson, W., and Wollin, E.: The rate of growth and apparent duration of untreated primary bronchial carcinoma. Cancer *16:* 694, 1963.

Gerle, R., and Felson, B.: Metastatic endobronchial hypernephroma. Dis. Chest *44:* 225, 1963.

Gibbs, A. R., and Seal, R. M. E.: Primary lymphoproliferative conditions of lung. Thorax *33:* 140, 1978.

Good, C. A., and Holman, C. B.: Cavitary carcinoma of the lung: roentgenologic features in 19 cases. Dis. Chest 37: 289, 1960.

Greene, R., McCloud, T. C., and Stark, P.: Other malignant tumors of the lung. Semin. Roentgenol. 12: 225, 1977.

Greenfield, H., and Gyepes, M. T.: Oval-shaped consolidations simulating new growth of the lung. A.J.R. 91: 125, 1964.

Hartweg, H.: Das Rontgenbild des Thorax bei den chronischen Leukosen Fortschr. Geb. Rontgenstr. 92: 477, 1960.

Havard, C. W. H., Nicholas, J. B., and Stansfeld, A. G.: Primary lymphosarcoma of the lung. Thorax 17: 190, 1962.

Heimlich, H. T., and Rubin, M.: Spontaneous pneumothorax as a presenting feature of primary carcinoma of the lung. Dis. Chest 27: 457, 1955.

Heitzman, E. R.: Bronchogenic carcinoma: radiologic-pathologic correlations. Semin. Roentgenol. 12: 165, 1977.

Herskovic, T., Andersen, H. A., and Bayrd, E. D.: Intrathoracic plasmacytomas. Presentation of 21 cases and review of the literature. Dis. Chest 47: 1, 1965.

Ikins, P. M., Berne, A. S., Straehley, C. J., Jr., and Bugden, W. F.: Carbon dioxide pneumomediastinography as an aid in the evaluation of the resectability of bronchogenic carcinoma. J. Thorac. Cardiovasc. Surg. 44: 793, 1962.

Iverson, R. E., and Straehley, C. J.: Pulmonary blastoma; long term survival of juvenile patient. Chest 63: 436, 1973.

Jacques, J. E., and Barclay, R.: The solid sarcomatous pulmonary artery. Br. J. Dis. Chest 54: 217, 1960.

Janower, M. L., and Blennerhasset, J. B.: Lymphangitic spread of metastatic cancer to the lung. Radiology 101: 267, 1971.

Johansson, L., and Soderlund, S.: Intrathoracic lipoma. Acta Chir. Scand. 126: 558, 1963.

Kalifa, L. G., Schimmel, D. H., and Gamsu, G.: Multiple chronic benign pulmonary nodules. Radiology 121: 275, 1976.

Keats, T. E., and Teates, C. D.: The roentgen manifestations of thoracic reticulum cell sarcoma. Radiol. Clin. North Am. 6: 143, 1968.

Kittredge, R. D., and Sherman, R. S.: Roentgen findings in terminal bronchiolar carcinoma. A.J.R. 87: 875, 1962.

Latour, A., and Shulman, H. S.: Thoracic manifestations of renal cell carcinoma. Radiology 121: 43, 1976.

Liavaag, K.: Chronic nonmalignant pulmonary lesions simulating bronchogenic carcinoma. Acta Chir. Scand. 99: 313, 1950.

Liebow, A. A.: Pathology of carcinoma of the lung as related to the roentgen shadow. A.J.R. 74: 383, 1955.

Loring, W. E., and Wolman, S. R.: Idiopathic multiple hemorrhagic sarcoma of the lung (Kaposi's sarcoma). N. Y. State J. Med. 65: 668, 1965.

Ludington, L. G., Verska, J. J., Howard, T., Kypridakis, G., and Brewer, L. A., III: Bronchiolar carcinoma (alveolar cell), another great imitator; review of 41 cases. Chest 61: 622, 1972.

Madewell, J. E., and Feigin, D. S.: Benign tumors of the lung. Semin. Roentgenol. 12: 175, 1977.

Mason, W. E., and Templeton, A. W.: Bronchographic signs useful in the diagnosis of lung cancer. Dis. Chest 49: 284, 1966.

McCorkle, R. G., Koerth, C. J., and Donaldson, J. M.: Thoracic lipomas. J. Thorac. Surg. 9: 568, 1940.

McNamara, J. J., Kingsley, W. B., Paulson, D. L., Arndt, J. H., Salinas-Izaquirre, S. F., and Urschel, H. C.: Alveolar cell (bronchiolar) carcinoma of the lung. J. Thorac. Cardiovasc. Surg. 57: 648, 1969.

McNamara, J. J., Paulson, D. L., Kingsley, W. B., Salinas-Izaquirre, S. F., and Urschel, H. C., Jr.: Primary leiomyosarcoma of the lung. J. Thorac. Cardiovasc. Surg. 57: 635, 1969.

Meade, J. B., Whitwell, F., Bickford, B. J., and Waddington J. K. B.: Primary hemangiopericytoma of lung. Thorax 29: 1, 1974.

Milne, E.: Circulation of primary and metastatic pulmonary neoplasms. A postmortem microarteriographic study. A.J.R. 100: 603, 1967.

Moffat, R. E., Chang, C. H., and Slaven, J. E.: Roentgen considerations in primary pulmonary artery sarcoma. Radiology 104: 283, 1972.

Molnar, W., and Riebel, F. A.: Bronchography: an aid in the diagnosis of peripheral pulmonary carcinoma. Radiol. Clin. North Am. 1: 303, 1963.

Morgan, A. D., Jepson, E. M., and Billimoria, J. D.: Intrathoracic hibernoma. Thorax 21: 186, 1966.

Nakata, H., Matsuura, K., and Russell, W. J.: Roentgenologic observations of lung carcinoma in the ABCC-JNIH adult health study, 1950–1968, Hiroshima Nagasaki. Radiology 95: 623, 1970.

Neuhof, H., Rabin, C. B., and Sarot, I. A.: Topographic classification of cancer of lung with special reference to surgical implications of circumscribed variety. J. Thorac. Surg. 11: 388, 1942.

Neuhof, H., Sussman, M. L., and Nabatoff, R. A.: Angiocardiography in differential diagnosis of pulmonary neoplasms. Surgery 25: 178, 1949.

Nofsinger, C. D., and Vinson, P. P.: Intrabronchial metastasis of hypernephroma simulating primary bronchial carcinoma. J.A.M.A. 119: 944, 1942.

Nohl, H. C.: An investigation into the lymphatic and vascular spread of carcinoma of the bronchus. Thorax 11: 172, 1956.

Olbert, V. F.: Seltene angiographische untersuchungsmethoden beim bronchuskarzinom. Versuch einer kritischen wertung. Fortschr. Med. 94: 775, 1976.

Papavasiliou, C. G.: Pulmonary metastases from cancer of the nasopharynx associated with hypertrophic osteoarthropathy. Br. J. Radiol. 36: 429, 1963.

Peabody, J. W., Rupnik, E. J., and Hanner, J. M.: Bronchial carcinoma masquerading as a thin-walled cyst. A.J.R. 77: 1051, 1957.

Peacock, M. J., and Whitwell, F.: Pulmonary blastoma. Thorax 31: 197, 1976.

Ramanathan, T.: Primary leiomyosarcoma of the lung. Thorax 29: 482, 1974.

Renner, R. R., Nelson, D. A., and Lozner, E. L.: Roentgenologic manifestations of primary macroglobulinemia (Waldenstrom). A.J.R. 113: 499, 1971.

Rigler, L. G.: A roentgen study of the evolution of carcinoma of the lung. J. Thorac. Surg. 34: 283, 1957.

Rigler, L. G., and Kelby, G. M.: Emphysema: an early roentgen sign of bronchogenic carcinoma. Radiology 49: 578, 1947.

Rigler, L. G.: The roentgen signs of carcinoma of the lung. A.J.R. 74: 415, 1955.

Rinker, C. T., Garrotto, L. J., Lee, K. R., and Templeton, A. W.: Bronchography. Diagnostic signs and accuracy in pulmonary carcinoma. A.J.R. 104: 802, 1968.

Rinker, C. T., Templeton, A. W., MacKenzie, J., Ridings, G. R., and Kiphart, R.: Combined superior vena cavography and azygography in patients with suspected lung carcinoma. Radiology 88: 441, 1967.

Samuels, M. L., Howe, C. D., Dodd, G. D., Jr., Fuller, L. M., Shullenberger, C. C., and Leary, W. L.: Endobronchial malignant lymphoma. Report of five cases in adults. A.J.R. 85: 87, 1961.

Sanders, D. E., Delarue, N. C., and Silverberg, S. A.: Combined angiography and mediastinoscopy in bronchogenic carcinoma. Radiology 97: 331, 1970.

Schapiro, R. L., and Evans, E. T.: Anaplastic carcinoma involving the mediastinum. Radiology 103: 545, 1972.

Sherman, R. S., and Malone, B. H.: A roentgen study of muscle tumors primary in the lung. Radiology 54: 507, 1950.

Siltzbach, L. E.: Carcinoma simulating pulmonary tuberculosis. Differential diagnosis in the presymptomatic stage in two cases. Am. Rev. Tuberc. 55: 170, 1947.

Simon, G.: Intrathoracic Hodgkin's disease; I. Less common intrathoracic manifestations of Hodgkin's disease. Br. J. Radiol. 40: 926, 1967.

Skinner, D. B., Dreyfuss, J. R., and Nardi, G. L.: Azygography in the evaluation of operability of pulmonary carcinoma. N. Engl. J. Med. 267: 232, 1962.

Smith, R. A., Nigam, B. K., and Thompson, J. M.: Second primary lung carcinoma. Thorax 31: 507, 1976.

Stackhouse, E. M., Harrison, E. G., Jr., and Ellis, F. H., Jr.: Primary mixed malignancies of lung: carcinosarcoma and blastoma. J. Thorac. Cardiovasc. Surg. 57: 385, 1969.

Steele, J. D.: The solitary pulmonary nodule. J. Thorac. Cardiovasc. Surg. 46: 21, 1963.

Steiner, P. E., and Frances, B. J.: Primary apical lung carcinoma. Am. J. Cancer 22: 776, 1934.

Stenseth, J. H., Clagett, O. T., and Woolner, L. B.: Hypertrophic pulmonary osteoarthropathy. Dis. Chest 52: 62, 1967.

Storey, C. F.: Bronchiolar carcinoma. Am. J. Surg. 89: 515, 1955.

Strickland, B.: Intra-thoracic Hodgkin's disease; II. Peripheral manifestations of Hodgkin's disease in the chest. Br. J. Radiol. 40: 930, 1967.

Theros, E. G.: Varying manifestations of peripheral pulmonary neoplasms: a radiologic-pathologic correlative study. A.J.R. 128: 893, 1977.

Trapnell, D. H.: Radiological appearances of lymphangitis carcinomatosa of the lung. Thorax 19: 251, 1964.

Ward, P.: Pulmonary and oesophageal presentation of pancreatic carcinoma. Br. J. Radiol. 37: 27, 1964.

Webb, W. R., and Gamsu, F.: Sclerosing hemangioma of the lung. Br. J. Radiol. 50: 213, 1977.

Woodruff, J. R., Jr., Ottoman, R. E., and Isaac, F.: Bronchiolar-cell carcinoma. Radiology 70: 335, 1958.

Yacoubian, H., Connolly, J. E., and Wylie, R. H.: Leiomyosarcoma of lung. Ann. Surg. 147: 116, 1958.

Yang, S.-P., and Lin, C.-C.: Lymphangitic carcinomatosis of the lungs. The clinical significance of its roentgenologic classification. Chest 62: 179, 1972.

MEDIASTINUM

Bakst, A. A.: Blind supradiaphragmatic thoracic duct cyst. Case report. Ann. Surg. 140: 250, 1954.

Baron, M. G.: Radiologic notes in cardiology: obscuration of the aortic knob in coarctation of the aorta. Circulation 43: 311, 1971.

Barrett, A. F., and Toye, D. K. M.: Sympathicoblastoma: Radiological findings in forty-three cases. Clin. Radiol. 14: 33, 1963.

Barsony, T., and Wald, B.: Das Rontgenbild der oberen-hinteren schwachen Stelle des Mediastinums. Der pravertebrale, retroösophageale Lungenteil; Mediastinumstudien. Röntgenpraxis 8: 88, 1936.

Bates, J. C., and Leaver, F. Y.: Pericardial celomic cysts. Radiology 57: 330, 1951.

Berdon, W., and Baker, D. H.: Plain film findings in azygos continuation of the inferior vena cava. A.J.R. 104: 452, 1968.

Berdon, W. E., and Baker, D. H.: Radiographic findings in esophageal atresia with proximal pouch fistula. Pediatr. Radiol. 3: 70, 1975.

Bergstrom, J. F., Yost, R. V., Ford, K. T., and List, R. M.: Unusual roentgen manifestations of bronchogenic cysts. Radiology 107: 49, 1973.

Berne, A. S., Gerle, R. D., and Mitchell, G. E.: The mediastinum: normal roentgen anatomy and radiologic technics. Semin. Roentgenol. 4: 3, 1969.

Bill, A. H., Jr., and Sumner, D. S.: A unified concept of lymphangioma and cystic hygroma. Surg. Gynecol. Obstet. 120: 70, 1965.

Blank, N., and Castellino, R. A.: Patterns of pleural reflections of the left superior mediastinum. Normal anatomy and distortions produced by adenopathy. Radiology 102: 585, 1972.

Boat, T. F., Sant'Agnese, P. A., Warwick, W. J., and Handwerger, S. A.: Pneumothorax in cystic fibrosis. J.A.M.A. 209: 1498, 1969.

Brijs, A.: Pneumomediastinum bei Neugeborenen Fortschr. Geb. Rontgenstr. 110: 687, 1969.

Carey, L. S., Ellis, F. H., Jr., Good, C. A., and Woolner, L. B.: Neurogenic tumors of the mediastinum: a clinicopathologic study. A.J.R. 84: 189, 1960.

Castellino, R. A., and Blank, N.: Adenopathy of the cardiophrenic angle (diaphragmatic) lymph nodes. A.J.R. 114: 509, 1972.

Castleman, B., Iverson, L., and Menendez, V. P.: Localized mediastinal lymph node hyperplasia resembling thymoma. Cancer 9: 822, 1956.

Celis, A., Pacheco, C. R., and del Castillo, H.: Angiocardiographic diagnosis of mediastinal tumors, with special reference to aortic aneurysms. Radiology 56: 31, 1951.

Chang, C. H. (Joseph), and Zinn, T. W.: Roentgen recognition of enlarged hilar lymph nodes: an anatomical review. Radiology 120: 291, 1976.

Chester, W.: Trachea in nonsyphilitic diseases of ascending aorta and aortic arch. A.J.R. 28: 795, 1932.

Christensen, E. E., Landay, M. J., Dietz, G. W., and Brinley, G.: Buckling of the innominate artery simulating a right apical lung mass. A.J.R. 131: 119, 1978.

Cicciarelli, F. E., Soule, E. H., and McGoon, D. C.: Lipoma and liposarcoma of the mediastinum: a report of 14 tumors including one lipoma of the thymus. J. Thorac. Cardiovasc. Surg. 47: 411, 1964.

Cornell, S. H.: Calcium in the fluid of mediastinal bronchogenic cyst: a new roentgenographic finding. Radiology 85: 825, 1965.

Cruikshank, D. G.: Primary intrathoracic neurogenic tumors. J. Fac. Radiol. 8: 369, 1957.

Cueto, J. C., McFee, A. S., and Bernstein, E. F.: Intrathoracic pheochromocytoma. Report of a case. Dis. Chest 48: 539, 1965.

Davis, J. G., and Simonton, J. H.: Mediastinal carinal bronchogenic cysts. Radiology 67: 391, 1956.

Davis, J. M., Mark, G. J., and Greene, R.: Benign blood vascular tumors of the mediastinum. Radiology 126: 581, 1978.

Dines, D. E., Payne, W. S., and Howard, P. H., Jr.: Von Recklinghausen's neurofibromatosis with plexiform mediastinal involvement. Dis. Chest 50: 437, 1966.

Doub, H. P., and Jones, H. C.: Hernia of mediastinum. A.J.R. 38: 297, 1937.

Dow, J.: Dissecting aneurysms of the aorta. Br. J. Radiol. 39: 315, 1966.

Doyle, F. H., Read, A. E., and Evans, K. T.: The mediastinum in portal hypertension. Clin. Radiol. 112: 114, 1961.

Dyer, N. H.: Cystic thymomas and thymic cysts. A review. Thorax 22: 408, 1967.

Edlin, P.: Mediastinal pseudocyst of pancreas; case report and discussion. Gastroenterology 17: 96, 1951.

Eklof, O., and Gooding, C. A.: Intrathoracic neuroblastoma. A.J.R. 100: 202, 1967.

Emerson, G. L.: Supradiaphragmatic thoracic duct cyst. N. Engl. J. Med. 242: 575, 1950.

Evans, J. A., and Smalldon, T. R.: Mediastinal emphysema. A.J.R. 64: 375, 1950.

Fechner, R. E.: Recurrence of noninvasive thymomas. Report of four cases and review of literature. Cancer 23: 1423, 1969.

Feigin, D. S., Fenoglio, J. J., McAllister, H. A., and Madewell, J. E.: Pericardial cysts. Radiology 125: 15, 1977.

Fell, S. C., Sprayregen, S., and Becker, N. H.: Bilateral carcinoid tumors of the mediastinum. Ann. Thorac. Surg. 2: 429, 1966.

Felson, B.: The mediastinum. Semin. Roentgenol. 4: 41, 1969.

Felson, B., et al.: Anomalous right subclavian artery. Radiology *54:* 340, 1950.

Felson, B., and Palayew, M. J.: Two types of right aortic arch. Radiology *81:* 745, 1963.

Ferguson, T. B., and Burford, T. H.: Mediastinal granuloma. A 15-year experience. Ann. Thorac. Surg. *1:* 125, 1965.

Feutz, E. T., Yune, H. Y., Mandelbaum, I., and Brasher, R. E.: Intrathoracic cystic hygroma. Radiology *108:* 61, 1973.

Figley, M. M.: Mediastinal minutae. Semin. Roentgenol. *4:* 22, 1969.

Fishbone, G., Robbins, D. I., Osborn, D. J., and Grnja, V.: Trauma to the thoracic aorta and great vessels. Radiol. Clin. North Am. *11:* 543, 1973.

Fleischner, F. G., Bernstein, C., and Levine, B. E.: Retrosternal infiltration in malignant lymphoma. Radiology *51:* 350, 1948.

Freed, T. A., Neal, M. P., Jr., and Vinik, M.: Roentgenographic findings in extracardiac injury secondary to blunt chest automobile trauma. A.J.R. *104:* 424, 1968.

Friedman, J.: Congenital atresia of esophagus with tracheo-esophageal fistula. A.J.R. *29:* 527, 1933.

Fifer, W. R., Woellner, R. C., and Gordon, S. S.: Mediastinal histoplasmosis. Report of three cases with dysphagia as the presenting complaint. Dis. Chest *47:* 518, 1965.

Gayola, G., Janis, M., and Weil, P. H.: Intrathoracic nerve sheath tumor of the vagus. J. Thorac. Cardiovasc. Surg. *49:* 412, 1965.

Gee, W., Foster, E. D., and Doheen, D. J.: Mediastinal pancreatic pseudocyst. Ann. Surg. *169:* 420, 1969.

Gladnikoff, H.: A roentgenographic study of the mediastinum in health and primary pulmonary carcinoma. Acta Radiol. Suppl. LXXIII, 1948.

Gleeson, J. A., and Stovin, P. G. I.: Mediastinal enterogenous cysts associated with vertebral anomalies. Clin. Radiol. *12:* 41, 1961.

Gomes, M., and Hufnagel, C. A.: Intrapericardial bronchogenic cysts. Am. J. Cardiol. *36:* 817, 1975.

Good, C. A.: Roentgenologic findings in myasthenia gravis associated with thymic tumor. A.J.R. *57:* 305, 1947.

Goodman, J., McClintock, J., Denton, G. R., and Stein, A.: Cystic hygromas in adults. Arch. Surg. *86:* 145, 1963.

Gross, R. E., and Hurwitt, E. S.: Cervicomediastinal and mediastinal hygromas. Surg. Gynecol. Obstet. *87:* 599, 1948.

Gunnells, J. C., Jr., Miller, D. E., Jacoby, W. J., Jr., and May, R. L.: Thymolipoma simulating cardiomegaly: opacification of the tumor by cineangiocardiography. Am. Heart J. *66:* 670, 1963.

Hache, L., Woolner, L. B., and Bernatz, P. E.: Idiopathic fibrous mediastinitis.

Dis. Chest *41:* 9, 1962.

Hammarskjold, B.: Contribution to knowledge of teratomas and dermoids in anterior mediastinum. Acta Radiol. *15:* 210, 1934.

Han, S. Y., Rudolph, A. J., and Teng, C. T.: Pneumomediastinum in infancy. J. Pediatr. *62:* 754, 1963.

Hanten, S. J., Keyes, T. F., and Meyer, R. R.: Spontaneous rupture of mediastinal dermoid cysts into the pleural cavity. Radiology *64:* 348, 1955.

Heimburger, L. L., and Battersby, J. S.: Primary mediastinal tumors of childhood. J. Thorac. Cardiovasc. Surg. *50:* 92, 1965.

Heitzman, E. R., Scrivani, J. V., Martino, J., and Moro J.: The azygos vein and its pleural reflections: I. Normal roentgen anatomy. Radiology *101:* 249, 1971; II. Applications in the radiological diagnosis of mediastinal abnormality. Radiology *101:* 259, 1971.

Herskovic, T., Andersen, H. A., and Bayrd, E. D.: Intrathoracic plasmacytomas. Presentation of 21 cases and review of the literature. Dis. Chest *47:* 1, 1965.

Heuer, G. J., and Andrus, W.: The surgery of mediastinal tumors. Am. J. Surg. *50:* 143, 1940.

Hewlett, T. H., Steer, A., and Thomas, D. E.: Progressive fibrosing mediastinitis. Ann. Thorac. Surg. *2:* 345, 1966.

Hillenius, L.: Intrathoracic meningocoele. Acta Med. Scand. *163:* 15, 1959.

Holmes Sellors, T., Thackray, A. C., and Thomson, A. D.: Tumours of the thymus. A review of 88 operation cases. Thorax *22:* 193, 1967.

Holt, J. F.: Epipericardial fat shadows in differential diagnosis. Radiology *48:* 472, 1947.

Hope, J. W., Borns, P. F., and Koop, C. E.: Radiologic diagnosis of mediastinal masses in infants and children. Radiol. Clin. North Am. *1:* 17, 1963.

Hutchin, P., and Mark, T. B. D.: Intrathoracic meningocoele not associated with neurofibromatosis. J. Thorac. Cardiovasc. Surg. *48:* 29, 1964.

Jacobson, G., Felson, B., Pendergrass, E. P., Flinn, R. H., and Lainhart, W. S.: Eggshell calcifications in coal and metal miners. Semin. Roentgenol. *2:* 276, 1967.

Jemelin, C., and Candardjis, G.: Retrosternal soft tissue: quantitative evaluation and clinical interest. Radiology *109:* 7, 1973.

Kaung, D. T., Cech, R. F., and Peterson, R. E.: Benign thymoma and erythroid hypoplasia. Cancer *22:* 445, 1968.

Keeffe, E., Jr., and Jones, C. F.: Pneumomediastinum in the newborn. Radiology *57:* 567, 1951.

Keene, R. J., Steiner, R. E., Olsen, E. J. G., and Oakley, C.: Aortic root aneurysm—radiographic and pathologic

features. Clin. Radiol. *22:* 330, 1971.

Kemp, F. H.: Factors influencing the mediastinal shadow in young children. Br. J. Radiol. *23:* 703, 1950.

Kemp, F. H., Morley, H. M. C., and Emrys-Roberts, E.: A sail-like triangular projection from the mediastinum; a radiographic appearance of the thymus gland. Br. J. Radiol. *21:* 618, 1948.

Kemp Harper, R. A., and Guyer, P. B.: The radiological features of thymic tumors. A review of sixty-five cases. Clin. Radiol. *16:* 97, 1965.

Koerner, H. J., and Donald, I-C. Sun: Mediastinal lipomatosis secondary to steroid therapy. A.J.R. *98:* 461, 1966.

Kountz, S. L., Connolly, J. E., and Cohn, R.: Seminoma-like (or seminomatous) tumors of the anterior mediastinum. J. Thorac. Cardiovasc. Surg. *45:* 289, 1963.

Laird, C. A., and Clagett, O. T.: Mediastinal pseudocyst of the pancreas in a child: report of a case. Surgery *60:* 465, 1966.

Lajos, T. Z., Charrette, E. J. P., and Farr, J. A.: Primary mediastinal seminoma. Chest *59:* 575, 1971.

Lane, E. J., Heitzman, E. R., and Dinn, W. M.: The radiology of the superior intercostal veins. Radiology *120:* 263, 1976.

Lee, W. J., and Fattal, G.: Mediastinal lipomatosis in simple obesity. Chest *70:* 308, 1976.

Legg, M. A., and Brady, W. J.: Pathology and clinical behavior of thymomas. Cancer *18:* 1131, 1965.

Leigh, T. F.: Mass lesions of the mediastinum. Radiol. Clin. North Am. *1:* 377, 1963.

Leigh, T. F., and Weens, H. S.: *The Mediastinum.* Charles C Thomas, Springfield, Ill., 1959.

LeRoux, B. T.: Intrathoracic duplication of the foregut. Thorax *17:* 357, 1962.

LeRoux, B. T., Rogers, M. A., and Gotsman, M. S.: Aneurysms of the thoracic aorta. Thorax *26:* 638, 1971.

Levin, B.: The continuous diaphragm sign. A newly-recognized sign of pneumomediastinum. Clin. Radiol. *24:* 337, 1973.

Levowitz, G. S., Khan, M. Y., Rand, E., and Hurwitz, A.: Thoracic vertebral chordoma presenting as a posterior mediastinal tumor. Ann. Thorac. Surg. *2:* 75, 1966.

Light, R. W., and George, R. B.: Incidence and significance of pleural effusion after abdominal surgery. Chest *69:* 621, 1976.

Lillard, R. L., and Allen, R. P.: The extrapleural air sign in pneumomediastinum. Radiology *85:* 1093, 1965.

Lillie, W. I., McDonald, J. R., and Clagett, O. T.: Pericardial celomic cysts and pericardial diverticuli. J. Thorac.

Surg. *20:* 494, 1950.

Lim, R. A., Divertie, M. B., Harrison, E. G., Jr., and Bernatz, P. E.: Cervicomediastinal cystic hygroma. Dis. Chest *40:* 265, 1961.

Lincoln, J. C. R., Deverall, P. B., Stark, J., Aberdeen, E., and Waterston, D. J.: Vascular anomalies compressing the oesophagus and trachea. Thorax *24:* 295, 1969.

Lipchik, E. O., and Robinson, K. E.: Acute traumatic rupture of the thoracic aorta. A.J.R. *104:* 408, 1968.

Loehr, W. M.: Pericardial cysts. A.J.R. *68:* 584, 1952.

Lowman, R. M., Bloor, C. M., and Newcomb, A. W.: Roentgen manifestations of thoracic extramedullary hematopoesis. Dis. Chest *44:* 154, 1963.

Lull, G. F., Jr.: Pericardial celomic cyst. A re-evaluation. Radiology *71:* 534, 1958.

Maier, H. C.: Lymphatic cysts of the mediastinum. A.J.R. *73:* 15, 1955.

McClenathan, J. E., and Brettschneider, L.: Traumatic thoracic aortic aneurysms. J. Thorac. Cardiovasc. Surg. *50:* 74, 1965.

McCort, J. J.: Intrathoracic goiter. Radiology *53:* 227, 1949.

Mendelow, H., and Slobodkin, M.: Aortic-body tumor (chemodectoma) of the mediastinum. Report of a case and review of the literature Cancer *10:* 1008, 1957.

Moncada, R., Shannon, M., Miller, R., White, H., Friedman, J., and Shuford, W. H.: The cervical aortic arch. A.J.R. *125:* 591, 1975.

Moncada, R., Warpeha, R., Pickleman, J., Spak, M., Cardoso, M., Berkow, A., and White, H.: Mediastinitis from odontogenic and deep cervical infection. Anatomic pathways of propagation. Chest *73:* 497, 1978.

Moseley, J. E.: Loculated pneumomediastinum in the newborn; a thymic "spinnaker sail" sign. Radiology *75:* 788, 1960.

Nanson, E. M.: Lymphangioma (cystic hygroma) of the mediastinum. J. Cardiovasc. Surg. *9:* 3, 1968.

Nelson, W. P., Lundberg, G. D., and Dickerson, R. B.: Pulmonary artery obstruction and cor pulmonale due to chronic fibrous mediastinitis. Am. J. Med. *38:* 279, 1965.

Neuhauser, E. B. D.: Roentgen diagnosis of double aortic arch and other anomalies of the great vessels. A.J.R. *56:* 1, 1946.

Neuhauser, E. B. D., Harris, G. B. C., and Berrett, A.: Roentgenographic features of neurenteric cysts. A.J.R. *79:* 235, 1958.

Newman, A., and Ko, S. K.: Bilateral neurofibroma of the intrathoracic vagus associated with Recklinghausen's disease. A.J.R. *112:* 389, 1971.

Oberman, H. A., and Libcke, J. H.: Malignant germinal neoplasms of the mediastinum. Cancer *17:* 498, 1964.

Ochsner, J. L., and Ochsner, S. F.: Congenital cysts of the mediastinum. Ann. Surg. *163:* 909, 1966.

O'Gorman, L. D., Cottingham, R. A., Sargent, E. N., and O'Loughlin, B. J.: Mediastinal emphysema in the newborn: a review and description of a new extrapleural gas sign. Dis. Chest *53:* 301, 1968.

Oliphant, M., Wiot, J. F., and Whalen, J. P.: The cervicothoracic continuum. Radiology *120:* 257, 1976.

Oosterwijk, W. M., and Swierenga, J.: Neurogenic tumours with an intrathoracic localization. Thorax *23:* 374, 1968.

Ozonoff, M. B.: Pneumomediastinum associated with asthma and pneumonia in children. A.J.R. *95:* 112, 1965.

Pachter, M. R., and Lattes, R.: Mediastinal cysts: a clinicopathologic study of twenty cases. Dis. Chest *44:* 416, 1963.

Pachter, M. R., and Lattes, R.: Mesenchymal tumors of the mediastinum: I. Tumors of fibrous tissue, adipose tissue, smooth muscle and striated muscle. Cancer *16:* 74, 1963; II. Tumors of blood vascular origin. Cancer *16:* 95, 1963: III. Tumors of lymph vascular origin. Cancer *16:* 108, 1963.

Pachter, M. R., and Lattes, R.: "Germinal" tumors of the mediastinum: a clinicopathologic study of adult teratomas, teratocarcinomas, choriocarcinomas and seminomas. Dis. Chest *3:* 301, 1963.

Papavasilou, C. G.: Tumor simulating extramedullary hematopoesis. Clinical and roentgenologic considerations. A.J.R. *93:* 695, 1965.

Pfister, R. C., Oh, K. S., and Ferrucci, J. T.: Retrosternal density. A radiological evaluation of the retrosternal-premediastinal space. Radiology *96:* 317, 1970.

Phemister, D. B., Steen, W. B., and Voldauer, J. C.: A roentgenologic criterion of dermoid cyst. A.J.R. *36:* 14, 1936.

Phillips, E. W.: Intrathoracic xanthogranulomatous new growths; report of 2 cases and collection of 3 similar cases in the literature. J. Thorac. Surg. *7:* 74, 1937.

Price, J. E., Jr., and Rigler, L. G.: Widening of the mediastinum resulting from fat accumulation. Radiology *96:* 497, 1970.

Raison, J. C. A.: Intrathoracic meningocoele. Thorax *11:* 334, 1956.

Rakower, J.: Sarcoidal bilateral hilar lymphoma (Lofgren's syndrome). A review of 31 cases. Am. Rev. Respir. Dis. *87:* 518, 1963.

Rakower, J., and Milwidsky, H.: Primary mediastinal echinococcus. Am. J. Med. *29:* 79, 1960.

Ranniger, K.: Retrograde azygography. Radiology *90:* 1097, 1968.

Raphael, M. J.: Mediastinal hematoma. A description of some radiological appearances. Br. J. Radiol. *36:* 921, 1963.

Reed, J. C., Hallet, K. K., and Geigin, D. S.: Neural tumors of the thorax: subject review from the AFIP. Radiology *126:* 9, 1978.

Ringertz, N., and Lidholm, S. O.: Mediastinal tumors and cysts. J. Thorac. Surg. *31:* 458, 1956.

Rogers, L. F., and Osmer, J. C.: Bronchogenic cyst. A review of 46 cases. A.J.R. *91:* 273, 1964.

Rogers, L. F., Puig, A. W., Dooley, B. N., and Cuello, L.: Diagnostic considerations in mediastinal emphysema: a pathophysiologic-roentgenologic approach to Boerhaave's syndrome and spontaneous pneumomediastinum. A.J.R. *115:* 495, 1972.

Rohlfine, B. M., Webb, W. R., and Schlobohm, R. M.: Ventilator-related extraalveolar air in adults. Radiology *121:* 25, 1976.

Roland, A. S.: The syndrome of benign thymoma and primary aregenerative anemia: an analysis of forty-three cases. Am. J. Med. Sci. *247:* 719, 1964.

Rudhe, U., and Ozonoff, M. B.: Pneumomediastinum and pneumothorax in the newborn. Acta Radiol. *4:* 193, 1966.

Rusby, N. L.: Dermoid cysts and teratomata of mediastinum. J. Thorac. Surg. *13:* 169, 1944.

Sandor, F.: Incidence and significance of traumatic mediastinal haematoma. Thorax *22:* 43, 1967.

Schillhammer, W. R., Jr., and Tyson, M. D.: Mediastinal thymic cysts. Arch. Surg. *85:* 72, 1962.

Schowengerdt, C. G., Suyemoto, R., and Main, F. B.: Granulomatous and fibrous mediastinitis. A review and analysis of 180 cases. J. Thorac. Cardiovasc. Surg. *57:* 365, 1969.

Schwarz, M. I., and Marmorstein, B. L.: A radiographic sign of left sided mediastinal lymph node enlargement. Chest *68:* 116, 1975.

Seltzer, R. A., Mills, D. S., Baddock, S. S., and Felson, B.: Mediastinal thymic cyst. Dis. Chest *53:* 186, 1968.

Sengpiel, G. W., Ruzicka, F. F., and Lodmell, E. A.: Lateral intrathoracic meningocoele. Radiology *50:* 515, 1948.

Shapiro, J. H., Jacobson, H. G., Stern, W. Z., and Poppel, M. H.: Posterior mediastinal goiter. Radiology *71:* 79, 1958.

Sherman, R. S., and Leaming, R.: Roentgen findings in neuroblastoma. Radiology *60:* 837, 1960.

Shuford, W. H., and Weems, H. S.: Azygos vein dilatation simulating mediastinal tumor. A.J.R. *80:* 225, 1958.

Shuford, W. H., Sybers, R. G., and Edwards, F. K.: The three types of right aortic arch. A.J.R. *109:* 67, 1970.

Shuford, W. H., Sybers, R. E., Milledge, R. D., and Brinsfield, D.: The cervical aortic arch. A.J.R. *116:* 519, 1972.

Simeone, J. F., Minagi, H., and Putman, C. E.: Traumatic disruption of the thoracic aorta: significance of the left apical pleural cap. Radiology *117:* 265, 1975.

Sowerbutts, J. G.: Mediastinal bronchogenic cysts. J. Fac. Radiol. *10:* 158, 1959.

Stevens, G. M.: Buckling of the aorta (pseudocoarctation, kinking): a roentgenographic entity. Radiology *70:* 62, 1958.

Stewart, J. R., Kincaid, O. W., and Edwards, J. E.: *An Atlas of Vascular Rings and Related Malformations of the Aortic Arch System.* Charles C Thomas, Springfield, Ill., 1964.

Stewart, J. R., Kincaid, O. W., and Titus, J. L.: Right aortic arch: plain film diagnosis and significance. A.J.R. *97:* 377, 1966.

Stoney, R. J., Roe, B. B., and Redington, J. V.: Rupture of thoracic aorta due to closed-chest trauma. Arch. Surg. *89:* 840, 1964.

Strickland, B., and Wolverson, M. K.: Intrathoracic vagus nerve tumors. Thorax *29:* 215, 1974.

Sweet, R. H.: Intrathoracic goiter located in posterior mediastinum. Surg. Gynecol. Obstet. *89:* 57, 1949.

Tausend, M. E., and Stern, W. Z.: Thymic patterns in the newborn. A.J.R. *95:* 125, 1965.

Tucker, D. H., Gaylor, D. H., Jacoby, W. J., Jr., and Sumner, R. G.: Prominence of the left epipericardial fat pad. A cause of apparent cardiomegaly. Am. J. Med. *38:* 268, 1965.

Wessler, H., and Greene, C. M.: Intrathoracic Hodgkin's disease: its roentgen diagnosis. J.A.M.A. *74:* 445, 1920.

Whalen, J. P., and Woodruff, C. L.: The cervical prevertebral fat stripe. A new aid in evaluating the cervical prevertebral soft tissue space. A.J.R. *109:* 445, 1970.

Whalen, J. P., Meyers, M. A., Oliphant, M., Caragol, W. J., and Evans, J. A.: The retrosternal line. A new sign of anterior mediastinal mass. A.J.R. *117:* 861, 1973.

Wilkinson, R., and Forgan-Smith, R.: Chemodectoma in relation to the aortic arch (aortic body tumour). Thorax *24:* 488, 1969.

Willis, R. A.: *Teratomas. Atlas of Tumor Pathology, Section III, Fascicle 9.* Armed Forced Institute of Pathology, Washington, D. C., 1951.

Wilson, R. F., Arbulu, A., Bassett, J. S., and Walt, A. J.: Acute mediastinal widening following blunt chest trauma. Arch. Surg. *104:* 551, 1972.

Wright, F. W.: Enlarged hilar and me-diastinal nodes (and especially lower right hilar node enlargement) as a sign of metastasis of a renal tumour. Clin. Radiol. *28:* 431, 1977.

Yacoub, M. H., and Thompson, V. C.: Chronic idiopathic pulmonary hilar fibrosis. Thorax *26:* 365, 1971.

Yeoh, C. B., Ford, J. M., Lattes, R., and Wylie, R. H.: Intrapulmonary thymoma. J. Thorac. Cardiovasc. Surg. *51:* 131, 1966.

Young, R., Pochaczevsky, R., Pollak, L., and Bryk, D.: Cervicomediastinal thymic cysts. A.J.R. *117:* 855, 1973.

Zavod, W. A.: Fibrin bodies in pelural space in case of artificial pneumothorax with necropsy. Am. Rev. Tuberc. *33:* 48, 1936.

THE PLEURA

Abo, S.: Roentgenographic detection of minimal pneumothorax in lateral decubitus position. A.J.R. *77:* 1066, 1957.

Abrams, W. B., and Small, M. J.: Current concepts of tuberculous pleurisy with effusion as derived from pleural biopsy studies. Dis. Chest *38:* 60, 1960.

Anton, H. C.: Multiple pleural plaques. Br. J. Radiol. *40:* 685, 1967.

Anton, H. C.: Multiple pleural plaques; II. Br. J. Radiol. *41:* 341, 1968.

Asch, T.: The case for pneumoperitoneum in the diagnosis of inflammatory disease about the diaphragm. Radiology *86:* 60, 1966.

Bachman, A. L., and Macken, J.: Pleural effusions following supervoltage radiation for breast carcinoma. Radiology *72:* 699, 1959.

Berne, A. S., and Heitzman, E. R.: The roentgenologic signs of pedunculated pleural tumors. A.J.R. *87:* 892, 1962.

Borow, M., Conston, A., Livornese, L., and Schalet, N.: Mesothelioma following exposure to asbestos: a review of 72 cases. Chest *64:* 641, 1973.

Bower, G.: Eosinophilic pleural effusion. A condition with multiple causes. Am. Rev. Respir. Dis. *95:* 746, 1967.

Bryk, D.: Infrapulmonary effusion. Effect of expiration on the pseudodiaphragmatic contour. Radiology *120:* 33, 1976.

Calvert, R. J., and Smith, E.: An analytical review of spontaneous haemopneumothorax. Thorax *10:* 64, 1955.

Campbell, G. D., and Ferrington, E.: Rheumatoid pleuritis with effusion. Dis. Chest *53:* 521, 1968.

Chamberlain, J. L., III: Spontaneous pneumothorax in the newborn. Clin. Pediatr. *4:* 732, 1965.

Christiansen, K. H., Morgan, S. W., Karich, A. F., and Takaro, T.: Pleural space following pneumonectomy. Ann. Thorac. Surg. *1:* 298, 1965.

Collins, T. F. B.: Pleural reaction associated with asbestos exposure. Br. J. Radiol. *41:* 655, 1968.

Crutcher, R. R., Waltuch, T. L., and Blue, M. E.: Recurring spontaneous pneumothorax associated with menstruation. J. Thorac. Cardiovasc. Surg. *54:* 599, 1967.

Dandy, W. E., Jr.: Incomplete pulmonary interlobar fissure sign. Radiology *128:* 21, 1978.

Darke, C. S., and Dewhurst, C. J.: Meig's syndrome with blood-stained pleural effusion. Thorax *11:* 41, 1956.

Davies, R.: Recurrent spontaneous pneumothorax concomitant with menstruation. Thorax *23:* 370, 1968.

Davis, S., Gardner, F., and Qvist, G.: The shape of a pleural effusion. Br. Med. J. *1:* 436, 1963.

Euphrat, E. J., and Beck, E.: Fibrin body following traumatic pneumothorax. A.J.R. *74:* 86, 1955.

Finby, N., and Steinberg, I.: Roentgen aspects of pleural mesothelioma. Radiology *65:* 169, 1955.

Fleischner, F. G.: Atypical arrangement of free pleural effusion. Radiol. Clin. North Am. *1:* 347, 1963.

Greene, R., McCloud, T. C., and Stark, P.: Pneumothorax. Semin. Roentgenol. *12:* 313, 1977.

Heller, R. M., Janower, M. L., and Weber, A. L.: The radiological manifestations of malignant pleural mesothelioma. A.J.R. *108:* 53, 1970.

Hessen, I.: Roentgen examination of pleural fluid: a study of the localization of free effusions, the potentialities of diagnosing minimal quantities of fluid and its existence under physiological conditions. Acta Radiol. Suppl. 86, 1951.

Hourihane, D. O'B., Lessof, L., and Richardson, P. C.: Hyaline and calcified pleural plaques as an index of exposure to asbestos—a study of radiological and pathological features of 100 cases with a consideration of epidemiology. Br. Med. J. *1:* 1069, 1966.

Janetos, G. P., and Ochsner, S. F.: Bilateral pneumothorax in metastatic osteogenic sarcoma. Am. Rev. Respir. Dis. *88:* 73, 1963.

Jones, D. B.: Basal pleural fluid accumulations resembling elevated diaphragm. Radiology *50:* 227, 1948.

Kaunitz, J.: Three zones of simple pleural effusions. A.J.R. *35:* 57, 1936.

Kautz, F. G., and Pinner, M.: Periapical empyema; report of 3 cases with necropsy findings. A.J.R. *37:* 446, 1937.

Klemperer, P., and Rabin, C. B.: Primary neoplasms of pleural. Arch. Pathol. *11:* 385, 1931.

Knies, P. T.: Paradoxical roentgen image in pneumothorax: result of pachypleuritis. A.J.R. *44:* 230, 1940.

Korol, E., and Scott, H. A.: Veiled air bubble in hydropneumothorax. A.J.R. *33:* 777, 1935.

Langston, H. T., Barker, W. L., and Graham, A. A.: Pleural tuberculosis. J. Thorac. Cardiovasc. Surg. *54:* 511, 1967.

Leroux, B. T.: Pleural tumors. Thorax *17:* 111, 1962.

Liberson, M.: Diagnostic significance of the mediastinal profile in massive unilateral pleural effusions. Am. Rev. Respir. Dis. *88:* 176, 1963.

Lowman, R. M., et al.: Traumatic chylothorax. A.J.R. *65:* 529, 1951.

Madan, S. C., Rosenthal, S. P., and Bochetto, J. F.: Pneumomediastinum and pneumothorax following lower neck surgery. Arch. Surg. *98:* 153, 1969.

Macewan, D. W., Dunbar, J. S., Smith, R. D., and Brown, B. S. J.: Pneumothorax in young infants—recognition and evaluation. J. Can. Assoc. Radiol. *22:* 264, 1971.

Meigs, J. V., and Cass, J. W.: Fibroma of the ovary with ascites and hydrothorax, with report of seven cases. Am. J. Obstet. Gynecol. *33:* 249, 1937.

Meyer, P. C.: Metastatic carcinoma of the pleura. Thorax *21:* 437, 1966.

Mulvey, R. B.: The effect of pleural fluid on the diaphragm. Radiology *84:* 1080, 1965.

Oosthuizen, S. F., Theron, C. P., and Sluis-Cremer, G. K.: Calcified pleural plaques in asbestosis. An investigation into their significance. Med. Proc. *10:* 406, 1964.

Pratt, H. J., and Shamblin, W. R.: Spontaneous hemothorax as a direct complication of hemoperitoneum. Ann. Surg. *167:* 867, 1968.

Rabinowitz, J. G., and Wolf, B. S.: Roentgen significance of the pulmonary ligament. Radiology *87:* 1013, 1966.

Rakower, J., and Milwidsky, H.: Hydatid pleural disease. Am. Rev. Respir. Dis. *90:* 623, 1964.

Raunio, V.: Occurence of unusual pleural calcification in Finland. Ann. Med. Int. Finn. *55:* Suppl. 47, 1966.

Rigler, L.: Roentgenologic observations on movement of pleural effusions. A.J.R. *25:* 220, 1931.

Roland, A. S., Merdinger, W. F., and Froeb, H. F.: Recurrent spontaneous pneumothorax. A clue to the diagnosis of histiocytosis X. N. Engl. J. Med. *270:* 73, 1964.

Rose, M. E., Howard, R., Sibley, J. J., and Reilly, Jr., H. F.: Pneumothorax directly resulting from perforated bronchogenic carcinoma. Ann. Thorac. Surg. *4:* 160, 1967.

Ross, J., and Farber, J. E.: Right-sided spontaneous pneumothorax complicating therapeutic pneumoperitoneum. Am. Rev. Tuberc. *63:* 67, 1951.

Rottenberg, L. A., and Golden, R.: Spontaneous pneumothorax: a study of 105 cases. Radiology *53:* 157, 1949.

Salmon, U. J.: Benign pelvic tumors associated with ascites and pleural effusion. J. Mt. Sinai Hosp. *1:* 169, 1934.

Sargent, E. N., Jacobson, G., and Gordonson, J. S.: Pleural plaques: a signpost of asbestos dust inhalation. Semin. Roentgenol. *12:* 287, 1977.

Scheff, S., Bednarz, W. W., and Levene, F.: Roentgenologic aspects of retropleural hematomas following sympathectomy. Radiology *68:* 224, 1957.

Selikoff, I. J., Churg, J., and Hammond, E. C.: Relation between exposure to asbestos and mesothelioma. N. Engl. J. Med. *272:* 560, 1965.

Sharma, O. P., and Gordonson, J.: Pleural effusion in sarcoidosis: a report of six cases. Thorax *30:* 95, 1975.

Sherman, R. S., and Brant, E. E.: An x-ray study of spontaneous pneumothorax due to cancer metastases to the lungs. Dis. Chest *26:* 328, 1954.

Stout, A. P., and Murray, M. R.: Localized pleural mesothelioma. Arch. Pathol. *34:* 951, 1942.

Swischuk, L.: Two lesser known but useful signs of neonatal pneumothorax. A.J.R. *127:* 623, 1976.

TenEyck, E. A.: Subpleural lipoma. Radiology *74:* 295, 1960.

Tivenius, L.: Benign pleural lesions simulating tumor. Thorax *18:* 39, 1963.

Walerk, W. C., and Wright, V.: Rheumatoid pleuritis. Ann. Rheum. Dis. *26:* 467, 1967.

Winslow, W. A., Ploss, L. N., and Loitman, B.: Pleuritis in systemic lupus erythematosus: its importance as early manifestations in diagnosis. Ann. Intern. Med. *49:* 70, 1958.

Wright, F. W.: Spontaneous pneumothorax and pulmonary malignant disease—a syndrome sometimes associated with cavitating tumours. Clin. Radiol. *27:* 211, 1976.

THE DIAPHRAGM

Ackermann, A. J.: Primary tumors of the diaphragm roentgenologically considered. A.J.R. *47:* 711, 1942.

Adkins, P. C., and Wesselhoeft, C. W., Jr.: Congenital diaphragmatic hernias. G. P. *39:* 78, 1969.

Brown, S., and Fine, A.: The diaphragm. Radiology *50:* 157, 1948.

Campbell, J. A.: The diaphragm in roentgenology of the chest. Radiol. Clin. North Am. *1:* 395, 1963.

Carter, B. N., Guiseffi, J., and Felson, B.: Traumatic diaphragmatic hernia. A.J.R. *65:* 56, 1951.

Davis, W. S., and Allen, R. P.: Accessory diaphragm. Duplication of the diaphragm. Radiol. Clin. North Am. *6:* 253, 1968.

Delario, A. J.: Subdiaphragmatic abscess. A.J.R. *31:* 177, 1934.

Efron, G., and Hyde, I.: Nonpenetrating traumatic rupture of the diaphragm. Clin. Radiol. *18:* 394, 1967.

Felder, M. E.: Intradiaphragmatic cyst. Am. J. Surg. *98:* 95, 1959.

Fleischner, F. G., Robins, S. A., and Abrams, M.: High renal extopy and congenital diaphragmatic hernia. Radiology *55:* 24, 1950.

Hislop, A., and Reid, L.: Persistent hypoplasia of the lung after repair of congenital diaphragmatic hernia. Thorax *31:* 450, 1976.

Hitzenberger, K.: *Das Zwerchfell im gesunden und kranken Zustand.* J. Springer, Vienna, 1927.

Kaye, M. D.: Pleuropulmonary complications of pancreatitis. Thorax *23:* 297, 1968.

Kirklin, B. R.: Roentgenologic characteristics of diaphragmatic hernia. A.J.R. *58:* 77, 1947.

Neveux, J. Y., Hazan, E., Levasseur, J. C., Galey, J. J., and Mathey, J.: Traumatic rupture of the diaphragm. Thorax *22:* 142, 1967.

Olafsson, G., Rausing, A., and Holen, O.: Primary tumors of the diaphragm. Chest *59:* 568, 1971.

Rabin, C. B.: Notes on subphrenic abscess. J. Mt. Sinai Hosp. *17:* 717, 1951.

Raichoudhury, R. C., Patnaik, S. C., Sahoo, M., Panda, K., and Patnaik, B. K.: Foramen of Bochdalek hernia in adults. Chest *64:* 259, 1971.

Sterns, L. P., Jensen, N. K., Schmidt, W. R., Garamella, J. J., and Lynch, M. F.: Diaphragmatic disruption in major trauma: a review of 16 cases. Can. J. Surg. *12:* 426, 1969.

Sutton, J. P., Carlisle, R. B., and Stephenson, S. E., Jr.: Traumatic diaphragmatic hernia. A review of 25 cases. Ann. Thorac. Surg. *3:* 136, 1967.

Swingle, J. D., Logan, R., and Juhl, J. H.: Inversion of the left hemidiaphragm. J.A.M.A. *208:* 863, 1969.

Wooler, G. H.: Subphrenic abscess. Thorax *11:* 211, 1956.

APPENDIX: CT OF THE CHEST

Crowe, J. K., Brown, L. R., and Muhm, J. R.: Computed tomography of the mediastinum. Radiology *128:* 78, 1978.

Heitzman, E. R., Goldwin, R. L., and Proto, A. V.: Radiologic analysis of the mediastinum utilizing computed tomography. Radiol. Clin. North Am. *15:* 309, 1977.

Jost, R. G., Sagel, S. S., Stanley, R. J., and Levitt, R. G.: Computed tomography of the thorax. Radiology *126:* 125, 1978.

Kollins, S. A.: Computed tomography of the pulmonary parenchyma and the chest wall. Radiol. Clin. North Am. *15:* 297, 1977.

Kreel, L.: Computed tomography of the thorax. Radiol. Clin. North Am. *16:* 575, 1978.

Muhm, J. R., Brown, L. R., and Crowe, J. K.: Use of computed tomography in the detection of pulmonary nodules. Mayo Clin. Proc. *52:* 345, 1977.

Schaner, E. G., Chang, A. E., Doppman, J. L., Conkle, D. M., Flye, M. W., and Rosenberg, S. A.: Comparison of computed and conventional whole lung tomography in detecting pulmonary nodules: A prospective radiologicpathologic study. A.J.R. *131:* 51, 1978.

Index